Overview

1. List of abbreviations

Singular:
A. = Arteria
Lig. = Ligamentum
M. = Musculus
N. = Nervus
Proc. = Processus
R. = Ramus
V. = Vena

Var. = variation
r. = right
l. = left

Plural:
Aa. = Arteriae
Ligg. = Ligamenta
Mm. = Musculi
Nn. = Nervi
Procc. = Processus
Rr. = Rami
Vv. = Venae

♀ = female
♂ = male

Percentages: In the light of the large variation in individual body measurements, the percentages indicating size should only be taken as approximate values.

2. General terms of direction and position

The following terms indicate the position of organs and parts of the body in relation to each other, irrespective of the position of the body (e.g. supine or upright) or direction and position of the limbs. These terms are relevant not only for human anatomy but also for clinical medicine and comparative anatomy.

General terms
anterior – posterior = in front – behind (e.g. anterior and posterior tibial artery)
ventral – dorsal = towards the belly – towards the back
superior – inferior = above – below (e.g. superior and inferior nasal concha)
cranial – caudal = towards the head – towards the tail
middle, intermediate = located between two other structures (e.g. the middle nasal concha is located between the superior and the inferior nasal concha)
median = located in the midline (anterior median fissure of the spinal cord). The median plane is a sagittal plane which divides the body into right and left halves.
medial – lateral = located near to the midline – located away from the midline of the body (e.g. medial and lateral inguinal fossa)
frontal = located in a frontal plane, but also towards the front (e.g. frontal process of the maxilla)
longitudinal = parallel to the longitudinal axis (e.g. superior longitudinal muscle of the tongue)
sagittal = located in a sagittal plane
transverse = located in a transverse plane/transverse direction (e.g. transverse process of a thoracic vertebra)

Terms of direction and position for the limbs
proximal – distal = located towards or away from the attached end of a limb or the origin of a structure (e.g. proximal and distal radio-ulnar joint)

For the upper limb:
radial – ulnar = on the radial side – on the ulnar side (e.g. ¬radial and ulnar artery)

For the hand:
palmar – dorsal = towards the palm of the hand – towards the back of the hand (e.g. palmar aponeurosis, dorsal interosseous muscle)

For the lower limb:
tibial – fibular = on the tibial side – on the fibular side (e.g. anterior tibial artery)

For the foot:
plantar – dorsal = towards the sole of the foot – towards the back of the foot (e.g. lateral and medial plantar artery, ¬dorsalis pedis *artery)*

3. Use of brackets

[ ]: Latin terms in square brackets refer to alternative terms.
( ): Round brackets are used in different ways:
- for terms also listed in round brackets in the Terminologia Anatomica
- for terms not included in the official nomenclature but which the editors consider important and clinically relevant, e.g. (zygomaticoalveolar crest)
- to indicate the origin of a given structure, e. g. spinal branch (vertebral artery)
- to indicate the right (r.) or left (l.) side of the body and the approximate reduction or magnification of size, e. g. (r., 70%).

4. Orientation diagrams

Most of the topographic illustrations are supplied with "compass roses", which refer to the numbers of the illustrations of the respective adjacent regions:

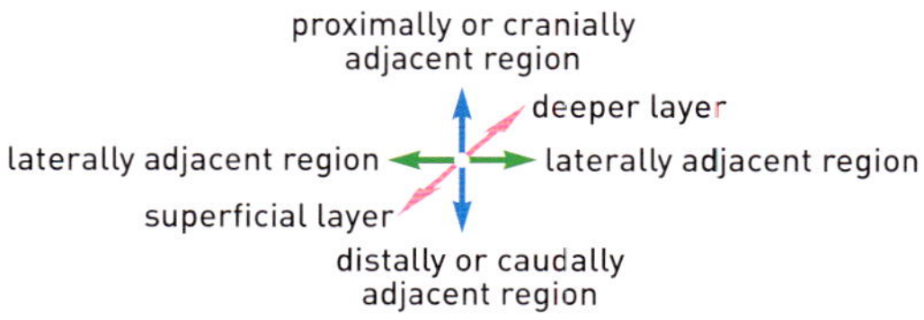

Sobotta

Atlas of Human Anatomy
One Volume Edition

Edited by R. Putz and R. Pabst
In collaboration with Renate Putz

**Head, Neck,
Upper Limb,
Thorax, Abdomen,
Pelvis, Lower Limb**

14th edition, newly edited
1431 colour plates with 1984 figures
Tables of muscles, joints and nerves

ELSEVIER
URBAN & FISCHER

URBAN & FISCHER
München · Jena

Correspondence and feedback should be addressed to:
Elsevier GmbH, Urban & Fischer Verlag, Department for Medical Student Information, Dr. Helmar Weiß, Karlstraße 45, 80333 München, Germany
e-mail: medizinstudium@elsevier.de

Addresses of the editors:

Professor Dr. med. Reinhard Putz
Vizepräsident der
Ludwig Maximilians-Universität
Geschwister-Scholl-Platz 1
80539 München
Germany
e-mail: putz@lmu.de

Professor Dr. med. Reinhard Pabst
Leiter der Abteilung
Funktionelle und Angewandte Anatomie
Medizinische Hochschule Hannover
Carl-Neuberg-Straße 1
30625 Hannover
Germany
e-mail: pabst.reinhard@mh-hannover.de

Bibliographic information published by Die Deutsche Bibliothek

Die Deutsche Bibliothek lists this publication in the Deutsche Nationalbibliografie; detailed bibliographic data is available in the Internet at http://dnb.ddb.de.

08 09 10 11 5 4 3 2 1

The contents of this edition are identical with the 22nd in two volumes. The order of the chapters has been changed.

Editorial staff at Elsevier: Dr. med. Dorothea Hennessen
Alexander Gattnarzik
Dr. Andrea Beilmann
Alexandra Frntic
Editorial staff and translation: Ulrike Kriegel, buchundmehr, Munich
Illustrators: Ulrike Brugger, Munich; Rüdiger Himmelhan, Heidelberg; Horst Ruß, Munich; Henriette Rintelen, Velbert
Book production: Renate Hausdorf, buchundmehr, Munich
Composed by: Mitterweger&Partner, Plankstadt
Printed and bound by: 1010 Printing International Limited

Cover design: Carsten Tschirner, Munich

Printed in China
ISBN 978-0-7020-3322-3

This atlas was founded by Johannes Sobotta†, former Professor of Anatomy and Director of the Anatomical Institute of the University of Bonn, Germany.

German Editions:
1st Edition: 1904–1907 J. F. Lehmanns Verlag, Munich
2nd–11th Edition: 1913–1944 J. F. Lehmanns Verlag, Munich
12th–20th Edition: 1948–1993 Urban & Schwarzenberg, Munich
13th Edition: 1953, editor H. Becher
14th Edition: 1956, editor H. Becher
15th Edition: 1957, editor H. Becher
16th Edition: 1967, editor H. Becher
17th Edition: 1972, editors H. Ferner and J. Staubesand
18th Edition: 1982, editors H. Ferner and J. Staubesand
19th Edition: 1988, editor J. Staubesand
20th Edition: 1993, editors R. Putz and R. Pabst
21st Edition: 2000, editors R. Putz and R. Pabst, Urban & Fischer Verlag, Munich
22nd Edition: 2006, editors R. Putz and R. Pabst, Elsevier GmbH, Munich

Foreign Editions:
Arabic Edition
Modern Technical Center, Damascus
Chinese Edition (complex characters)
Ho-Chi Book Publishing Co, Taiwan
Chinese Edition (simplified Chinese edition)
Elsevier, Health Sciences Asia, Singapore
Croatian Edition
Naklada Slap, Jastrebarsko
Dutch Edition
Bohn Stafleu van Loghum, Houten
English Edition (with nomenclature in English)
Atlas of Human Anatomy
Lippincott Williams & Wilkins
English Edition (with nomenclature in Latin)
Atlas of Human Anatomy
Elsevier GmbH, Urban & Fischer
French Edition
Atlas d'Anatomie Humaine
Tec & Doc Lavoisier, Paris
Greek Edition (with nomenclature in Greek)
Maria G. Parissianos, Athens
Greek Edition (with nomenclature in Latin)
Maria G. Parissianos, Athens
Hungarian Edition
az ember anatómiájának atlasza
Alliter Kiadái, Budapest
Indonesian Edition
Atlas Anatomi Manusia
Penerbit Buku Kedokteran EGC, Jakarta
Italian Edition
Atlante di Anatomia Umana
UTET, Torino
Japanese Edition
Igaku Shoin Ltd., Tokyo
Korean Edition
ShingHeung MedScience, Seoul
Polish Edition
Atlas anatomii cztowieka
Urban & Partner, Wroclaw
Portuguese Edition (with nomenclature in English)
Atlas de Anatomia Humana
Editora Guanabara Koogan, Rio de Janeiro
Portuguese Edition (with nomenclature in Latin)
Atlas de Anatomia Humana
Editora Guanabara Koogan, Rio de Janeiro
Spanish Edition
Atlas de Anatomia Humana
Editorial Medica Panamericana, Buenos Aires/Madrid
Turkish Edition
Insan Anatomisi Atlasi
Beta Basim Yayim Dagitim, Istanbul

Current information by www.elsevier.com and www.elsevier.de

Contents

Preface

It was just over a hundred years ago that Johannes Sobotta set out to publish the first edition of his Atlas of Human Anatomy. Since then, this piece of work has evolved step by step as a result of the constant interaction between students, lecturers and editors. It has not only been the most modern basis for the complex subject of macroscopic anatomy throughout many generations of doctors, but has also developed into a lasting work of reference for both clinical training and advanced medical education. All in all, it has become a book for a medical doctor's life. Once again, in this new edition the additional figures have been drawn strictly on the basis of original specimens.

The 14th edition has been particularly designed to meet the demands of a reformed medical curriculum, emphasizing the integration of clinical medicine into the preclinical curriculum. For this purpose, the new edition has been extended to include the following features:

- Surface anatomy including projection of internal organs (45 colour photos)
- Anatomical diagrams next to imaging figures
- Integration of imaging techniques to a greater extent (ultrasound, X-ray, CT, MRI; 119 figures)
- Endoscopic, intraoperative colour images and figures exemplifying techniques of puncture and examination (54 figures)
- Images of patients presenting with typical palsies
- Diagrams of the most important arterial variations (93 figures)
- Frequent variations in the location of internal organs (24 figures)
- Integration of histology at low magnification of important internal organs (intestine, liver, kidney, etc.)

In order to improve the presentation of the knowledge, the following features have been introduced:

- Clear-cut arrangement of the chapters according to the different regions of the body
- Thematically corresponding figures presented on double pages
- The appendix contains tables of muscles, joints and nerves

One particular aim of the new edition is to facilitate finding of specific structures. The SOBOTTA depicts anatomical structures precisely without the reader loosing the greater picture. Therefore, specific didactic tools have been improved and new aspects included:

- Each chapter has been allocated to a particular colour
- A "menu bar" on each double page ensures precise orientation within a given chapter
- The number of outlines depicting spatial orientation has been significantly increased (270 figures)
- Overviews of total body regions ensure general orientation
- New diagrams of particular muscles clarify their location and course (24 figures)
- Confusion is kept to a minimum by only depicting limbs of the right side of the body
- "Compass roses" point to adjacent figures, thus facilitating following a given structure over several pages
- Continuous leader lines facilitate finding of structures
- Coloured dots at the end of leader lines in topographic diagrams mark arteries, veins, nerves, and muscles
- The larger dimensions of the book improve clarity

With the exception of discussions about the general concept of the atlas and mutual correction, the editors have worked separately on individual chapters, with the work divided as follows:

R. Putz: General anatomy, upper limb, brain, eye, ear, back, lower limb;
R. Pabst: Head, neck, thoracic and abdominal walls, thoracic, abdominal and pelvic viscera.

The inclusion of a large number of new figures is the result of the extraordinary capability of the following medical illustrators: Ulrike Brugger, Rüdiger Himmelhan and Horst Ruß. It is to their credit that the classic "SOBOTTA style" has been retained. Several of the diagrams have been generated on the computer by Henriette Rintelen. We also gratefully acknowledge our clinical colleagues for making clinical illustrations available to us (see picture credits). We owe a debt of gratitude to our colleagues from the institutes for their understanding and helpful suggestions. Dr. N. Sokolov and A. Buchhorn have put meticulous efforts into generating the specimen preparations. S. Fryk and G. Hoppmann have supported us in text processing.

The staff of the editorial office of Elsevier publishers, in particular Dr. D. Hennessen and A. Gattnarzik, has our sincere thanks. Some of the creative development of the work is a result of very fruitful discussions. We would also like to thank R. Hausdorf for tremendous efforts in the production of the atlas. R. Putz together with G. Meier were responsible for the proofreading and simplification of page design and legends. Our special thanks go to Dr. U. Osterkamp-Baust for generating the index, and all others involved in the corrections. With our joint efforts, the SOBOTTA has been once more modernized both in contents and design.

We have included many of the helpful suggestions made over the years by students and colleagues, and would therefore ask all readers of this edition to pass on to us any criticism or suggestions on the new format of this atlas.

Munich and Hannover, September 2005
R. Putz and R. Pabst

Univ.-Prof. Dr. med. Reinhard Putz

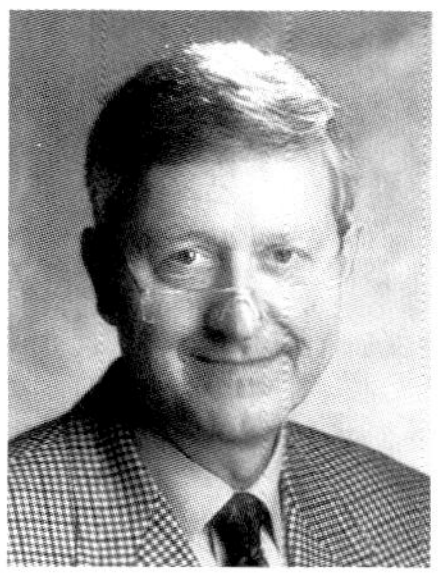

Born in Innsbruck/Austria

1962–1968	Studied medicine at the Leopold-Franzens-University of Innsbruck
1968	Received a doctorate
1968–1982	University assistant at the Institute of Anatomy at the University of Innsbruck
1978	Lecturer in anatomy
1979	Consultant for anatomy
1982–1989	Chair of the Anatomical Institute at the Albert-Ludwigs-University of Freiburg
since 1989	Chair of the Anatomical Institute at the Ludwig-Maximilians-University of Munich
1992–1994	President of the European Association of Clinical Anatomists
1993	Registration to practise medicine
1998–1999	Chairman of the Anatomical Society
1999	Member of the Akademie der Naturforscher und Ärzte (Leopoldina)
2002	Dr. h.c. of the University of Constanta, Romania
2003	Prorector I of the Ludwig-Maximilians-University of Munich

Research and fields of interest

- Functional anatomy of the passive locomotor system
- Evolution and functional anatomy of the vertebral column
- Form-function-relations of joints
- Applied anatomy (anatomical basics of orthopaedics, surgery, radiology)
- Questions about the contents and organisation of the medical curriculum
- Development of didactic training programmes at universities

Univ.-Prof. Dr. med. Reinhard Pabst

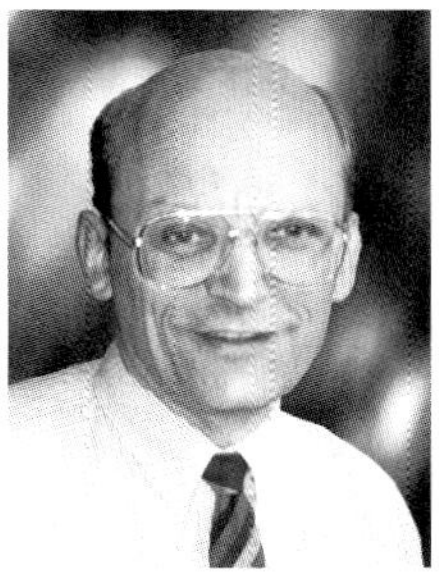

Born in Posen, grown up in Lüneburg

1965–1970	Studied medicine at the Hannover Medical School, and in Glasgow/Scotland
1970	University degree and doctorate
1971	Registration to practise medicine
1971–76	Scientific associate in the Department of Clinical Physiology, University of Ulm
1976	Lecturer for Clinical Physiology, University of Ulm, and new lectureship at the Hannover Medical School
1976–80	Senior assistant in the Department of Functional and Applied Anatomy, Hannover Medical School
1978	Extension of the Venia legendi to include anatomy
1980–1992	Head of the Department of Topographic Anatomy and Biomechanics
since 1992	Head of the Department of Functional and Applied Anatomy, Hannover Medical School
1986–1990	Prorector for studies and education, Hannover Medical School
1993–1997	Dean of the Hannover Medical School
1997–1998	Chairman of the Anatomical Society
1999–2003	Prorector of Research of the Hannover Medical School
2001	Member of the Akademie der Naturforscher und Ärzte (Leopoldina)

Research and fields of interest

- Functional anatomy of lymphatic organs
- Proliferation and migration of lymphocytes
- Development of the intestinal immune system
- Function of the pulmonary immune system
- Questions of a clinically orientated anatomy in the medical curriculum
- Evaluation of teaching

Picture credits

The editors sincerely thank all clinical colleagues that made ultrasound, computed tomographic and magnetic resonance images as well as endoscopic and intraoperative pictures available:

Prof. Altaras, Centre for Radiology, University of Gießen (Fig. 741, 763, 764)
Dr. Baumeister, Department of Radiology, University of Freiburg (Fig. 889)
PD Dr. Burgkardt, Orthopaedic Clinic, Technical University of Munich (Fig. 1163)
Prof. Brückmann & Dr. Linn, Neuroradiology, Institute for Diagnostic Radiology, University of Munich (Fig. 1367, 1431 a, b, 1432 a, b)
Prof. Daniel, Department of Cardiology, University of Erlangen (Fig. 631, 632, 633, 705)
Prof. Degenhardt, Bielefeld (Fig. 865, 867)
Prof. Galanski & Dr. Kirchhoff, Department of Diagnostic Radiology, Hannover Medical School (Fig. 944, 945, 994, 996)
Prof. Galanski & Dr. Schäfer, Department of Diagnostic Radiology, Hannover Medical School (Fig. 603 a, b, 659, 703, 723, 926, 936, 939, 941)
Prof. Gebel, Department of Gastroenterology, Hepatology and Endocrinology, Hannover Medical School (Fig. 242, 749, 758, 759, 770, 771, 806, 824)
Dr. Goei, Radiology, Heerlen, The Netherlands (Fig. 882, 883) (with permission from Radiology 173; 137–141: 1989)
Dr. Greeven, St.-Elizabeth-Hospital, Neuwied (Fig. 150, 970)
Prof. Hoffmann & PD Dr. Bektas, Clinic for Abdominal and Transplantation Surgery, Hannover Medical School (Fig. 772, 960)
Prof. Hohlfeld, Clinic for Pneumology, Hannover Medical School (Fig. 661, 662)
Prof. Jonas, Urology, Hannover Medical School (Fig. 834 a, b, 835)
Prof. Kampik & Prof. Müller, Ophthalmology, University of Munich (Fig. 1362)
Dr. Kirchhoff & Dr. Weidemann, Department of Diagnostic Radiology, Hannover Medical School (Fig. 773, 825, 834, 928, 930, 932, 934, 937)
Prof. Kremers, Department for Restorative Dentistry and Periodontology, University of Munich (Fig. 169)
Prof. Kunze, von Haunersches Children's Hospital, University of Munich (Fig. 327–330)
Dr. Meyer, Department of Gastroenterology, Hepatology and Endocrinology, Hannover Medical School (Fig. 676, 719 a, b, 724, 877, 878)
Prof. Müller-Vahl, Neurology, Hannover Medical School (Fig. 128 a, b)
Prof. Pfeifer, Radiology, Institute for Diagnostic Radiology, University of Munich (Fig. 293, 294, 310, 312, 449, 451, 501–504, 539–542, 987, 1018, 1019, 1049, 1050)
PD Dr. Rau, Department of Radiology, University of Freiburg (Fig. 644, 657, 658)
Prof. Ravelli †, formerly Institute of Anatomy, University of Innsbruck (Fig. 499)
PD Dr. Rieger, Radiology, Institute for Diagnostic Radiology, University of Munich (Fig. 1127)
Prof. Reich, Orofacial Surgery, University of Bonn (Fig. 113 a, b)
Prof. Reiser & Dr. Wagner, Institute for Diagnostic Radiology, University of Munich (Fig. 436, 449, 451, 453, 524, 1276, 1277, 1278, 1281, 1282)
Prof. Rudzki-Janson, Department of Orthodontics, University of Munich (Fig. 72, 73)
Dr. Scheibe, Department of Surgery, Rosman Hospital, Breisach (Fig. 1011 a–c)
Prof. Scheumann, Clinic for Abdominal and Transplantation Surgery, Hannover Medical School (Fig. 243, 244, 245)
Prof. Schillinger, Department of Gynaecology, University of Freiburg (Fig. 866)
Prof. Schliephake, Orofacial Surgery, Göttingen (Fig. 152, 196, 197)
Prof. Schlösser, Centre for Gynaecology, Hannover Medical School (Fig. 864 a, b, 872, 873, 910)
Prof. Schumacher, Neuroradiology, Department of Radiology, University of Freiburg (Fig. 1166 a, b)
Dr. Sommer & PD Dr. Bauer, Radiologists, Munich (Fig. 1022–1024, 1367)
Prof. Stotz, Paediatrics, University of Munich (Fig. 971, 972)
PD Dr. Vogl, Radiology, University of Munich (Fig. 436, 453, 1349, 1350)
Prof. Vollrath, Ear-Nose-Throat Department, Mönchengladbach (Fig. 229, 230, 231)
Prof. Wagner †, Diagnostic Radiology II, Hannover Medical School (Fig. 684, 796, 797, 801, 804, 884)
Prof. Wenz, formerly Department of Radiology, University of Freiburg (Fig. 500)
Prof. Witt, Department of Neurosurgery, University of Munich (Fig. 405)
Dr. Willführ, formerly Clinic for Abdominal and Transplantation Surgery, Hannover Medical School (Fig. 783)
PD Dr. Wimmer, Department of Radiology, University of Freiburg (Fig. 531)

Additional illustrations were obtained from the following textbooks:

Benninghoff-Drenckhahn: Anatomie, Band 1 (Drenckhahn D., Hrsg.), 16. Aufl., Urban & Fischer, München 2003 (Fig. 555, 556, 580, 581, 582)
Welsch, U.: Lehrbuch Histologie, Urban & Fischer, München 2003 (Fig. 654, 752, 829, 854, 855)
Welsch, U. (Hrsg.): Sobotta, Atlas Histologie, 6. Aufl., Urban & Fischer, München 2002 (Fig. 857 a, b, 869, 917)
Wicke, L.: Atlas der Röntgenanatomie, 3. Aufl., Urban & Schwarzenberg, München–Wien–Baltimore 1985 (Fig. 675 a, b)

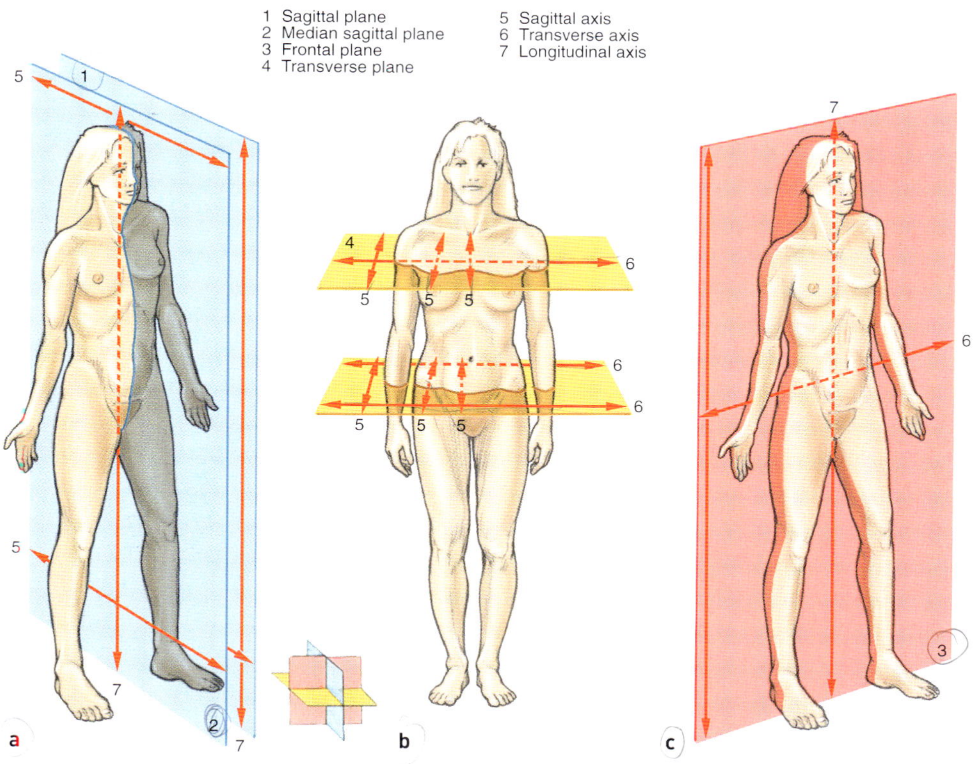

Fig. 1 a–c Planes and axes.
a Sagittal plane, sagittal and longitudinal axes
b Transverse plane (= horizontal plane), transverse and sagittal axes
c Frontal plane (= coronal plane), longitudinal and transverse axes

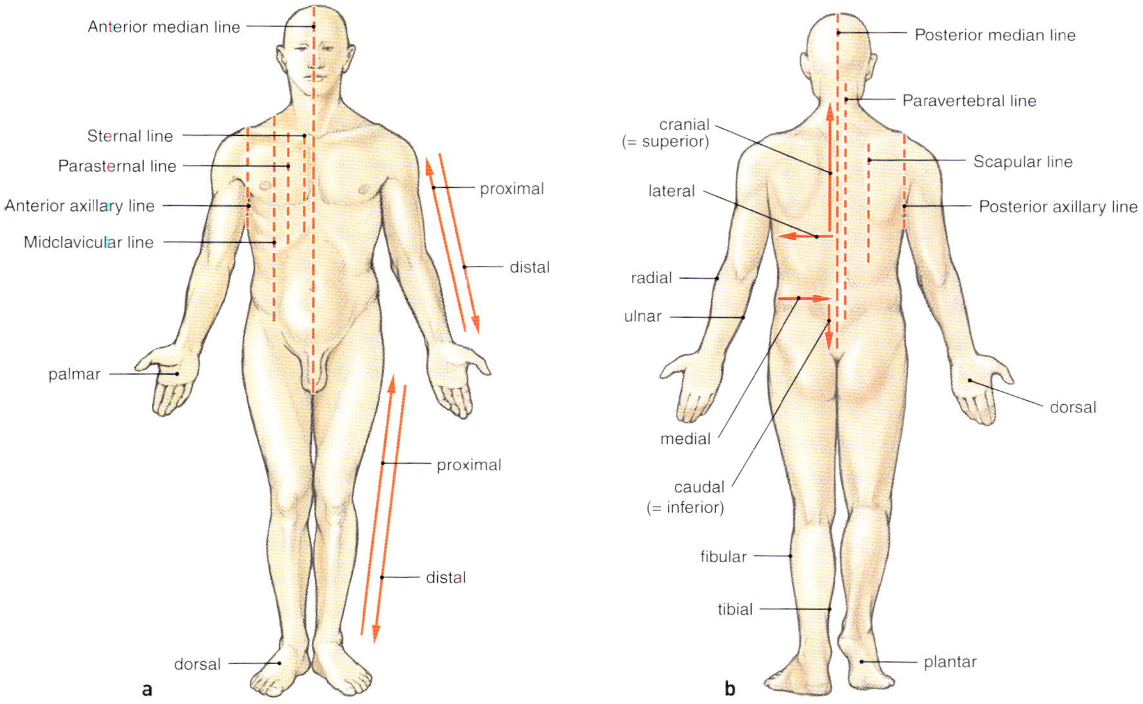

Fig. 2 a, b Orientation lines of the human body and terms of direction and position.
a Ventral view (ventralis, anterior)
b Dorsal view (dorsalis, posterior)

Parts of the human body

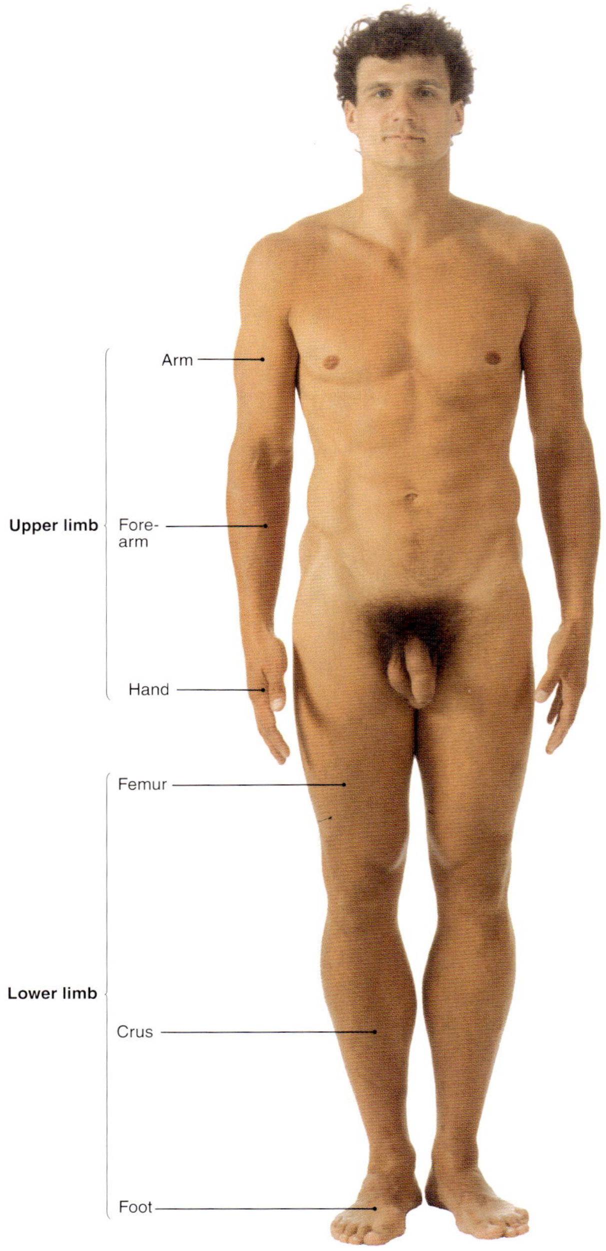

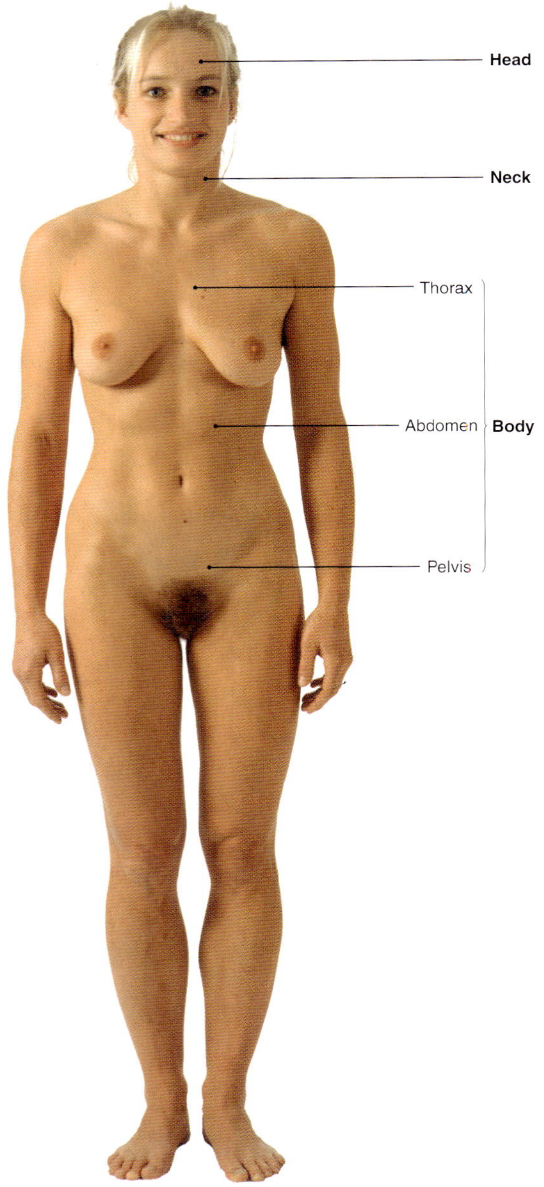

Fig. 3 Surface anatomy of the male.

Fig. 4 Surface anatomy of the female.

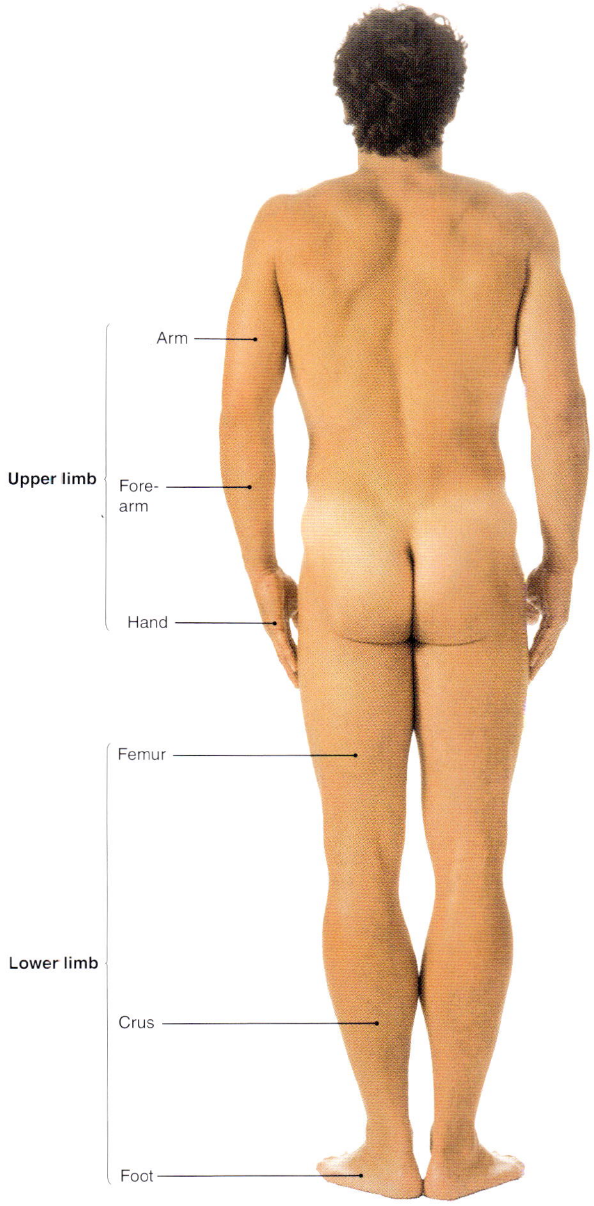

Fig. 5 Surface anatomy of the male.

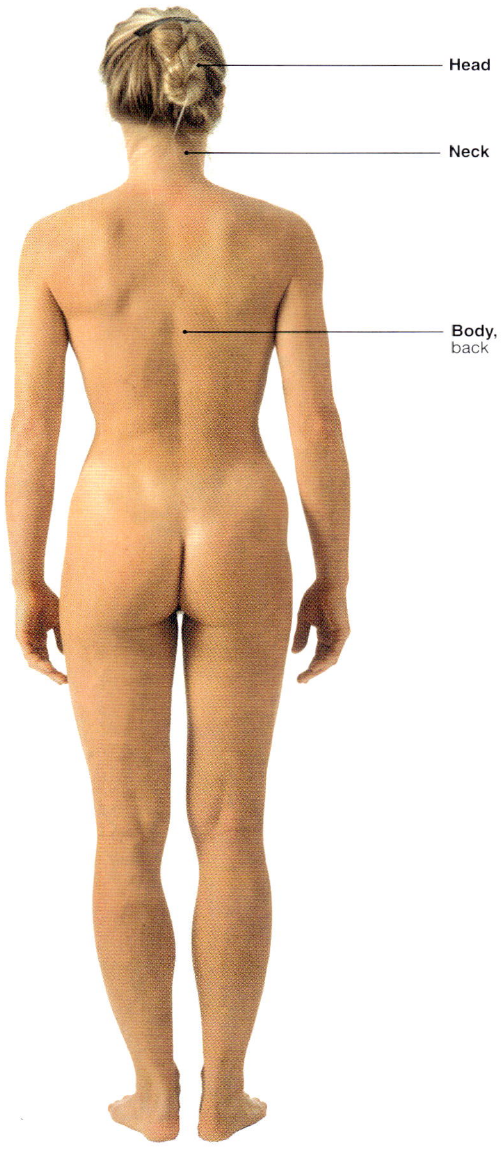

Fig. 6 Surface anatomy of the female.

Regions of the human body

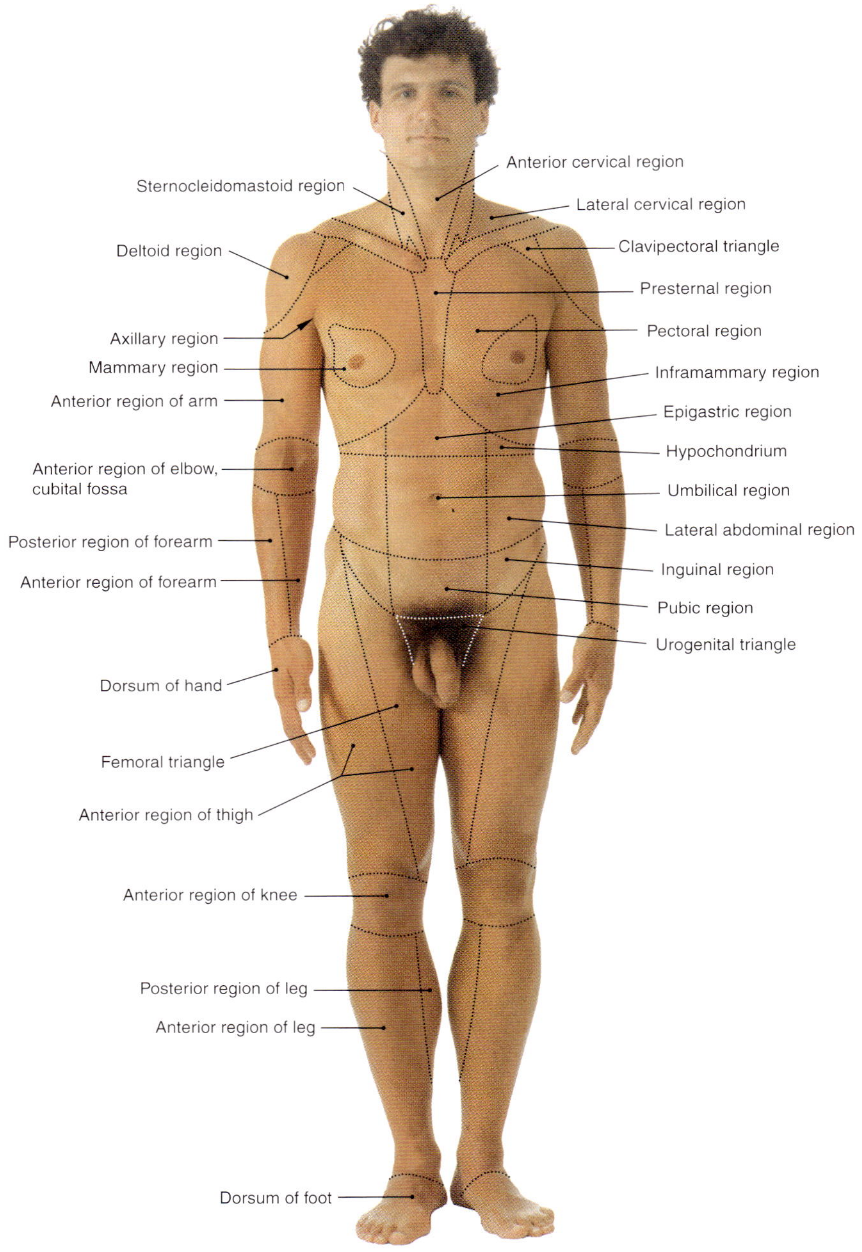

Fig. 7 Regions of the human body.

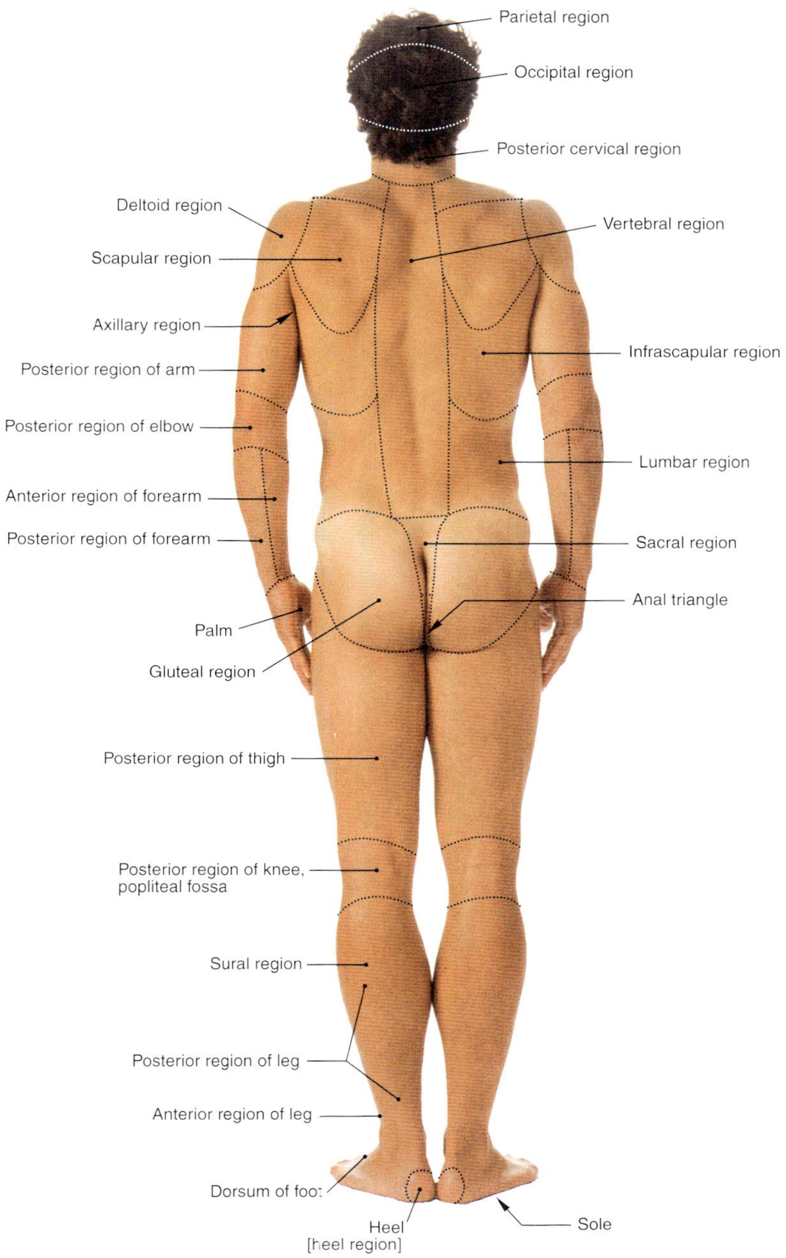

Fig. 8 Regions of the human body.

Skeleton

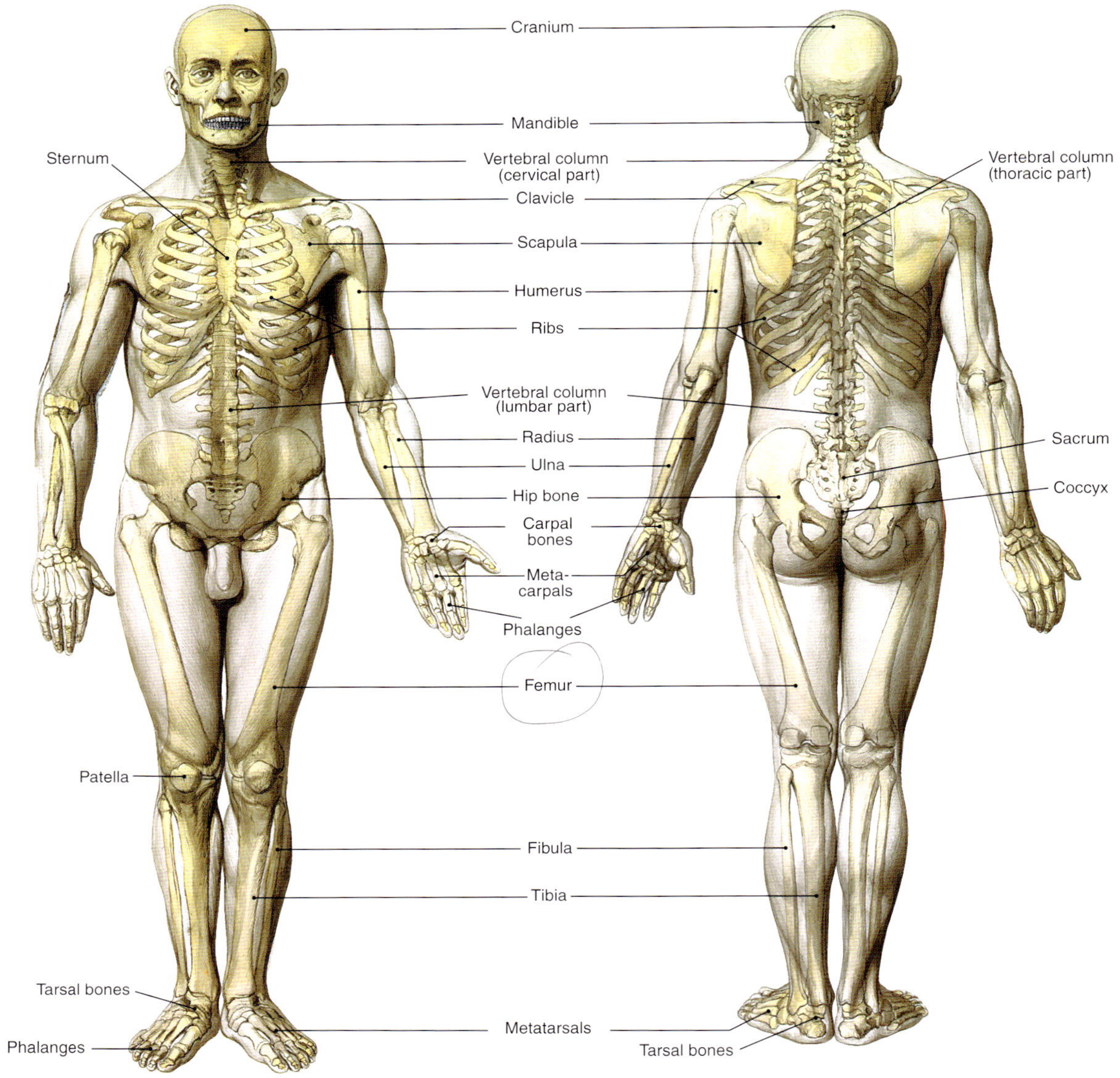

Fig. 9 Overview of the skeleton.

Fig. 10 Overview of the skeleton.

Parts of the human body

Head

Neck

Trunk
Thorax
Abdomen
Pelvis

Upper limb
Shoulder girdle
Arm

Lower limb
Pelvic girdle
Leg

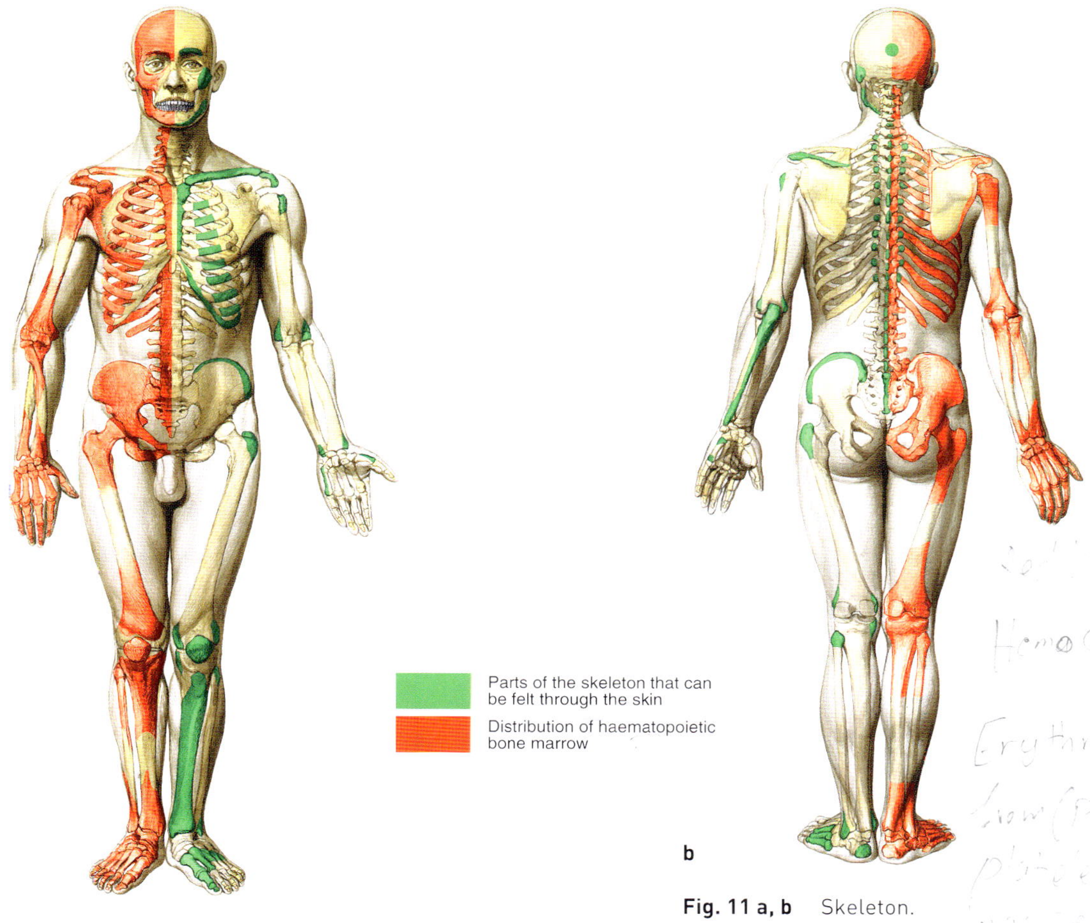

Fig. 11 a, b Skeleton.

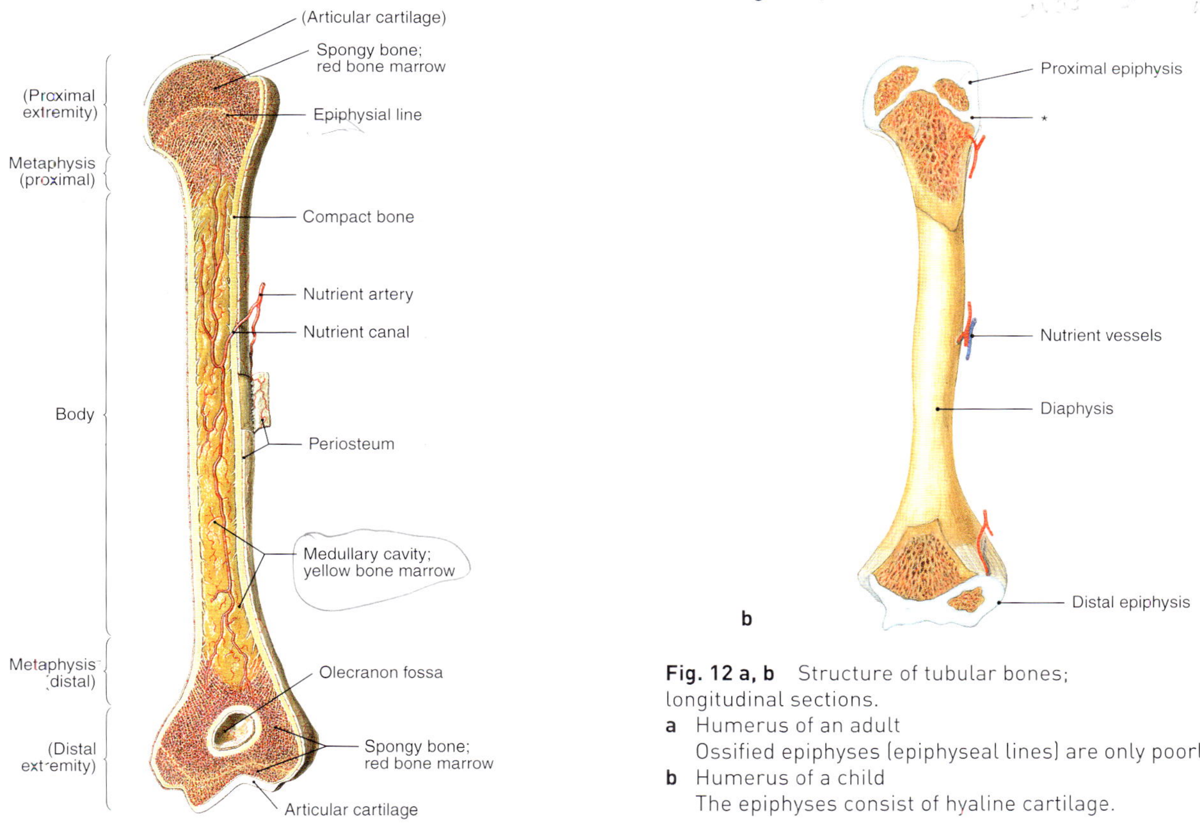

Fig. 12 a, b Structure of tubular bones; longitudinal sections.
a Humerus of an adult
Ossified epiphyses (epiphyseal lines) are only poorly visible.
b Humerus of a child
The epiphyses consist of hyaline cartilage.

* Epiphysis, epiphyseal plate

Bone development

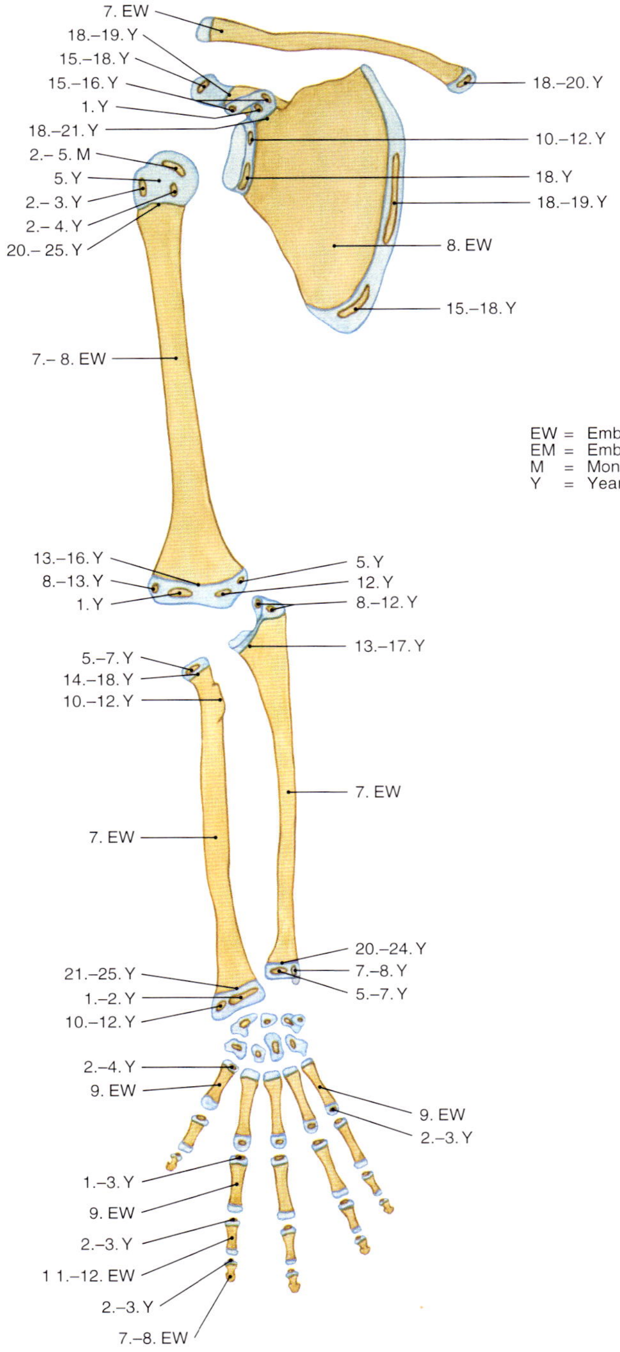

Scaphoid 3.– 6. M
Lunate 3.– 6. Y
Trapezium 3.– 8. Y
Trapezoid 3.– 7. Y

Pisiform 8.– 12. Y
Triquetrum 1.– 4. Y
Hamate 2.– 5. M
Capitate 2.– 4. M

EW = Embryonic week
EM = Embryonic month
M = Month of life
Y = Year of life

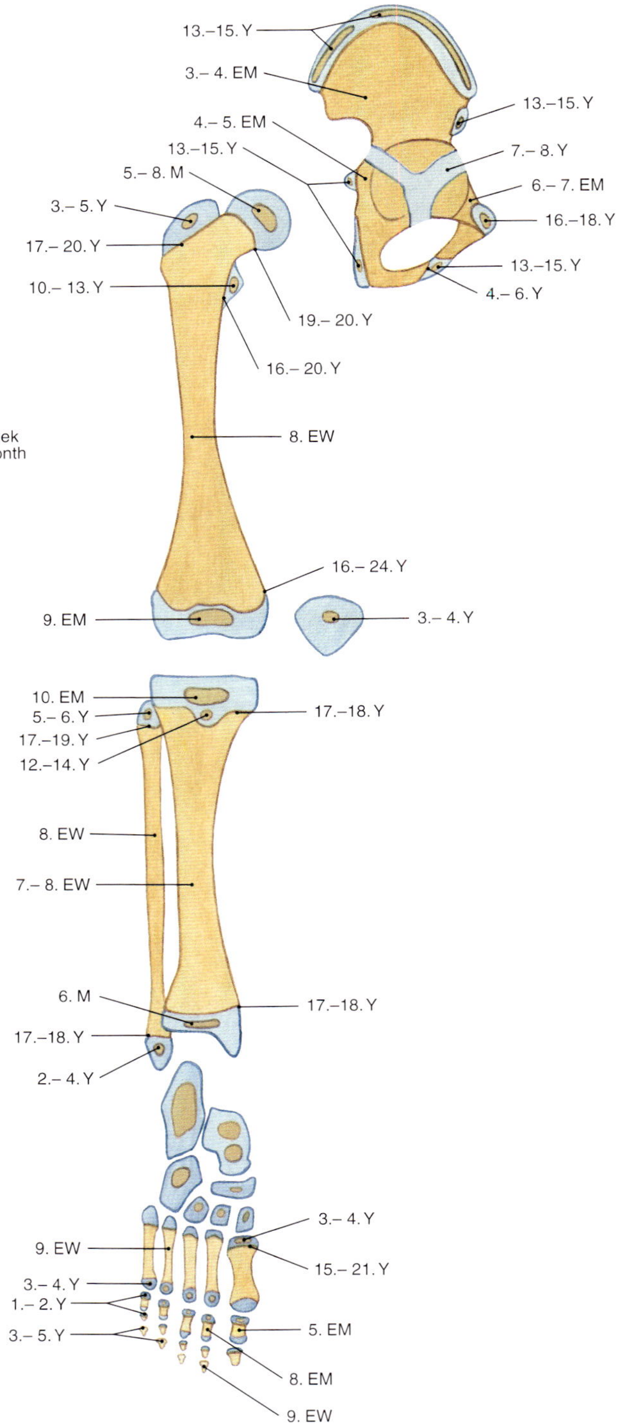

Talus 7. M
Calcaneus 5.– 6. M
Navicular 4. Y
Cuboid 10. M

Medial cuneiform 2.– 3. Y
Intermediate cuneiform 3.– 4. Y
Lateral cuneiform 12. M

Fig. 13 Appearance of ossification centres and synossification at the epiphyses of the upper limb (means according to v. LANZ, 1956; EXNER, 1990; HEUCK and BAST, 1994).

Fig. 14 Appearance of ossification centres and synossification at the epiphyses of the lower limb (means according to v. LANZ, 1956; EXNER, 1990; HEUCK and BAST, 1994).

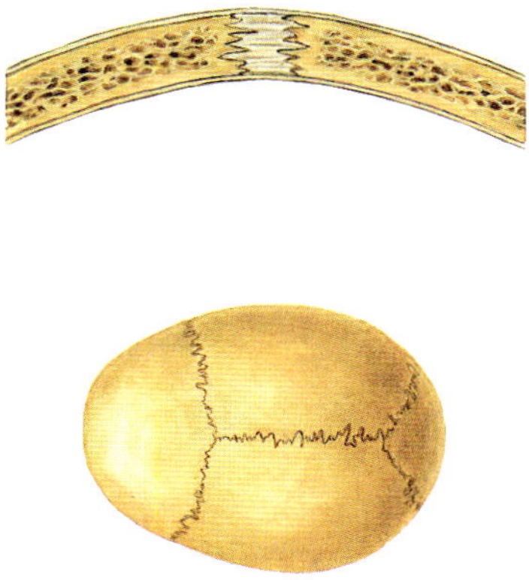

Fig. 15 Fibrous joint, exemplified by the sutures of the skull.

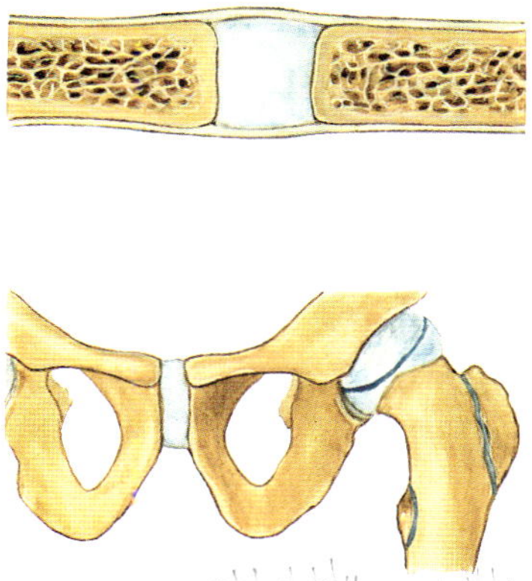

Fig. 16 Cartilaginous joint, exemplified by the pubic bone symphysis.

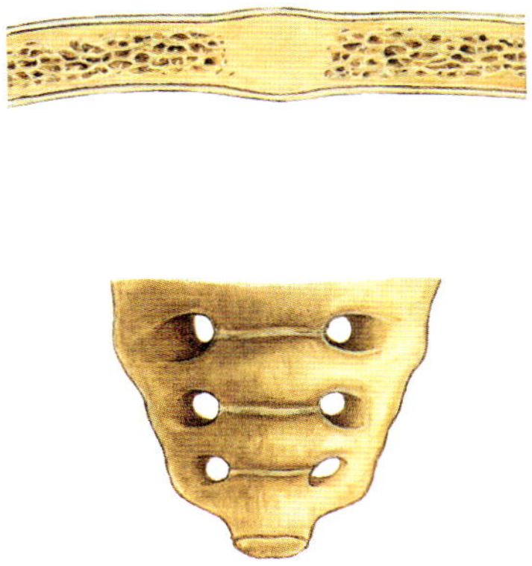

Fig. 17 Osseous joint, exemplified by the sacrum.

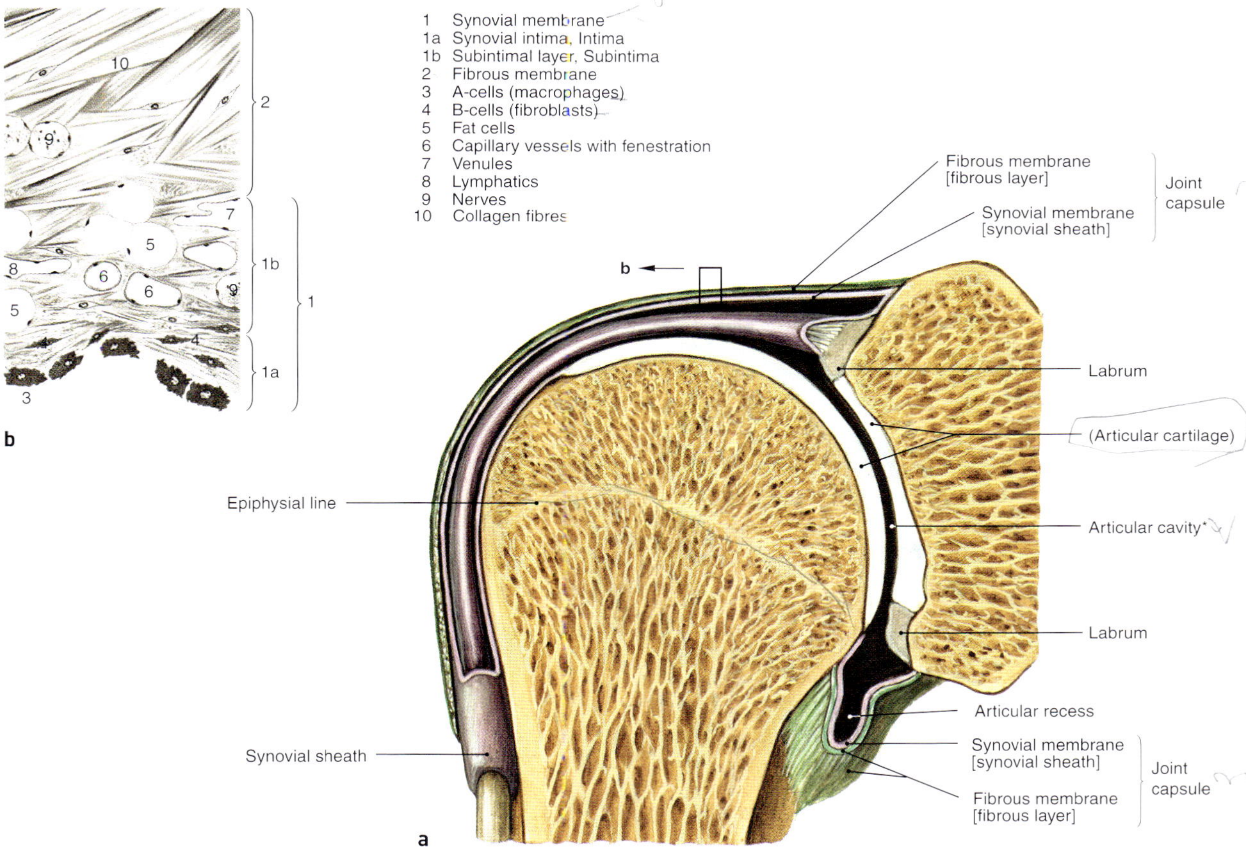

Fig. 18 Synovial joint, exemplified by the shoulder joint.
a Section in the scapular plane
b Structure of the joint capsule

* The joint cavity is illustrated broader to enhance visibility.

Joints

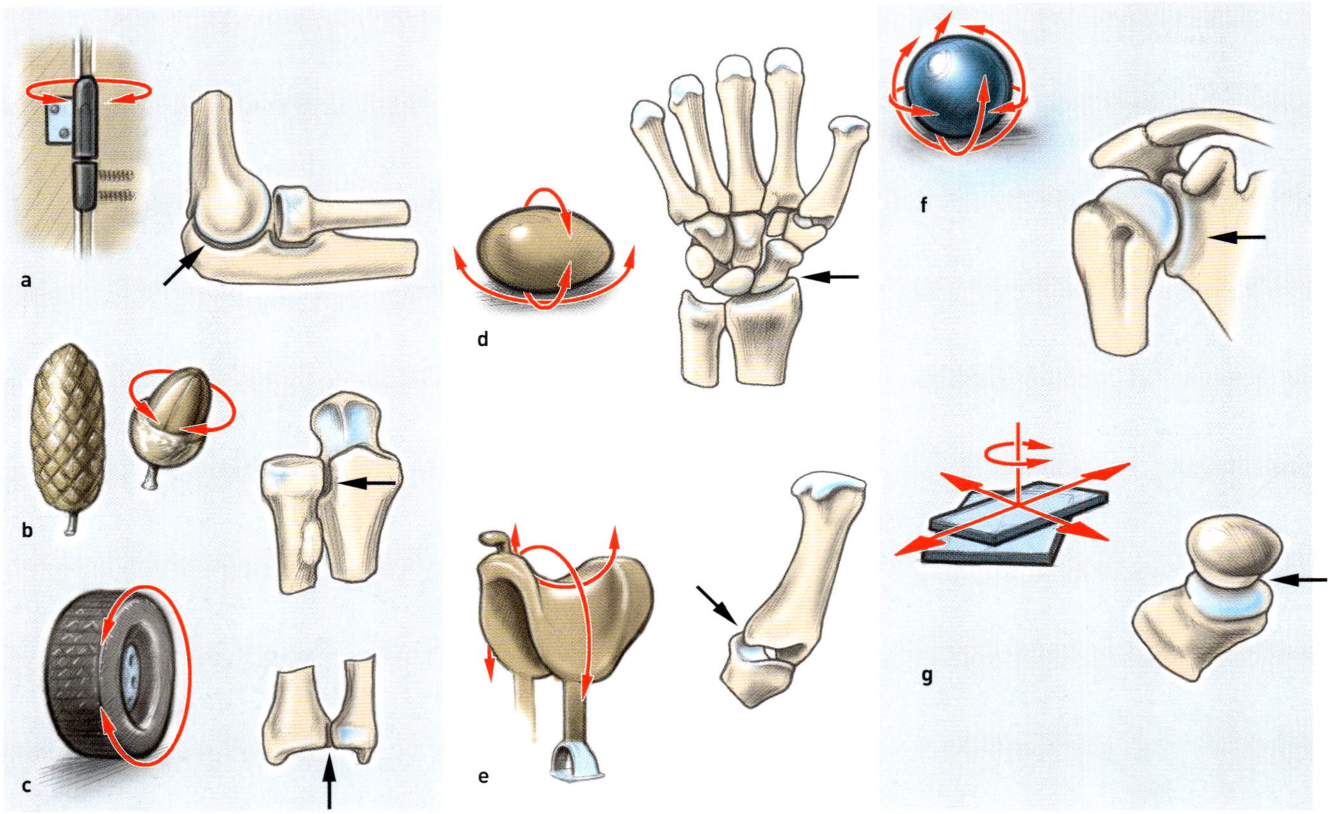

Fig. 19 a–g Joints.
a Hinge joint elbow and knee
b Conoid joint
c Pivot joint
d Condylar joint
e Saddle joint
f Spheroidal joint
g Plane joint

carbal bone of wrist
tarasal bone of ankle

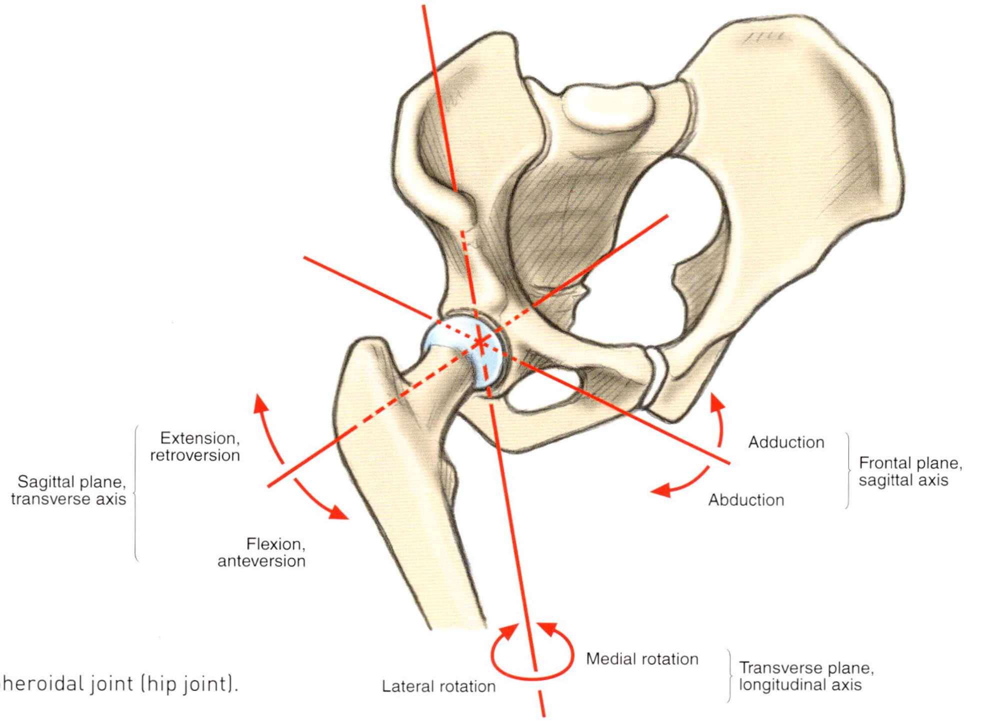

Fig. 20 Spheroidal joint (hip joint).

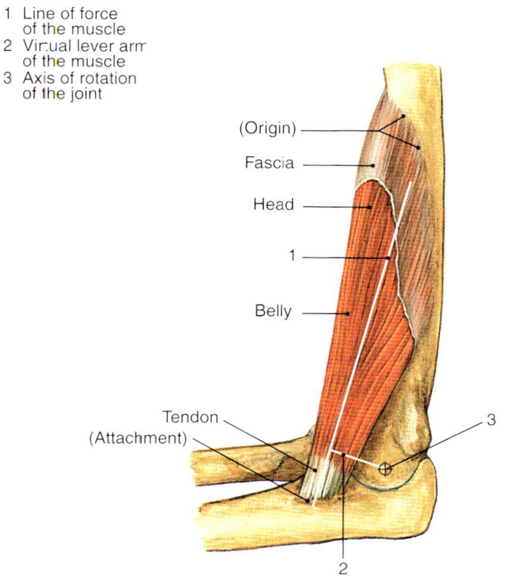

Fig. 21 Organisation principle of skeletal muscles, exemplified by the brachial muscle.

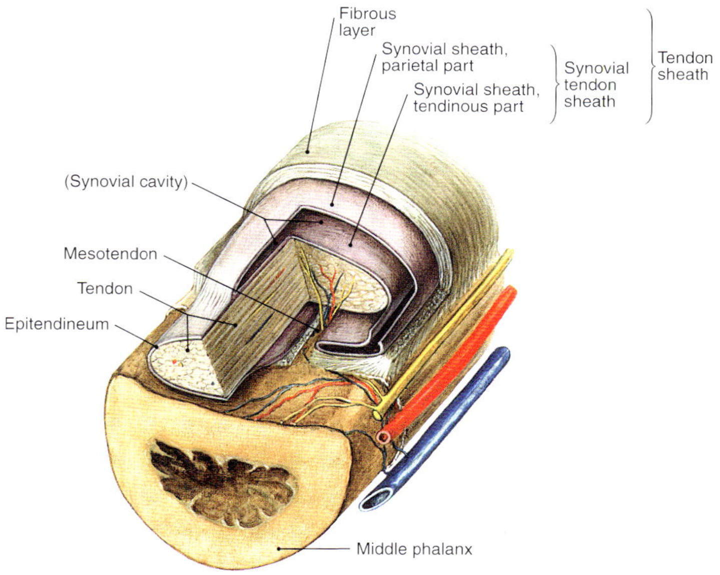

Fig. 22 Structure of a tendon sheath, exemplified by a finger.

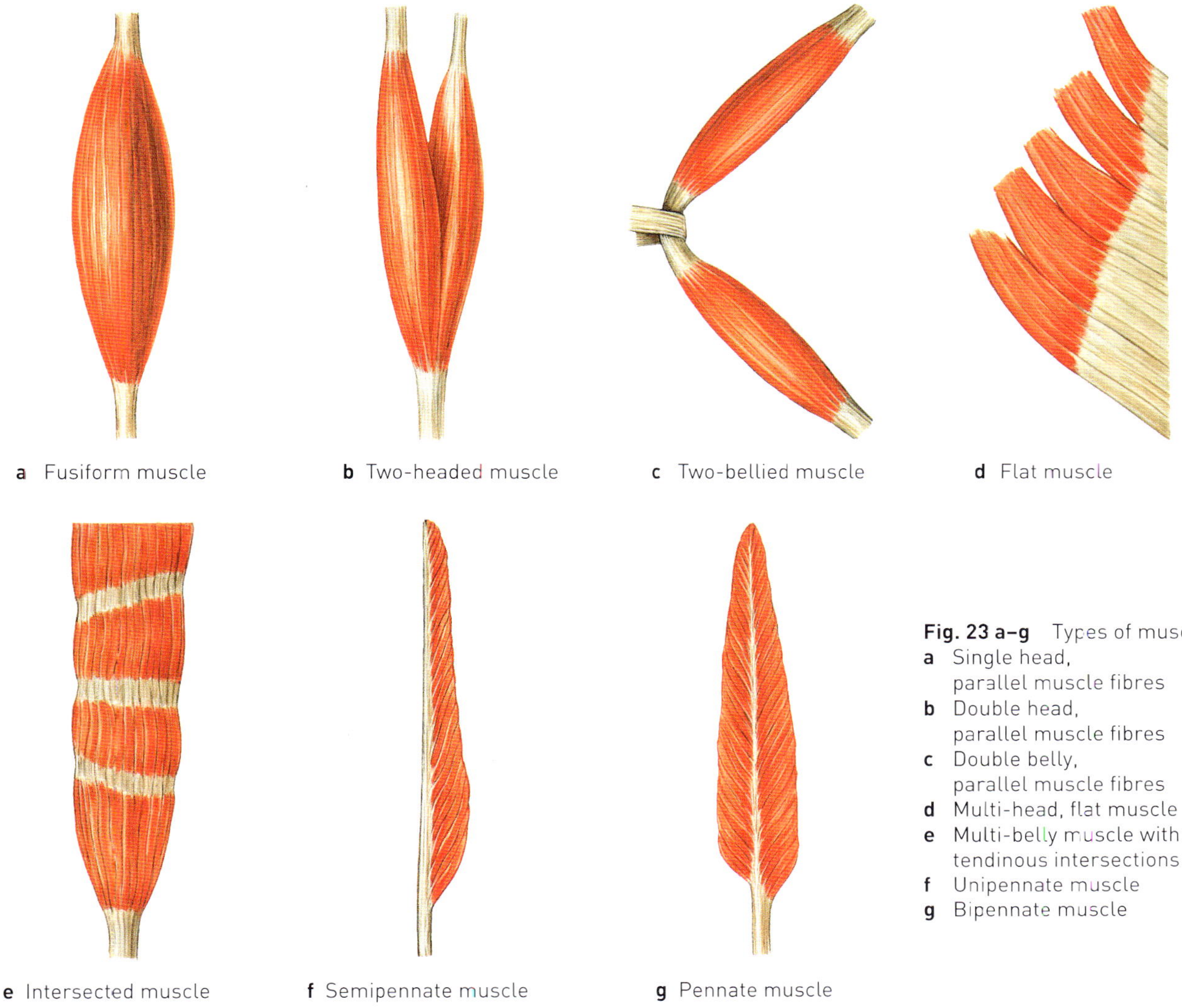

Fig. 23 a–g Types of muscles.

a Single head, parallel muscle fibres
b Double head, parallel muscle fibres
c Double belly, parallel muscle fibres
d Multi-head, flat muscle
e Multi-belly muscle with tendinous intersections
f Unipennate muscle
g Bipennate muscle

Skeletal muscles

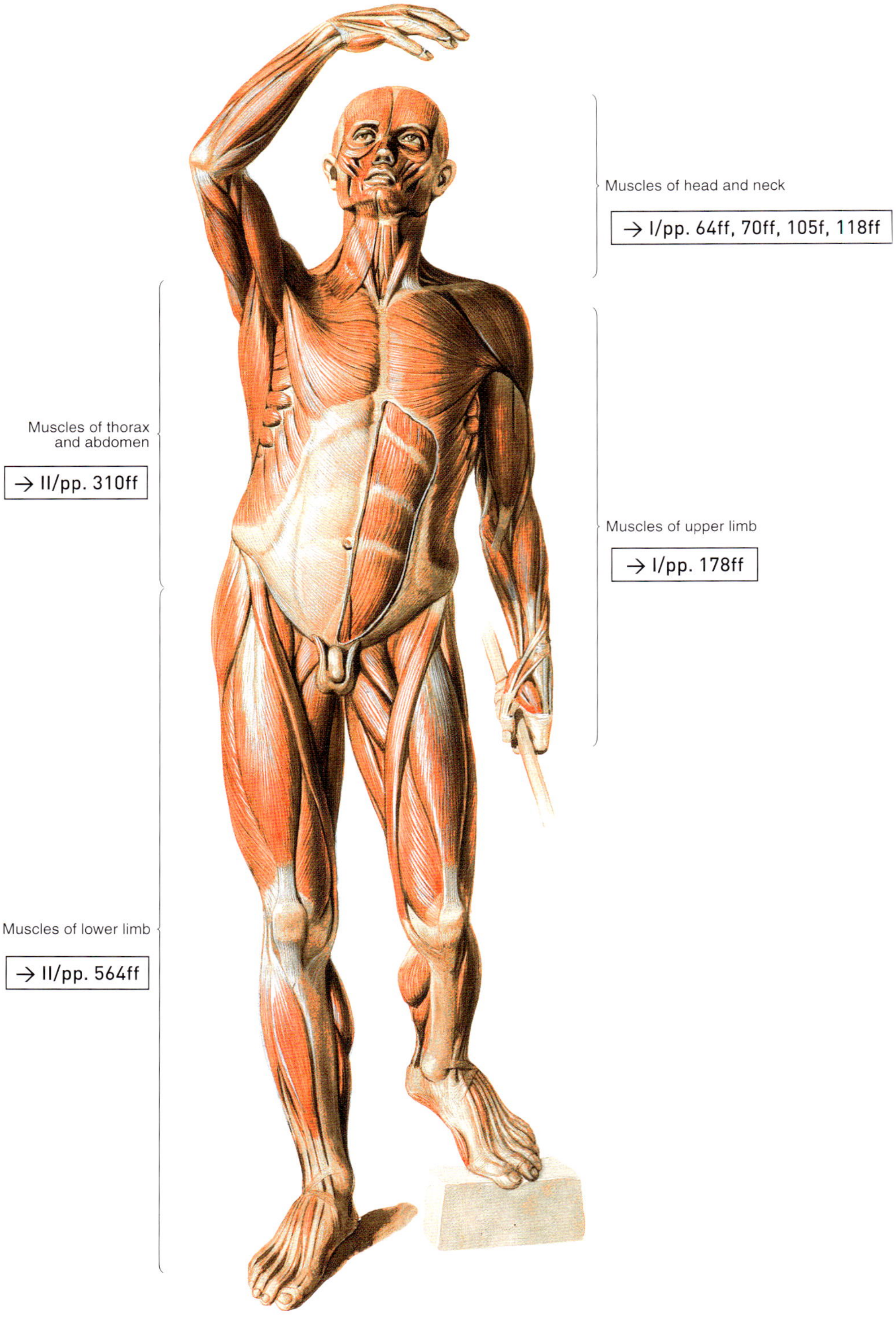

Fig. 24 Overview of the skeletal muscles.

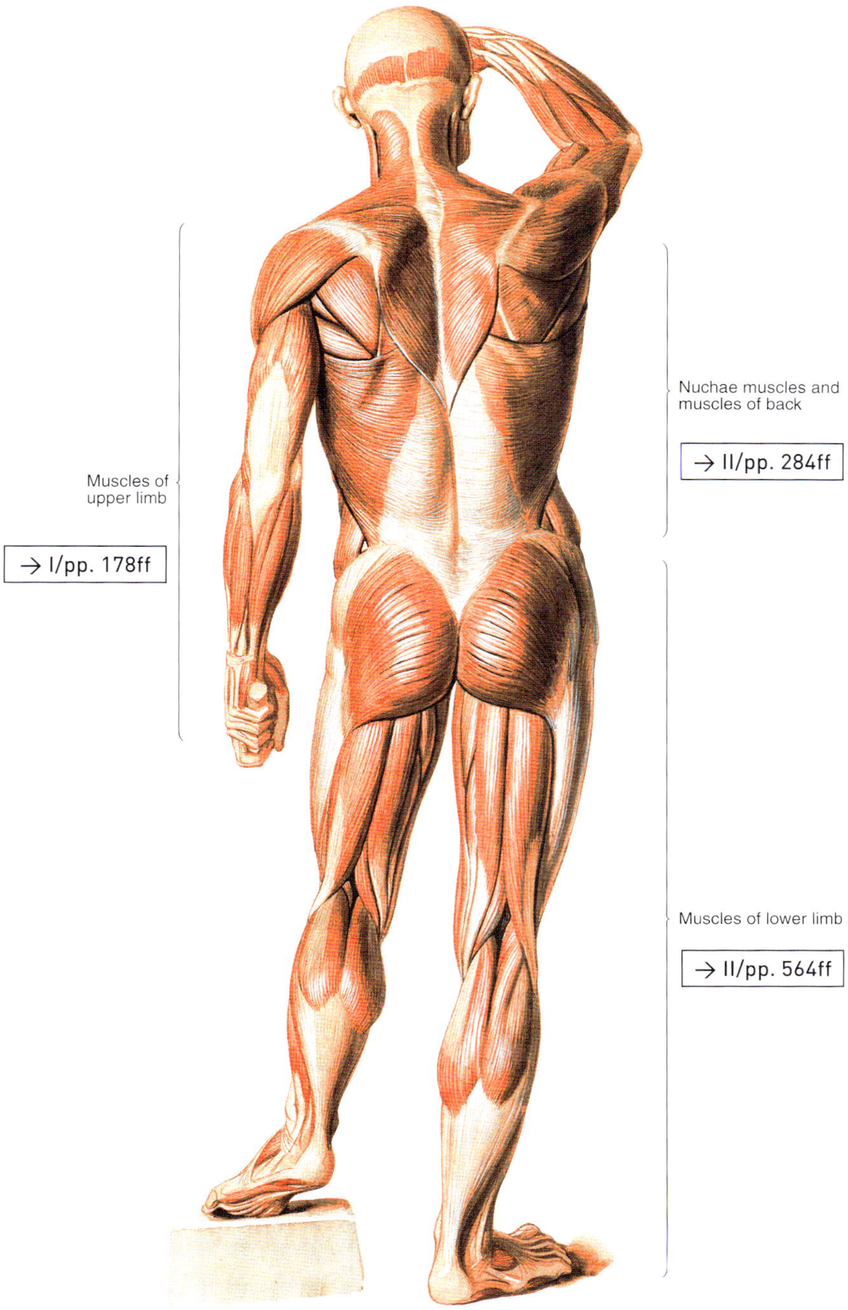

Fig. 25 Overview of the skeletal muscles.

Digestive and respiratory system

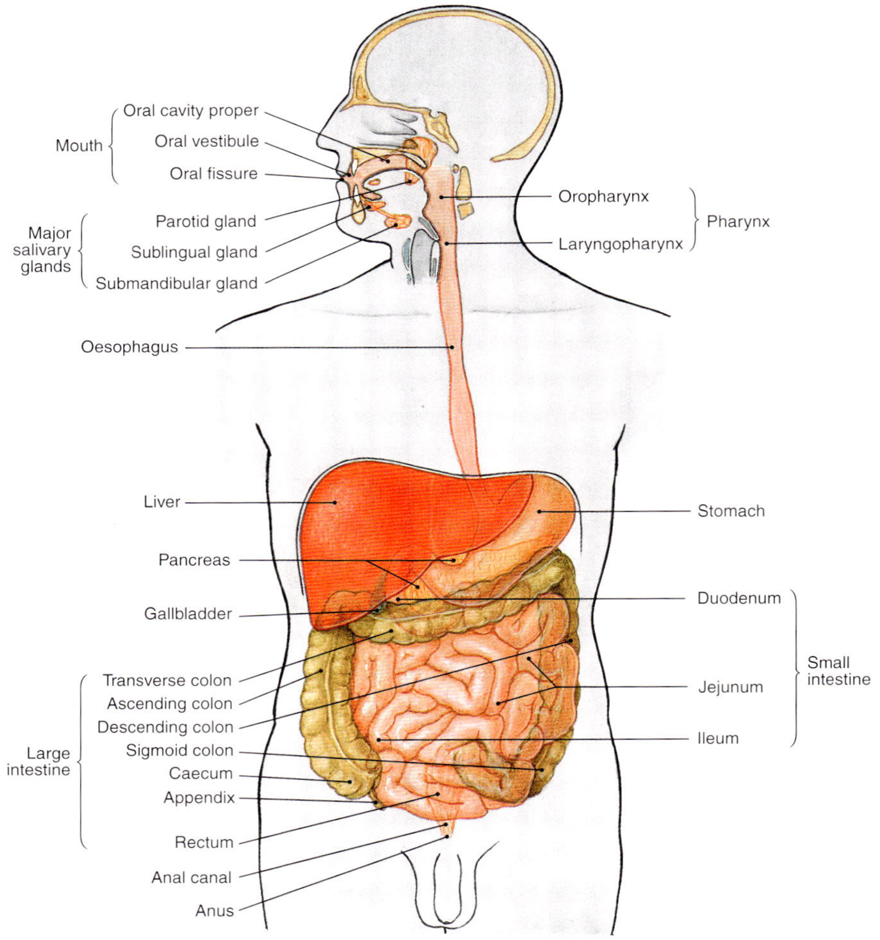

Fig. 26 Overview of the digestive system.

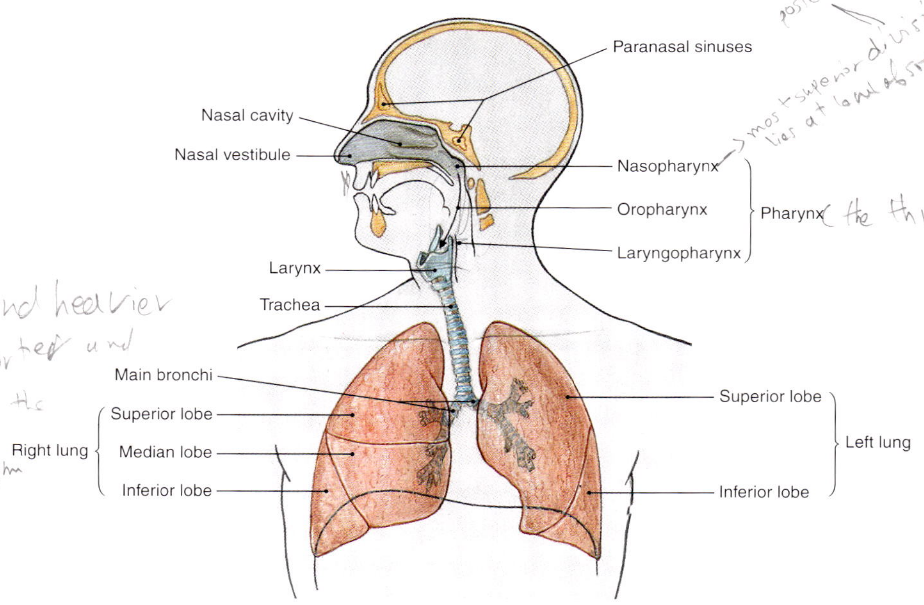

Fig. 27 Overview of the respiratory system.

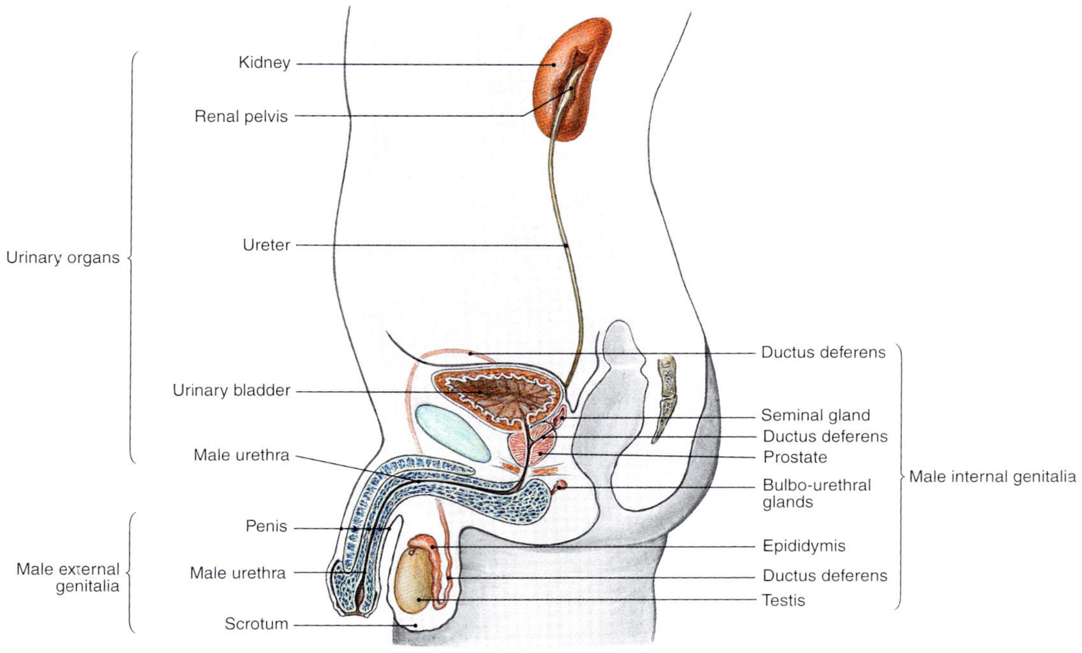

Fig. 28 Overview of the urinary and genital system of the male.

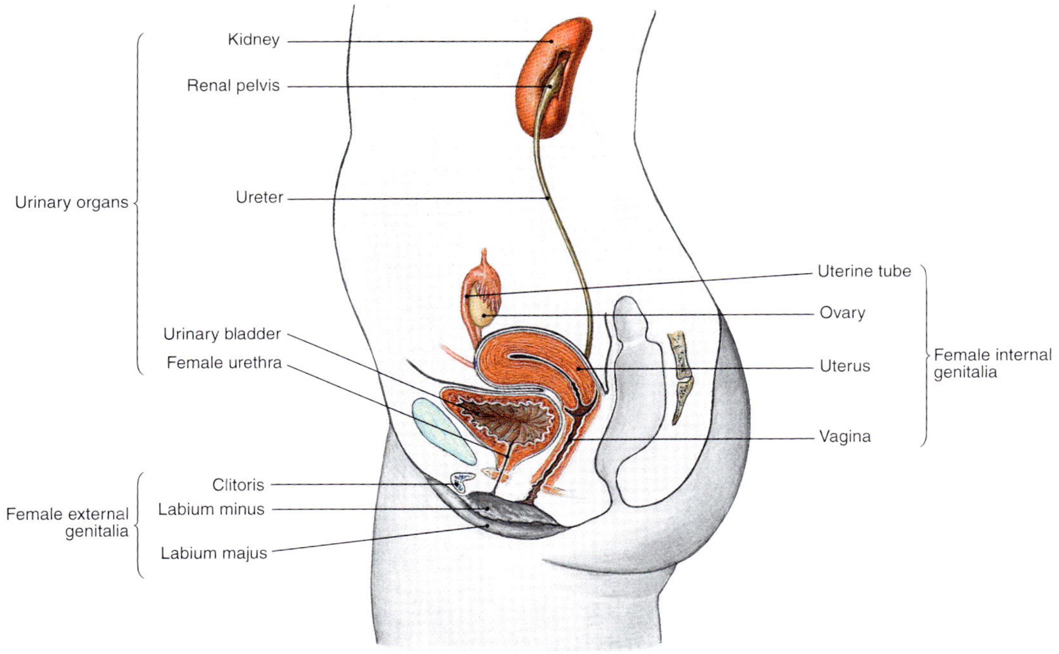

Fig. 29 Overview of the urinary and genital system of the female.

Internal organs, projection

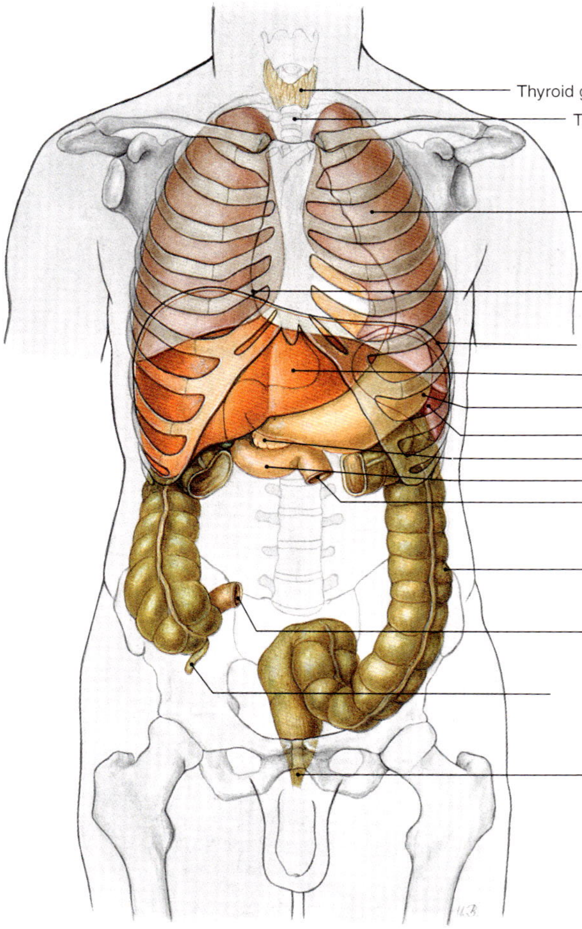

Fig. 30 Projection of the internal organs onto the surface of the body.

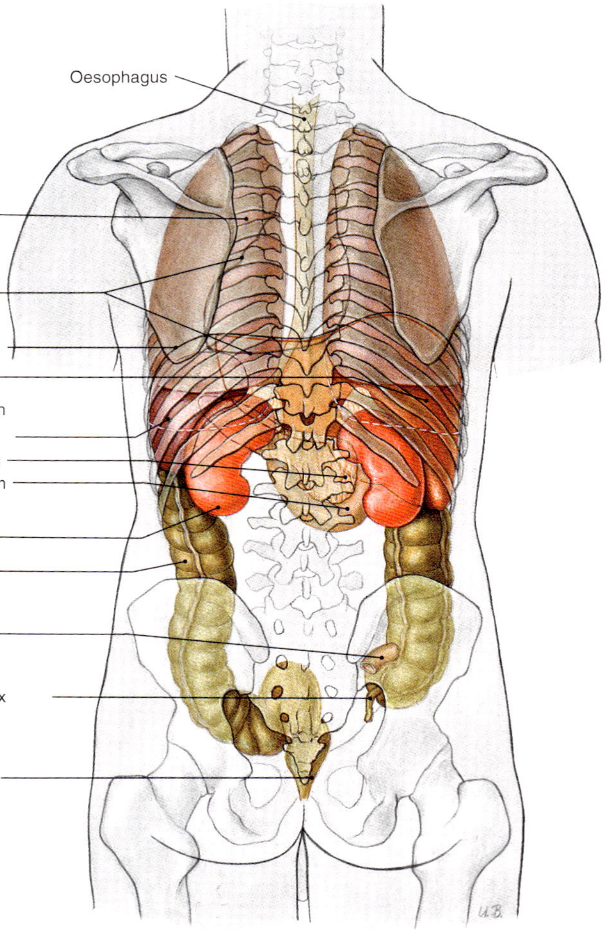

Fig. 31 Projection of the internal organs onto the surface of the body.

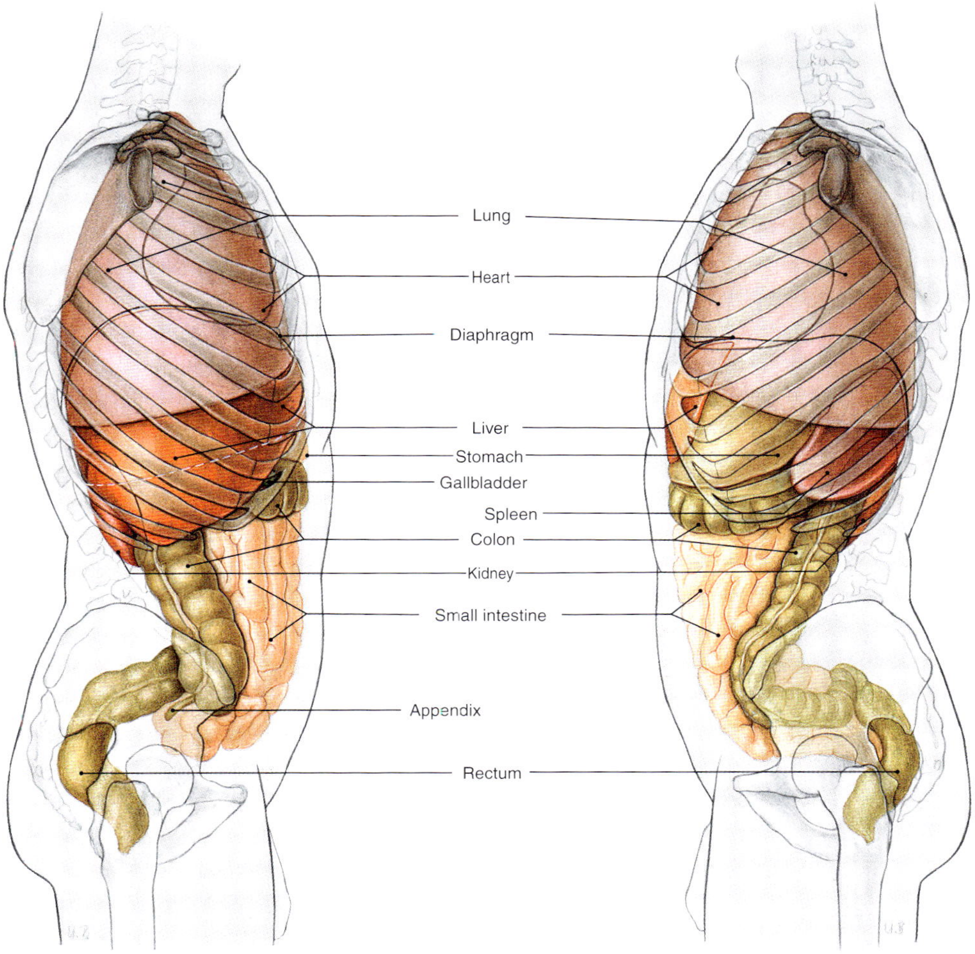

Fig. 32 Projection of the internal organs onto the surface of the body.

Fig. 33 Projection of the internal organs onto the surface of the body.

Arteries

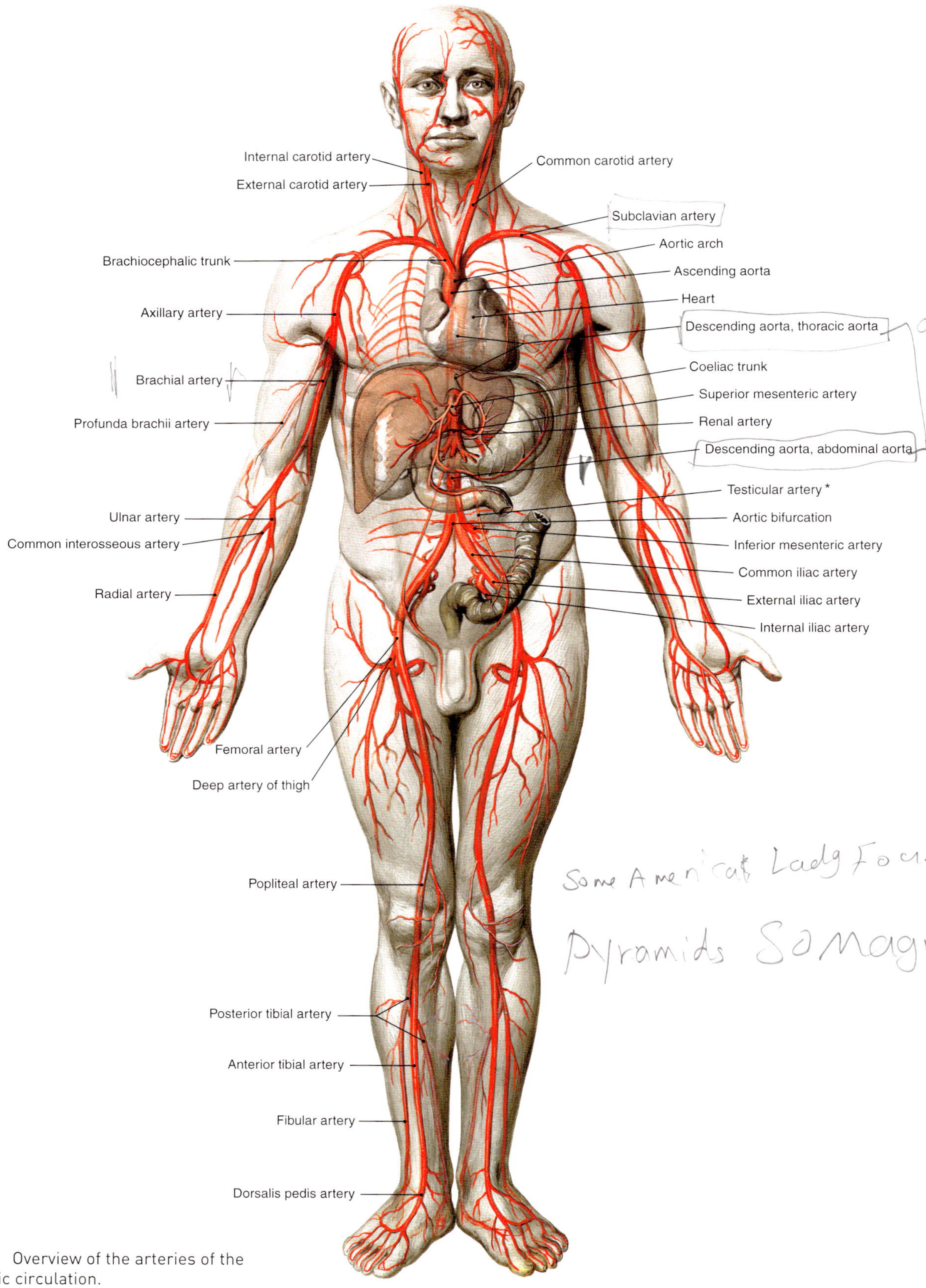

ascend from T4 to T12

T12–L4

Some American Lady Found Our Pyramids So magnificent

Fig. 34 Overview of the arteries of the systemic circulation.

* In the female: ovarian artery

Arteries

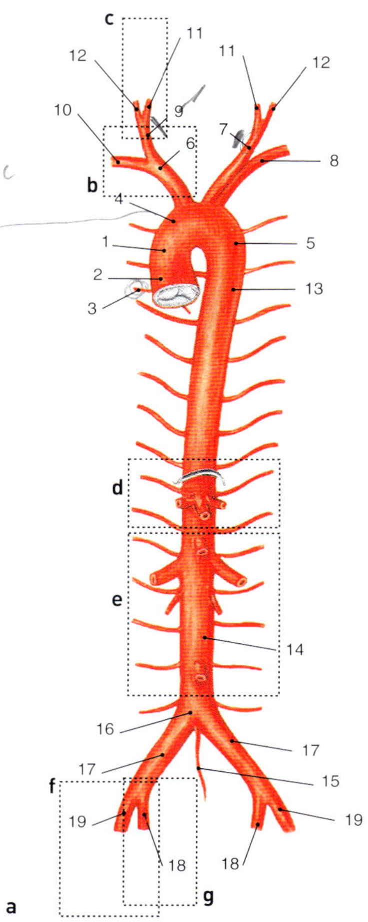

a

1 Ascending aorta
2 Aortic bulb
3 Coronary arteries
4 Aortic arch
5 Aortic isthmus
6 Brachiocephalic trunk
7 Left common carotid artery
8 Left subclavian artery
9 Right common carotid artery
10 Right subclavian artery
11 Internal carotid artery
12 External carotid artery
13 Thoracic aorta
14 Abdominal aorta
15 Median sacral artery
16 Aortic bifurcation
17 Common iliac artery
18 Internal iliac artery
19 External iliac artery

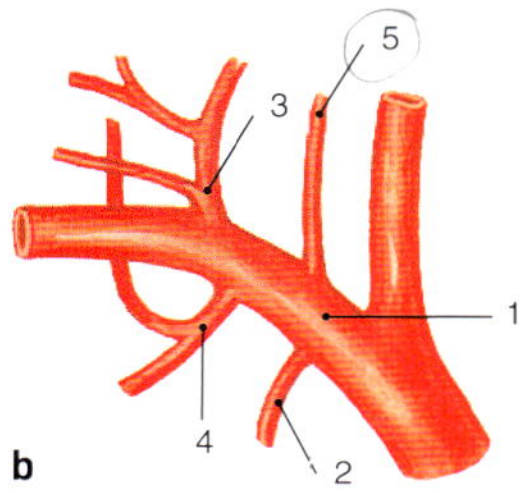

b

1 Subclavian artery
2 Internal thoracic artery
3 Thyrocervical trunk
4 Costocervical trunk
5 Vertebral artery

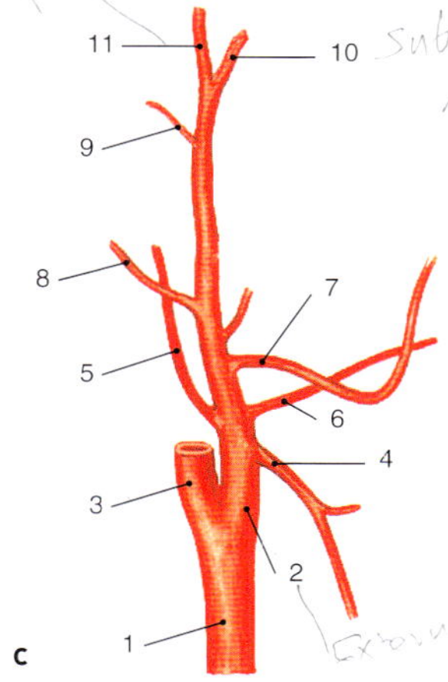

c

1 Common carotid artery
2 External carotid artery
3 Internal carotid artery
4 Superior thyroid artery
5 Ascending pharyngeal artery
6 Lingual artery
7 Facial artery
8 Occipital artery
9 Posterior auricular artery
10 Superficial temporal artery
11 Maxillary artery

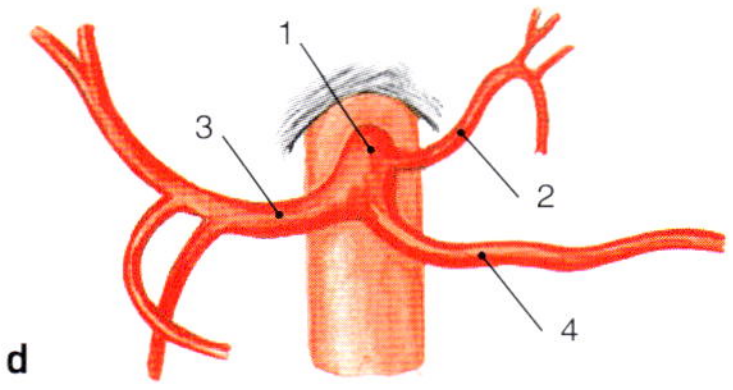

d

1 Coeliac trunk
2 Left gastric artery
3 Common hepatic artery
4 Splenic artery

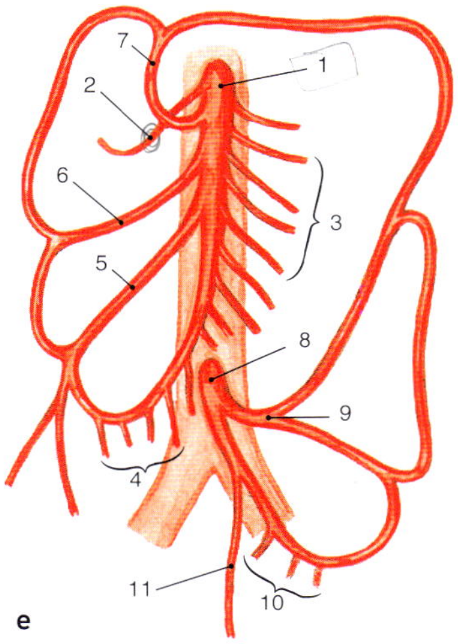

e

1 Superior mesenteric artery
2 Inferior pancreatico-duodenal artery
3 Jejunal arteries
4 Ileal arteries
5 Ileocolic artery
6 Right colic artery
7 Middle colic artery
8 Inferior mesenteric artery
9 Left colic artery
10 Sigmoid arteries
11 Superior rectal artery

Fig. 35 a–g Aorta and greater arteries; schema of the branching pattern.
a Aorta
b Subclavian artery
c External carotid artery
d Coeliac trunk
e Superior and inferior mesenteric artery
f External iliac artery
g Internal iliac artery

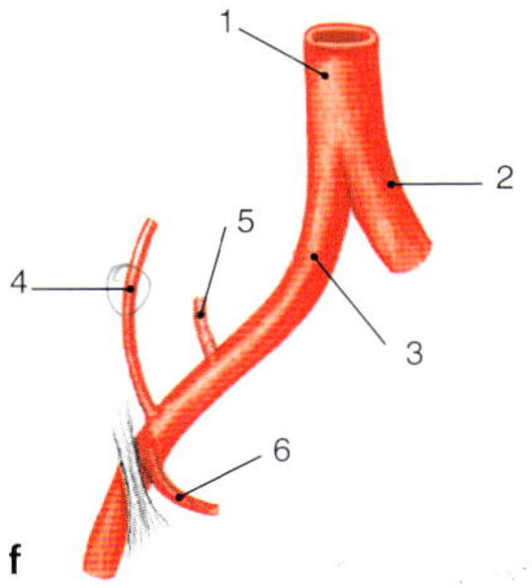

f

1 Common iliac artery
2 Internal iliac artery
3 External iliac artery
4 Inferior epigastric artery
5 Deep circumflex iliac artery
6 Pubic branch

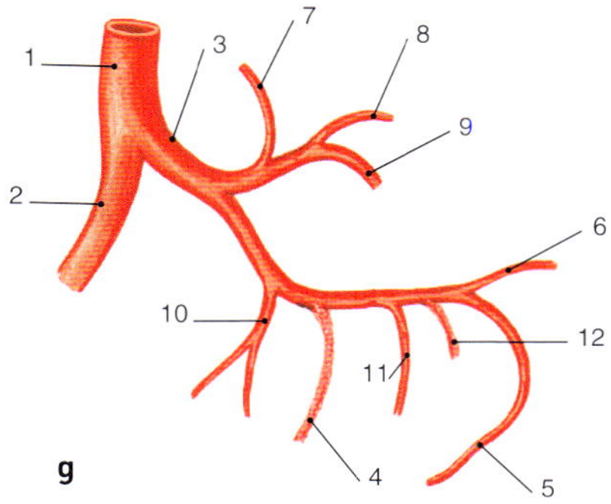

g

1 Common iliac artery
2 External iliac artery
3 Internal iliac artery
4 Obturator artery
5 Internal pudendal artery
6 Inferior gluteal artery
7 Iliolumbar artery
8 Lateral sacral arteries
9 Superior gluteal artery
10 Umbilical artery, patent part
11 Inferior vesical artery
12 Middle rectal artery

Veins

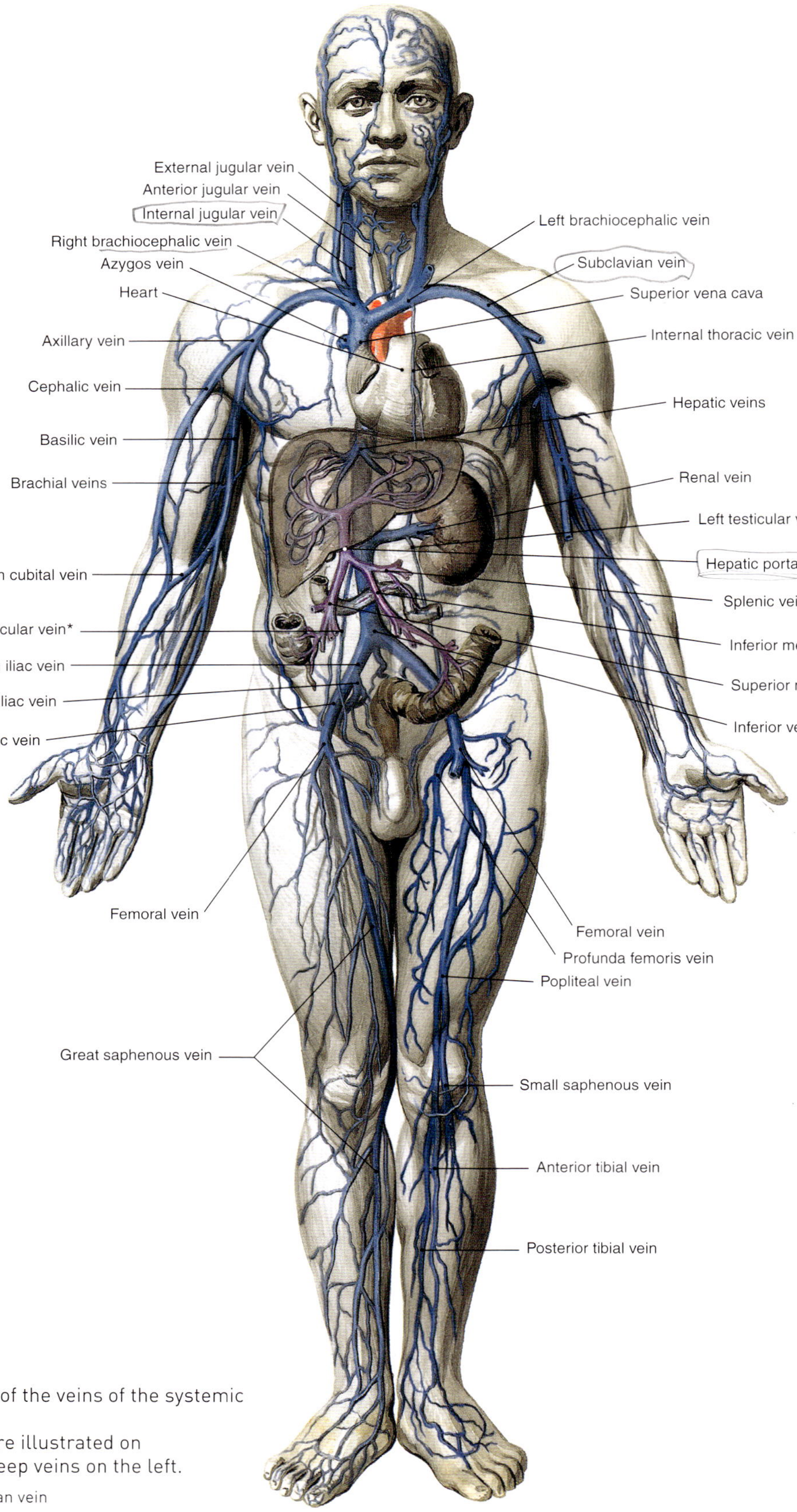

Fig. 36 Overview of the veins of the systemic circulation.
Superficial veins are illustrated on the right leg and deep veins on the left.

* In the female: ovarian vein

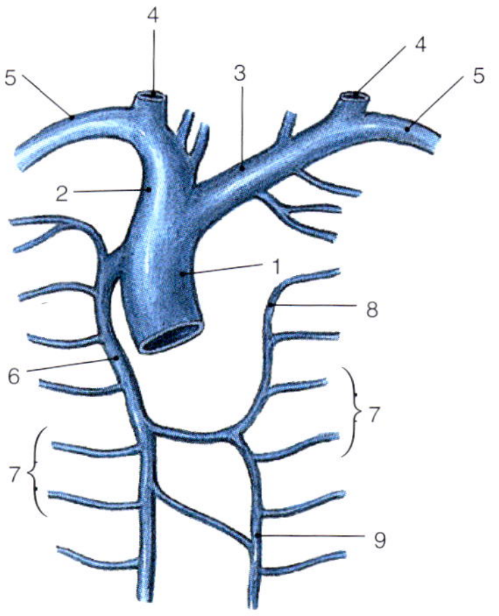

1 Superior vena cava
2 Right brachiocephalic vein
3 Left brachiocephalic vein
4 Internal jugular vein
5 Subclavian vein
6 Azygos vein
7 Posterior intercostal veins
8 Accessory hemi-azygos vein
9 Hemi-azygos vein

Fig. 37 Superior vena cava; schema of the tributaries.

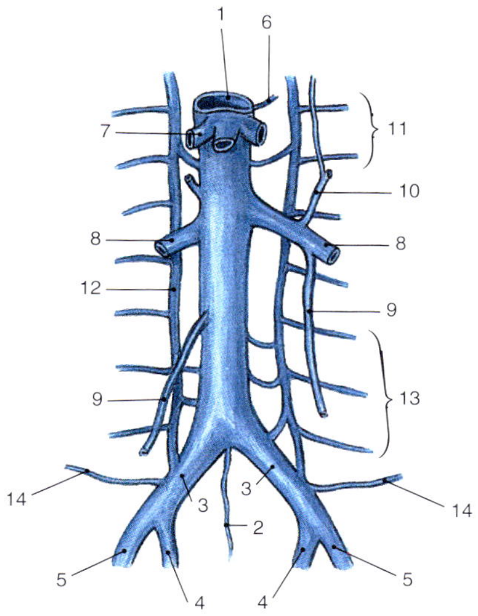

1 Inferior vena cava
2 Median sacral vein
3 Common iliac vein
4 Internal iliac vein
5 External iliac vein
6 Inferior phrenic veins
7 Hepatic veins
8 Renal vein
9 Testicular/ovarian vein
10 Suprarenal vein
11 Posterior intercostal veins
12 Ascending lumbar vein
13 Lumbar veins
14 Iliolumbar vein

Fig. 38 Inferior vena cava; schema of the tributaries.

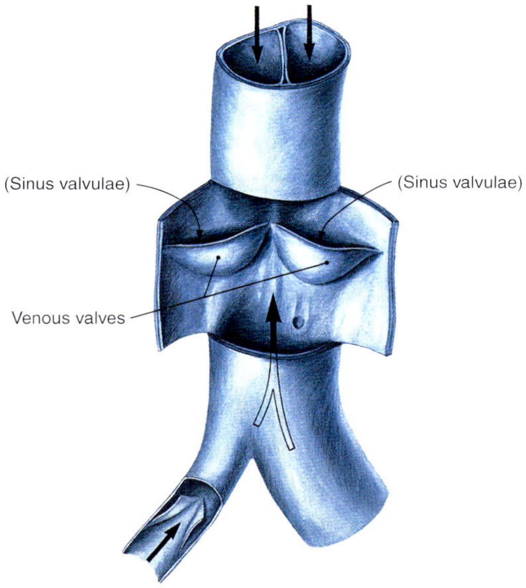

Fig. 39 Functional principle of venous valves. The arrows pointing upwards indicate the flow of blood. The valves close upon backflow of the blood (arrows pointing downwards).

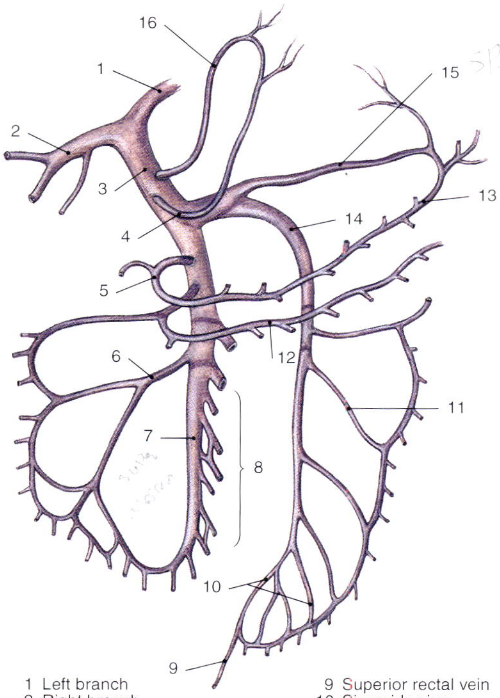

1 Left branch
2 Right branch
3 Hepatic portal vein
4 Right gastric vein
5 Right gastro-omental vein
6 Right colic vein
7 Superior mesenteric vein
8 Jejunal and ileal veins
9 Superior rectal vein
10 Sigmoid veins
11 Left colic vein
12 Middle colic vein
13 Left gastro-omental vein
14 Inferior mesenteric vein
15 Splenic vein
16 Left gastric vein

Fig. 40 Hepatic portal vein.

Foetal circulation

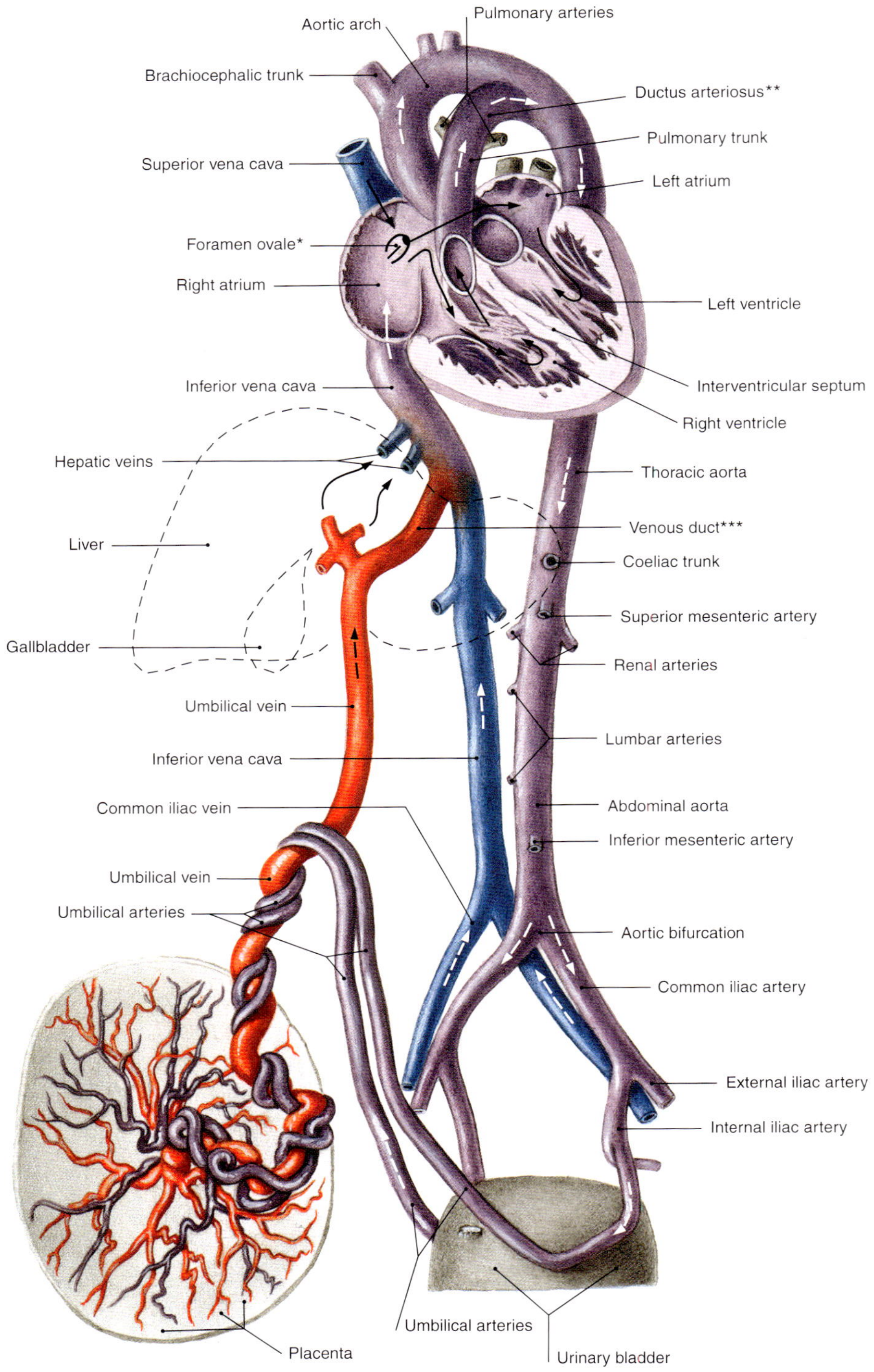

Fig. 41 Schema of foetal circulation.
The different colours indicate the oxygen content in the blood:
red = rich in oxygen,
blue = poor in oxygen,
purple = mixed blood.
Arrows indicate the direction of the blood flow.

* Short-circuit between the right and the left atrium
** Short-circuit between the pulmonary trunk and the arch of aorta
*** Short-circuit between the umbilical vein and the inferior vena cava

Conversion from foetal to postnatal circulation:

* The valve-like connection between the right and the left atrium via the foramen ovale is passively closed at the onset of respiratory activity in the lungs.
** The ductus arteriosus (BOTALLO), on the other hand, closes only during the first months of life as its lumen gradually obliterates by epithelial proliferation and increased tension of the wall.
*** The ductus venosus (ARANTIUS) obliterates after birth and becomes the ligamentum venosum in the portal area of the liver.

Lymph nodes: are small oval bodies enclosed in fibrous capsules.

Lymphatic system

* lymph node contains phagocytic cortical tissue (reticular tissue) adapted to filter lymph.

* Specialized band of CT called Trabeculae, divide the lymph

Subcapsular sinus through cortical sinus into superficial cortex and para cortex

Vessiles

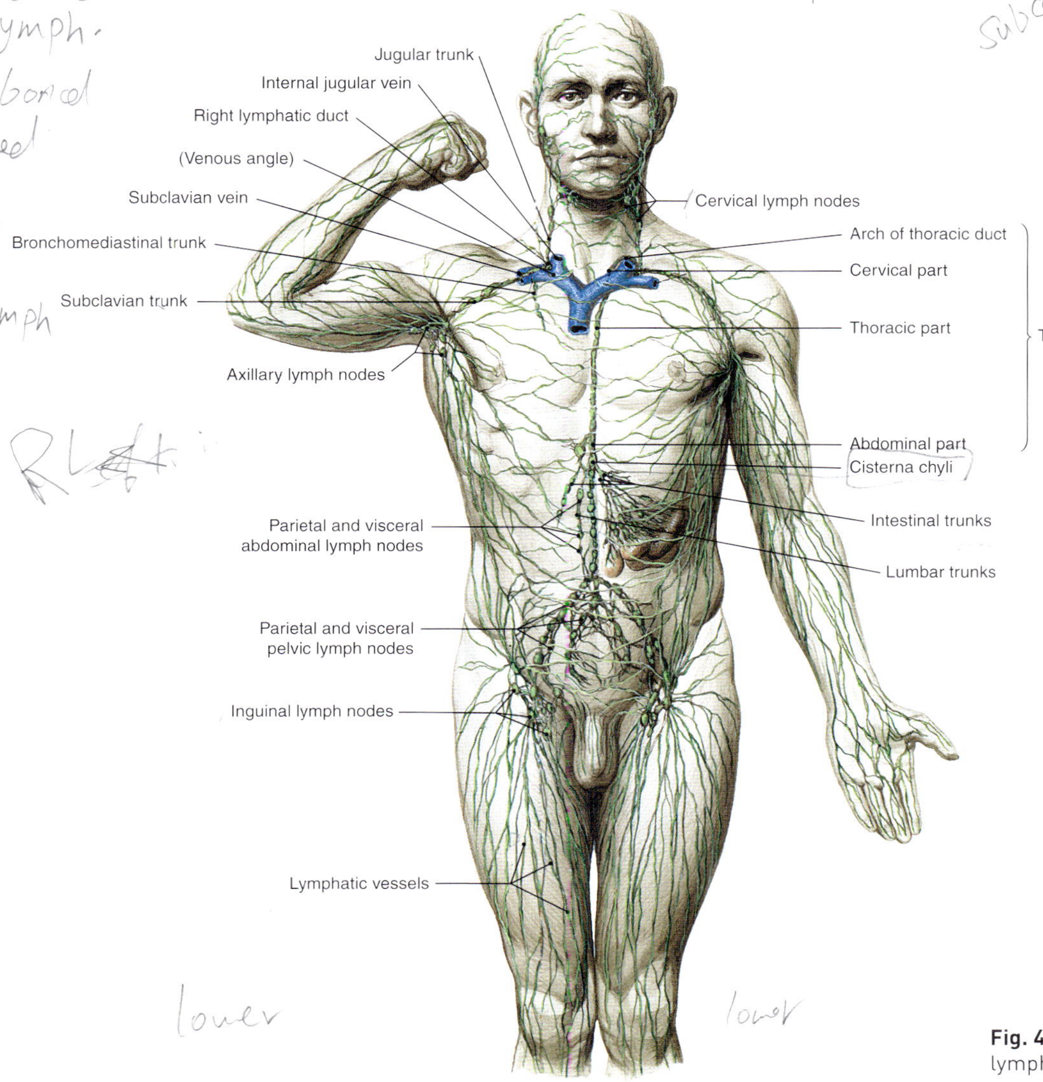

Fig. 42 Overview of the lymphatic system.

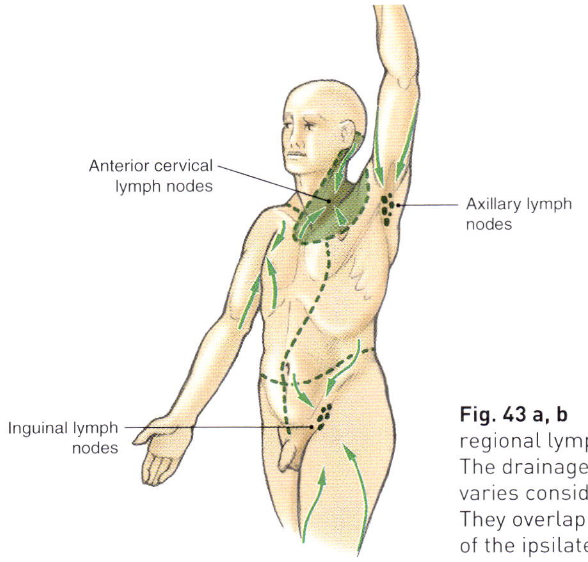

a

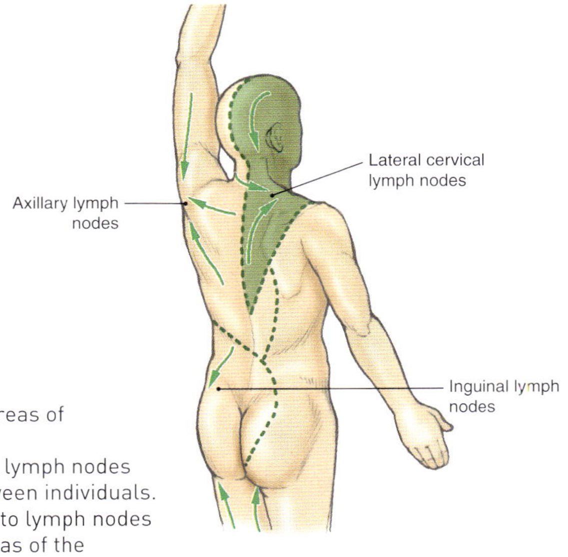

b

Fig. 43 a, b Drainage areas of regional lymph nodes.
The drainage of regional lymph nodes varies considerably between individuals. They overlap in draining to lymph nodes of the ipsilateral as well as of the contralateral side of the body.

Nervous system

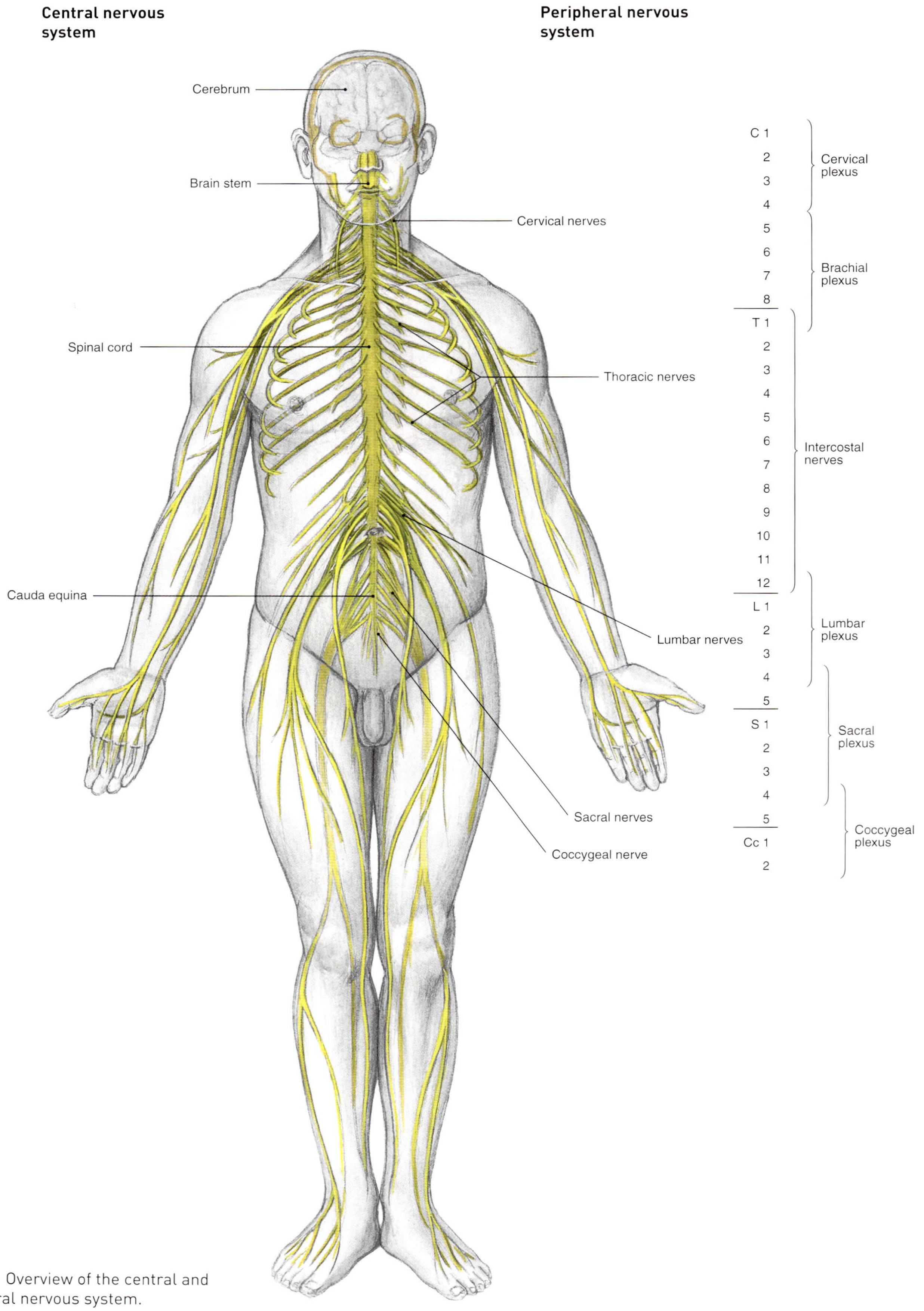

Fig. 44 Overview of the central and peripheral nervous system.

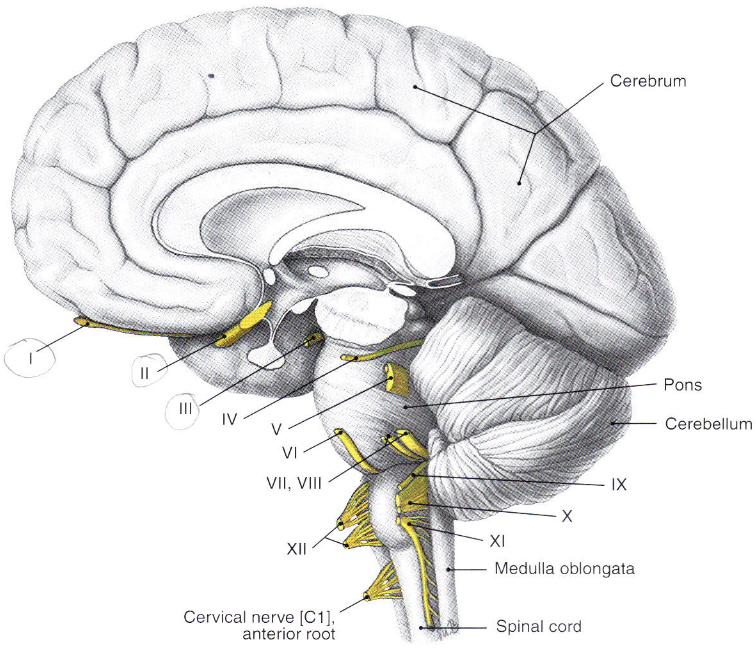

Cranial nerves	
I	Olfactory nerves
II	Optic nerve
III	Oculomotor nerve
IV	Trochlear nerve
V	Trigeminal nerve
VI	Abducent nerve
VII	Facial nerve
VIII	Vestibulocochlear nerve
IX	Glossopharyngeal nerve
X	Vagus nerve
XI	Accessory nerve
XII	Hypoglossal nerve

Fig. 45 Overview of the brain and the cranial nerves.

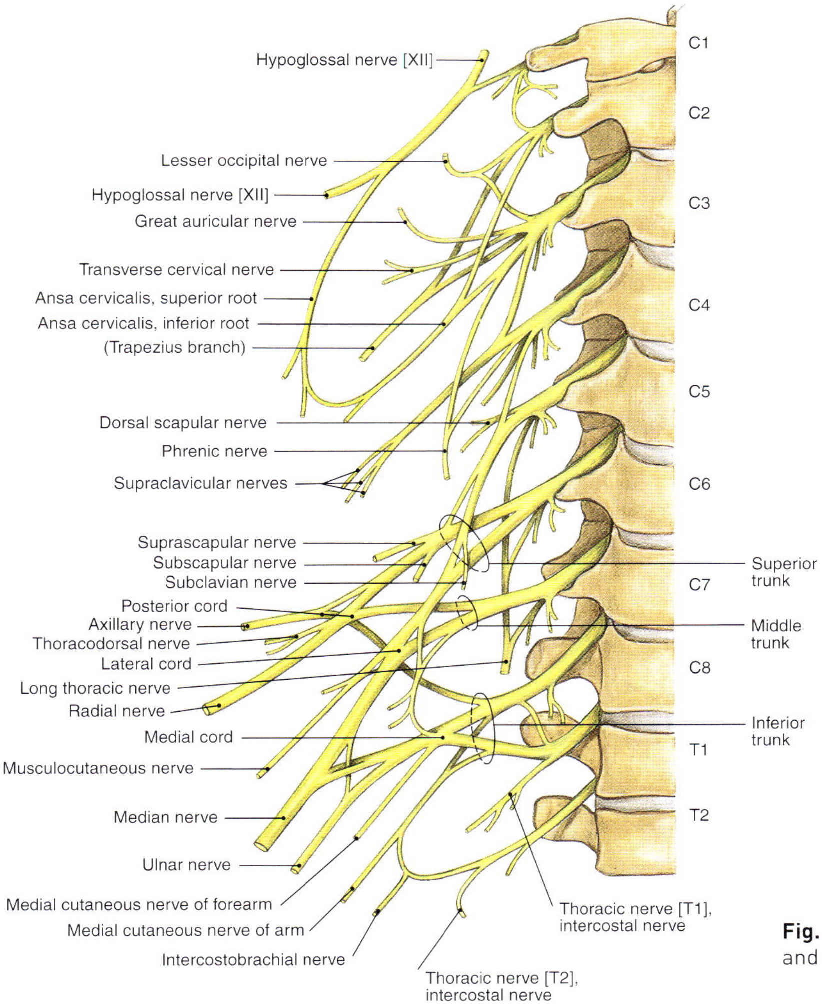

Fig. 46 Overview of the cervical and brachial plexus.

Peripheral nervous system

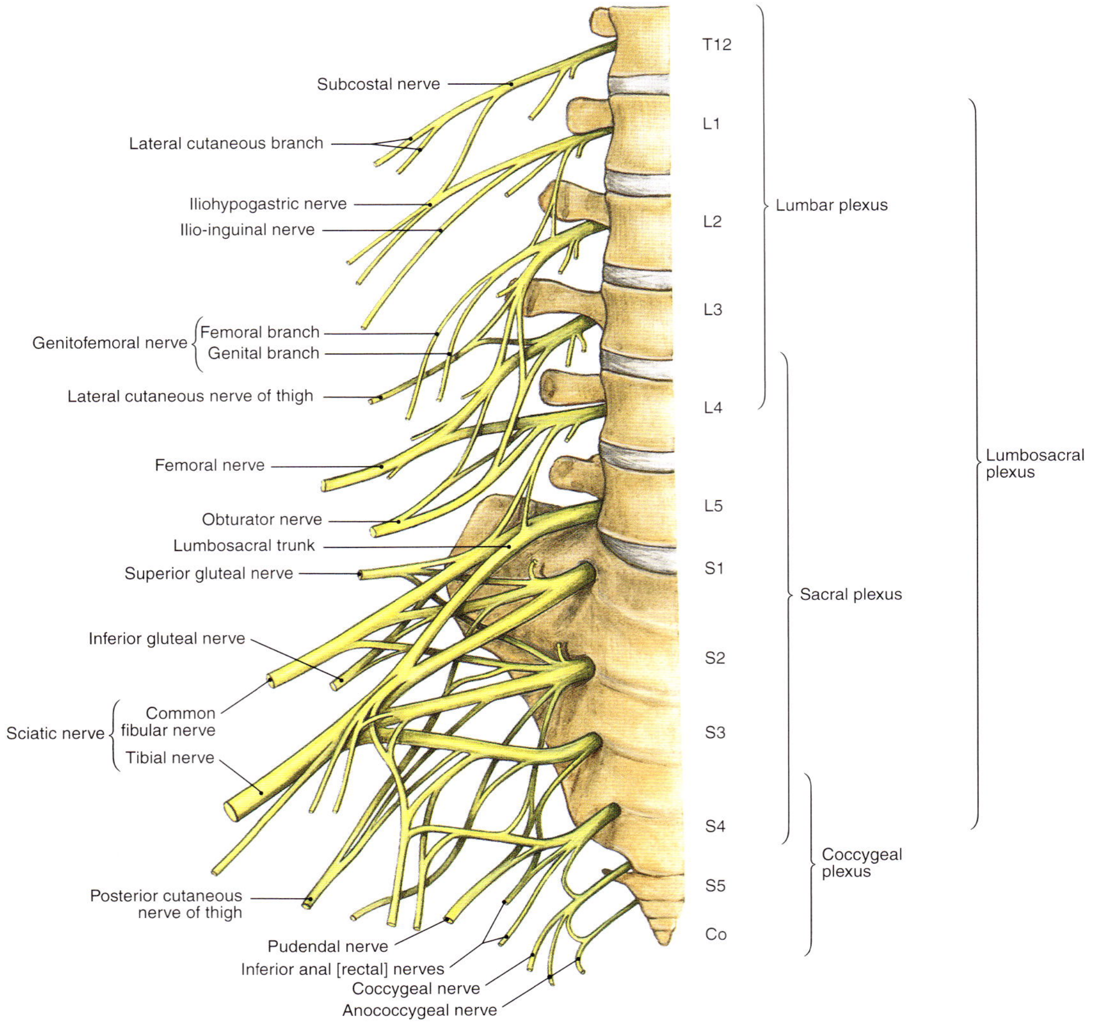

Fig. 47 Overview of the lumbosacral plexus and the coccygeal plexus.

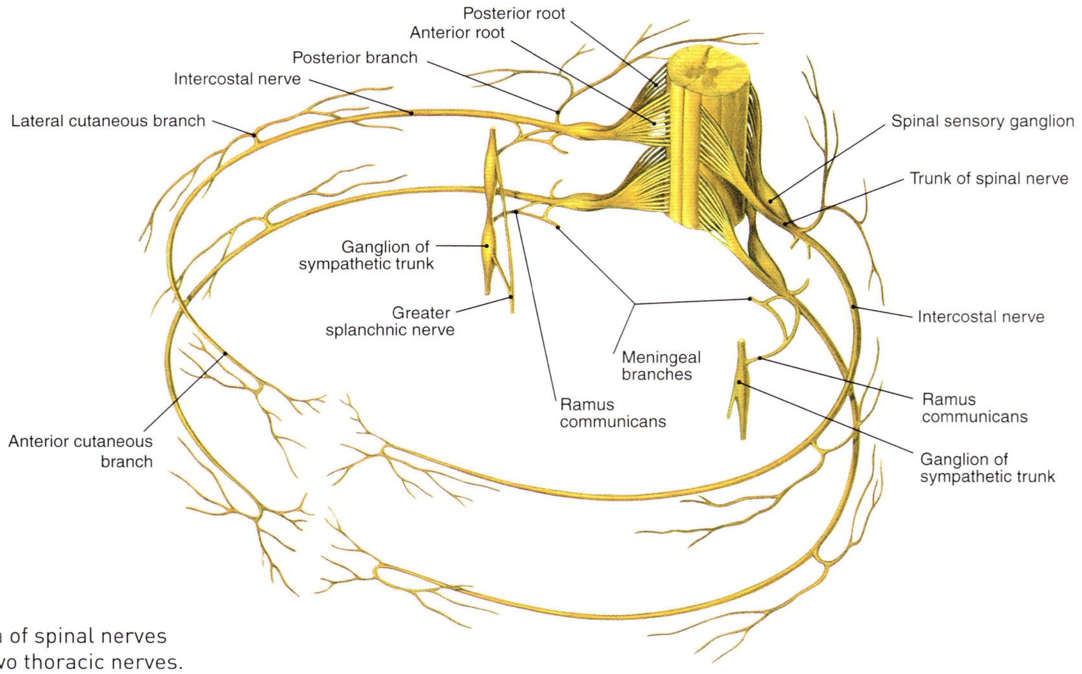

Spinal nerves

- Cervical nerves
- Thoracic nerves
- Lumbar nerves
- Sacral nerves
- Coccygeal nerves

Fig. 48 Schema of spinal nerves exemplified by two thoracic nerves.

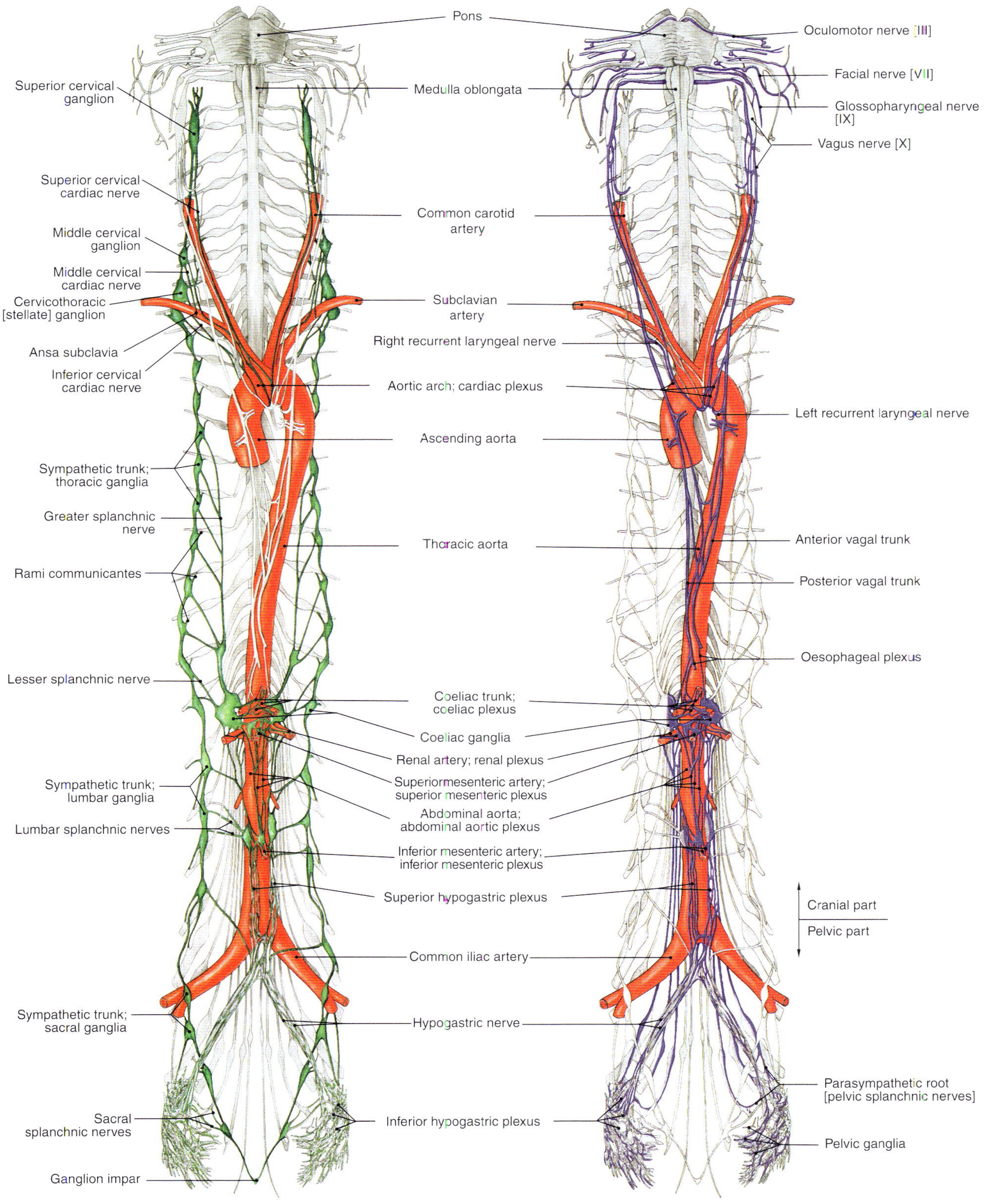

Fig. 49 Sympathetic part of the autonomous nervous system.
The entire system of sympathetic ganglia and their connections located along the vertebral column are referred to as sympathetic trunk (green).

Fig. 50 Parasympathetic part of the autonomous nervous system.
Parasympathetic fibres (violet) usually travel along with other nerve fibres.

Autonomous nervous system

Sympathetic part

Parasympathetic part

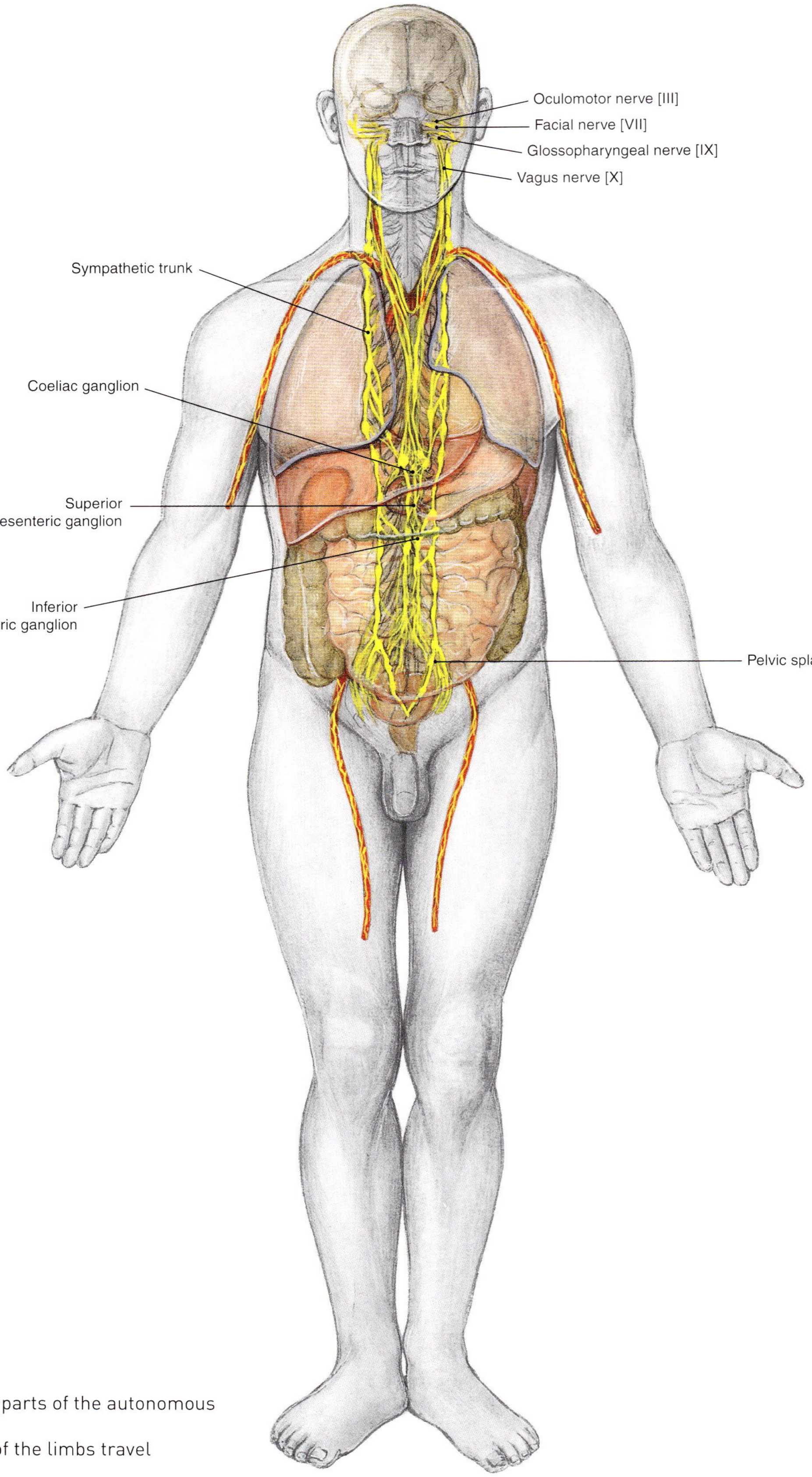

Fig. 51 Peripheral parts of the autonomous nervous system.
Sympathetic fibres of the limbs travel along with arteries.

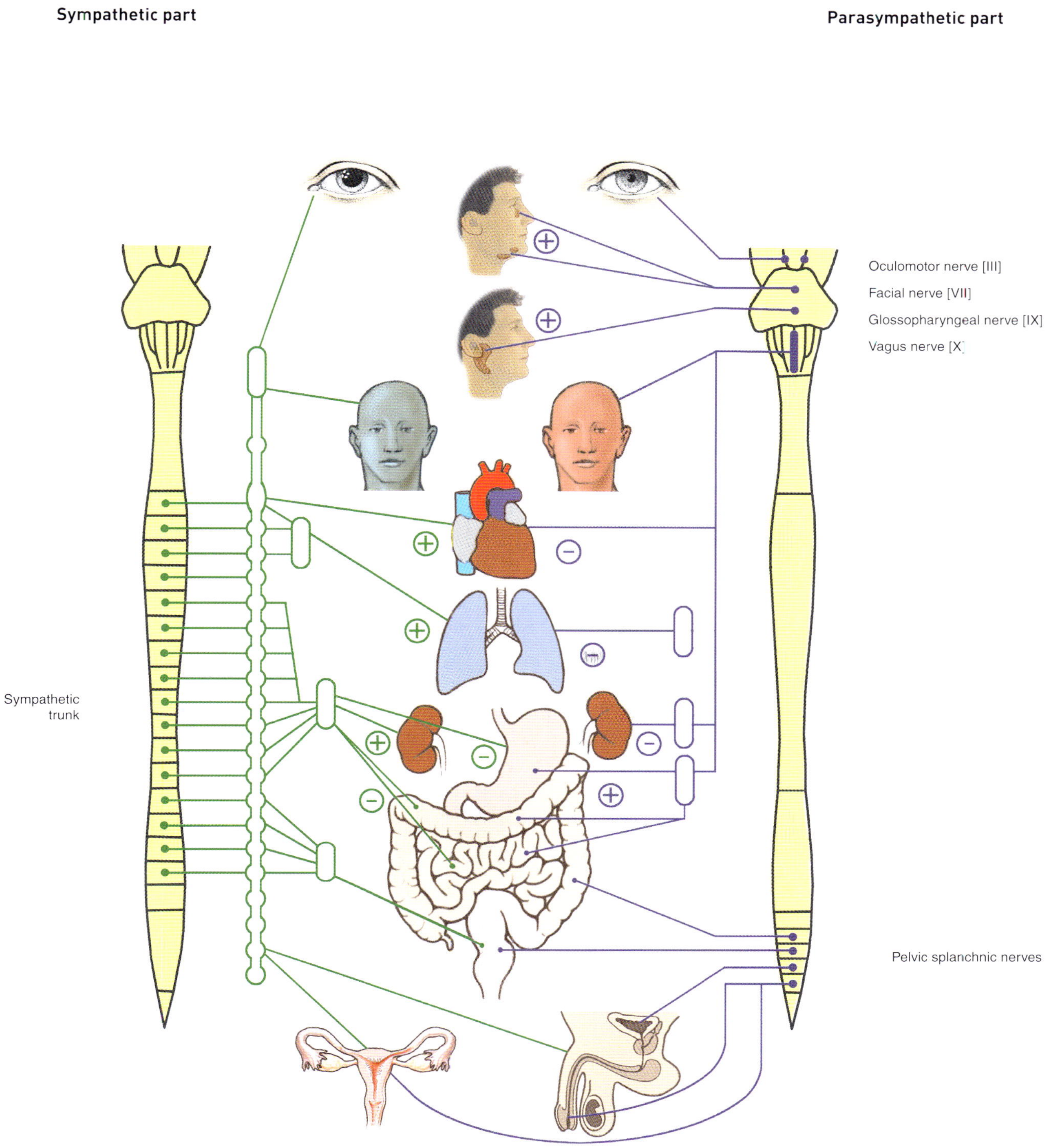

Fig. 52 Overview of the functions of the autonomous nervous system.

Endocrine organs

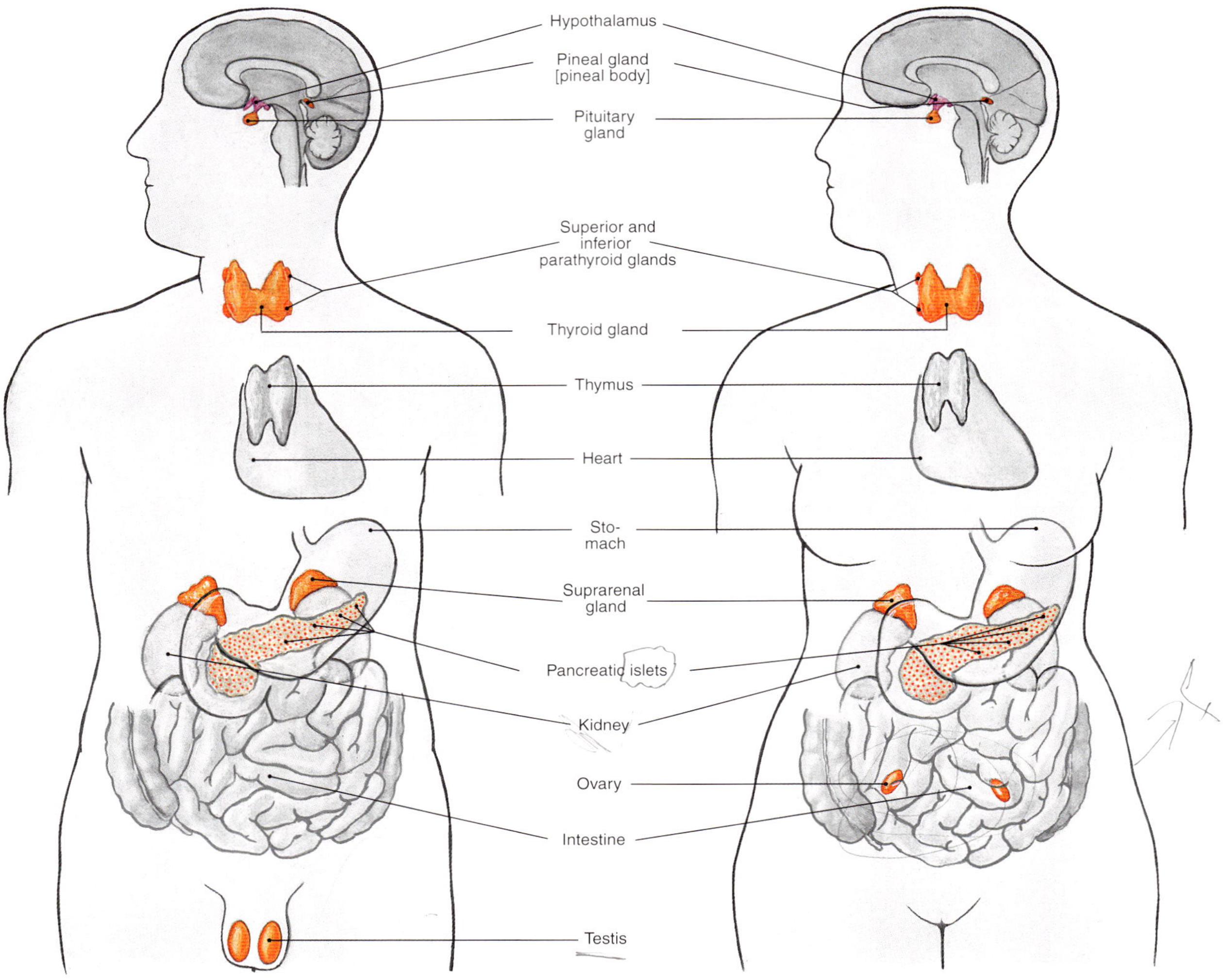

Fig. 53 Endocrine organs of the male.

Fig. 54 Endocrine organs of the female.

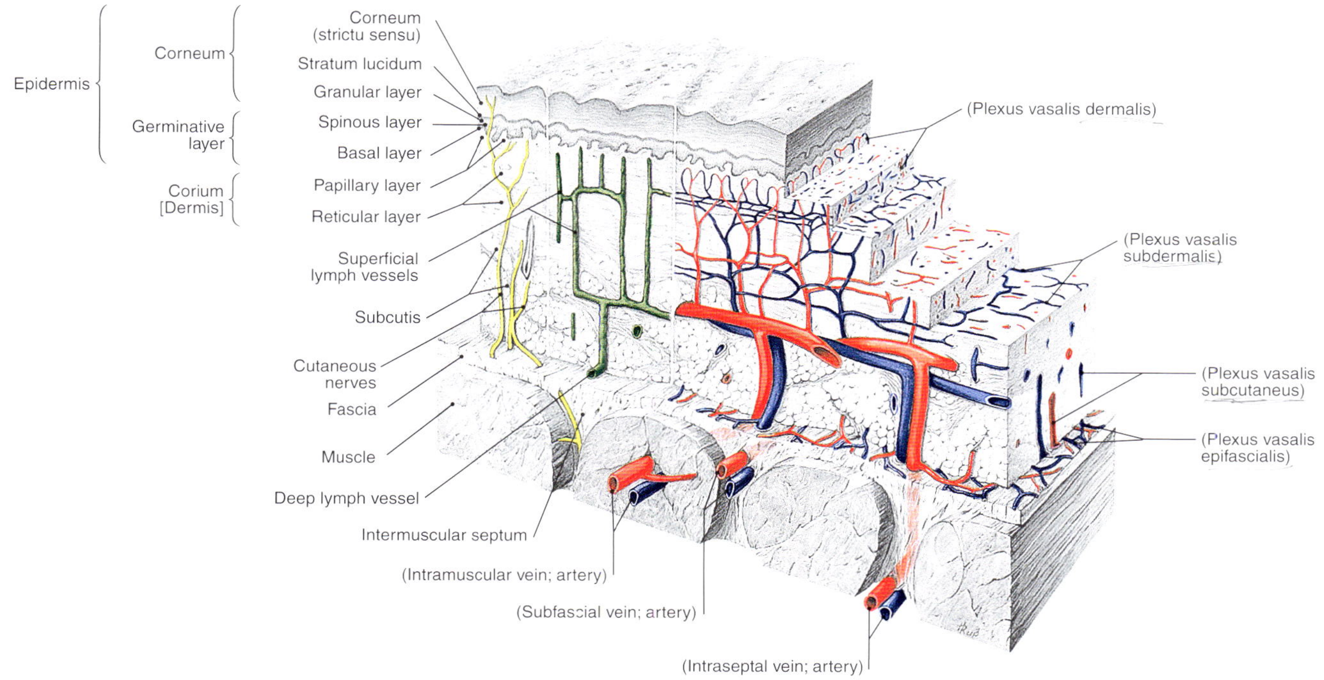

Fig. 55 Section through the skin; approximately 11-fold magnification.

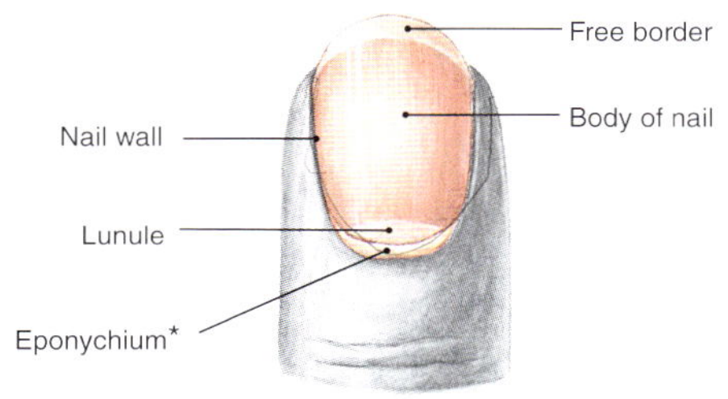

Fig. 56 Distal phalanx of a digit with fingernail.

* The epidermis of the nail is also known as cuticle.

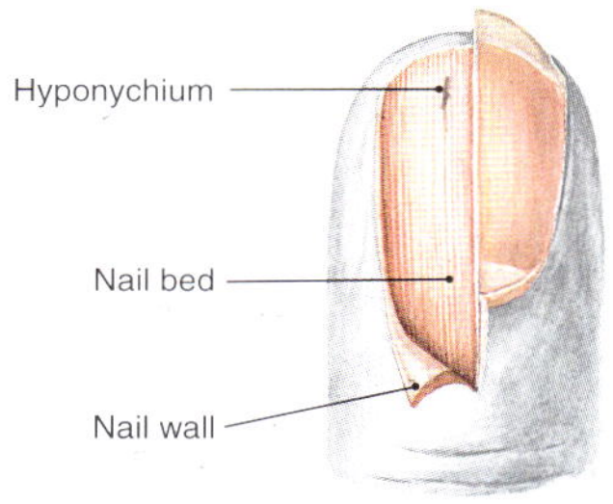

Fig. 57 Distal phalanx of a digit; the nail has been partly removed.

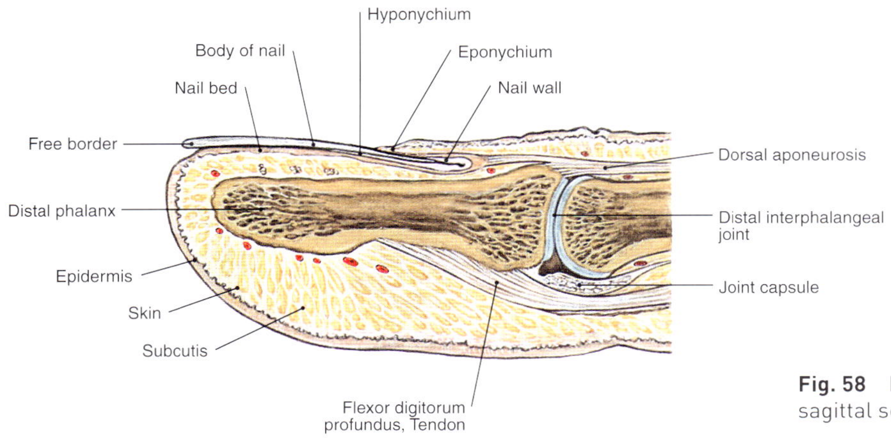

Fig. 58 Distal phalanx of a digit; sagittal section.

Regions

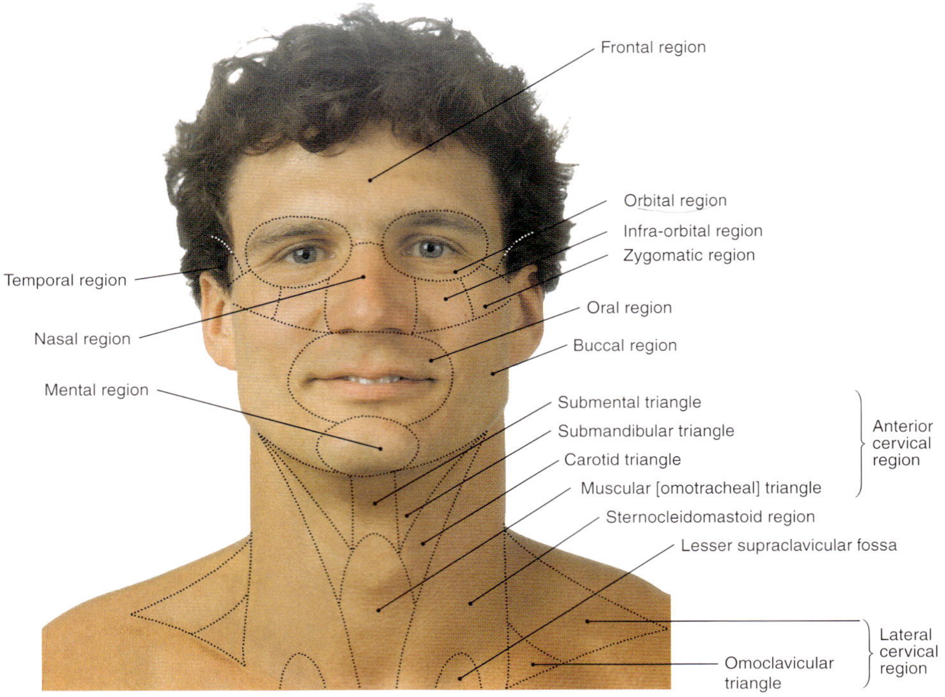

Fig. 59 Regions of the head and the neck.

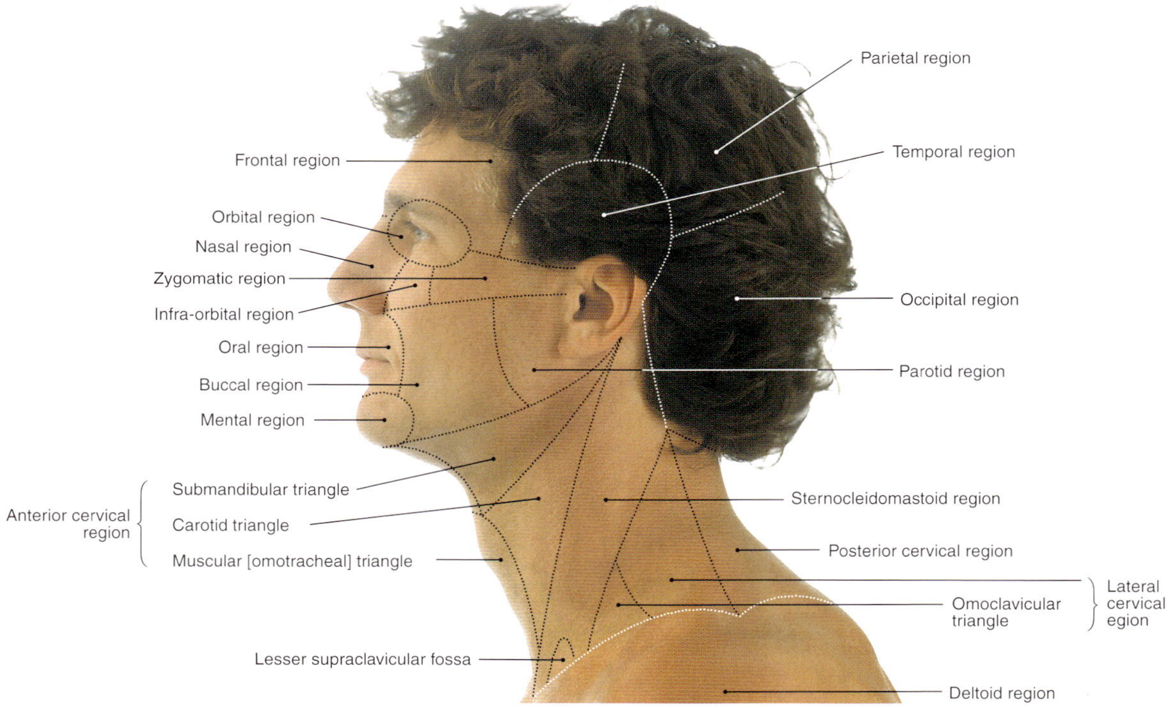

Fig. 60 Regions of the head and the neck.

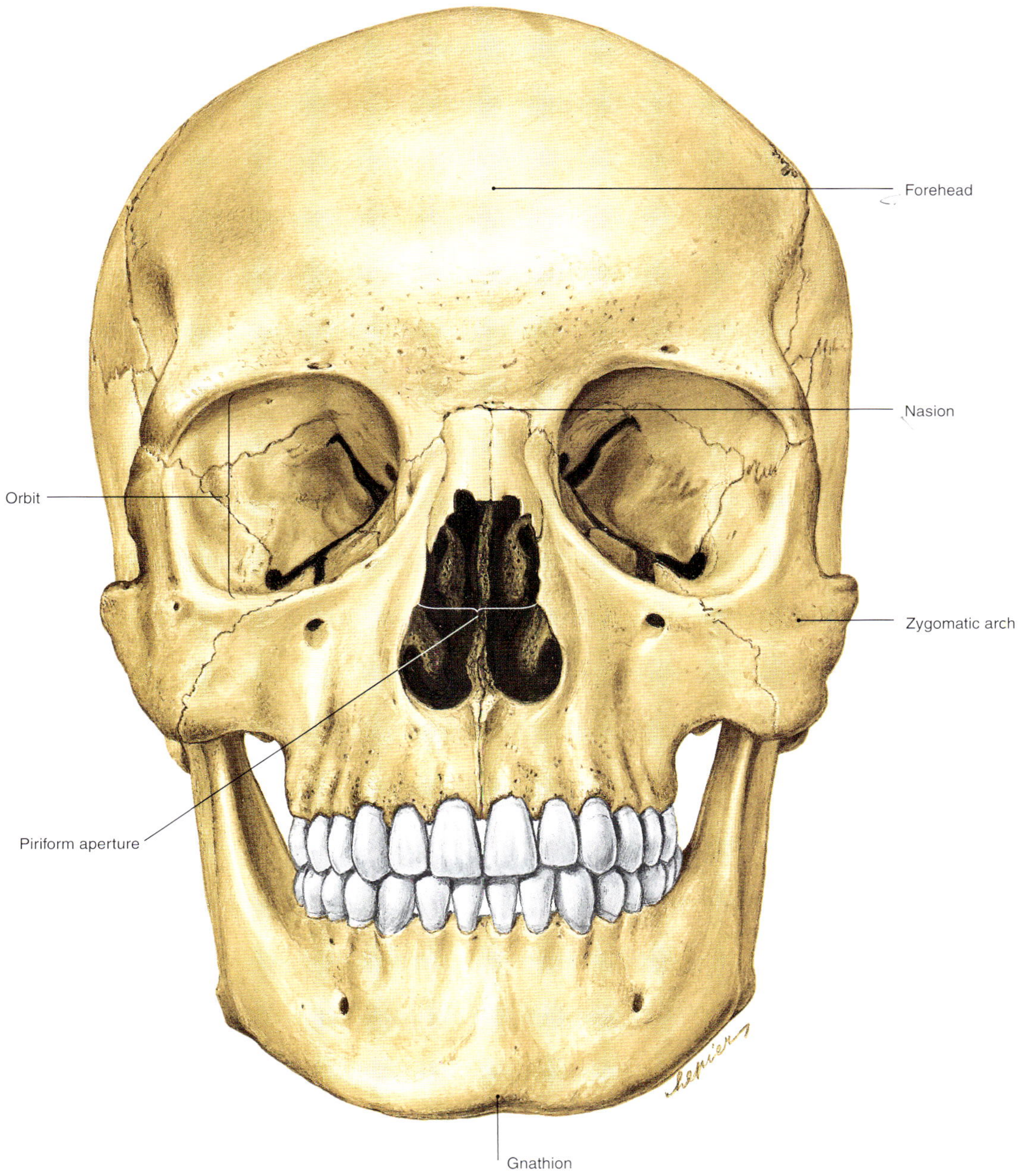
Forehead
Nasion
Orbit
Zygomatic arch
Piriform aperture
Gnathion

Fig. 61 Skull.

Bones of the skull

Viscerocranium (facial skeleton)
Consist of 15 irregular bones

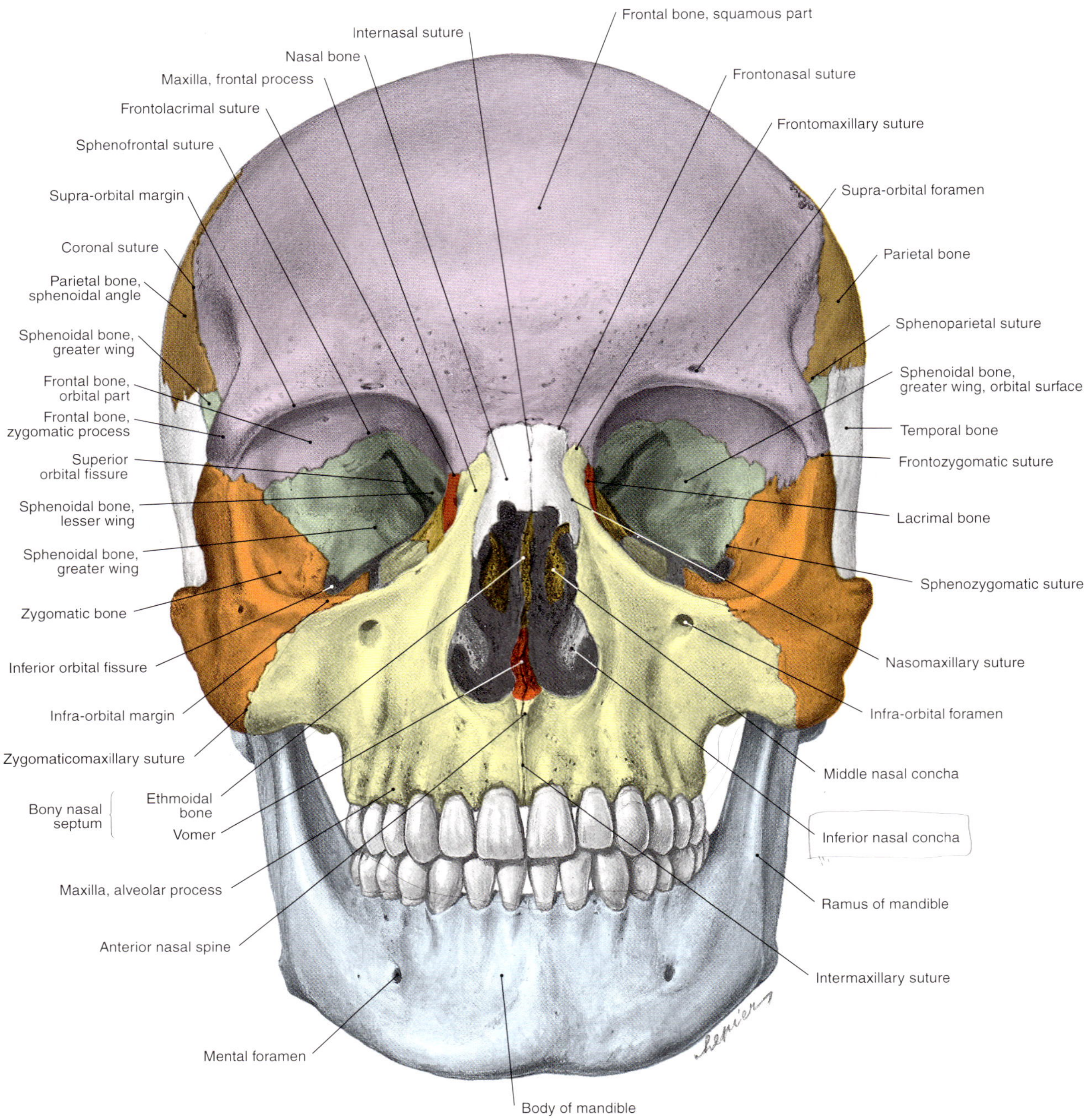

Frontal bone	Temporal bone	Vomer
Nasal bone	Inferior nasal concha	Ethmoidal bone
Maxilla	Mandible	Parietal bone
Zygomatic bone	Lacrimal bone	Sphenoidal bone

* 6 bones as bilateral pairs
· Maxilla
· inferior nasal conchae
· Zygomatic
· palatine
· Nasal
· lacrimal

* Several bones of Cranium
· frontal
· Temporal

Fig. 62 Bones of the skull.

· Sphenoid
· Ethmoid

3 single bones on the mid line
· Vomer
· mandible
· Ethmoidal

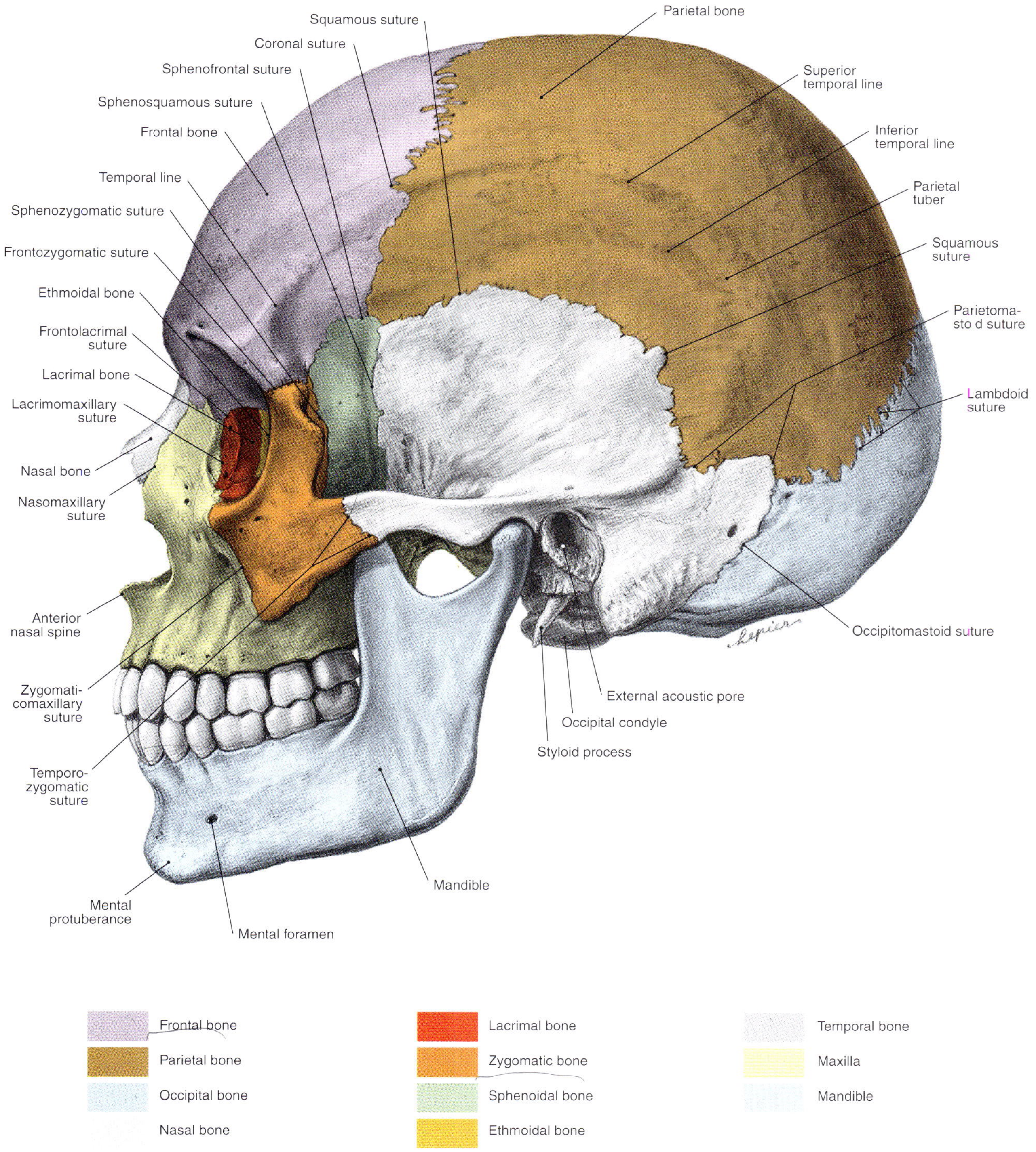

Fig. 63 Bones of the skull.

Bones of the skull

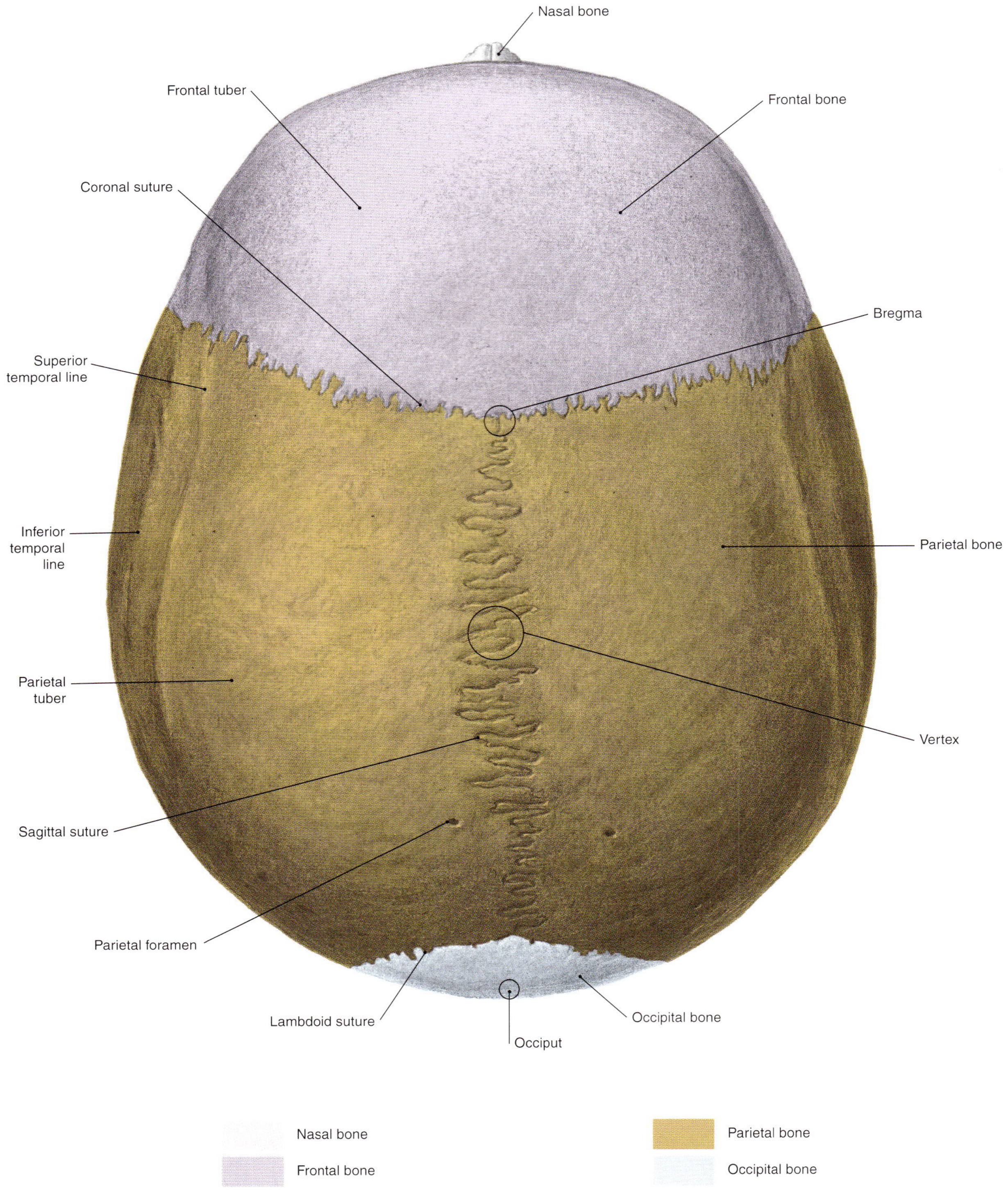

Fig. 64 Bones of the skull; superior view.

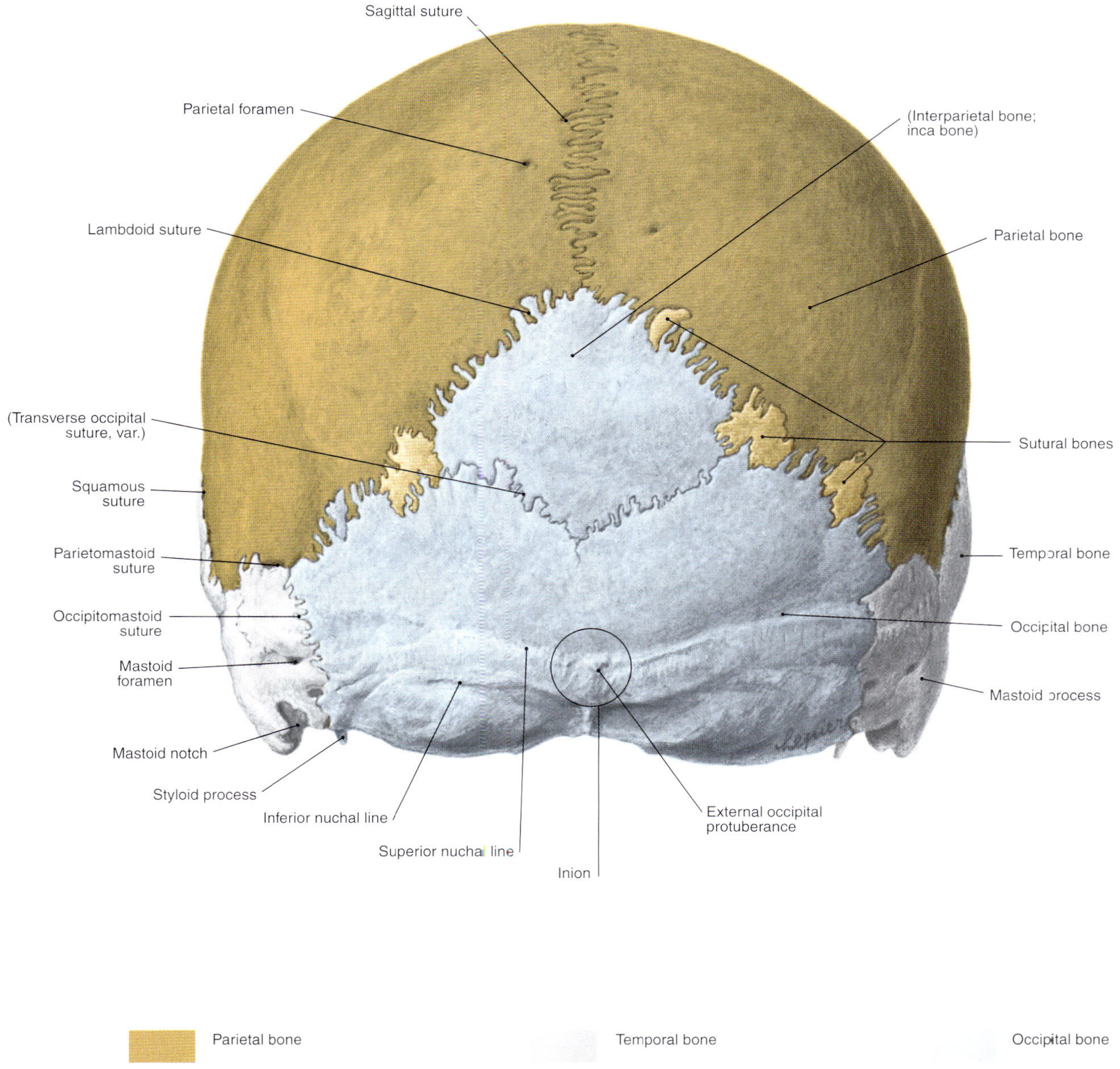

Fig. 65 Bones of the skull; posterior view.

Bones of the skull

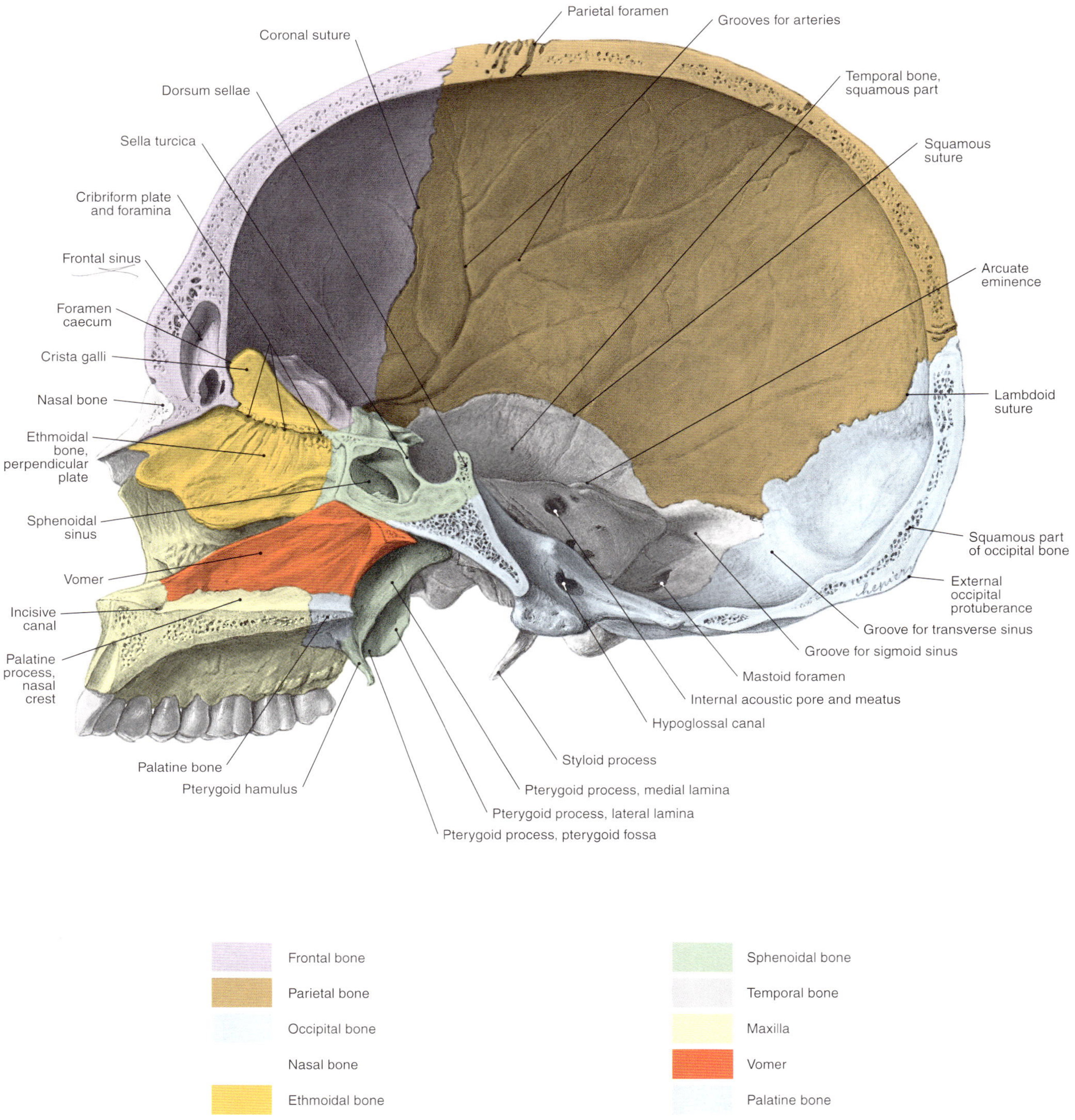

Fig. 66 Bones of the skull; medial view.

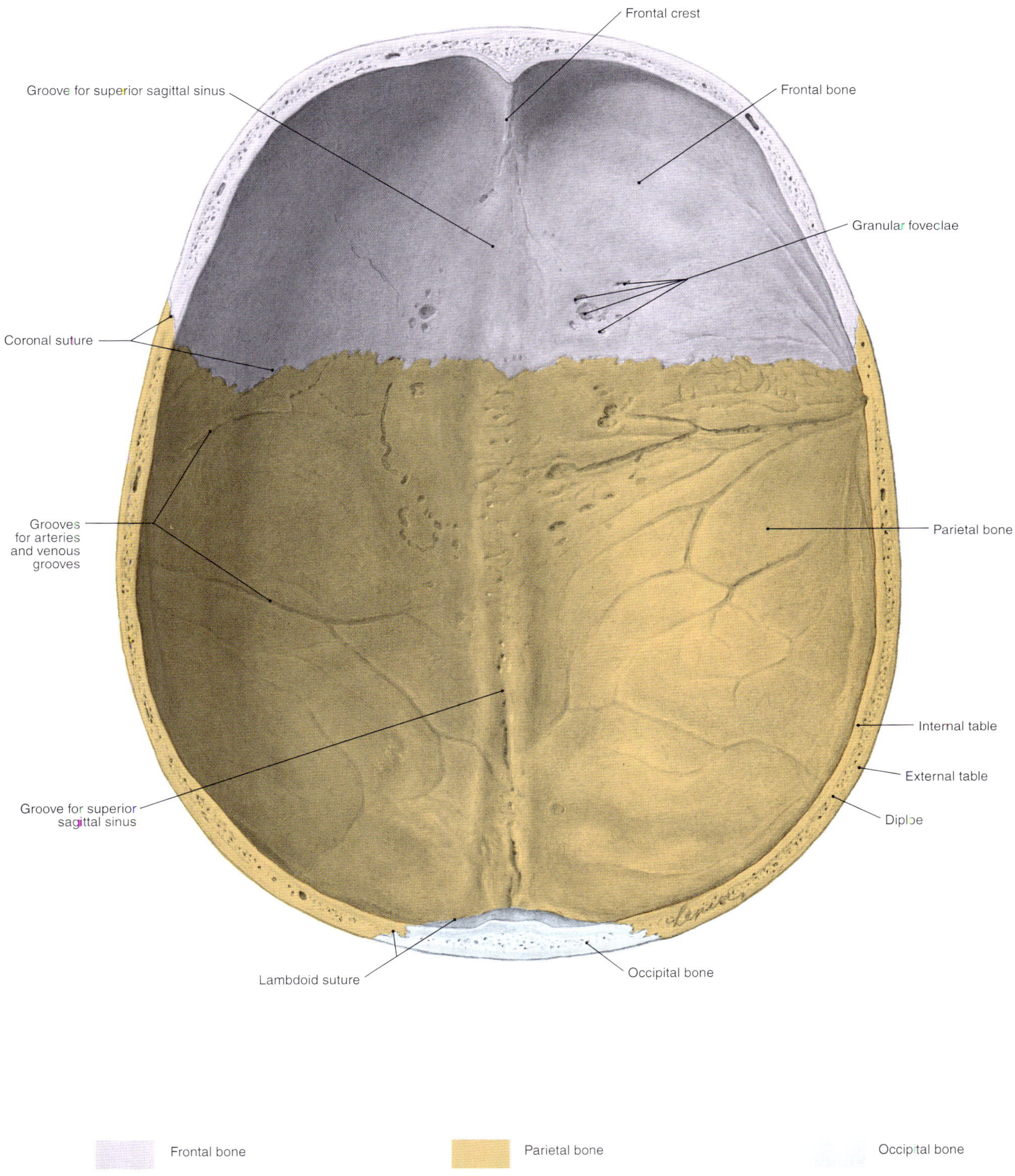

Fig. 67 Calvaria; internal aspect.

Bones of the skull

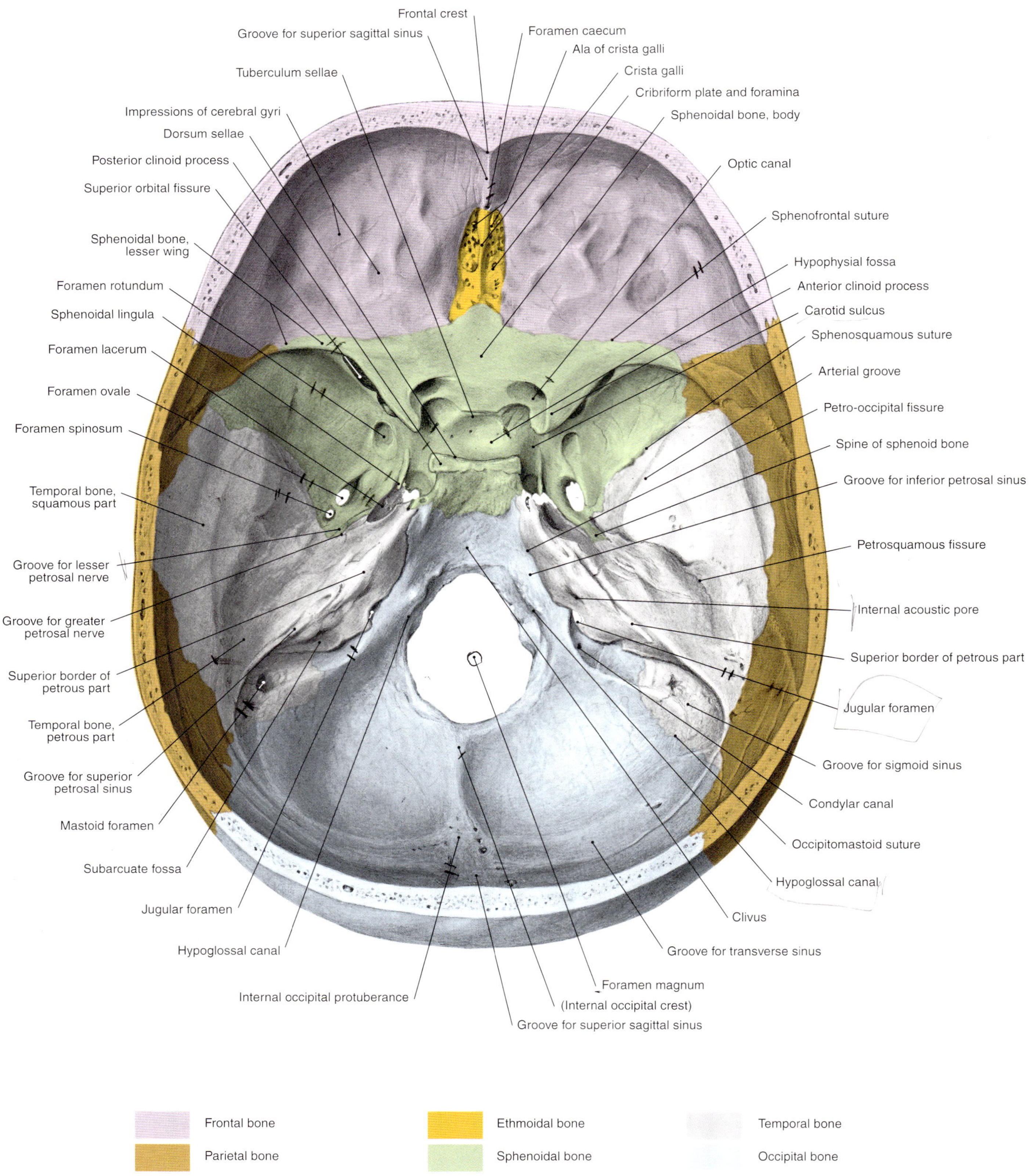

Fig. 68 Internal surface of the base of the skull.

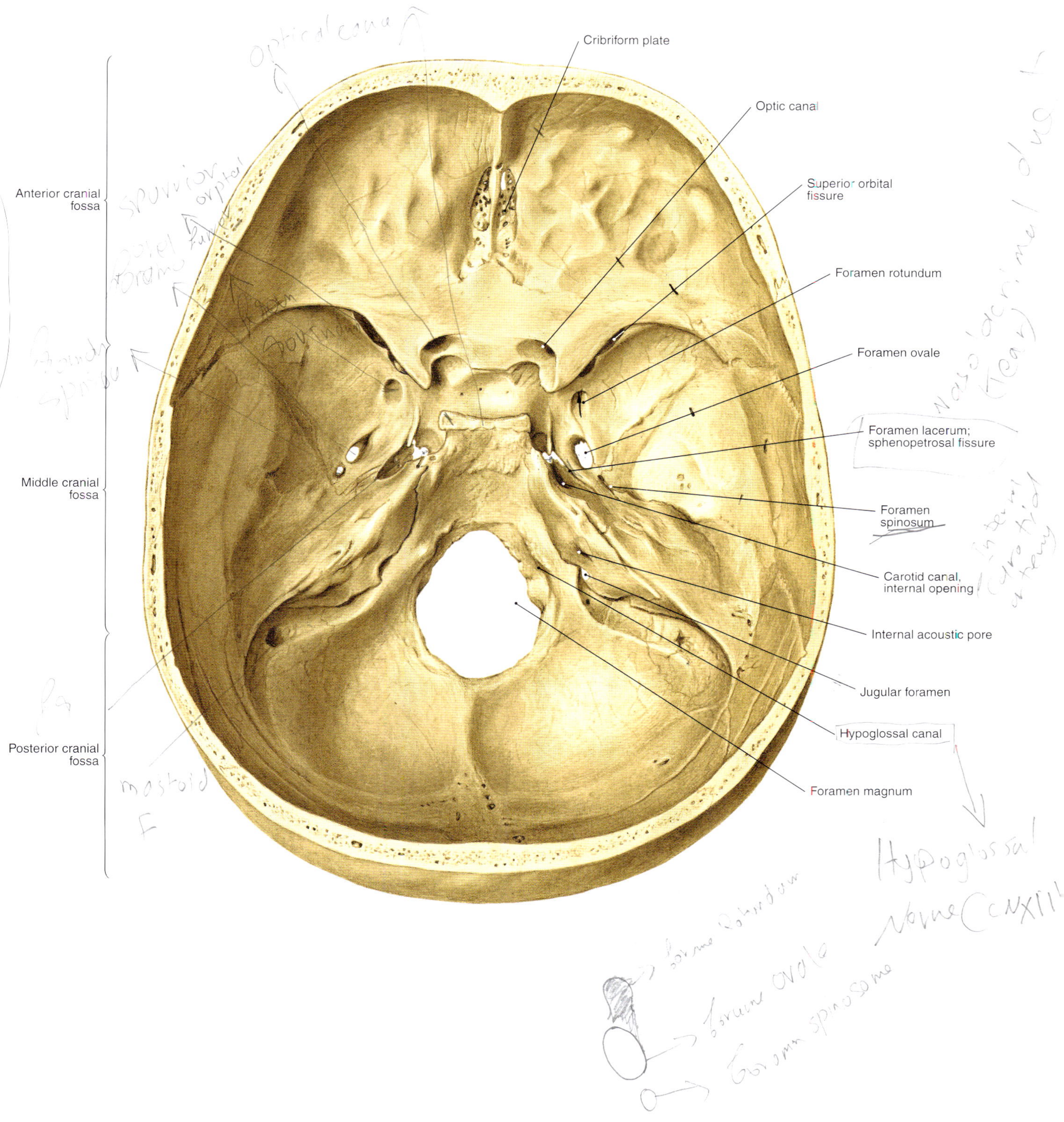

Fig. 69 Internal surface of the base of the skull and foramina.

→ 1173

Bones of the skull

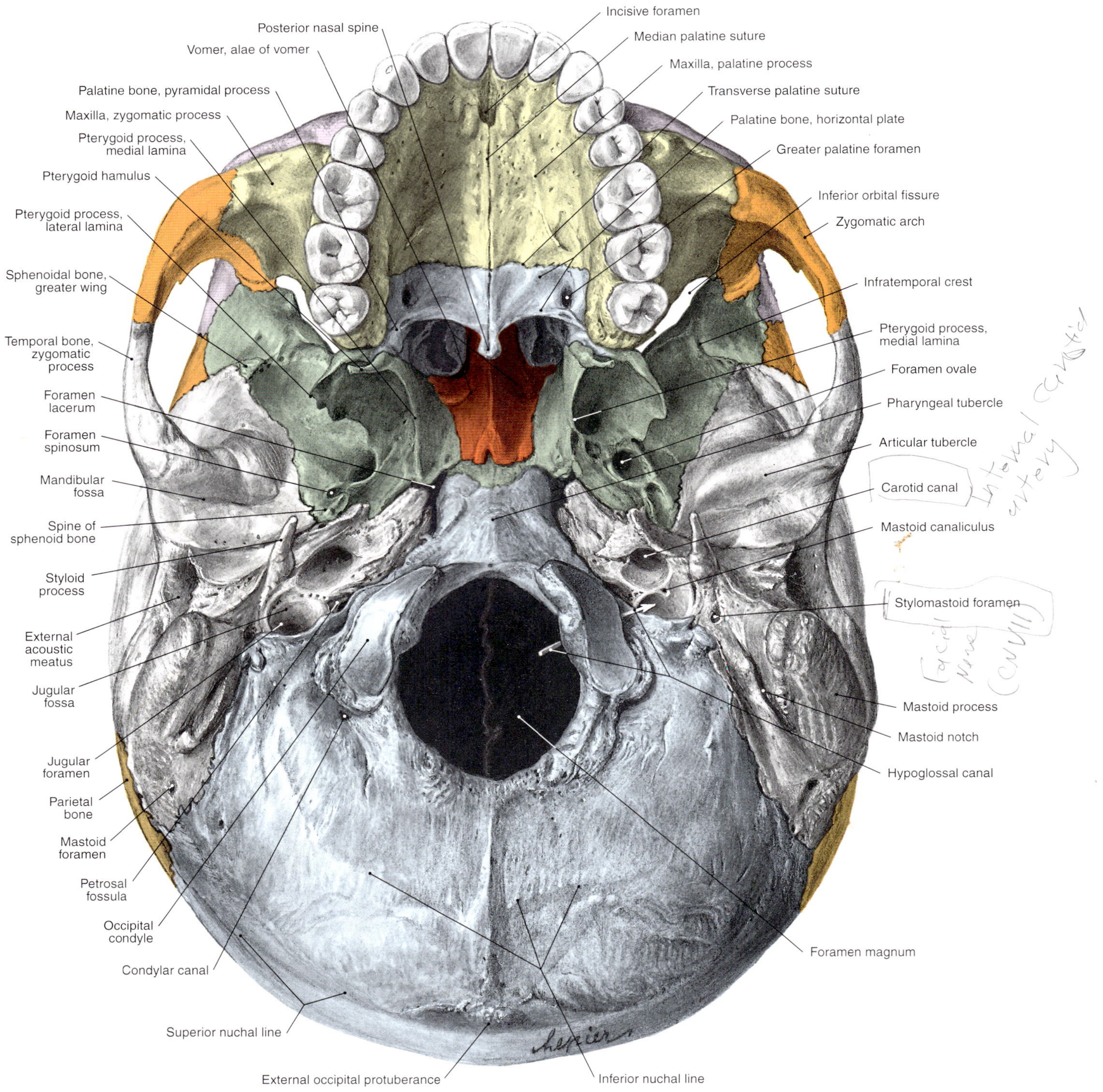

- Maxilla
- Frontal bone
- Parietal bone
- Palatine bone
- Vomer
- Zygomatic bone
- Sphenoidal bone
- Temporal bone
- Occipital bone

Fig. 70 External surface of the base of the skull.

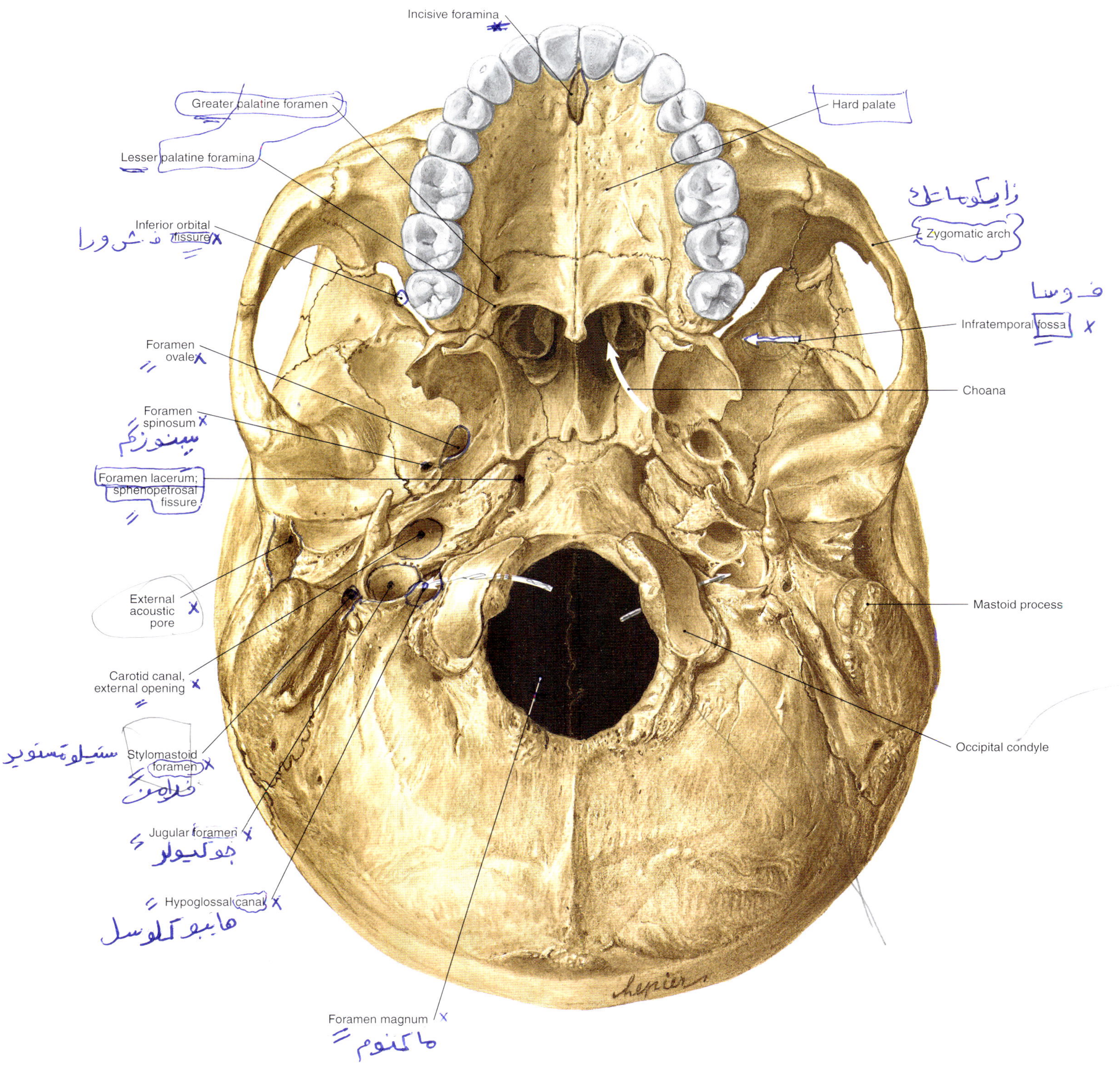

Fig. 71 External surface of the base of the skull and foramina.

→ 1172

Skull, radiography

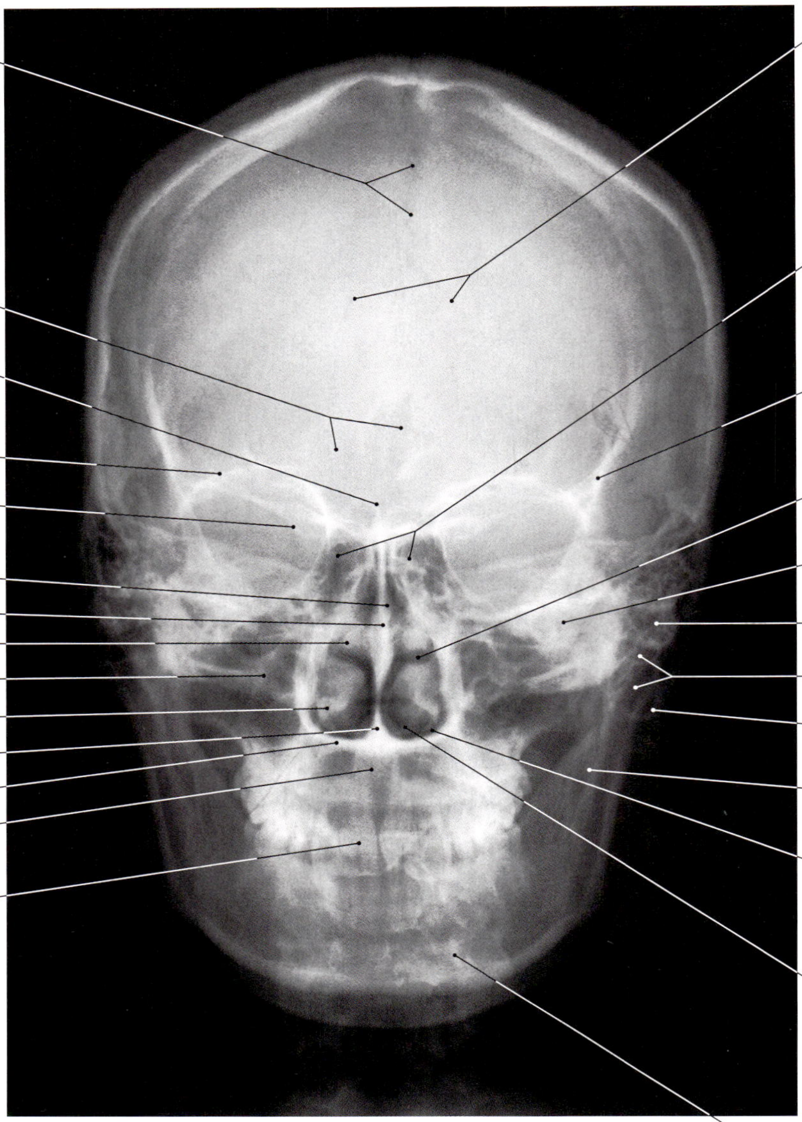

Fig. 72 Skull;
AP-teleradiograph.

* Innominate line, a projection line without anatomical correlate

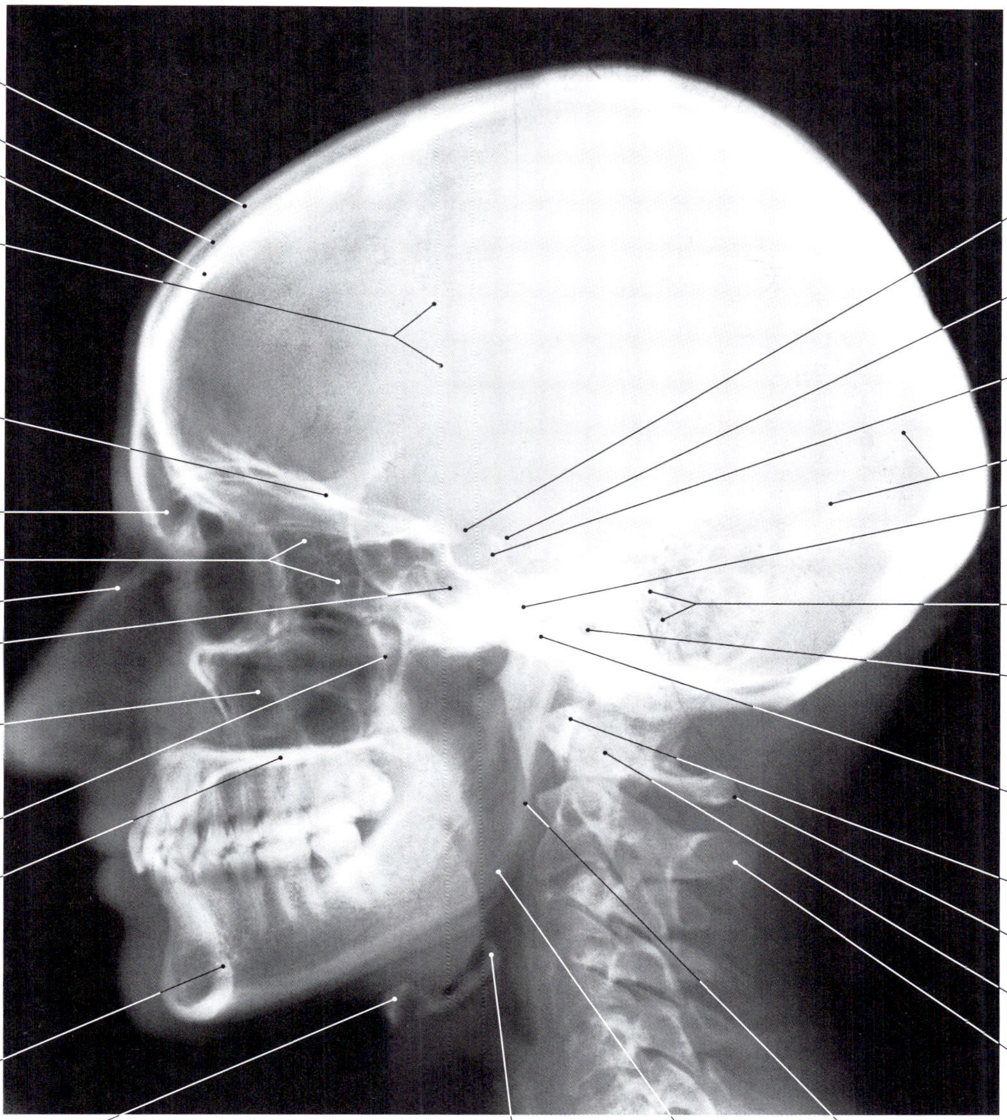

Fig. 73 Skull;
lateral teleradiograph.

* Posterior wall of the maxillary sinus

Skull, development

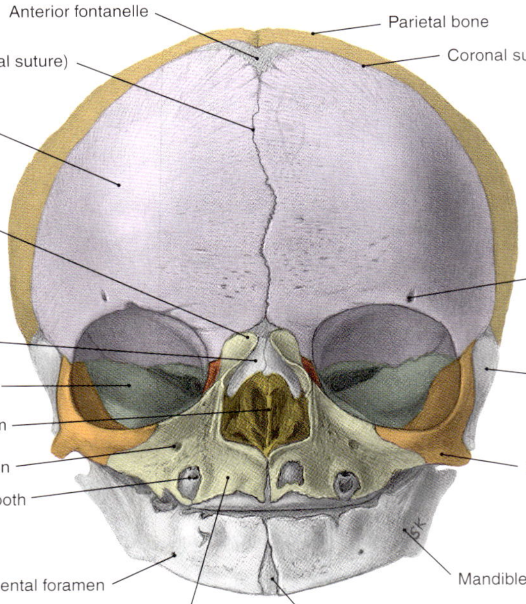

Fig. 74 Skull of a neonate.

- Lacrimal bone
- Frontal bone
- Parietal bone
- Occipital bone
- Maxilla, incisive bone
- Zygomatic bone
- Ethmoidal bone
- Sphenoidal bone
- Nasal bone, temporal bone, mandible

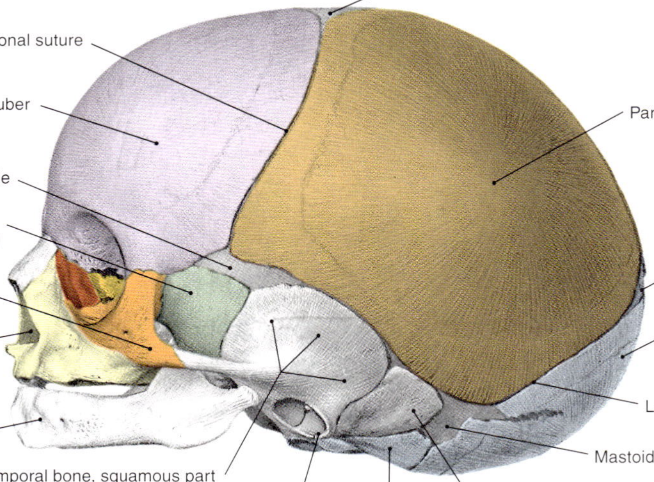

Fig. 75 Skull of a neonate.

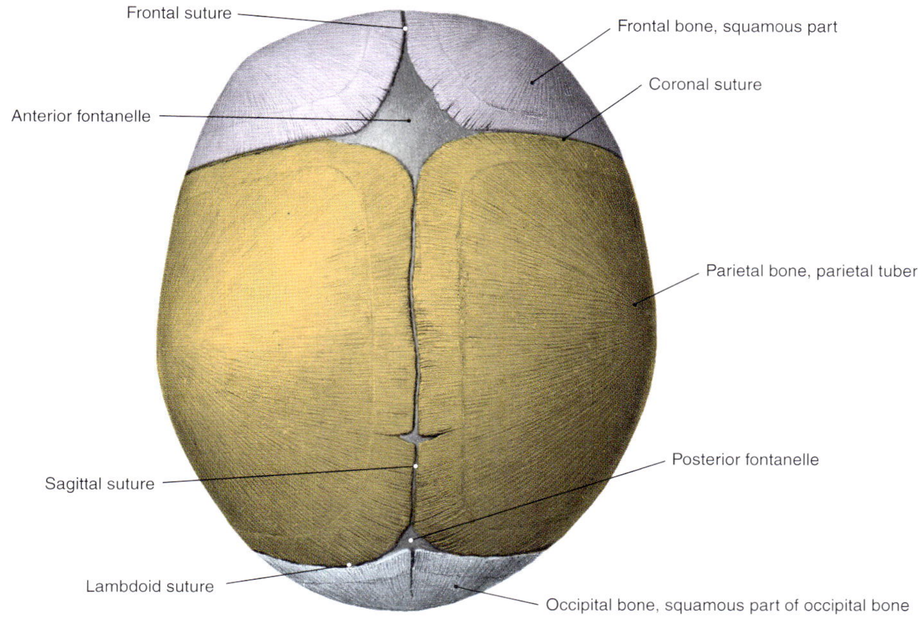

Fig. 76 Skull of a neonate.

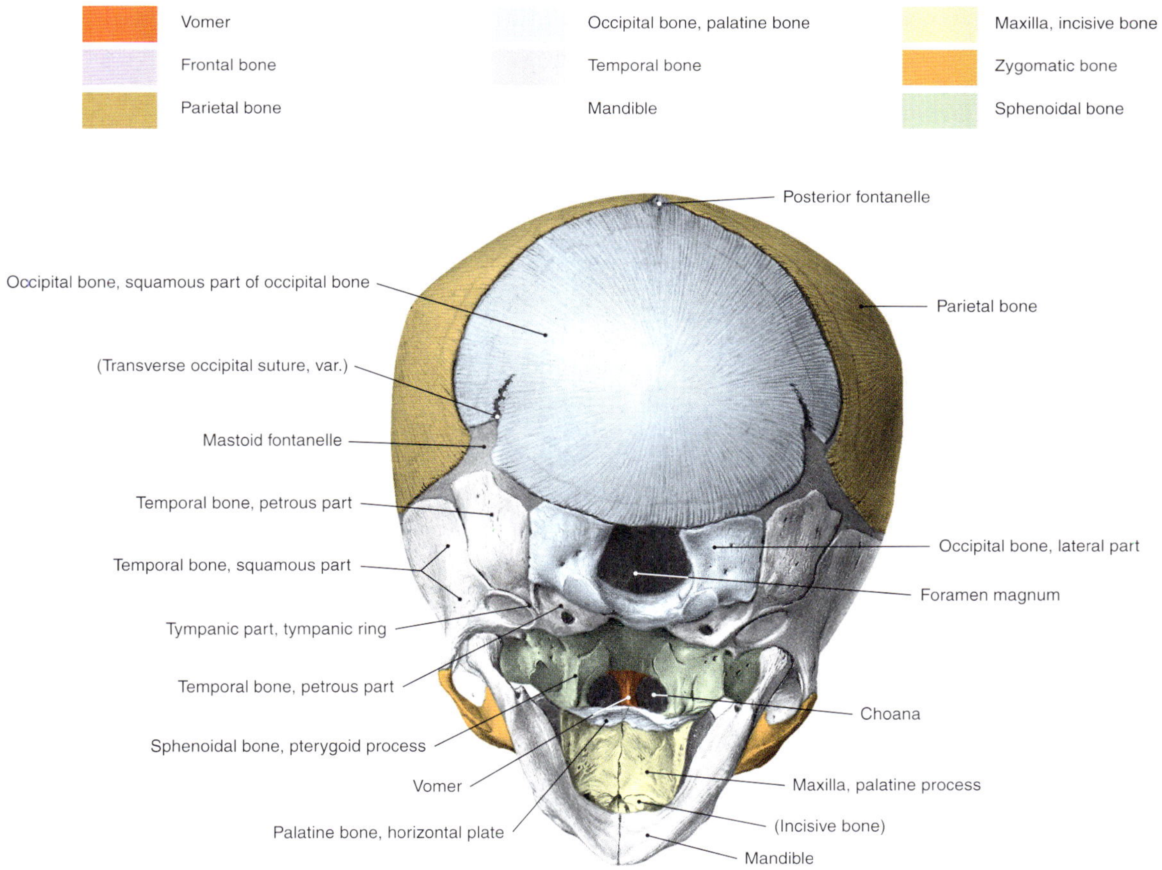

Fig. 77 Skull of a neonate.

Frontal and ethmoidal bone

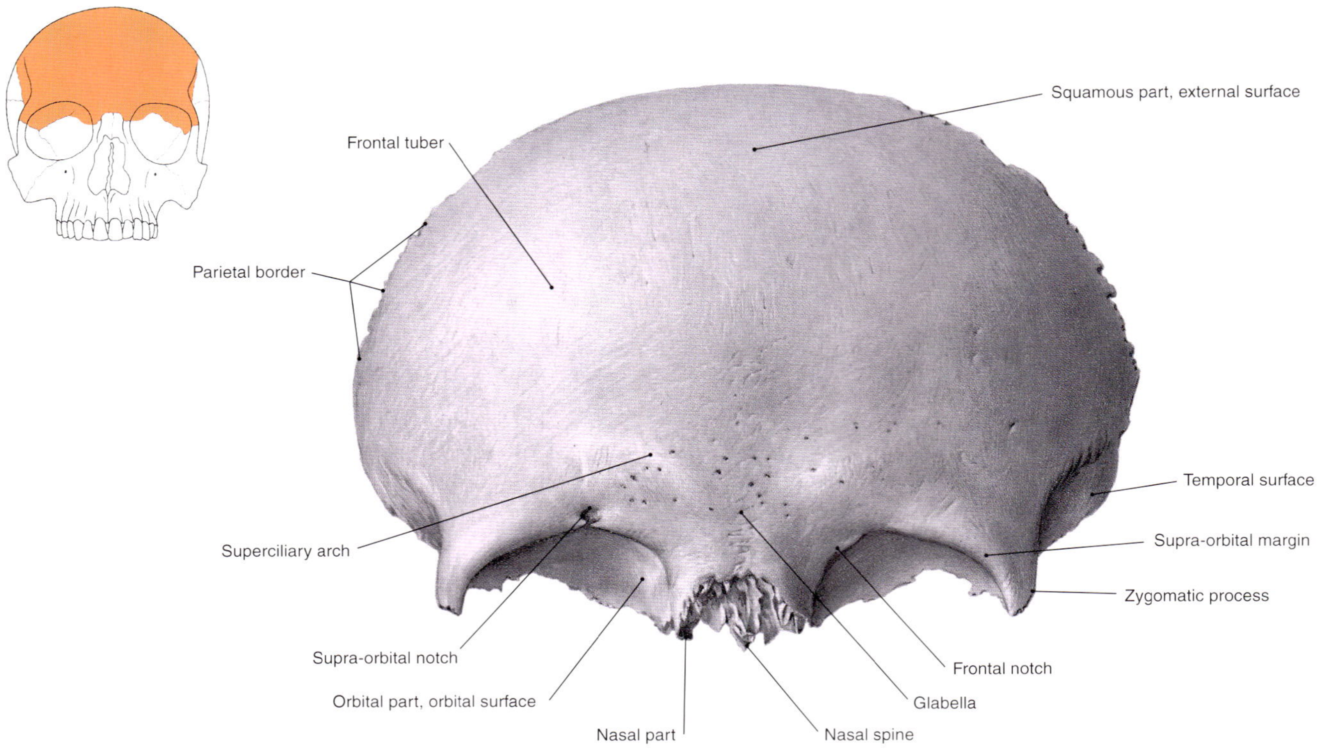

Fig. 78 Frontal bone.

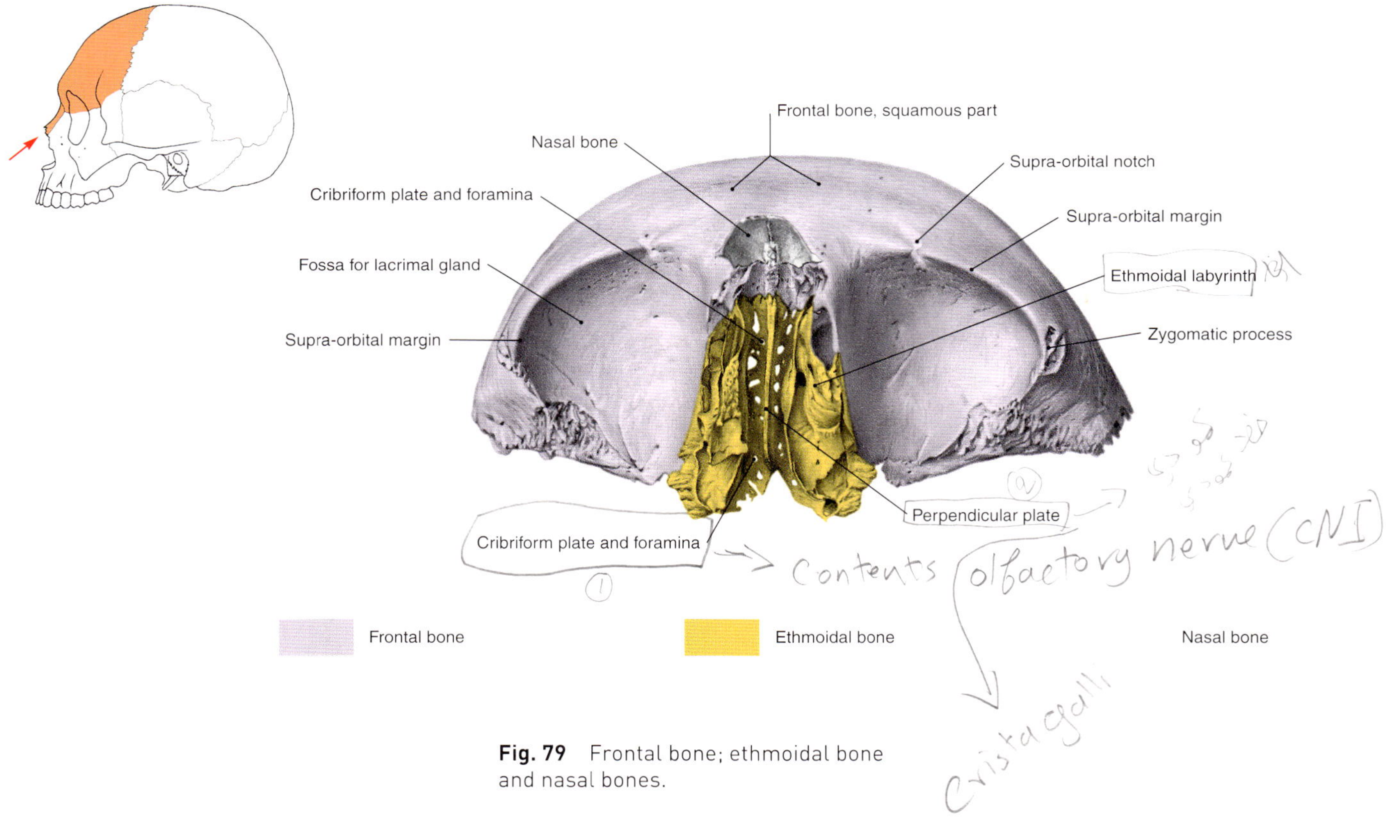

Fig. 79 Frontal bone; ethmoidal bone and nasal bones.

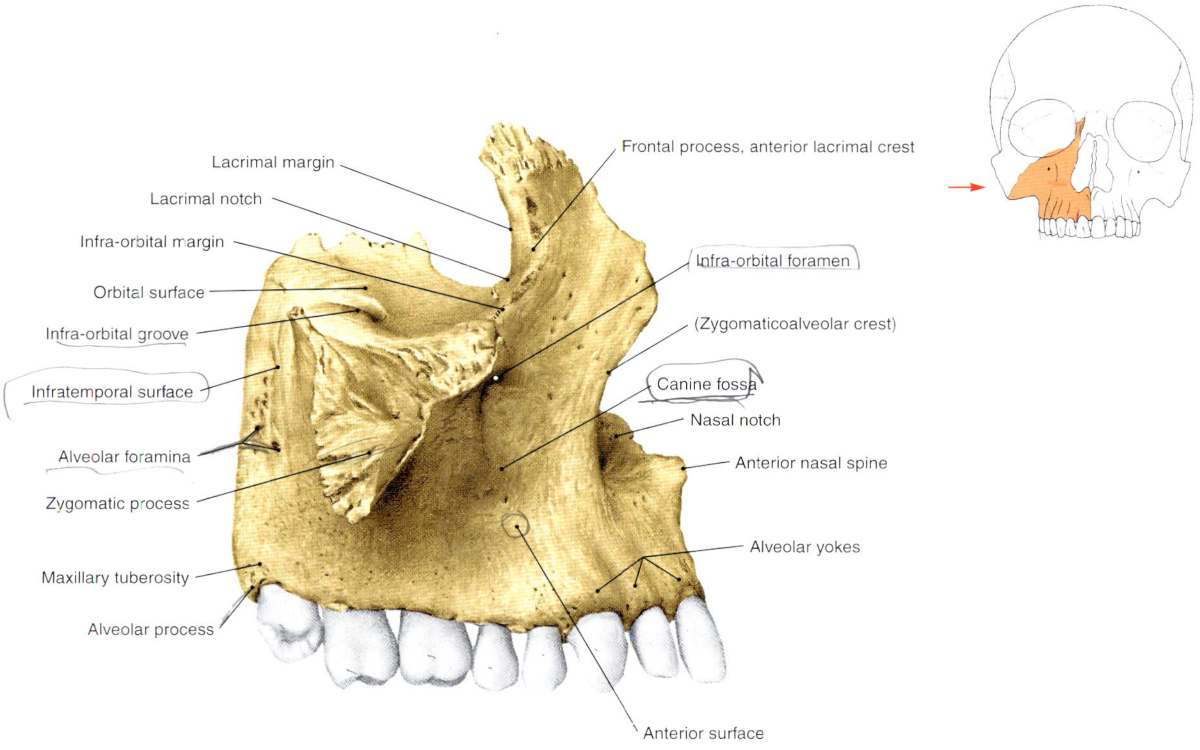

Fig. 80 Maxilla.

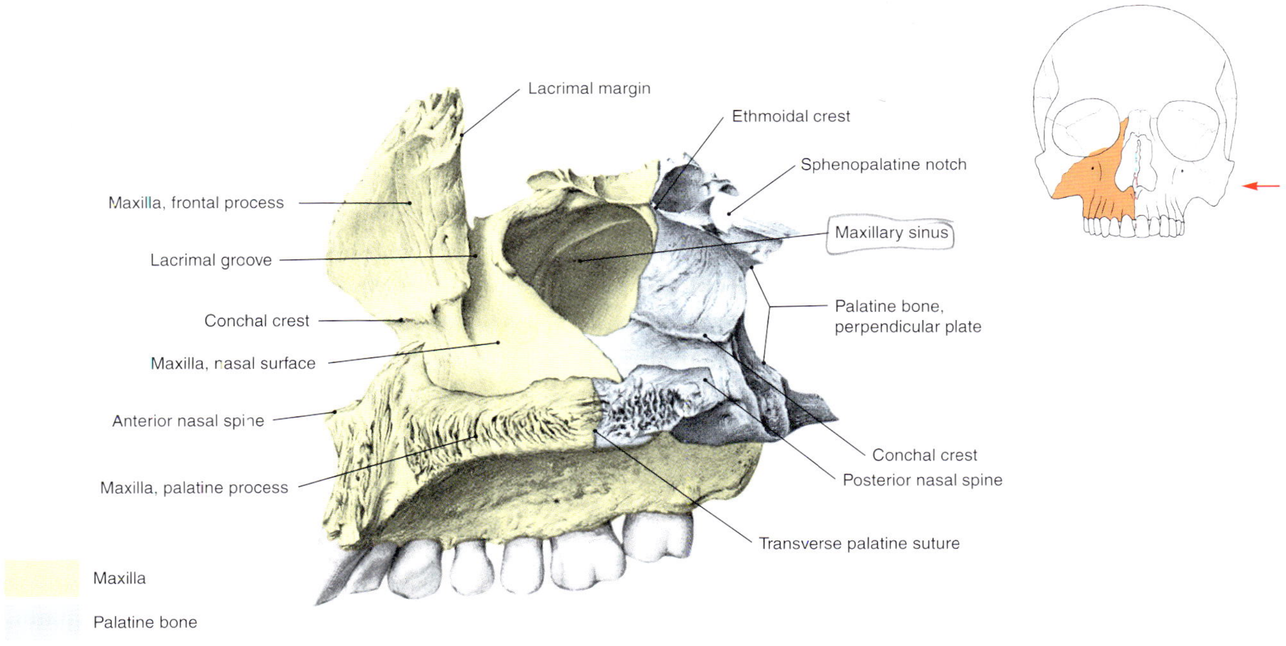

Fig. 81 Maxilla and palatine bone.

Nasal cavity

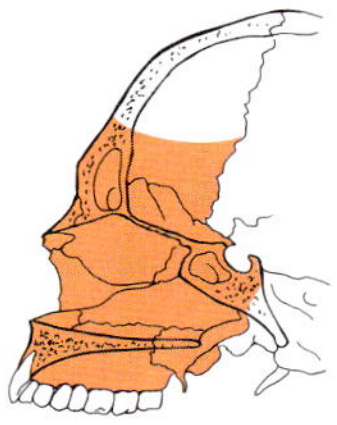

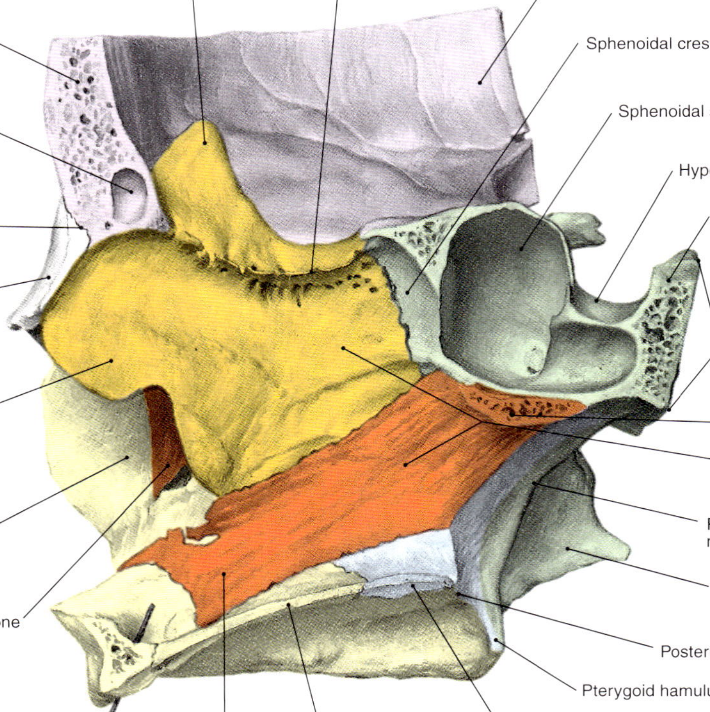

* Superior meatus: lies below and lateral to superior concha. The superior meatus Receives openings of the Posterior Ethmoidal Sinuses

*Inferior meatus: lies below and lateral to the inferior concha It Recievos the Opening of the Nasolacrimal duct It drains lacrimal fluid from surface of eye into the meatus for evaportion during inspiration.

- Maxilla
- Frontal bone
- Nasal bone
- Sphenoidal bone
- Palatine bone
- Ethmoidal bone
- Vomer
- Lacrimal bone

Fig. 82 Bony nasal septum.

* Middle meatus: lies below and lateral to Middle concha. It Recieves the opening of Frontal, Maxillary, anterior and middle ethmoidal sinuses.

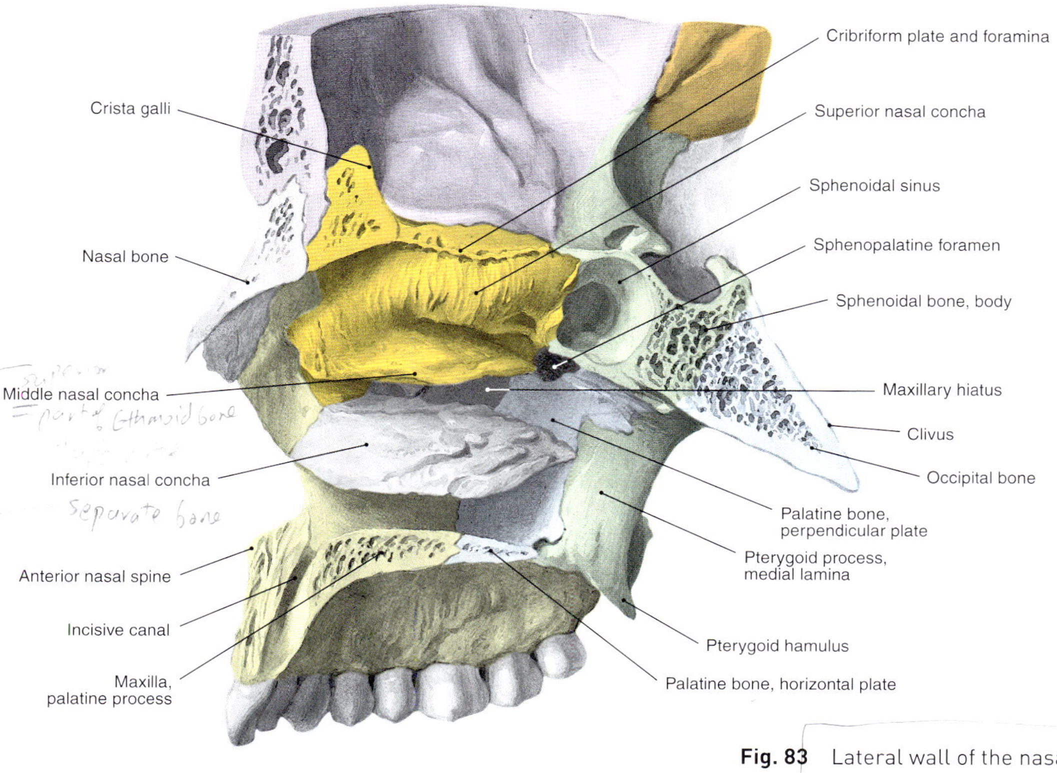

Fig. 83 Lateral wall of the nasal cavity.

No Vomer bone

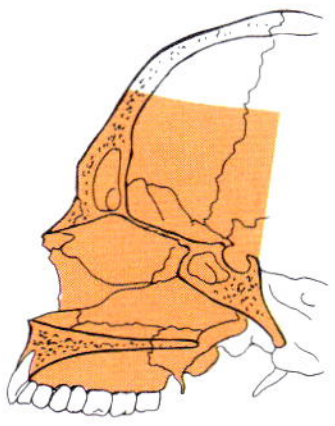

	Parietal bone		Inferior nasal concha		
	Maxilla		Sphenoidal bone		
	Frontal bone		Occipital bone		Ethmoidal bone
	Nasal bone		Palatine bone		Lacrimal bone

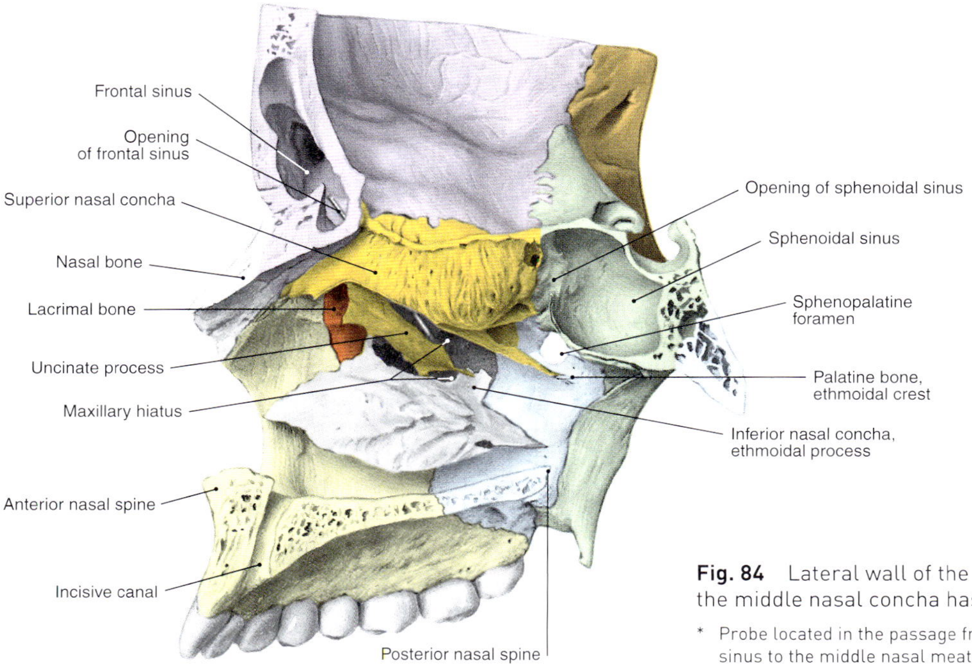

Fig. 84 Lateral wall of the nasal cavity; the middle nasal concha has been removed.

* Probe located in the passage from the frontal sinus to the middle nasal meatus

Hard palate

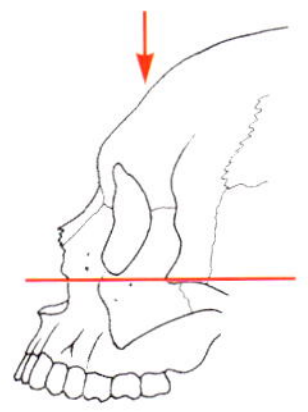

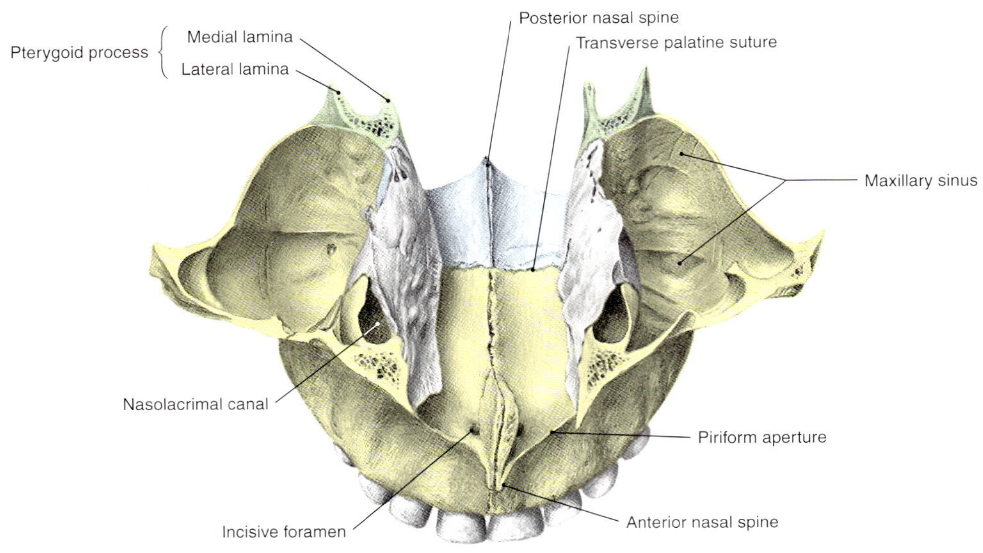

Fig. 85 Hard palate; maxillary sinus and inferior nasal concha.

Maxilla
Palatine bone
Sphenoidal bone
Inferior nasal concha

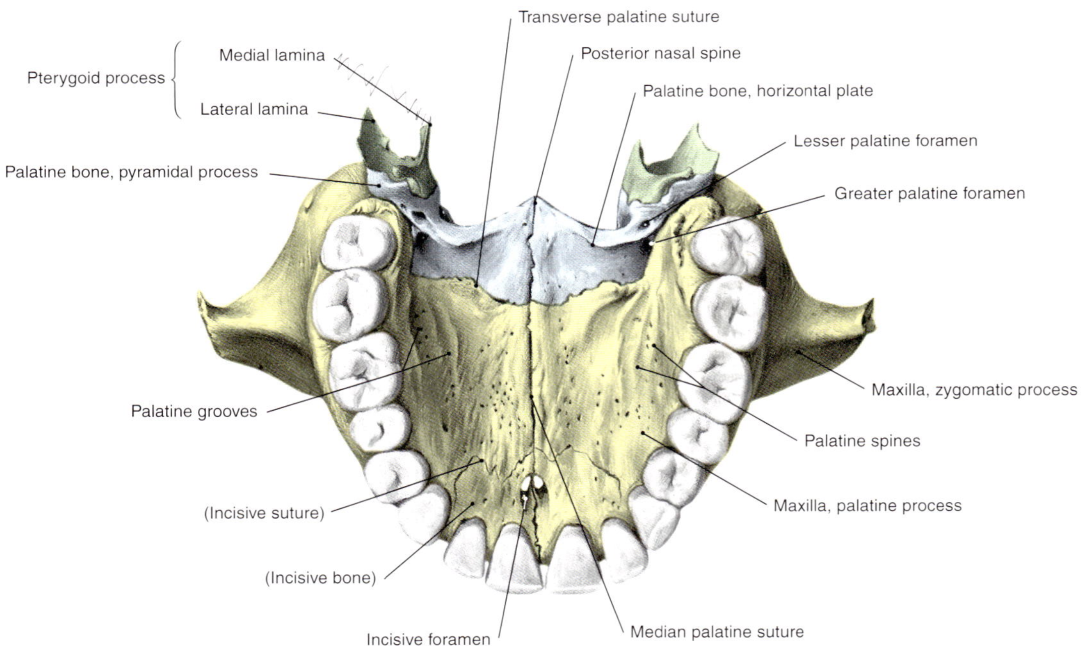

Fig. 86 Hard palate.

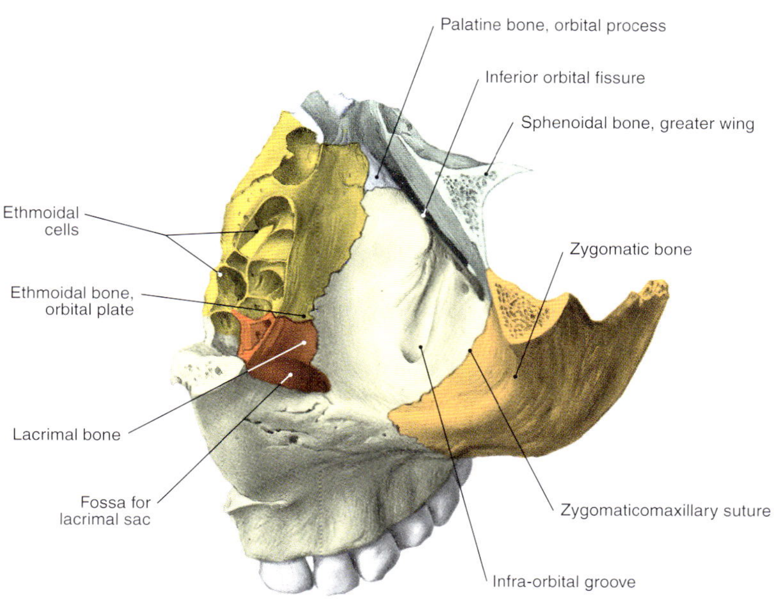

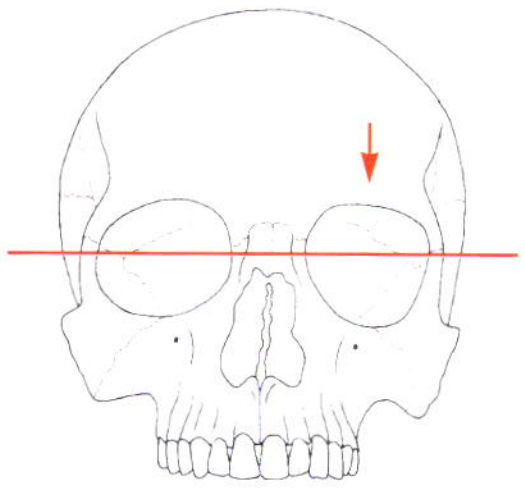

Fig. 87 Base of the orbit.

* This fossa contains the maxillary artery and nerve and their branches arising here (the infraorbital and sphenopalatine arteries)
The Maxillary division of Trigeminal nerve and branches. (pterygopalatine ganglion)

- Zygomatic bone
- Temporal bone
- Palatine bone
- Sphenoidal bone
- Maxilla
- Lacrimal bone
- Ethmoidal bone
- Frontal bone

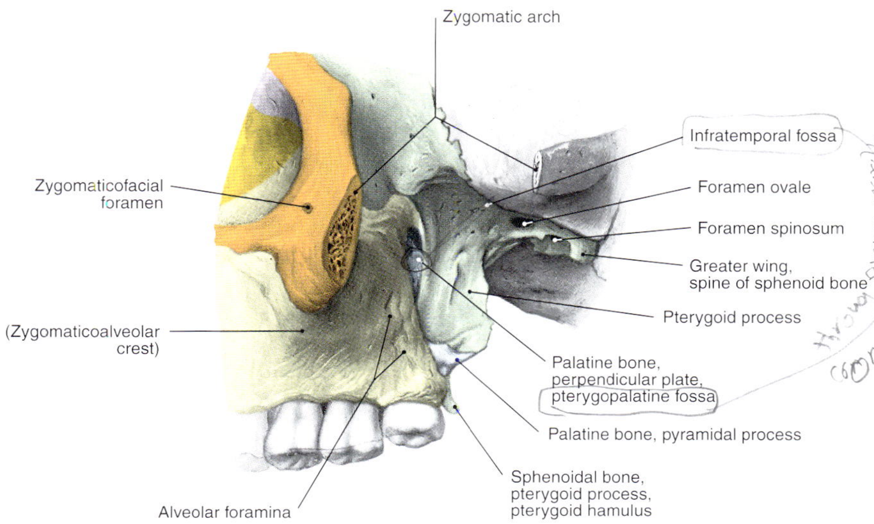

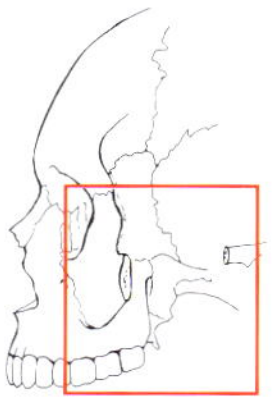

Fig. 88 Pterygopalatine fossa.

Orbit

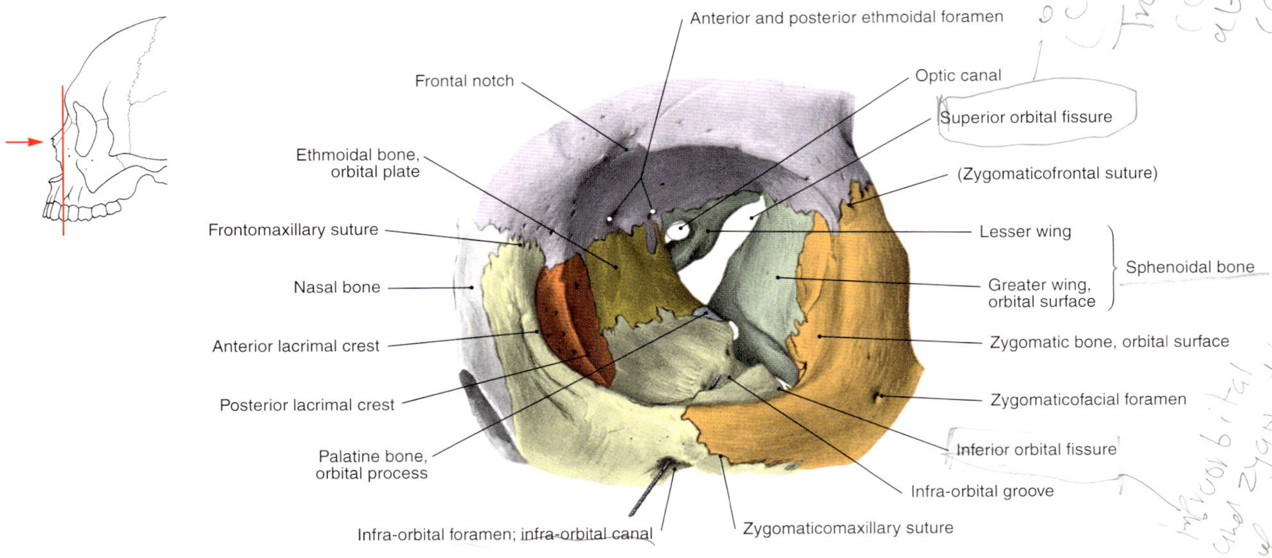

Fig. 89 Orbit; probe located in the infra-orbital canal.

- Nasal bone
- Frontal bone
- Palatine bone
- Ethmoidal bone
- Vomer
- Zygomatic bone
- Maxilla
- Temporal bone
- Inferior nasal concha
- Sphenoidal bone
- Lacrimal bone

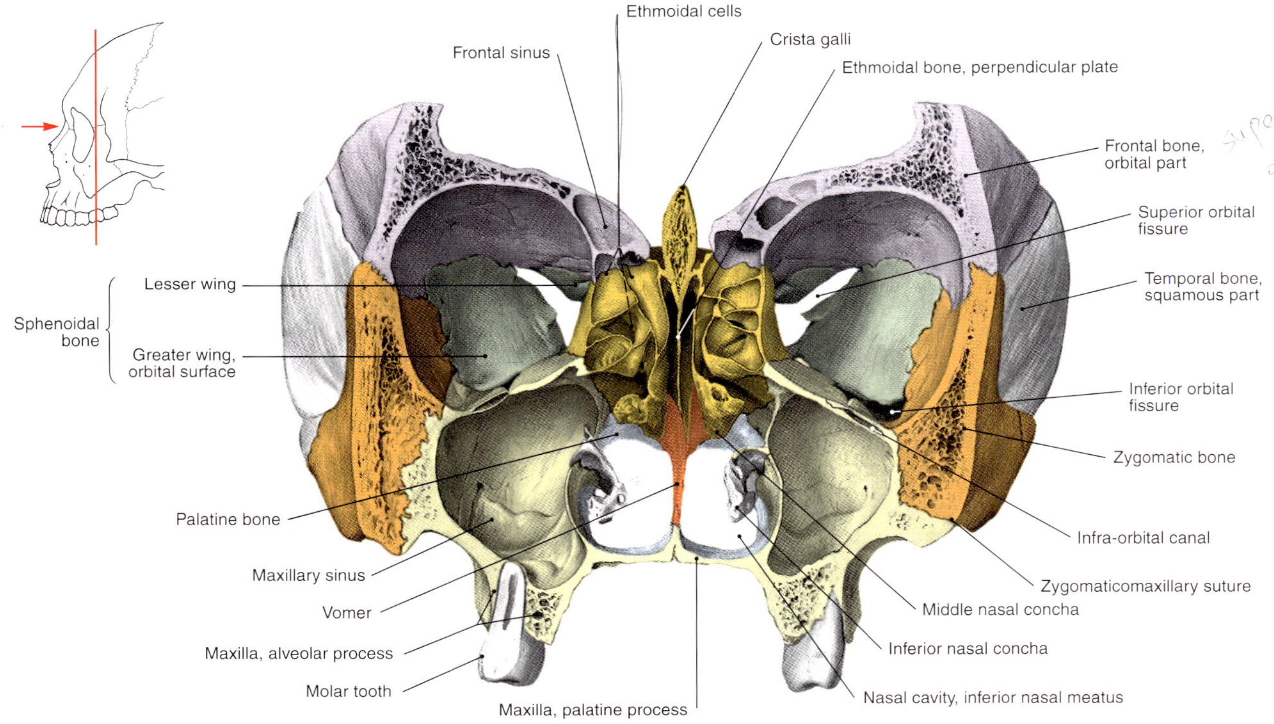

Fig. 90 Facial skeleton; frontal section.

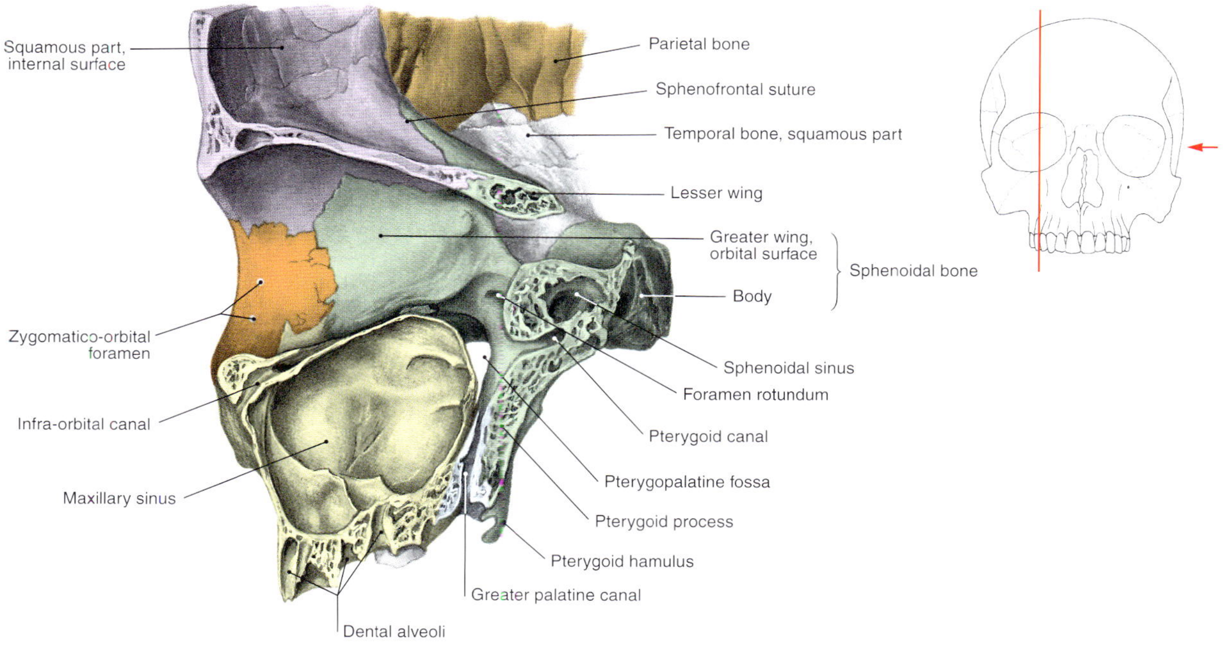

Fig. 91 Orbit;
lateral wall.

	Frontal bone		Nasal bone		Maxilla
	Lacrimal bone		Palatine bone		Temporal bone
	Sphenoidal bone		Ethmoidal bone		Zygomatic bone

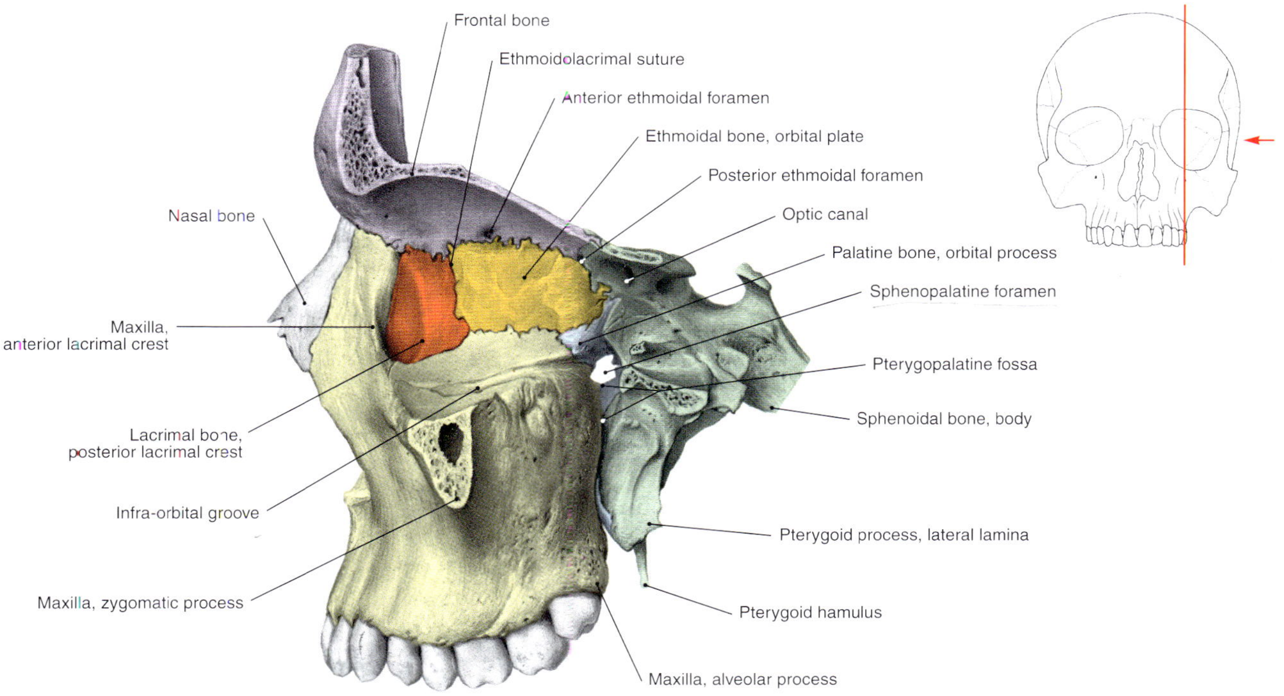

Fig. 92 Orbit;
medial wall.

Sphenoidal bone

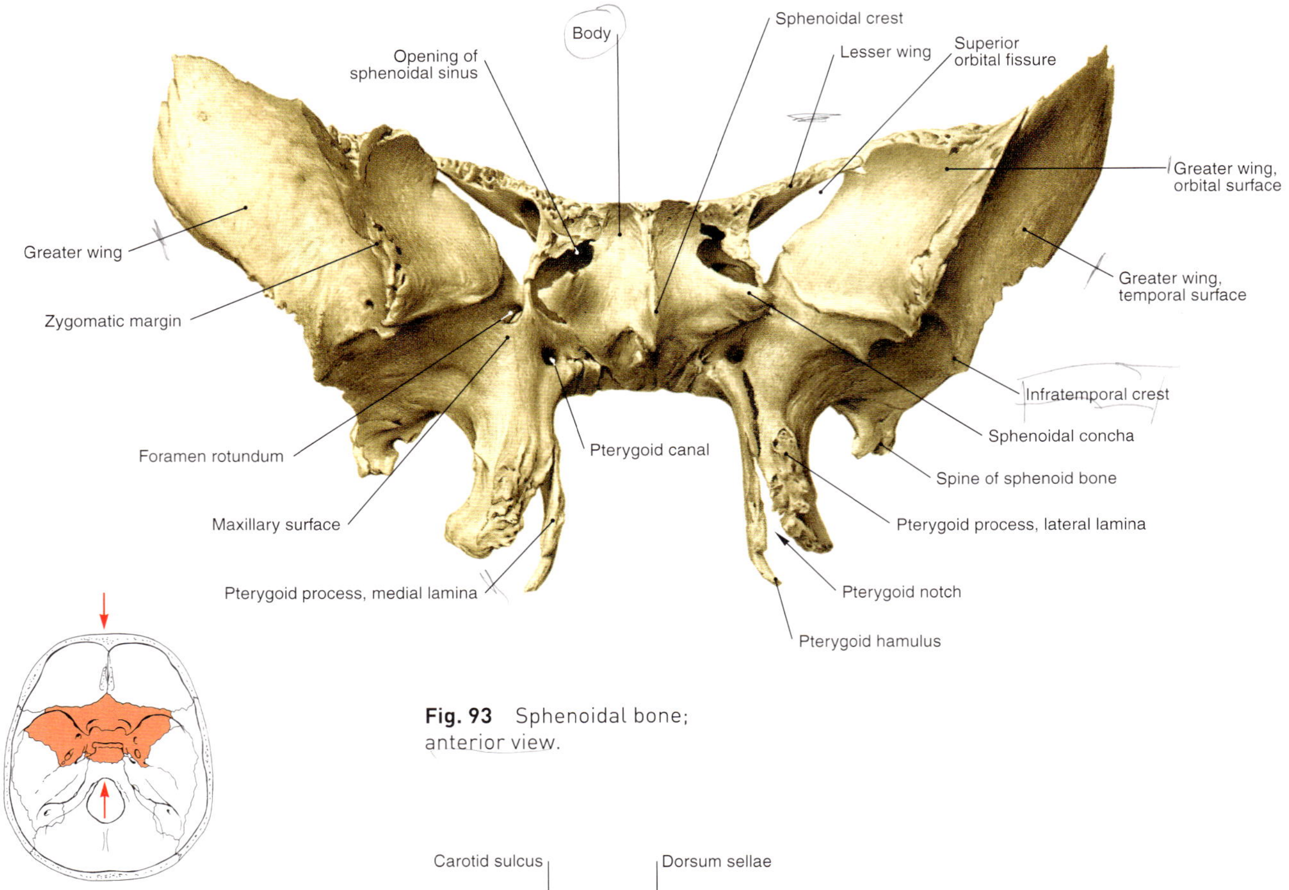

Fig. 93 Sphenoidal bone; anterior view.

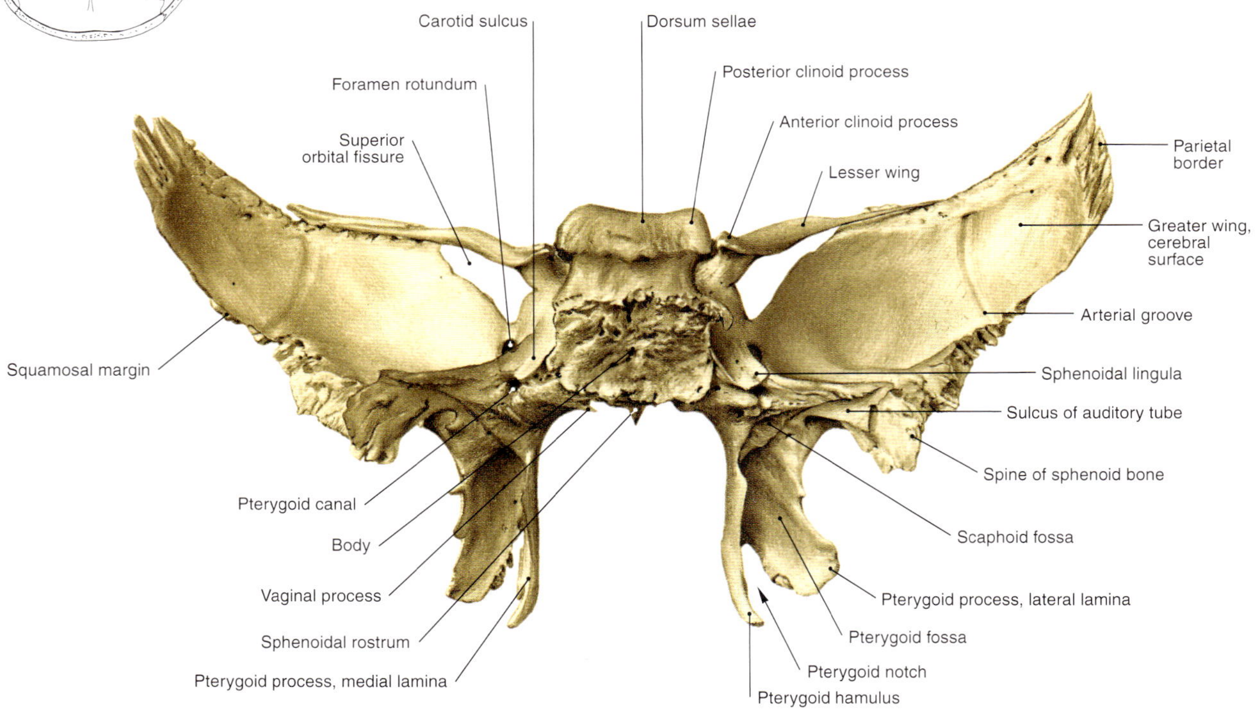

Fig. 94 Sphenoidal bone; posterior view.

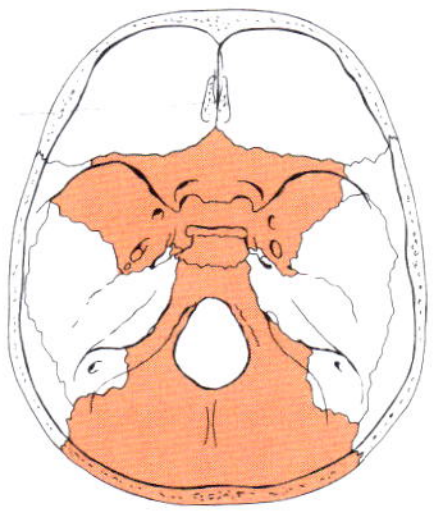

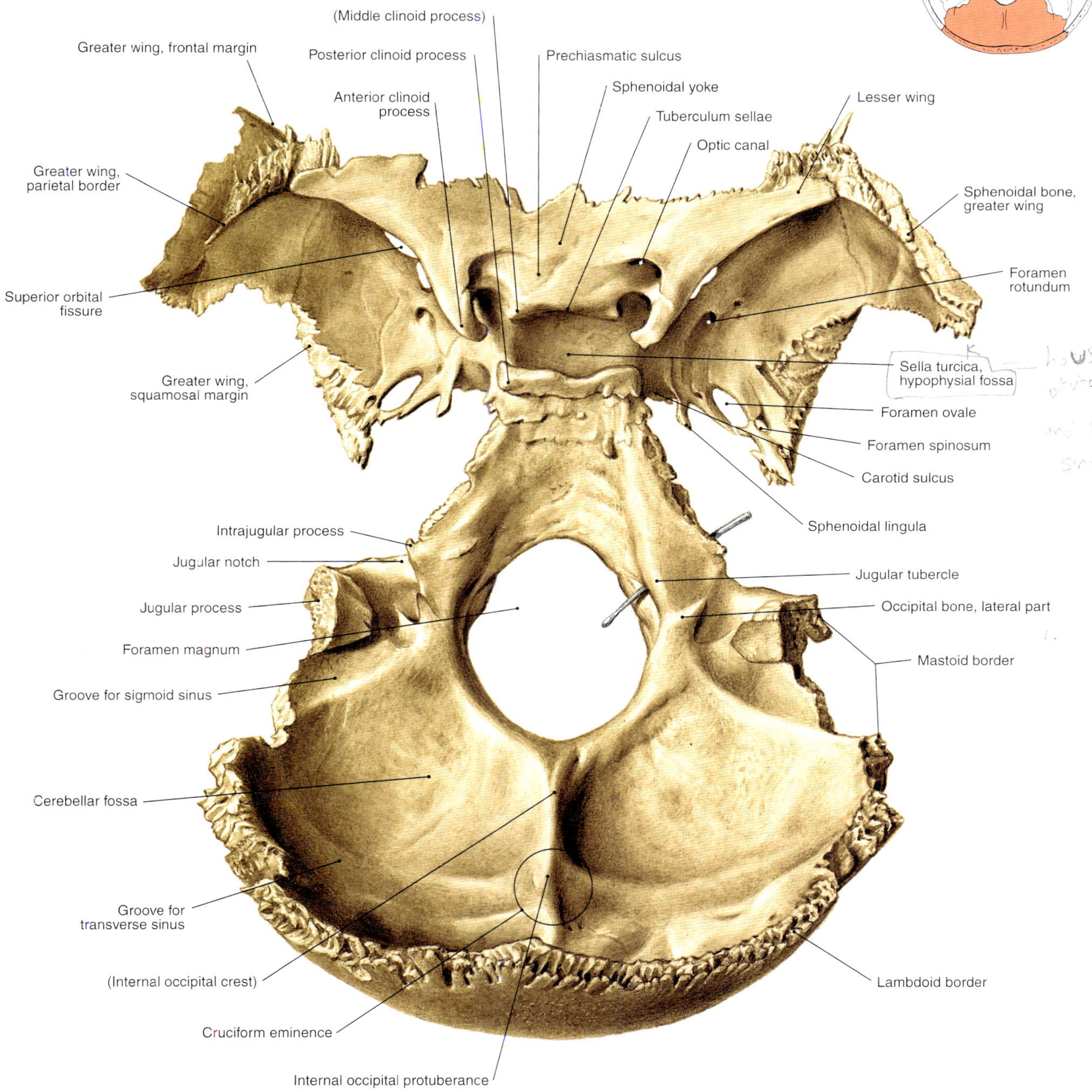

Fig. 95 Occipital bone and sphenoidal bone.

Temporal bone

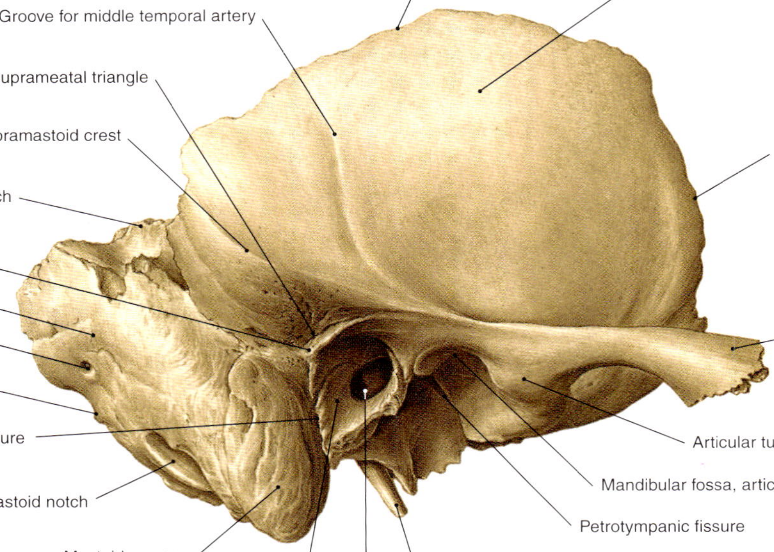

Fig. 96 Temporal bone.

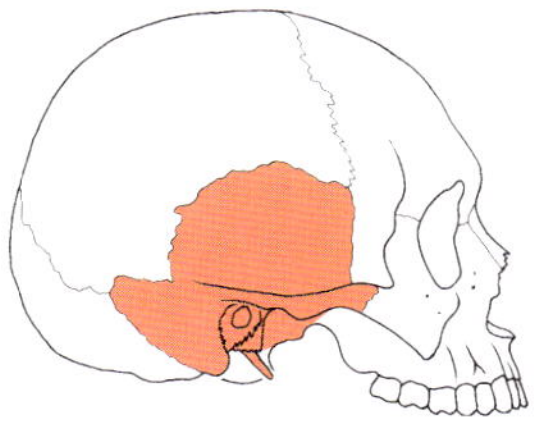

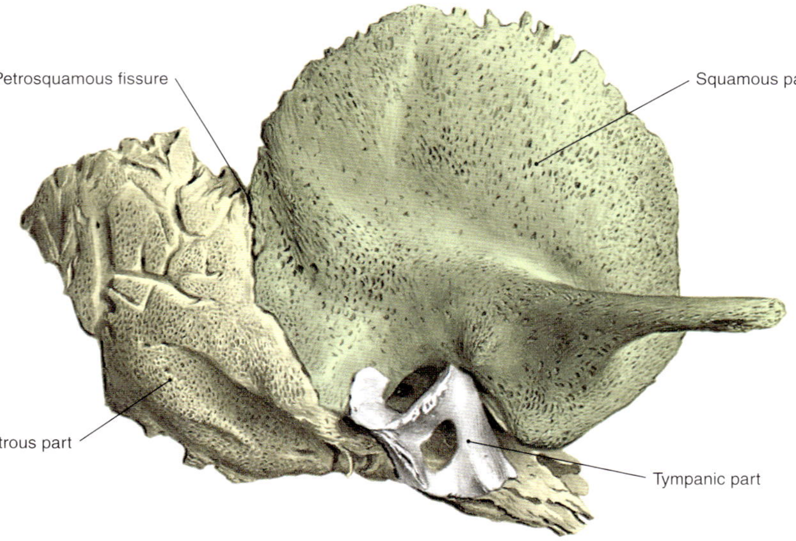

Fig. 97 Temporal bone of a neonate.

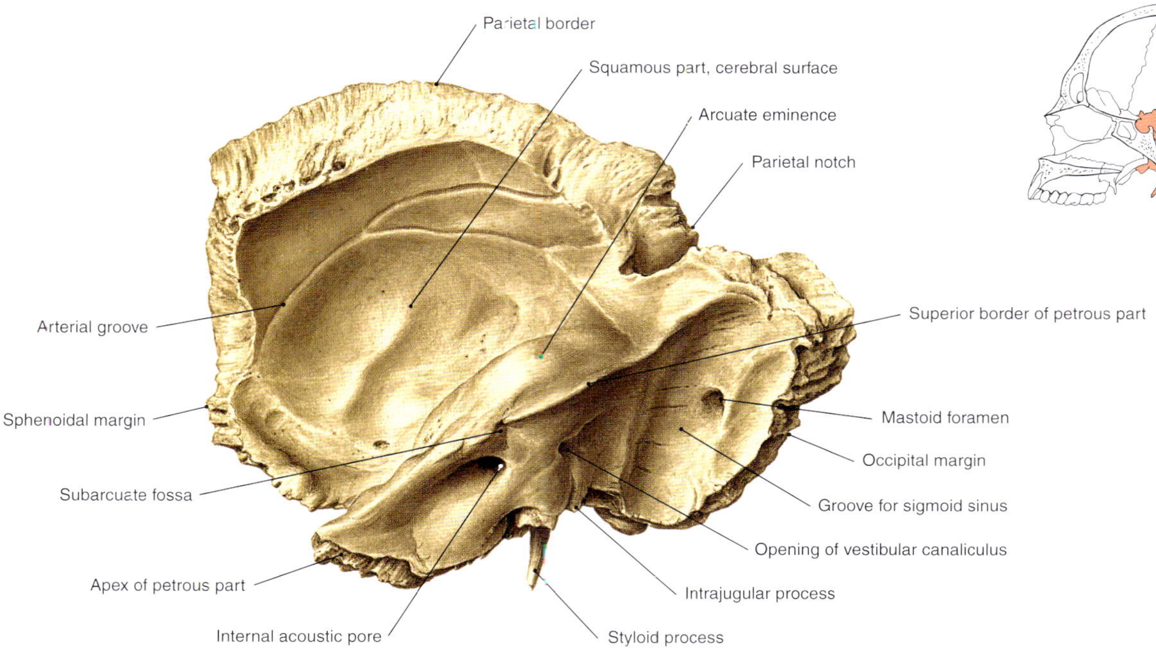

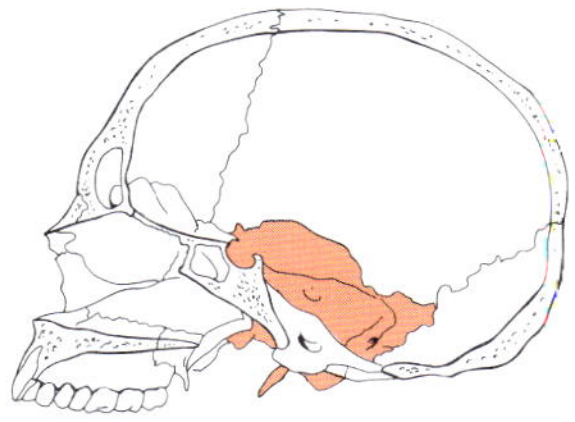

Fig. 98 Temporal bone.

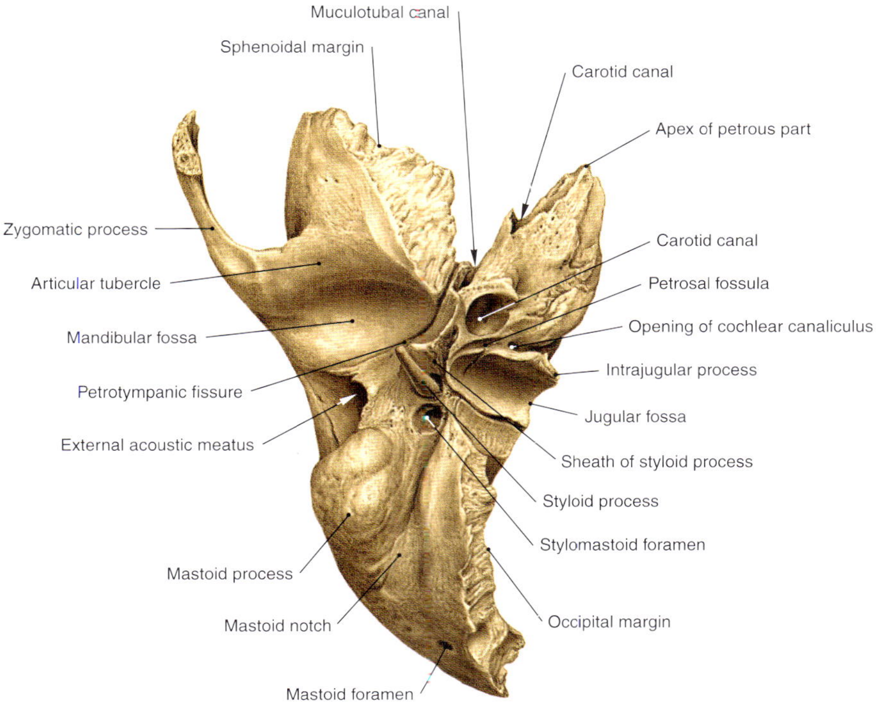

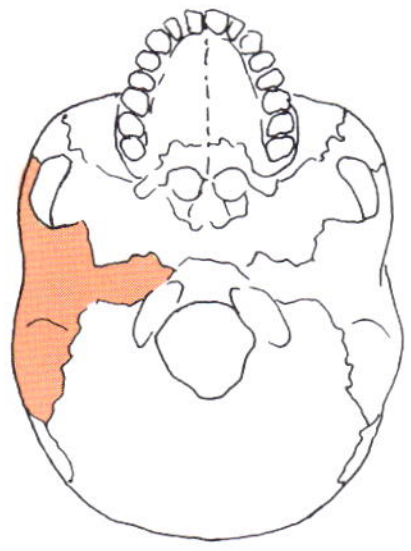

Fig. 99 Temporal bone.

Mandible

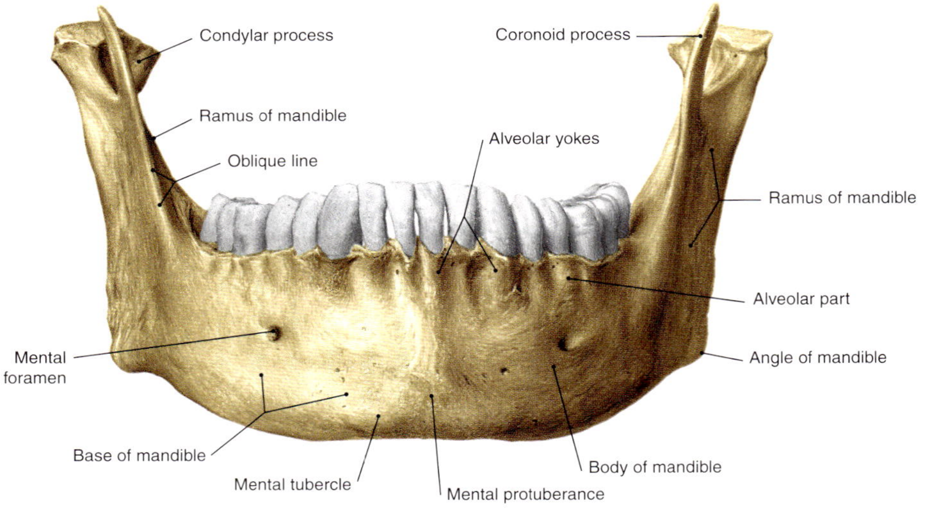

Fig. 100 Mandible.

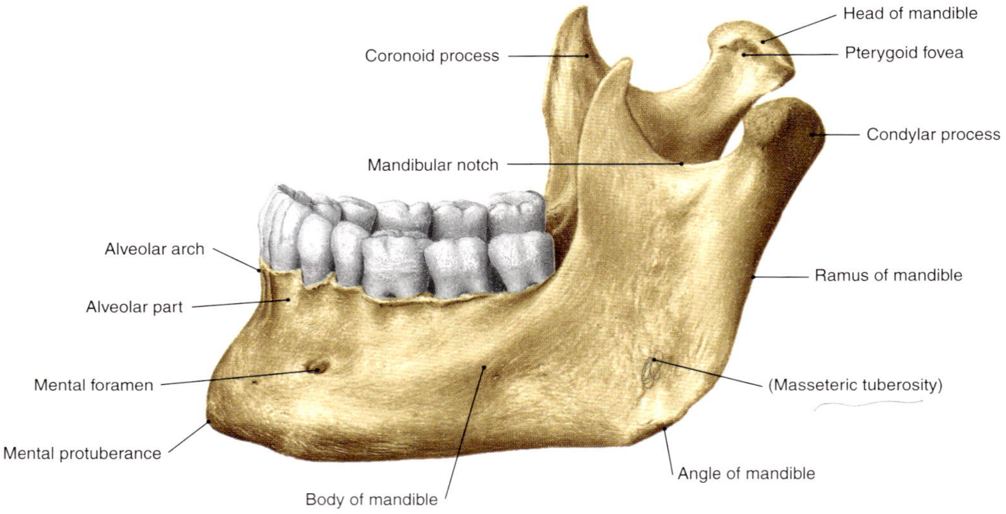

Fig. 101 Mandible.

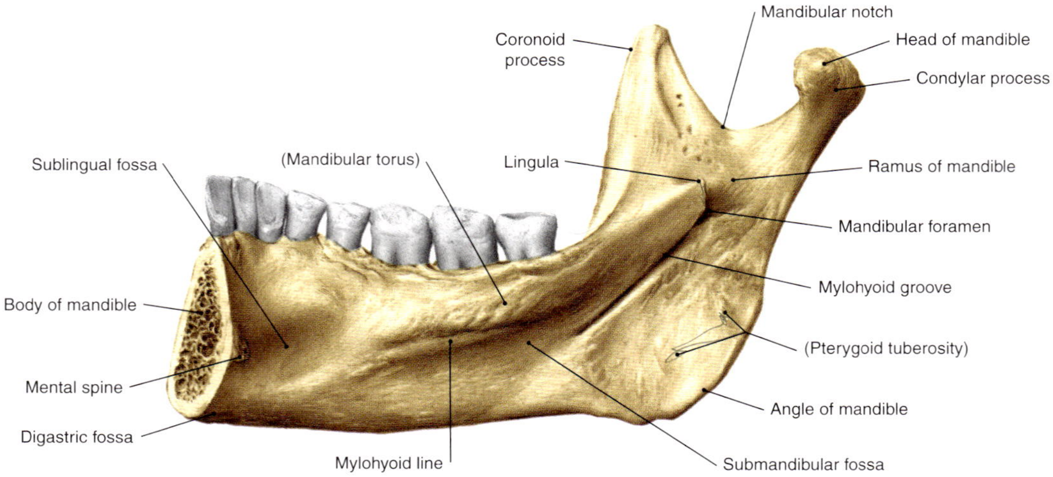

Fig. 102 Mandible.

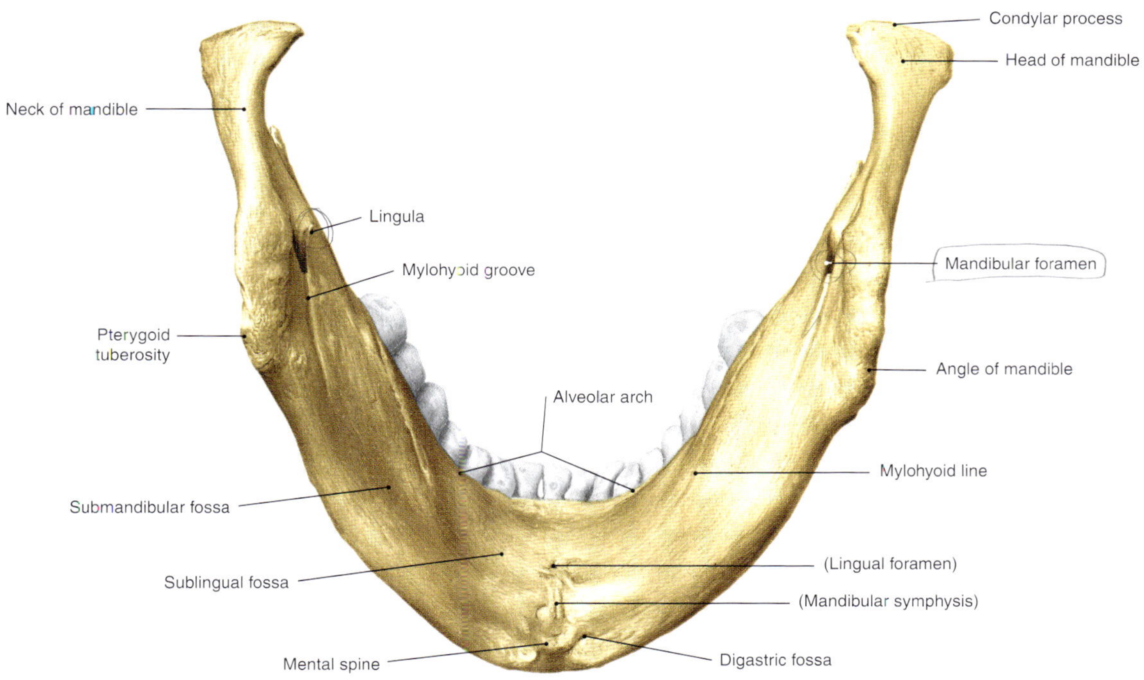

Fig. 103 Mandible.

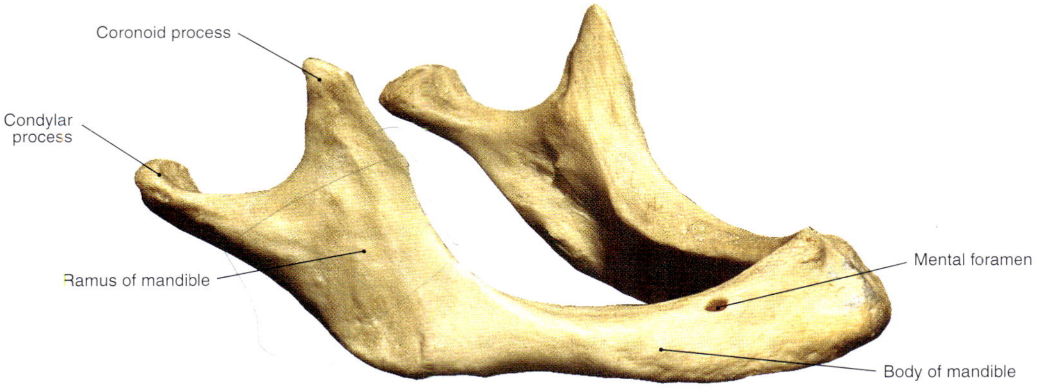

Fig. 104 Mandible of an elderly individual.

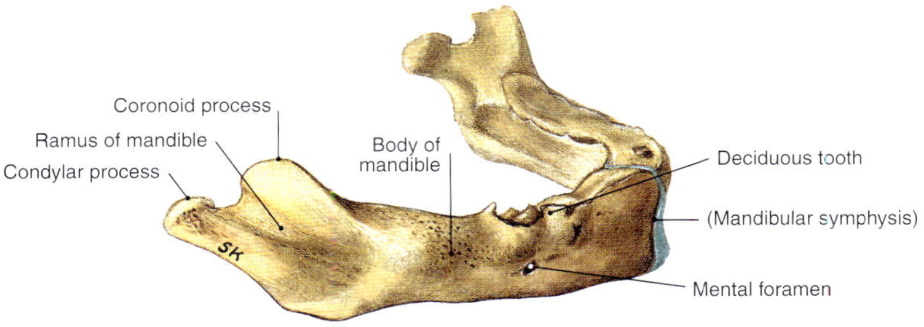

Fig. 105 Mandible of a neonate.

Temporomandibular joint

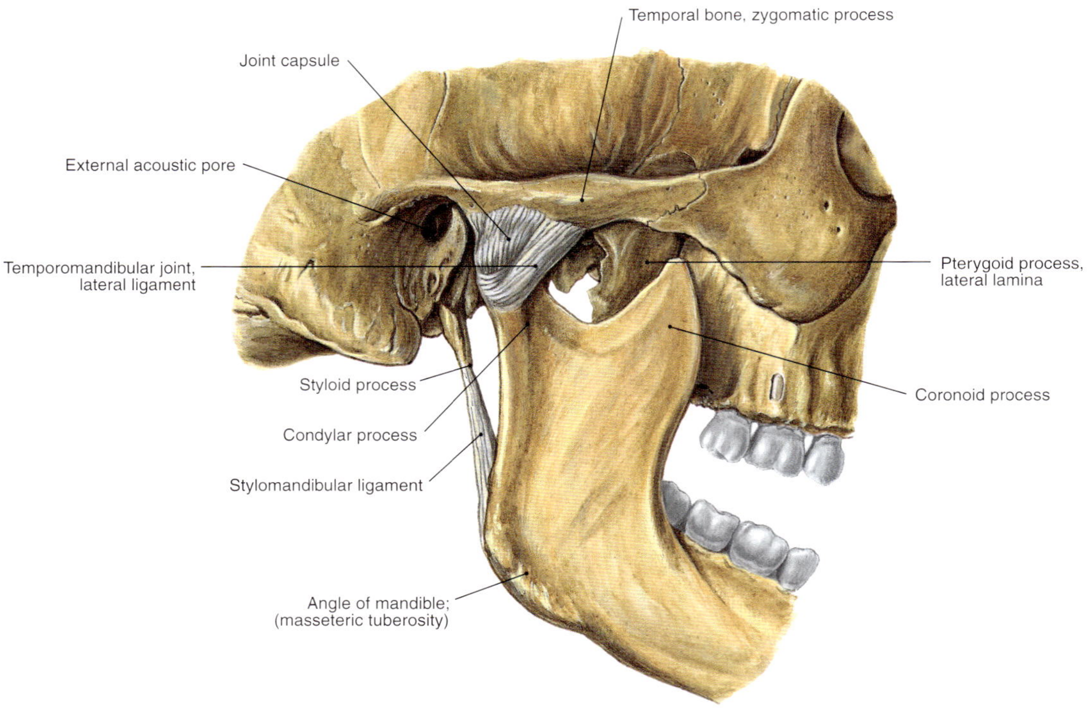

Fig. 106 Temporomandibular joint.

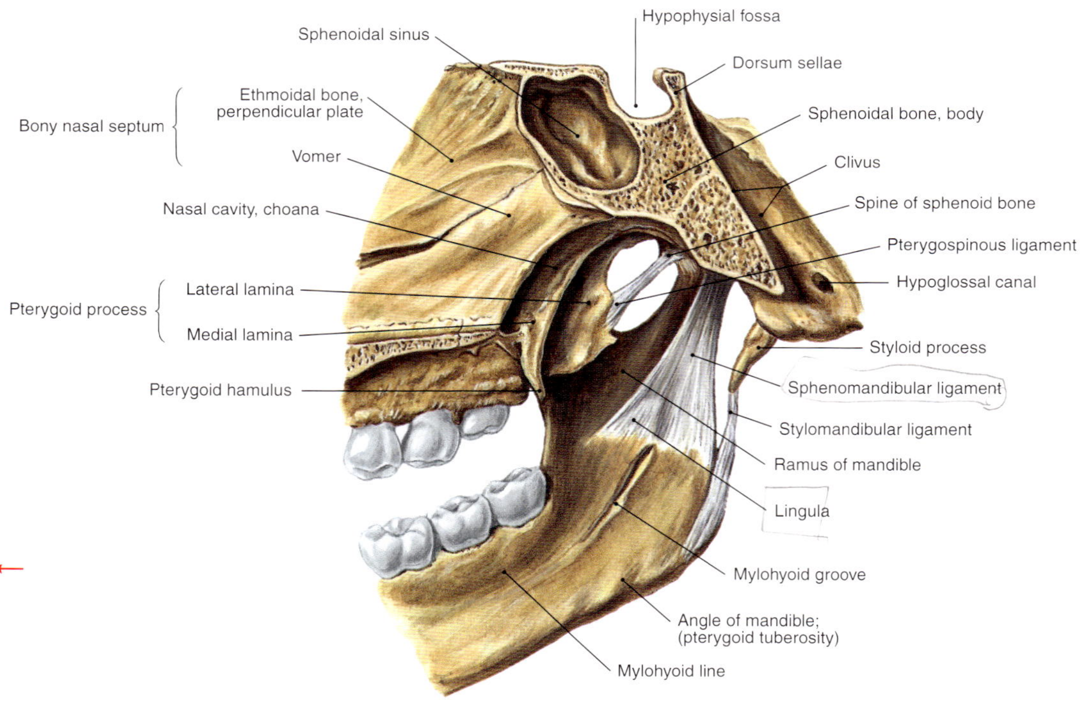

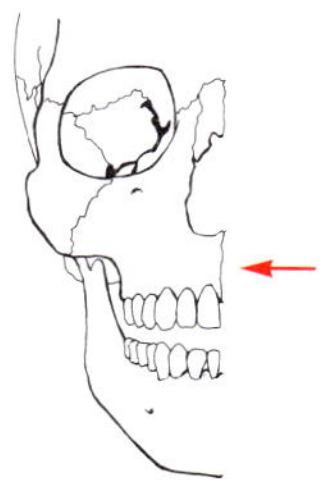

Fig. 107 Pterygospinous and sphenomandibular ligaments.

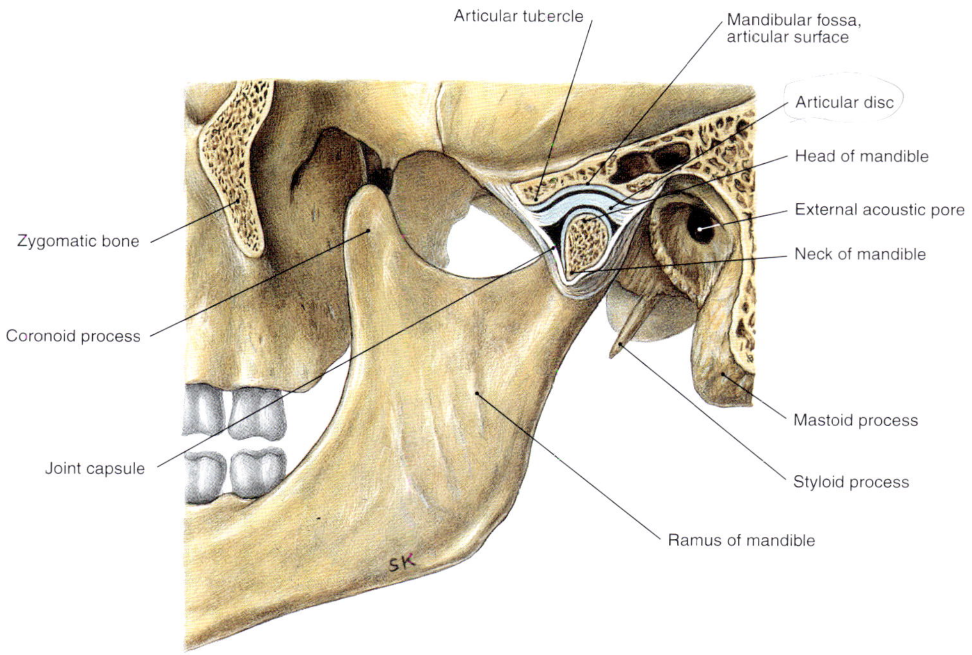

Fig. 108 Temporomandibular joint; sagittal section; mouth almost closed.

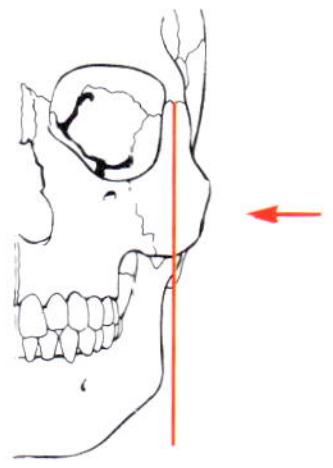

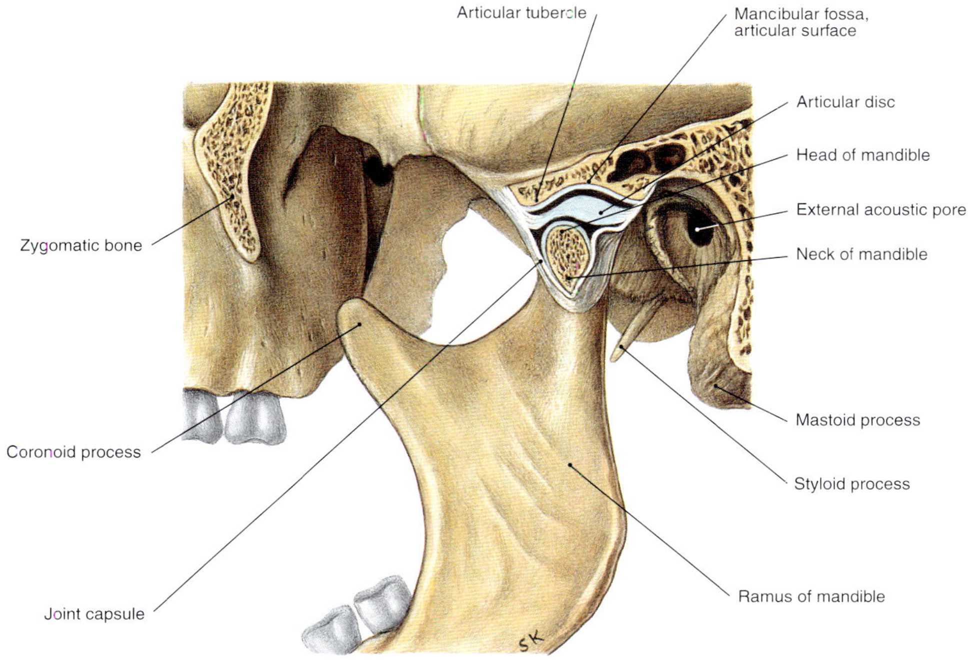

Fig. 109 Temporomandibular joint; sagittal section; mouth opened.

Temporomandibular joint and masticatory muscles

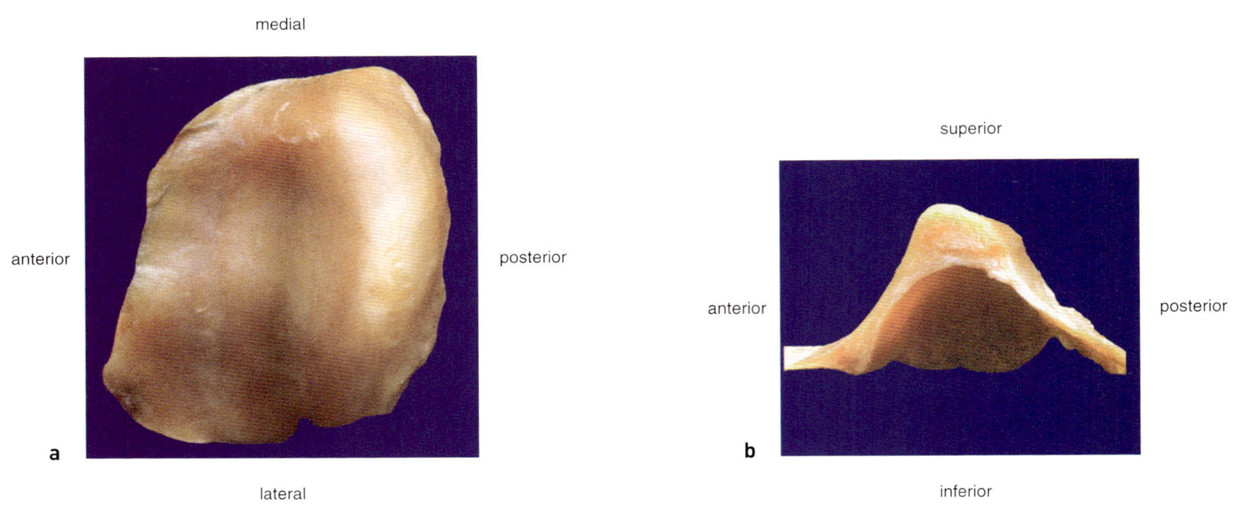

Fig. 110 a, b Articular disc of the temporomandibular joint.
a Superior view
b Lateral view.

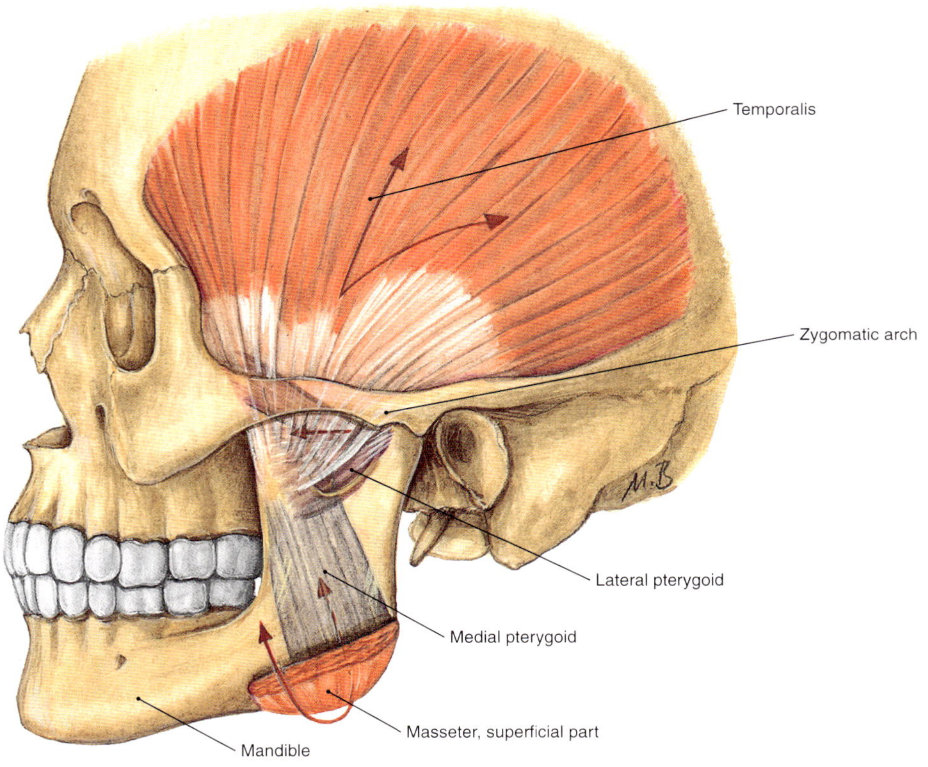

→ T 4

Fig. 111 Masticatory muscles.
Arrows indicate the direction of muscle traction when closing the mouth.

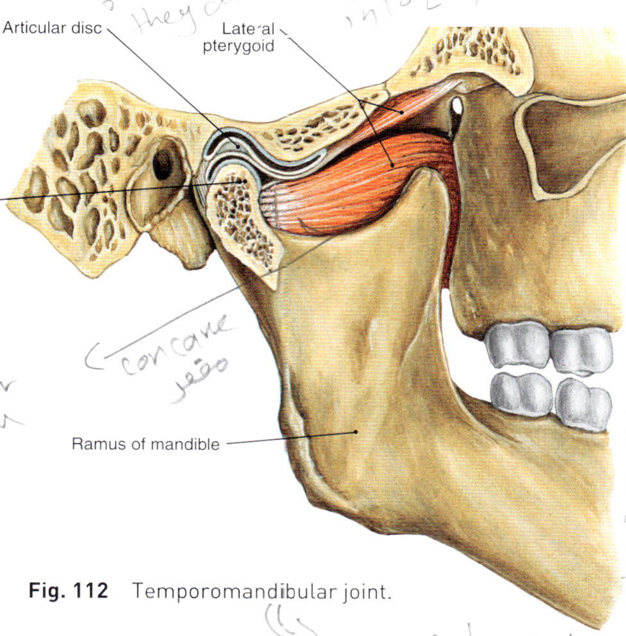

Fig. 112 Temporomandibular joint.

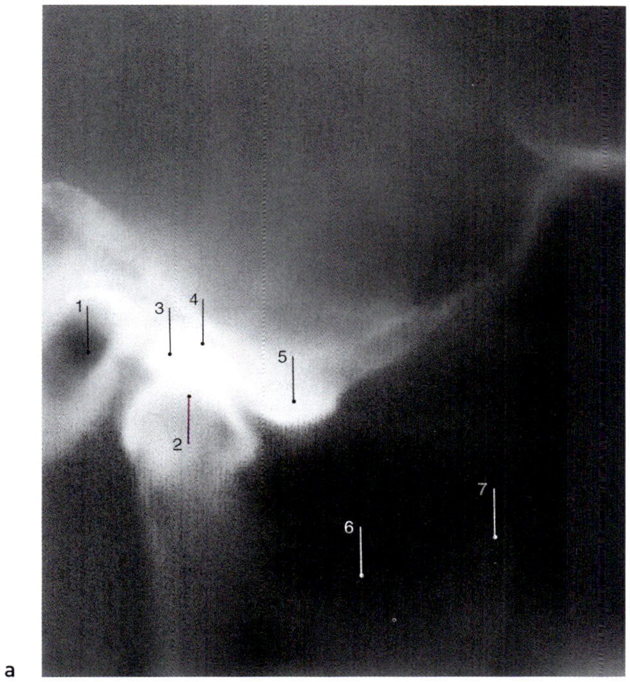

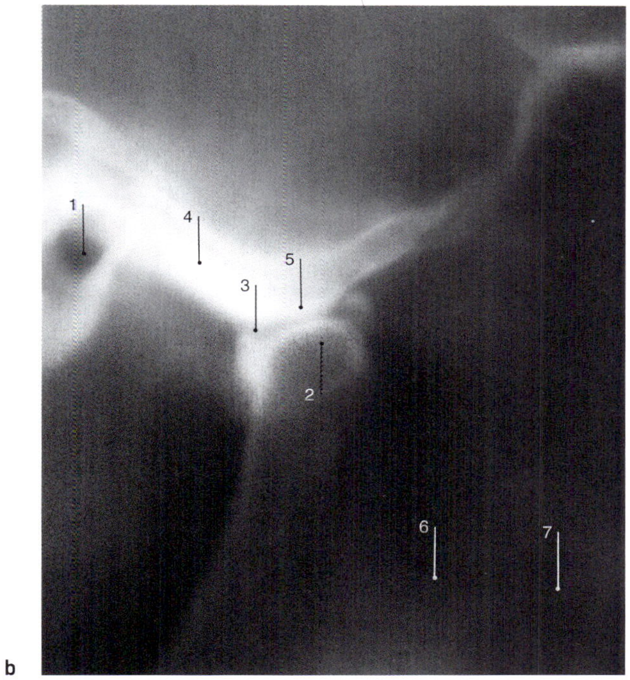

1 External acoustic meatus
2 Condylar process
3 Articular disc
4 Temporal bone, mandibular fossa
5 Temporal bone, articular tubercle
6 Mandibular notch
7 Coronoid process

Fig. 113 a, b Temporomandibular joint; tomography; lateral projection after injection of a contrast medium into the joint cavity (arthrography).
a Mouth closed
b Mouth opened

The articular disc shifts forward during opening of the mouth.

→ 108, 109

Masticatory muscles

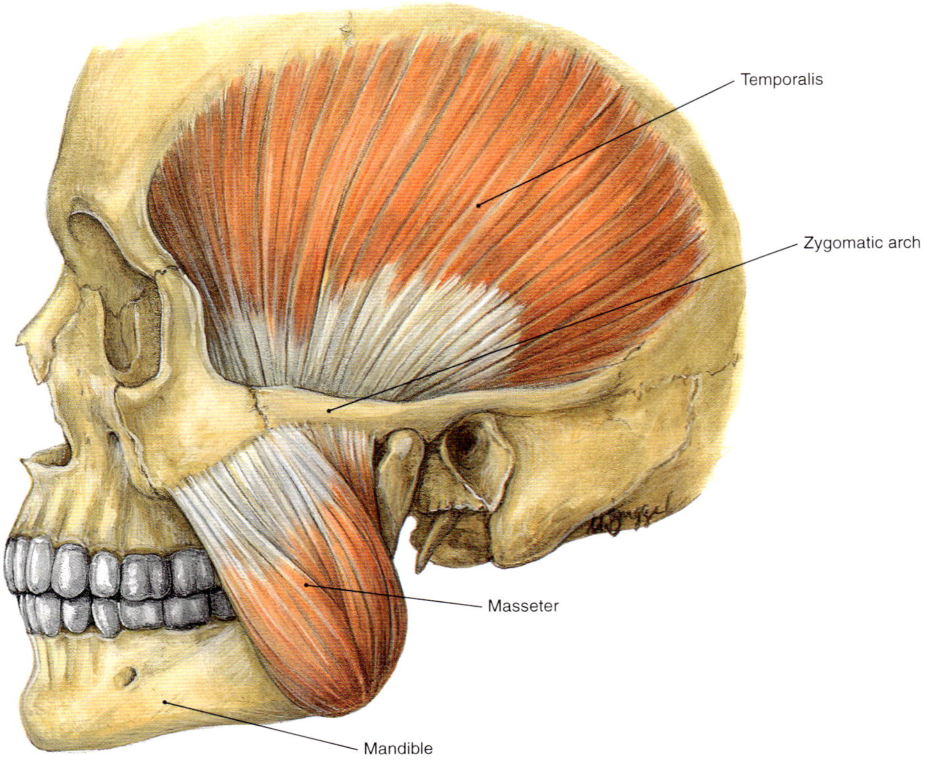

→ T 4

Fig. 114 Masseter and temporal muscle.

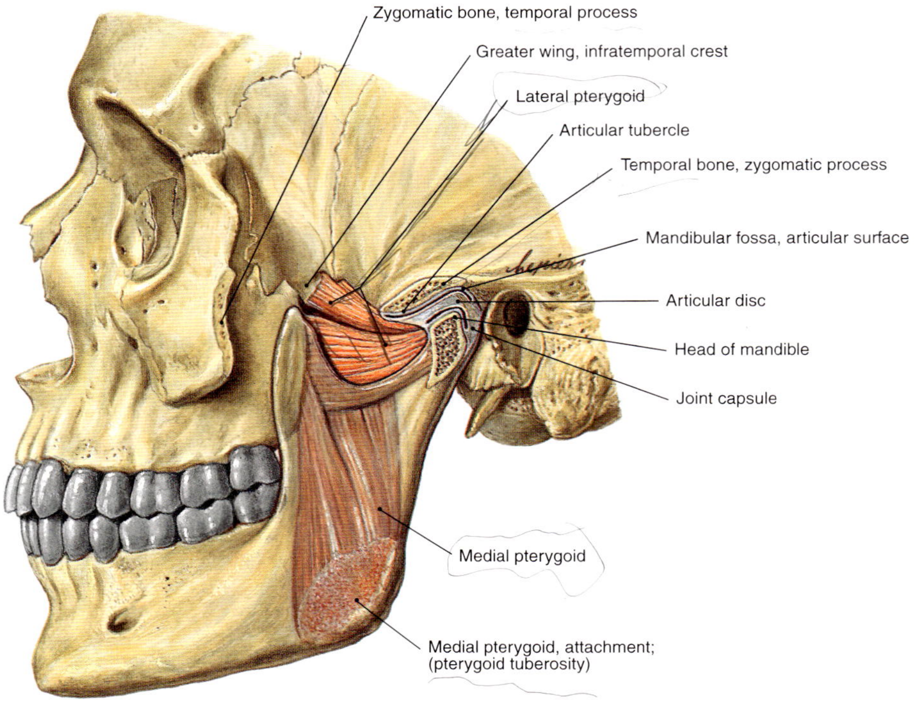

→ T 4

Fig. 115 Temporomandibular joint; medial and lateral pterygoid muscles.

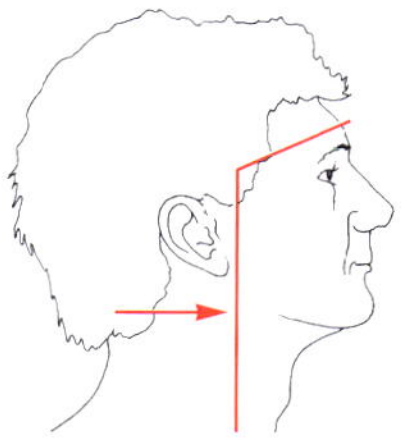

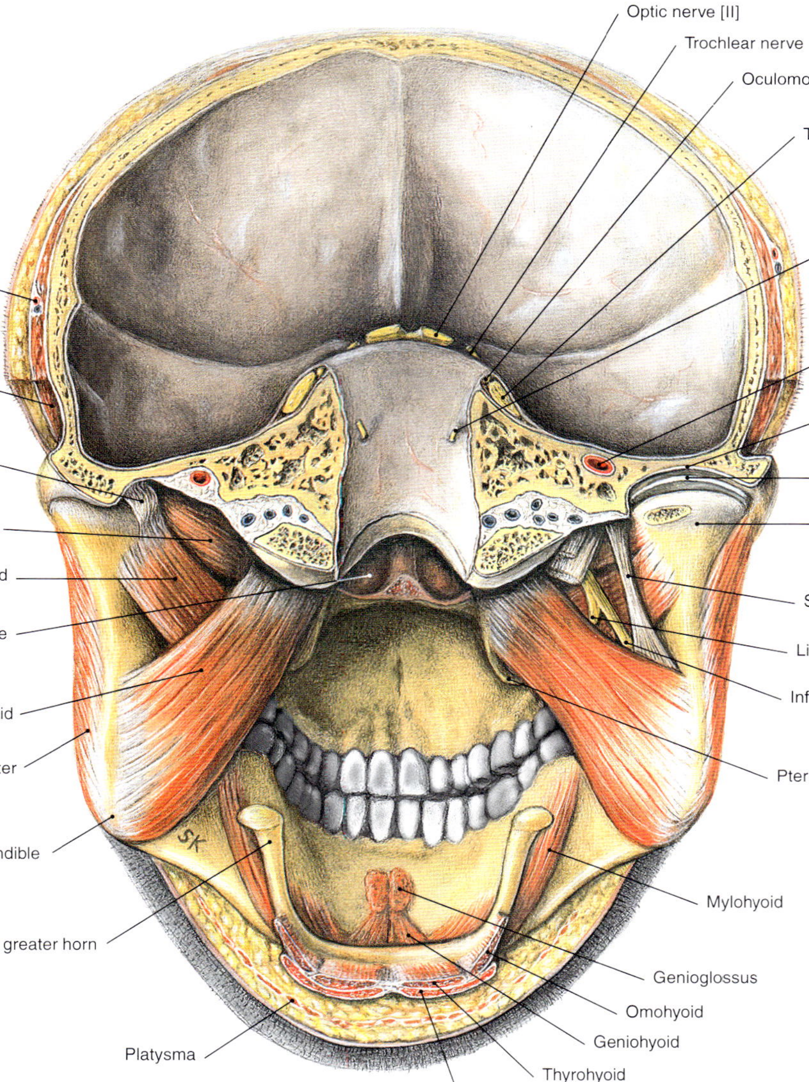

Fig. 116 Masticatory muscles;
frontal section through the temporomandibular joint
and horizontal section through the calvaria;
posterior view.

→ T 4

Masticatory muscles

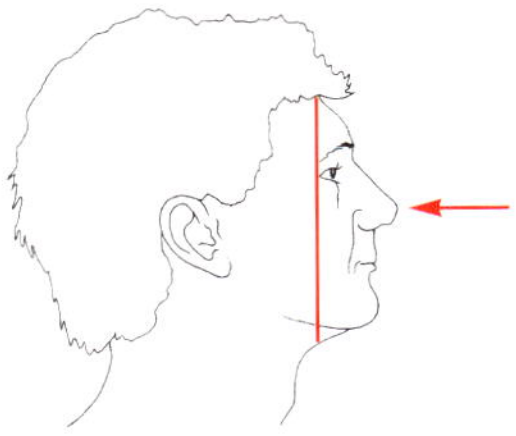

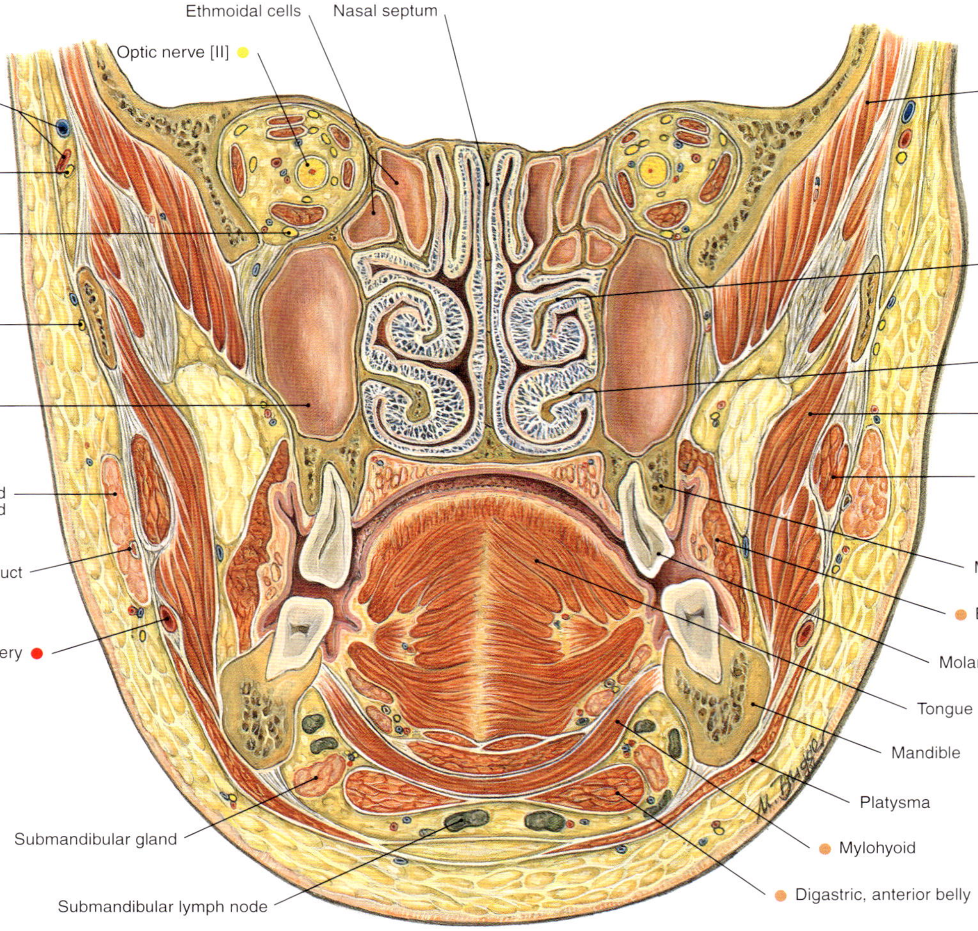

→ T 4

Fig. 117 Masticatory muscles; frontal section; anterior view.

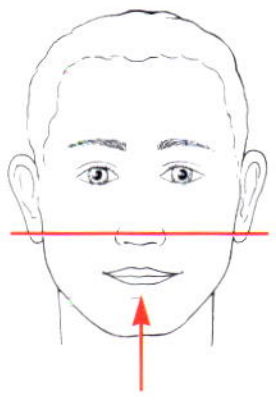

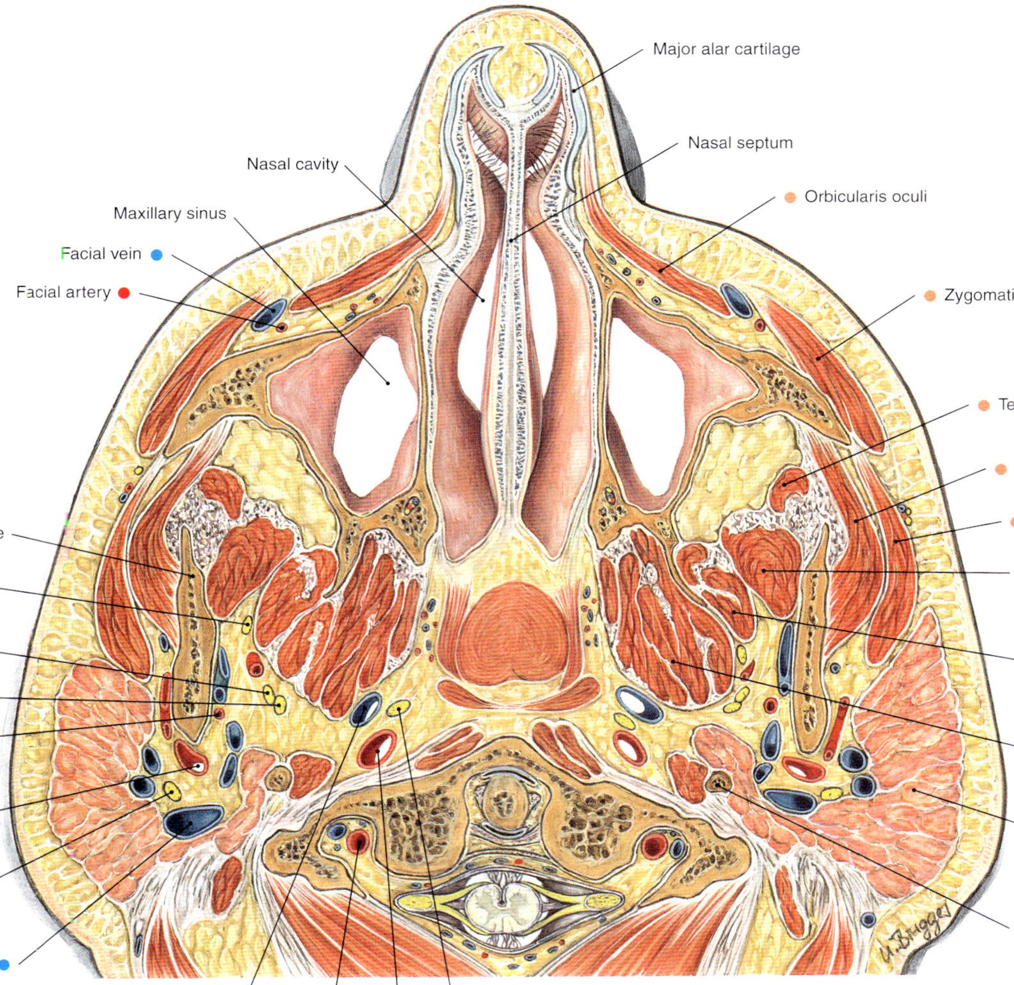

Fig. 118 Masticatory muscles; horizontal section.

→ T 4

Facial and masticatory muscles

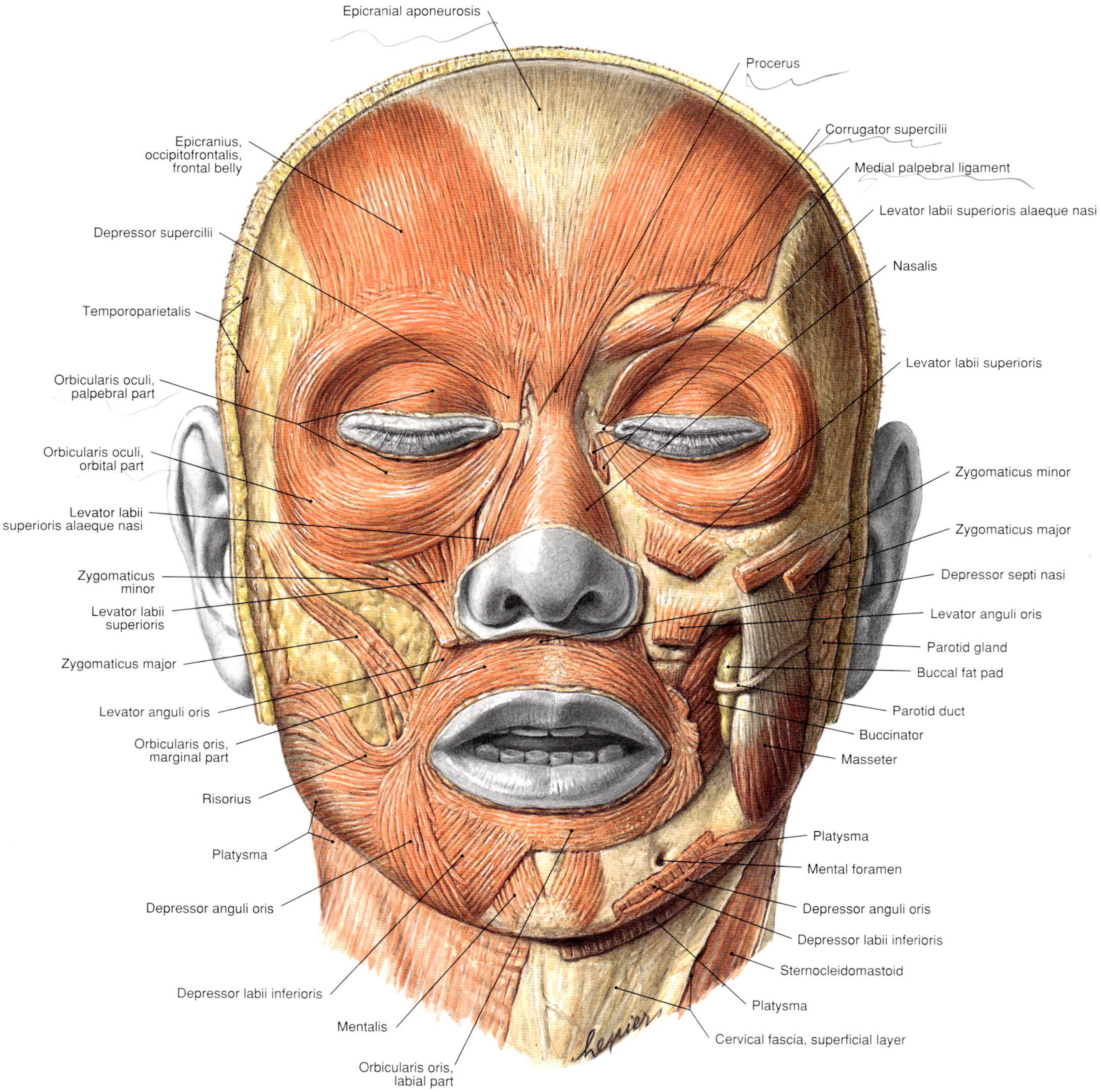

→ T 1 a, c–f, T 4

Fig. 119 Facial muscles and masticatory muscles.

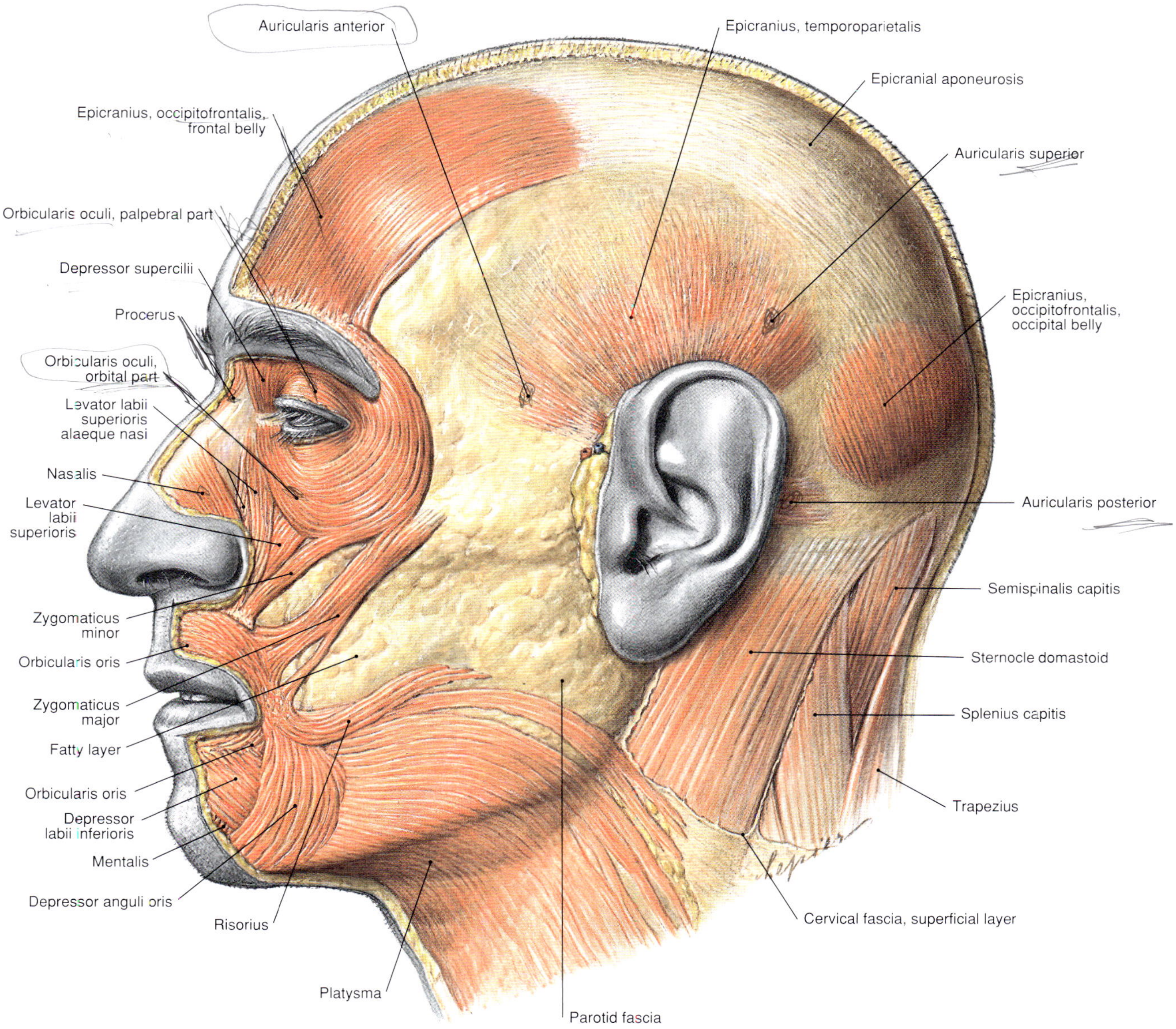

→ T 1

Fig. 120 Facial muscles.

121
253

Facial and masticatory muscles

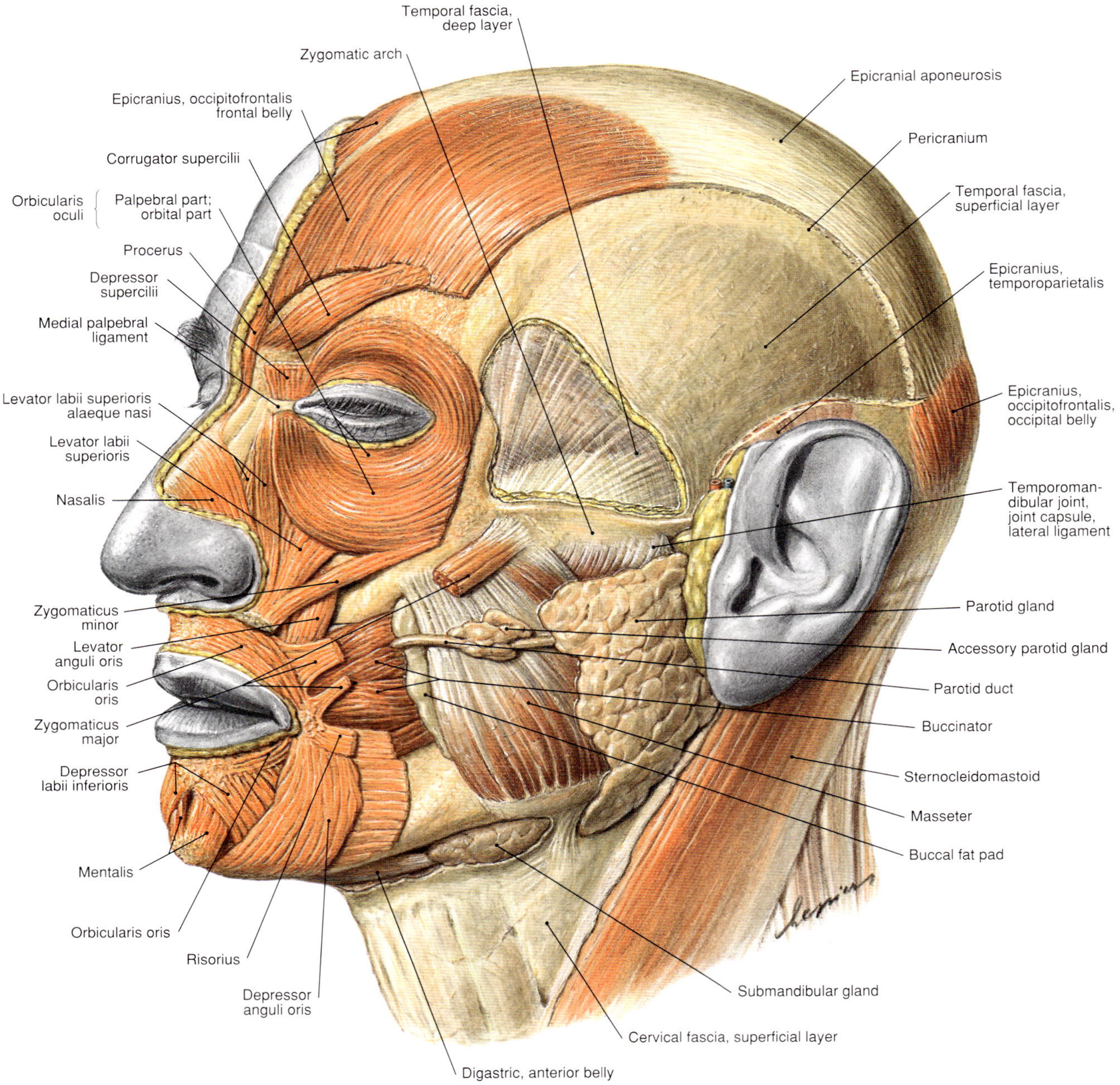

→ T 1, T 4

122
120
206

Fig. 121 Facial muscles and masticatory muscles.

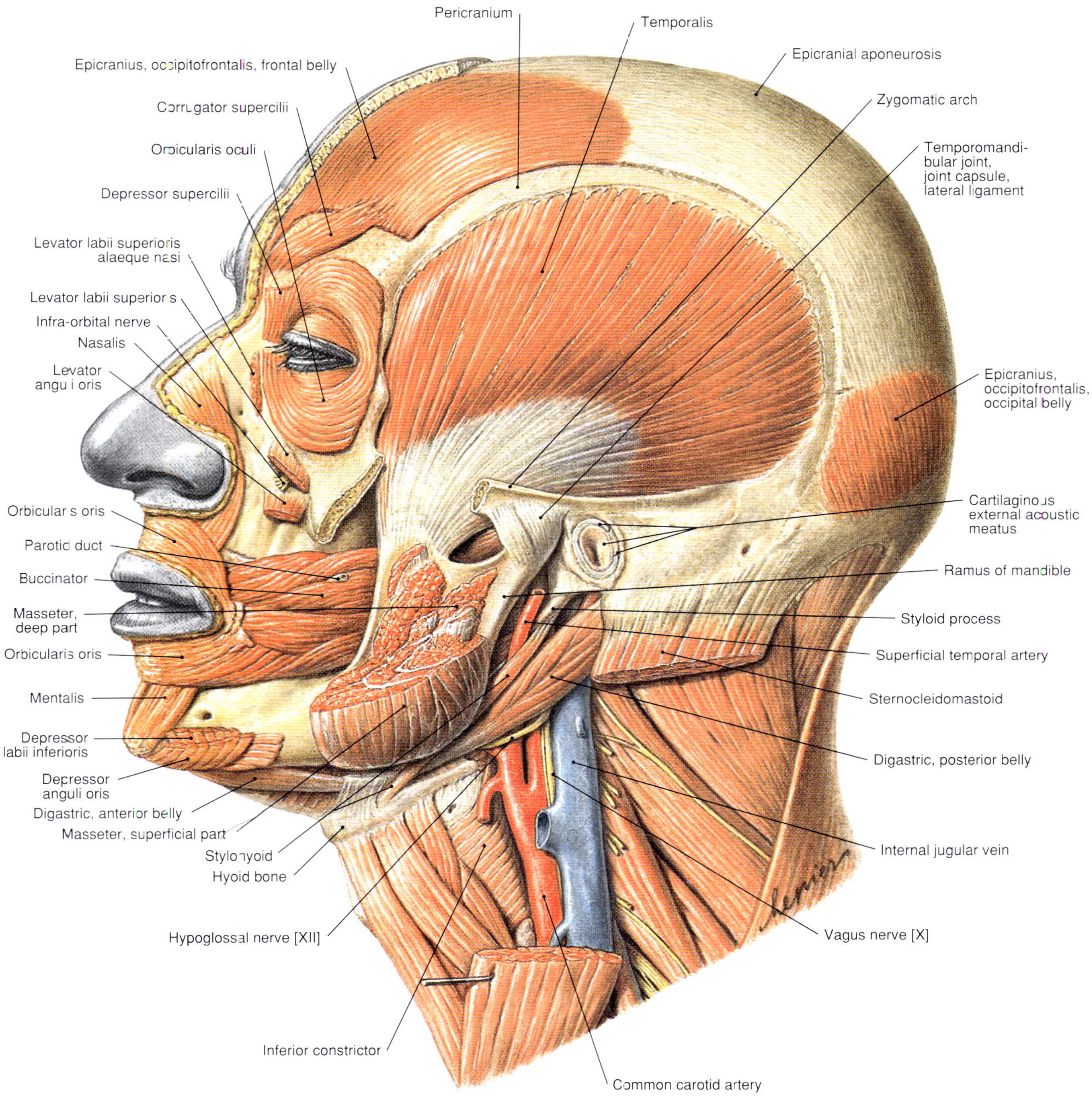

→ T 1, T 4

Fig. 122 Facial muscles and masticatory muscles.

121
256

Arteries of the head

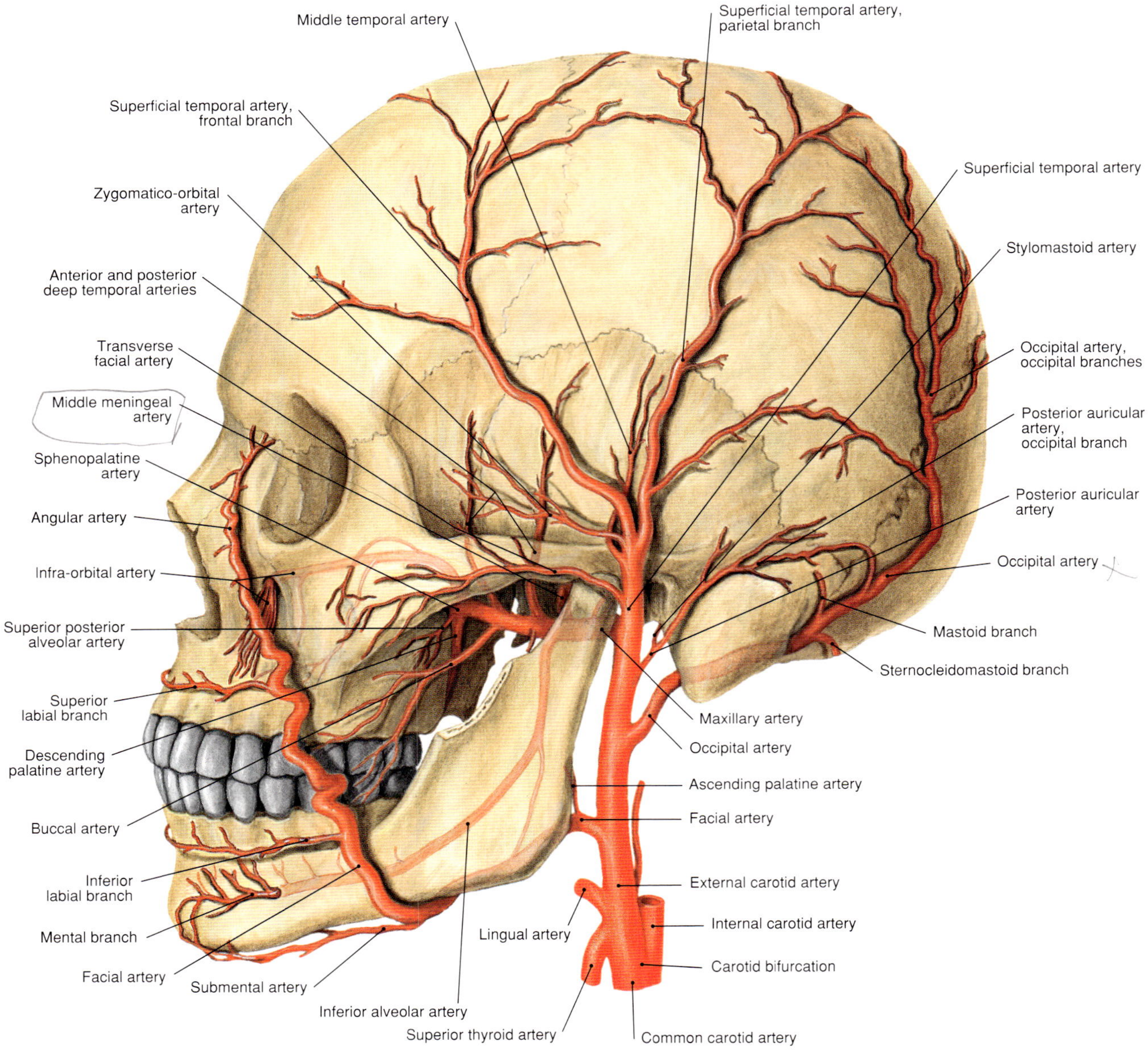

→ 264

Fig. 123 External carotid artery.

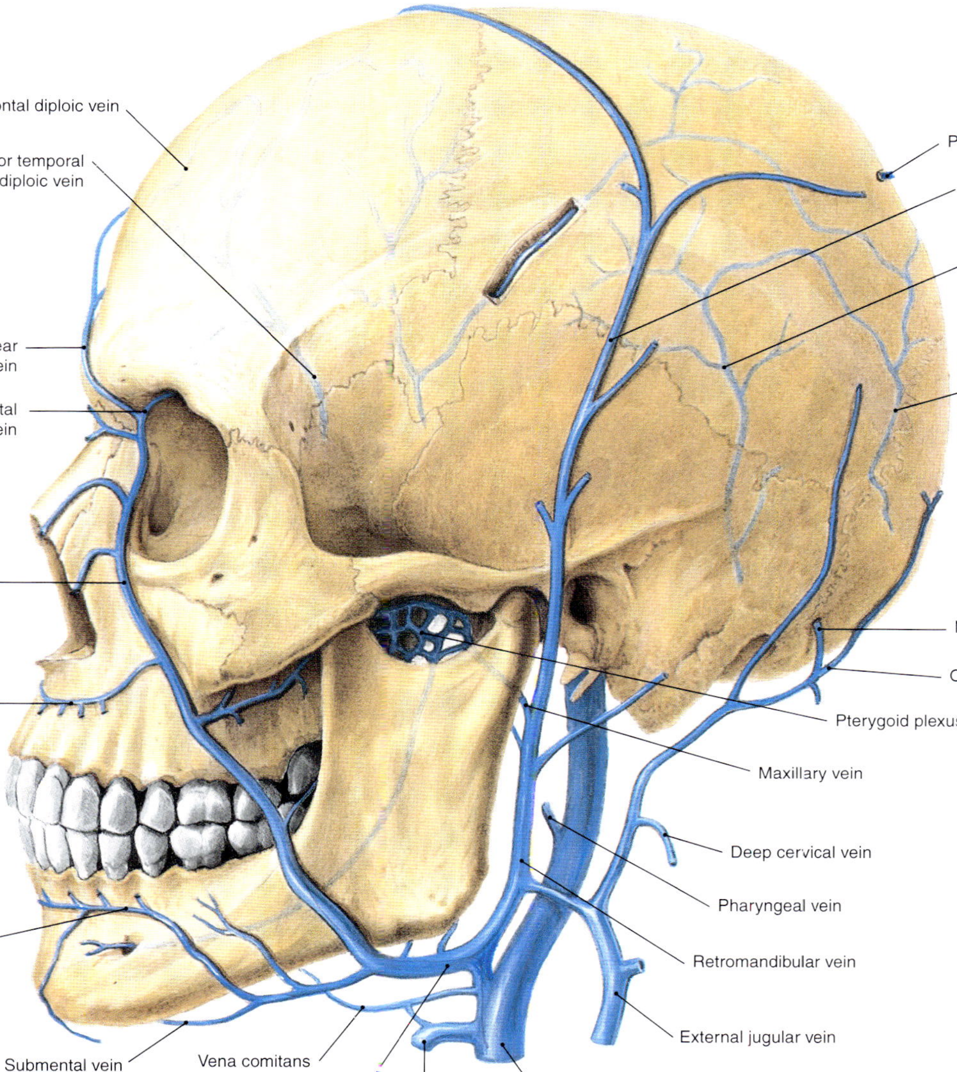

Fig. 124 Internal jugular vein.

→ 259

Lymphatics of the head and the neck

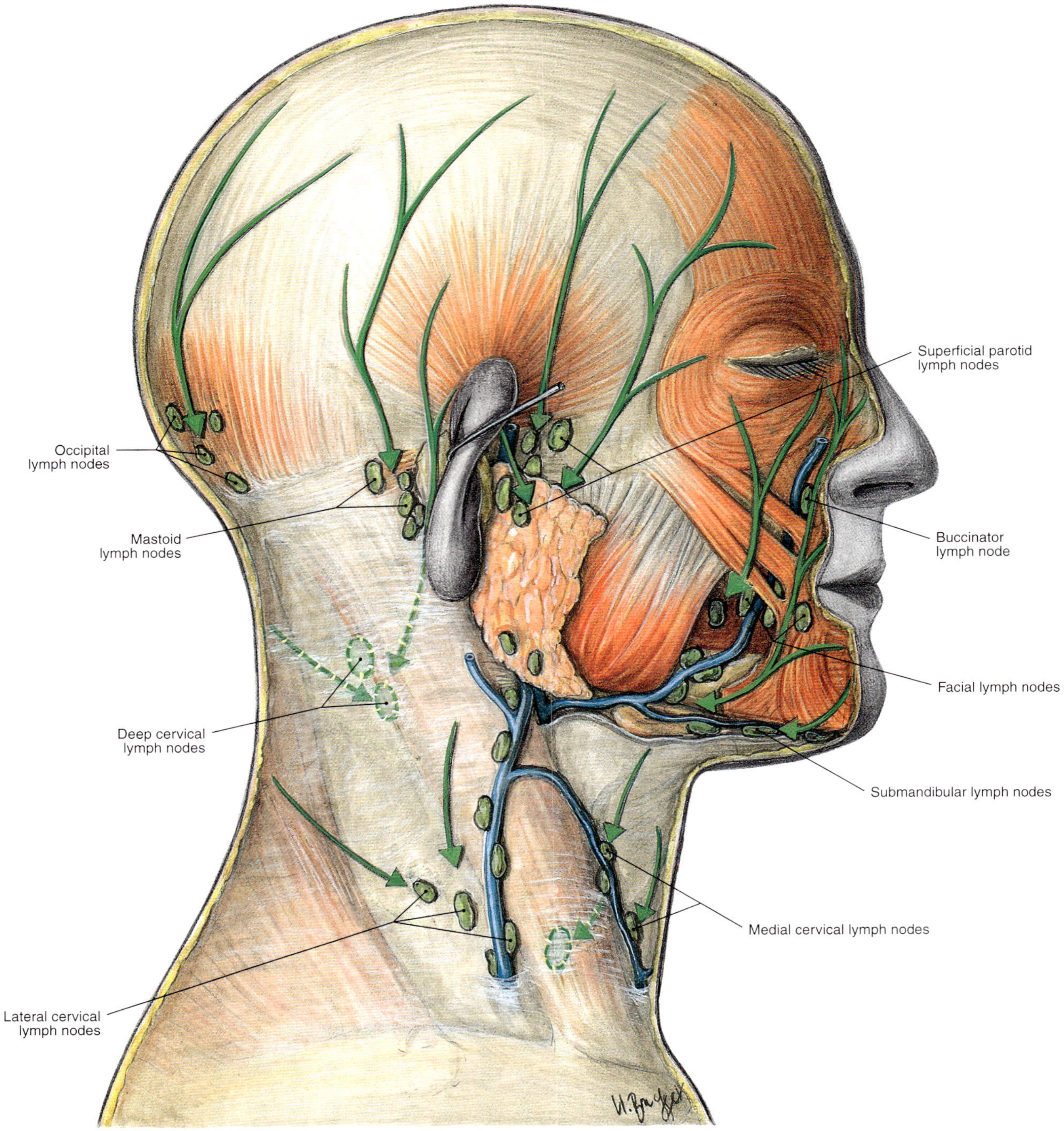

→ 261, 414

Fig. 125 Lymph nodes and lymphatics of the head and the neck; arrows indicate drainage areas.

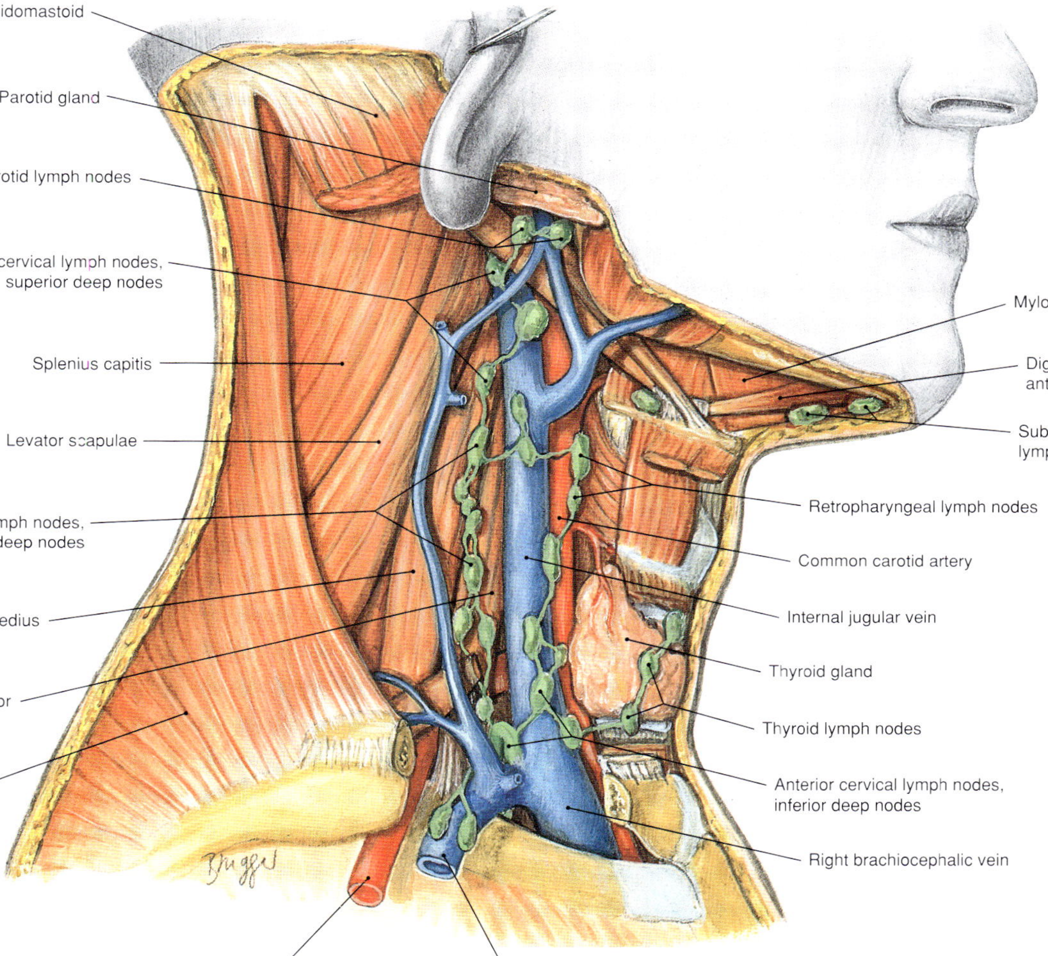

Fig. 126 Deep lymph nodes of the neck.

Facial nerve

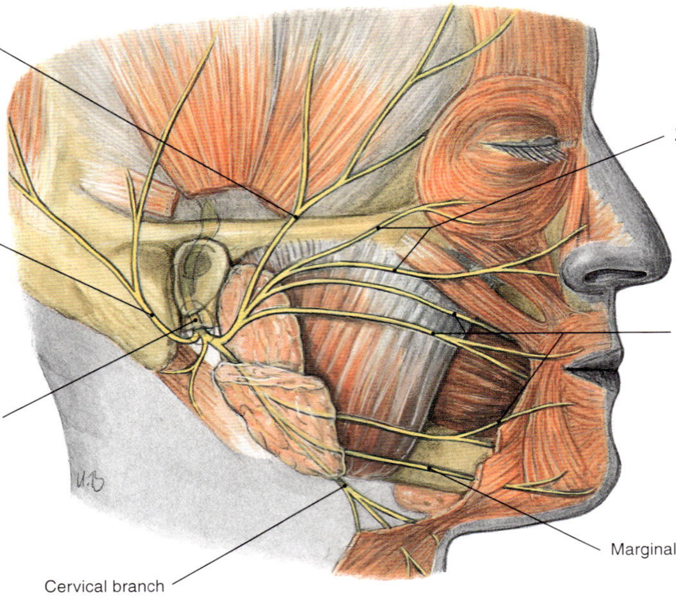

Fig. 127 Facial nerve.

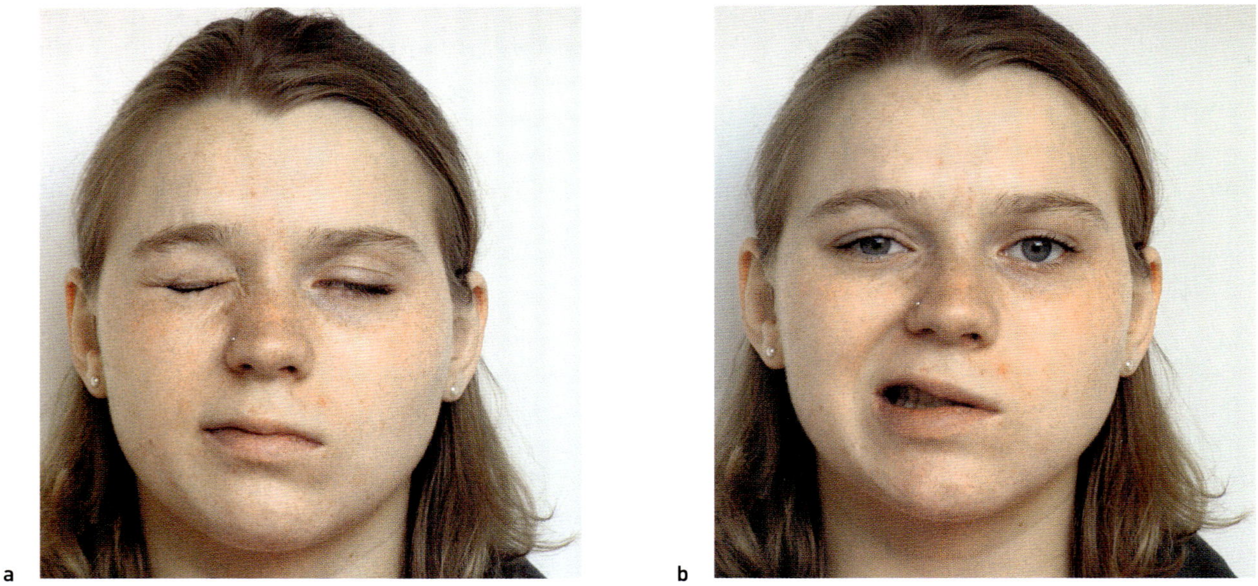

→ 1182

Fig. 128 a, b Palsy of the left facial nerve.

a The concerned eye cannot be closed upon request (lagophthalmus).

b The teeth of the concerned side cannot be shown upon request.

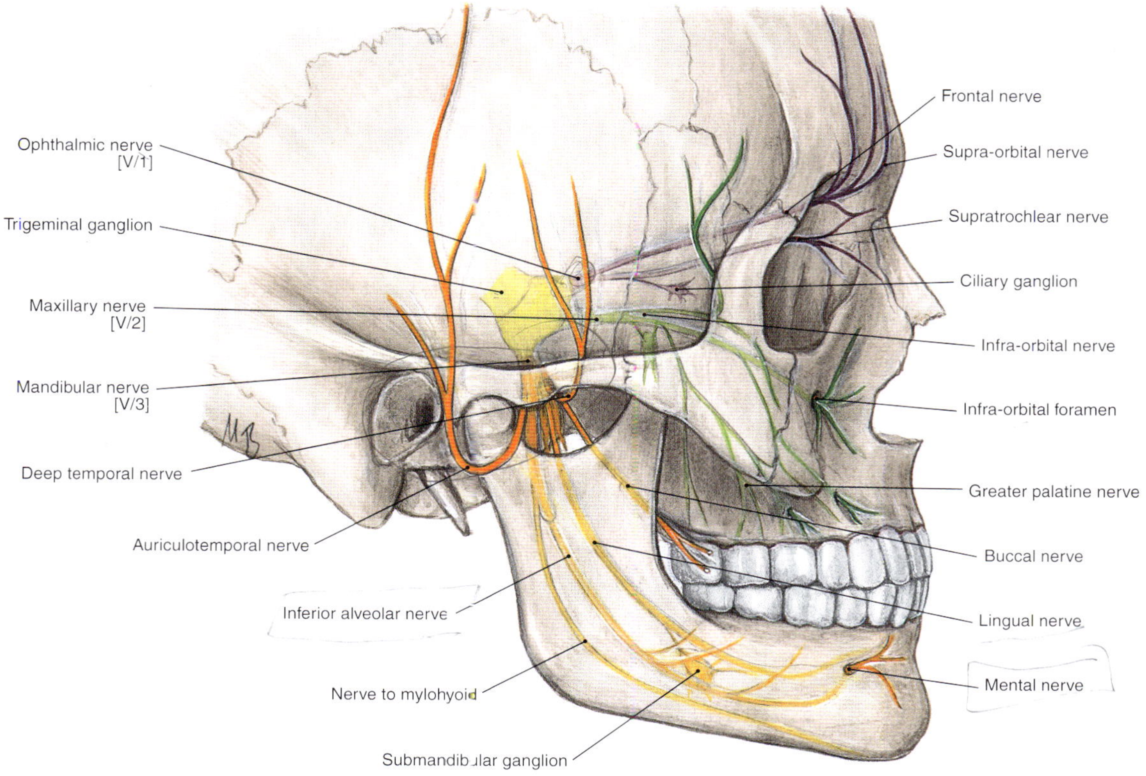

Fig. 129 Trigeminal nerve.

→ 472–475

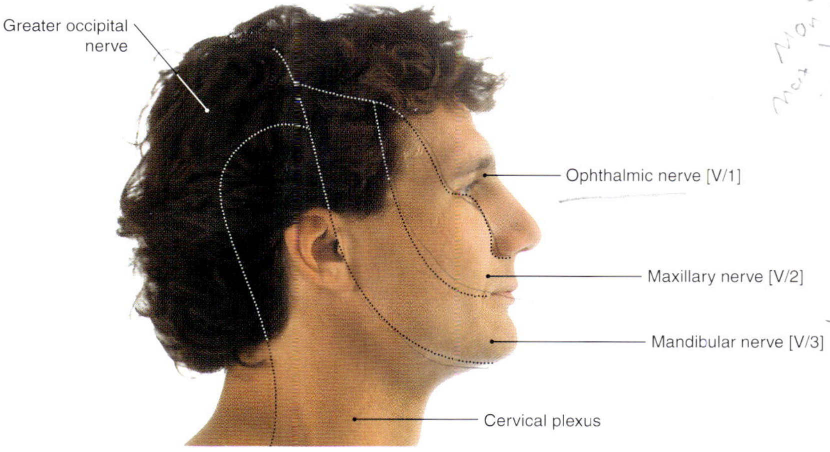

Fig. 130 Cutaneous innervation of the head and the neck.

Vessels and nerves of the head and the neck

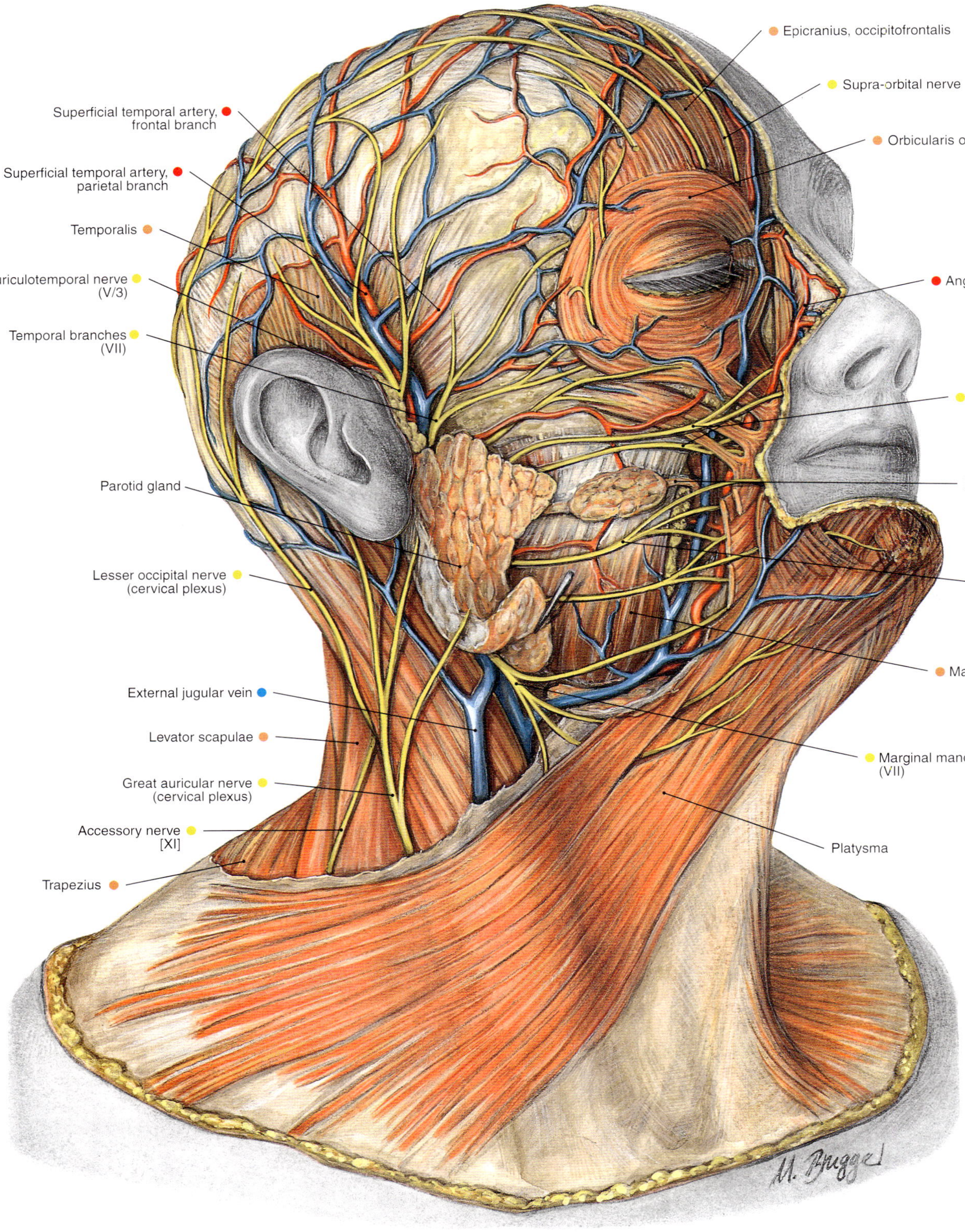

132
254

Fig. 131 Vessels and nerves of the head and the neck; superficial lateral regions.

Vessels and nerves of the head and the neck

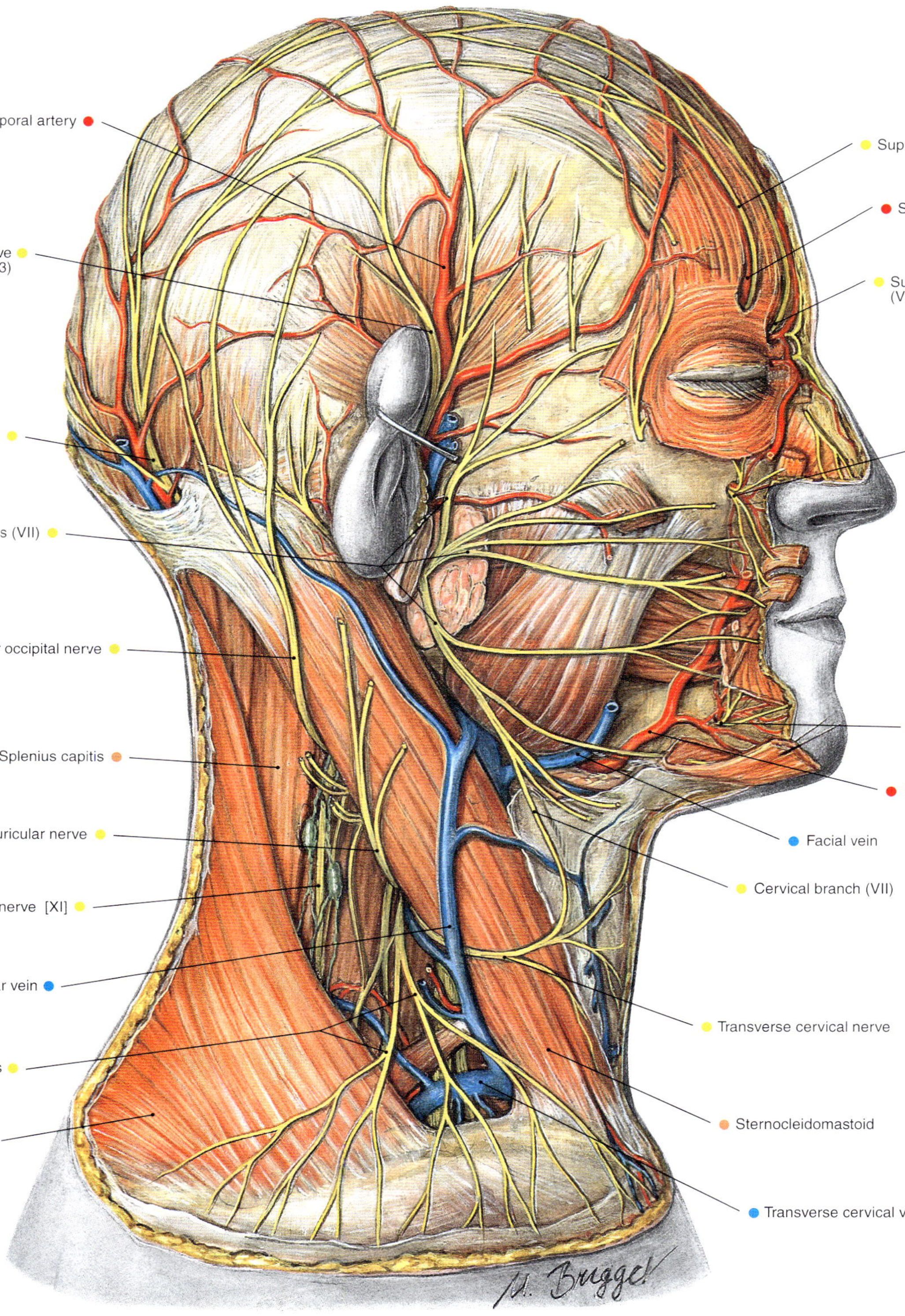

133
256
131

Fig. 132 Vessels and nerves of the head and the neck; deep lateral regions.

Lateral region of the face

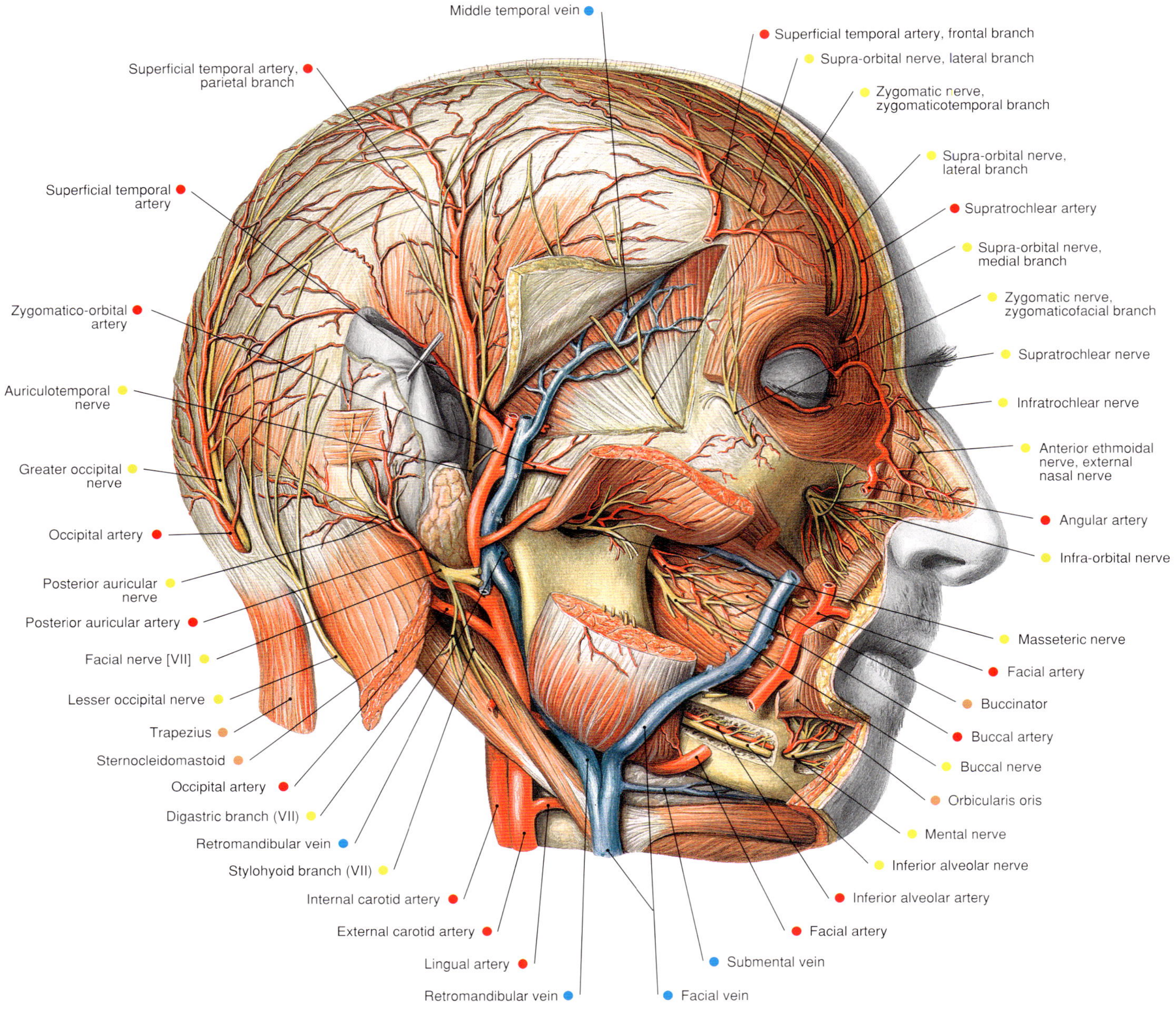

134
132
262

Fig. 133 Vessels and nerves of the head; deep lateral regions.

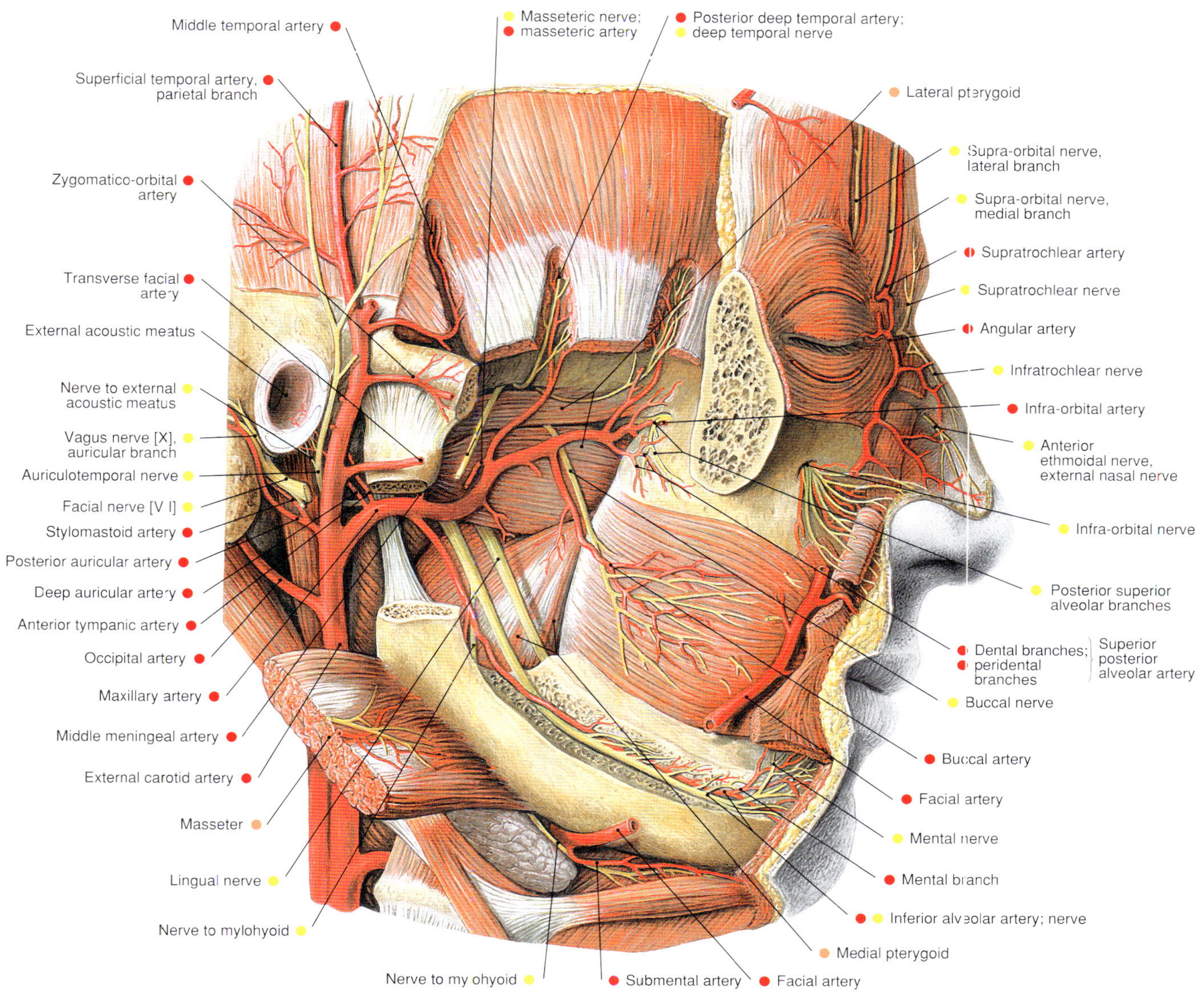

136
133
255

Fig. 134 Arteries and nerves of the head; deeper lateral regions.

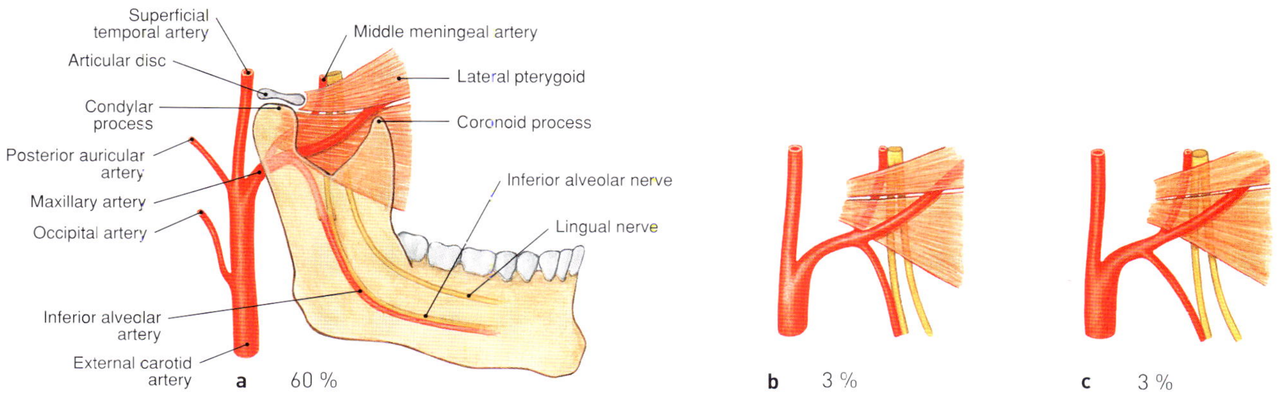

Fig. 135 a–c Variations of the middle meningeal artery.

a The middle meningeal artery branches off proximal to the inferior alveolar artery.

b The middle meningeal artery branches off across from the inferior alveolar artery.

c The middle meningeal artery branches off distal to the inferior alveolar artery.

Lateral region of the face

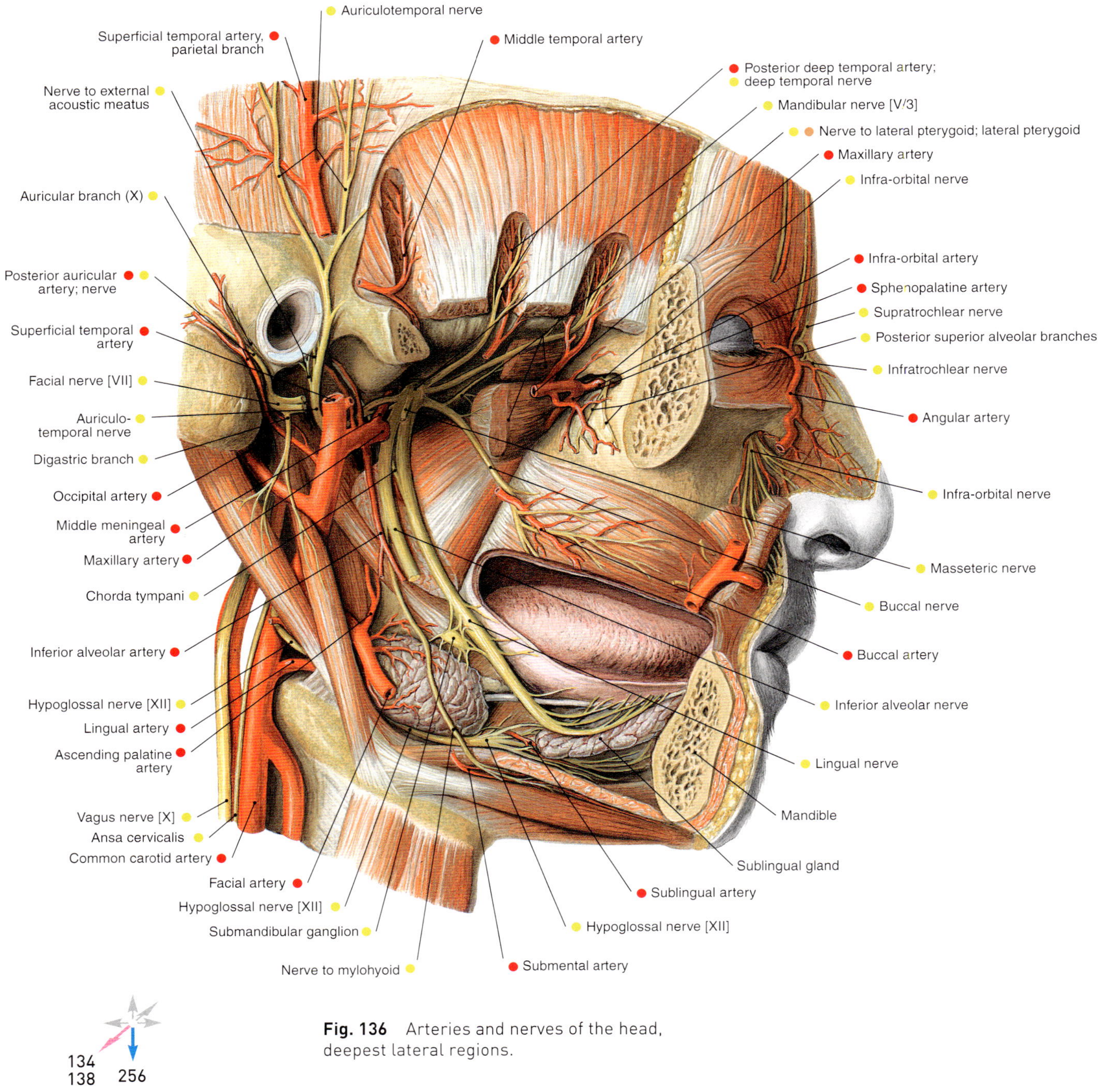

Fig. 136 Arteries and nerves of the head, deepest lateral regions.

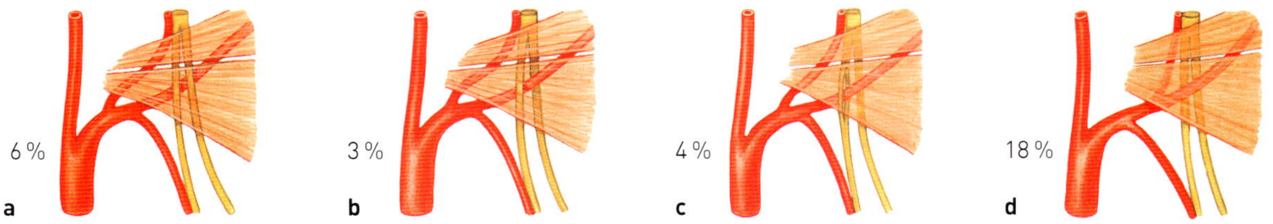

Fig. 137 a–d Variations in the course of the maxillary artery.

a The maxillary artery passes medially to the lateral pterygoid muscle, the lingual nerve and the inferior alveolar nerve.
b The maxillary artery passes between the lingual nerve and the inferior alveolar nerve.
c The maxillary artery passes through a loop formed by the inferior alveolar nerve.
d The middle meningeal artery branches off distal to the inferior alveolar artery.

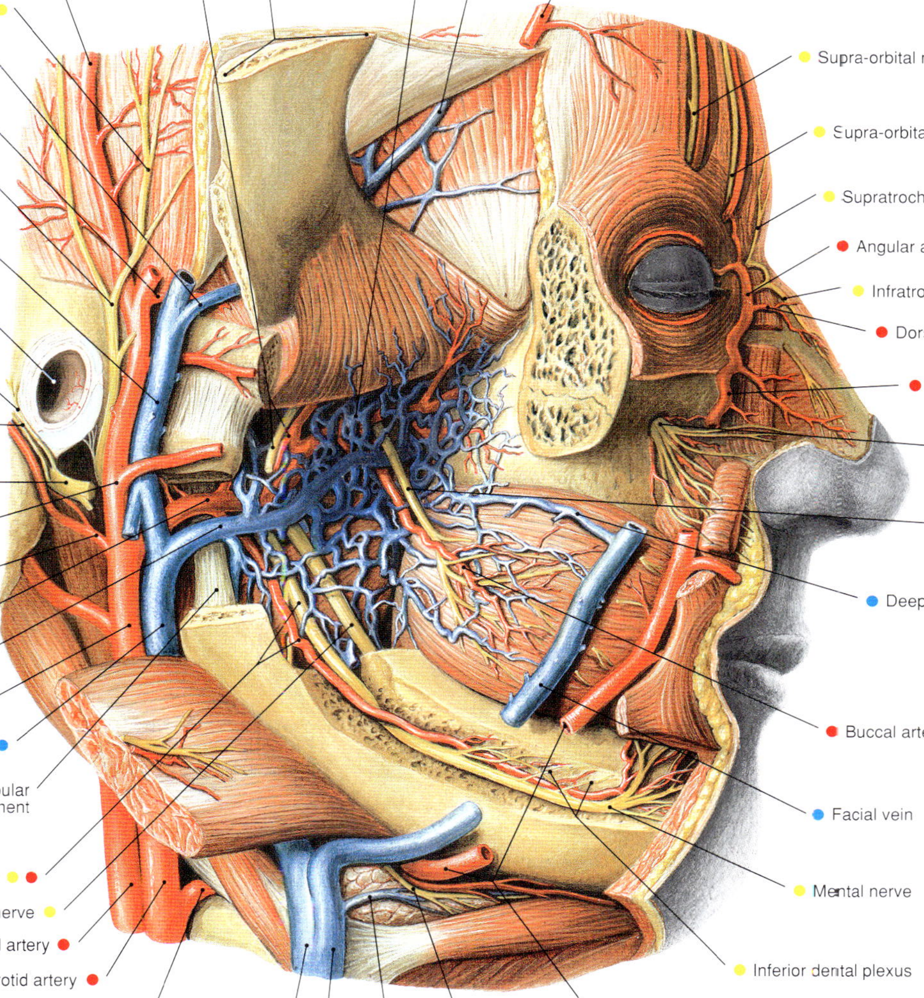

Fig. 138 Vessels and nerves of the head; deeper lateral regions.

136
133
255

Skeleton of the nose

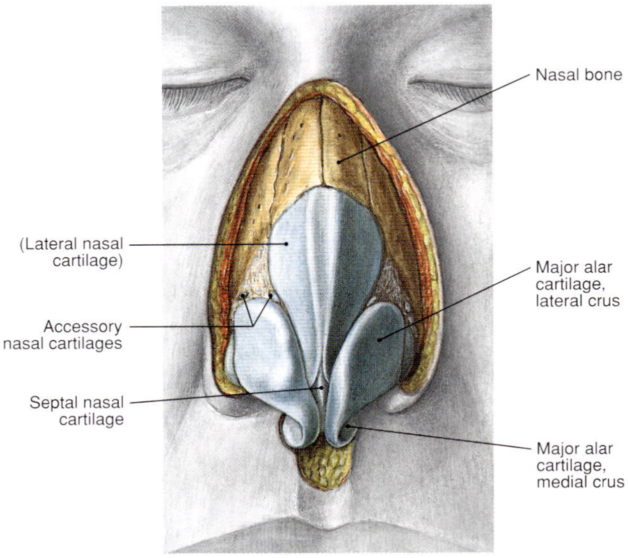

Fig. 139 Skeleton of the nose.

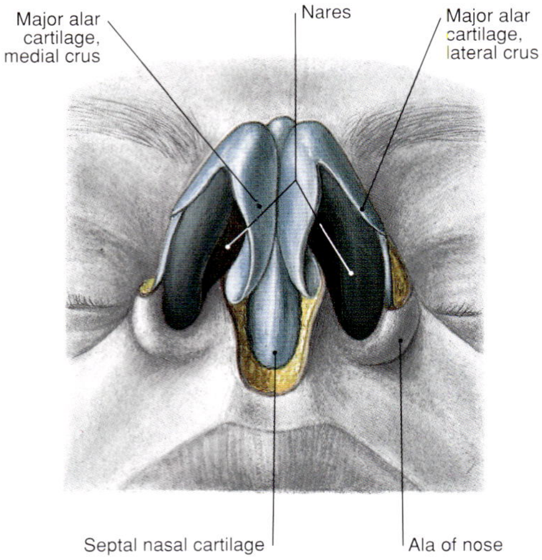

Fig. 140 Nasal cartilages.

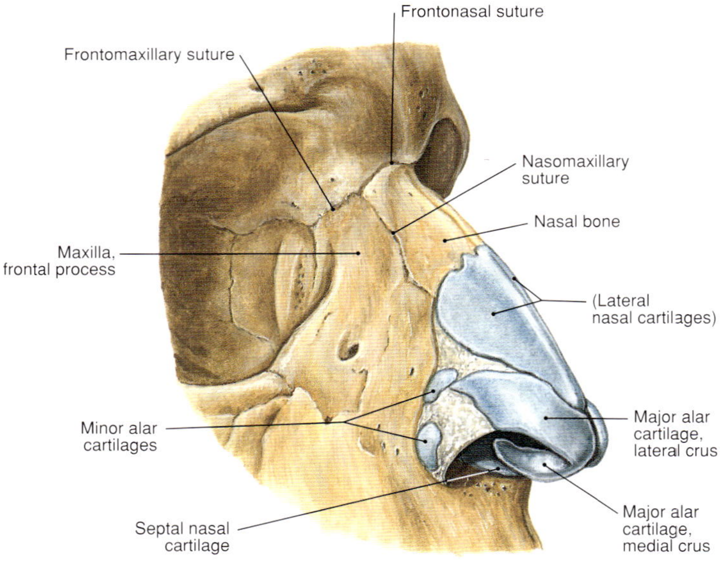

Fig. 141 Skeleton of the nose.

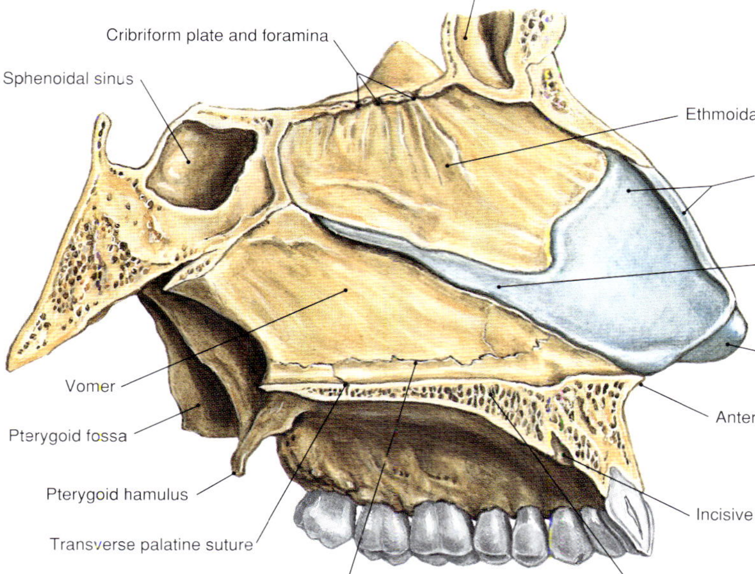

Fig. 142 Nasal septum.

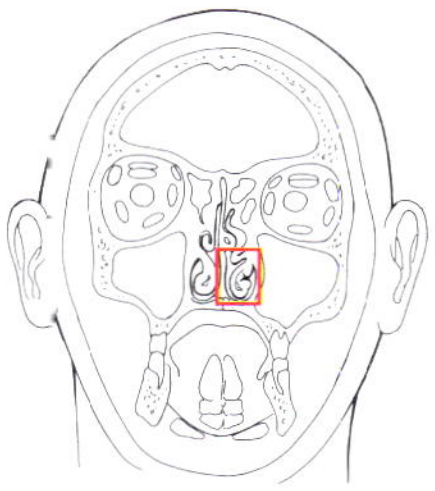

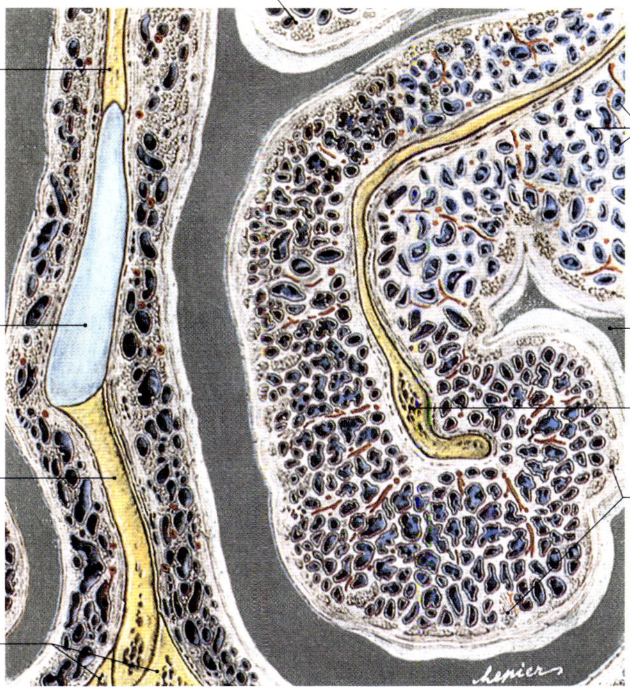

Fig. 143 Inferior nasal concha.

Nasal cavity

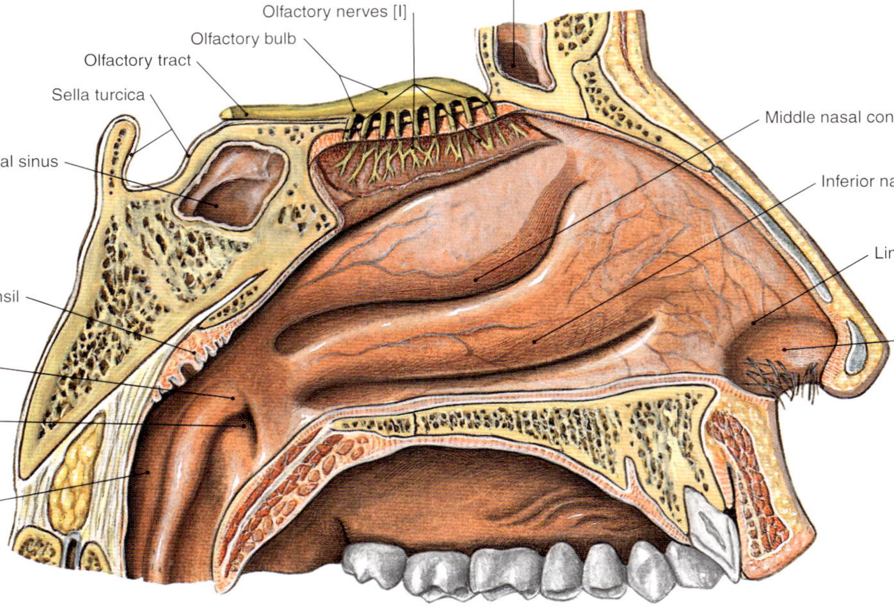

Fig. 144 Lateral wall of the nasal cavity.

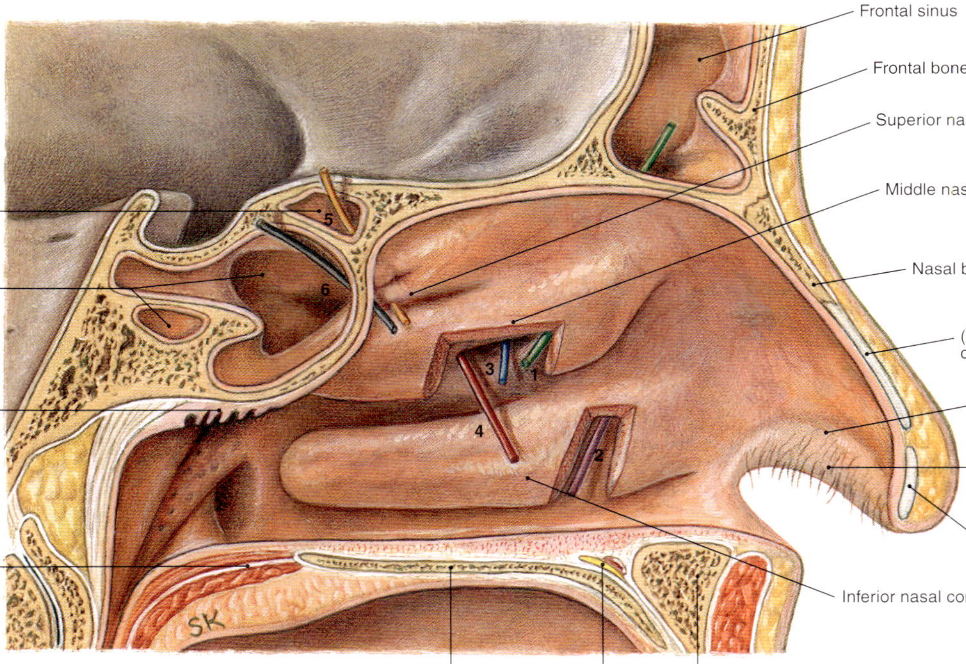

Openings of:
1 Sinus frontalis
2 Nasolacrimal duct
3 Anterior ethmoidal cells
4 Maxillary sinus
5 Posterior ethmoidal cells
6 Sphenoidal sinus

Fig. 145 Nasal cavity and openings of the paranasal sinuses.

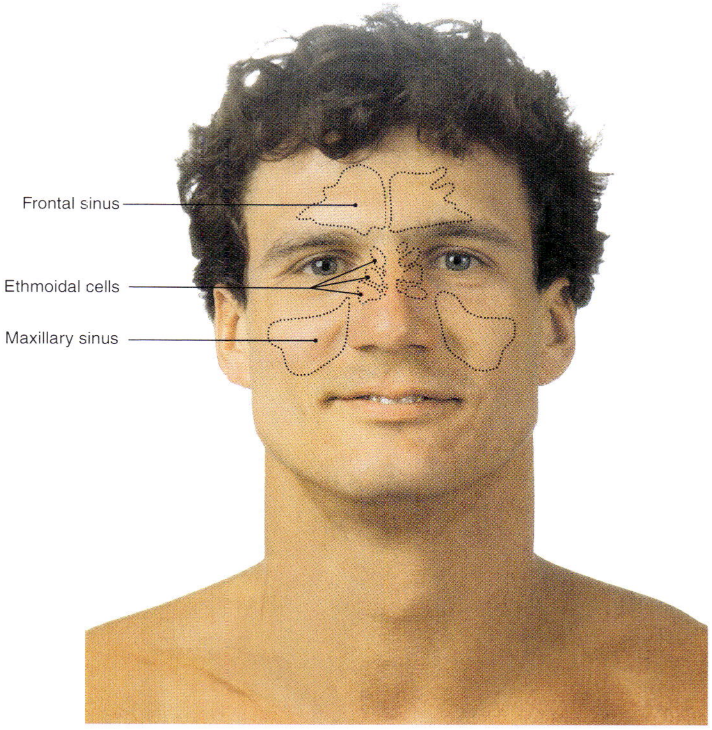

Fig. 146 Prcjection of the paranasal sinuses.

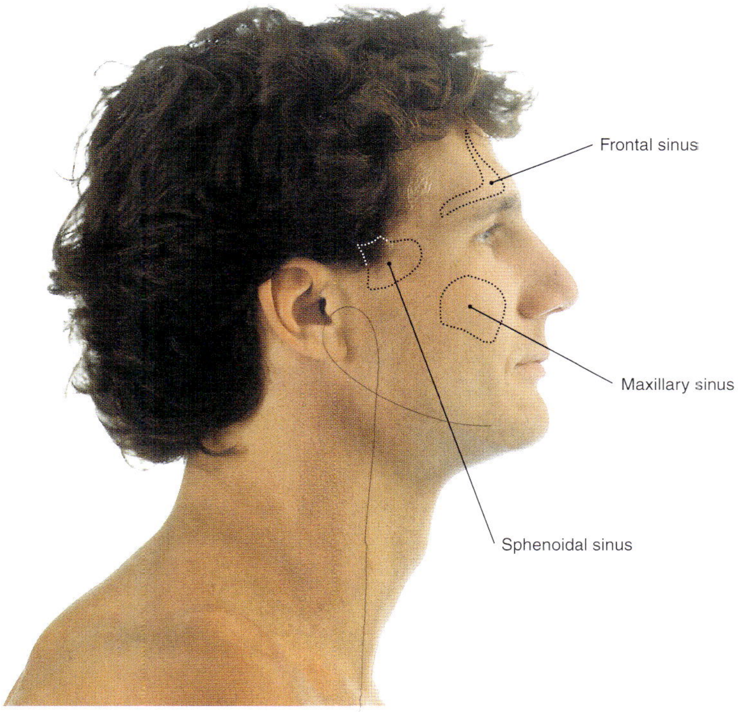

Fig. 147 Projection of the paranasal sinuses.

Paranasal sinuses

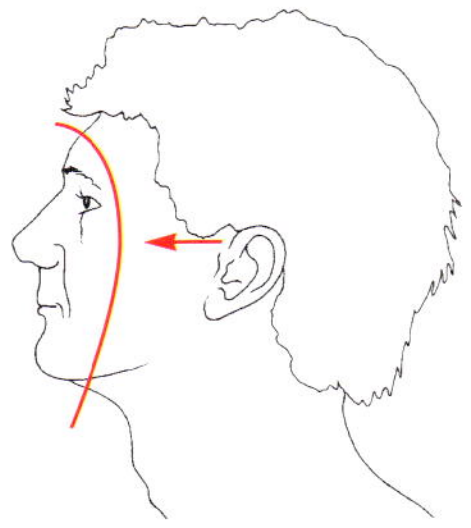

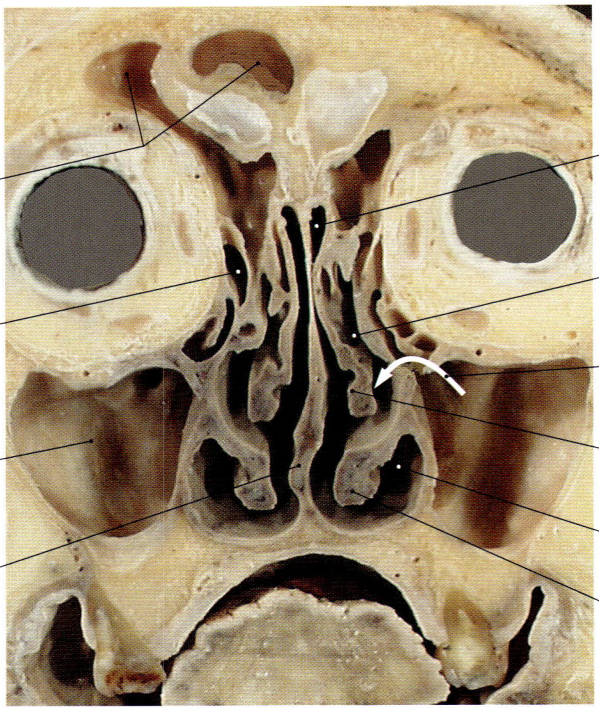

Fig. 148 Paranasal sinuses.

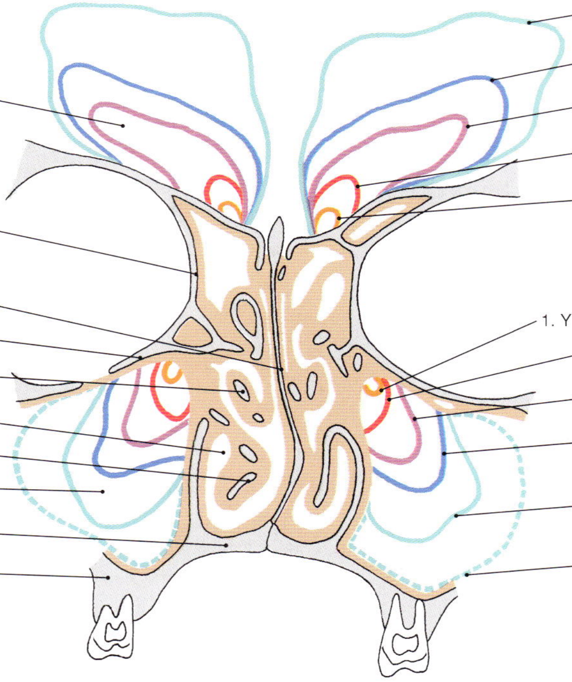

Fig. 149 Development of the maxillary and frontal sinuses.
Y – year of life

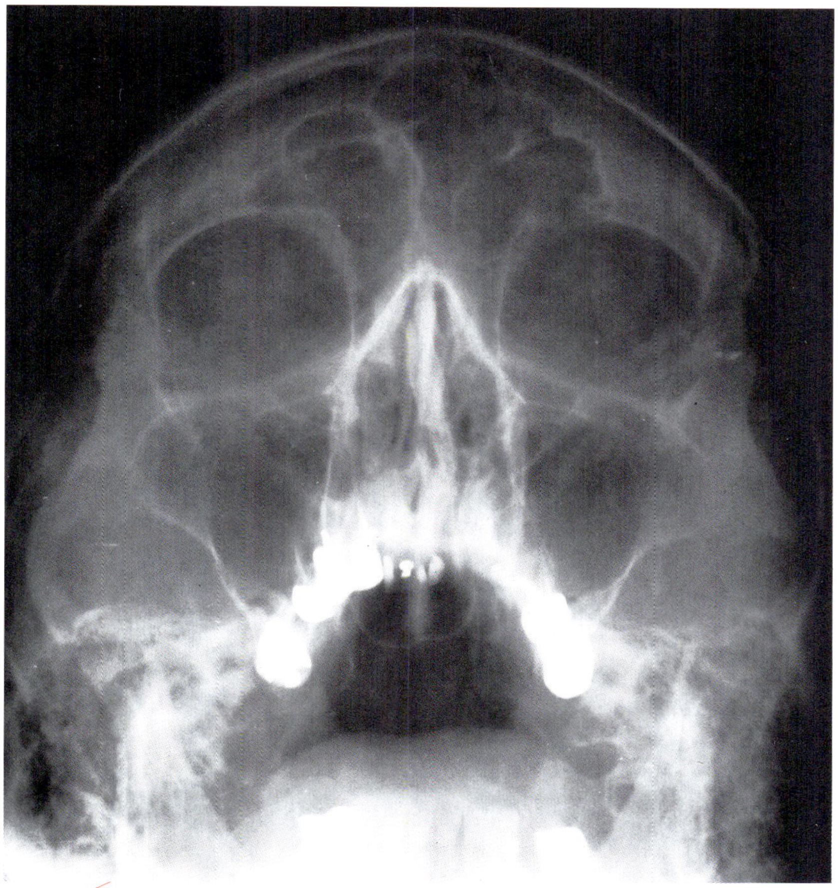

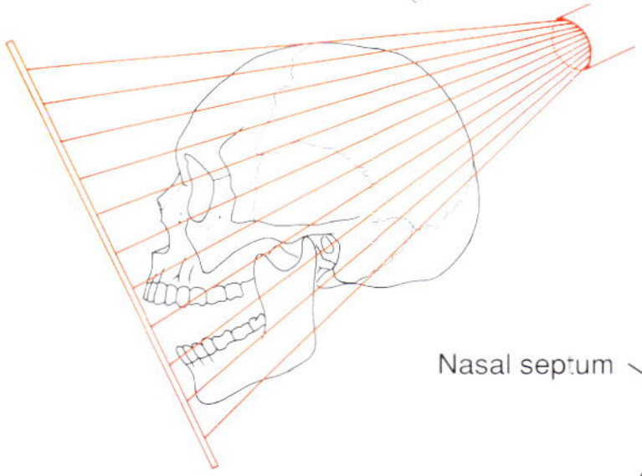

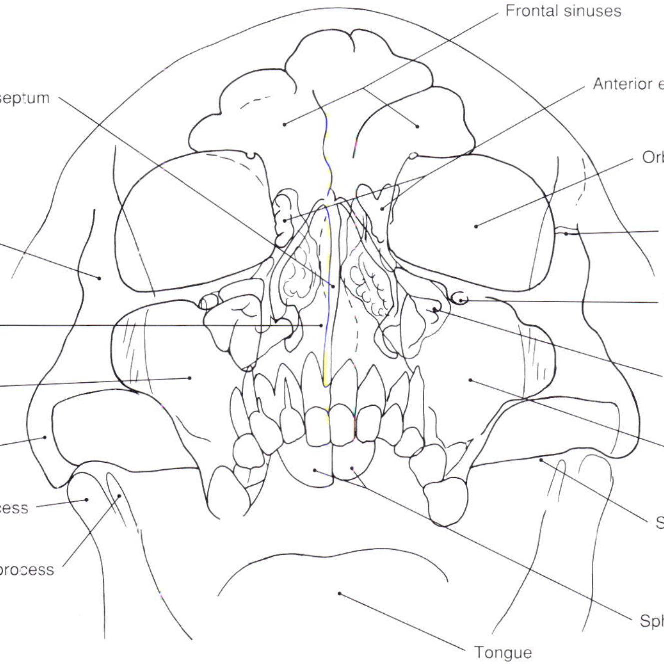

Fig. 150 Paranasal sinuses; PA-radiograph.

Oral cavity

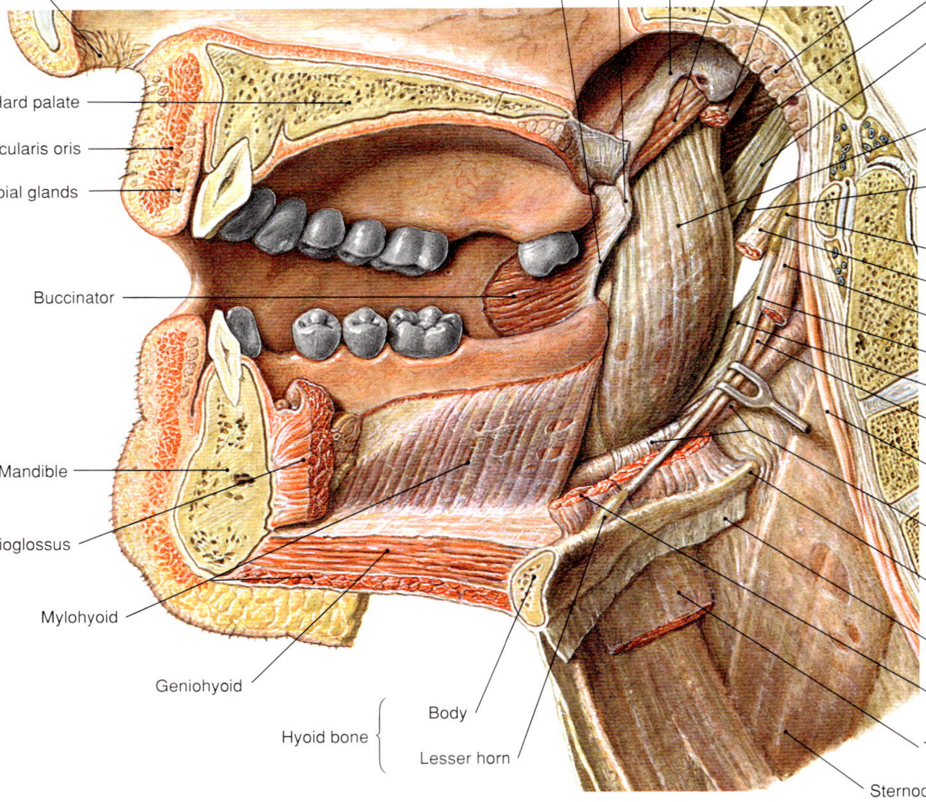

Fig. 151 Oral cavity.

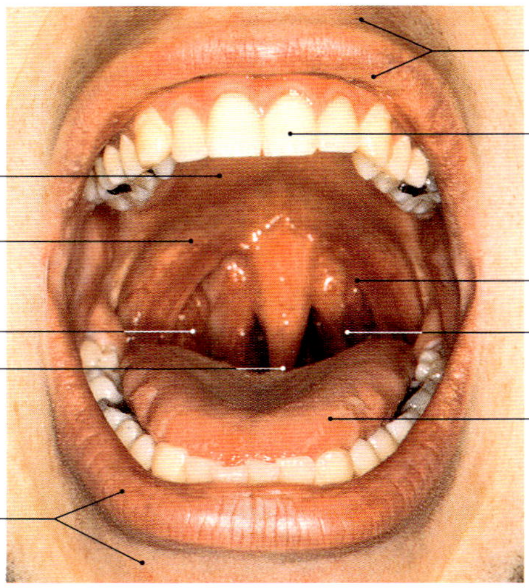

Fig. 152 Oral cavity.

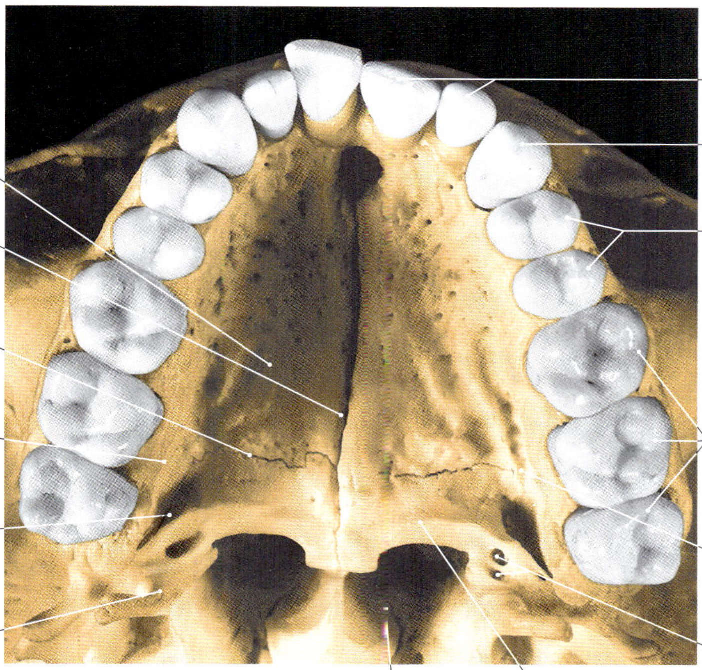

Fig. 153 Upper dental arcade and bony palate.

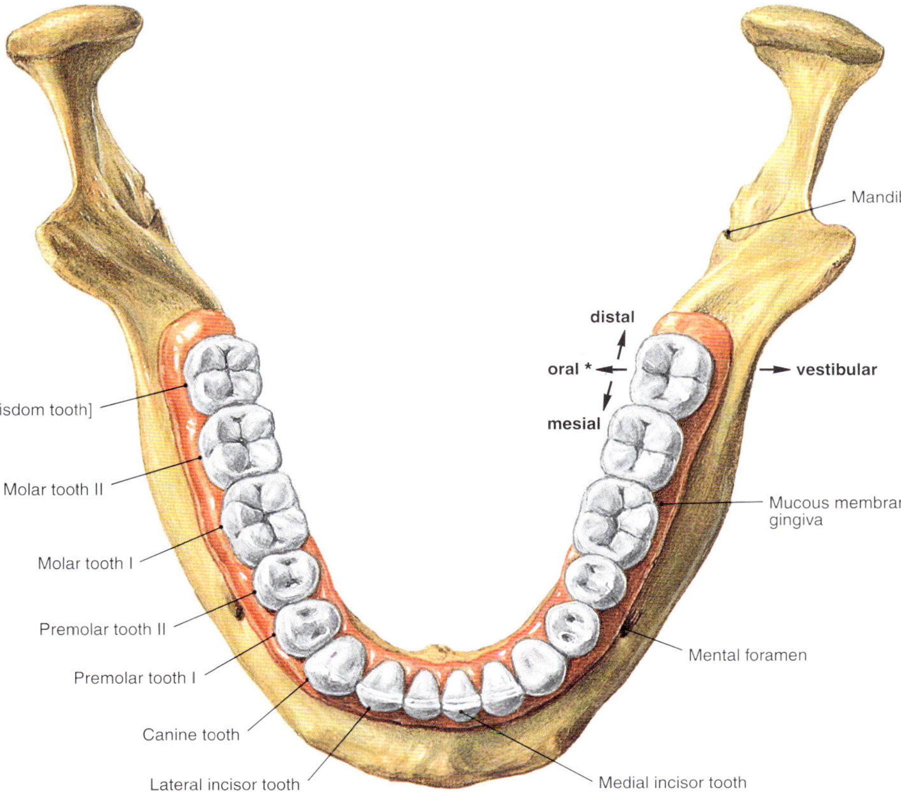

Fig. 154 Lower dental arcade.

* In the mandible oral is synonymous with lingual, and in the maxilla it is synonymous with palatinal.

Teeth, structure

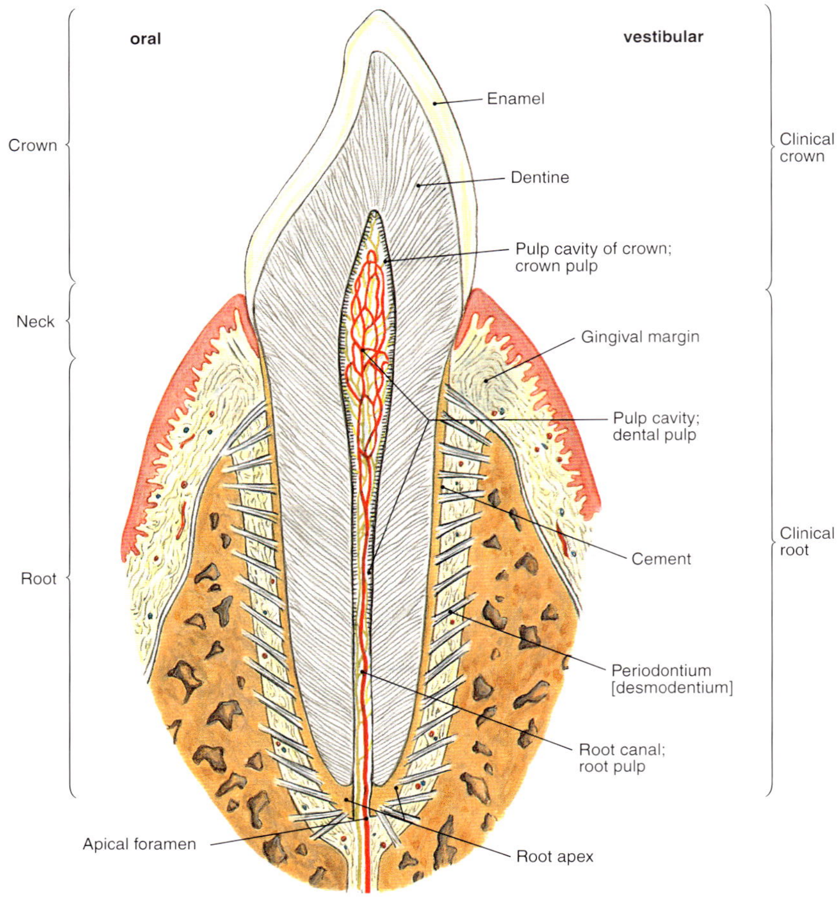

Fig. 155 Incisor tooth.

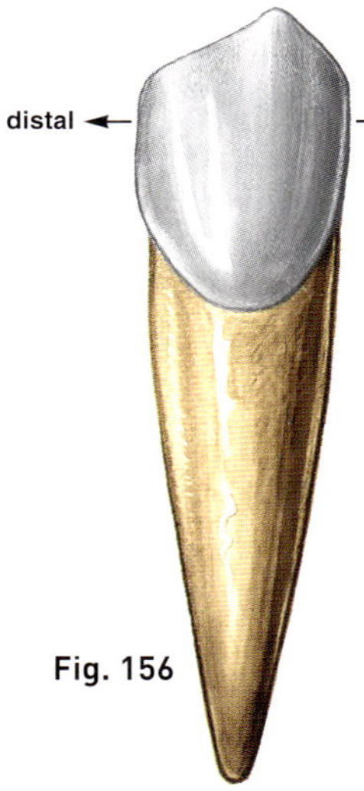

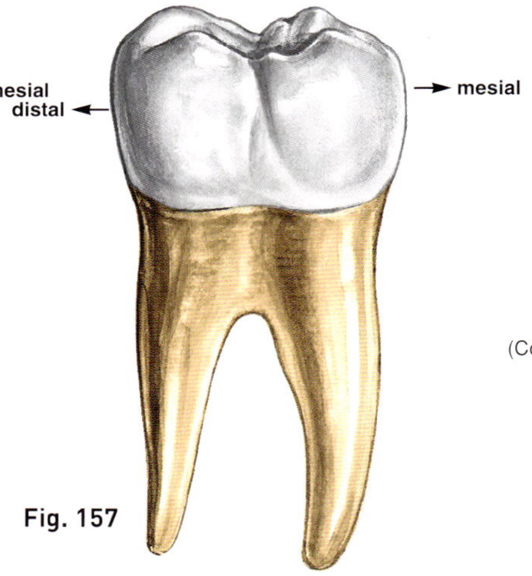

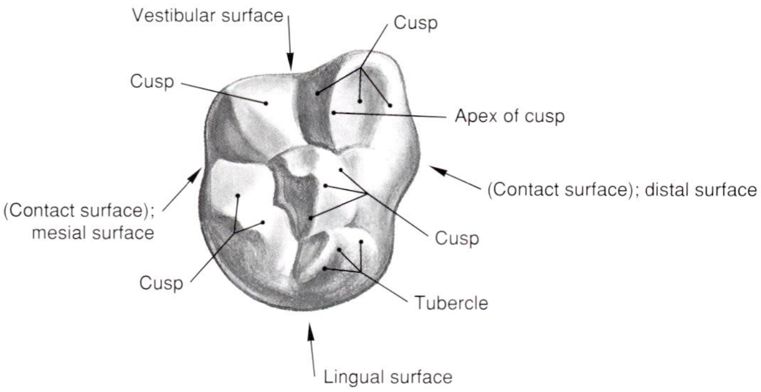

Fig. 156 Permanent lower canine tooth.

Fig. 157 Deciduous second molar tooth.

Fig. 158 Permanent upper first molar tooth.

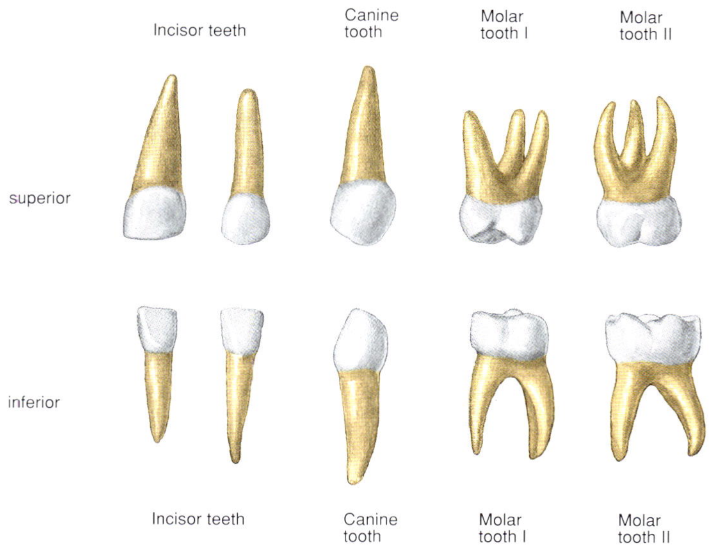

Fig. 159 Deciduous teeth of a 3-year-old child; vestibular view.

Maxilla

right	55	54	53	52	51	61	62	63	64	65	left
	85	84	83	82	81	71	72	73	74	75	

Mandible

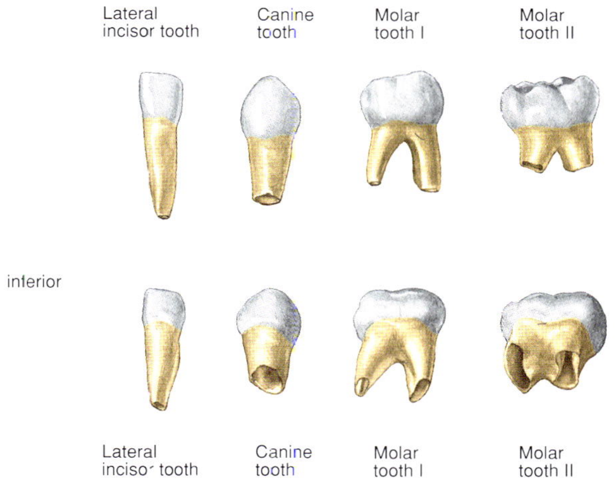

Fig. 160 Deciduous teeth of a 2-year-old child; top row viewed from vestibular; bottom row viewed obliquely from inferior.

Teeth

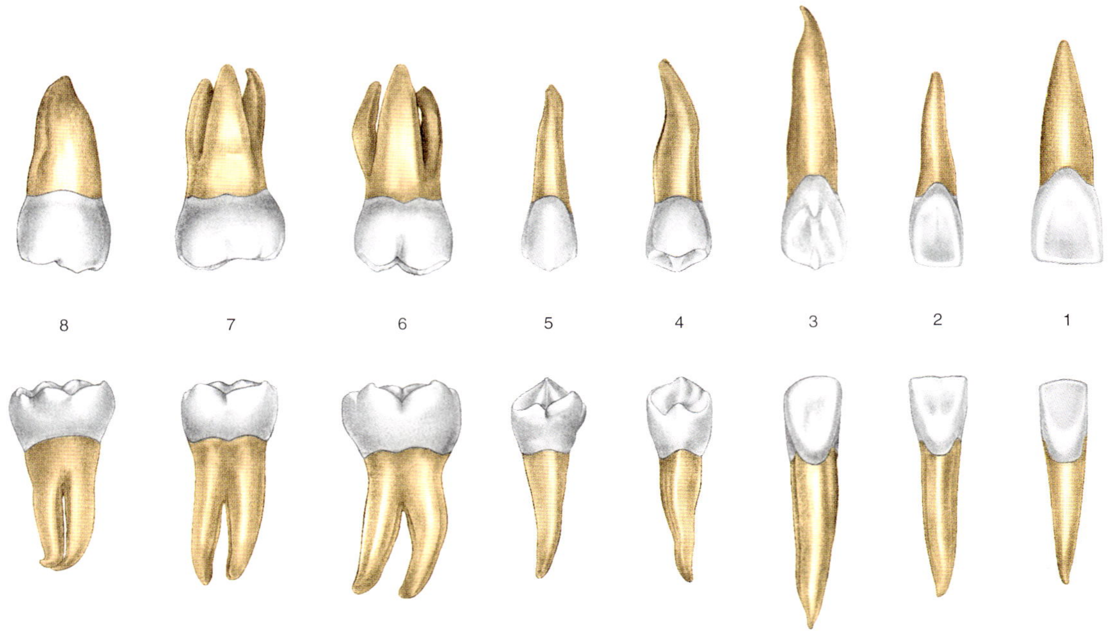

Fig. 161 Permanent teeth;
oral view.
(See p. 97 for identification of the numbers.)

Maxilla

right	18	17	16	15	14	13	12	11	21	22	23	24	25	26	27	28	left
	48	47	46	45	44	43	42	41	31	32	33	34	35	36	37	38	

Mandible

Adult dentition

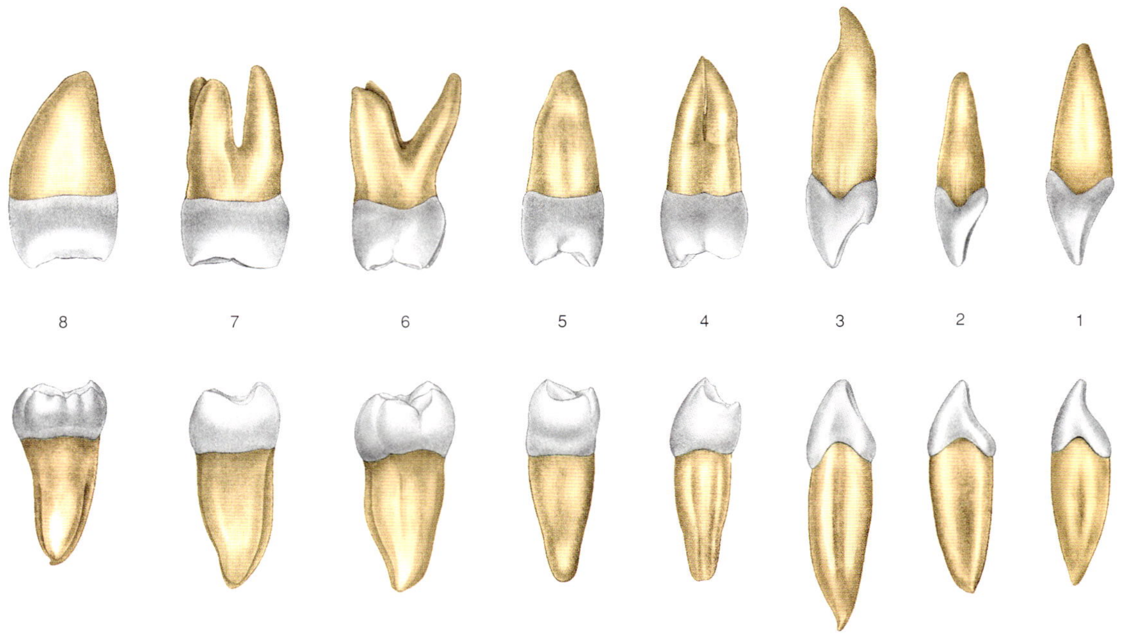

Fig. 162 Permanent teeth;
distal view.
(See p. 97 for identification of the numbers.)

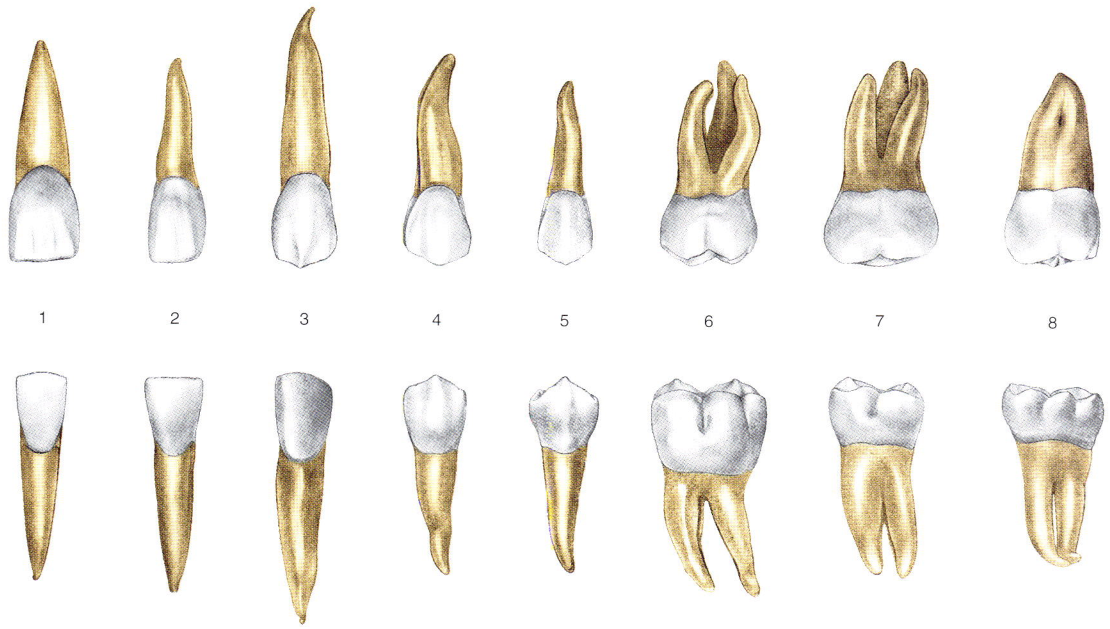

Fig. 163 Permanent teeth; vestibular view.

1 Incisor tooth I
2 Incisor tooth II
3 Canine tooth
4 Premolar tooth I
5 Premolar tooth II
6 Molar tooth I
7 Molar tooth II
8 Molar tooth III [wisdom tooth]

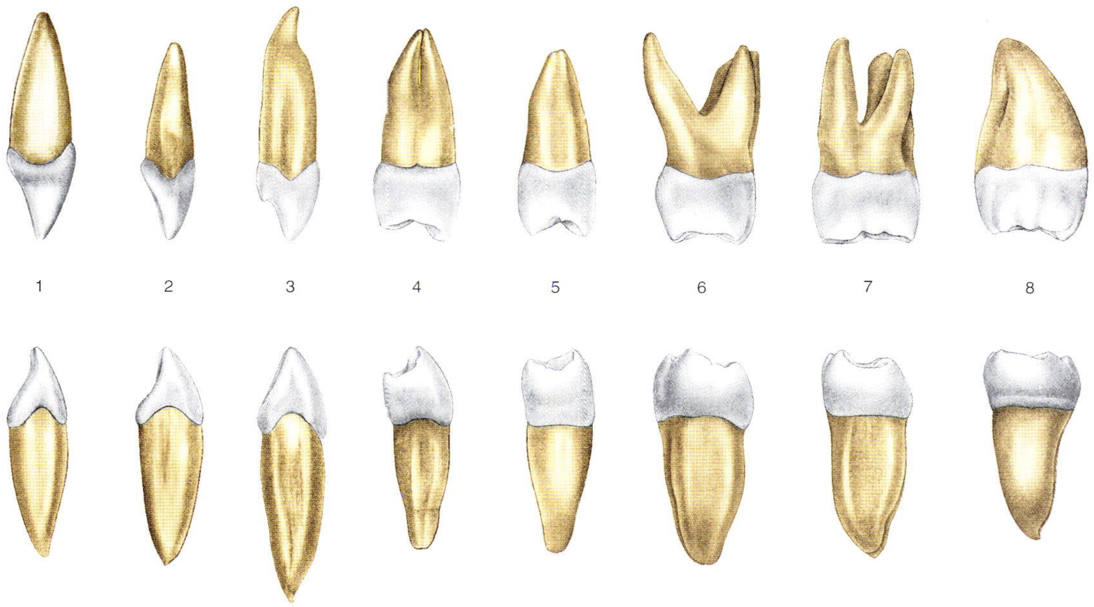

Fig. 164 Permanent teeth; mesial view.

Teeth, development

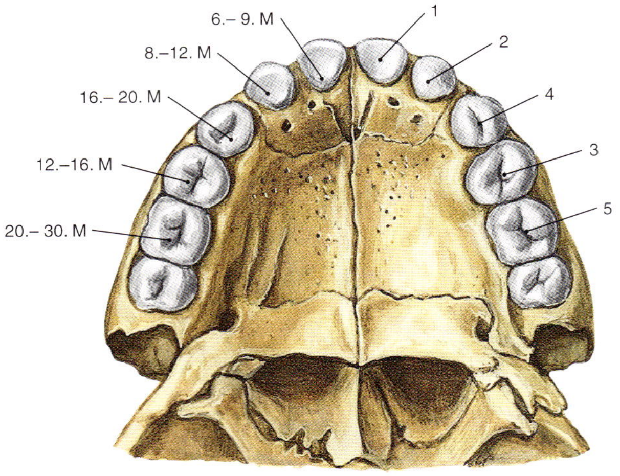

Fig. 165 Maxilla with deciduous teeth and the first permanent tooth;
left: median time of eruption in months (M);
right: order of eruption.

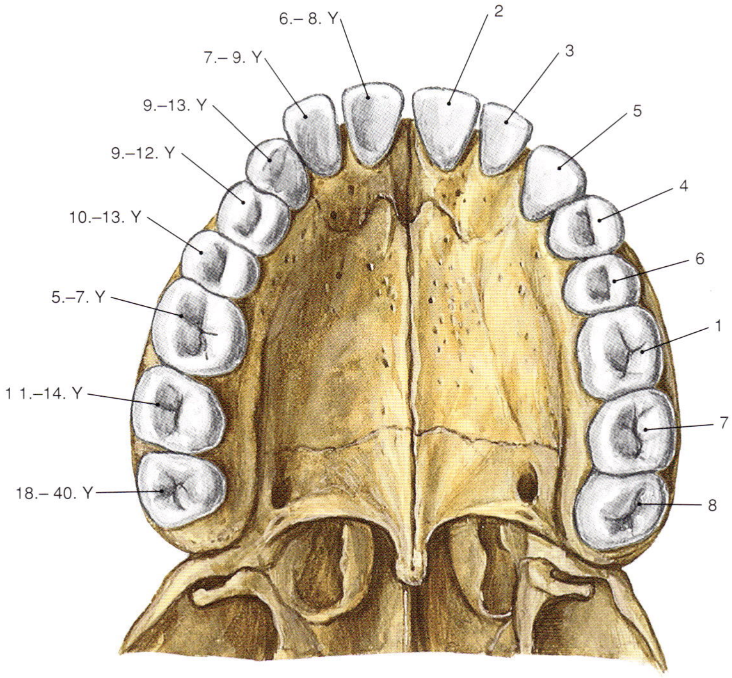

Fig. 166 Maxilla with permanent teeth;
left: median time of eruption in years (Y);
right: order of eruption.

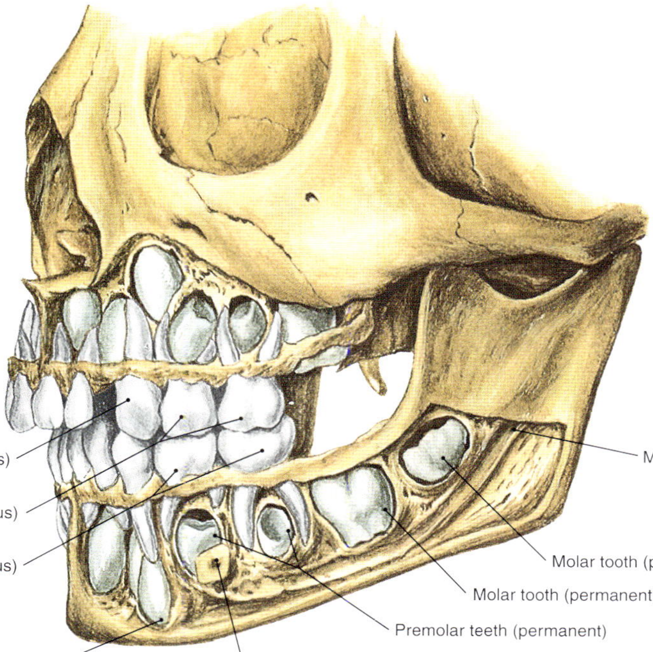

Fig. 167 Maxilla and mandible of a 5-year-old child; deciduous teeth and anlage of permanent teeth.

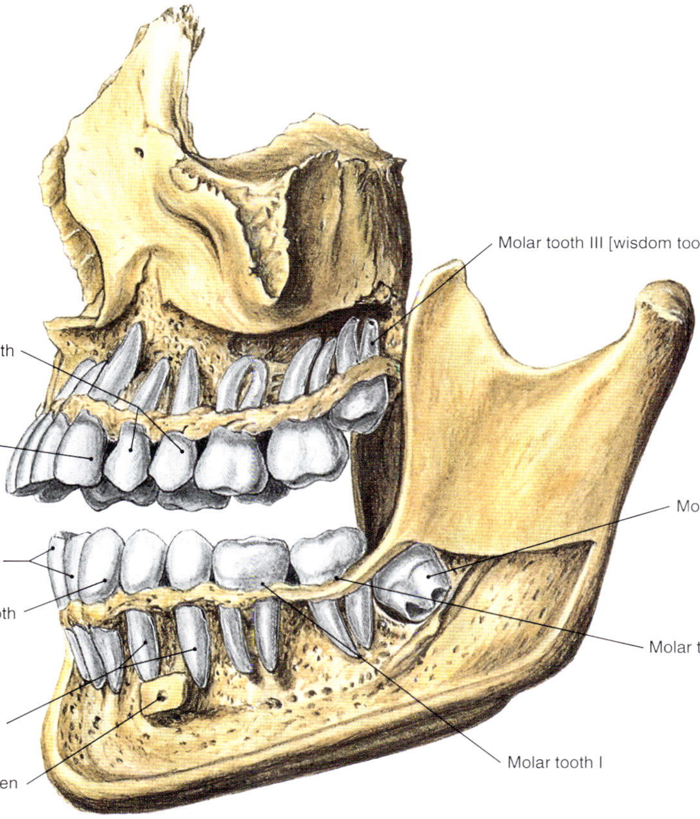

Fig. 168 Maxilla and mandible of a 20-year-old male.

Teeth, radiography

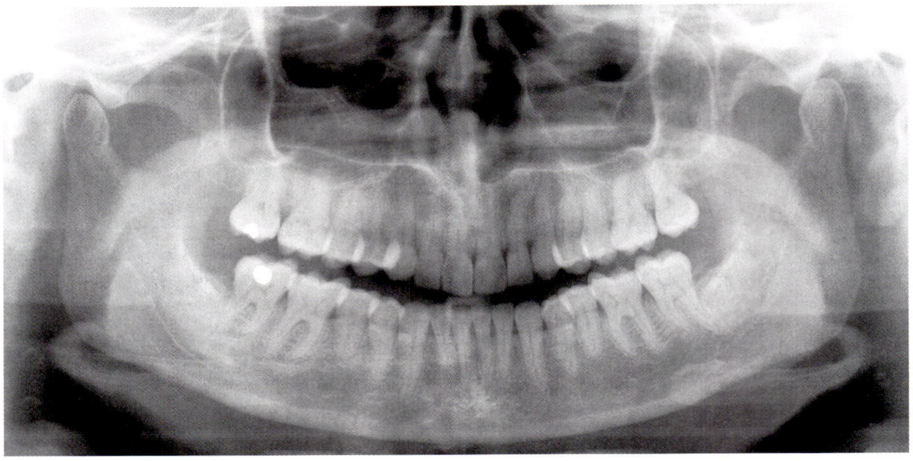

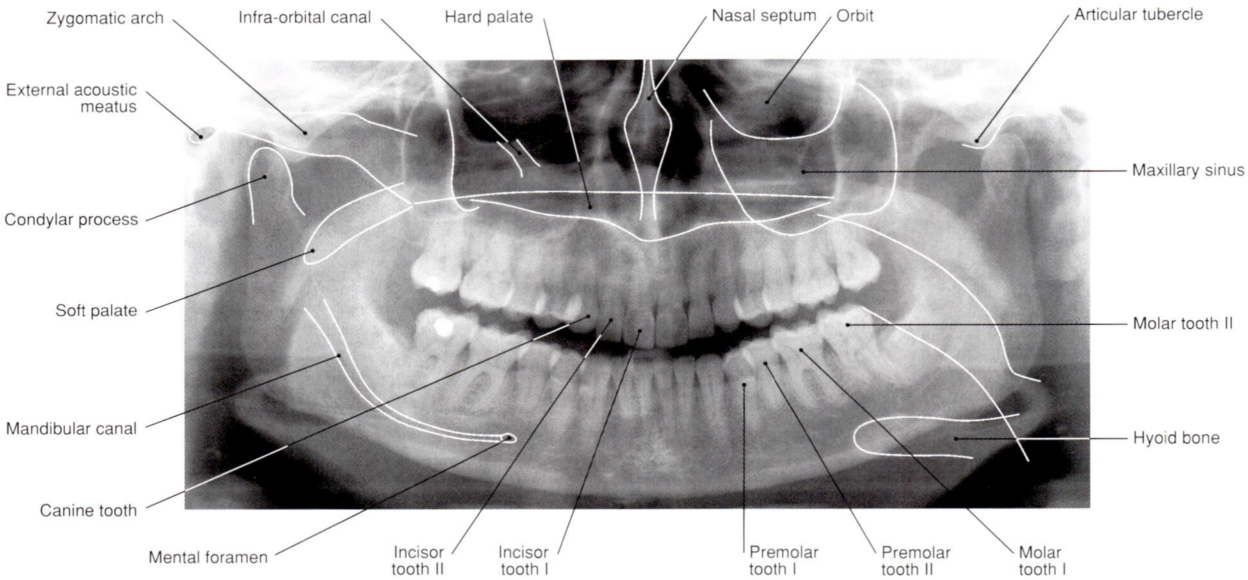

Fig. 169 Maxilla and mandible; panoramic radiograph; without wisdom teeth.

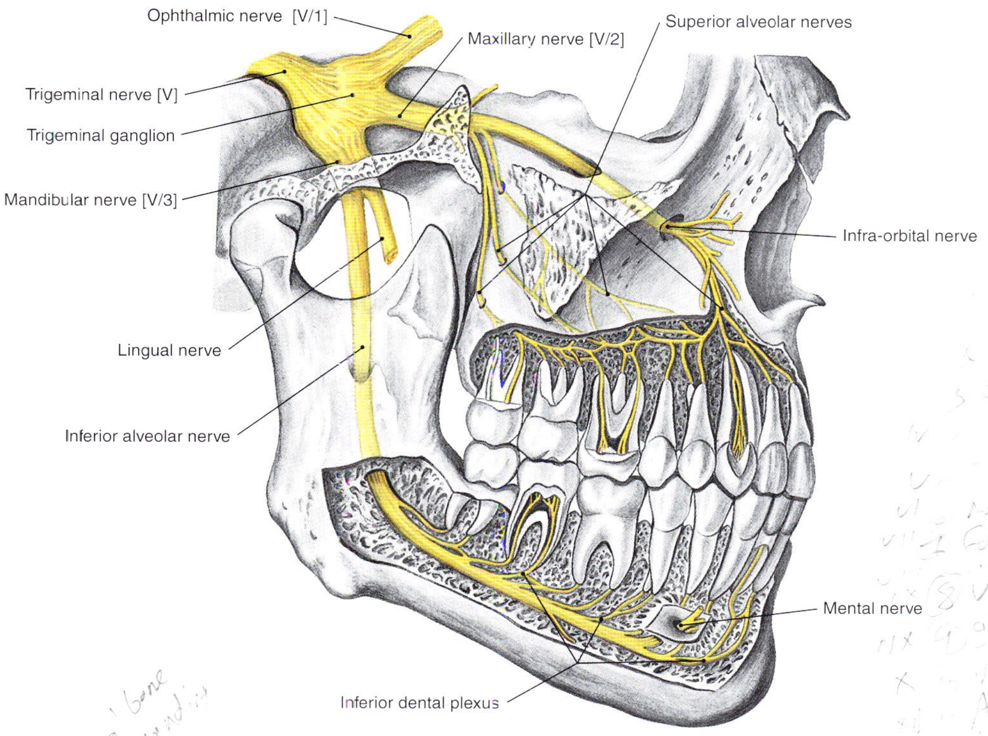

Fig. 170 Maxillary and mandibular nerve.

→ 1178, 1179

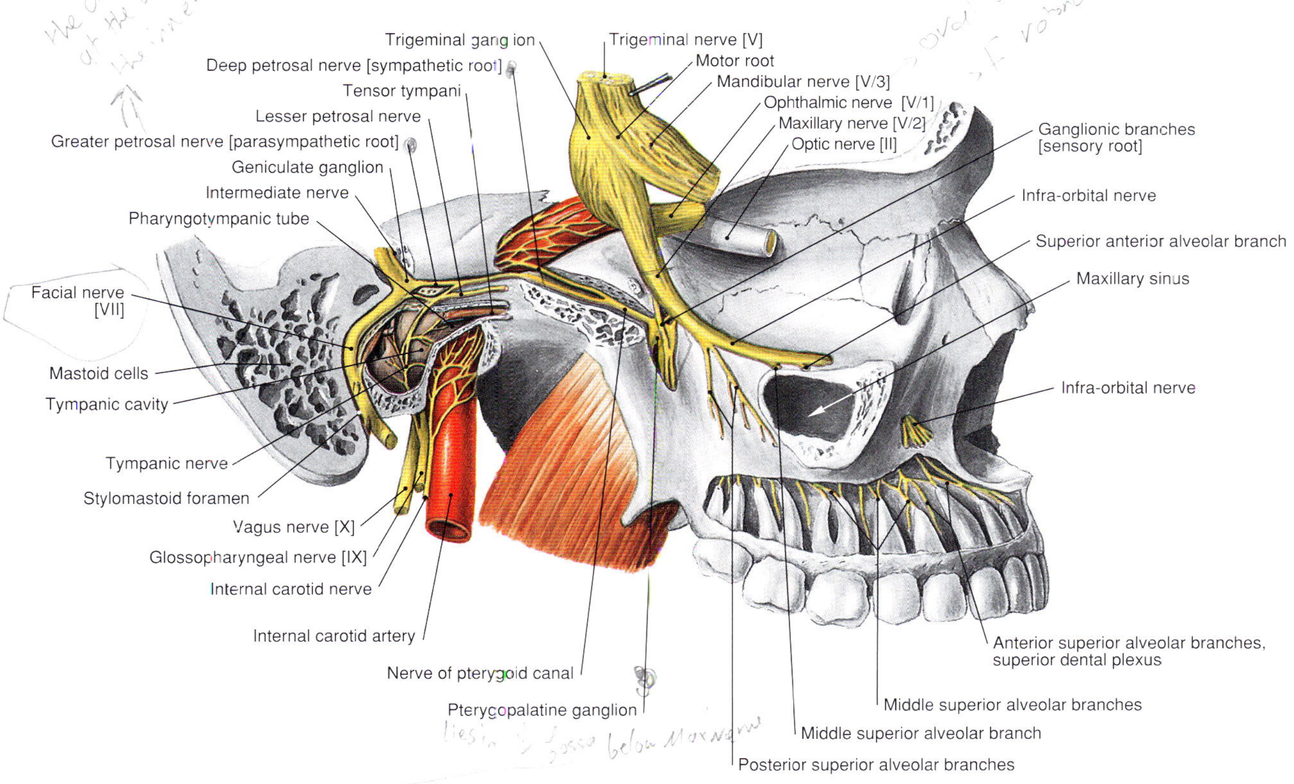

Fig. 171 Pterygopalatine ganglion.

Receives preganglionic parasympathetic fibers from Facial Nerve VII by Greater petrosal nerve

Palate

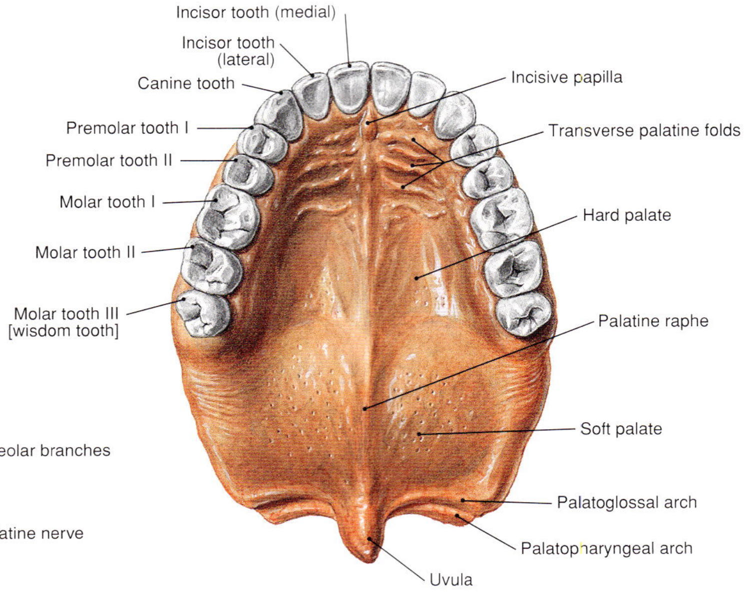

Fig. 172 Hard and soft palate; inferior view.

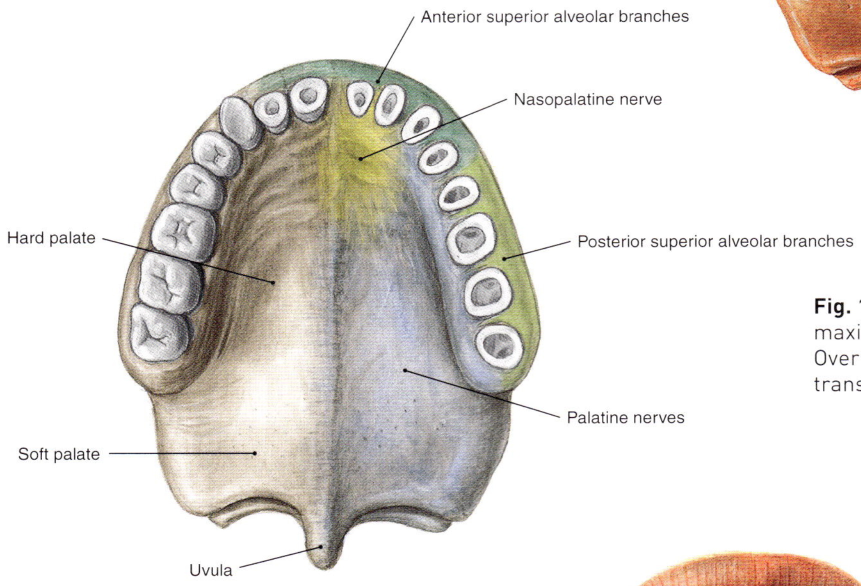

Fig. 173 Sensible innervation of the palate and maxilla.
Overlapping areas of innervation are indicated by transition of colours.

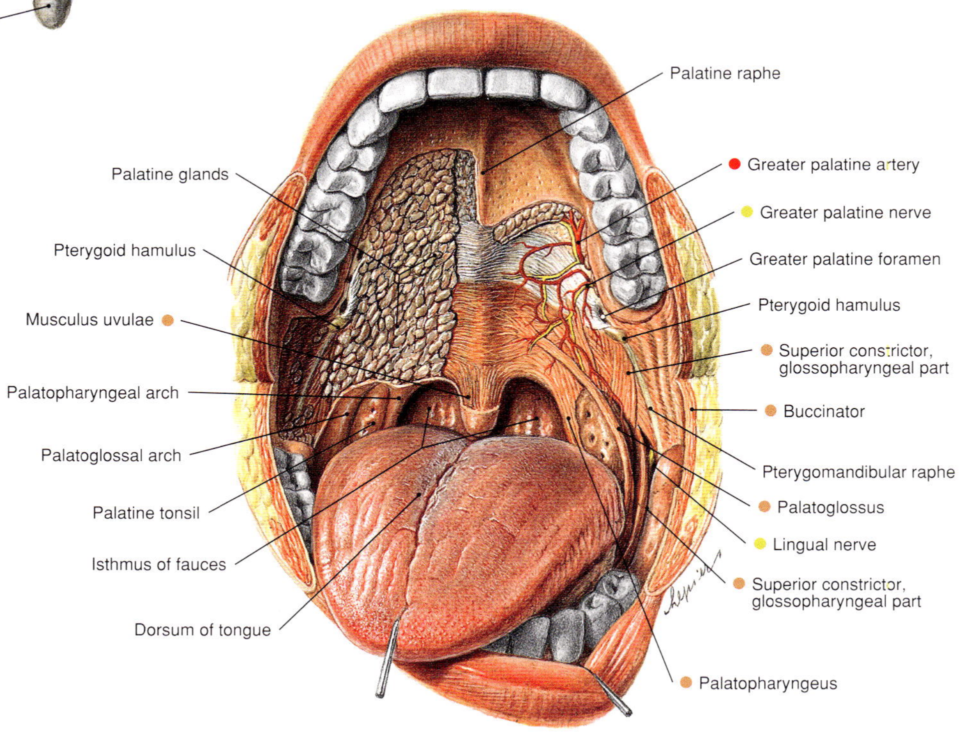

→ T 3

Fig. 174 Oral cavity and muscles of the palate.

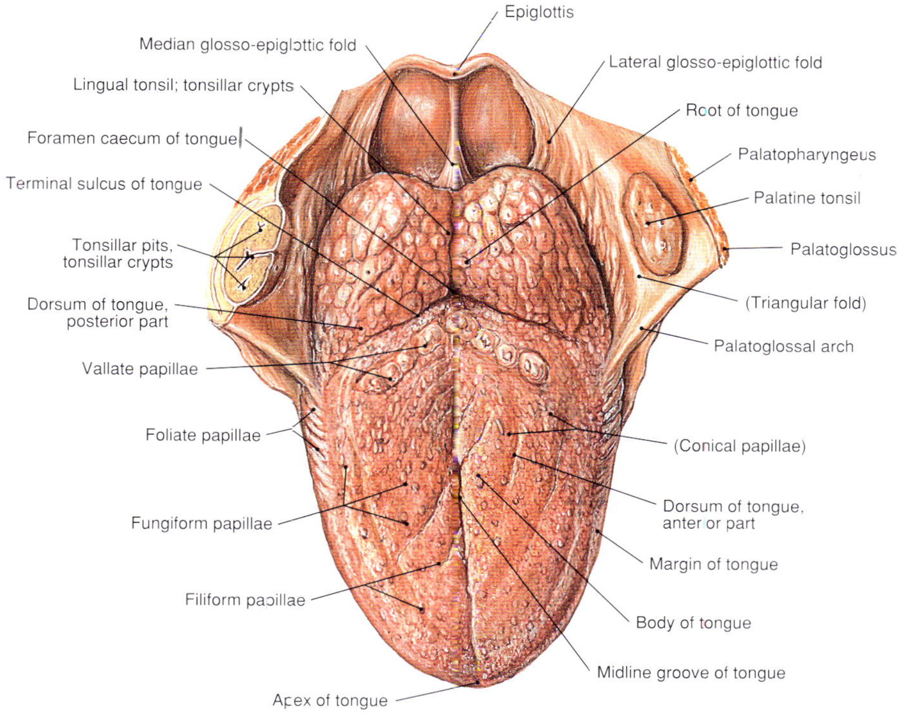

Fig. 175 Tongue.

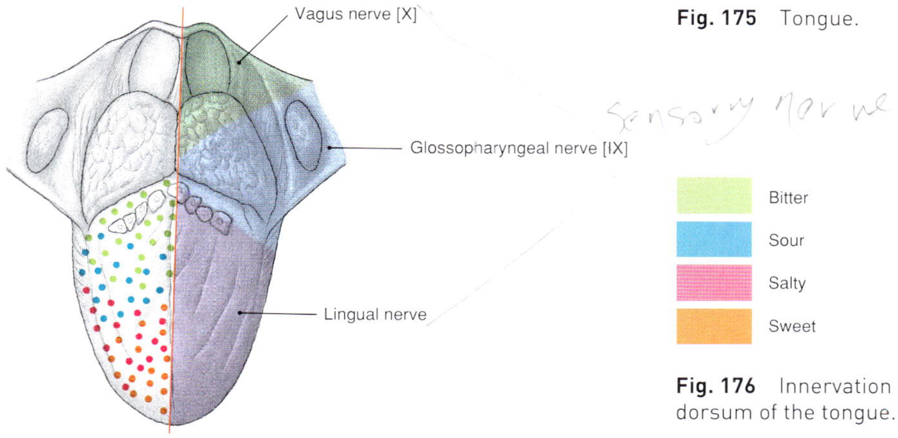

Fig. 176 Innervation and taste categories at the dorsum of the tongue.

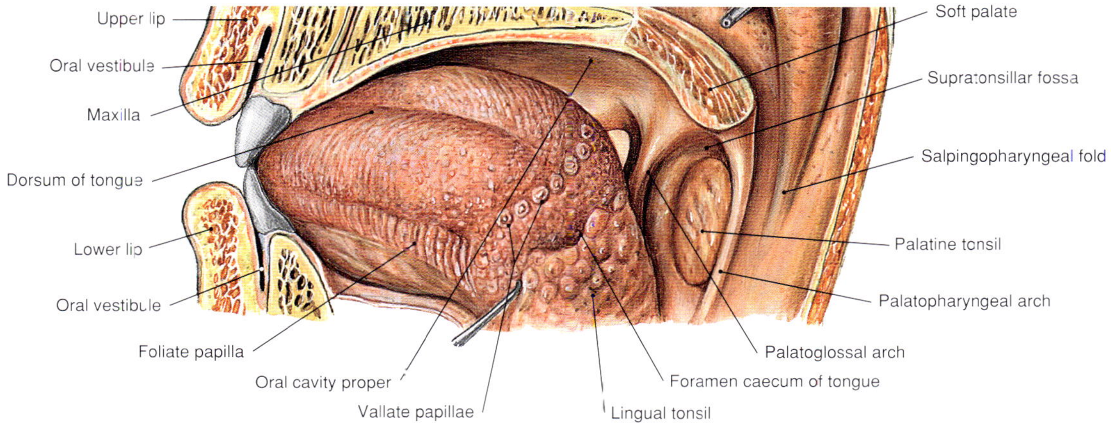

Fig. 177 Oral cavity.

Muscles of the tongue

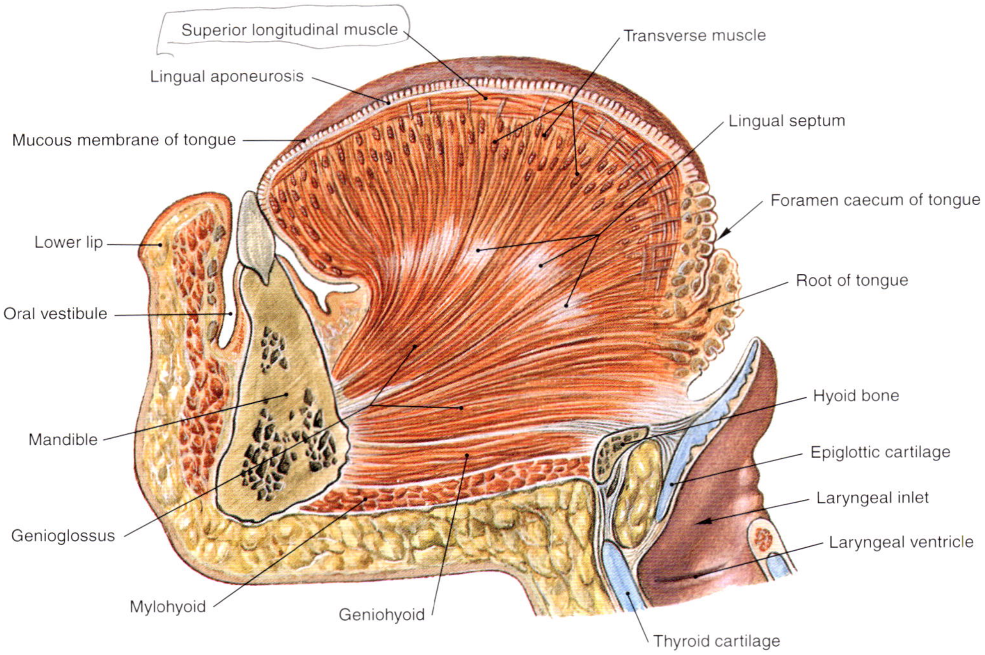

→ T 2a

Fig. 178 Tongue and muscles of the tongue; median section.

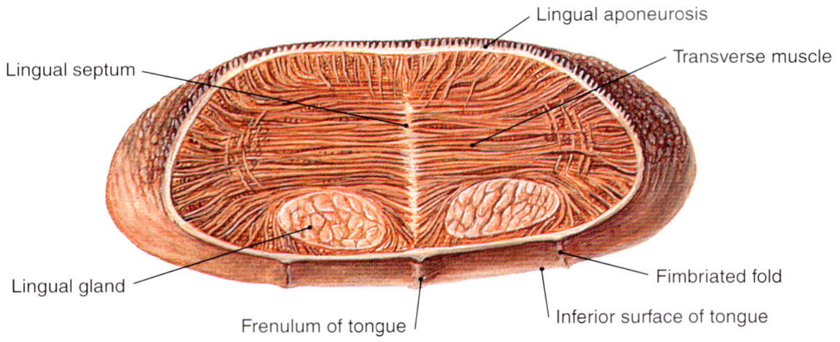

→ T 2a

Fig. 179 Tongue and muscles of the tongue; cross-section through the tip of the tongue.

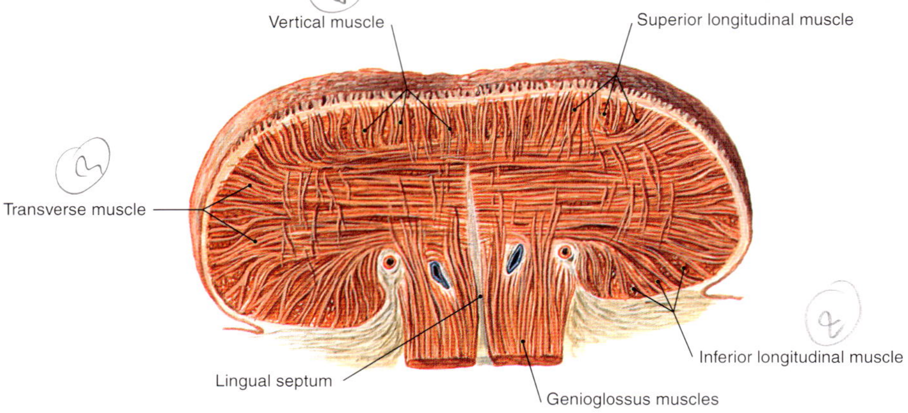

→ T 2a

Fig. 180 Tongue, and muscles of the tongue; cross-section at the level of the middle of the tongue.

Hyoid bone and infra- and suprahyoid muscles

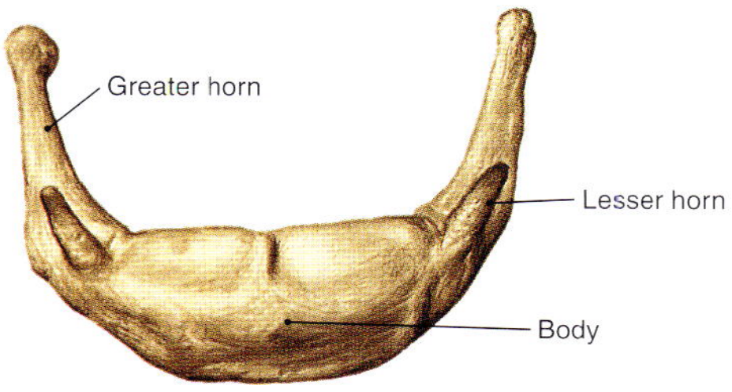

Fig. 181 Hyoid bone.

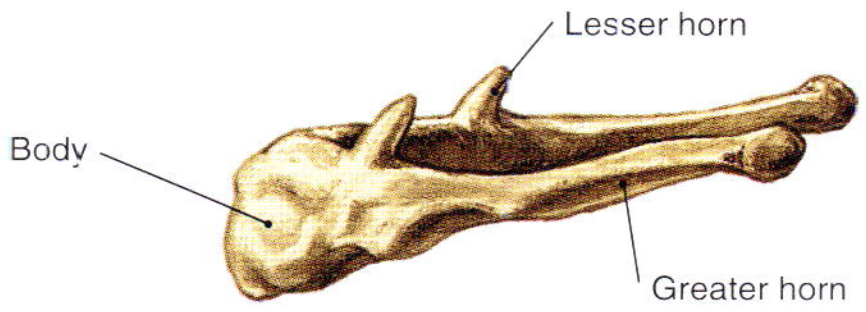

Fig. 182 Hyoid bone.

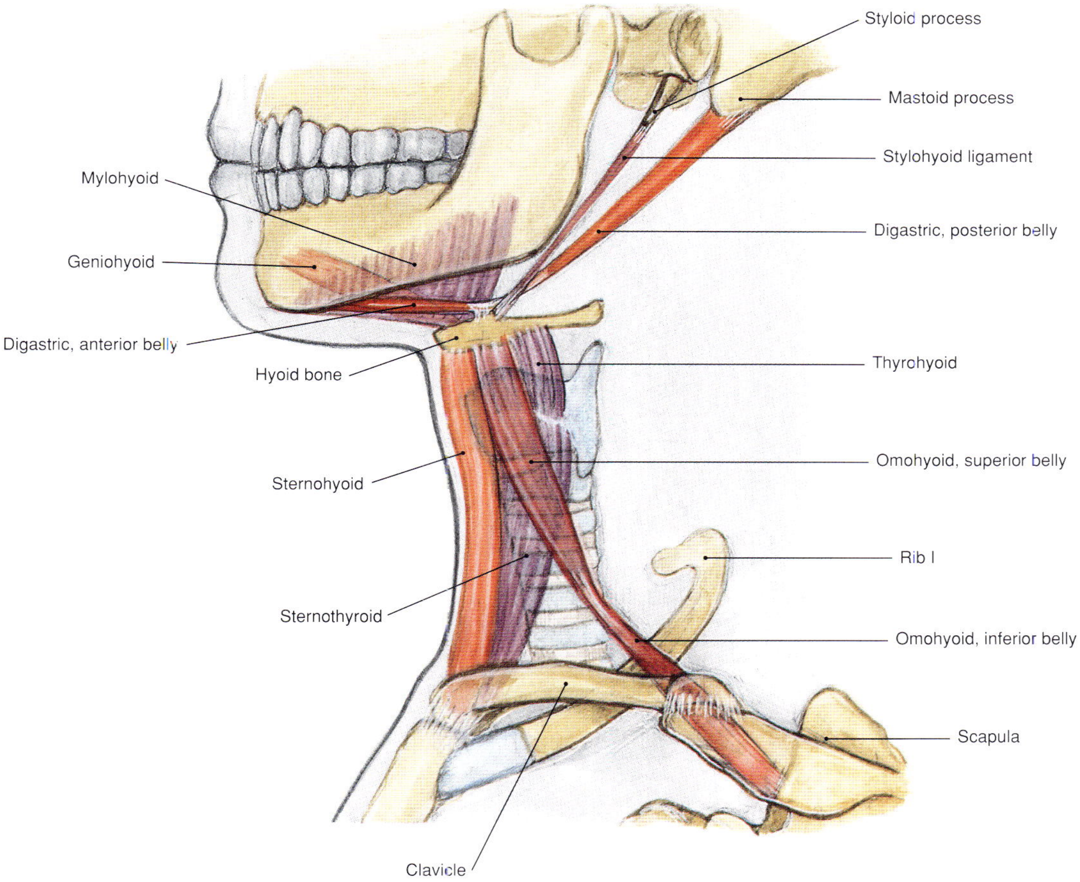

Fig. 183 Muscular suspension of the hyoid bone.

→ T 9, T 10

Suprahyoid muscles

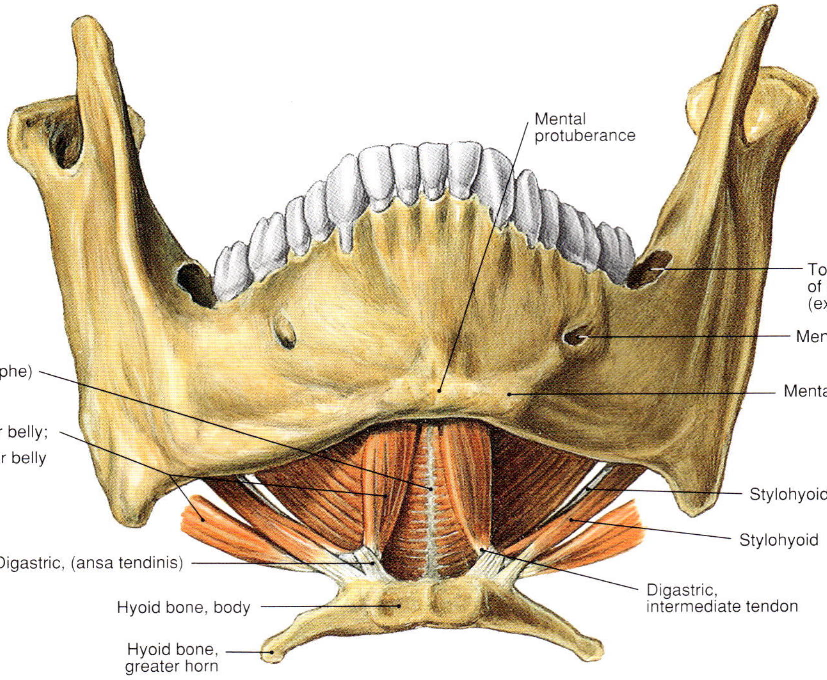

→ T 9

Fig. 184 Mandible and suprahyoid muscles.

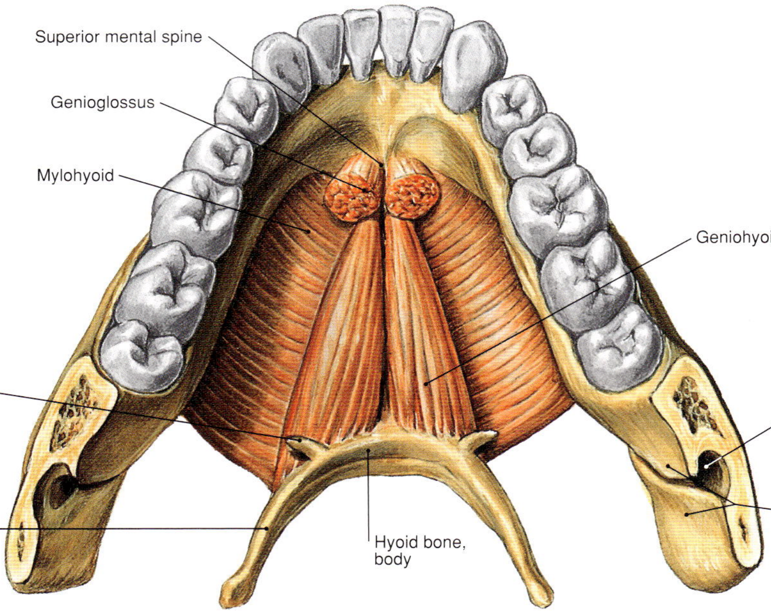

→ T 9

Fig. 185 Mandible; suprahyoid muscles and hyoid bone.

Muscles of the tongue

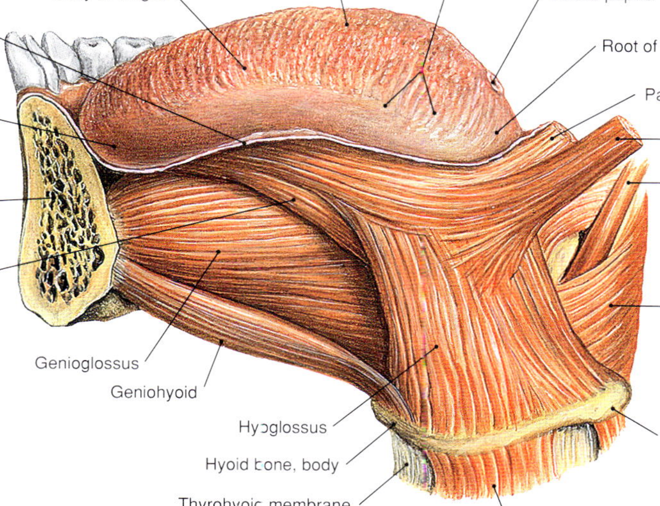

Fig. 186 Tongue and muscles of the tongue.

→ T 2b

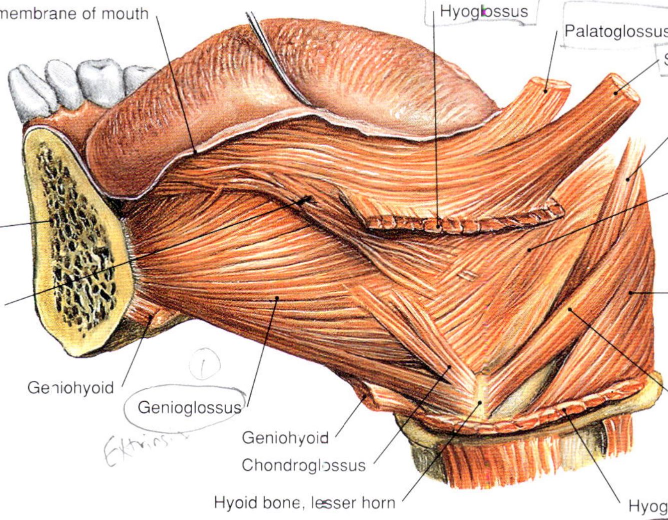

Fig. 187 Tongue and muscles of the tongue.

→ T 2b

Muscles of the tongue and the pharynx

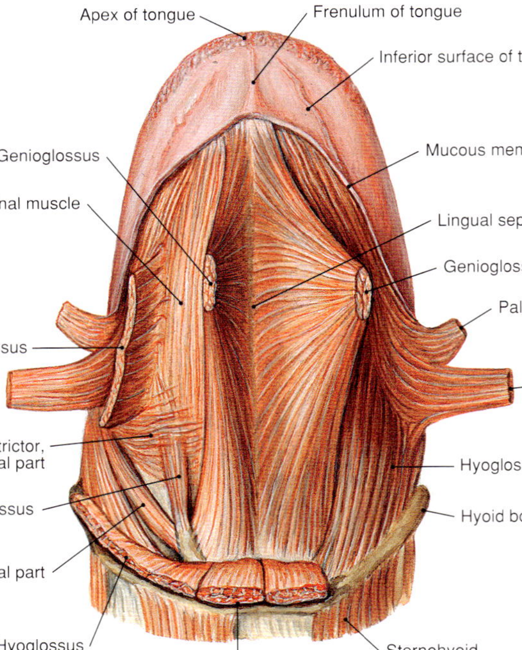

→ T 2b

Fig. 188 Muscles of the tongue.

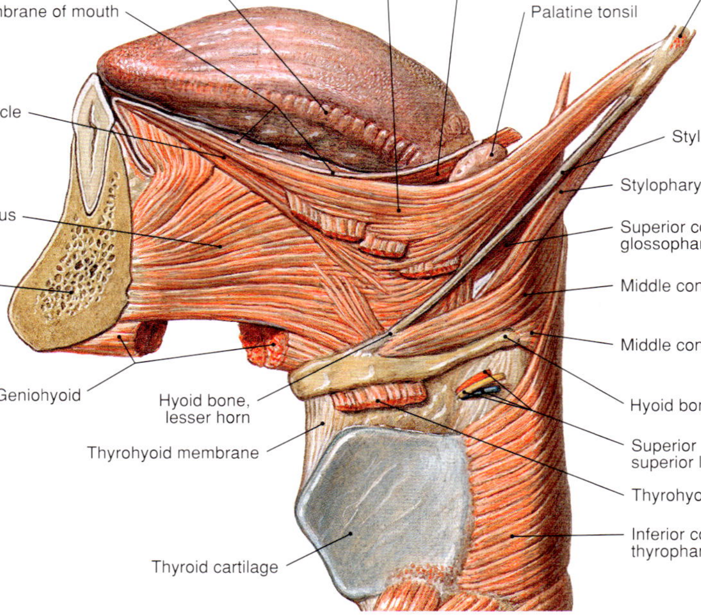

→ T 2b, T 5

Fig. 189 Muscles of the tongue and muscles of the pharynx.

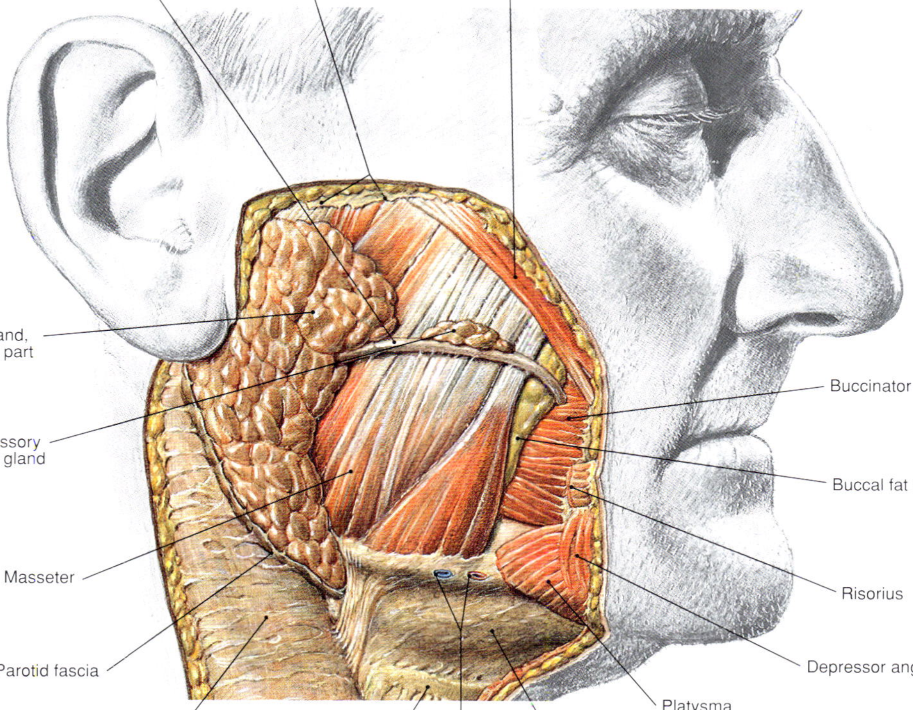

Fig. 190 Parotid gland.

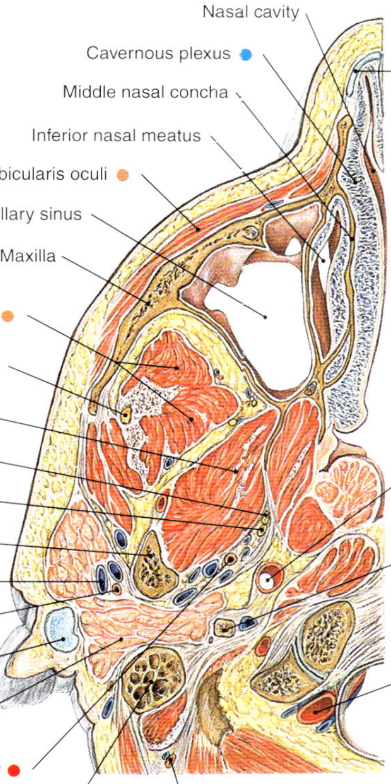

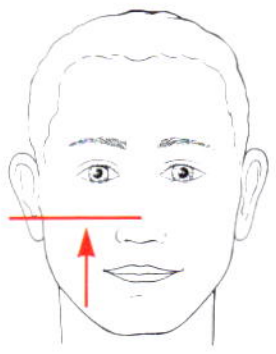

Fig. 191 Parotid gland and masticatory muscles; horizontal section; inferior view.

Submandibular gland

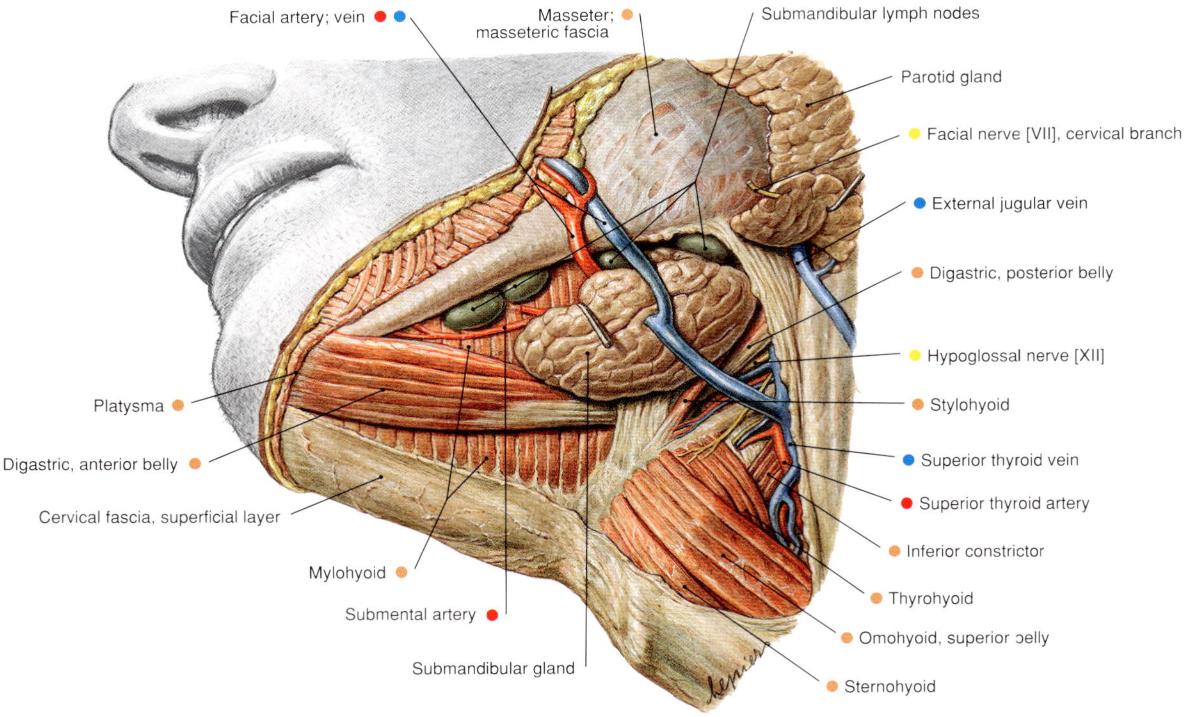

Fig. 192 Submandibular gland.

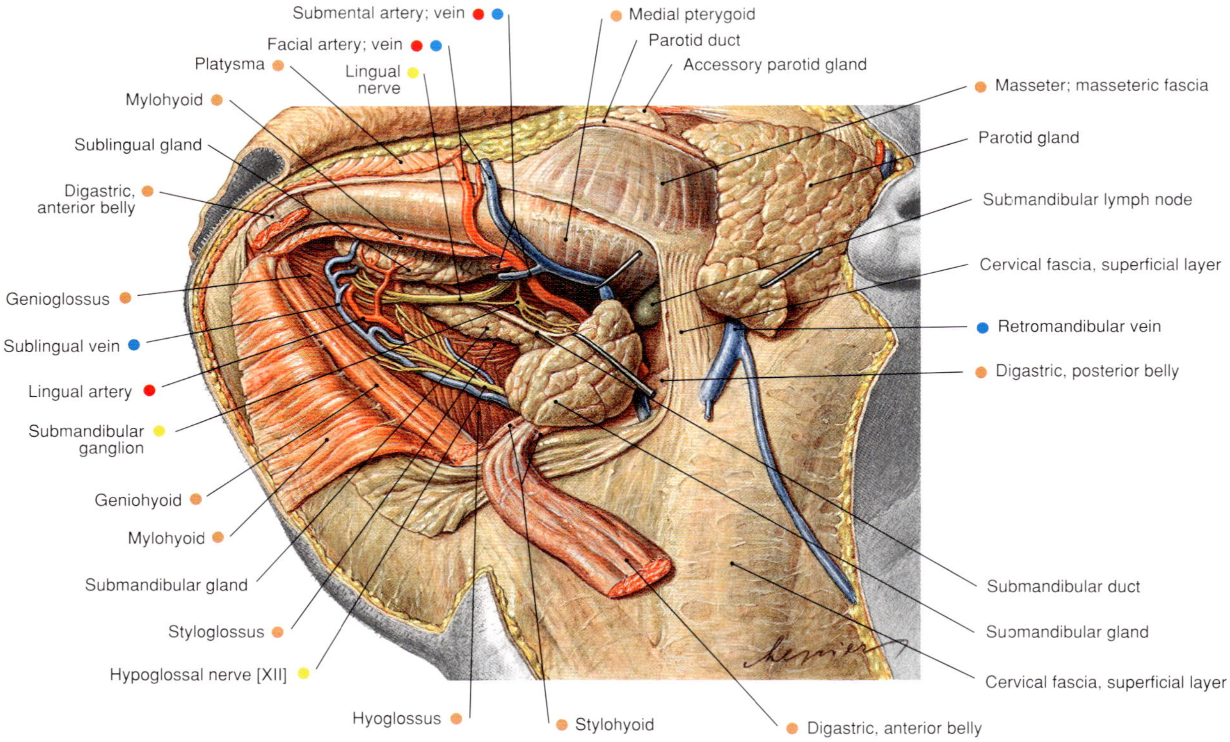

Fig. 193 Major salivary glands; inferolateral view.

Submandibular and sublingual gland

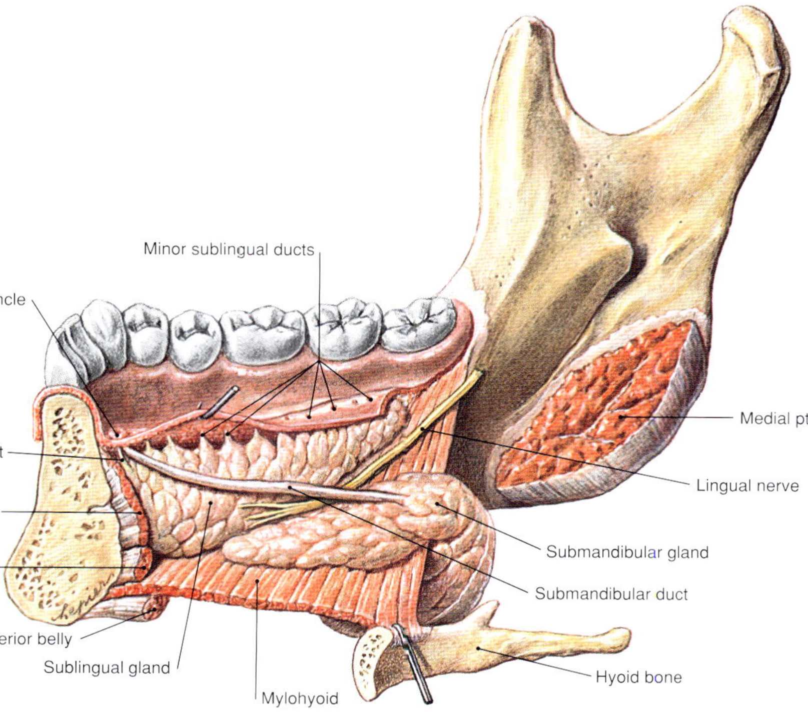

Fig. 194 Submandibular gland and sublingual gland.

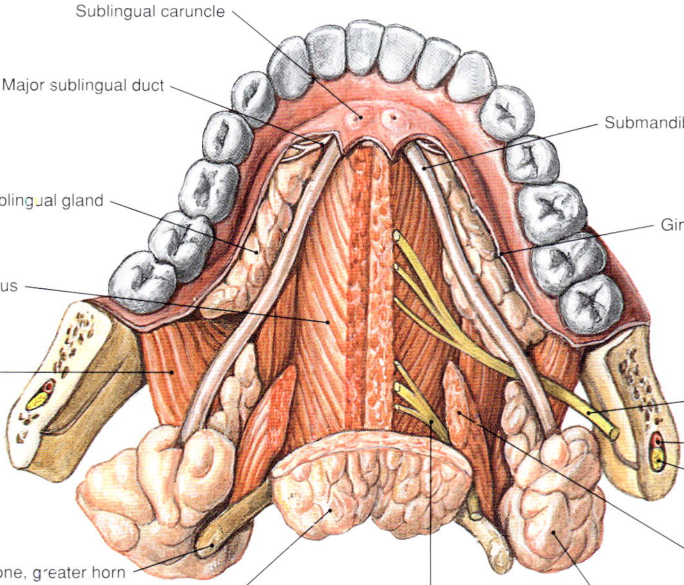

Fig. 195 Sublingual gland and submandibular gland; superior view.

Openings of the salivary glands

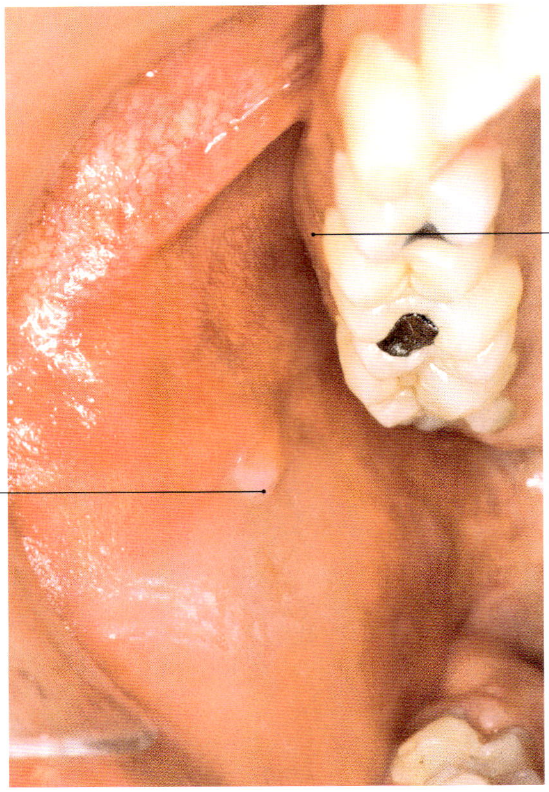

Fig. 196 Opening of the excretory duct of the parotid gland.

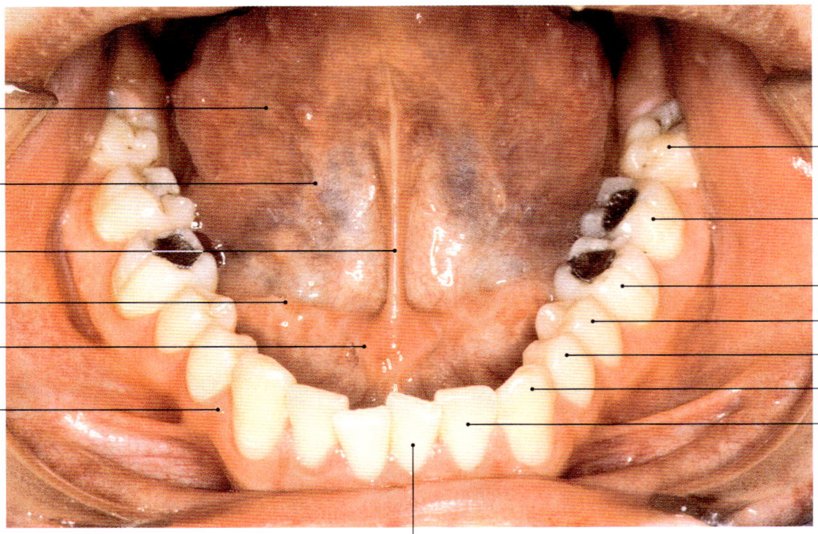

→ 154

Fig. 197 Opening of the excretory duct of the submandibular gland.

Arteries and nerves of the oral cavity

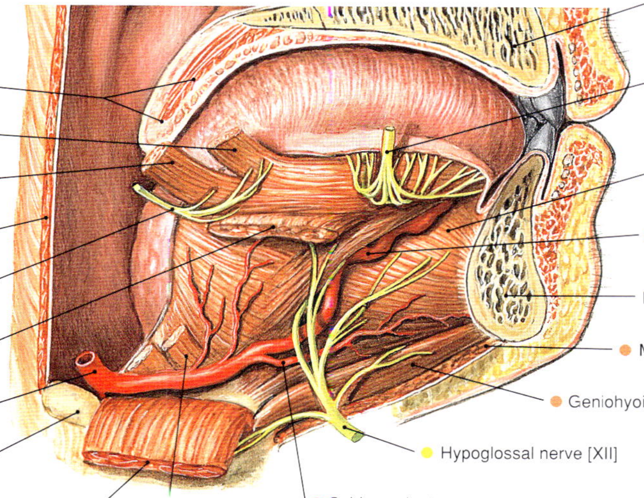

Fig. 198 Arteries and nerves of the tongue; medial view.

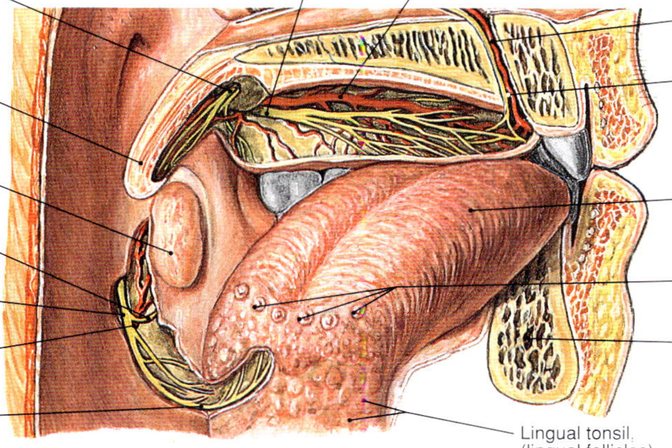

Fig. 199 Arteries and nerves of the palate and the root of the tongue; medial view.

Vessels and nerves of the tongue and the larynx

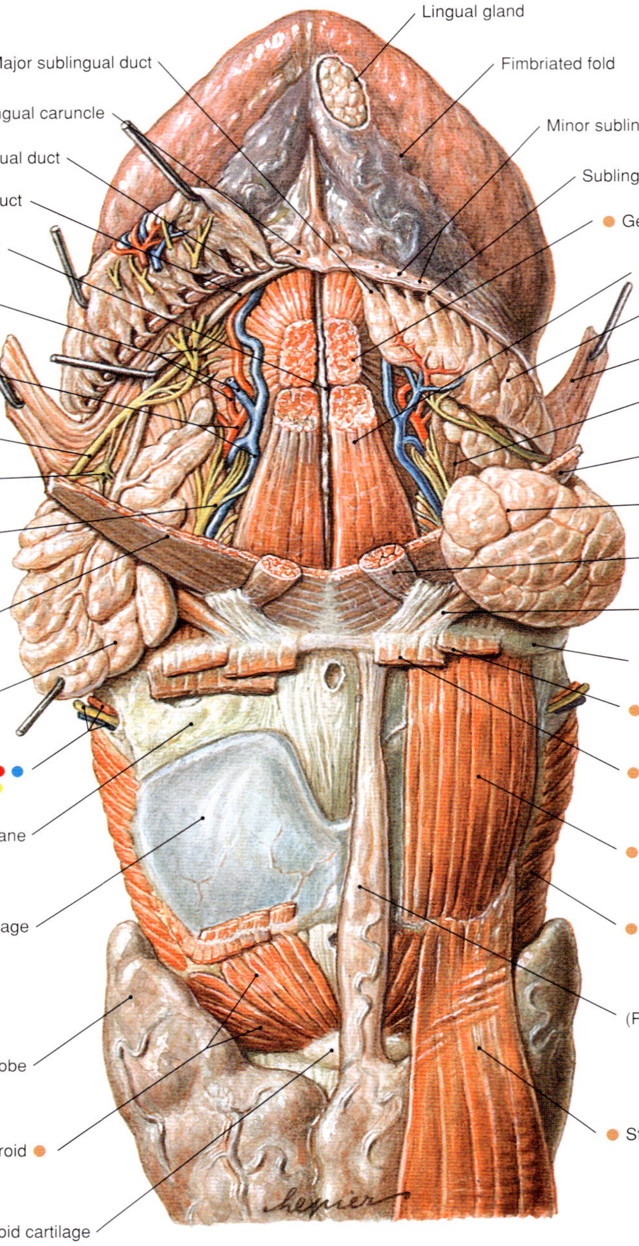

→ 204, 218, 234, 237

Fig. 200 Vessels and nerves of the tongue; major salivary glands and larynx; anterior-inferior view.

Vessels and nerves of the tongue and the thyroid gland

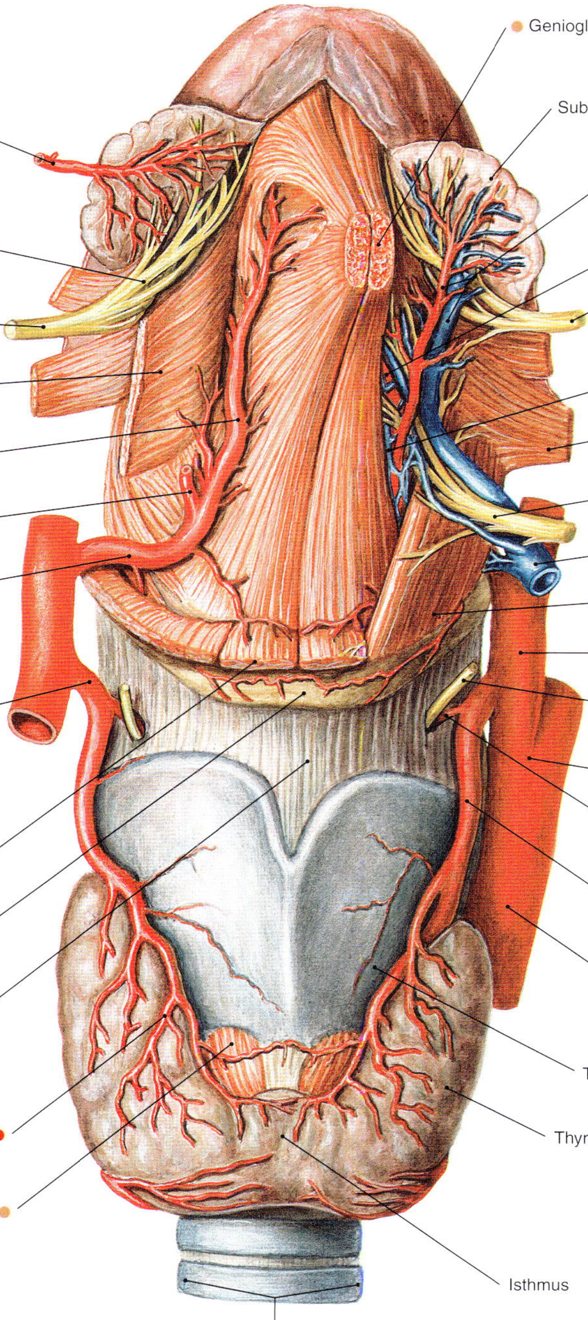

Fig. 201 Vessels and nerves of the tongue and the thyroid gland; anterior-inferior view.

→ 238, 264

Head, frontal section

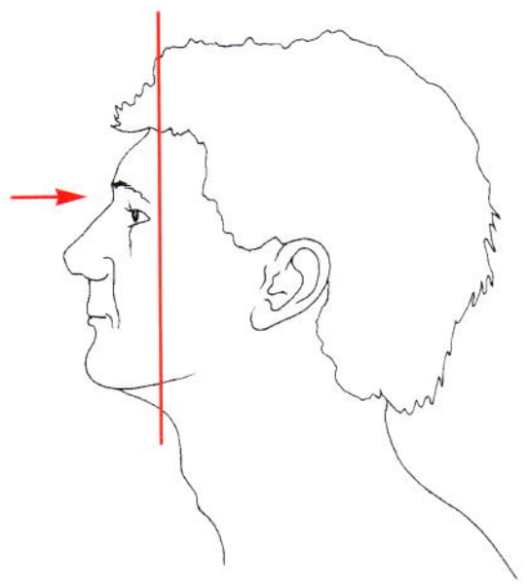

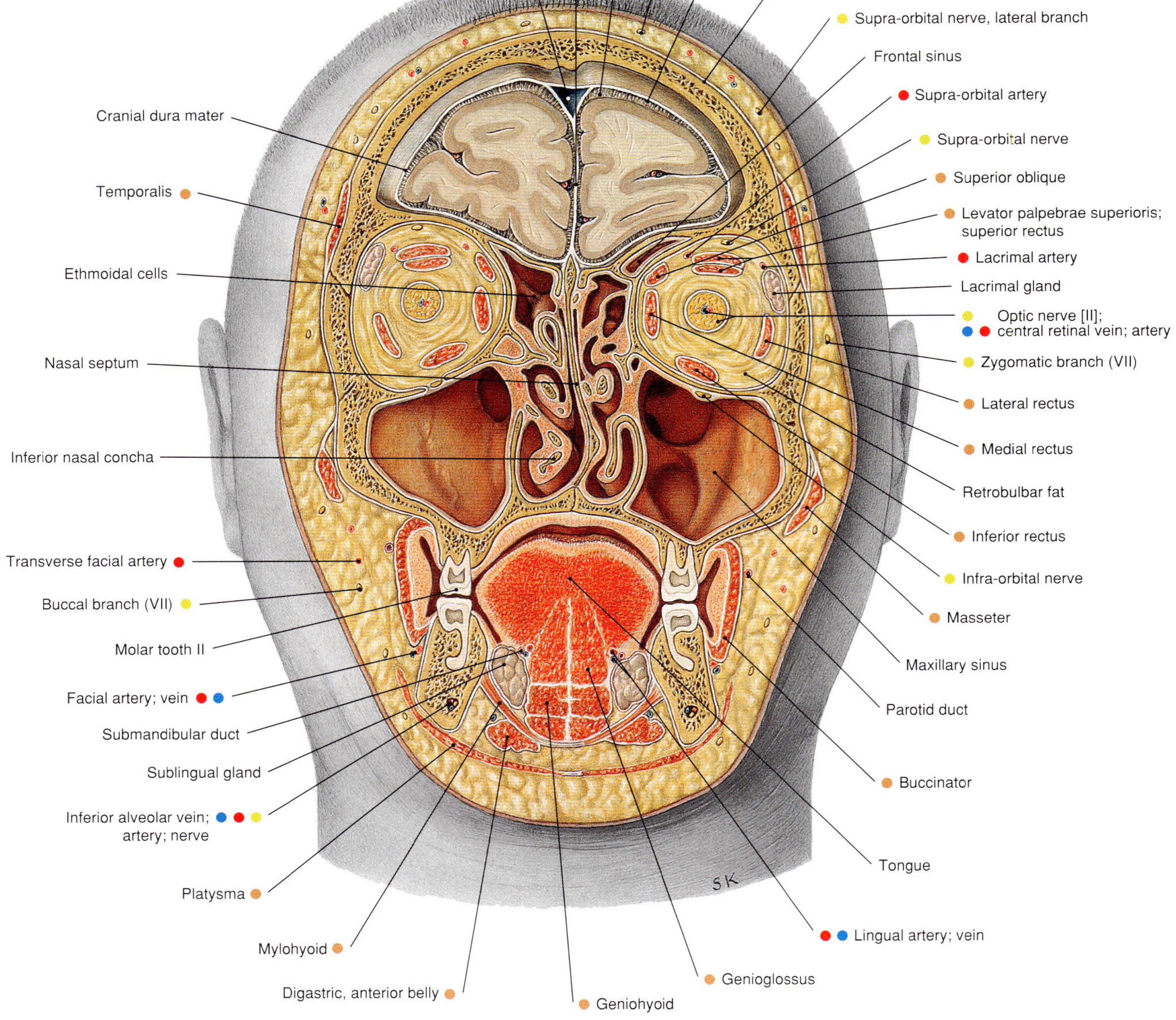

Fig. 202 Frontal section through the head of a 48-year-old male at the level of the second upper molar tooth; anterior view.

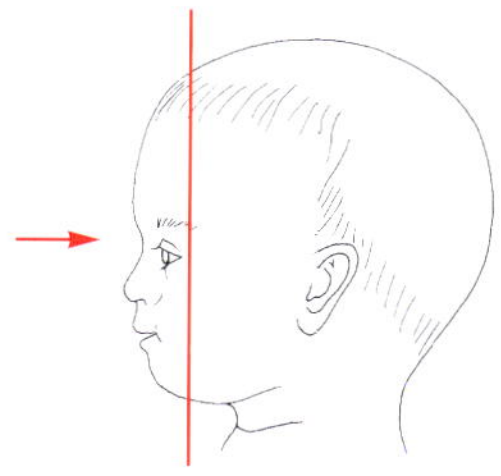

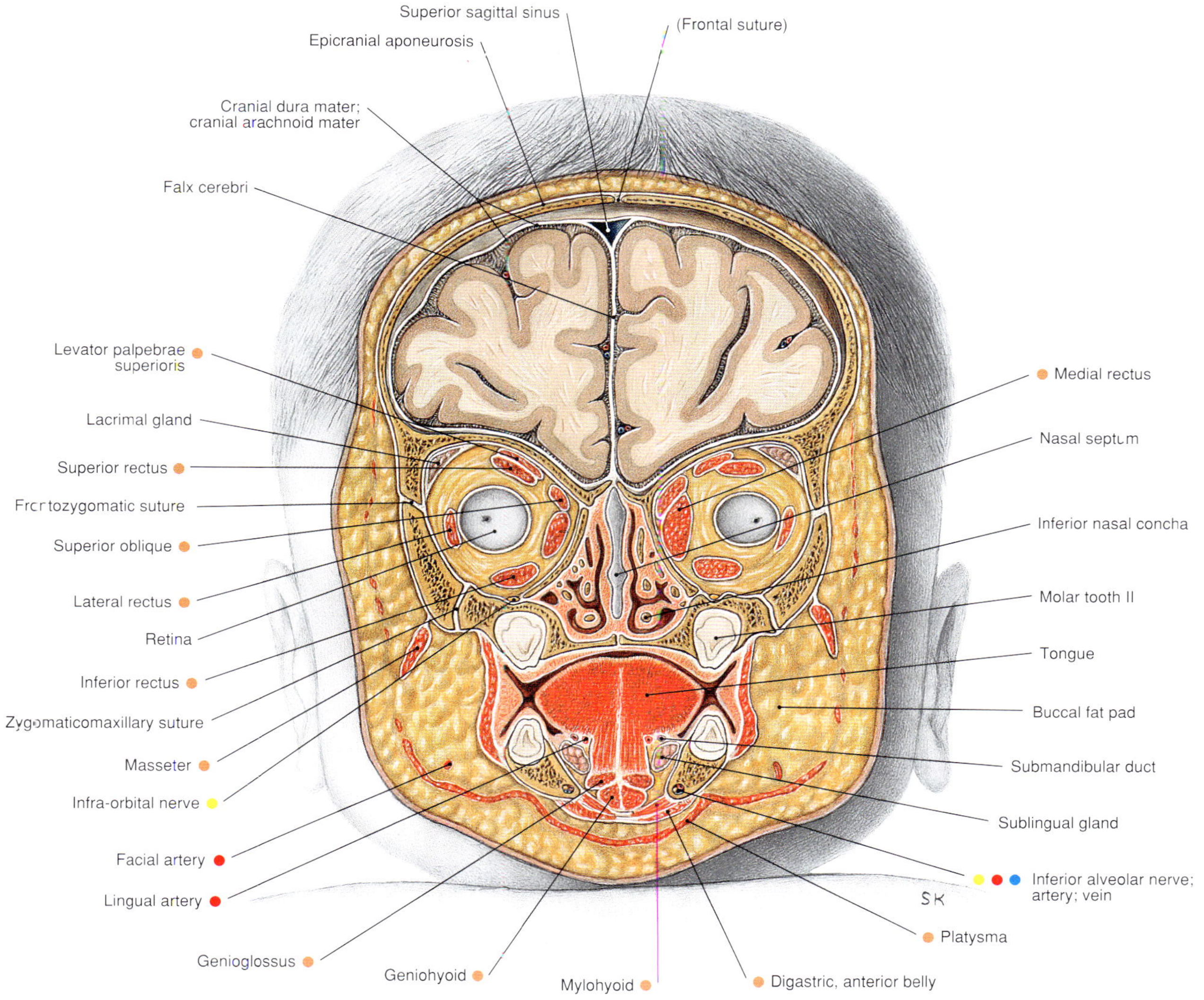

Fig. 203 Frontal section through the head of a neonate at the level of the second upper molar tooth; anterior view.
Note the absence of the maxillary sinus and the close proximity of the tooth anlage to the orbit.

▸▸ Surface p. 32 | Skeleton p. 264 ff.

Muscles of the neck and tracheotomy

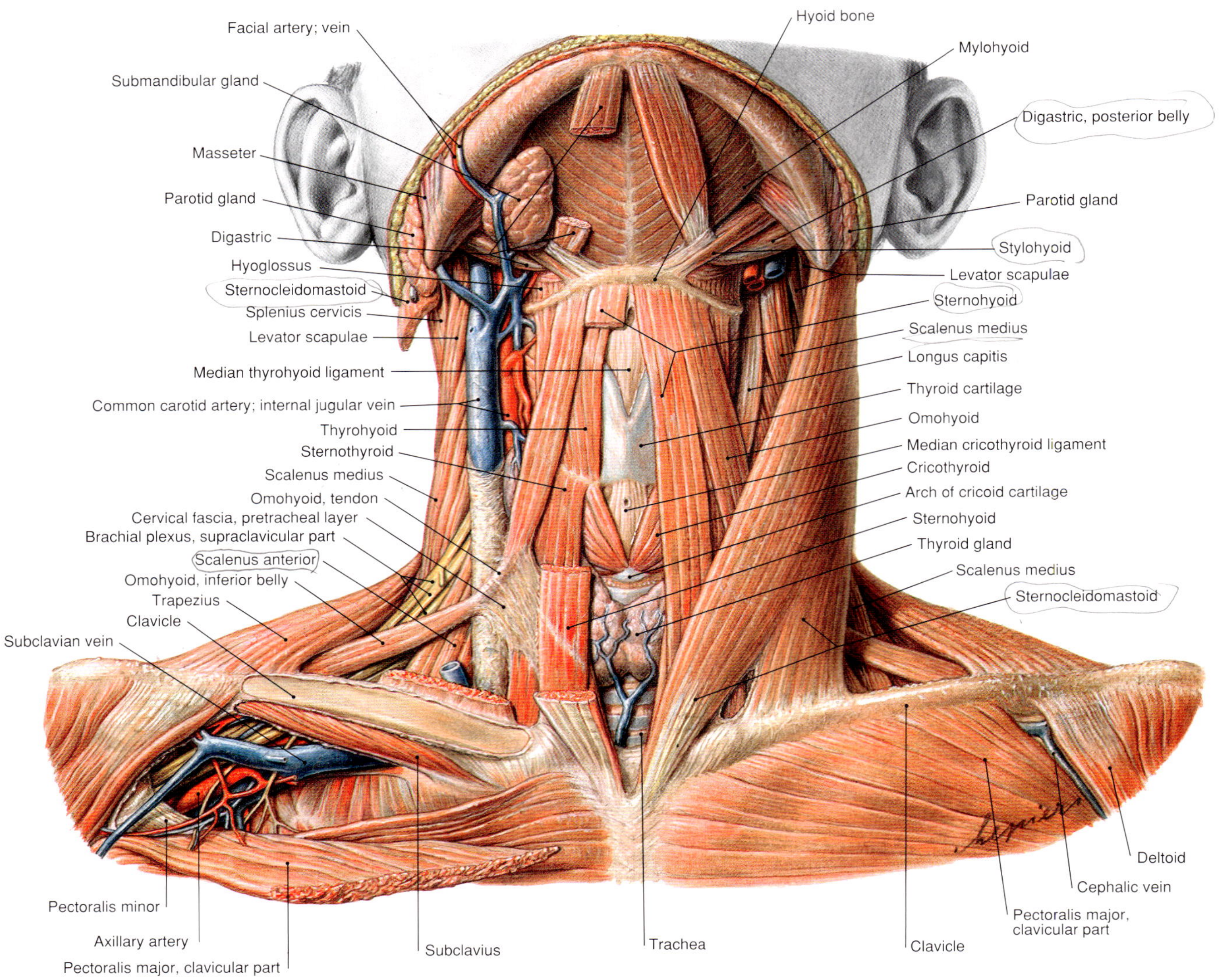

→ T 8, T 9, T 10, T 11

Fig. 204 Muscles of the neck.

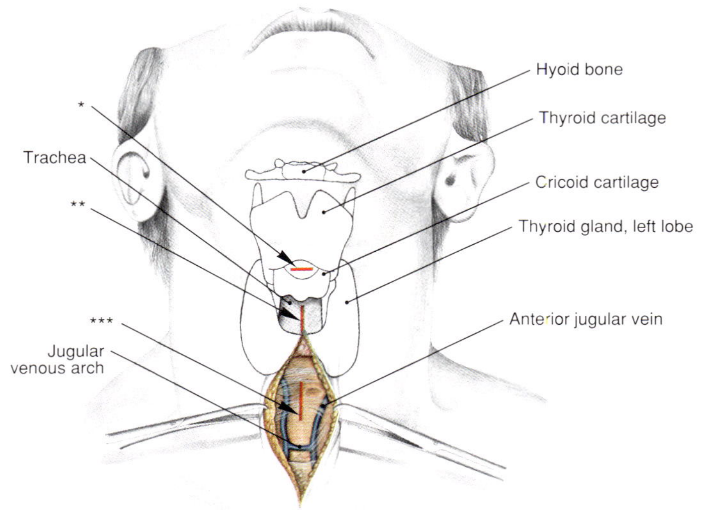

Fig. 205 Surgical access to the trachea with the neck hyperextended.

* Coniotomy
** Upper tracheotomy (above the isthmus of the thyroid gland)
*** Lower tracheotomy (below the isthmus of the thyroid gland)

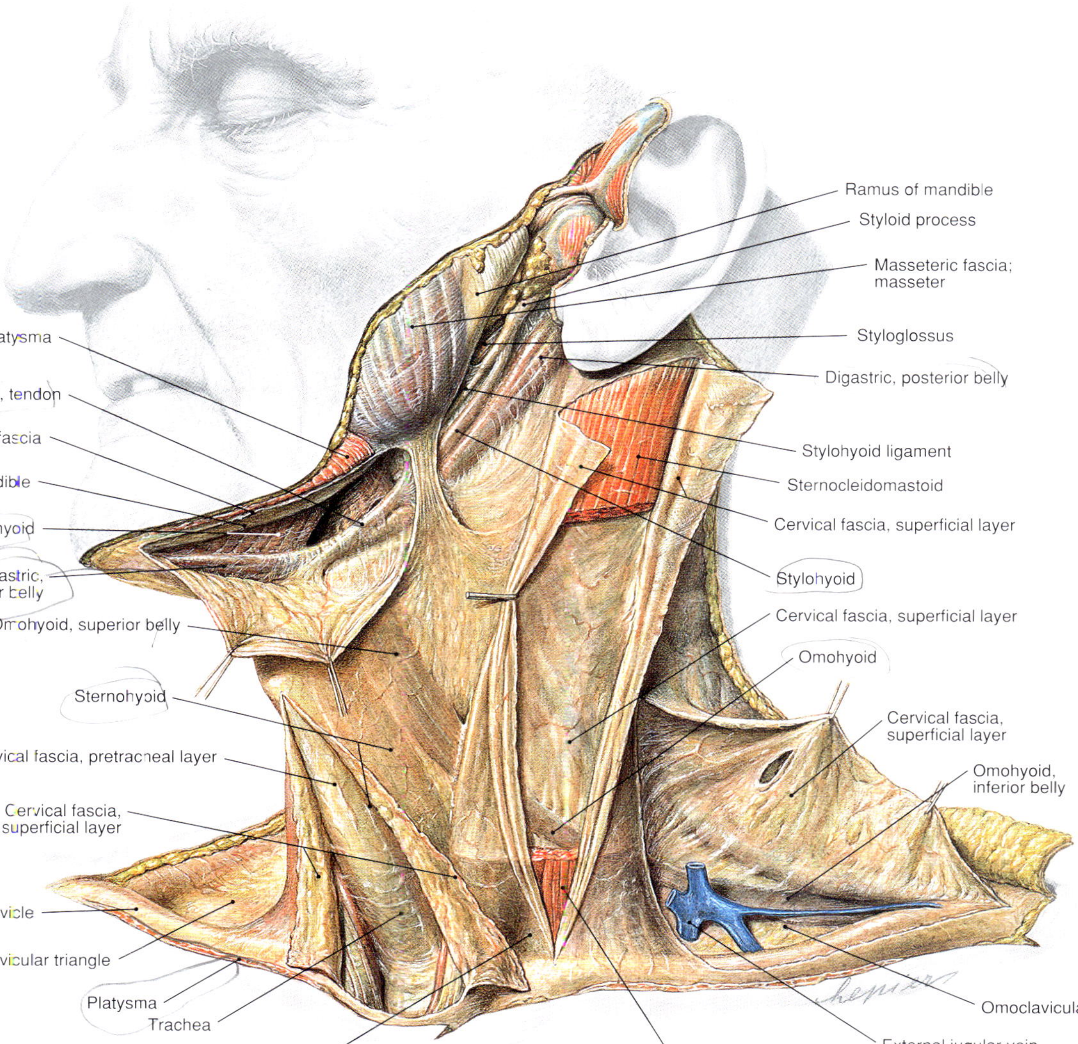

Fig. 206 Cervical fascia.

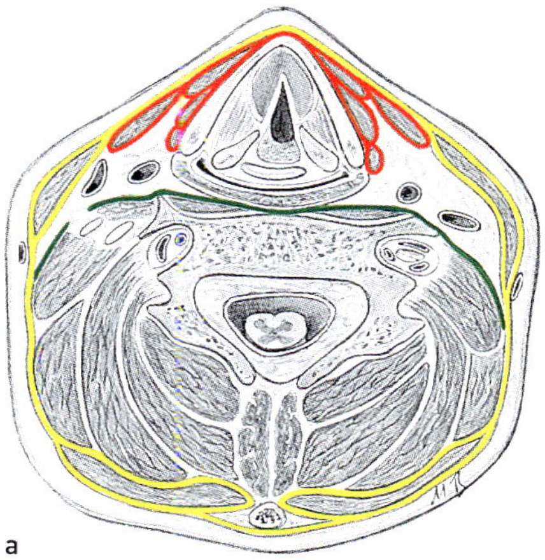

Cervical fascia

Yellow: Superficial layer

Red: Pretracheal layer

Green: Prevertebral layer

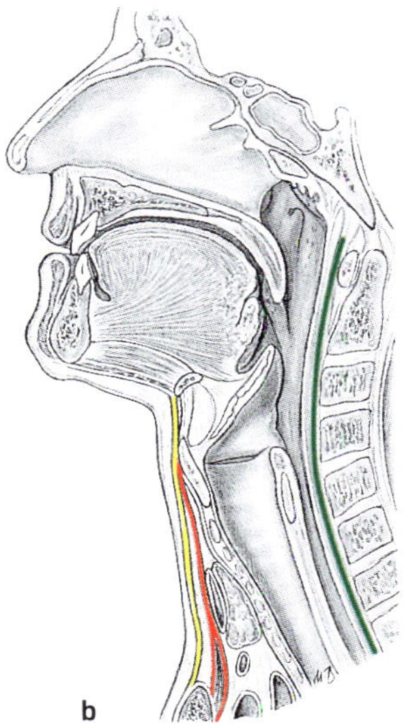

Fig. 207 Schema of the cervical fascia.

a Transverse section → 269

b Median section → 246

▸▸ Surface p. 32 | Skeleton p. 264 ff.

Muscles of the neck

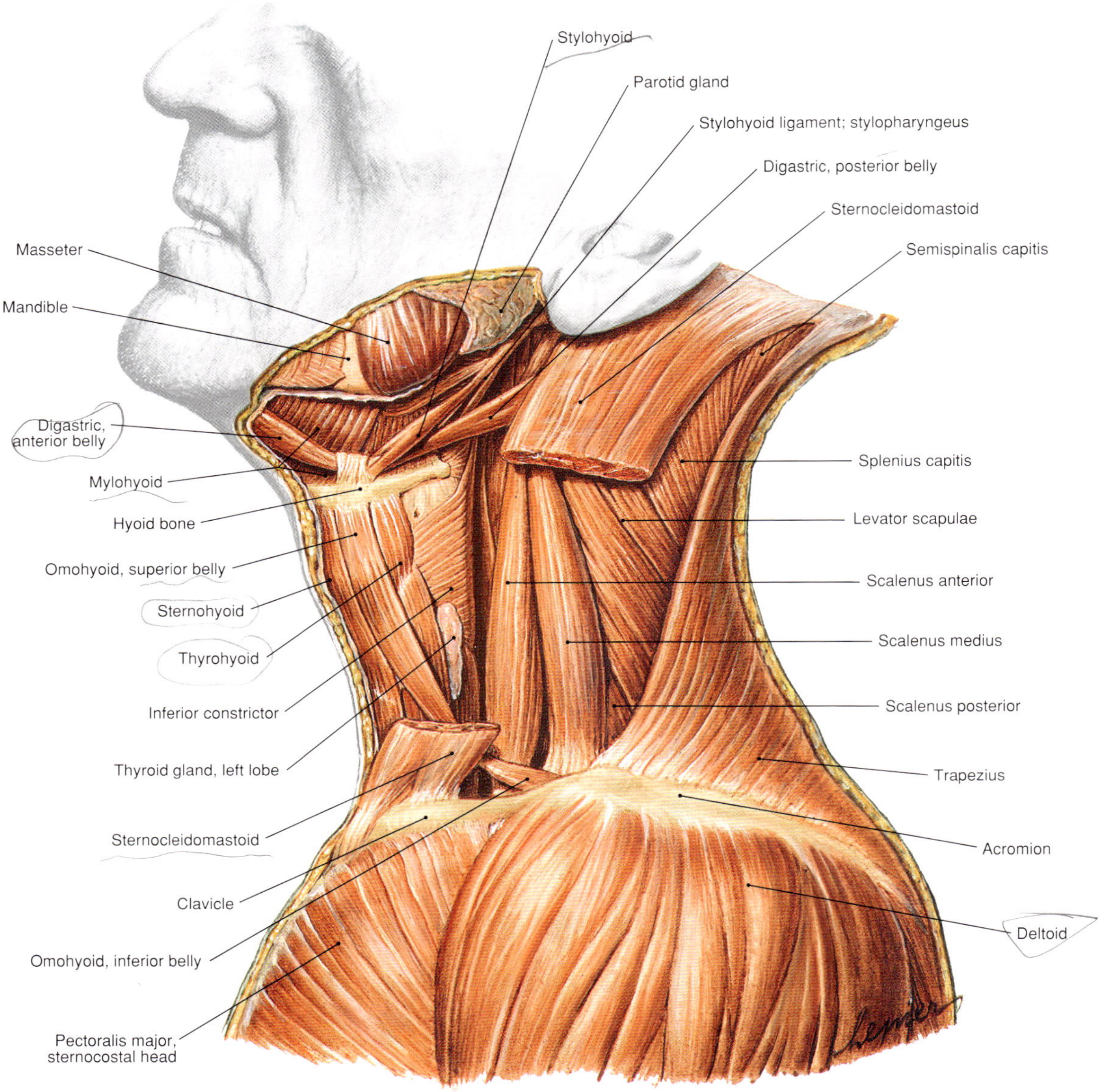

→ T 8, T 9, T 10, T 11

184
209
204 527

Fig. 208 Muscles of the neck.

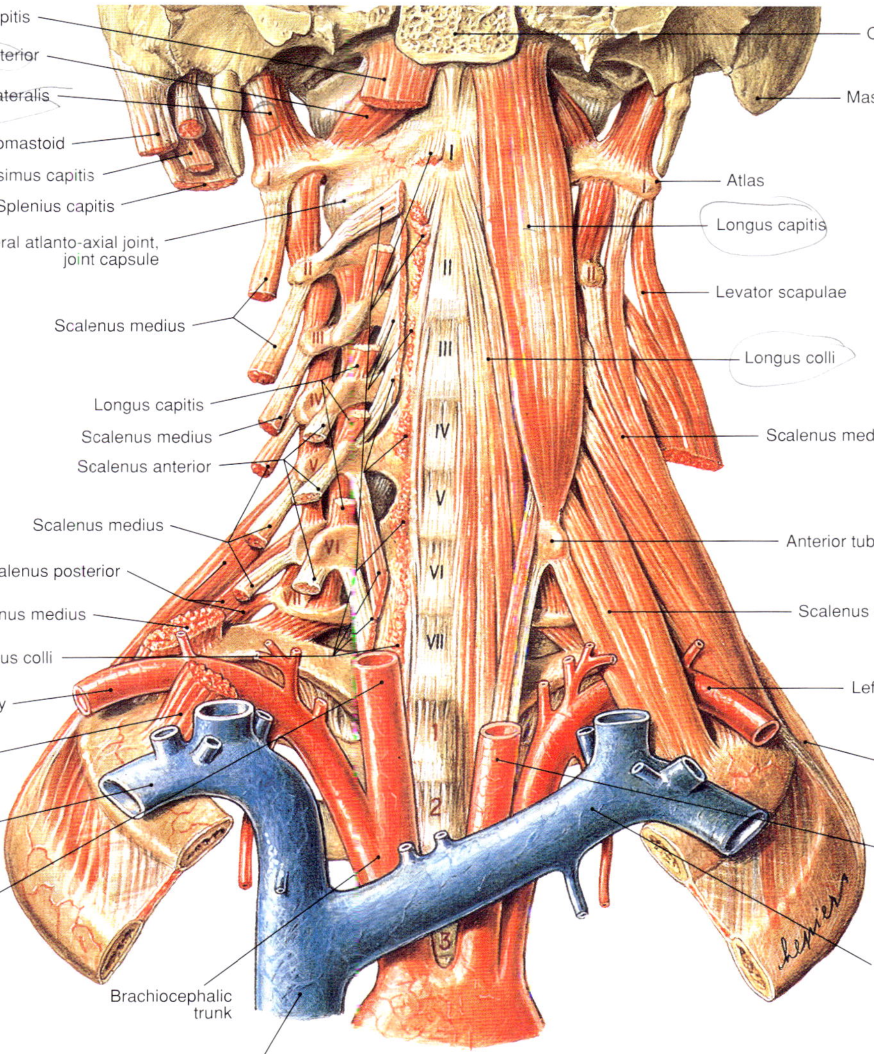

Fig. 209 Prevertebral muscles and scalenus muscles.
I – VII = First to seventh cervical vertebra
1 – 3 = First to third thoracic vertebra

→ T 11, T 12

Skeleton of the larynx

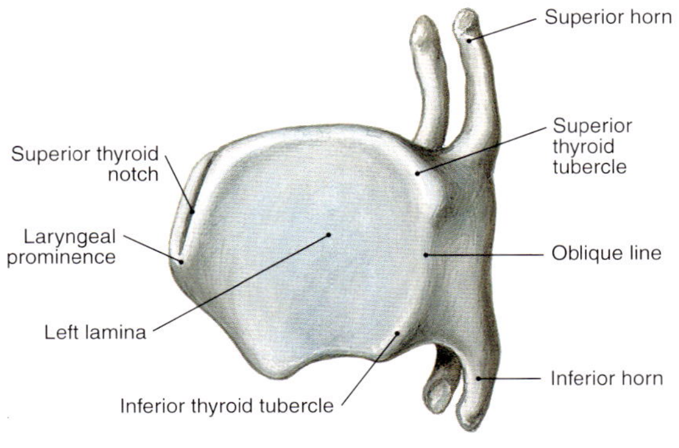

Fig. 210 Thyroid cartilage; viewed from the left.

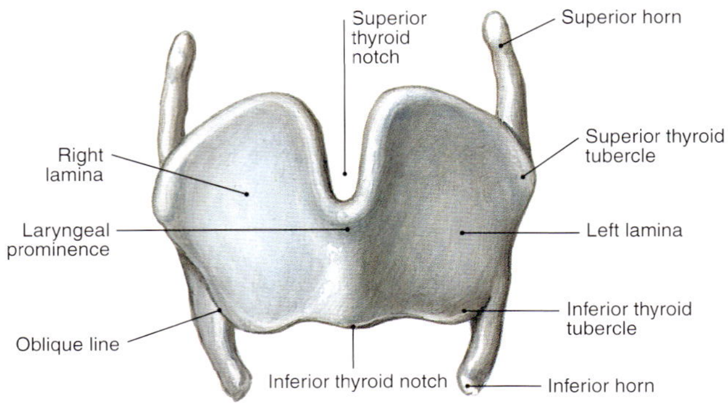

Fig. 211 Thyroid cartilage; ventral view.

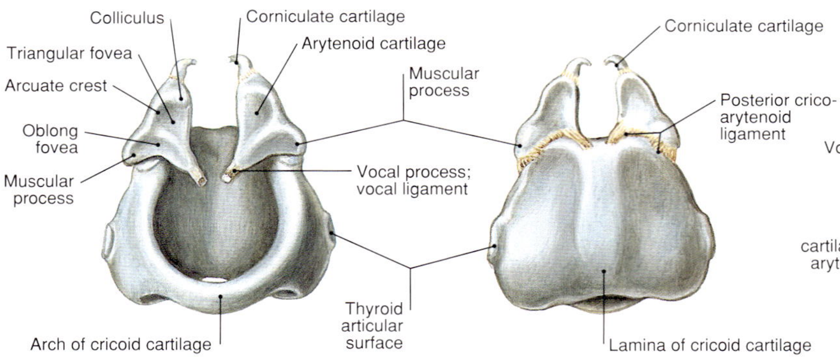

Fig. 212 Cartilages of the larynx; ventrosuperior view.

Fig. 213 Cartilages of the larynx; dorsal view.

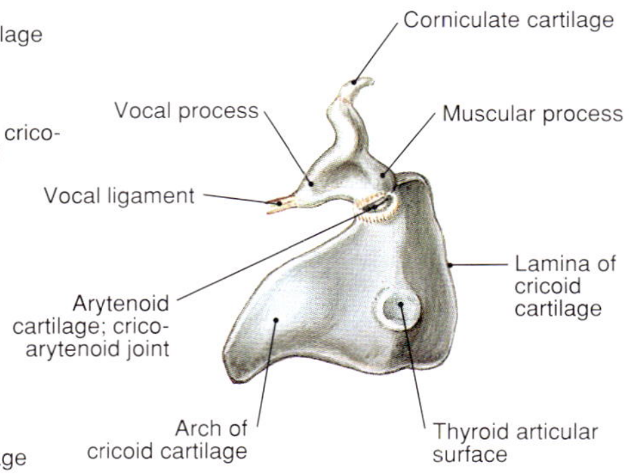

Fig. 214 Cartilages of the larynx; viewed from the left.

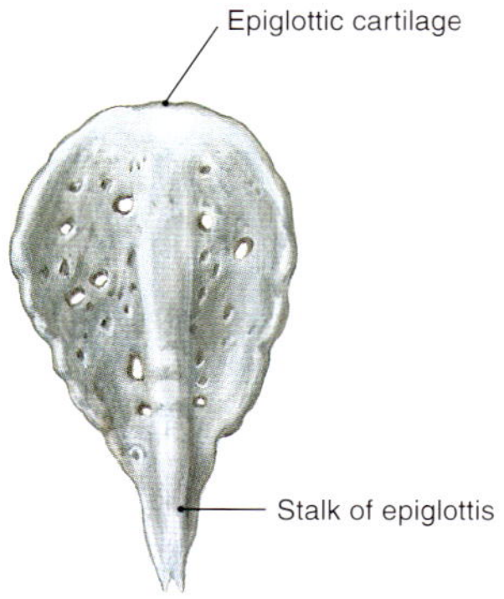

Fig. 215 Epiglottic cartilage; dorsal view.

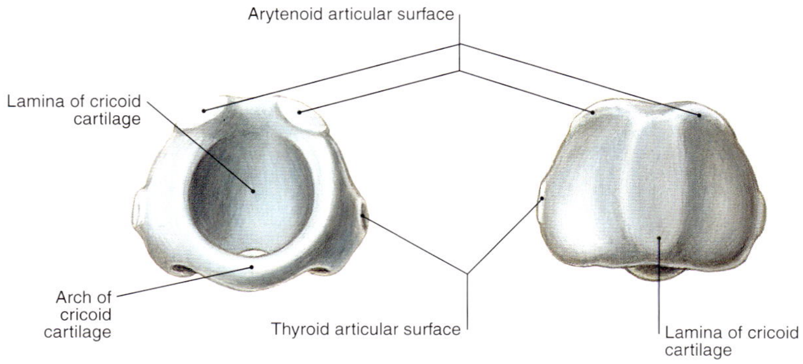

Fig. 216 Cricoid cartilage; ventrosuperior view.

Fig. 217 Cricoid cartilage; dorsal view.

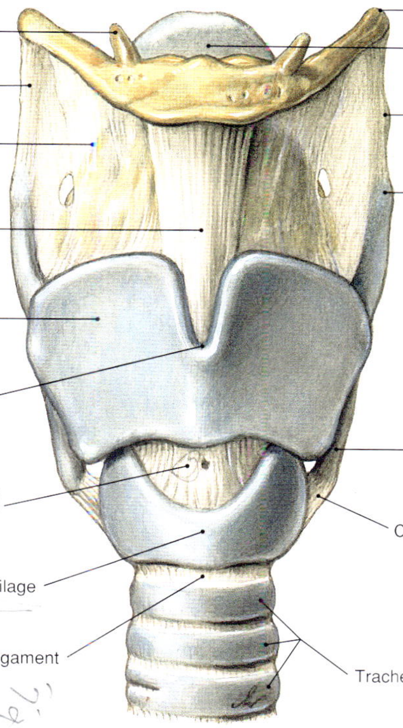

Fig. 218 Larynx and hyoid bone; ventral view.

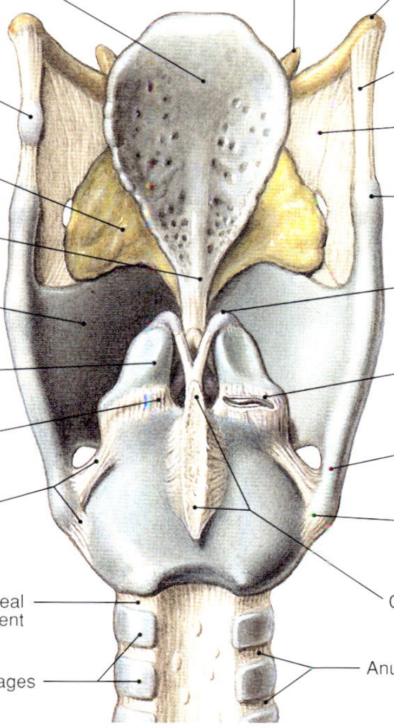

Fig. 219 Cartilages of the larynx and hyoid bone; dorsal view.

Hyoid bone and skeleton of the larynx

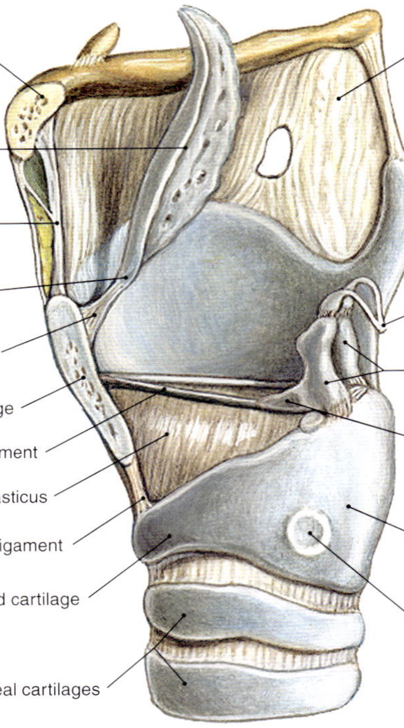

Fig. 220 Larynx and hyoid bone; viewed from the left.

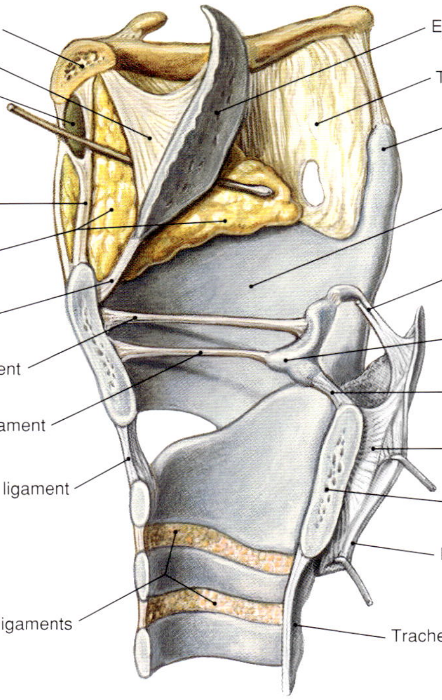

Fig. 221 Larynx and hyoid bone; median section; medial view.

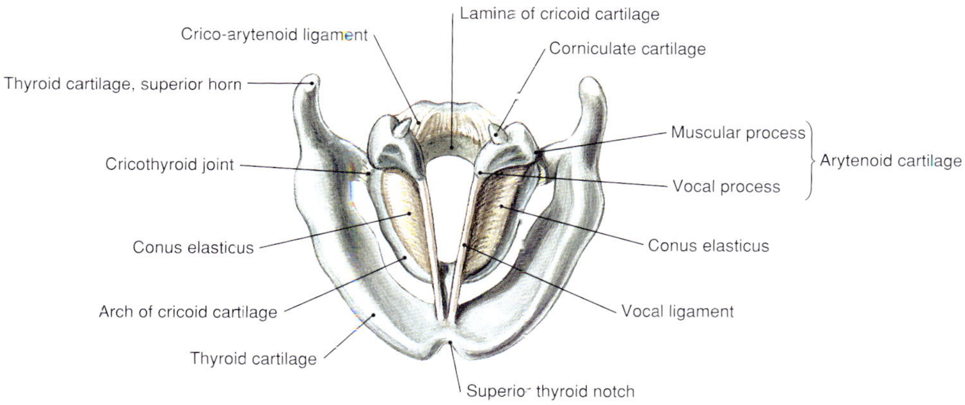

Fig. 222 Cartilages of the larynx and vocal ligament; ventrosuperior view.

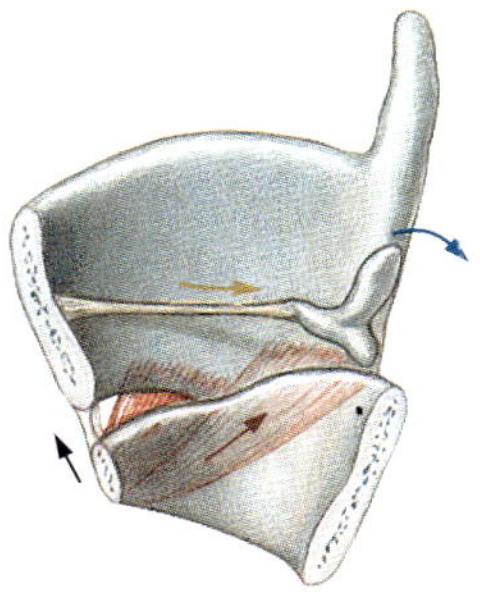

a Cricothyroid muscle

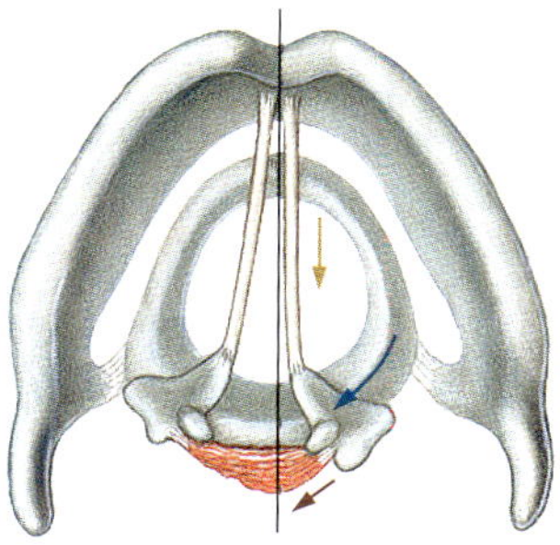

b Oblique and transverse arytenoid muscles

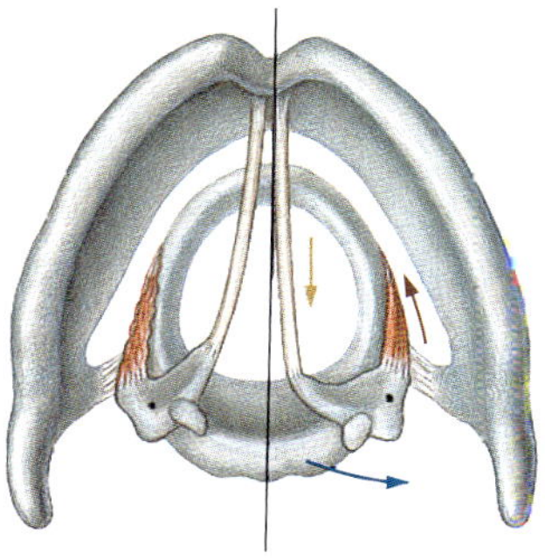

c Lateral crico-arytenoid muscle

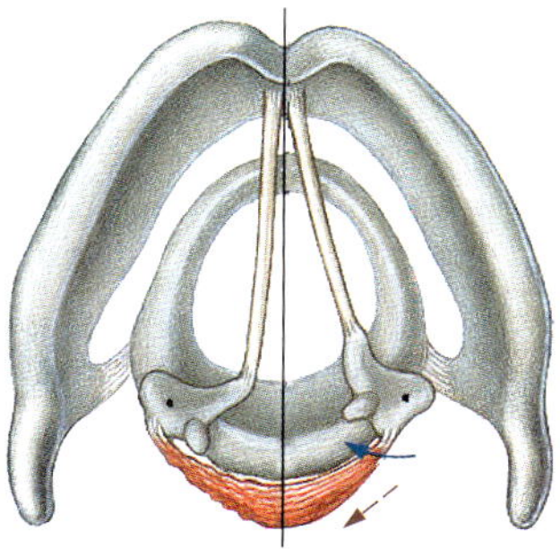

d Posterior crico-arytenoid muscle

Fig. 223 a–d Schema showing the functions of the laryngeal muscles;
yellow arrows: tension of the vocal ligament;
red arrows: muscle contraction;
blue arrows: direction of rotation;
the muscles on the left are relaxed; those on the right are contracted;
superior view.

Hyoid bone and skeleton of the larynx

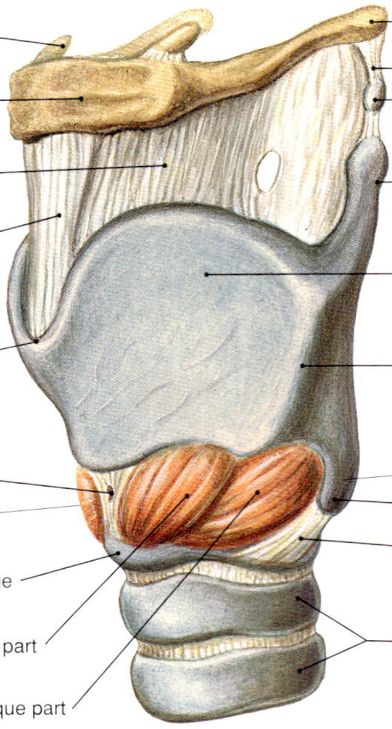

→ T 6

Fig. 224 Cricothyroid muscle; ventral view from the left.

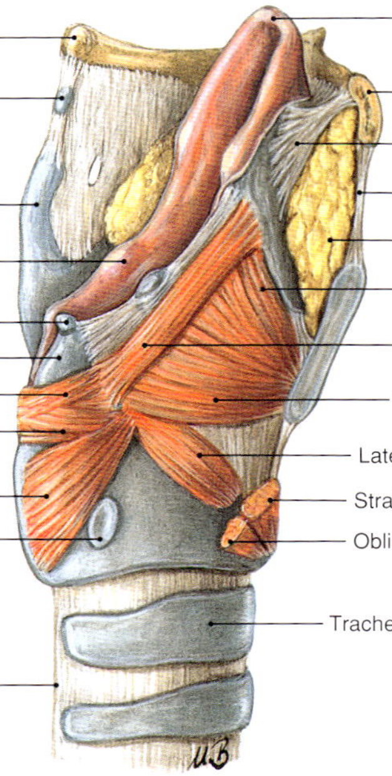

→ T 6

Fig. 225 Laryngeal muscles; dorsal view from the right.

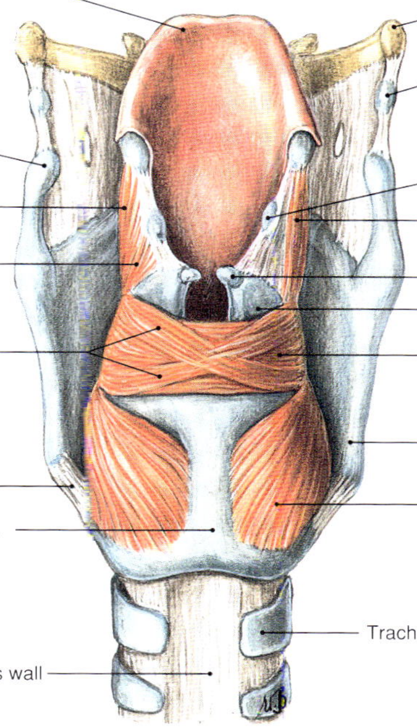

Fig. 226 Laryngeal muscles;
dorsal view.

→ T 6

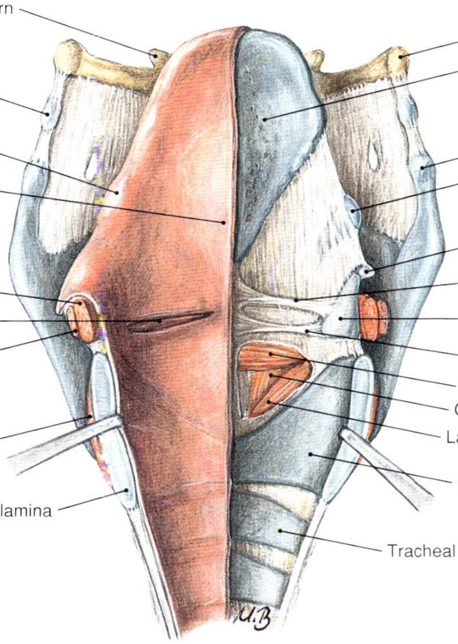

Fig. 227 Larynx;
sectioned from dorsal in the median plane and separated with hooks;
dorsal view.

→ T 6

Laryngoscopy

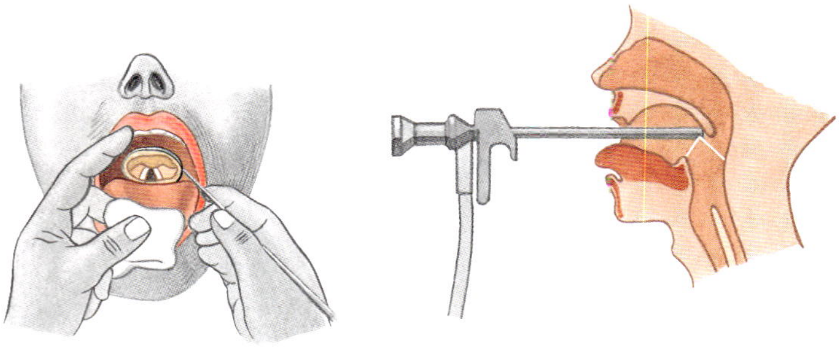

a b

Fig. 228 a, b Laryngoscopy.
a Indirect laryngoscopy
b Direct, endoscopic laryngoscopy

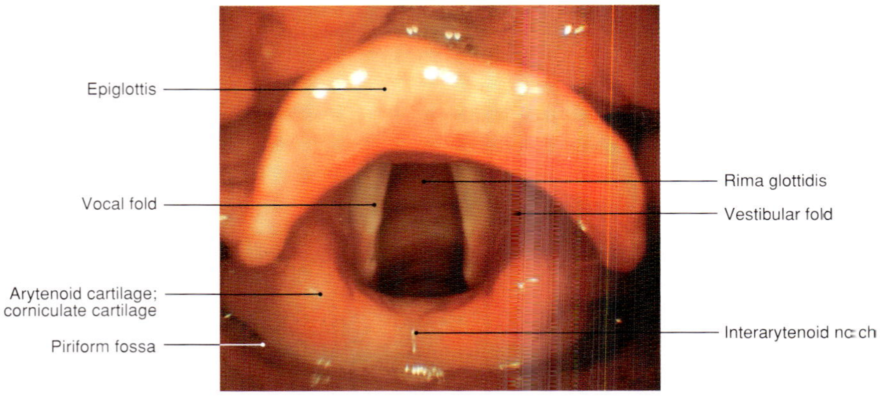

Fig. 229 Direct laryngoscopy; respiratory position.

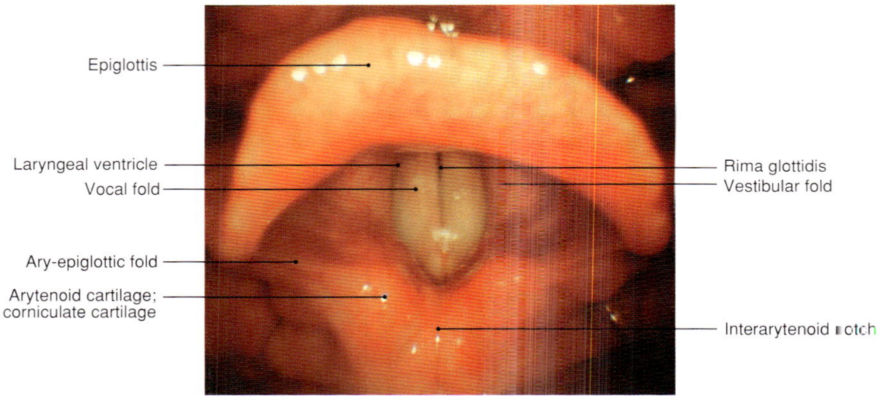

Fig. 230 Direct laryngoscopy; phonation position.

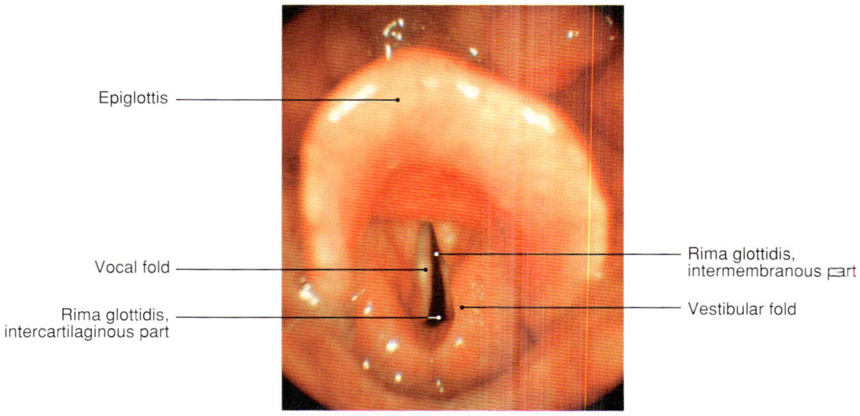

Fig. 231 Direct laryngoscopy; whispering position.

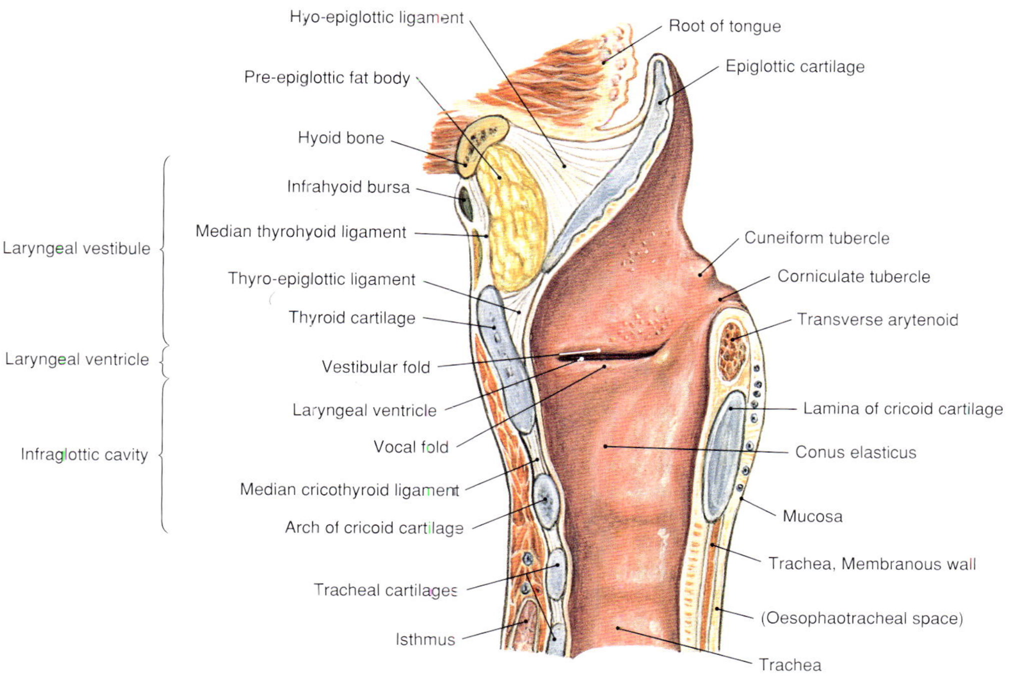

Fig. 232 Larynx.

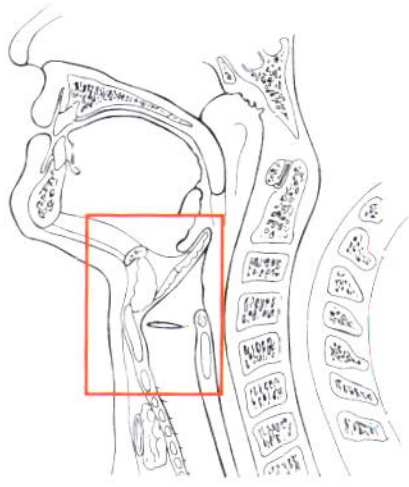

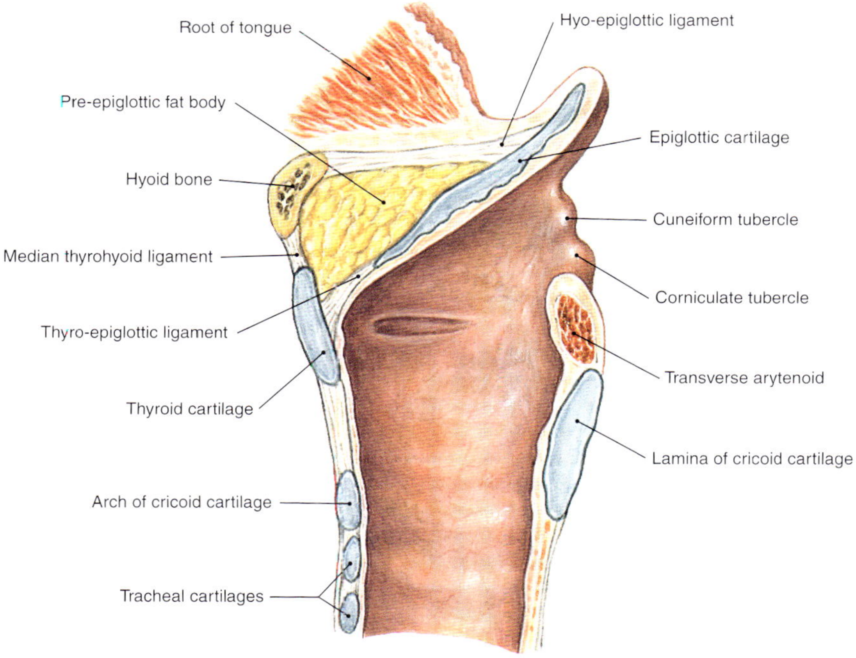

Fig. 233 Larynx;
position of the epiglottis during swallowing.

Arteries and nerves of the larynx

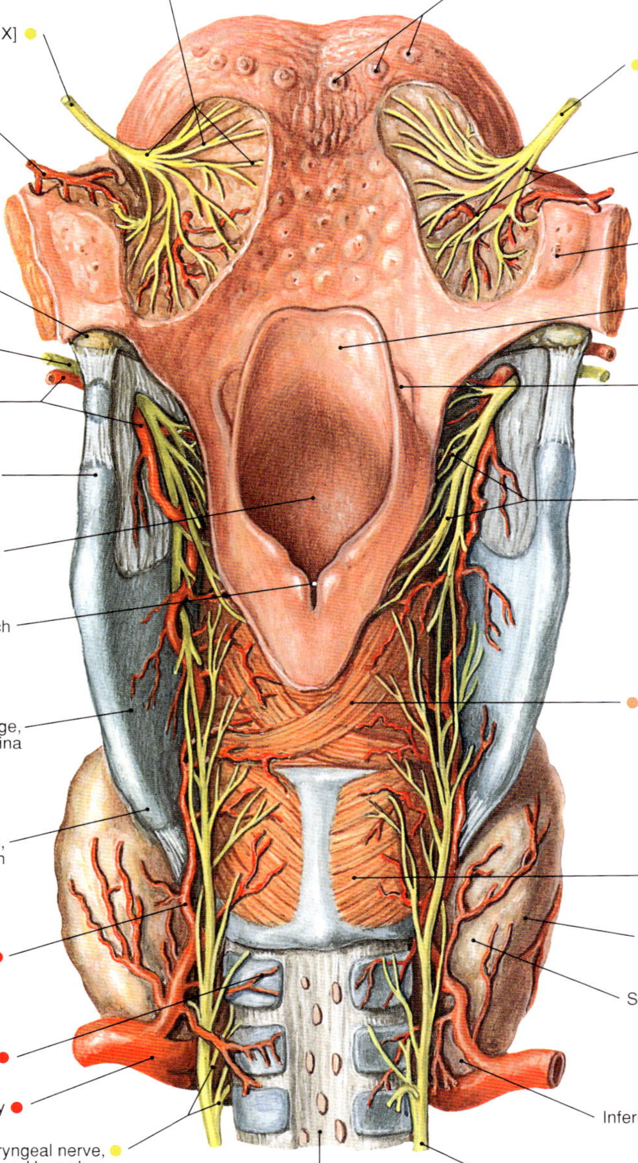

→ 252

Fig. 234 Arteries and nerves of the larynx and the root of the tongue.

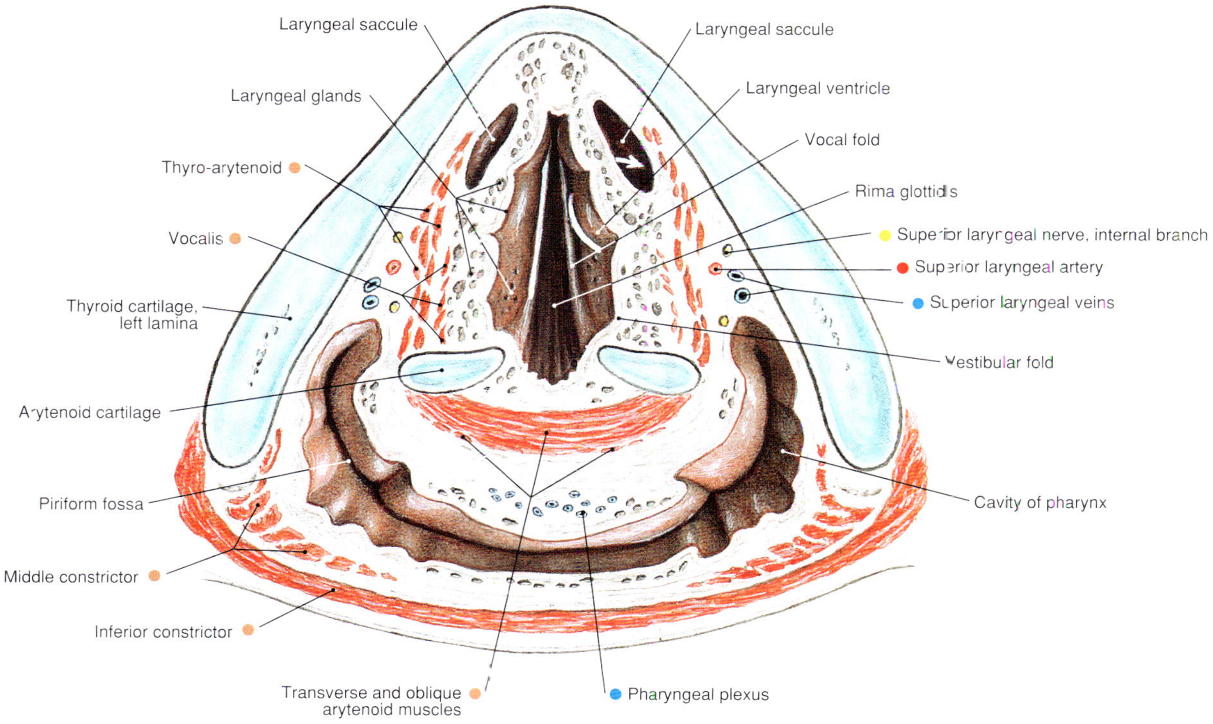

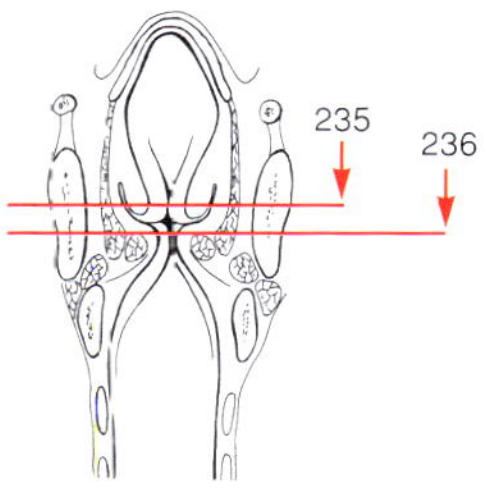

Fig. 235 Larynx.
The white arrow indicates the connection between the laryngeal ventricle and the laryngeal saccule.

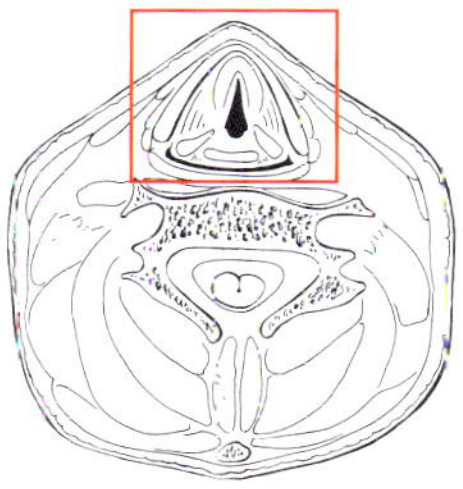

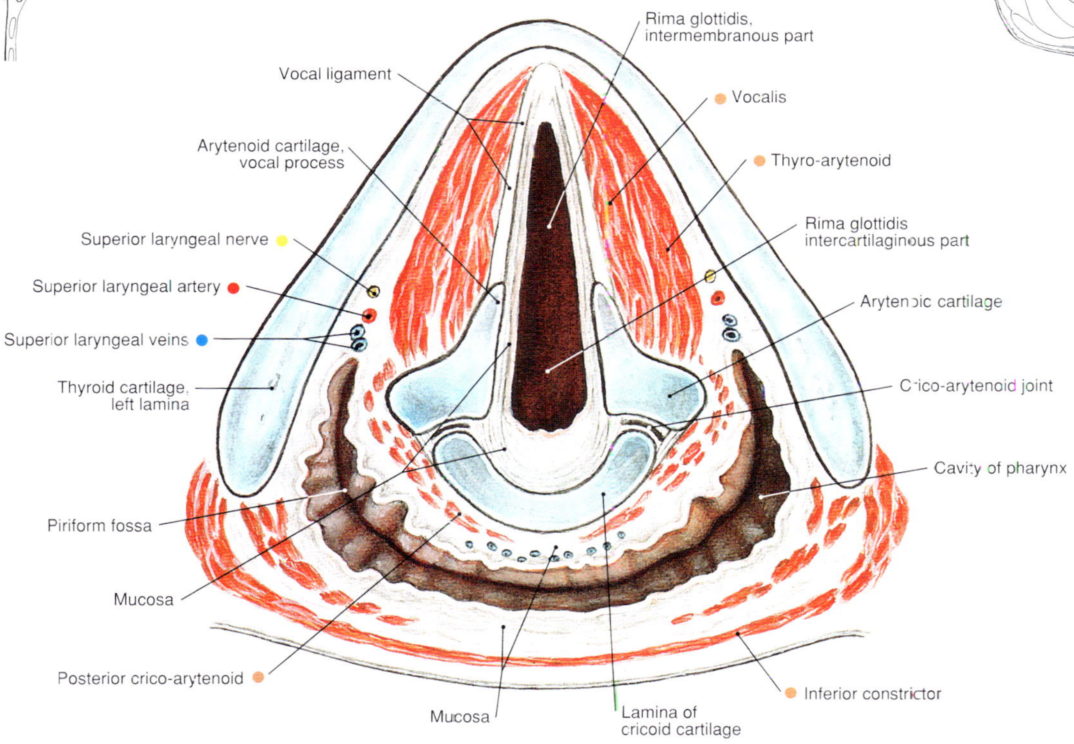

Fig. 236 Larynx.

Thyroid gland

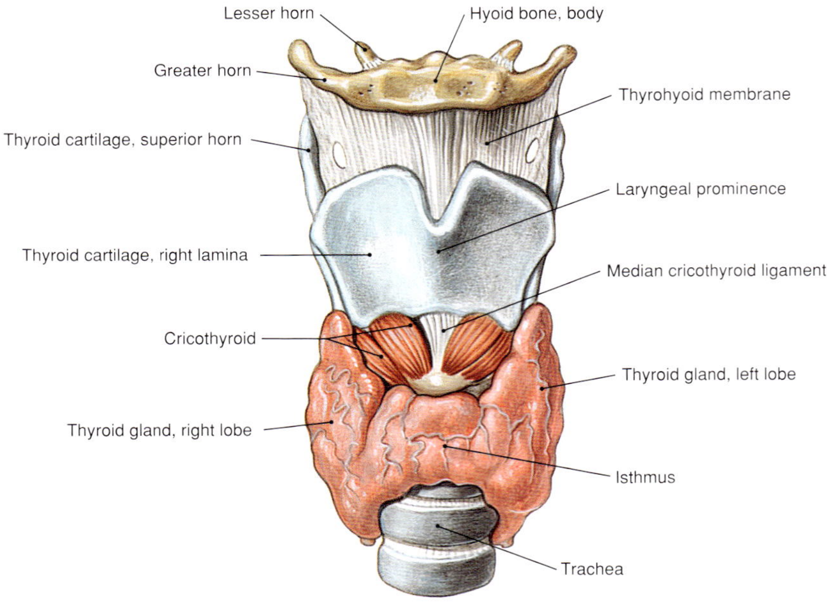

→ 205

Fig. 237 Thyroid gland and larynx.

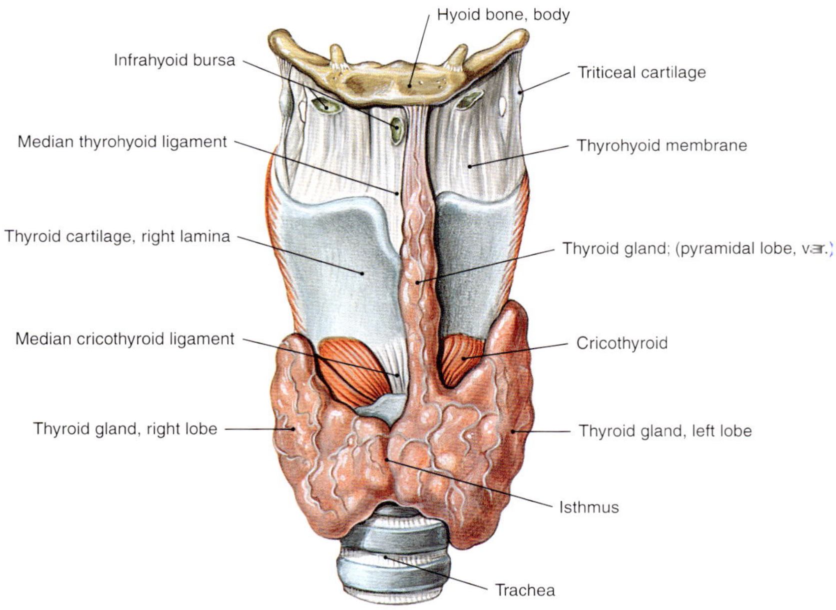

Fig. 238 Thyroid gland and larynx.

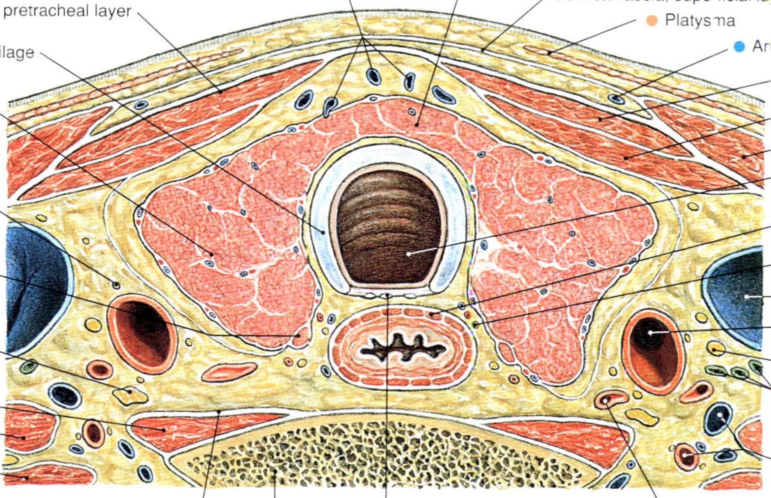

Fig. 239 Thyroid gland; horizontal section.

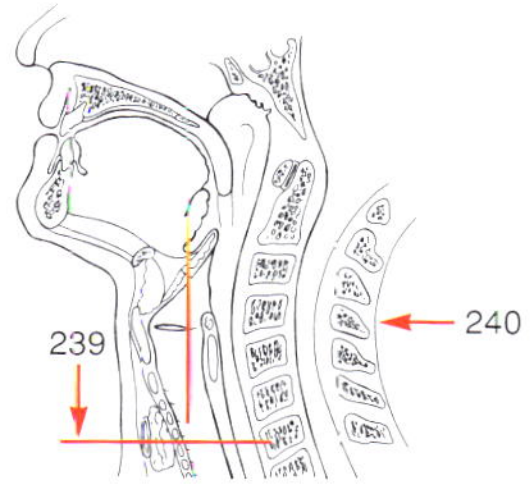

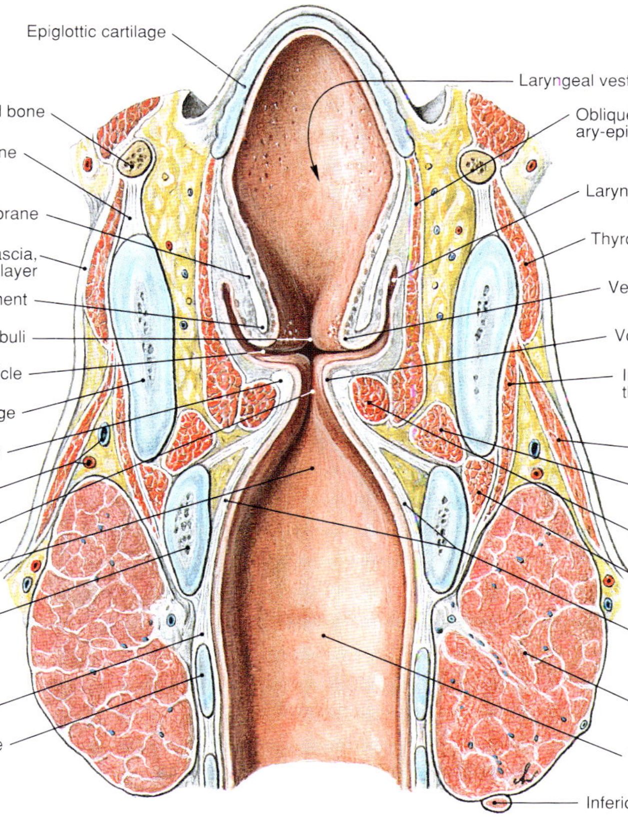

Fig. 240 Thyroid gland; frontal section.

Arterial supply of the thyroid gland

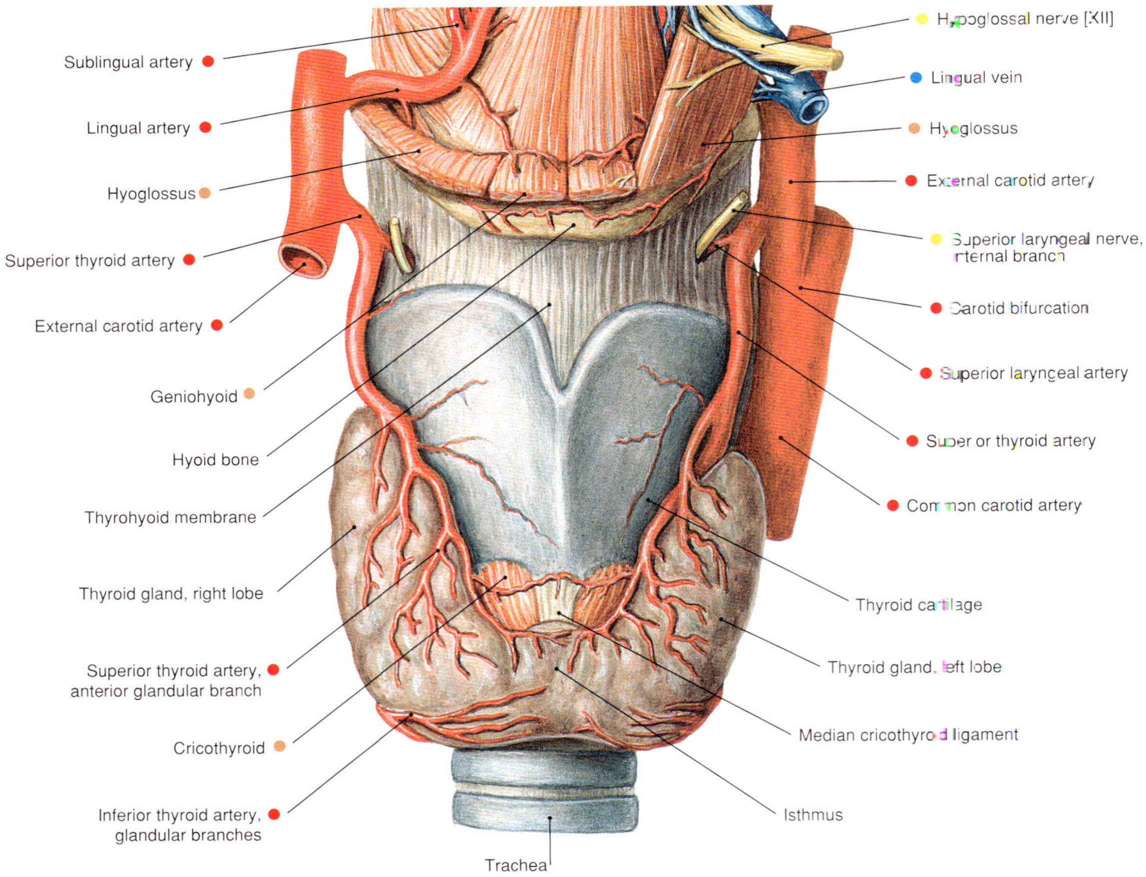

Fig. 241 Vessels and nerves of the thyroid gland and the larynx.

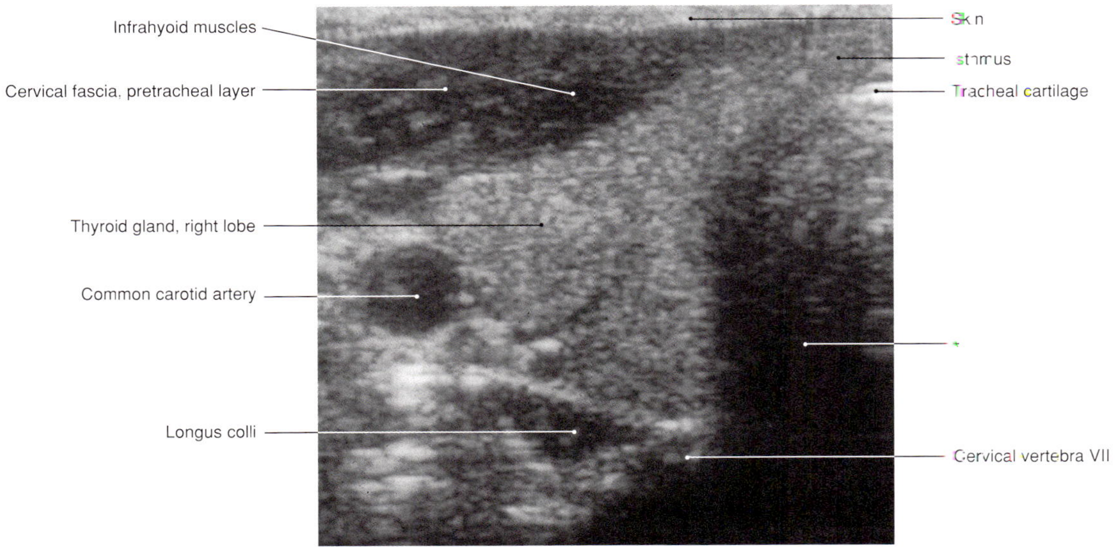

Fig. 242 Thyroid gland; oblique ultrasound image in ventrodorsal direction; inferior view (right, 200%).

* Ultrasound shadow of the trachea

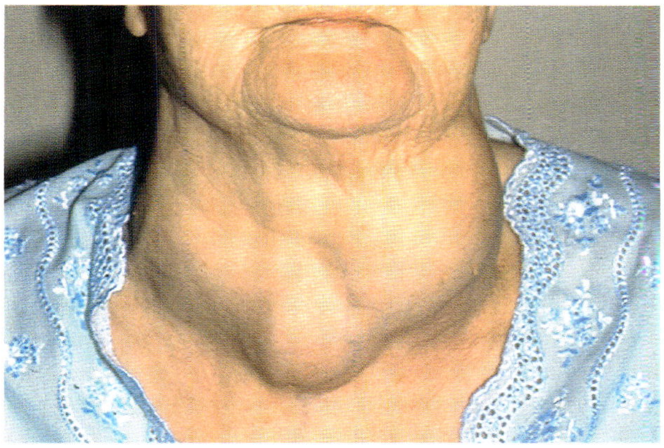

Fig. 243 Thyroid gland;
enlargement of the thyroid gland with three obvious nodes, Struma nodosa.

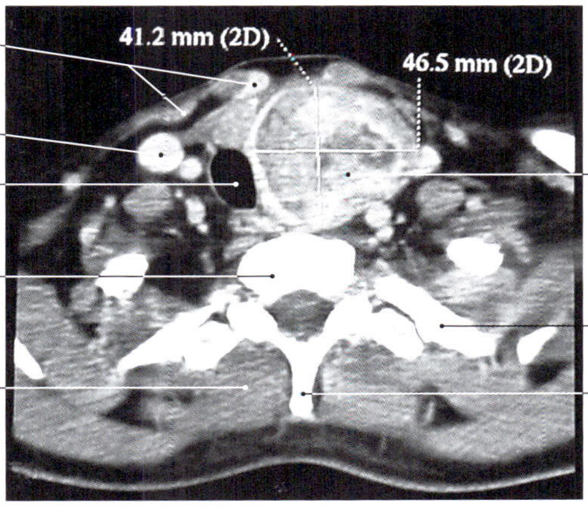

Fig. 244 Neck;
computed tomographic (CT) section;
inferior view.
The trachea is displaced towards the right by a pathologically enlarged node of the thyroid gland.

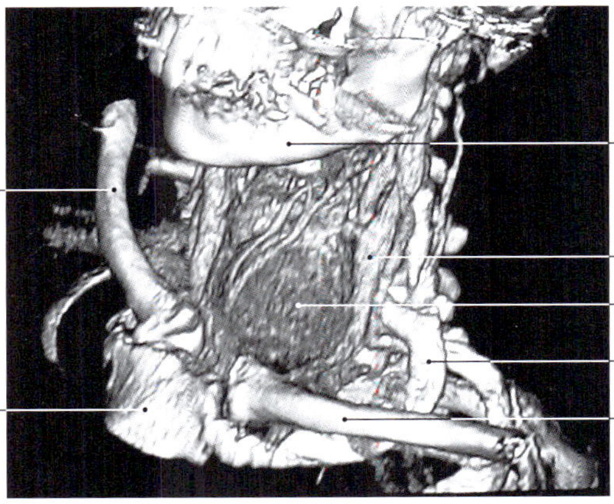

Fig. 245 Neck;
3-dimensional reconstruction from computed tomographic (CT) sections showing a heavily enlarged left lobe of the thyroid gland;
same patient as in Fig. 244.

Nasal and pharyngeal cavity, paramedian section

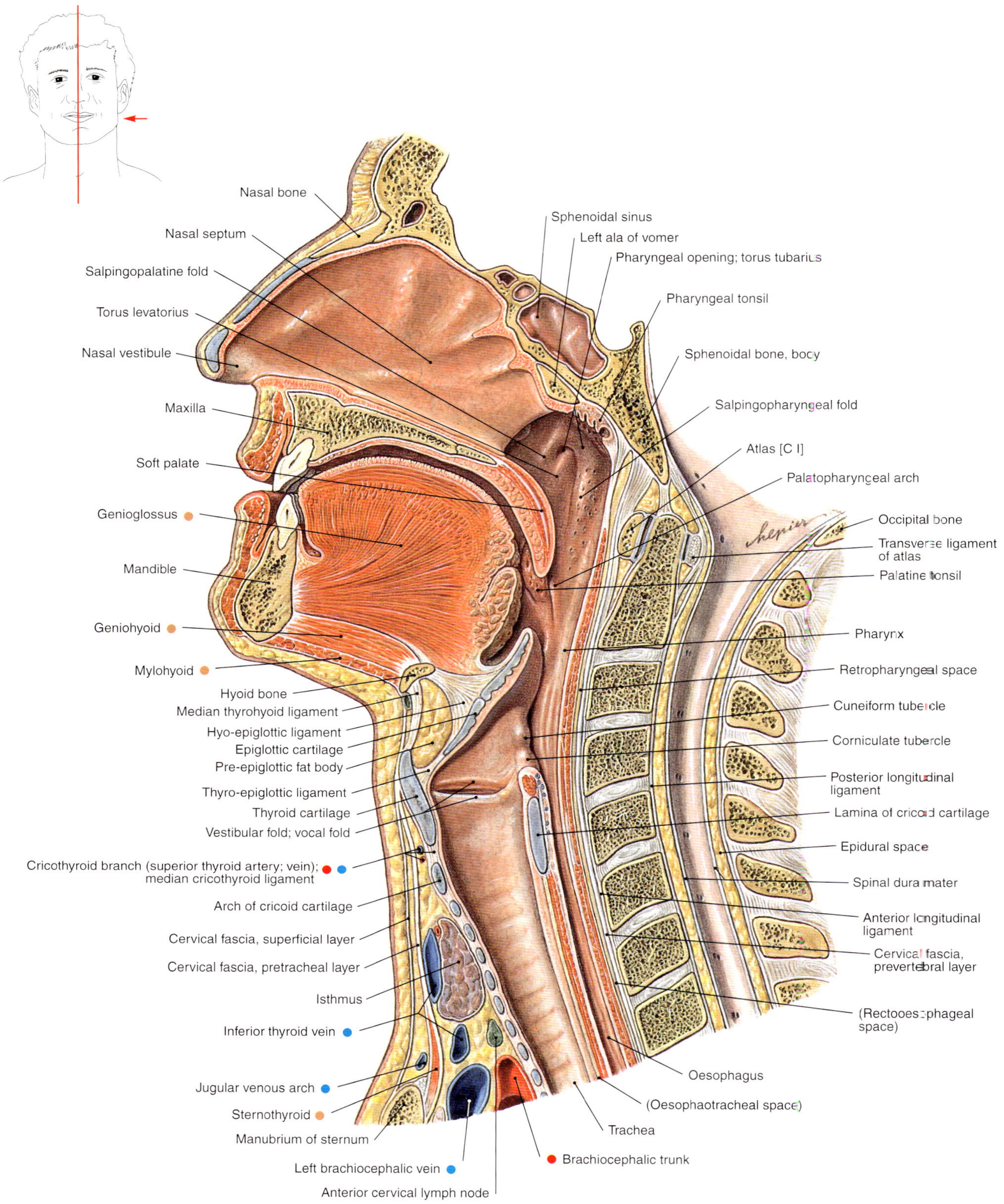

→ 271

Fig. 246 Nasal cavity; oral cavity; pharynx and larynx; paramedian section.

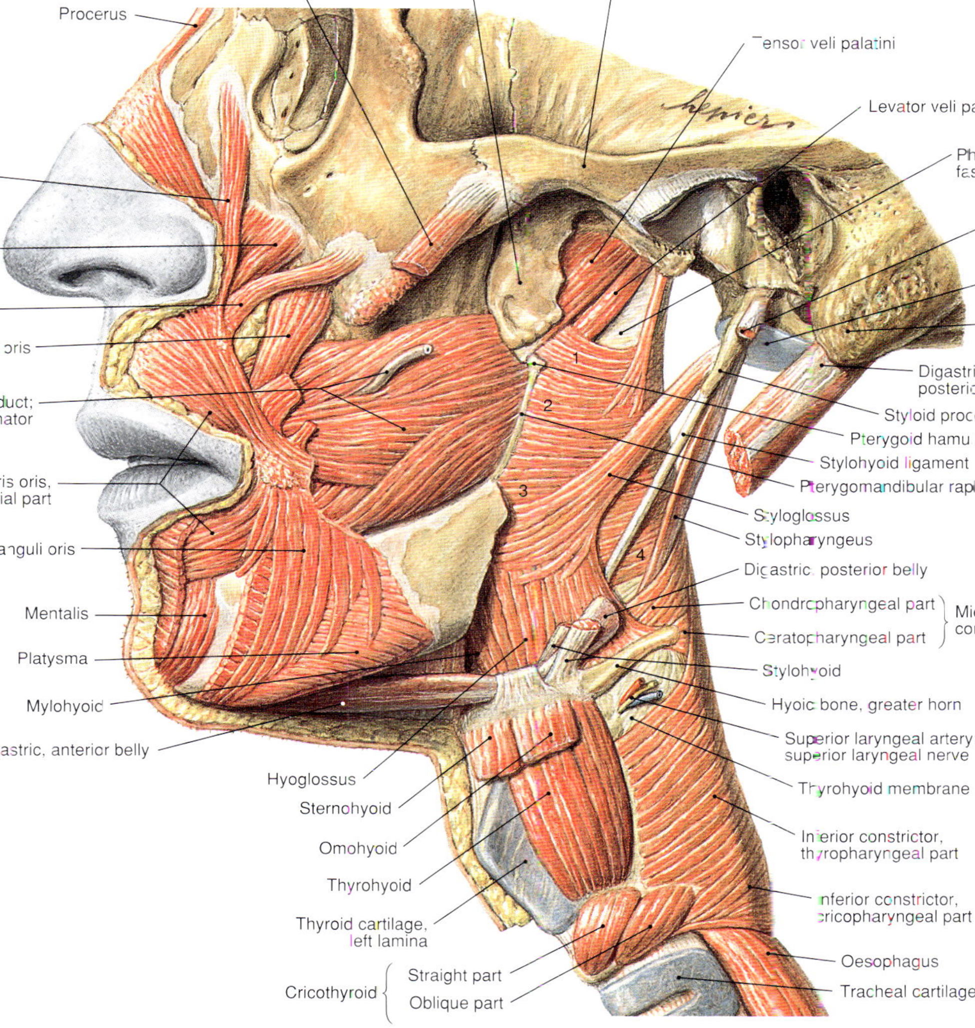

1 Pterygopharyngeal part
2 Buccopharyngeal part
3 Mylopharyngeal part
4 Glossopharyngeal part
} Superior constrictor

Fig. 247 Pharyngeal muscles and facial muscles.

→ T 1e, f, T 5

Pharyngeal muscles

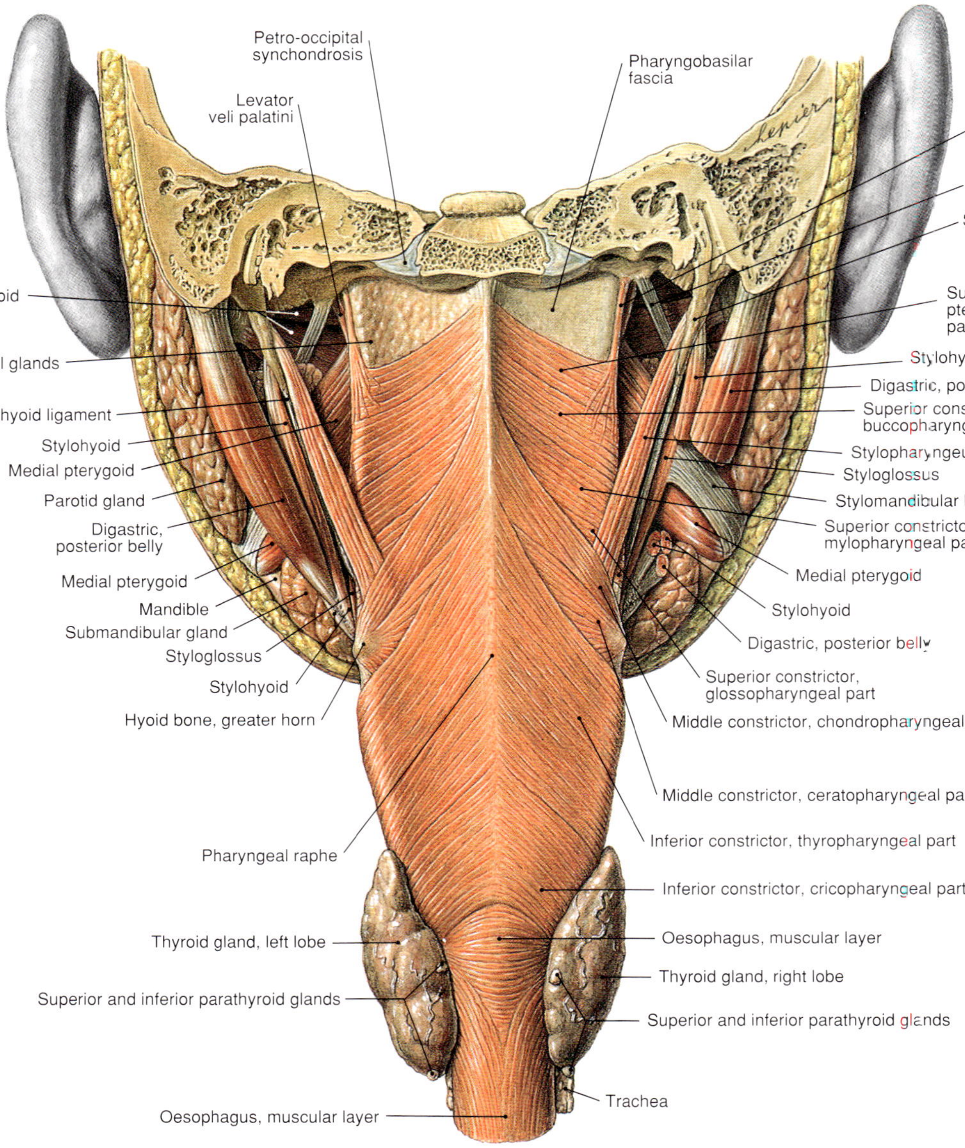

→ T 5

Fig. 248 Pharyngeal muscles.

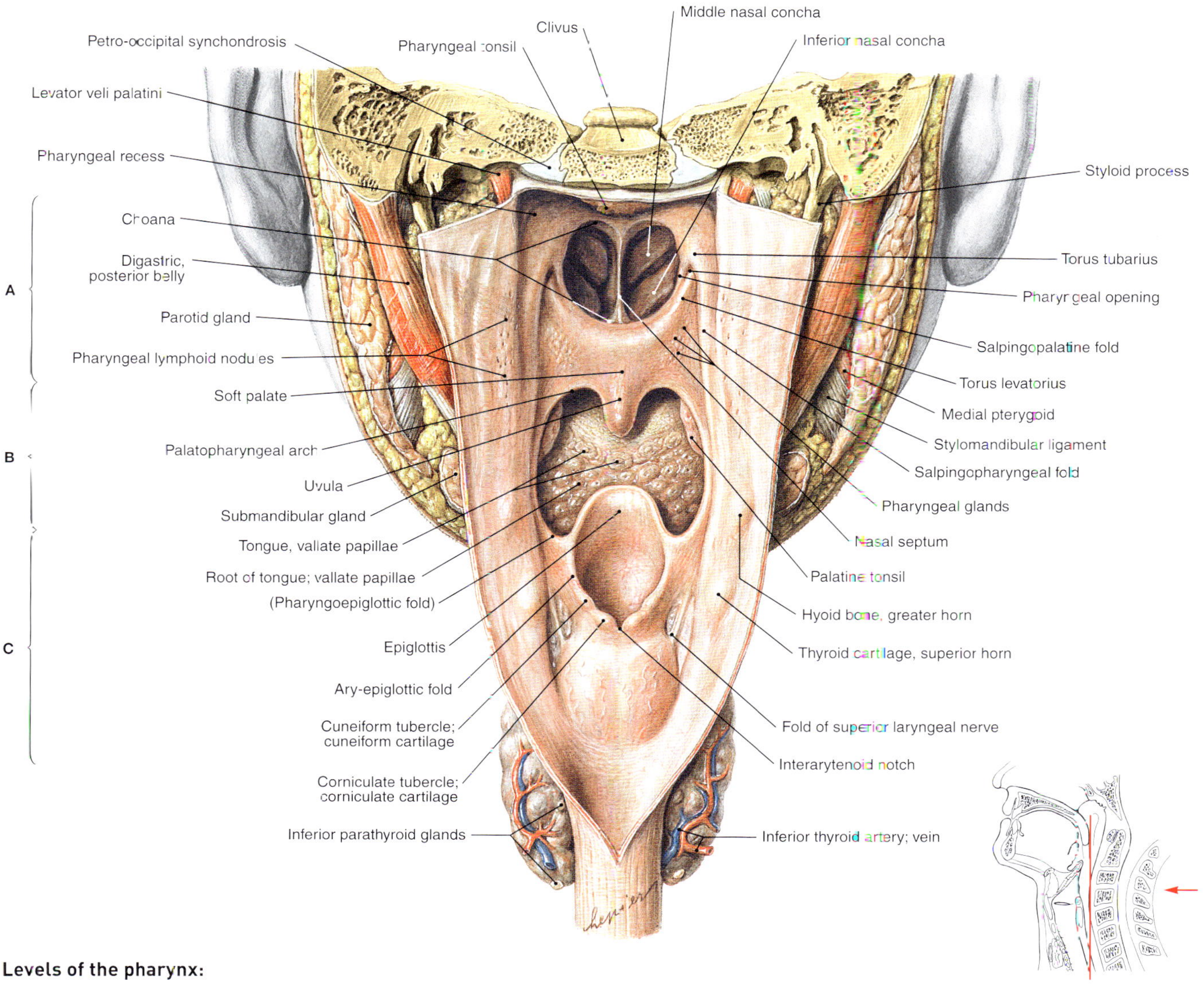

Levels of the pharynx:

A Nasopharynx
B Oropharynx
C Laryngopharynx, hypopharynx

Fig. 249 Pharynx.

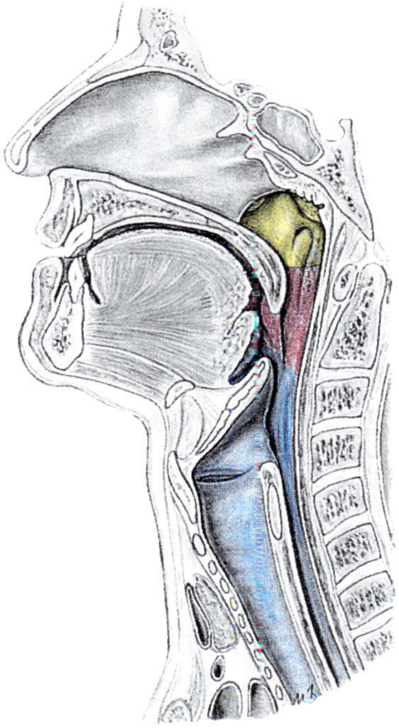

Maxillary nerve [V/2]
Glossopharyngeal nerve [IX]
Vagus nerve [X]

Fig. 250 Sensible innervation of the pharynx.

▸▸ Surface p. 32 | Skeleton p. 264 ff.

Vessels and nerves of the parapharyngeal space

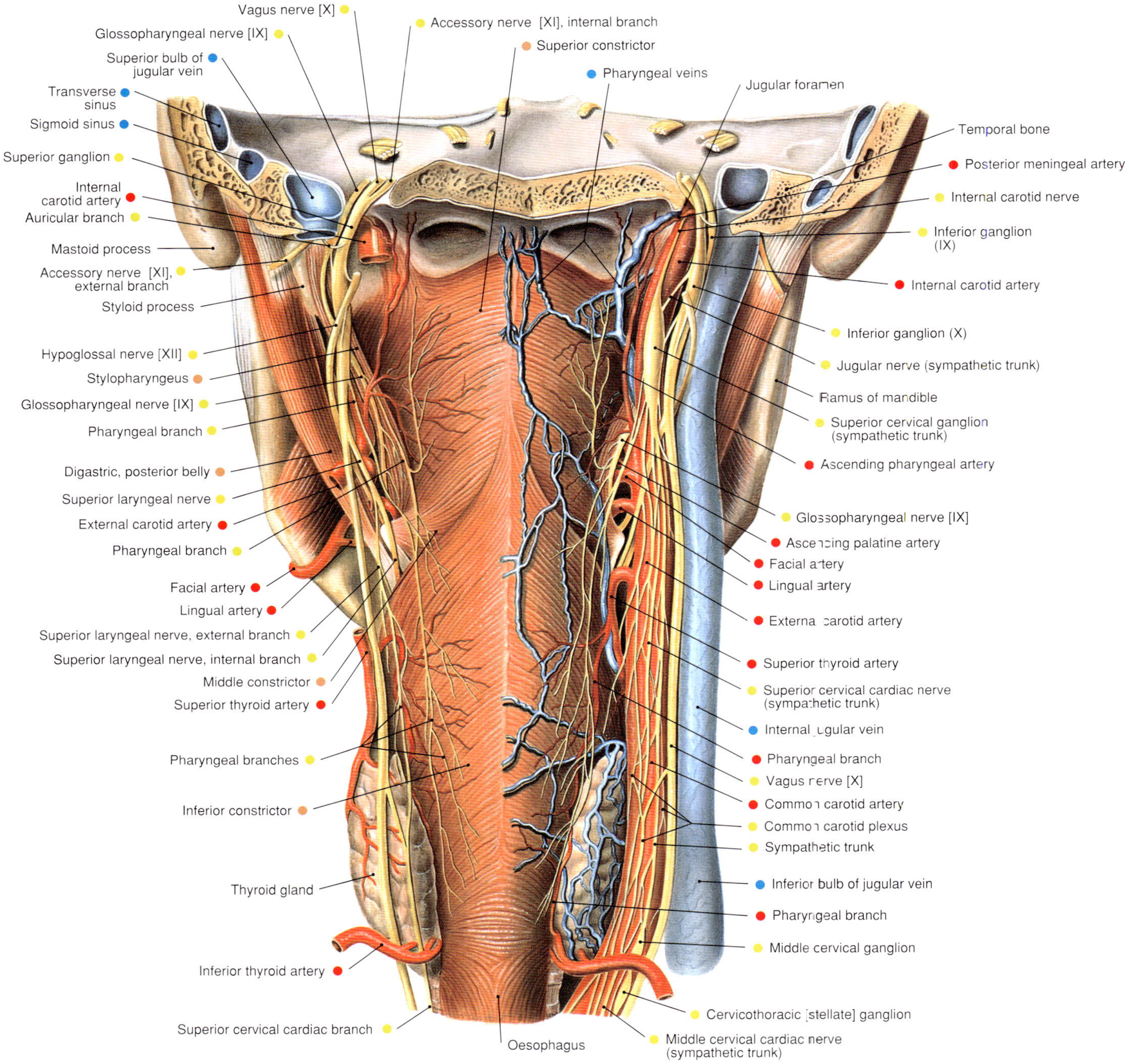

252
669

Fig. 251 Vessels and nerves of the pharynx and the parapharyngeal space.

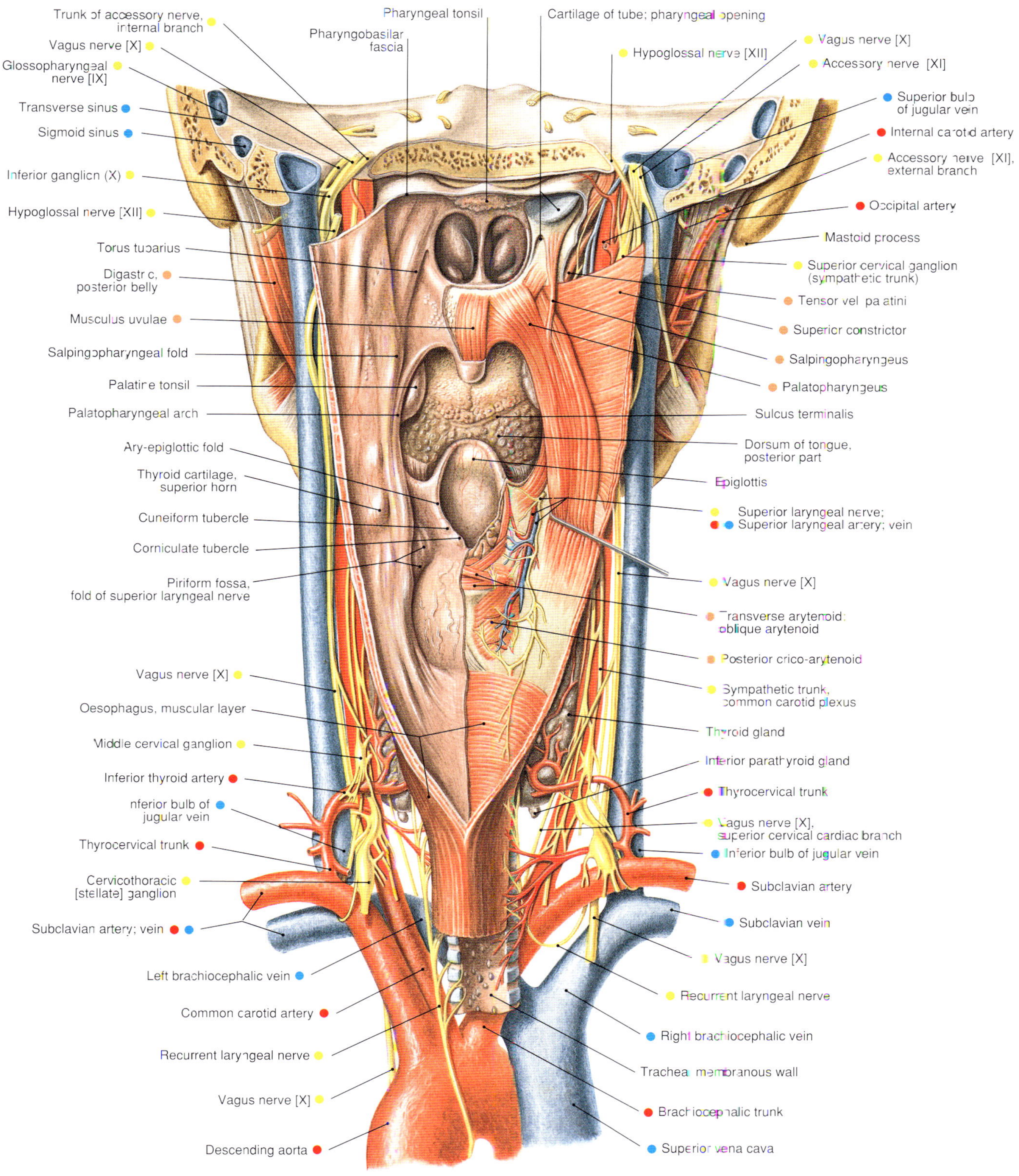

Fig. 252 Vessels and nerves of the pharynx and the parapharyngeal space.

234
251
669

Vessels and nerves of the neck

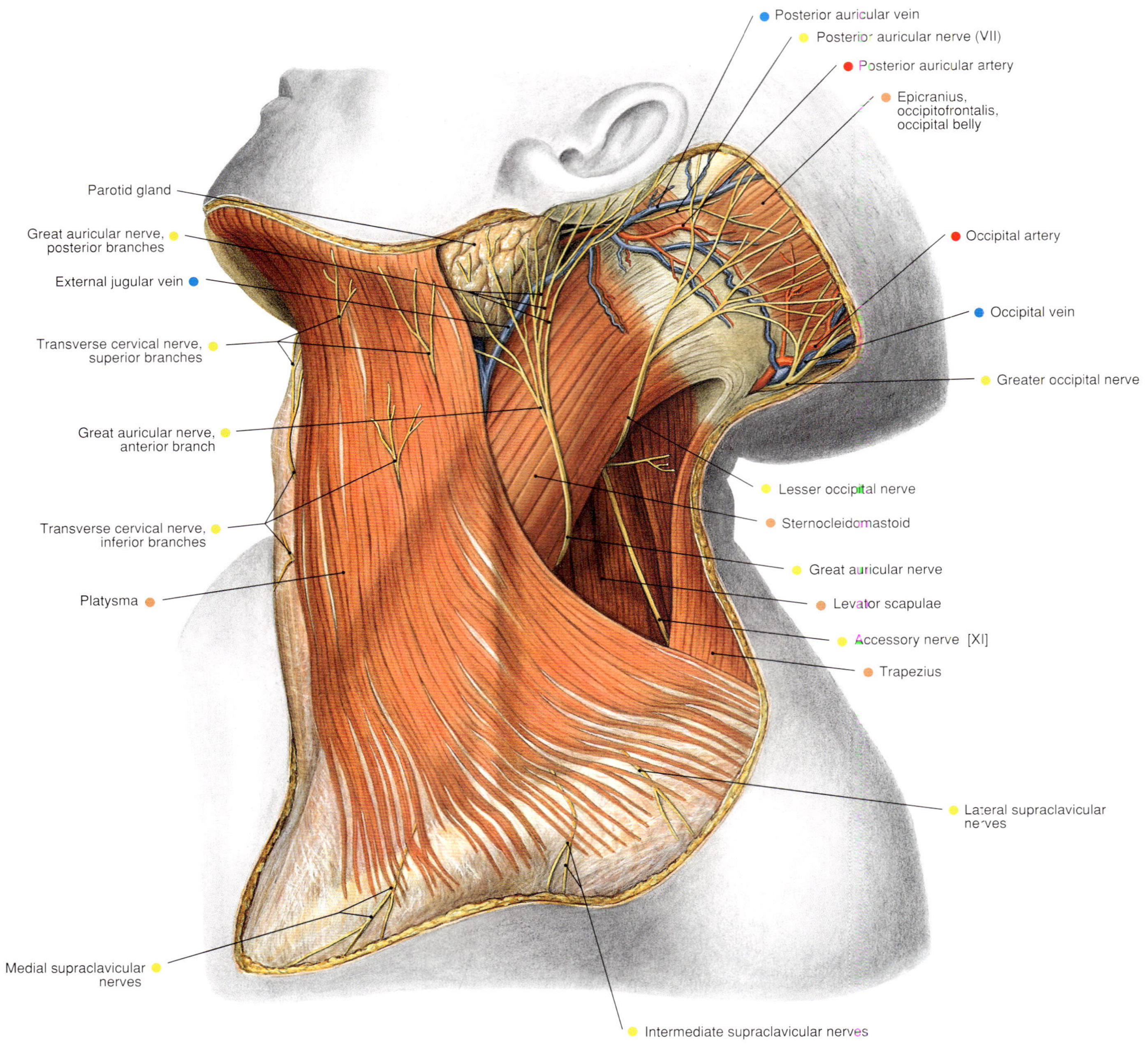

→ 46, T 7

Fig. 253 Vessels and nerves of the anterior and the lateral region of the neck; superficial layer.

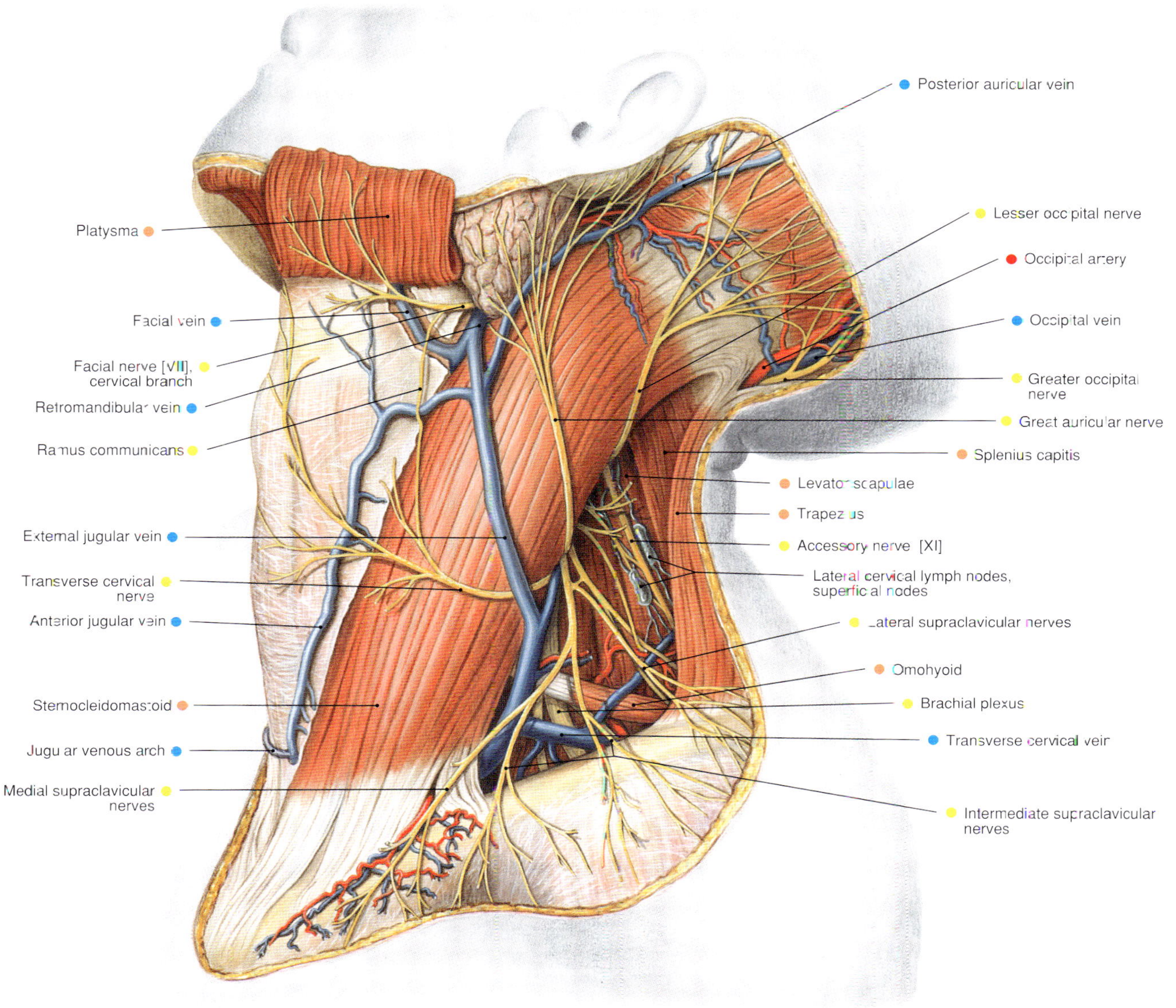

→ 46, T 7

121
255
253

Fig. 254 Vessels and nerves of the lateral region of the neck; parts of the platysma have been reflected cranially and the superficial layer of the cervical fascia has been largely removed.

Vessels and nerves of the neck

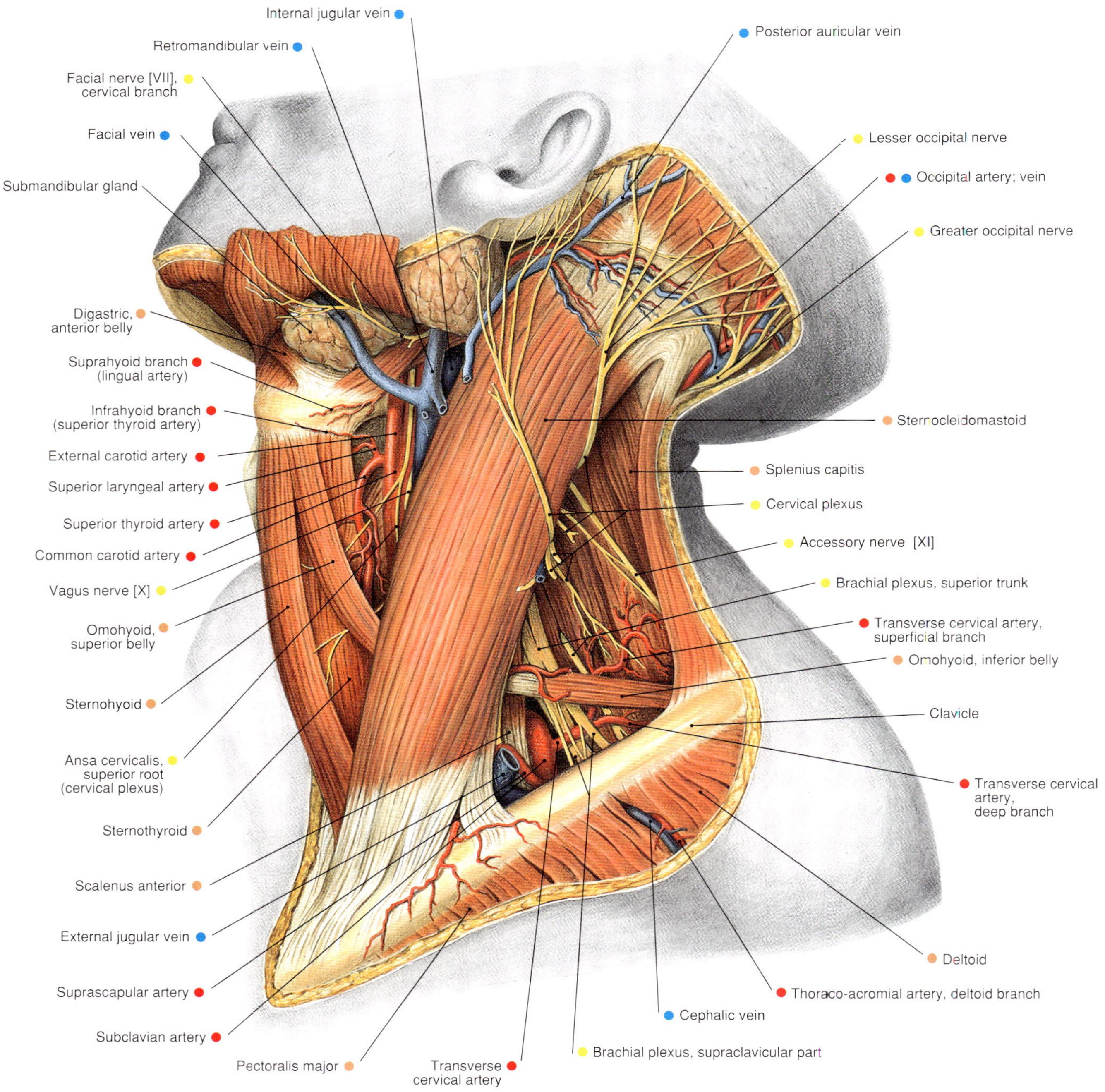

→ 46, T 7

121
254

Fig. 255 Vessels and nerves of the anterior and the lateral region of the neck; the superficial and the middle layer of the cervical fascia have been removed.

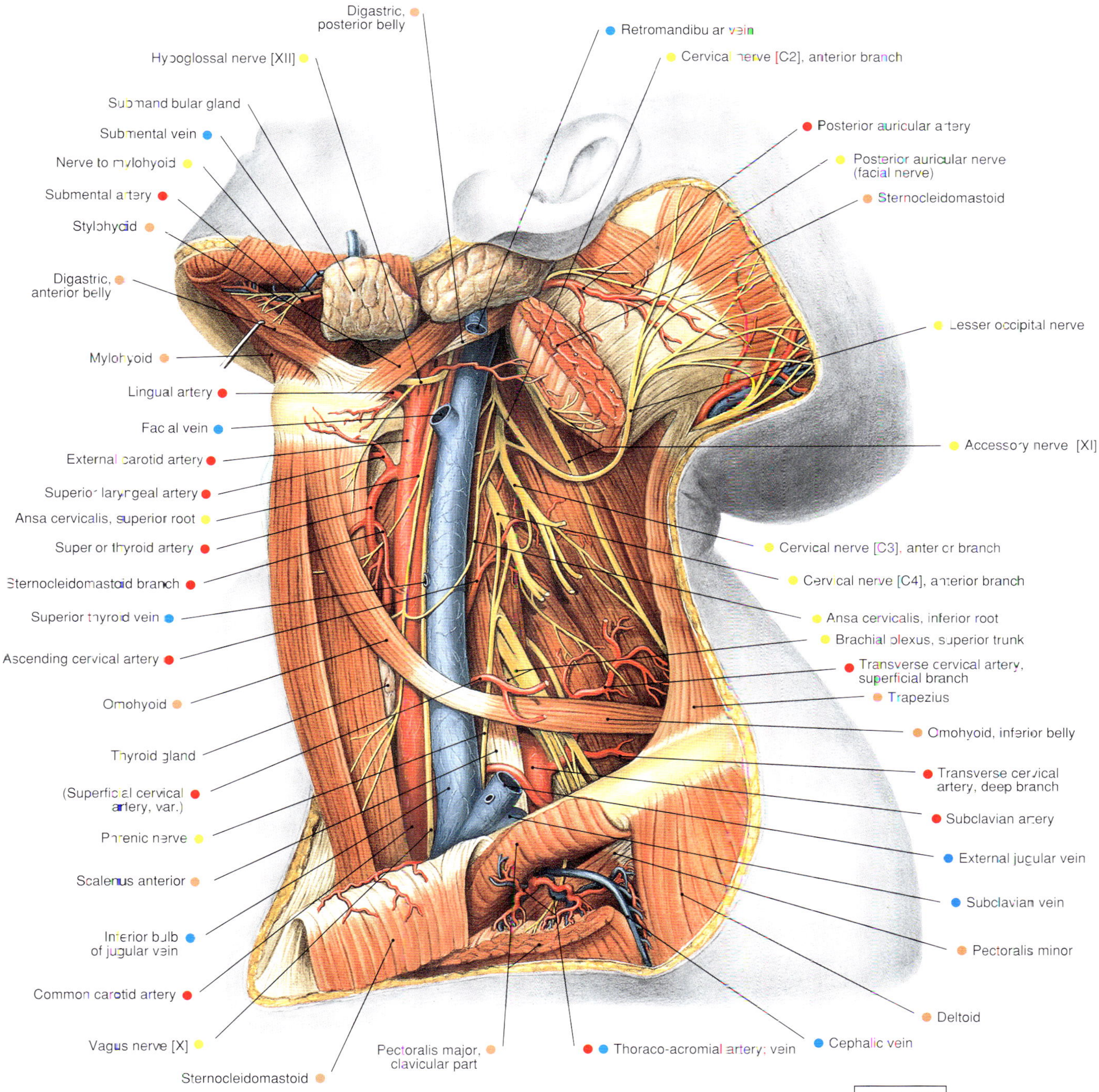

→ 46, T 7

Fig. 256 Vessels and nerves of the lateral region of the neck; after almost complete removal of the sternocleidomastoid muscle.

257
255

Vessels and nerves of the neck

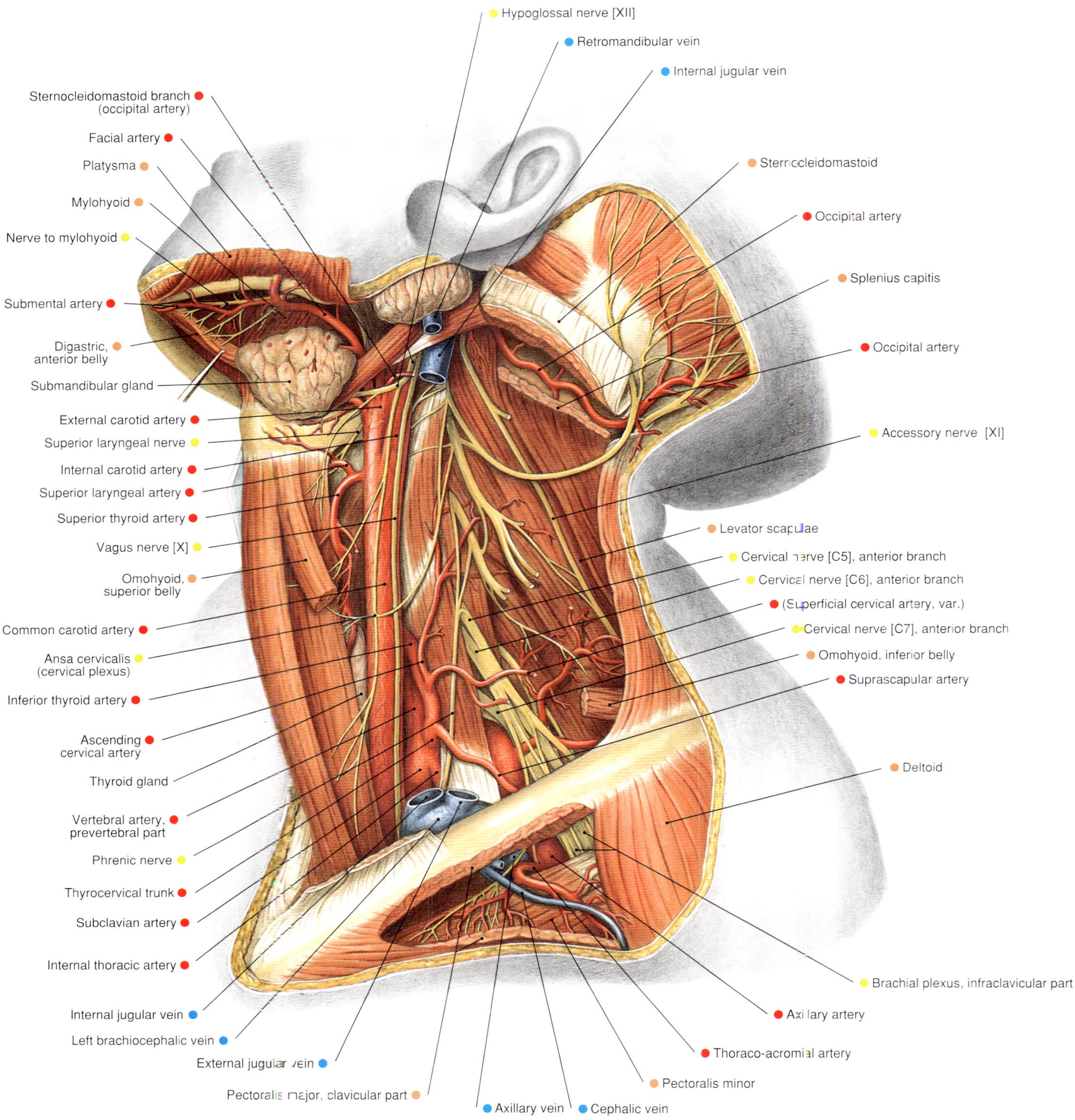

→ 46, T 7

258
256

Fig. 257 Vessels and nerves of the lateral region of the neck; deep layer.

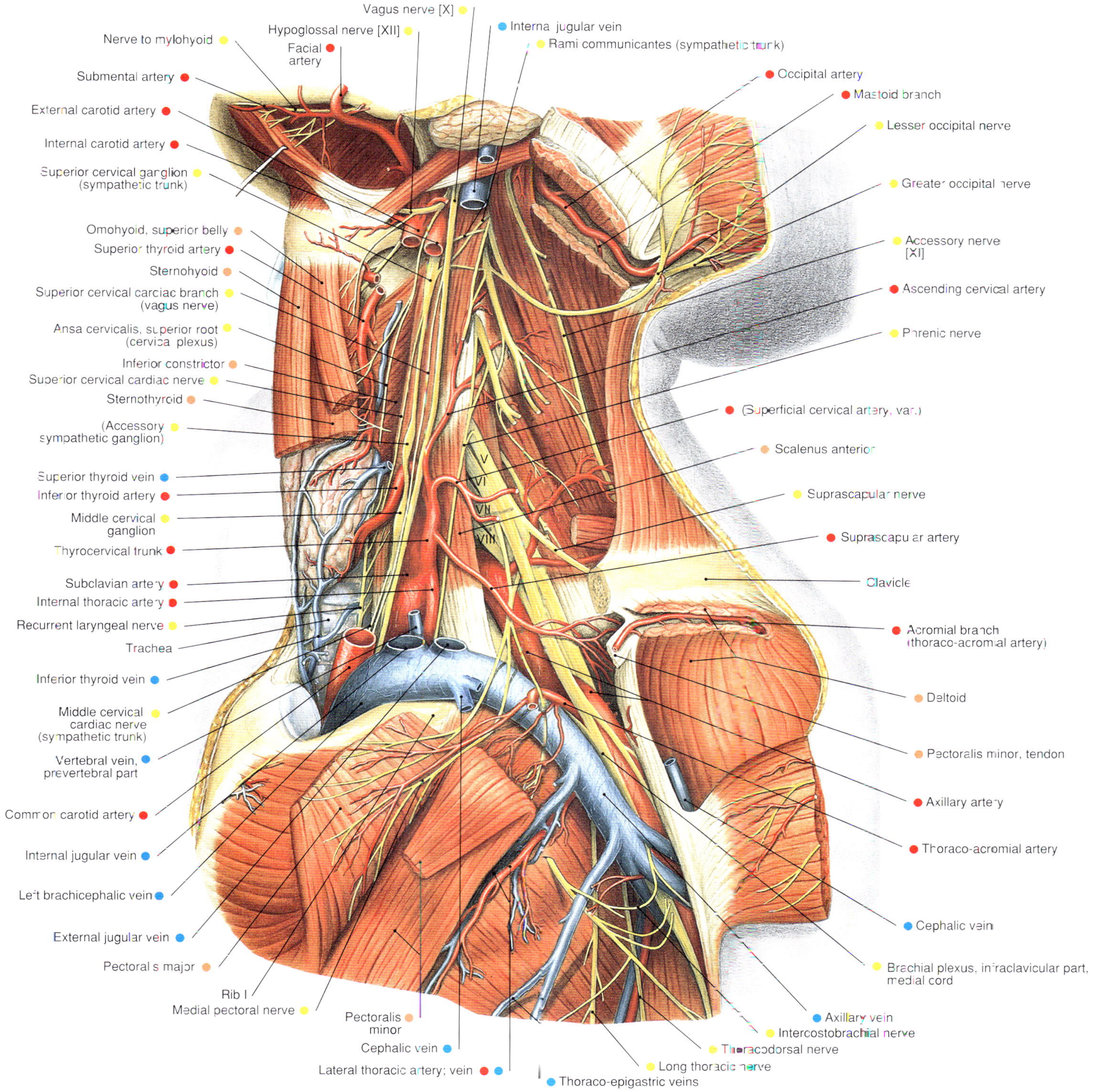

→ 46, T 7

Fig. 258 Vessels and nerves of the lateral region of the neck and the axillary region.
The numbers V–VIII indicate ventral branches of the corresponding cervical nerves

257 413

▸▸ Surface p. 32 | Skeleton p. 264 ff.

Veins of the neck

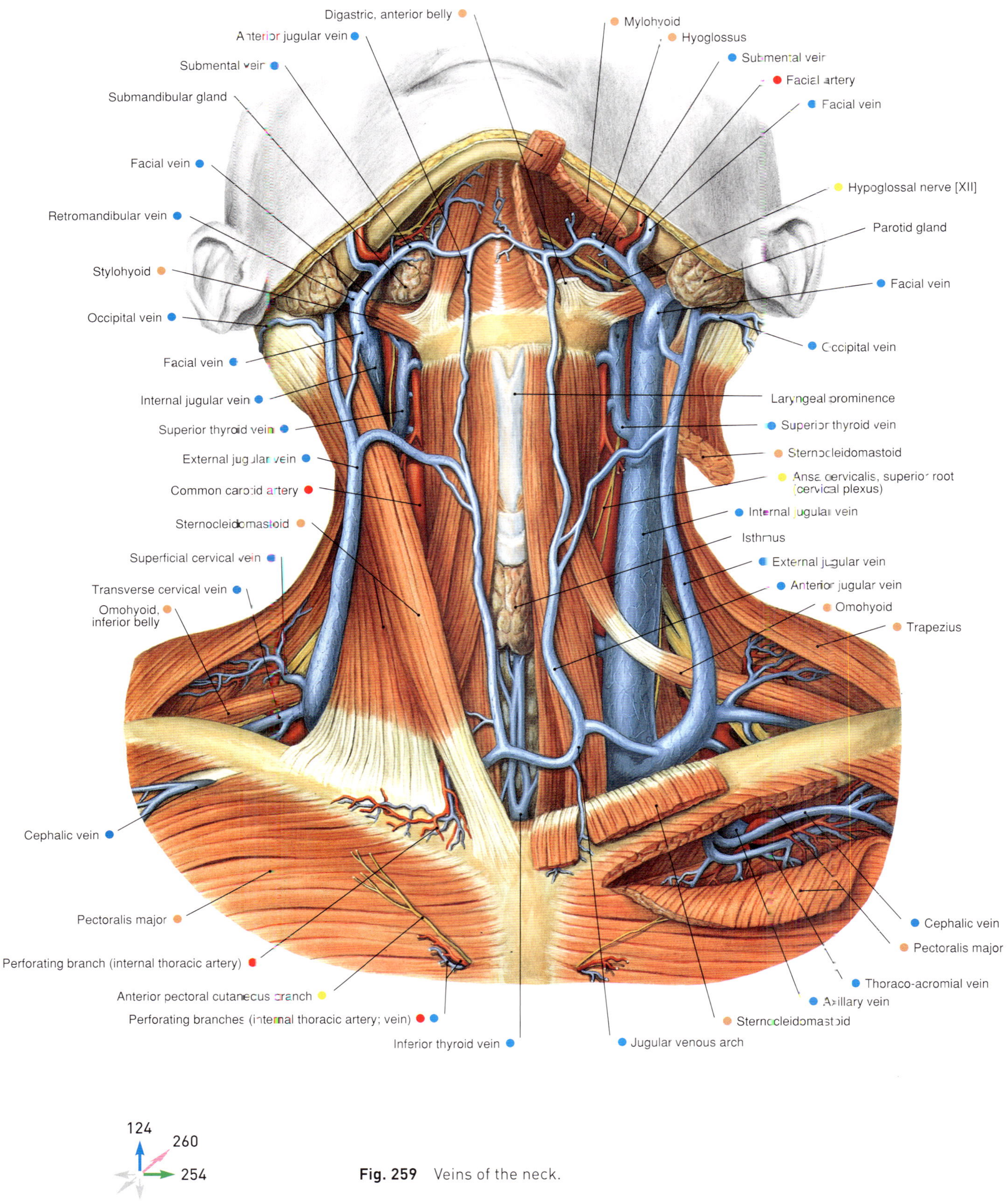

Fig. 259 Veins of the neck.

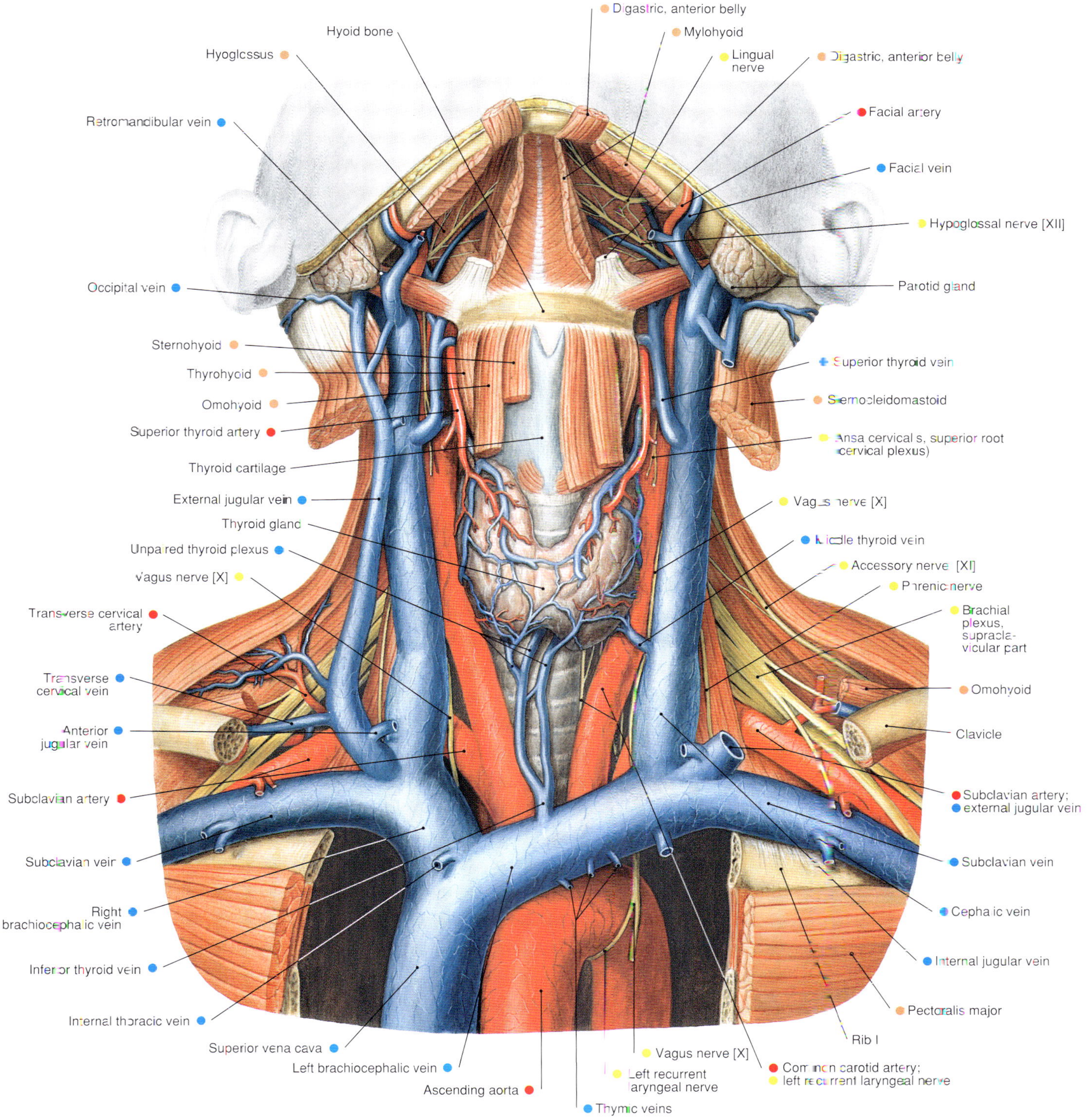

Fig. 260 Vessels and nerves of the neck and the upper thoracic aperture.

133
258
259

Lymphatics of the neck

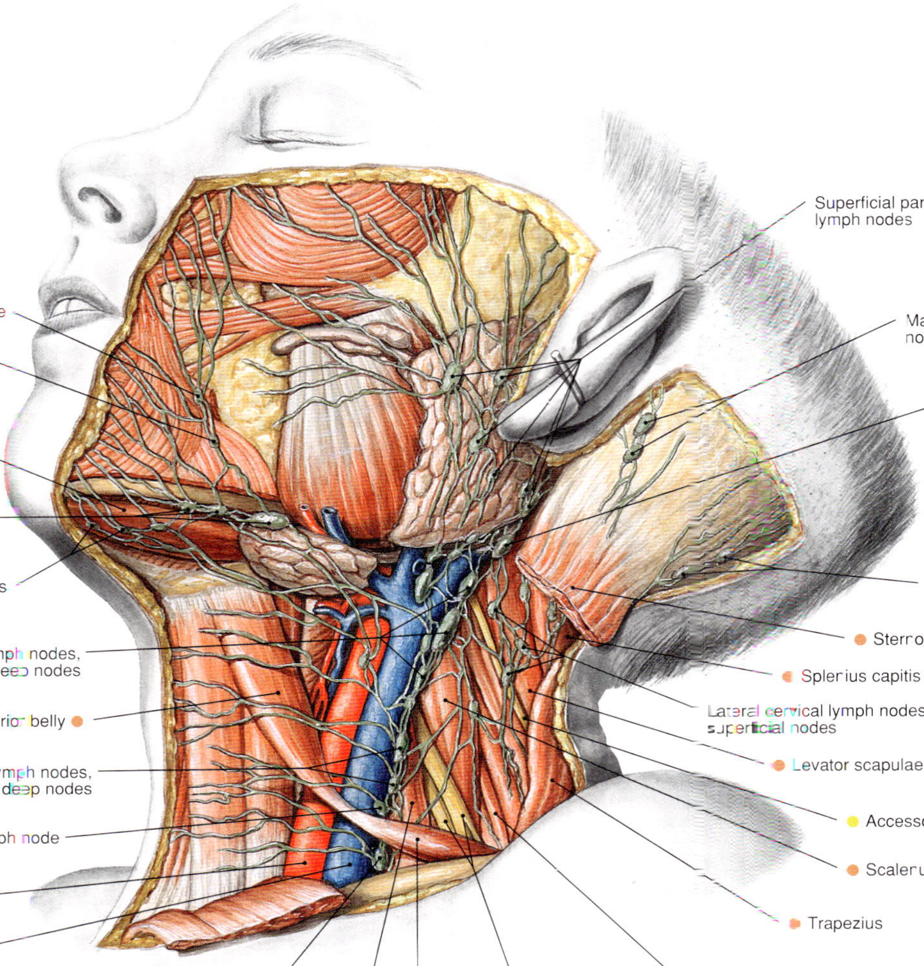

→ 125, 126

Fig. 261 Superficial lymphatics and lymph nodes of the head and the neck of an 8-year-old child.

Vessels and nerves of the submandibular triangle

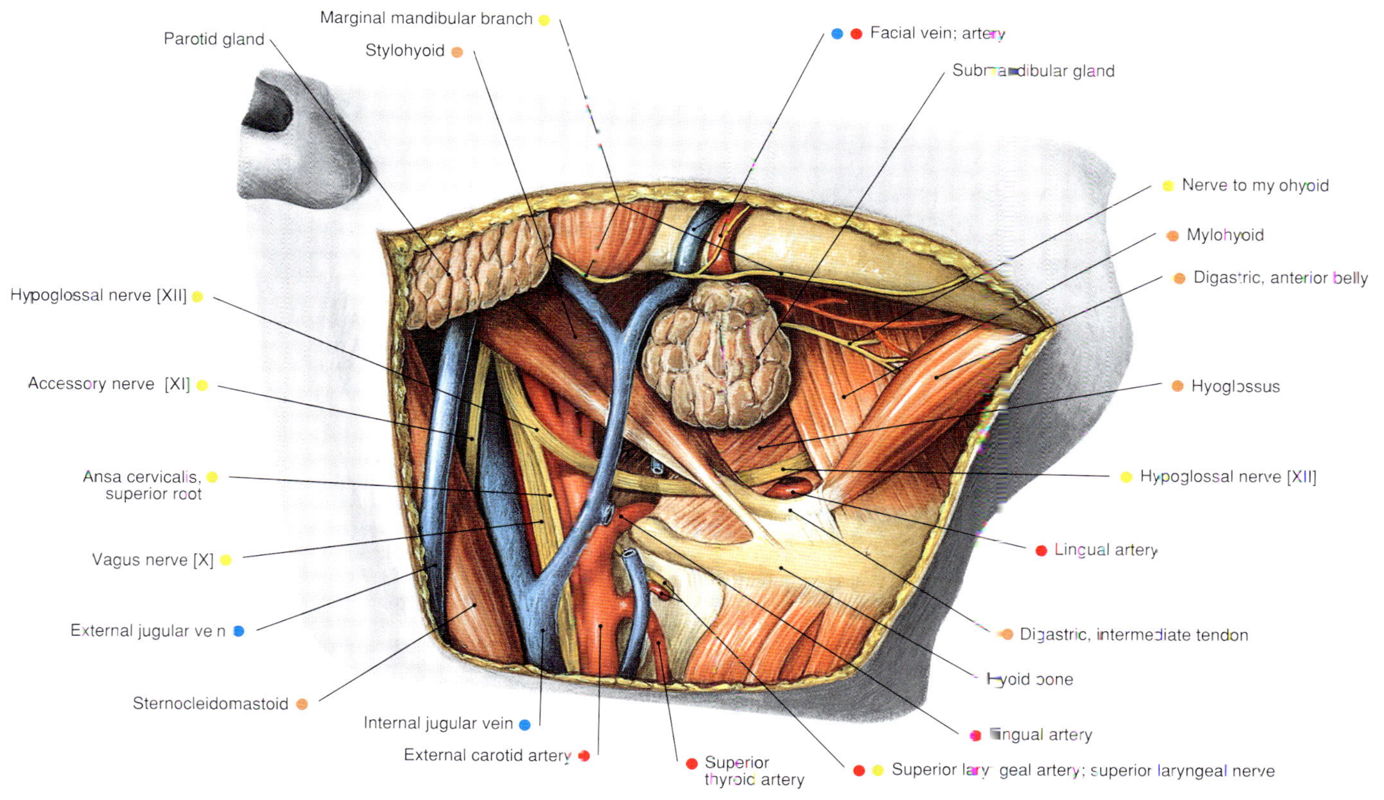

Fig. 262 Vessels and nerves of the submandibular triangle.

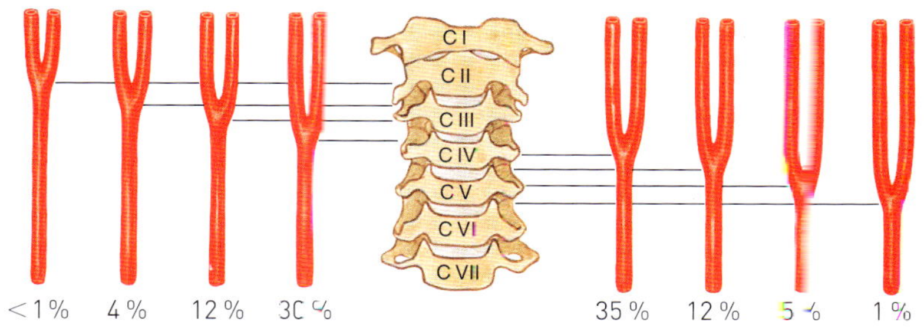

Fig. 263 Level of the bifurcation of the common carotid artery in relation to the cervical vertebrae.

▸▸ Surface p. 32 | Skeleton p. 264 ff.

Subclavian artery

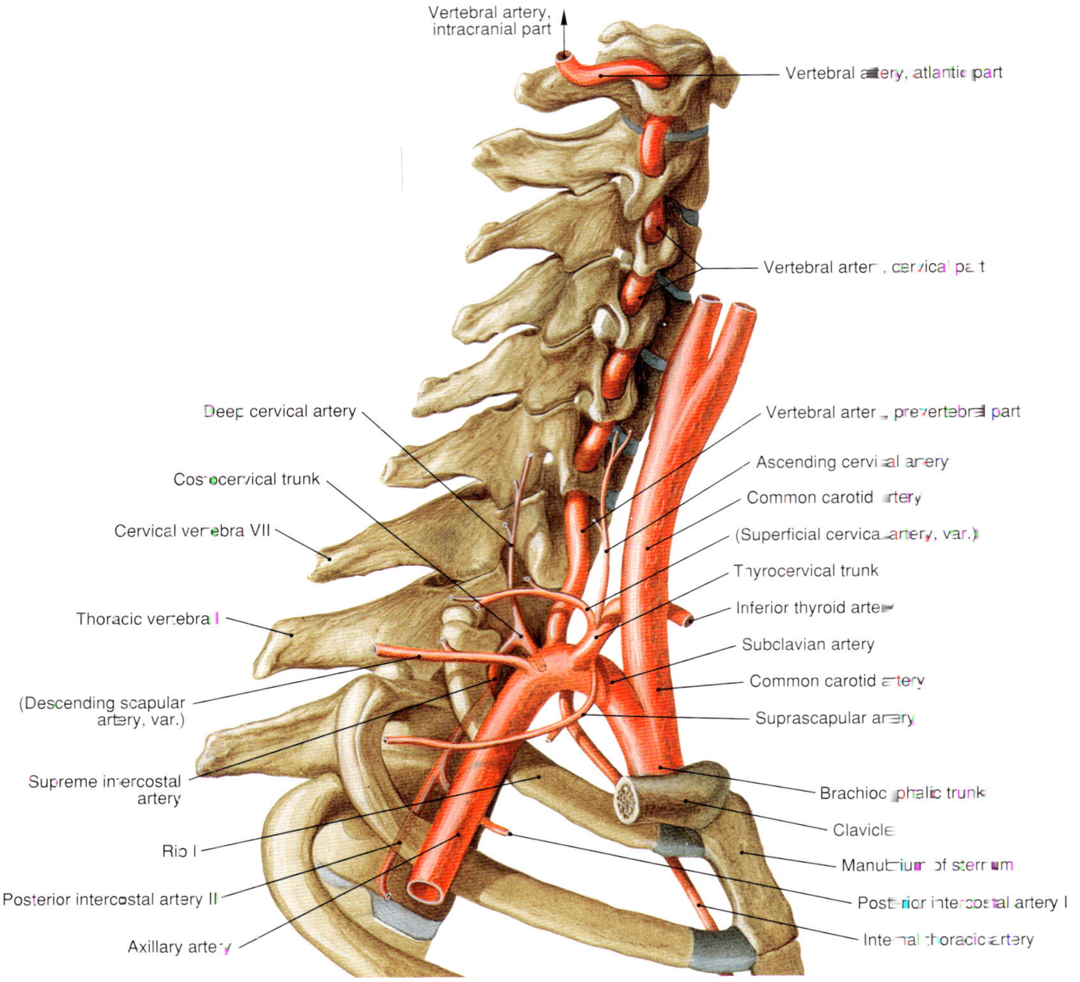

Fig. 264 Subclavian artery.

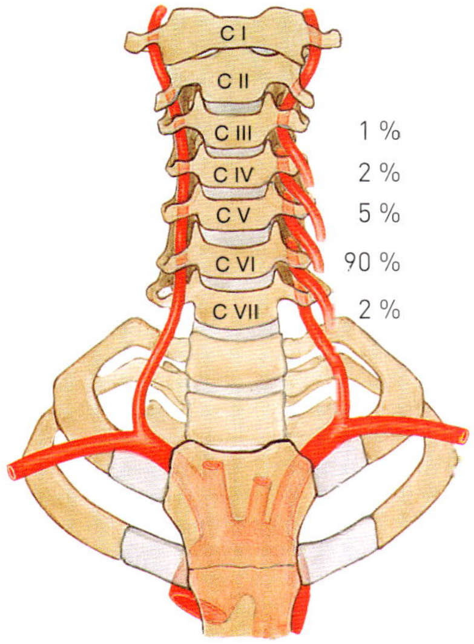

Fig. 265 Level of the entry of the vertebral artery into the transverse foramina.

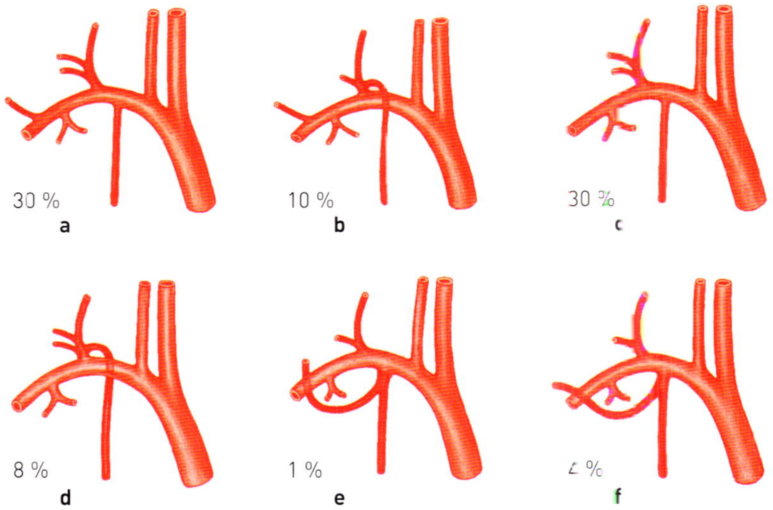

Fig. 266 a–f Variations in the truncus formed by the inferior thyroid artery, the suprascapular artery, the transverse cervical artery and the internal thoracic artery, when the vertebral artery branches off separately from the costocervical truncus.

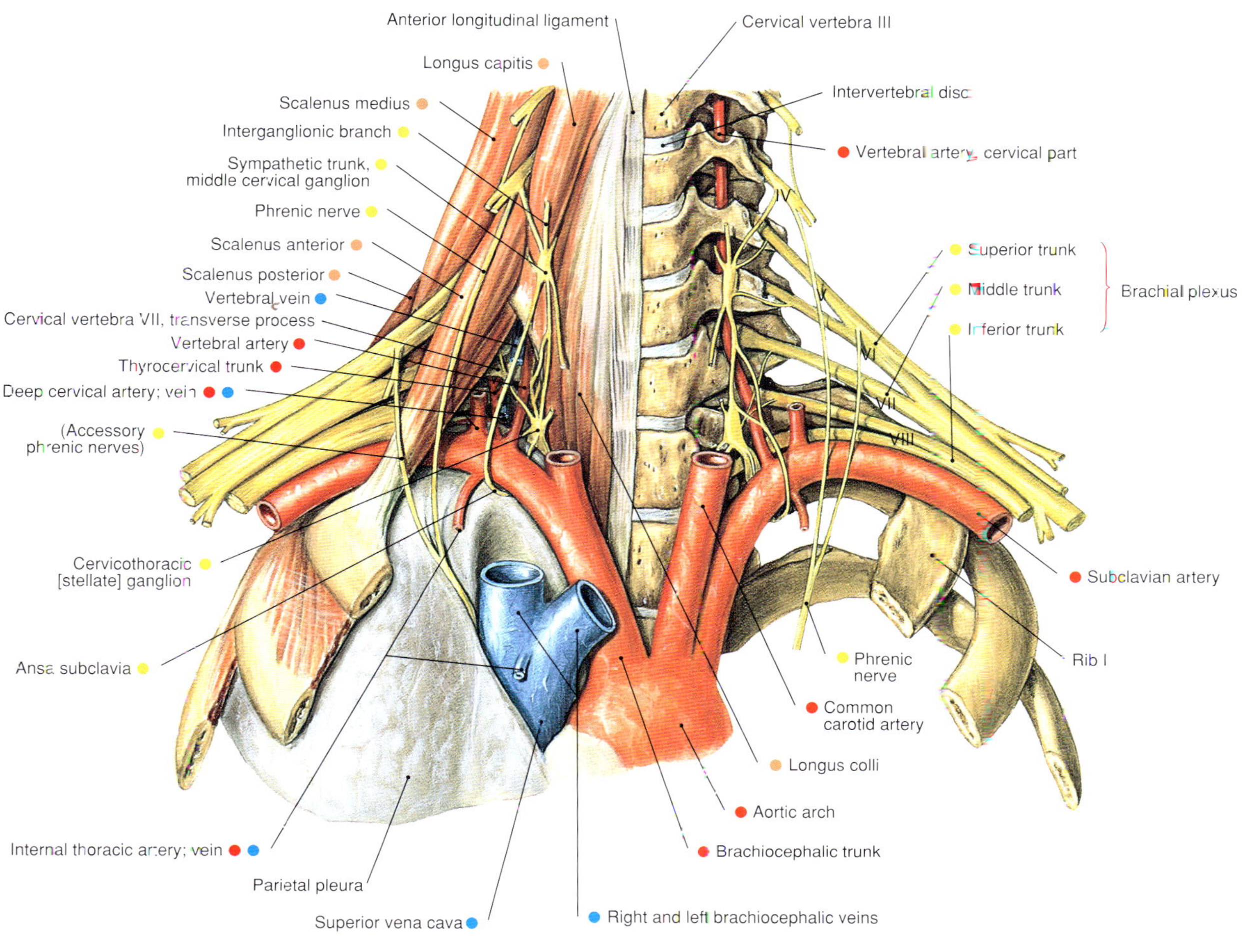

Fig. 267 Vessels and nerves at the transition from the neck to the thorax.
The numbers IV–VIII indicate ventral branches of the corresponding spinal nerves.

→ 46, 386, T 7, T 24

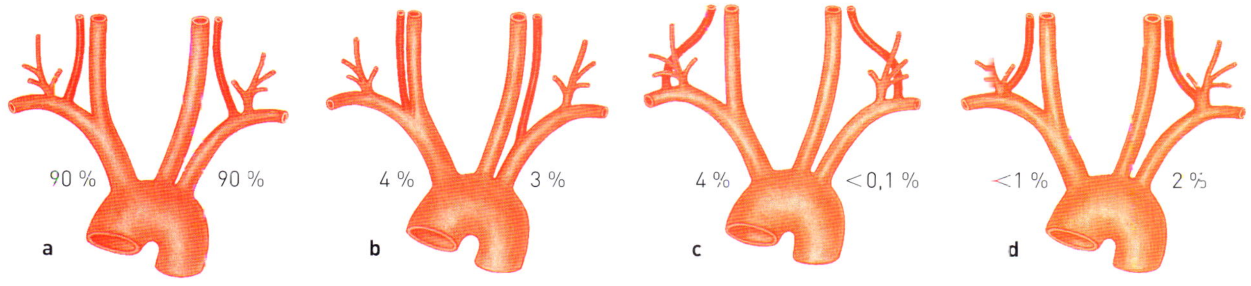

Fig. 268 a–d Variations in the origin of the vertebral artery.

▸▸ Surface p. 32 | Skeleton p. 264 ff.

Neck, transverse section

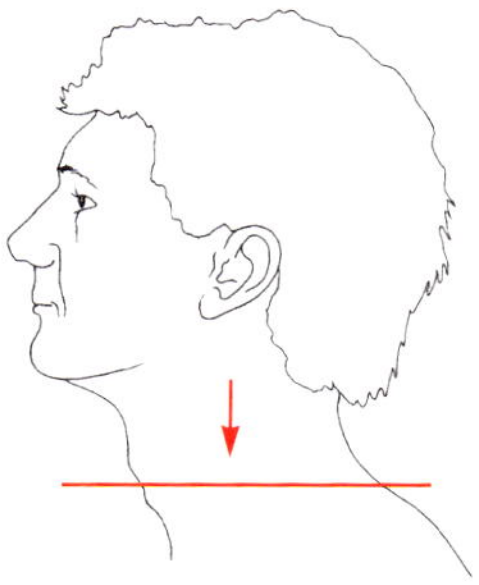

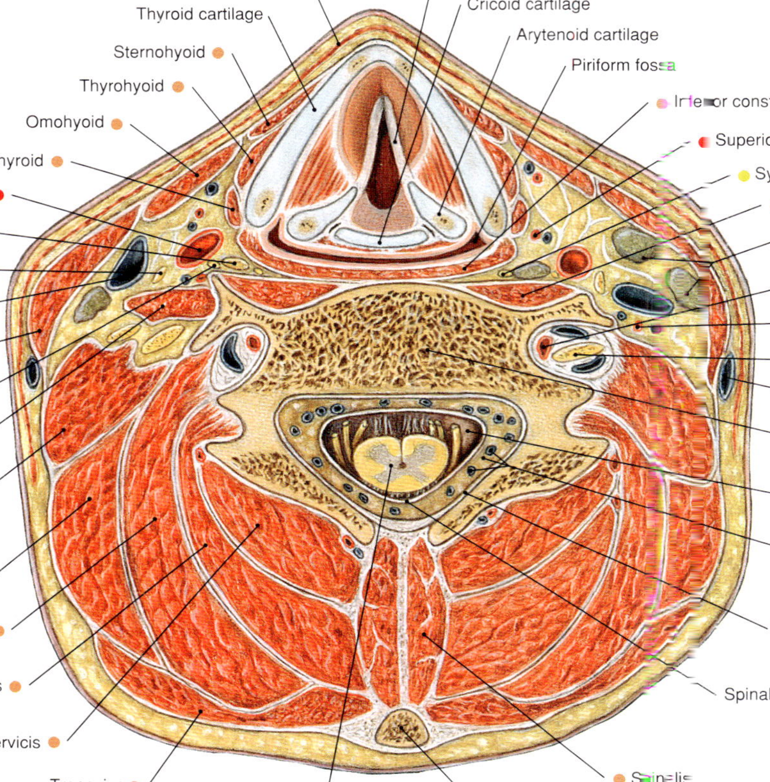

→ 236

Fig. 269 Neck;
transverse section at the level of the vocal cord.

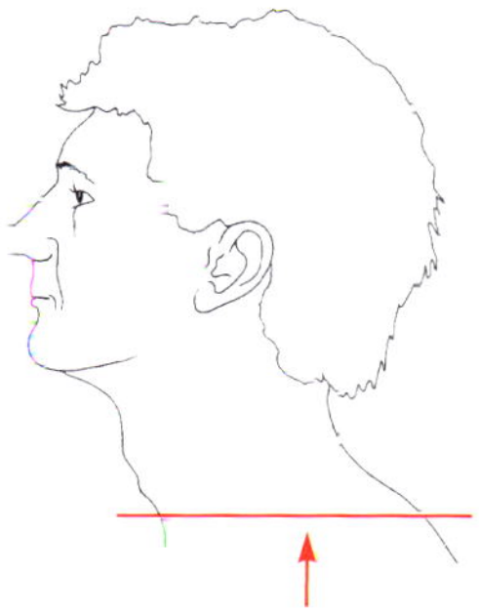

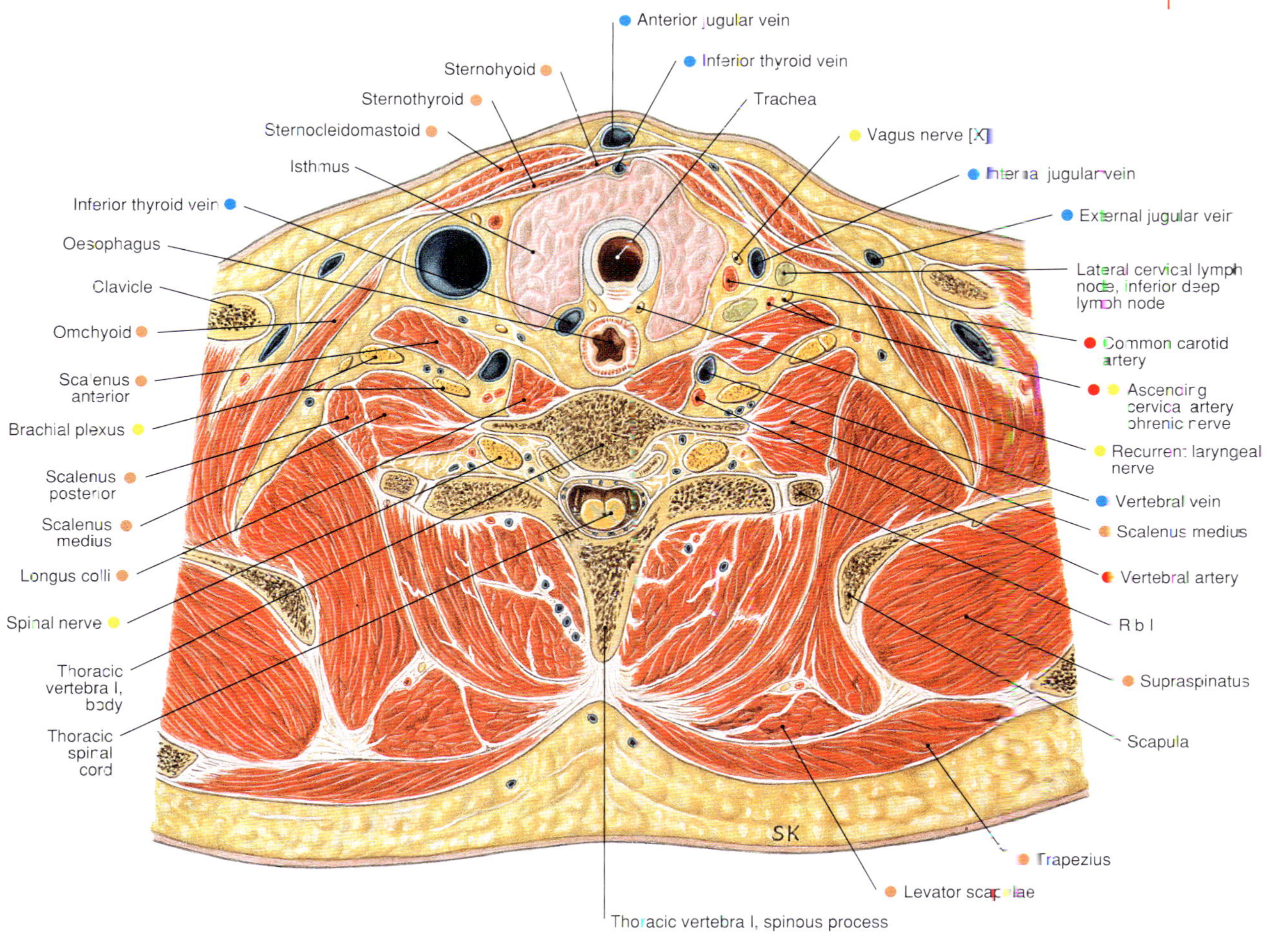

Fig. 270 Neck;
transverse section at the level of the first thoracic vertebra.

→ 239

Oral cavity and pharynx, median section

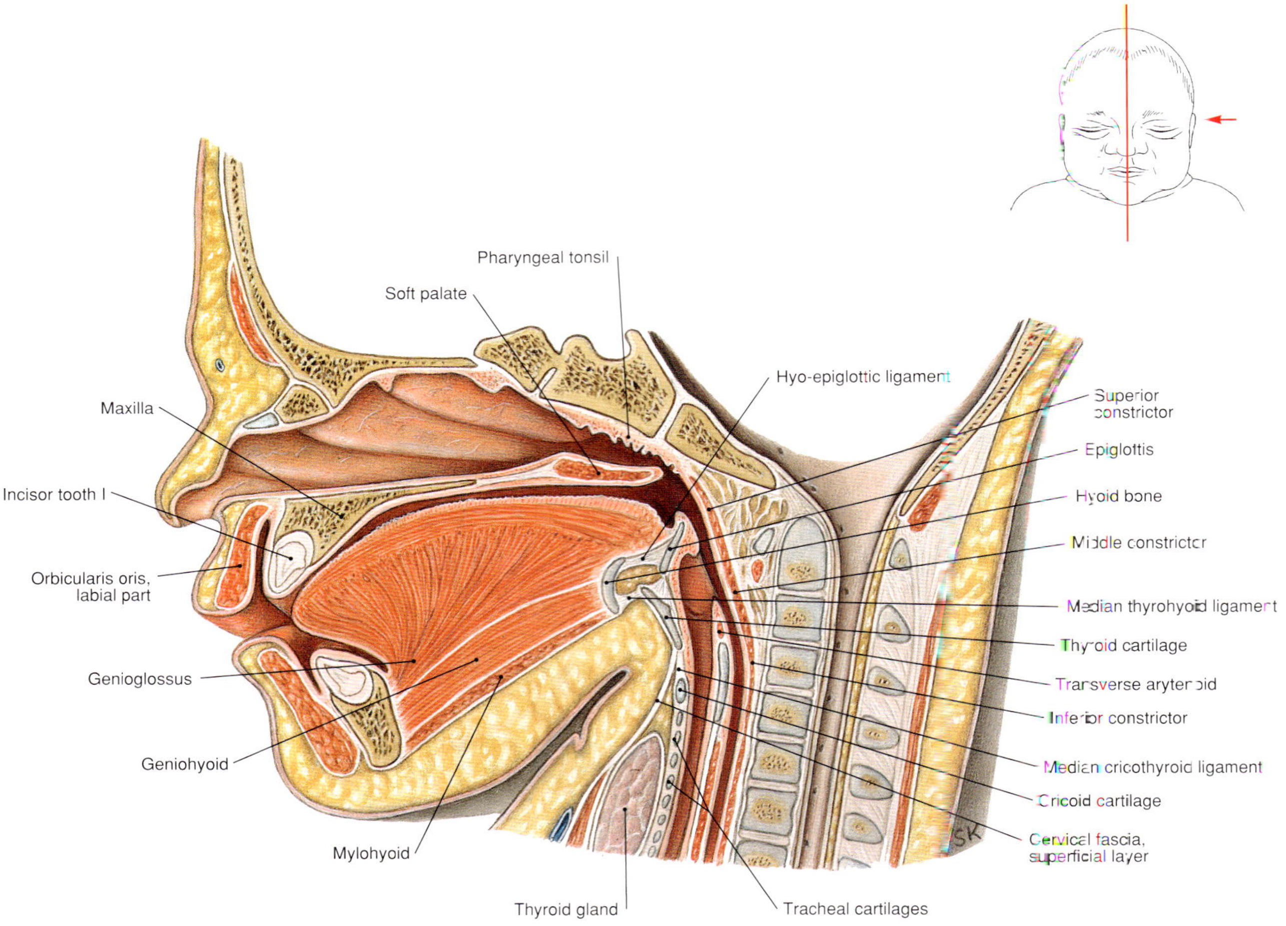

→ 246

Fig. 271 Facial part of the head and neck; median section through the head of a neonate.

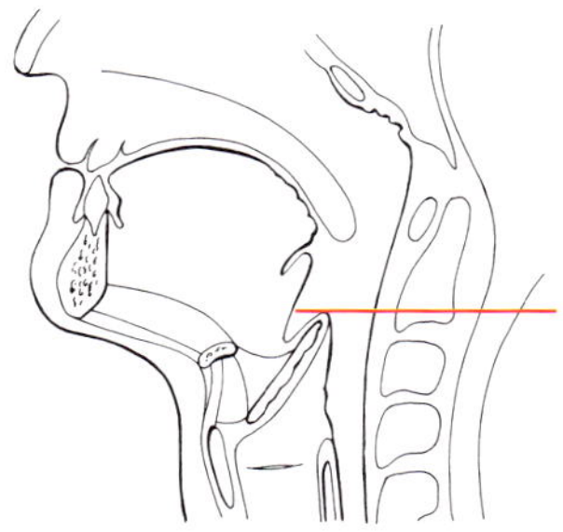

Fig. 272 Schema illustrating the distance between the root of the tongue and the epiglottis in the adult.

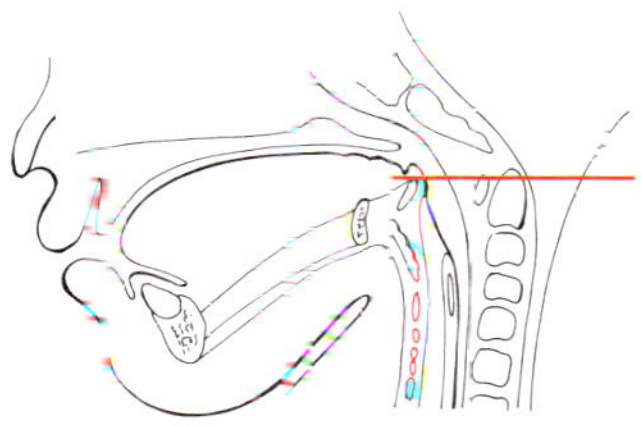

Fig. 273 Schema illustrating that the larynx in the neonate is positioned considerably higher than in the adult.

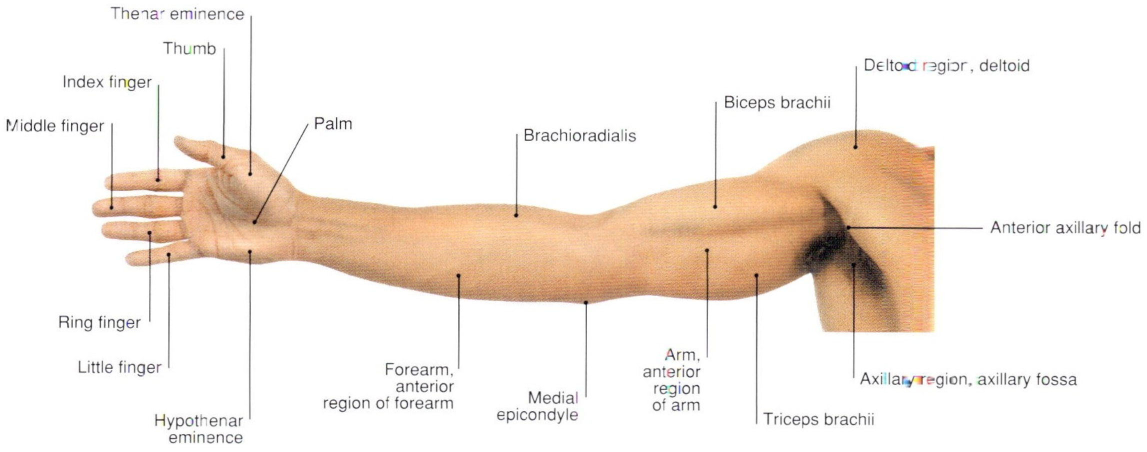

Fig. 274 Upper limb.

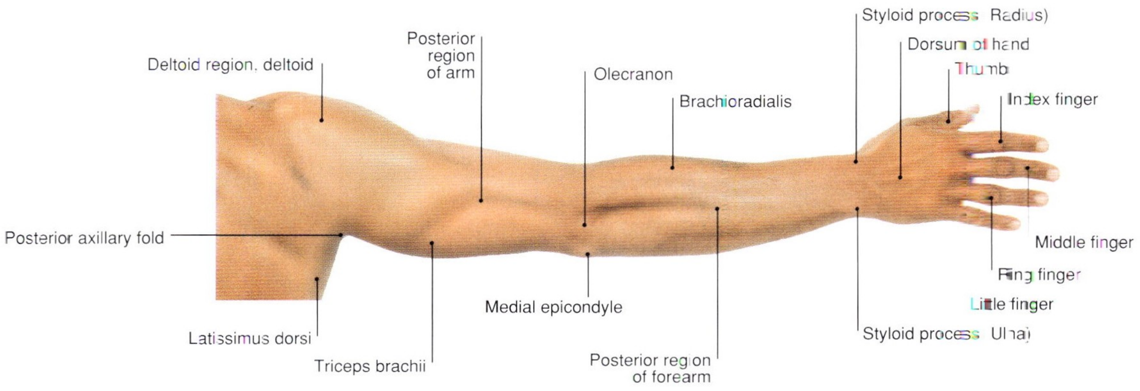

Fig. 275 Upper limb.

Skeleton of the upper limb

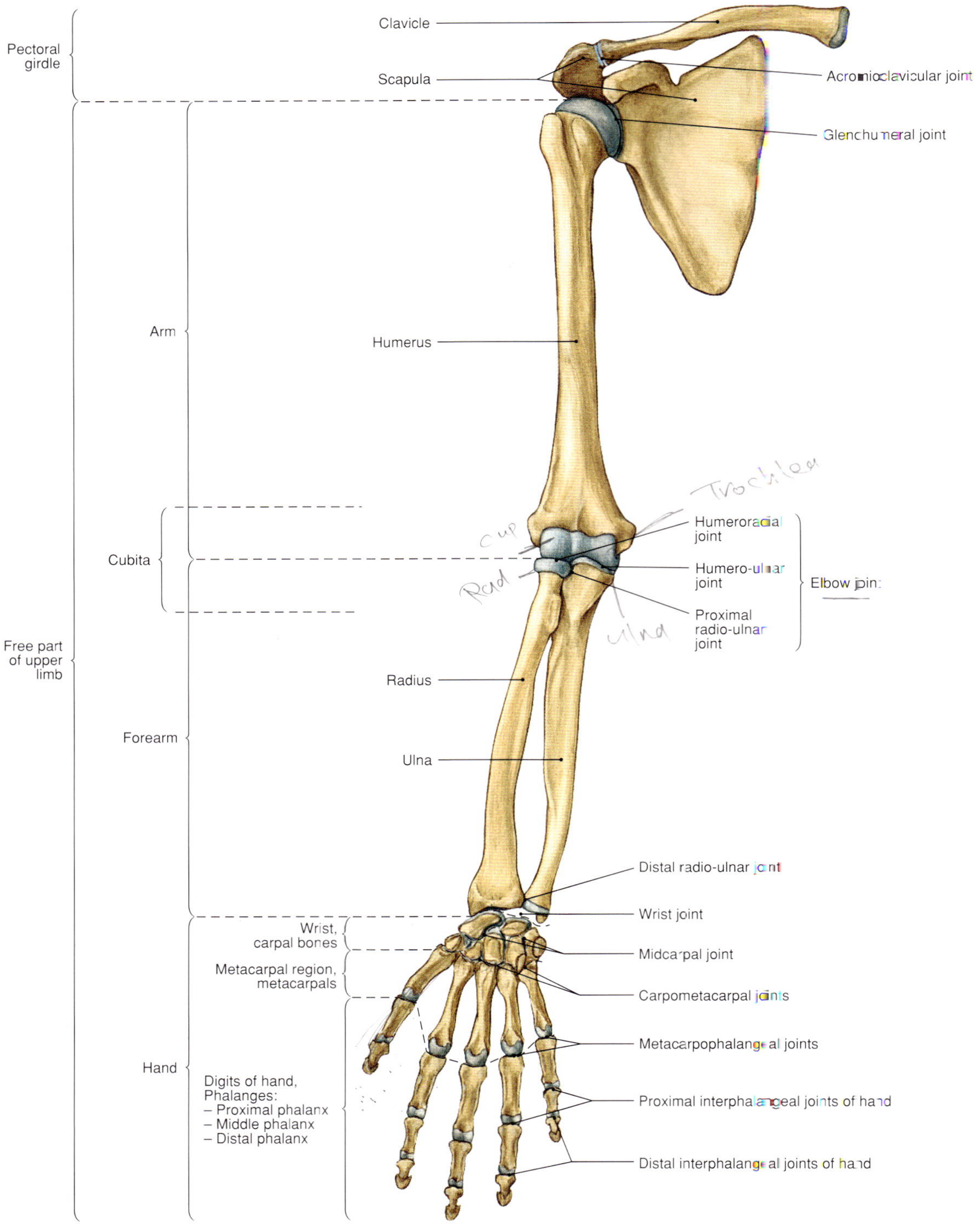

Fig. 276 Upper limb; overview, bones and joints.

Clavicle

Connects to the manubrium of sternum and to acromion of scapula

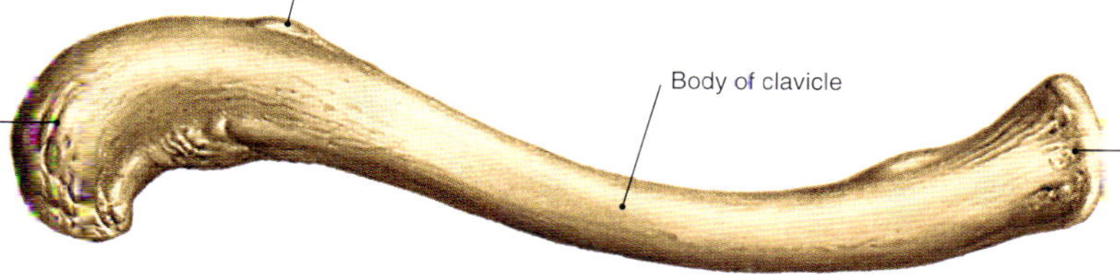

Fig. 277 Clavicle; superior view.

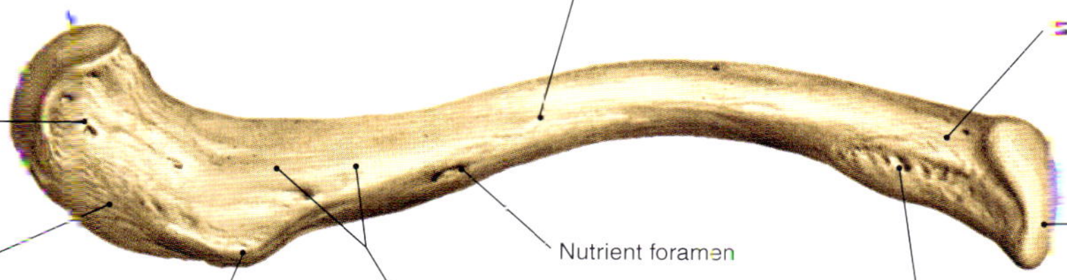

Fig. 278 Clavicle; inferior view.

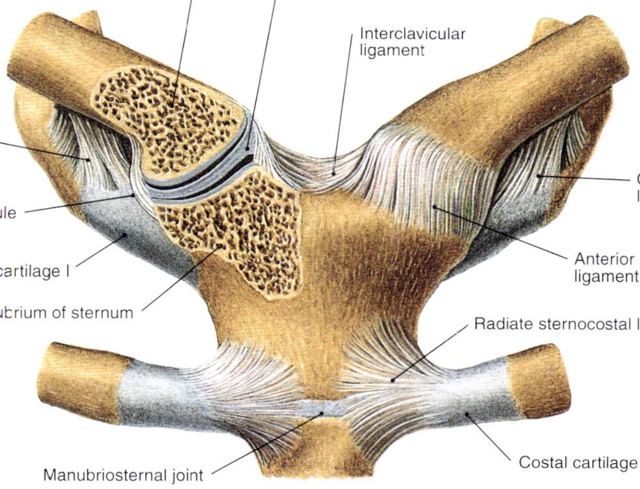

Fig. 279 Sternoclavicular joint; ventral view.

Scapula (Shoulder blade)

The Glenoid cavity is the lateral edge of scapula. and is the socket portion of the ball and socket joint of shoulder.
The Acromion of scapula connects to the clavicle.

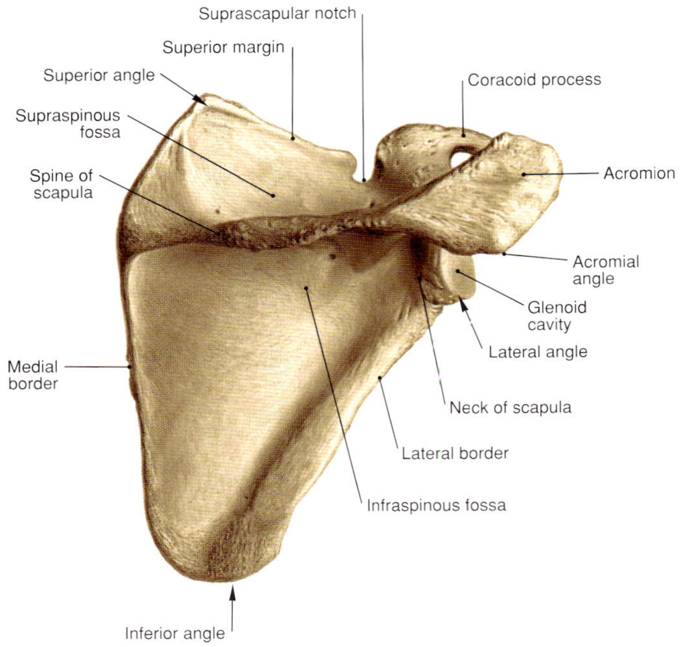

Fig. 280 Scapula; dorsal view.

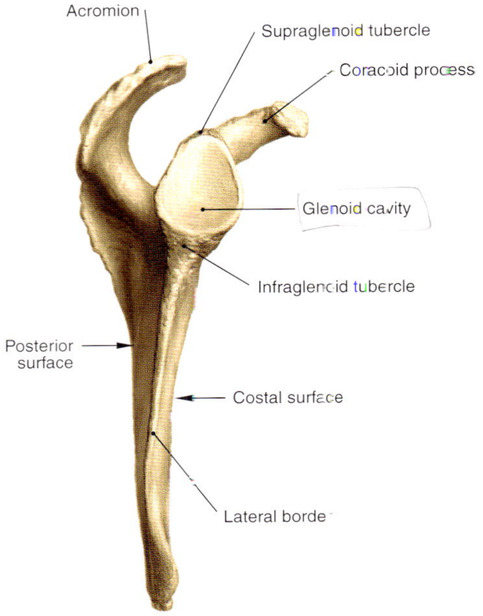

Fig. 281 Scapula; lateral view.

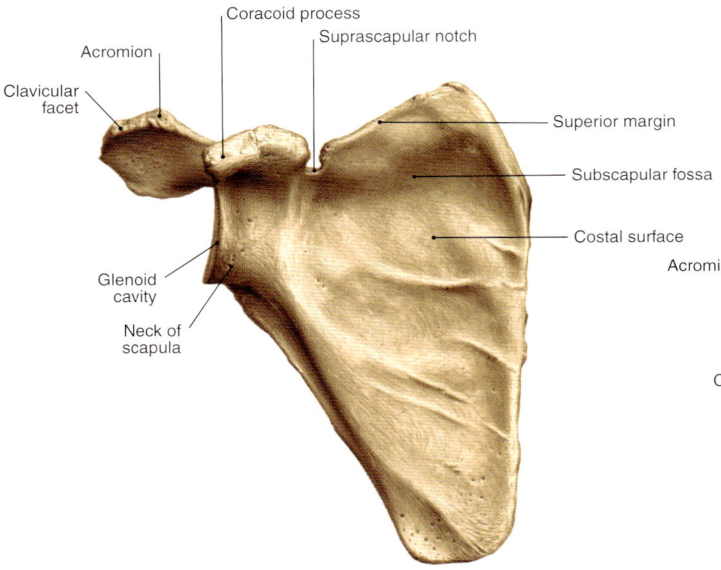

Fig. 282 Scapula; ventral view.

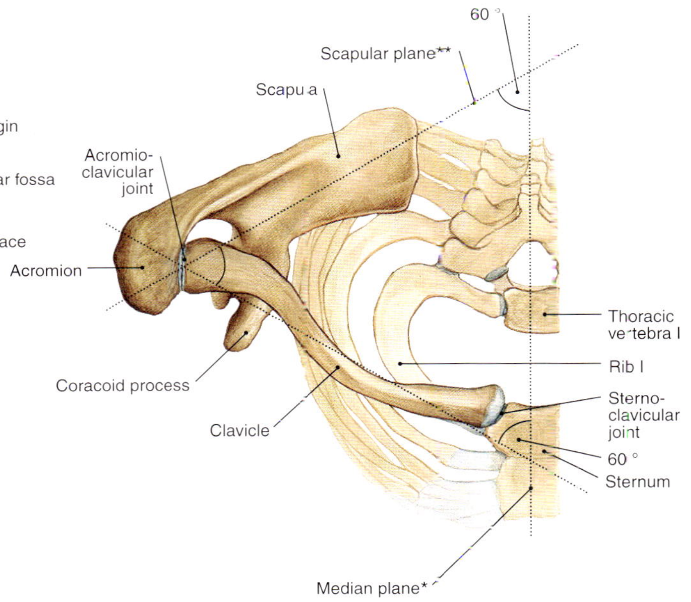

Fig. 283 Shoulder girdle; superior view.
The angles refer to the average relations in the adult.

* Median plane
** Scapular plane

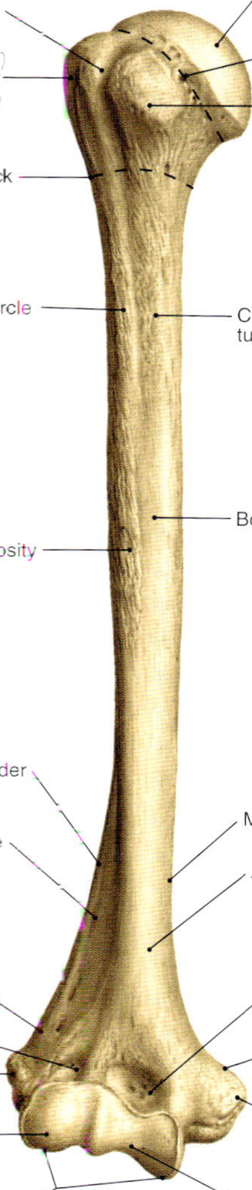

Fig. 284 Humerus;
ventral view.

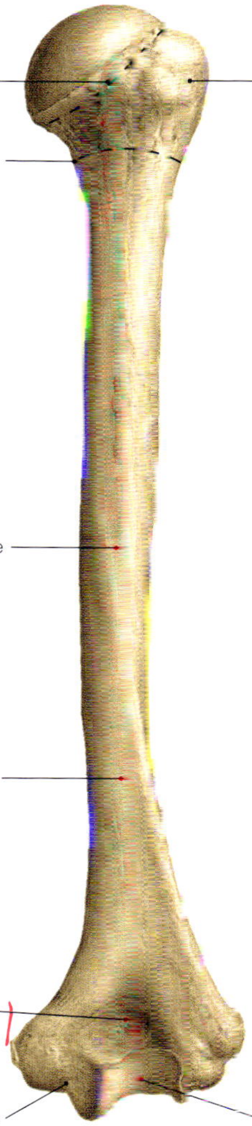

Fig. 285 Humerus;
dorsal view.

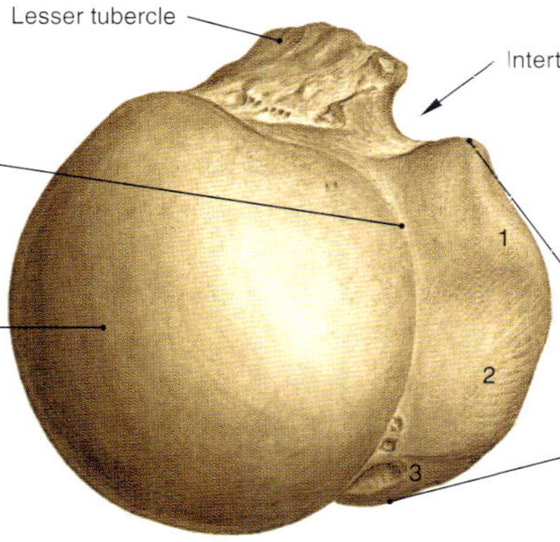

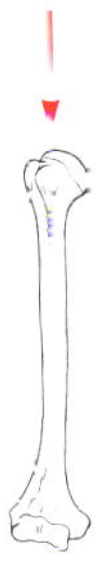

Fig. 286 Humerus;
proximal view.

Shoulder joint

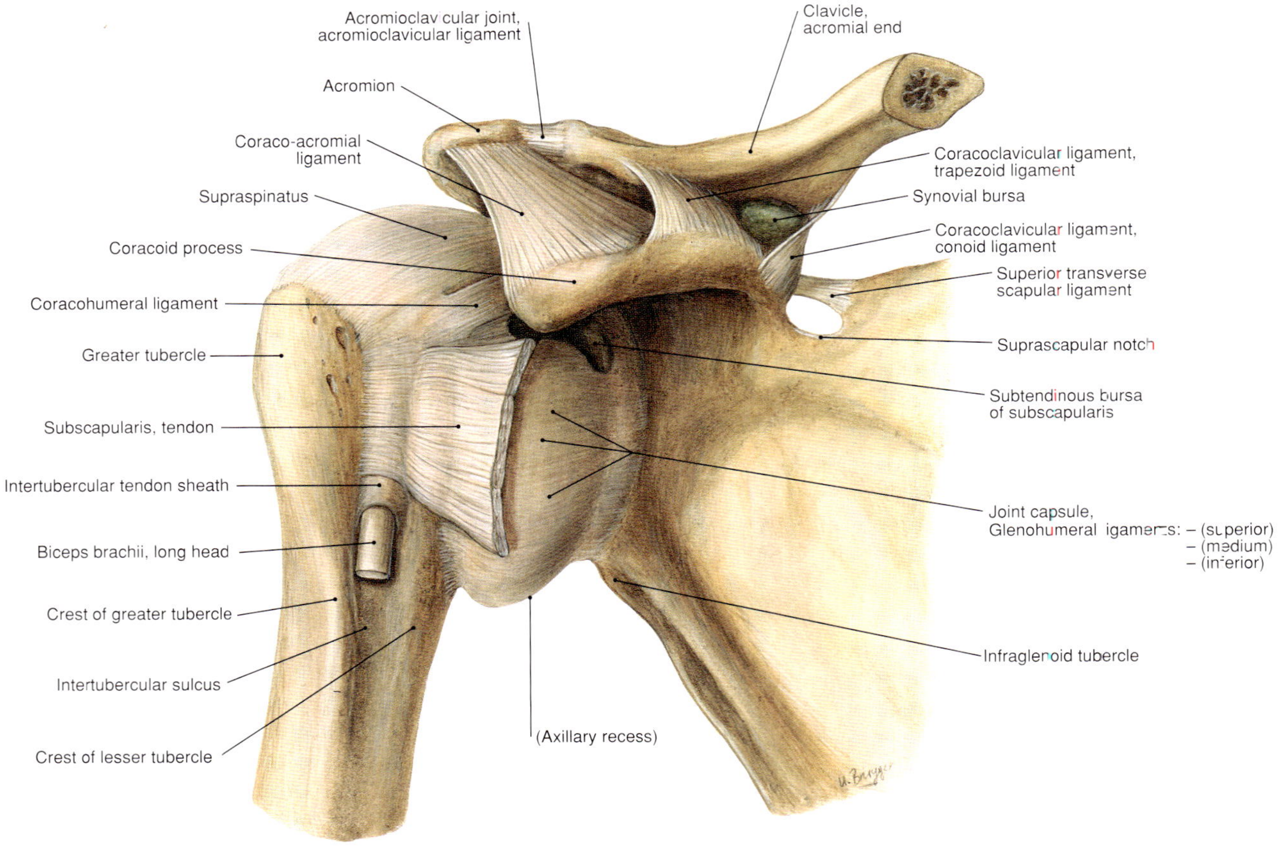

Fig. 287 Shoulder joint; ventral view.

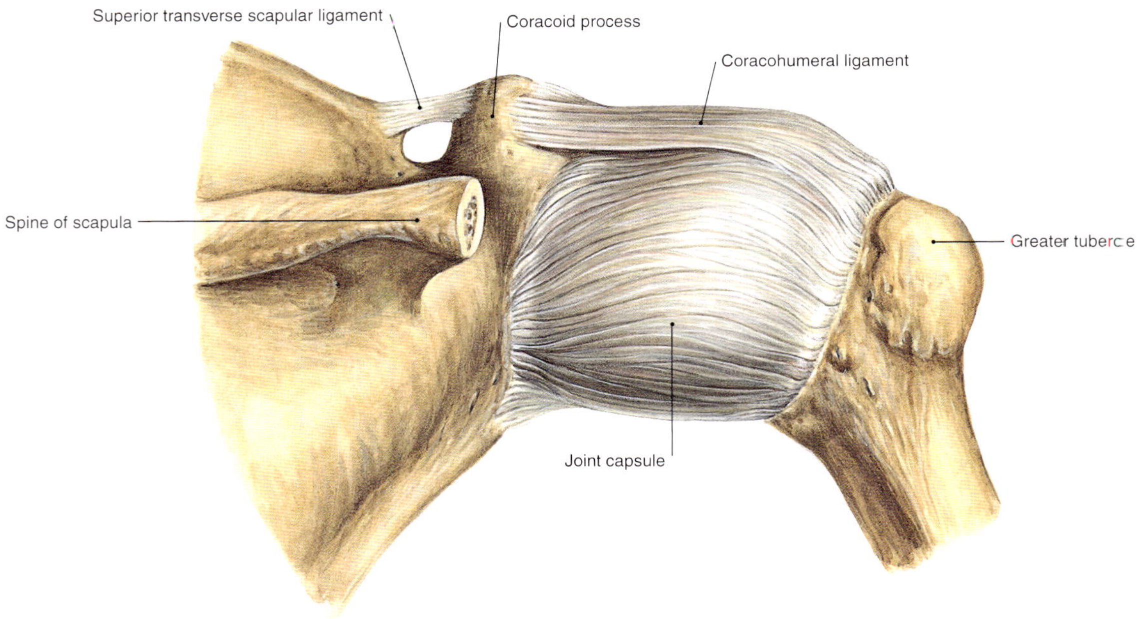

Fig. 288 Shoulder joint; the acromion has been removed; dorsal view.

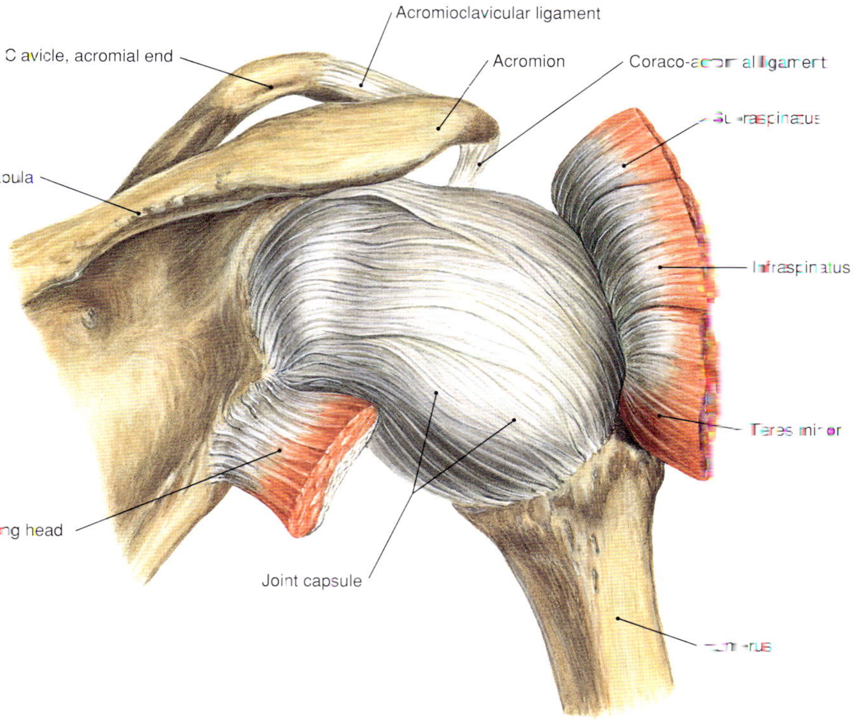

Fig. 289 Shoulder joint;
dorsal view.

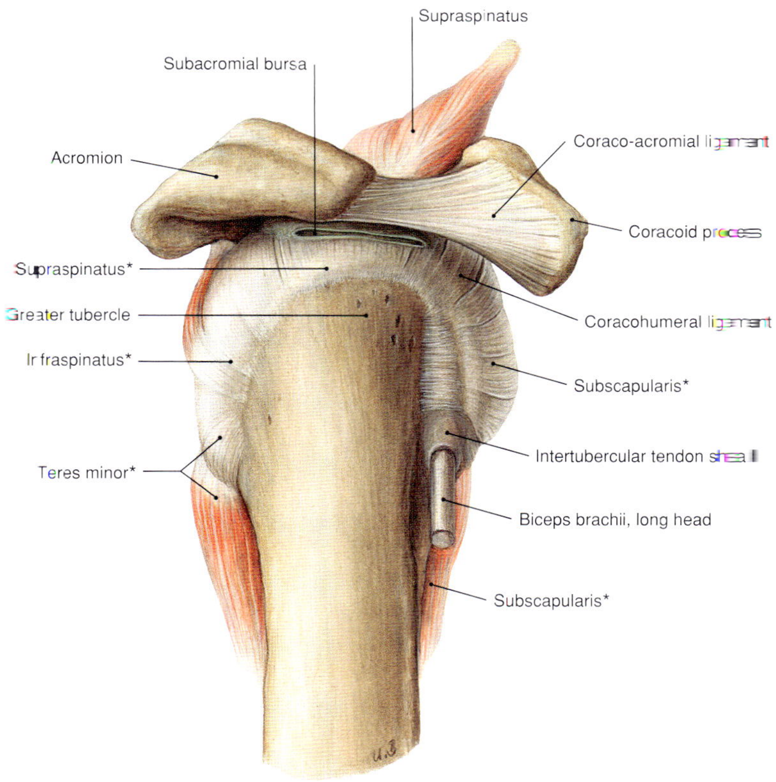

Fig. 290 Shoulder joint;
lateral view.

Together, the muscle tendons marked with * form the so-called rotator cuff.

Shoulder joint

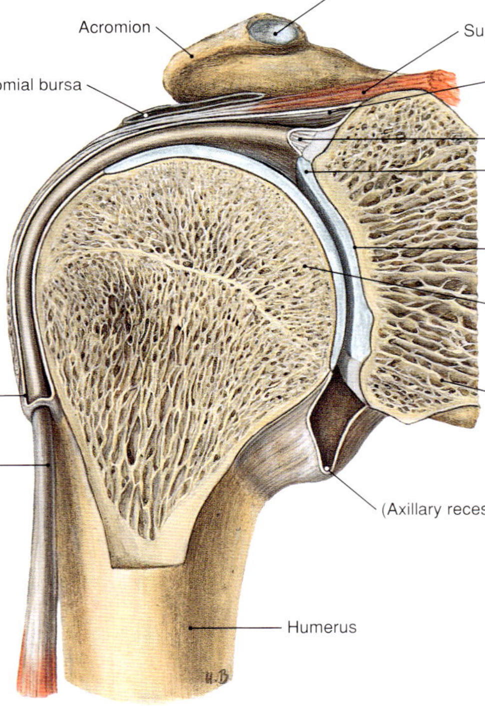

Fig. 291 Shoulder joint; section at the level of the scapula; ventral view.

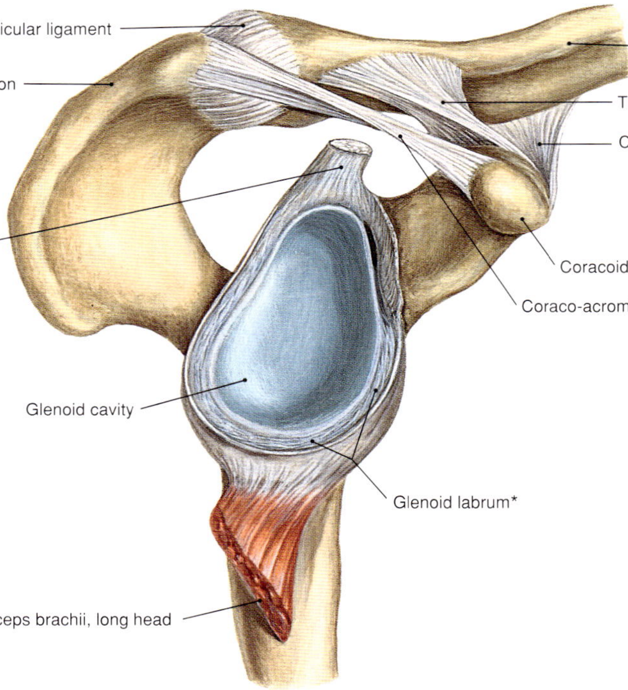

Fig. 292 Shoulder joint; lateral view.
Next to its origin at the supraglenoidal tubercle, the tendon of the biceps muscle is predominantly attached to the glenoid labrum.

* It forms a fibrocartilaginous collar around the glenoid cavity.

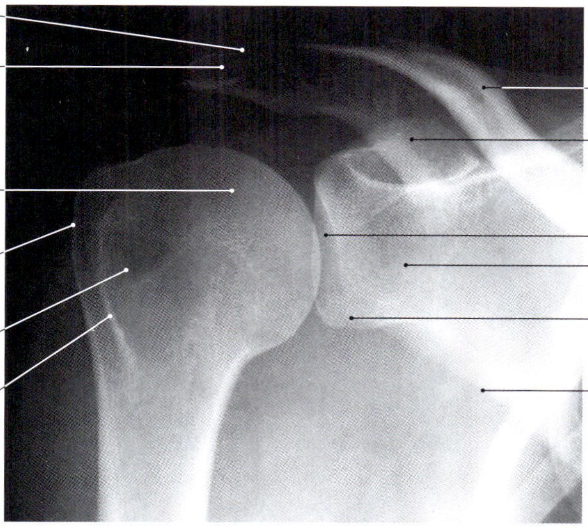

Fig. 293 Shoulder joint;
AP-radiograph.

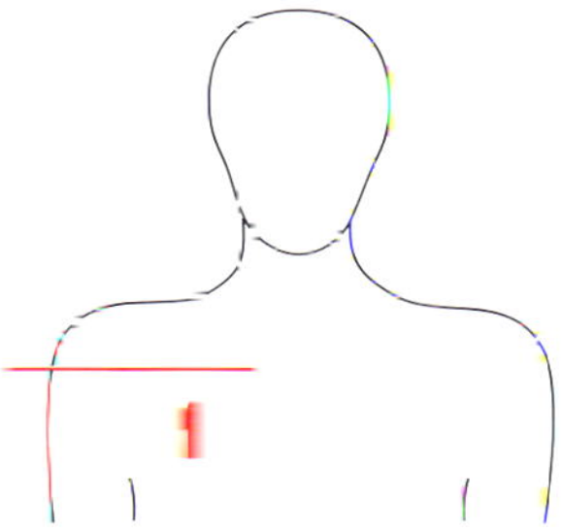

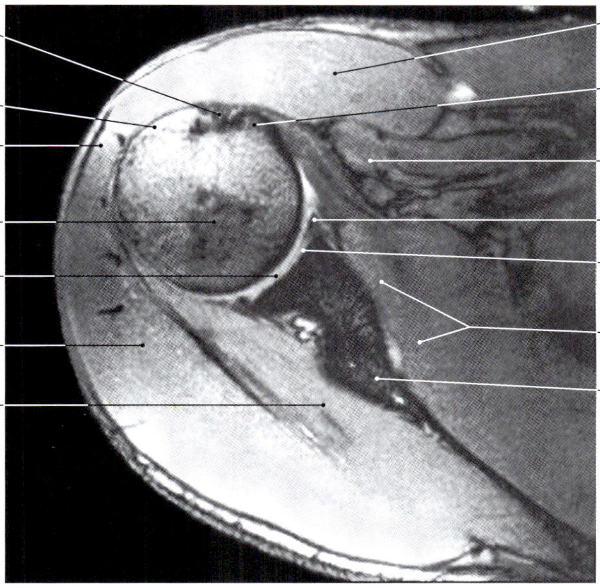

Fig. 294 Shoulder joint;
computed tomographic (CT) cross-section;
the joint cavity is filled with air (pneumo-CT);
inferior view.

Ulna

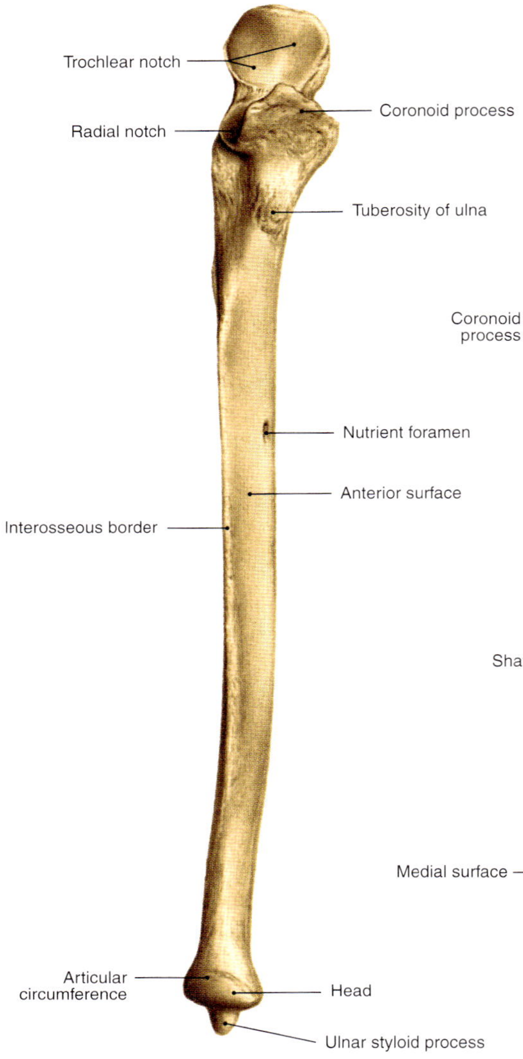

Fig. 295 Ulna; ventral view.

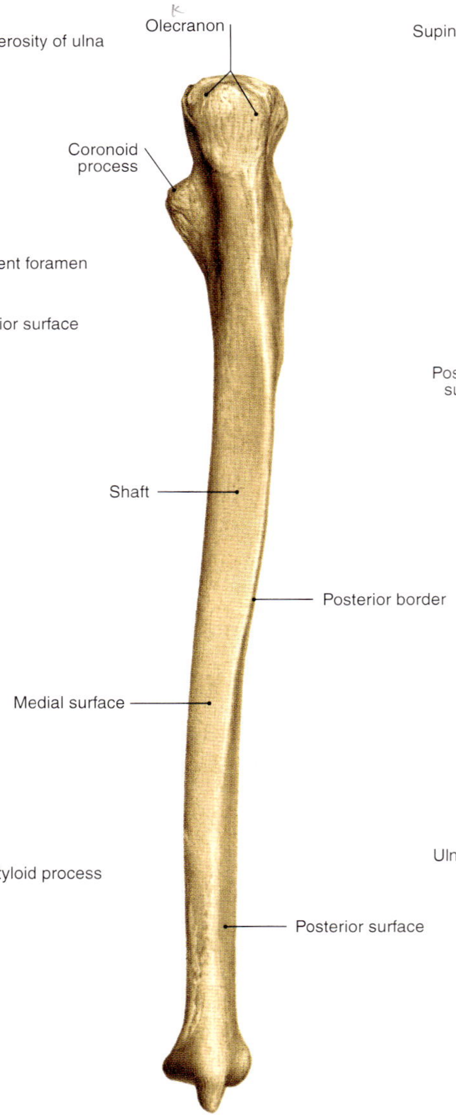

Fig. 296 Ulna; dorsal view.

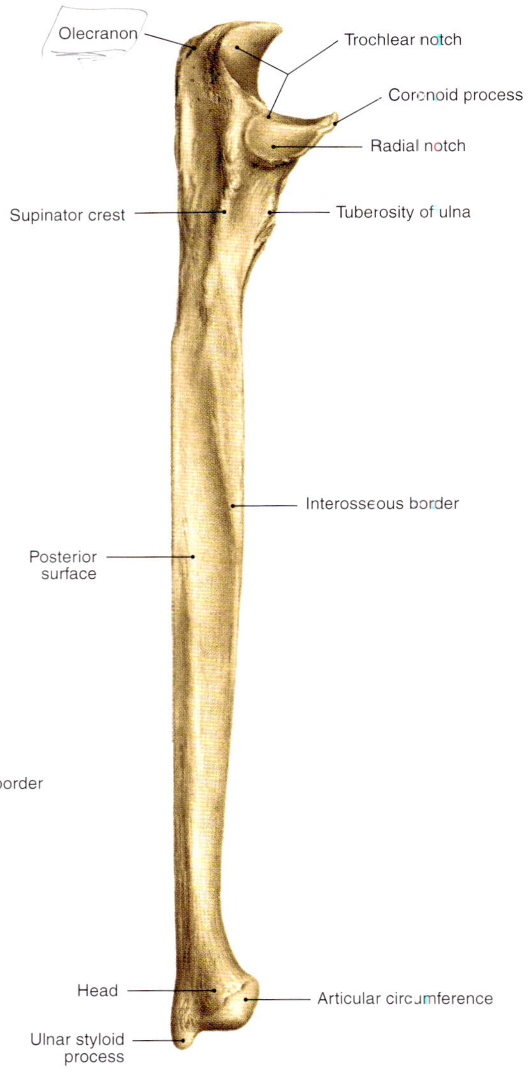

Fig. 297 Ulna; radial view.

when the hand is in supinate position (dorsal) the Radius and ulna are parallel to each other — is the lateral bone

when the hand is pronated the Radius crosses over the ulna

The head of radius pivots on the capitulum

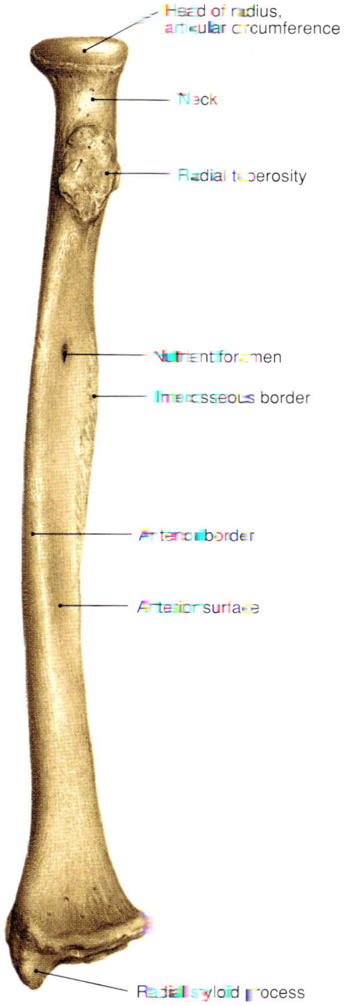

Fig. 298 Radius; ventral view.

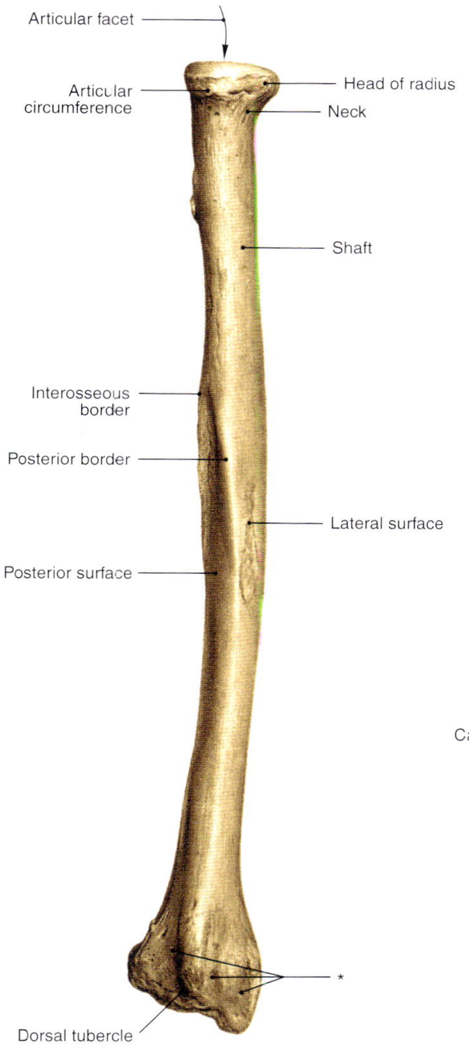

Fig. 299 Radius; dorsal view.

* Grooves and crests for the attachment of the extensor tendons

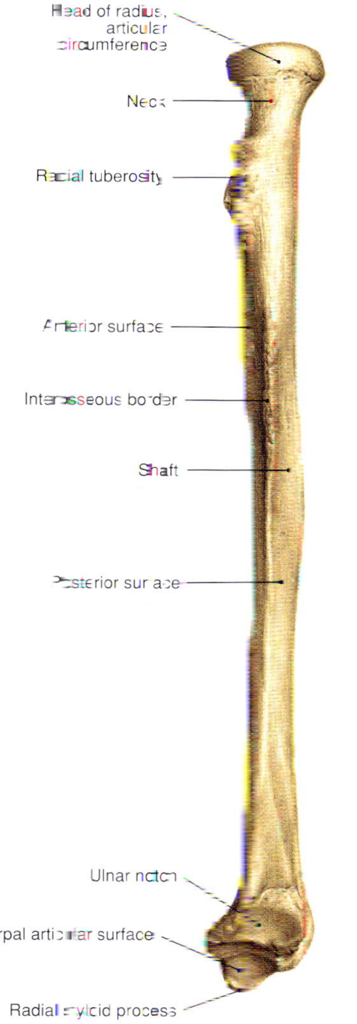

Fig. 300 Radius; ulnar view.

Elbow joint

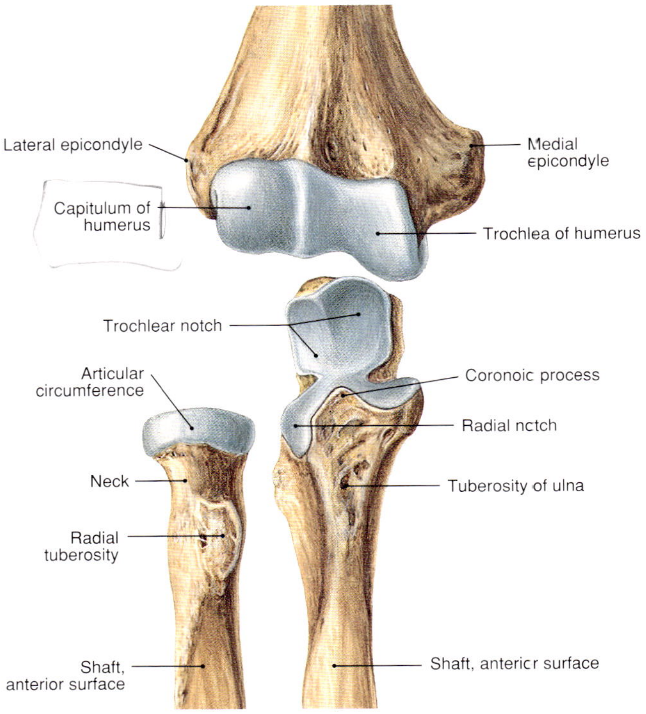

Fig. 301 Elbow joint; ventral view.

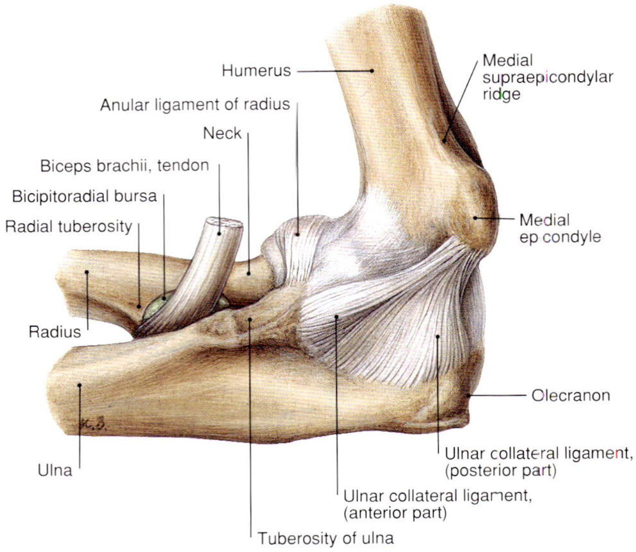

Fig. 302 Elbow joint in 90° flexion and 90° supination; medial view.

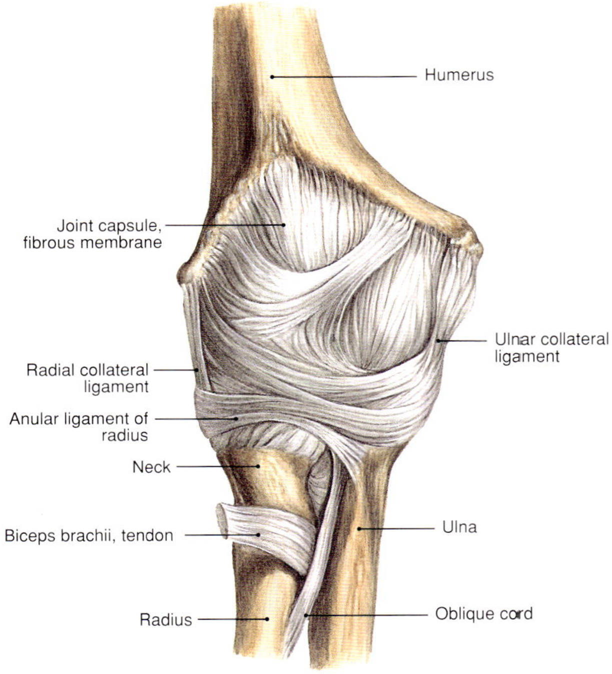

Fig. 303 Elbow joint; ventral view.

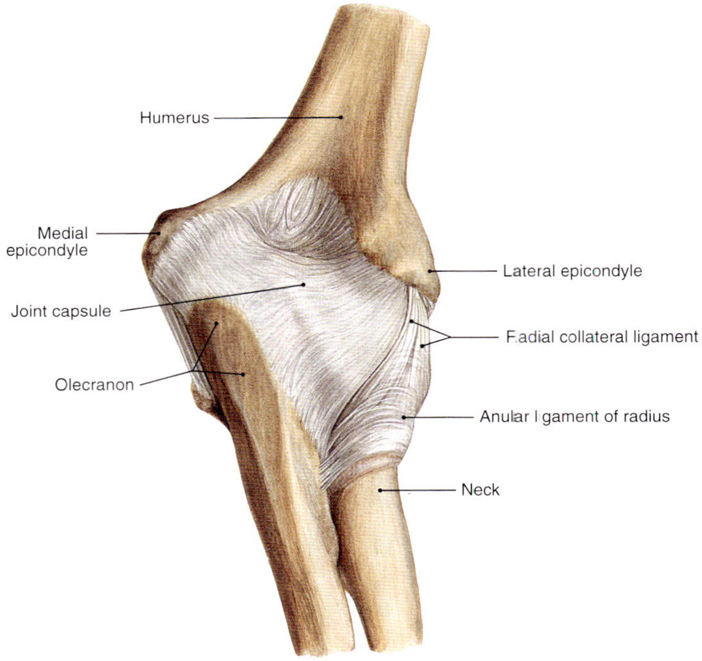

Fig. 304 Elbow joint; dorsal view.

Junctions of the bones of the forearm

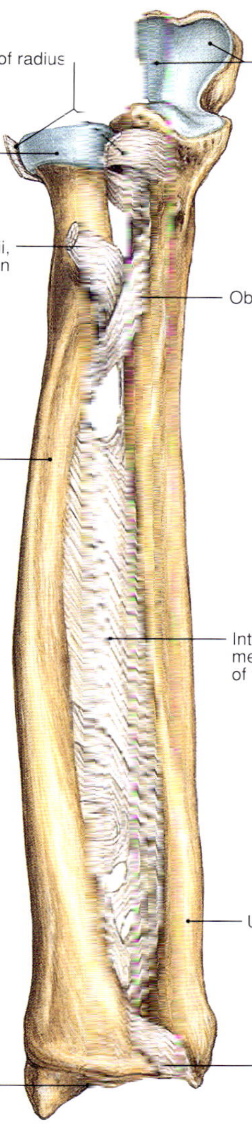

Fig. 305 Junctions of the bones of the forearm; in supination; ventral view.

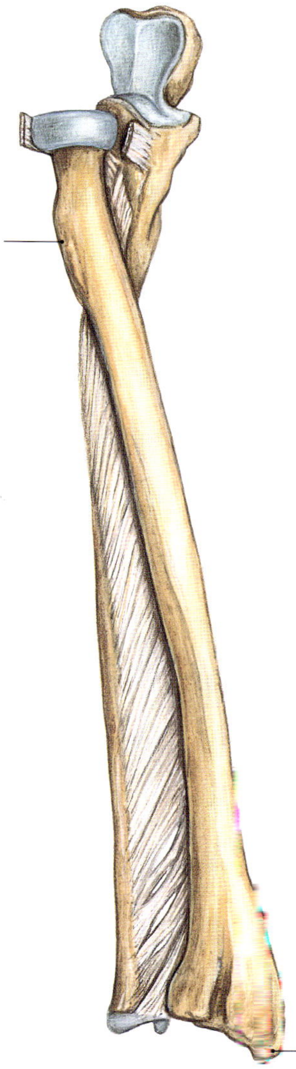

Fig. 306 Junctions of the bones of the forearm; in pronation; ventral view of the ulna, dorsal view of the radius.

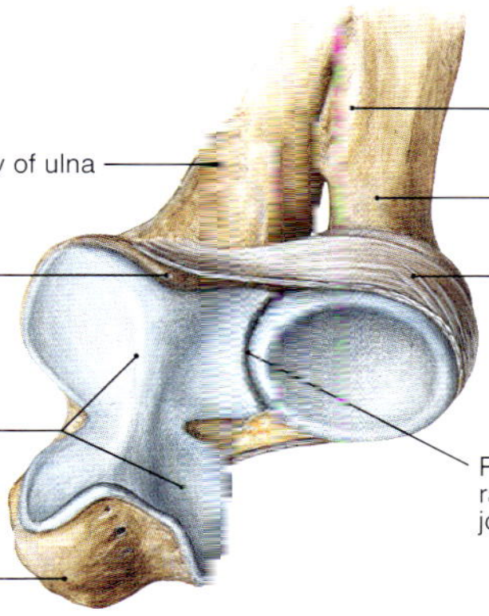

Fig. 307 Proximal radio-ulnar joint; ventroproximal view.

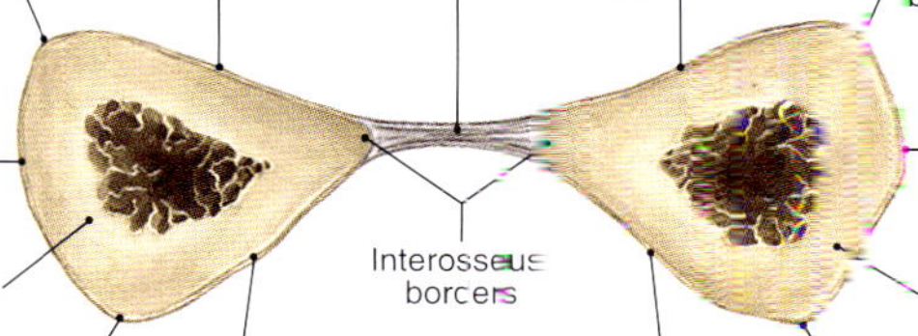

Fig. 308 Cross-section through the bones of the forearm; distal view.

Elbow joint, sections and radiography

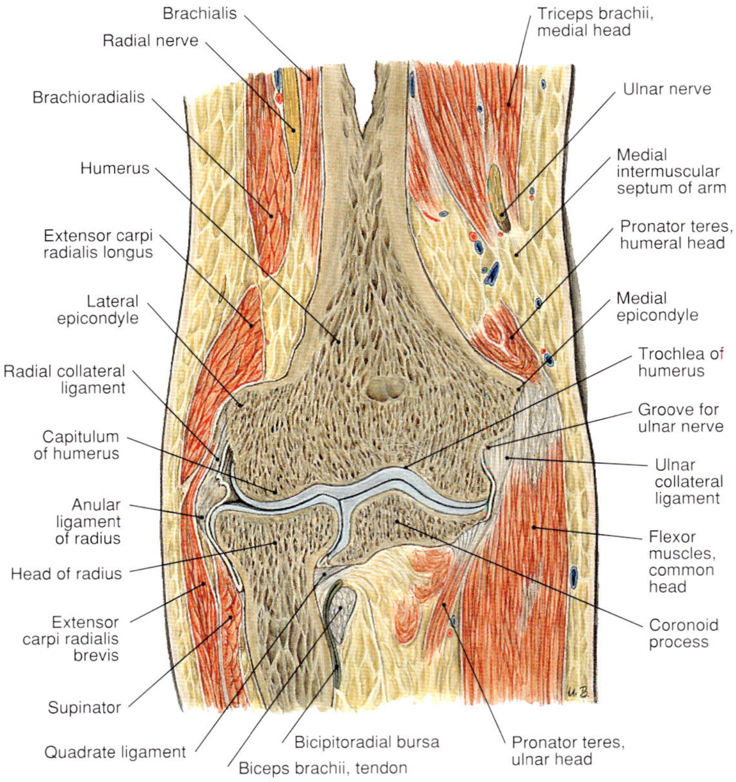

Fig. 309 Elbow joint; frontal section.

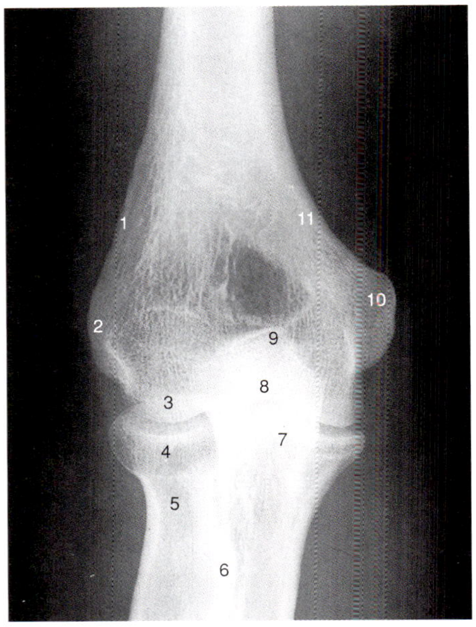

1 Lateral supraepicondylar ridge
2 Lateral epicondyle
3 Capitulum of humerus
4 Head of radius
5 Neck
6 Radial tuberosity
7 Coronoid process
8 Trochlea of humerus
9 Olecranon
10 Medial epicondyle
11 Medial supraepicondylar ridge

Fig. 310 Elbow joint; AP-radiograph.

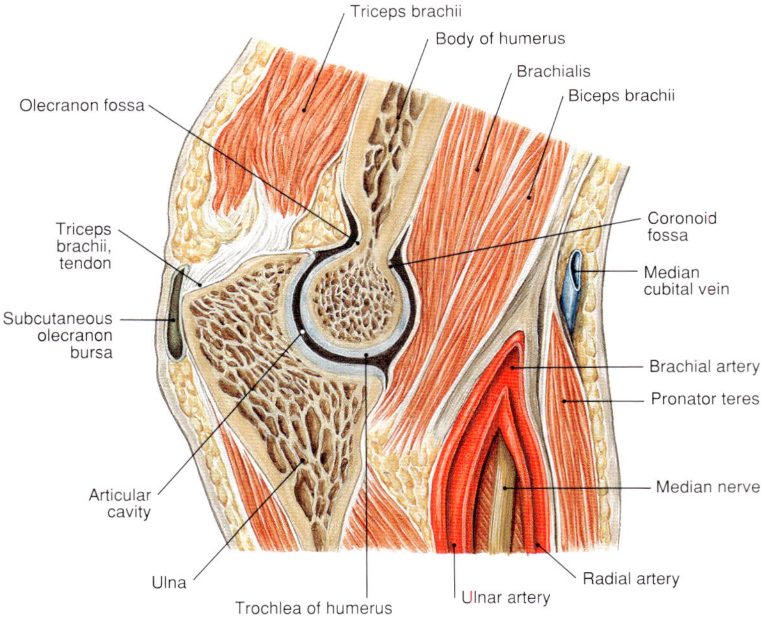

Fig. 311 Elbow joint; sagittal section.

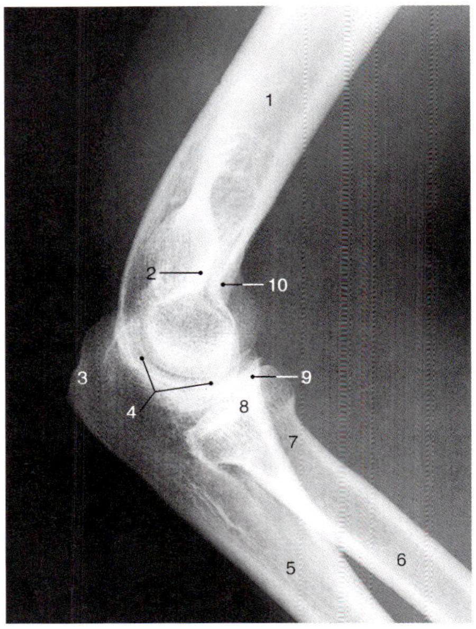

1 Humerus
2 Olecranon fossa
3 Olecranon
4 Trochlear notch
5 Ulna
6 Radius
7 Neck
8 Head of radius
9 Coronoid process
10 Coronoid fossa

Fig. 312 Elbow joint; lateral radiograph.

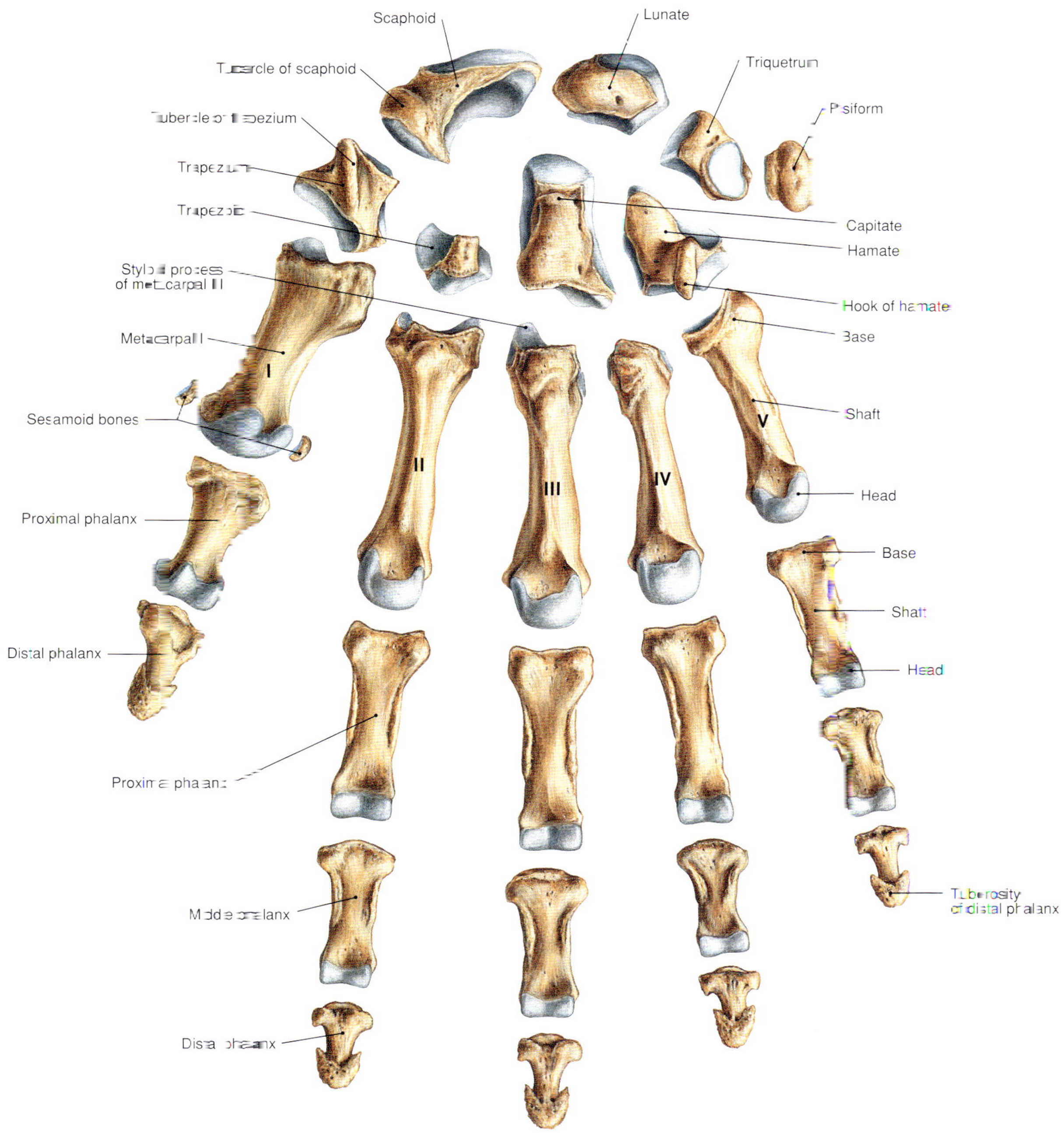

I Thumb
II Index finger
III Middle finger
IV Ring finger
V Little finger

Fig. 313 Bones of the hand; palmar view.

Skeleton of the hand

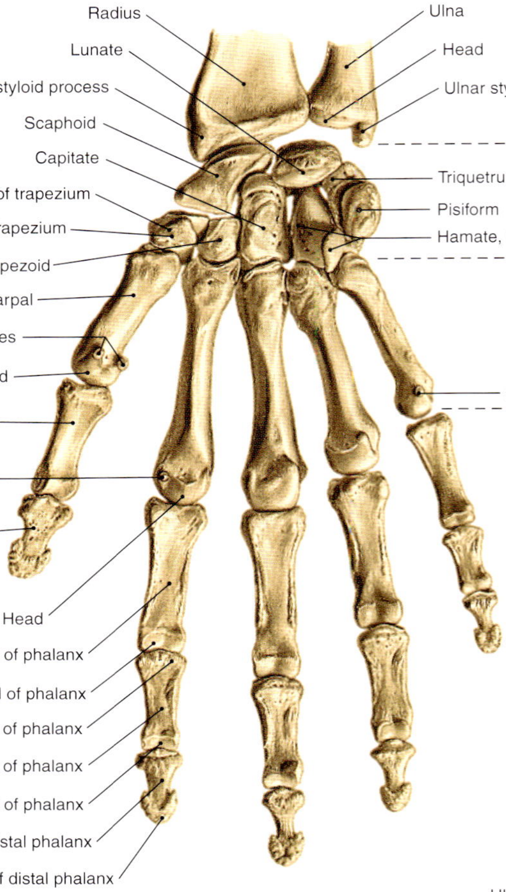

Fig. 314 Bones of the hand; palmar view.

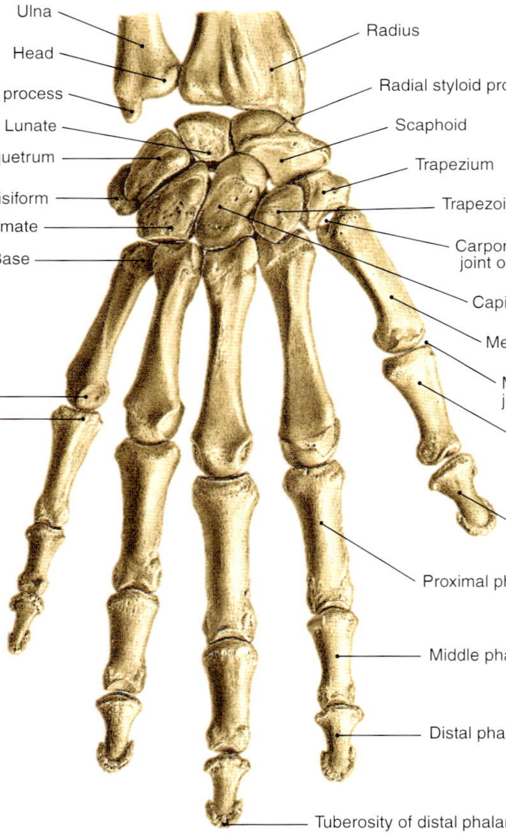

Fig. 315 Bones of the hand; dorsal view.

* Also: saddle joint of the thumb
** Also: proximal phalangeal joint of the thumb

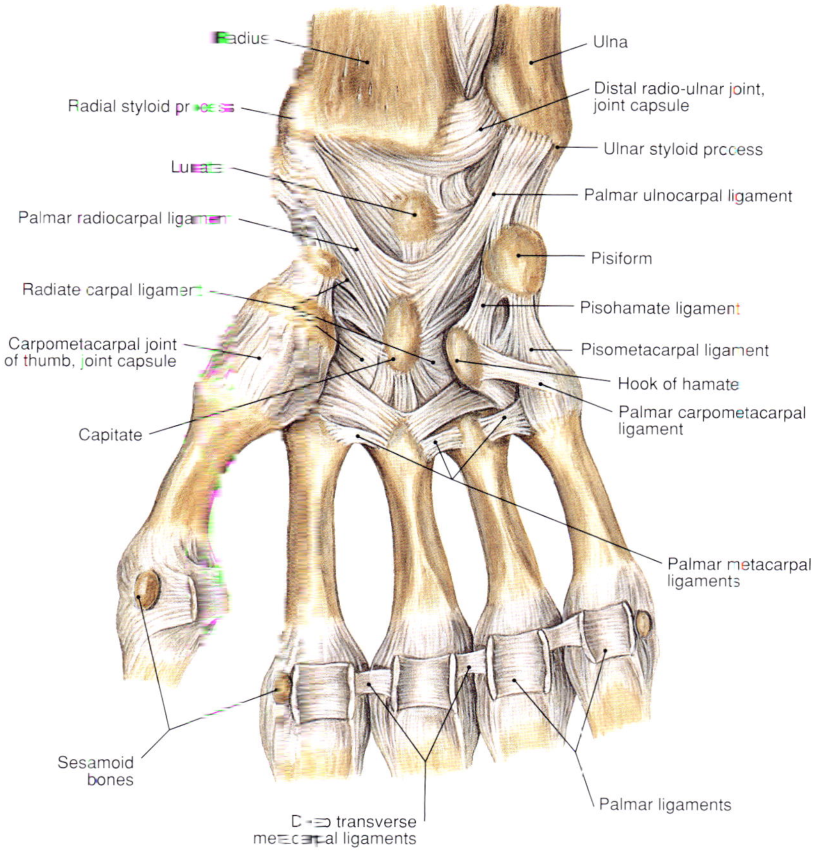

Fig. 316 Joints and ligaments of the hand; palmar view.

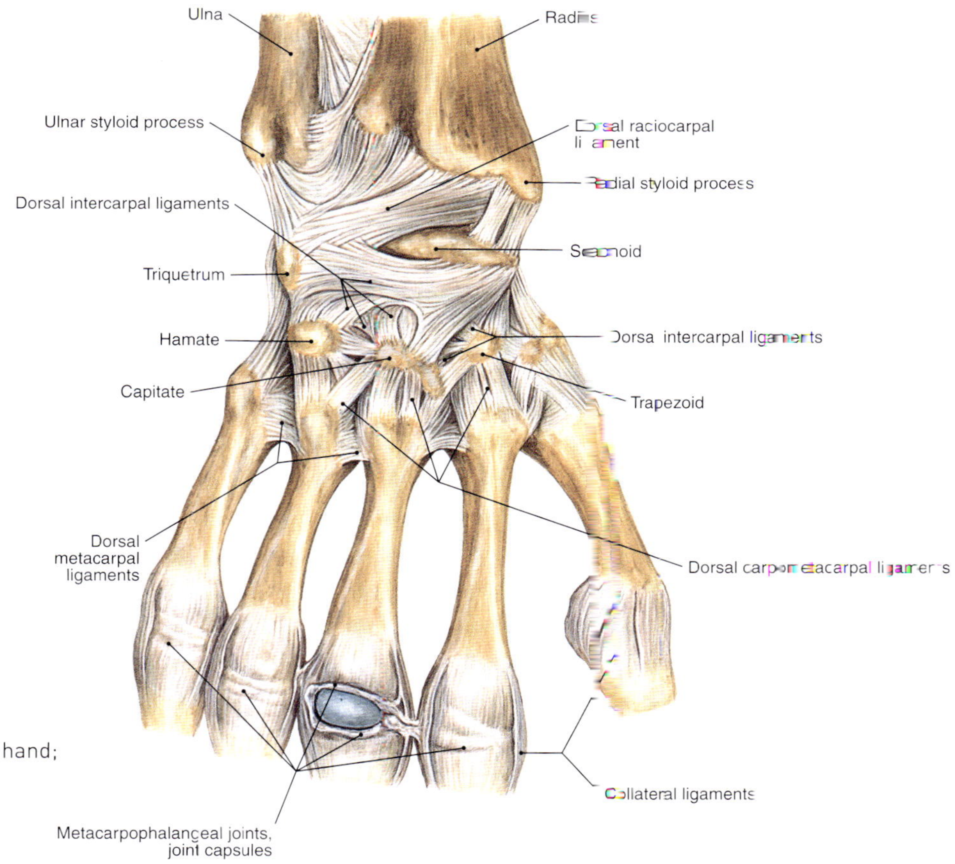

Fig. 317 Joints and ligaments of the hand; dorsal view.

Joints of the hand

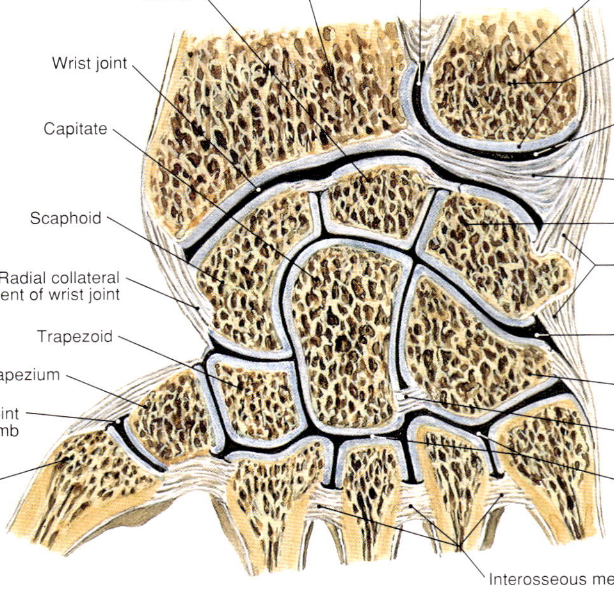

Fig. 318 Carpal joints;
longitudinal section parallel to the dorsum of the hand.

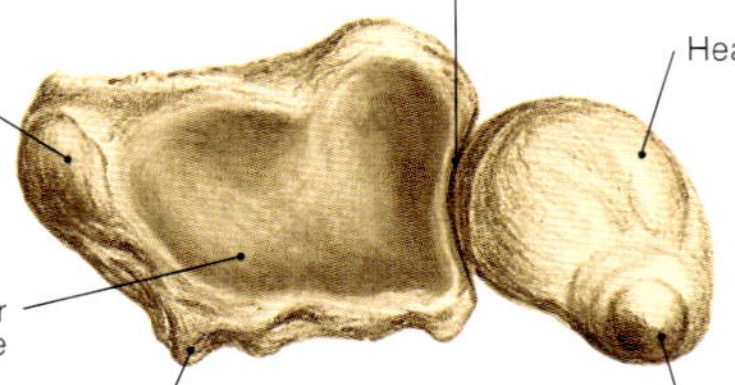

Fig. 319 Ulna and radius;
distal view.

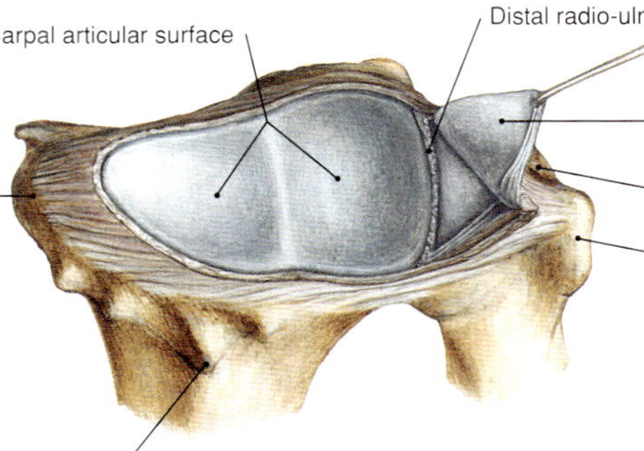

Fig. 320 Distal radio-ulnar joint;
distal-dorsal view.

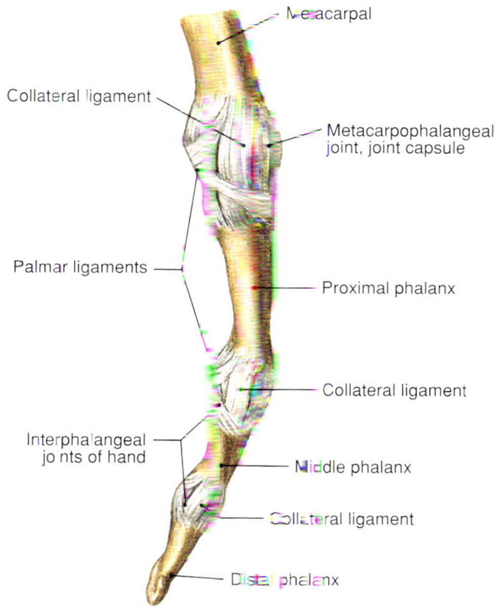

Fig. 321 Finger joints; lateral view.

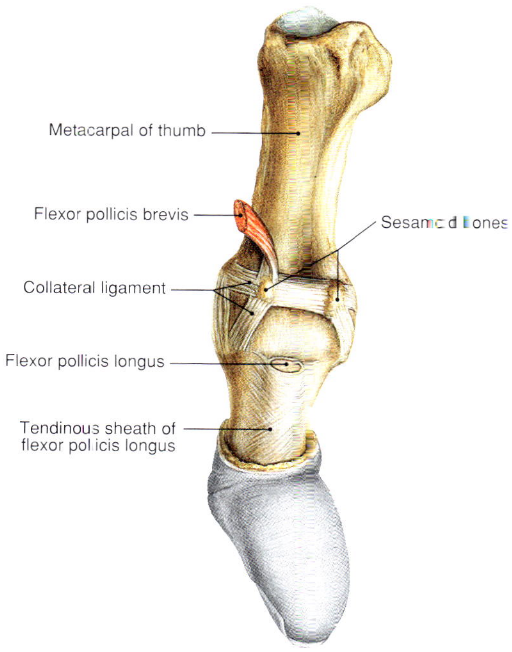

Fig. 322 Metacarpophalangeal joint of the thumb; radial-palmar view.

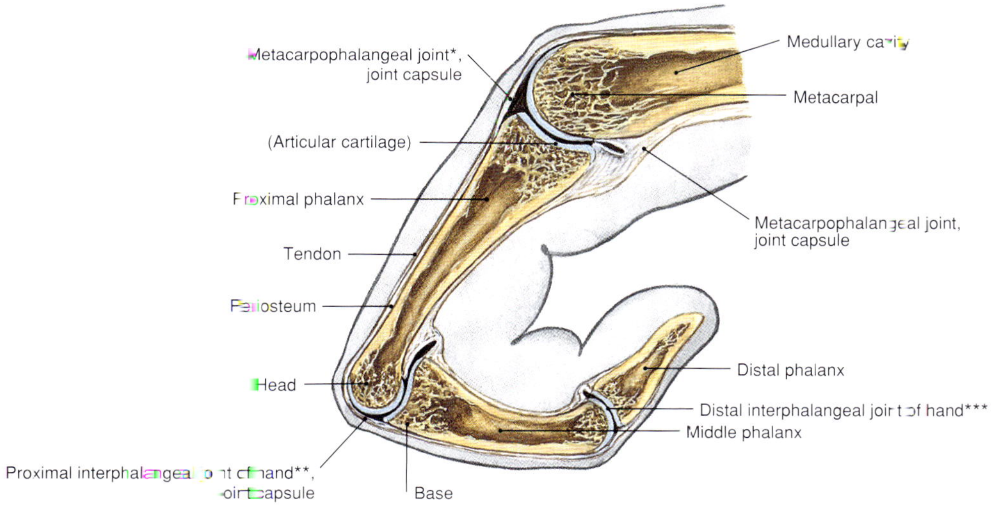

Fig. 323 Finger joints; sagittal section; lateral view.

* Clinical term: **MP** (= **m**etacarpo**p**halangeal joint)
** Clinical term: **PIP** (= **p**roximal **i**nter**p**halangeal joint)
*** Clinical term: **DIP** (= **d**istal **i**nter**p**halangeal joint)

Wrist, radiography

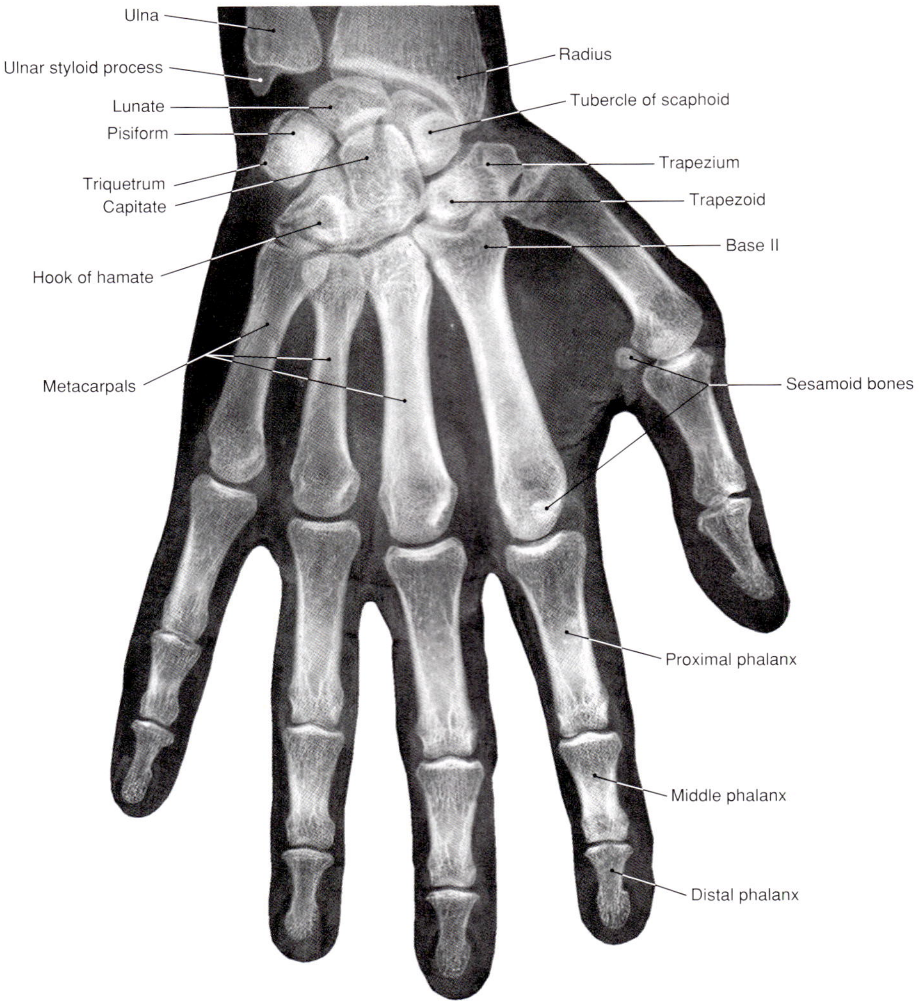

Fig. 324 Hand;
PA-radiograph.
Note: The pisiform bone is projected onto the triquetral bone.

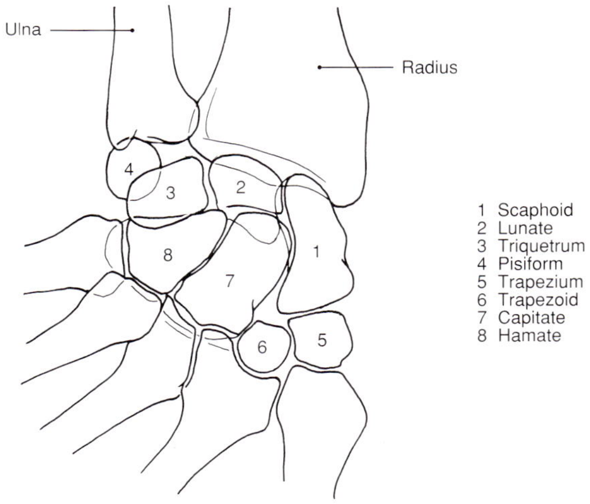

Fig. 325 Ulnar abduction of the hand;
schema of a PA-radiograph.

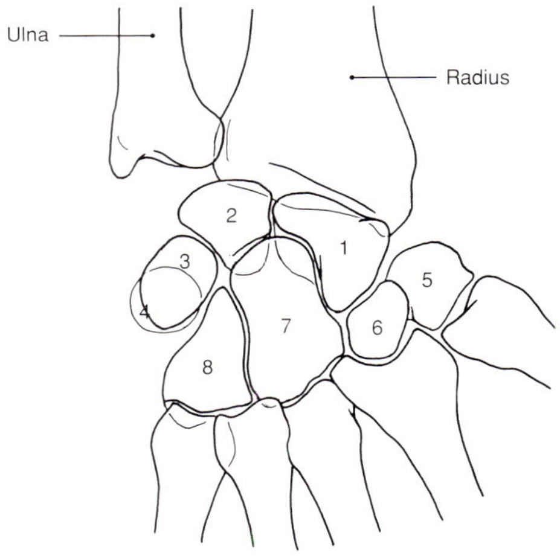

Fig. 326 Radial abduction of the hand;
schema of a PA-radiograph.

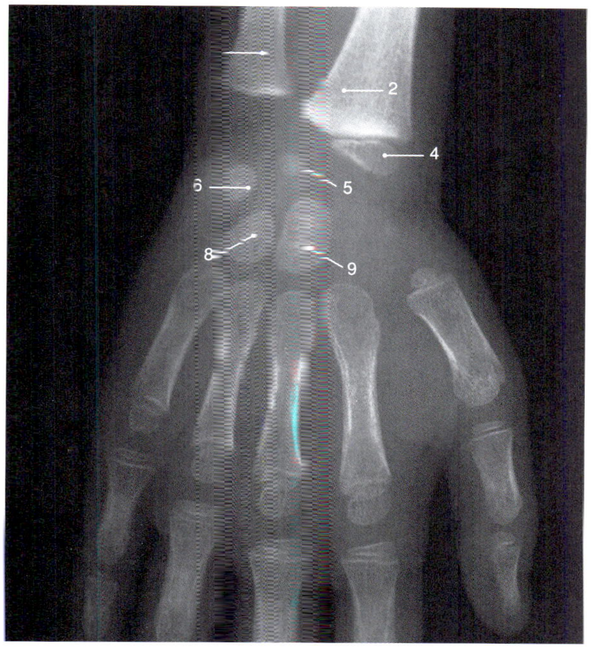

Fig. 327 PA-radiograph of the hand of a 41/2-year-old boy.

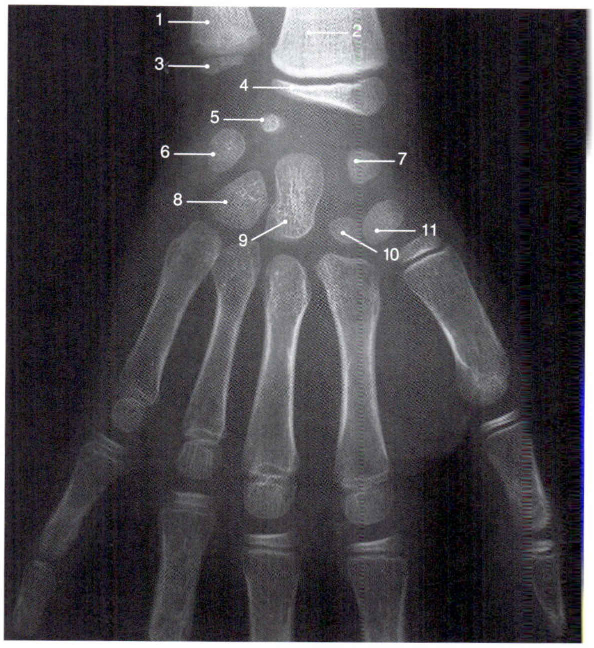

Fig. 328 PA-radiograph of the hand of a 7-year-old boy.

1 Ulna, diaphysis
2 Radius, diaphysis
3 Ulna, distal epiphysis
4 Radius, distal epiphysis
5 Lunate
6 Triquetrum
7 Scaphoid
8 Hamate
9 Capitate
10 Trapezoid
11 Trapezium
12 Pisiform

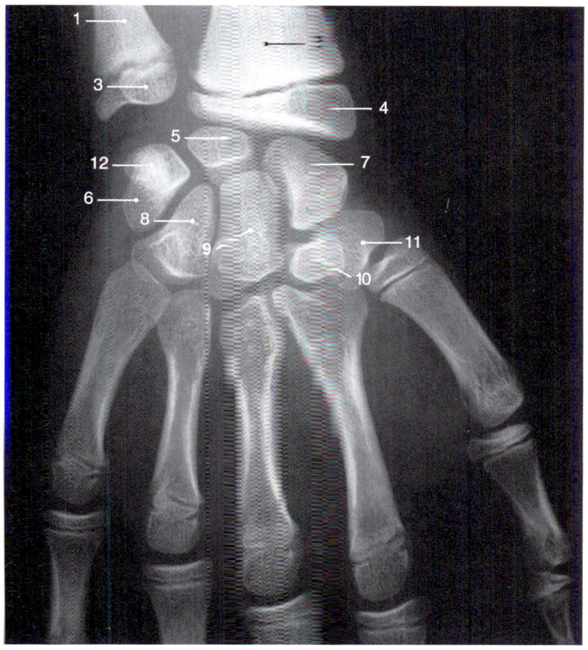

Fig. 329 PA-radiograph of the hand of an 11-year-old boy.

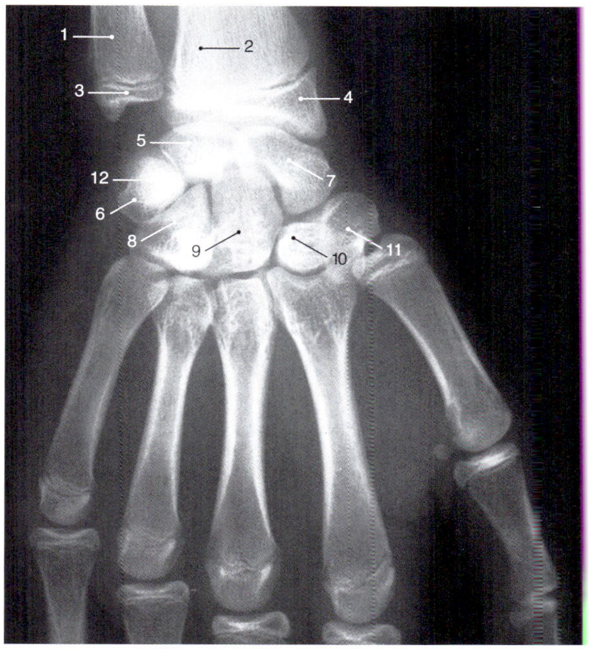

Fig. 330 PA-radiograph of the hand of a 13-year-old boy.

Fascia of the upper limb

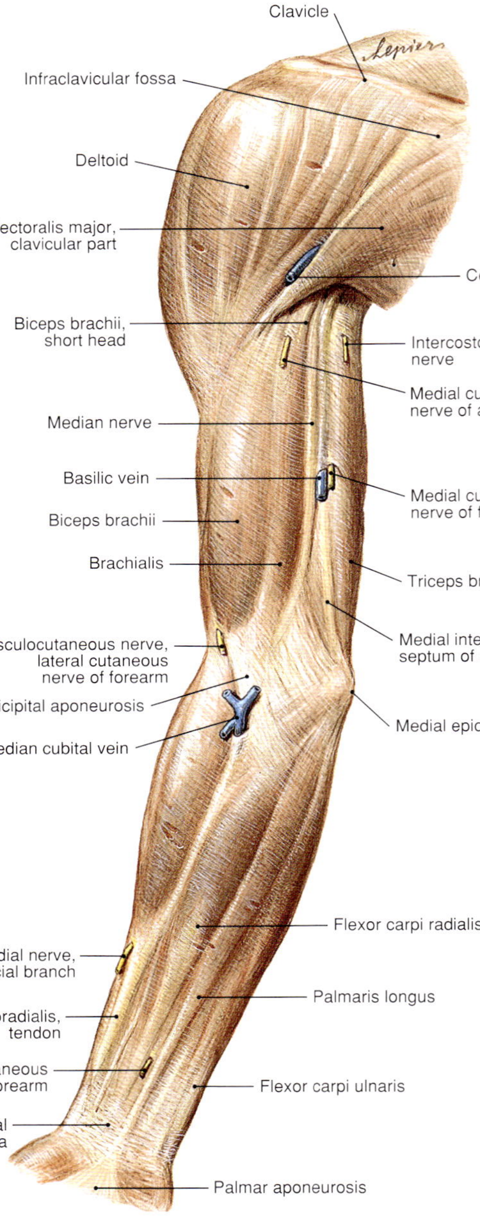

Fig. 331 Fascia of the flexor aspect of the upper limb.

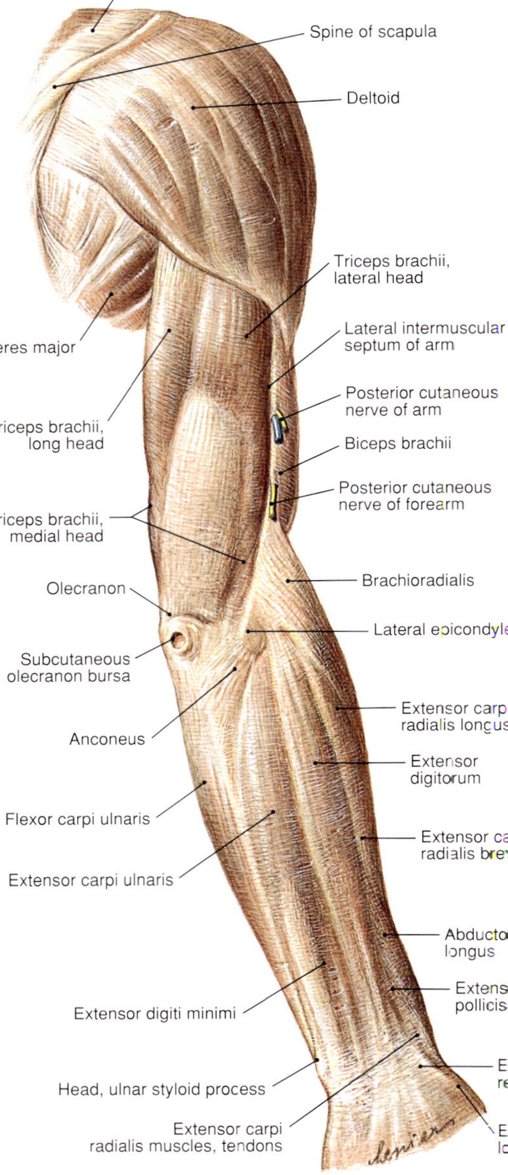

Fig. 332 Fascia of the extensor aspect of the upper limb.

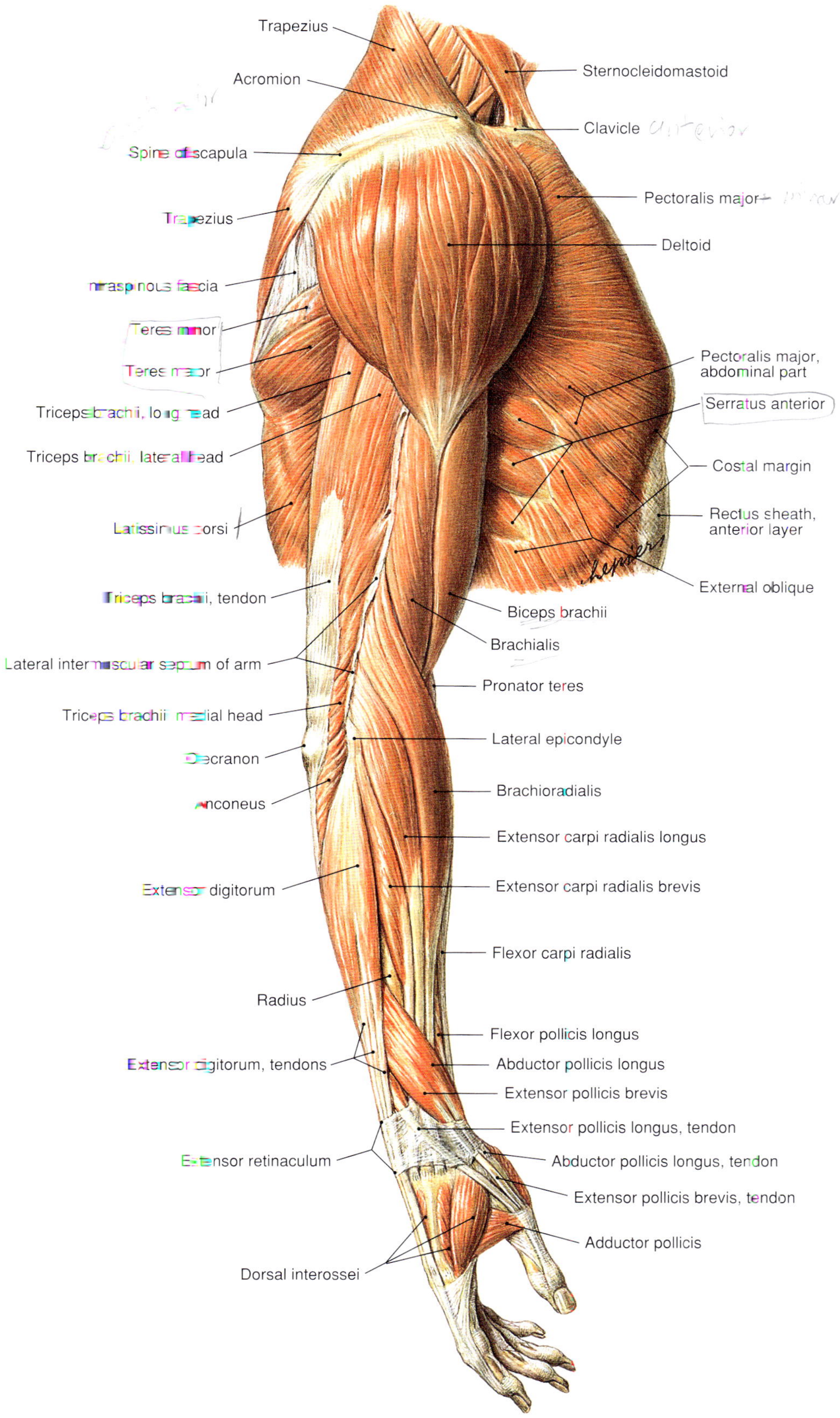

Fig. 333 Muscles of the upper limb, the thorax and the inferior region of the neck.

→ T 26–T 38

Muscles of the upper limb

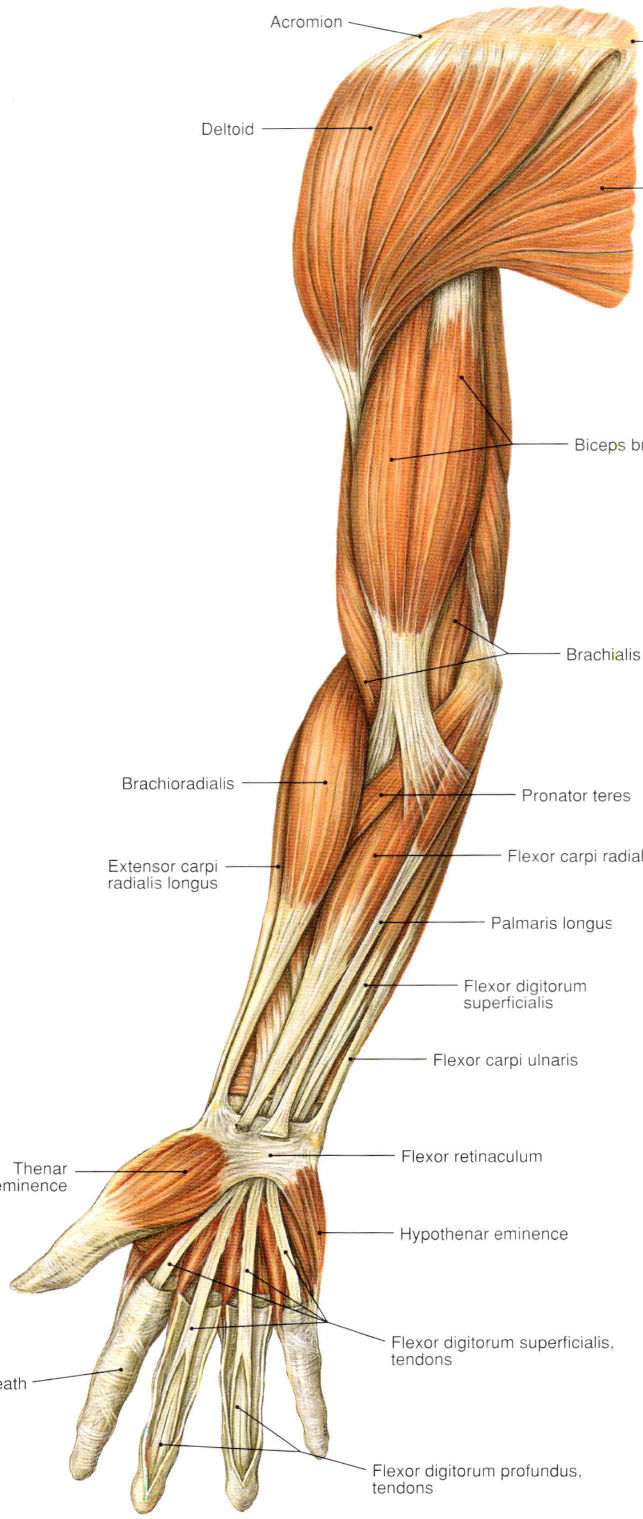

→ T 26–T 38

Fig. 334 Muscles of the flexor aspect of the upper limb.

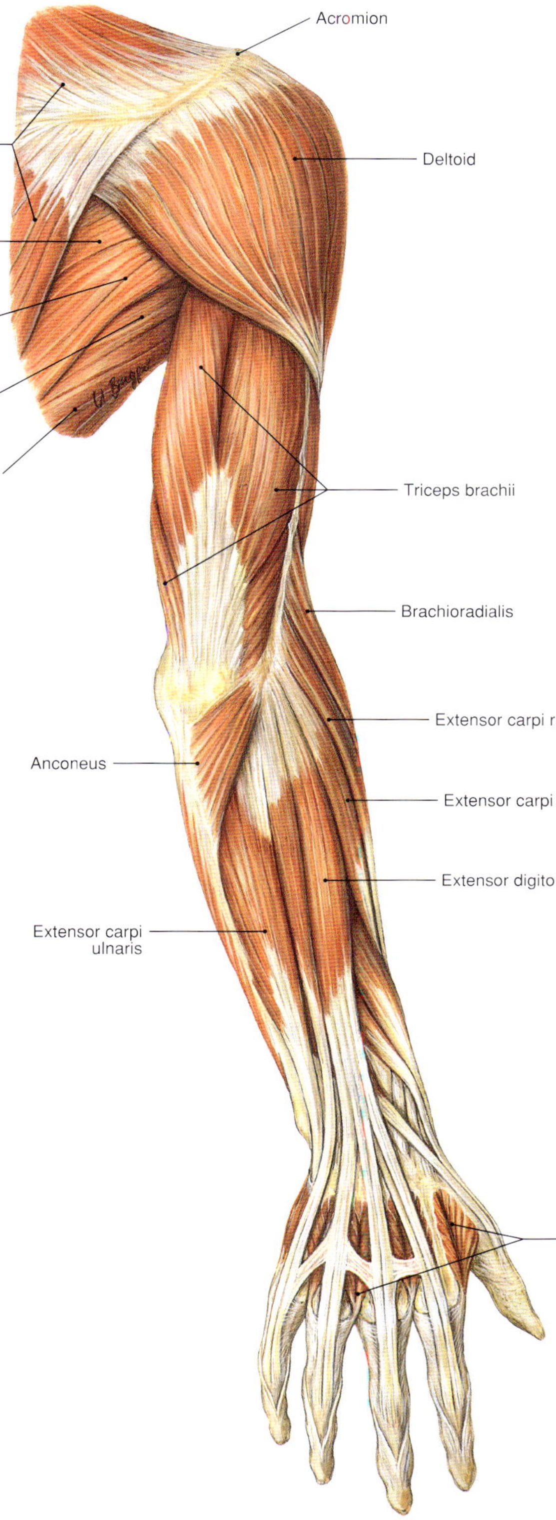

Fig. 335 Muscles of the extensor aspect of the upper limb.

→ T 26–T 38

Muscles of the shoulder

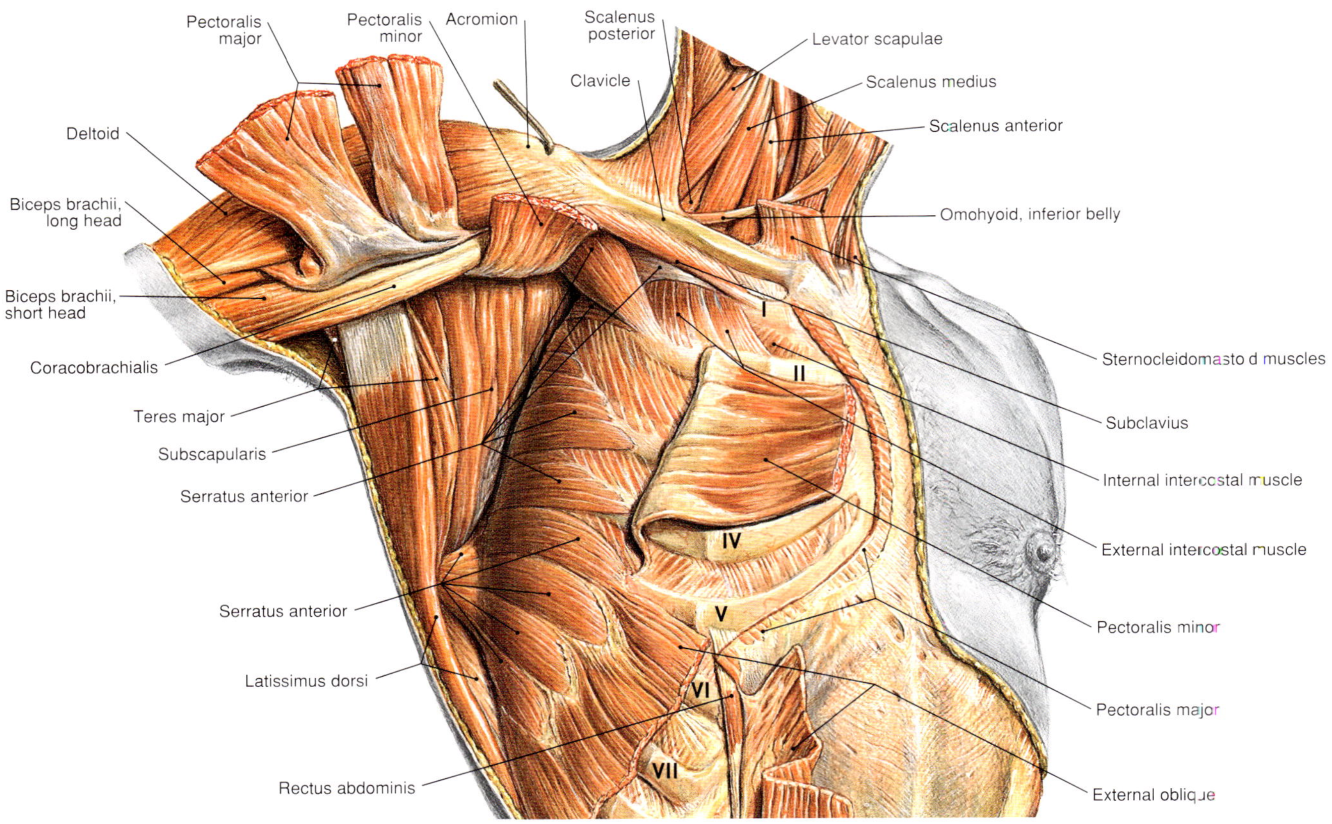

→ 204, 570, 571

Fig. 336 Muscles of the arm, the thorax and the inferior region of the neck.
I, II, IV–VII indicate the corresponding ribs.

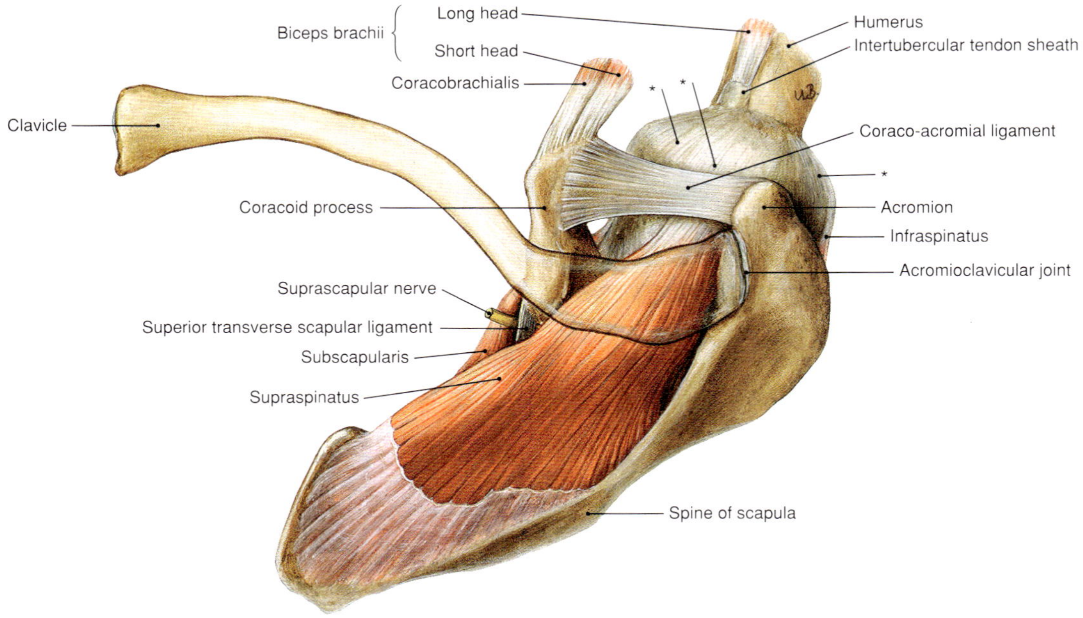

→ T 27

Fig. 337 Shoulder and muscles of the shoulder. Together, the muscle tendons marked with * form the so-called rotator cuff.

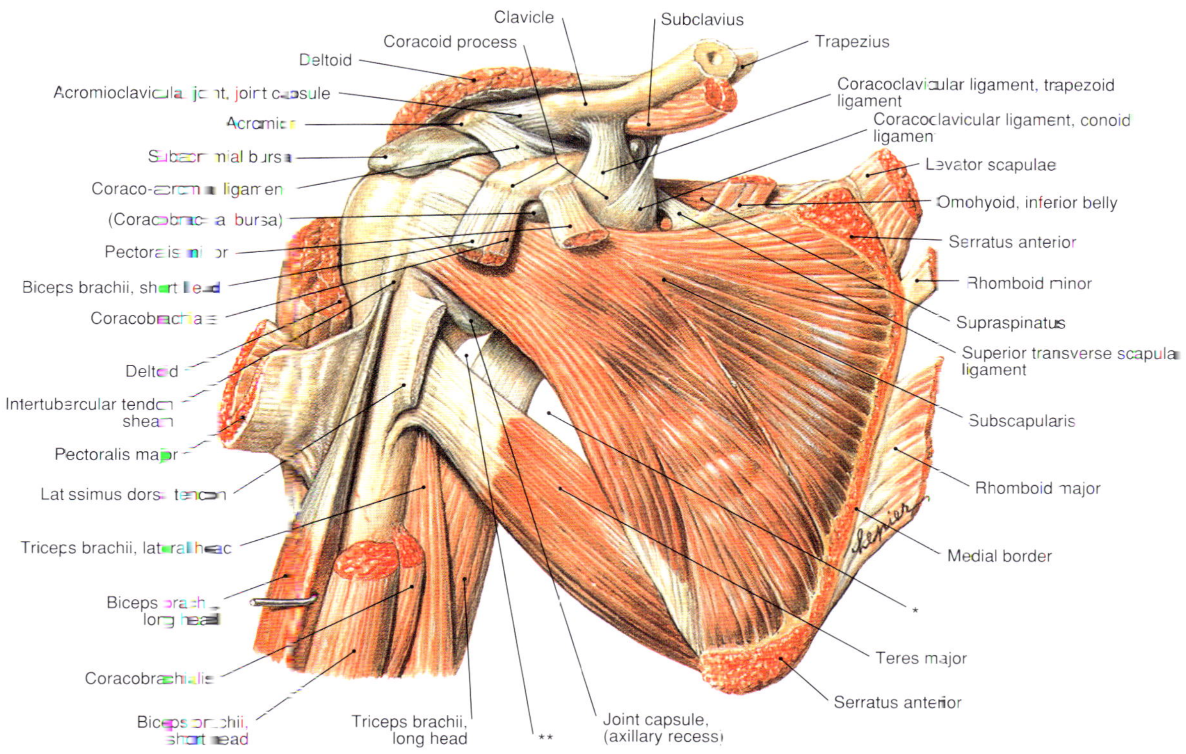

Fig. 338 Shoulder and muscles of the shoulder.

→ T 26

* Triangular space
** Quadrangular space

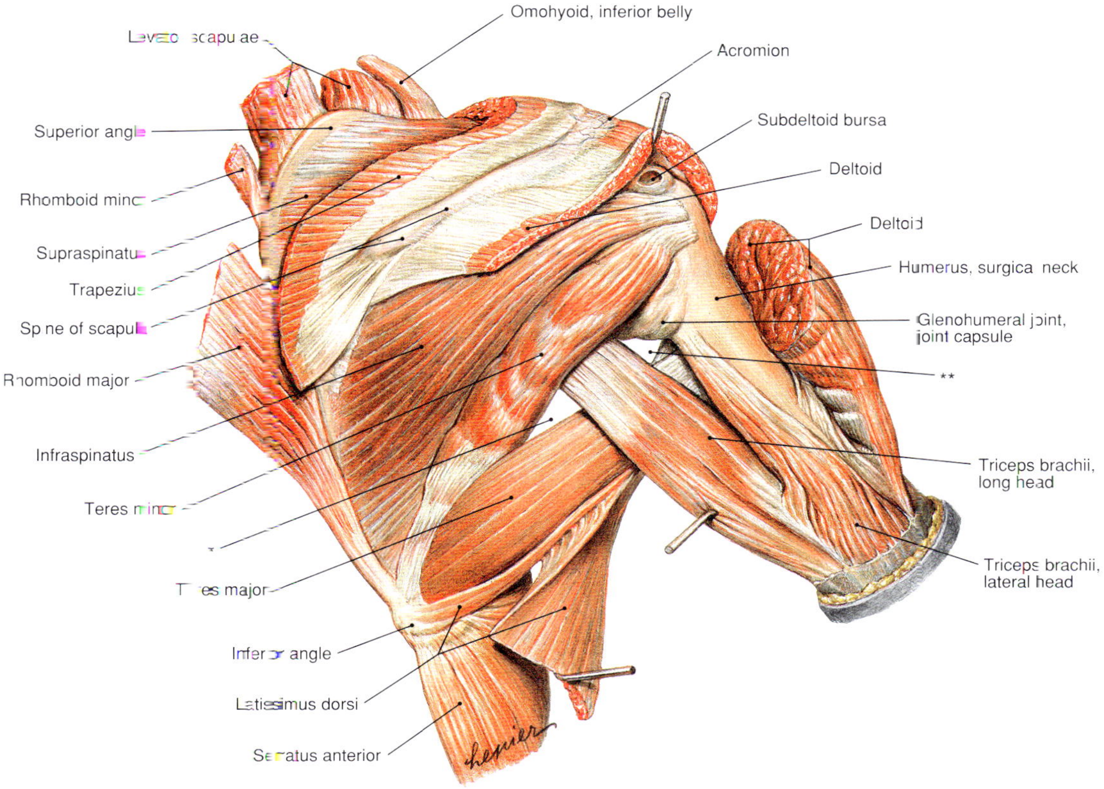

Fig. 339 Shoulder and muscles of the shoulder.

→ T 28

* Triangular space
** Quadrangular space

Muscles of the shoulder

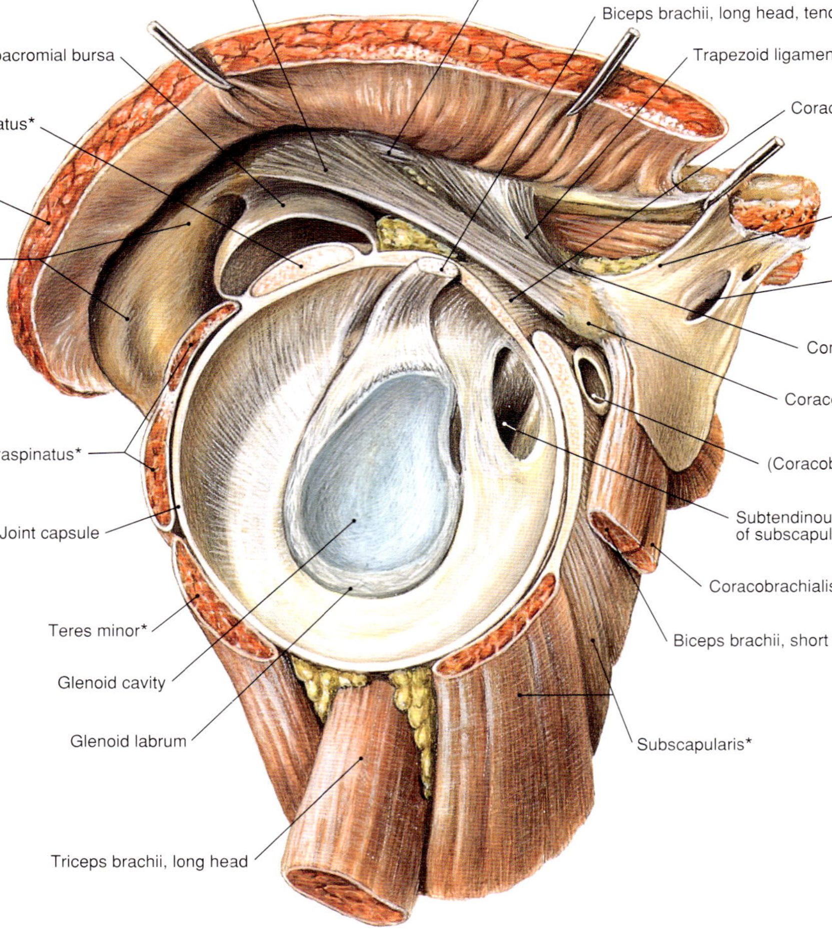

→ T 26–T 28

Fig. 340 Shoulder joint;
lateral view.
Together, the muscle tendons marked with * form the so-called rotator cuff.

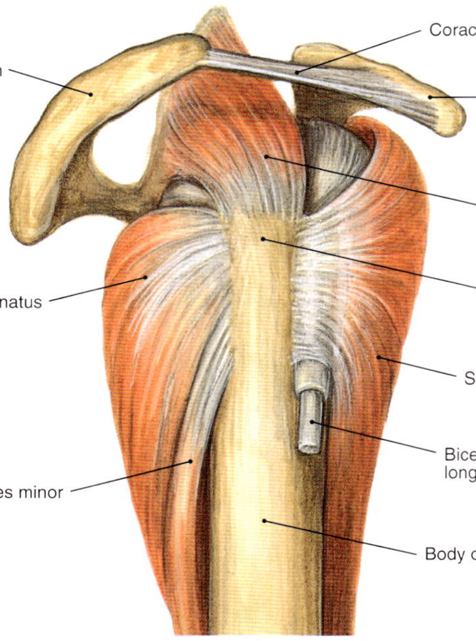

→ T 26–T 28

Fig. 341 Muscles of the so-called rotator cuff;
lateral view.

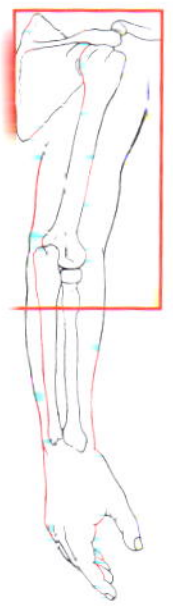

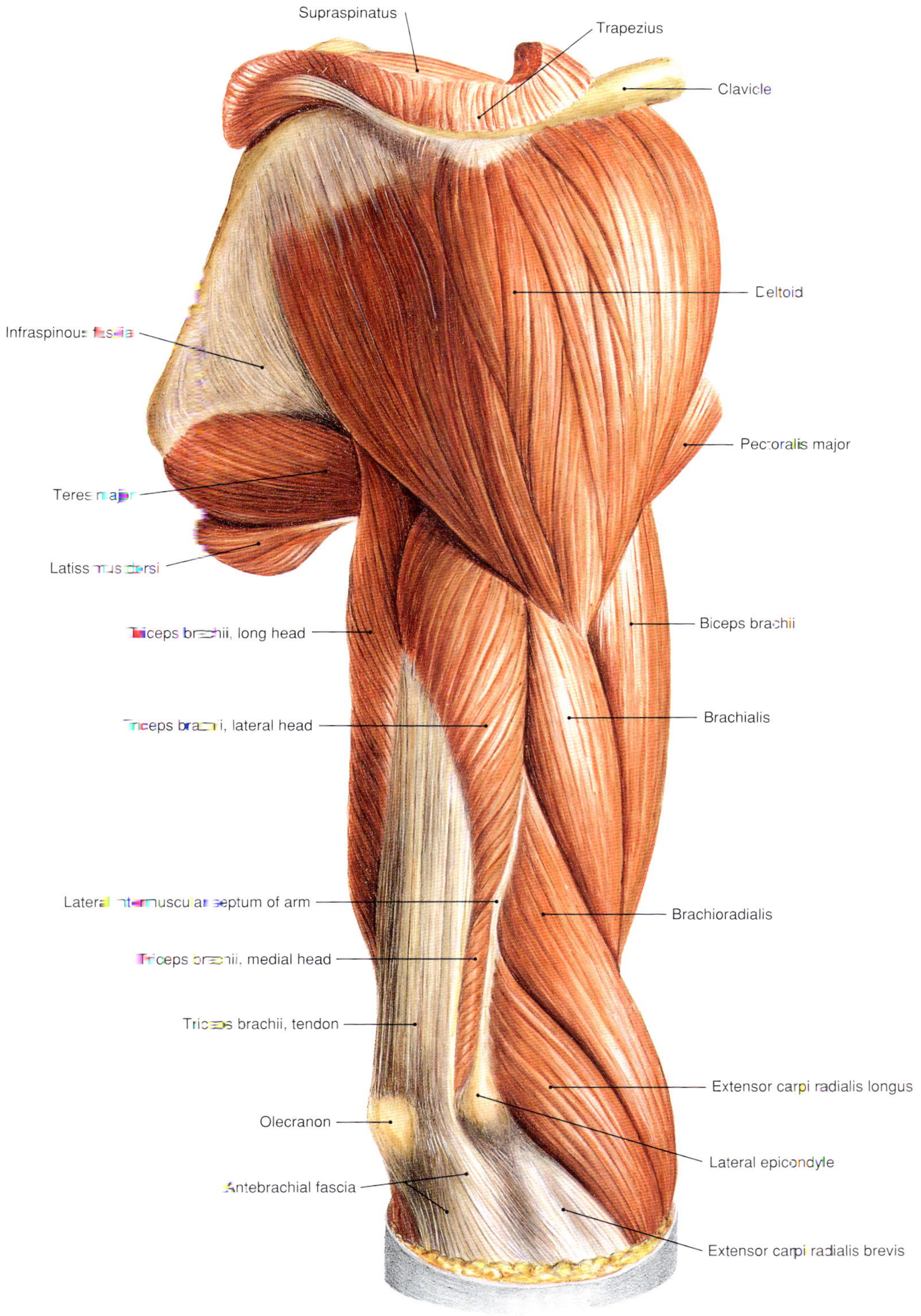

Fig. 342 Muscles of the arm;
superficial layer;
dorsolateral view.

→ T 27, T 30

Origins and insertions of the muscles of the shoulder and the arm

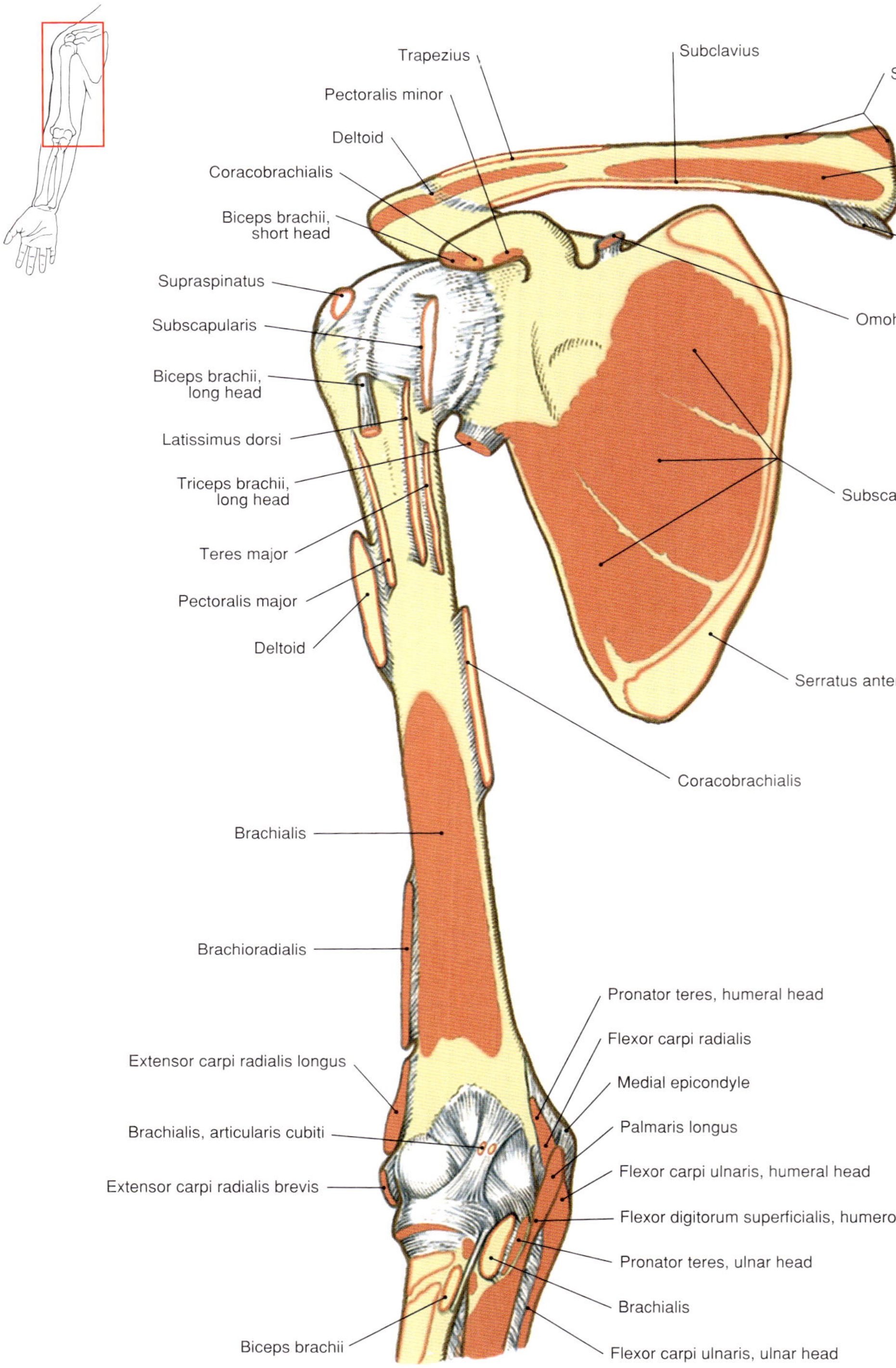

→ T 26–T 30

Fig. 343 Origins and insertions of the muscles at the clavicle, the scapula and the humerus (as well as ulnar origins of multi-head muscles).

Origins and insertions of the muscles of the shoulder and the arm

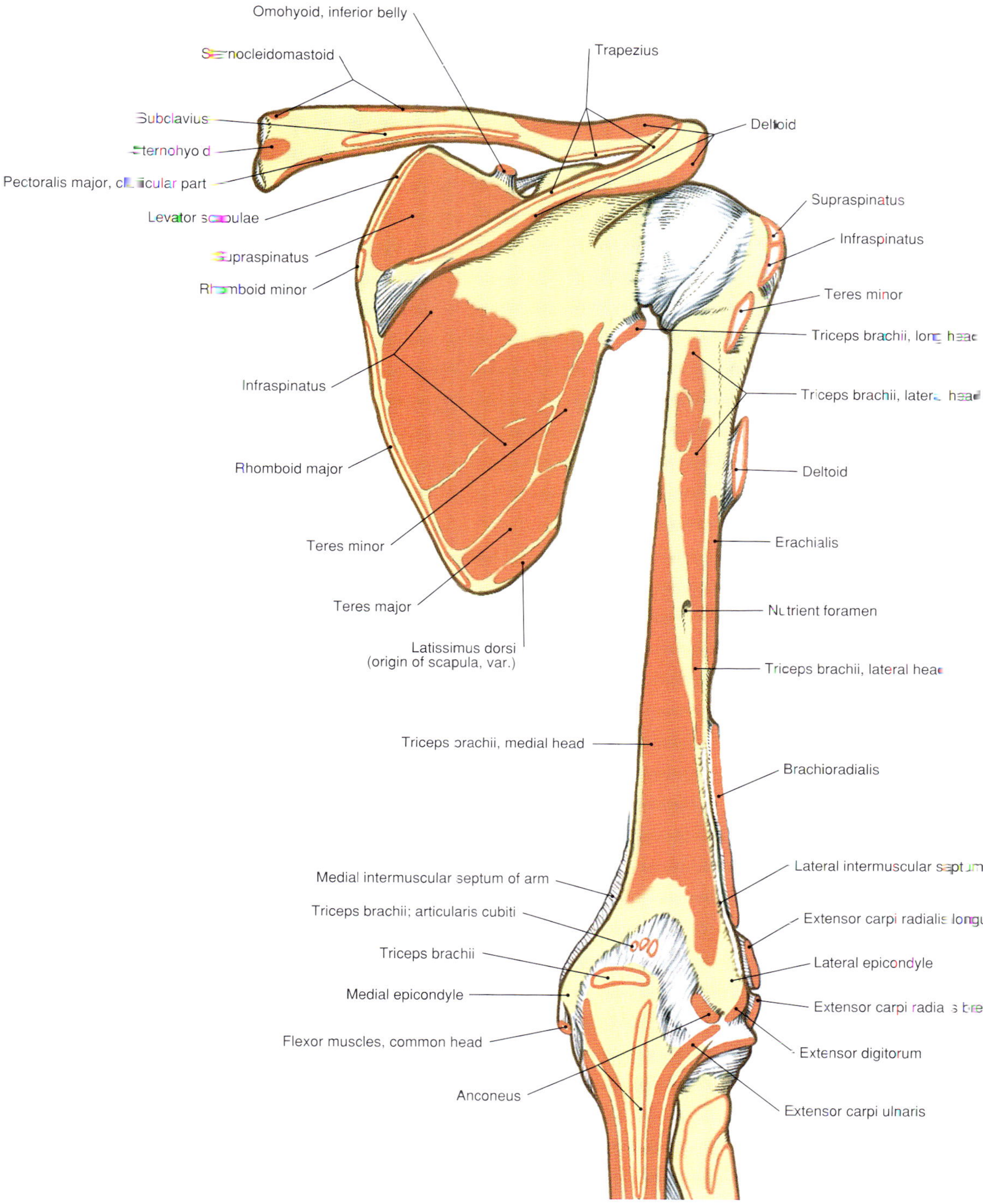

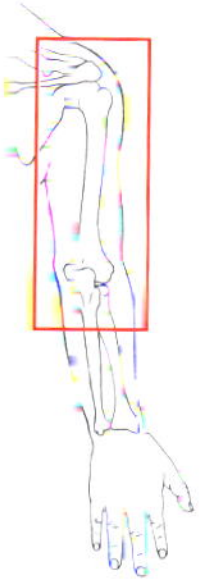

Fig. 344 Origins and insertions of the muscles at the clavicle, the scapula and the humerus (as well as ulnar origins of multi-head muscles).

→ T 26–T 30

Muscles of the arm

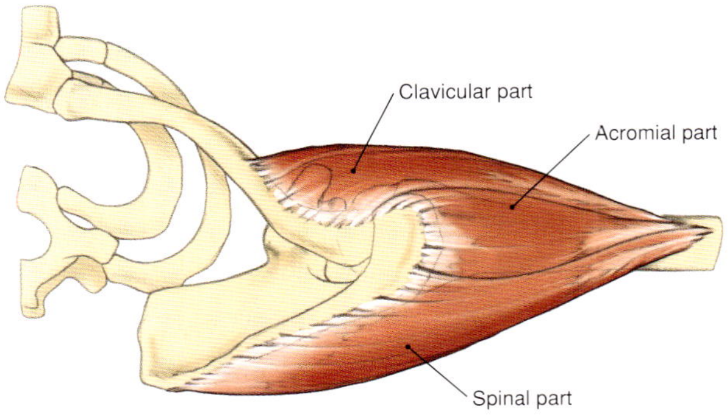

Fig. 345 Deltoid muscle.

→ T 27

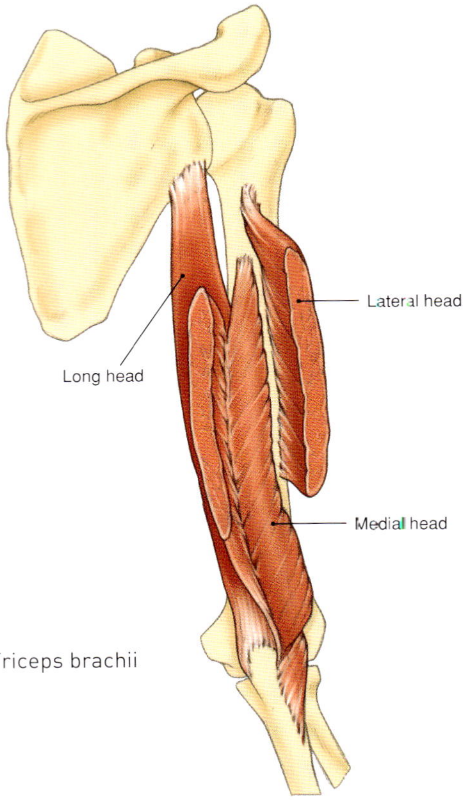

Fig. 346 Triceps brachii muscle.

→ T 30

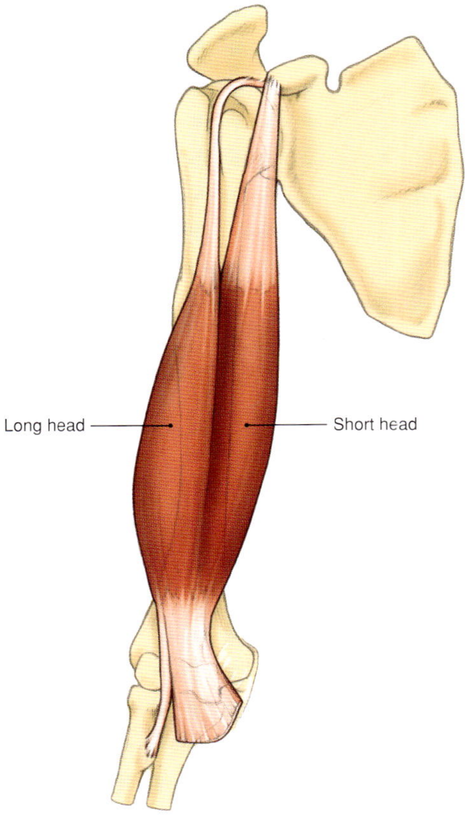

Fig. 347 Biceps brachii muscle.

→ T 29

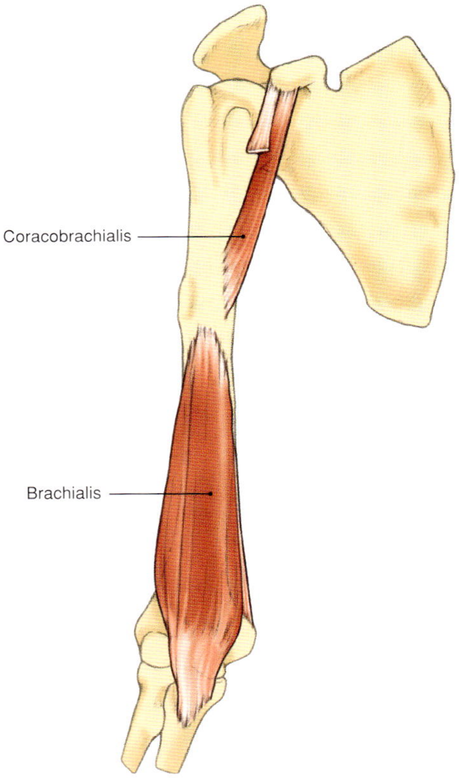

Fig. 348 Brachial and coracobrachial muscles.

→ T 29

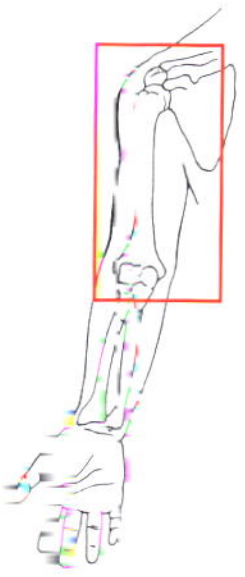

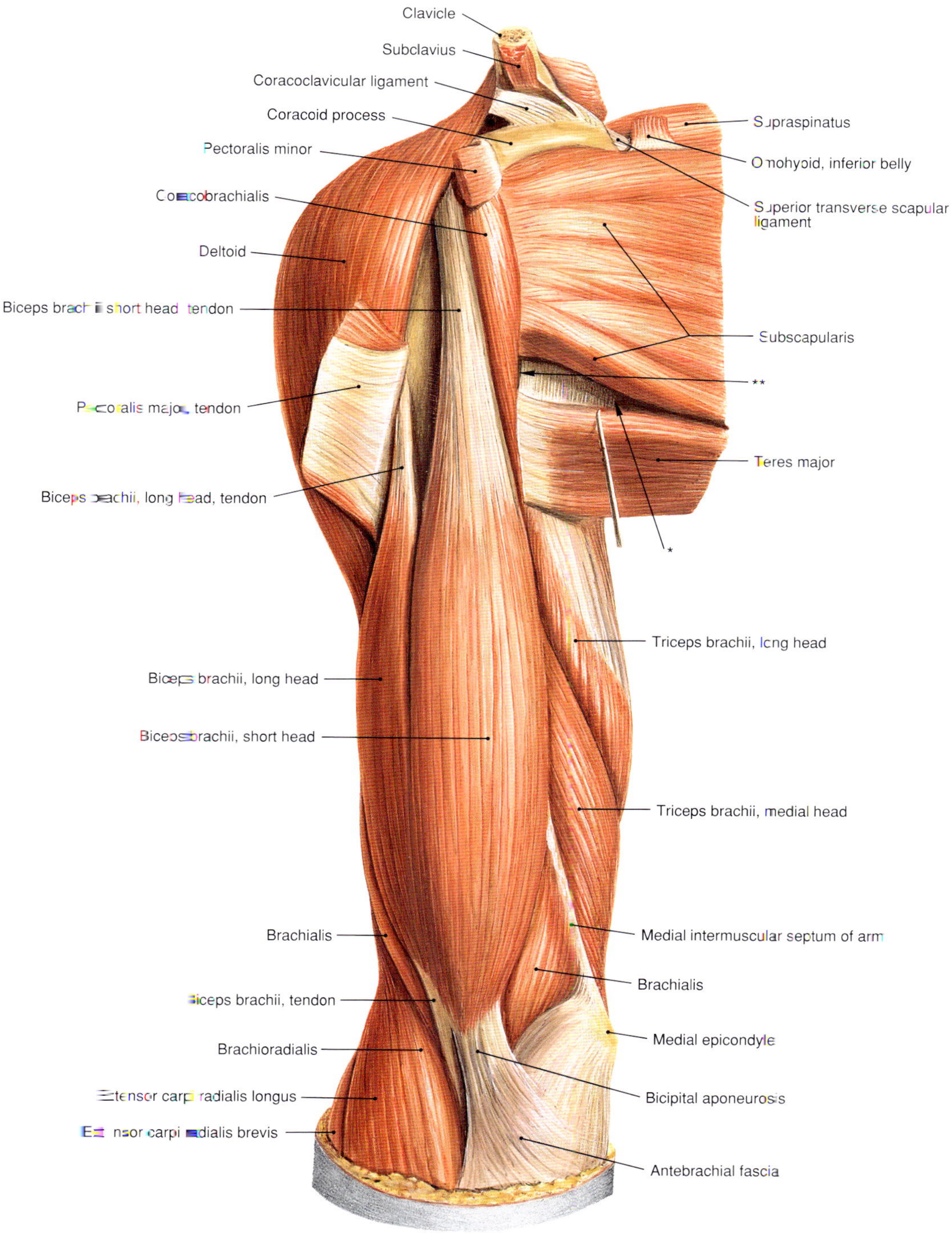

Fig. 349 Muscles of the arm; flexor aspect, superficial layer.

* Triangular space
** Quadrangular space

→ T 29

Muscles of the arm

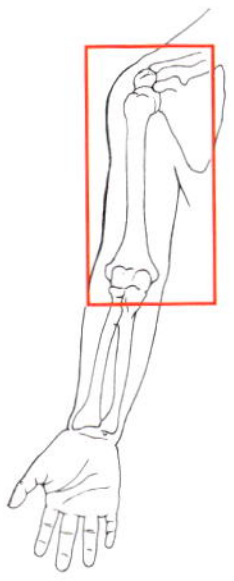

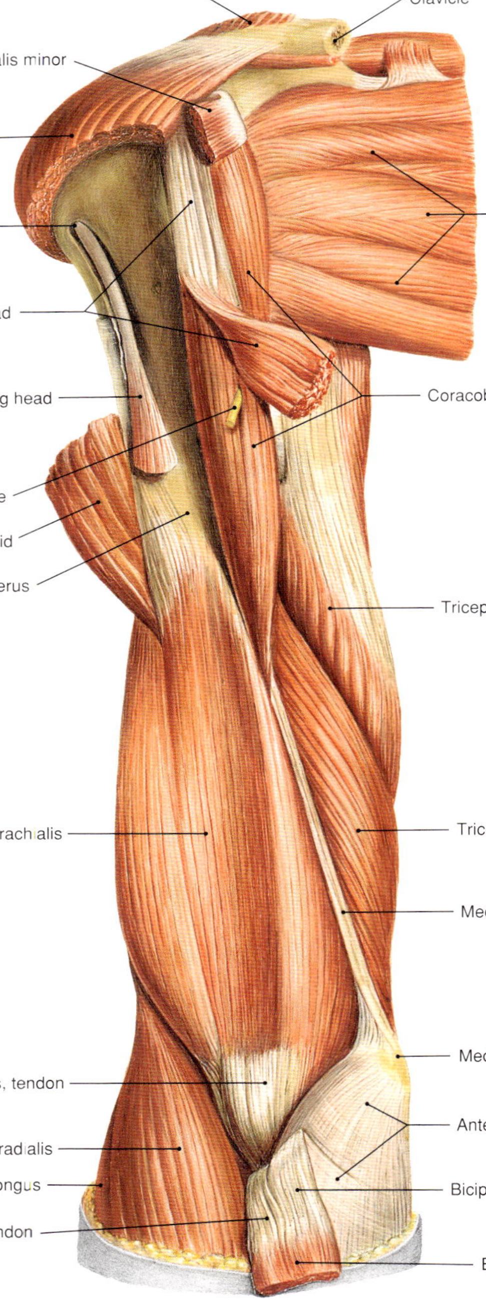

→ T 29

Fig. 350 Muscles of the arm; flexor aspect, deep layer.

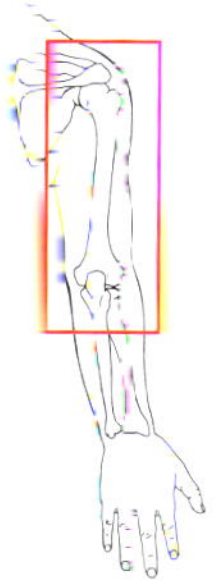

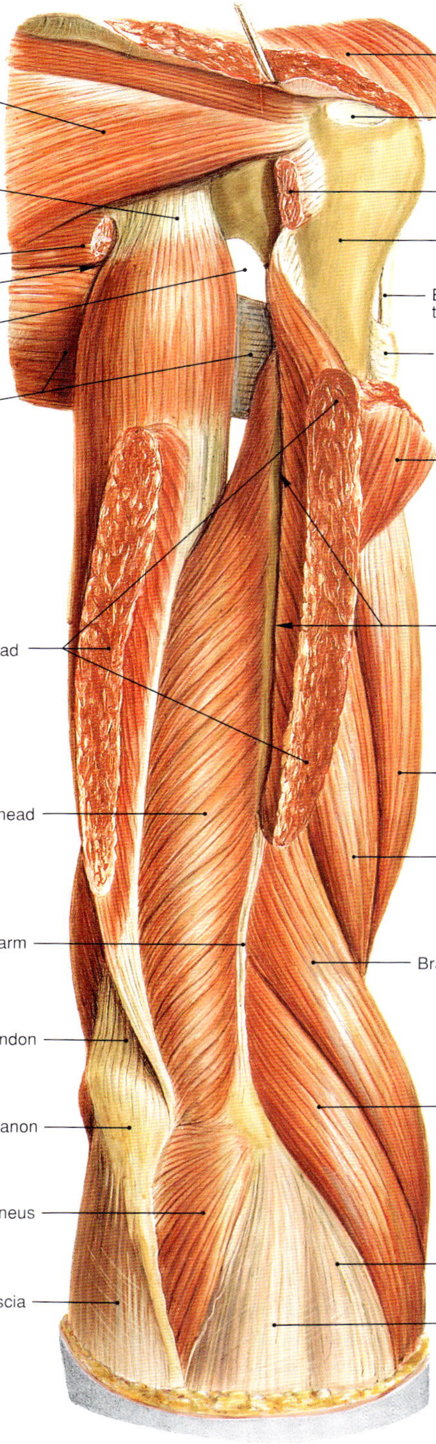

Fig. 351 Muscles of the arm; extensor aspect, deep layer.

→ T 30

* Triangular space
** Quadrangular space

Origins and insertions of the ventral muscles of the forearm

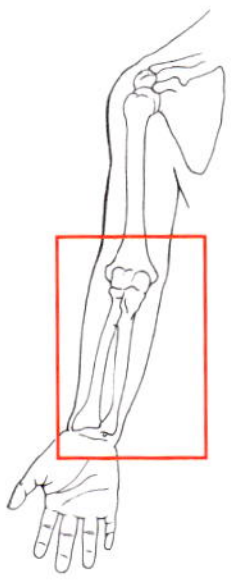

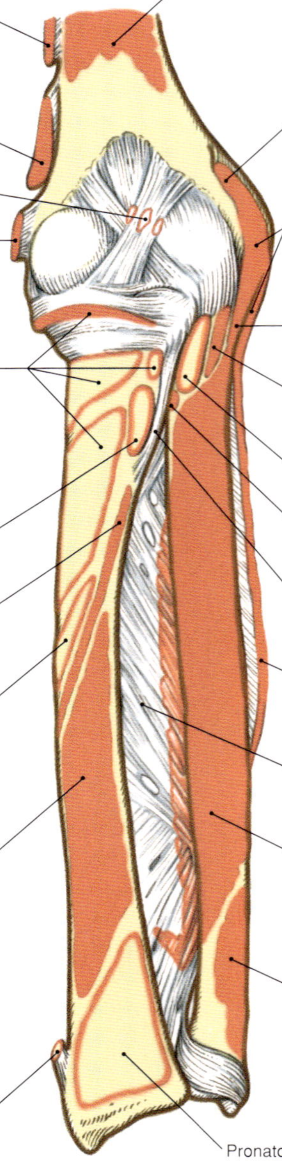

→ T 31–T 33

Fig. 352 Origins and insertions of the muscles at the radius, the ulna and the distal part of the humerus.

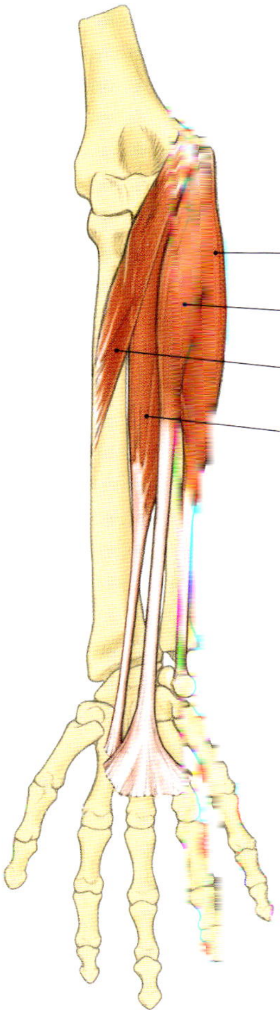

Fig. 353 Ventral muscles of the forearm; superficial layer.

→ T 31

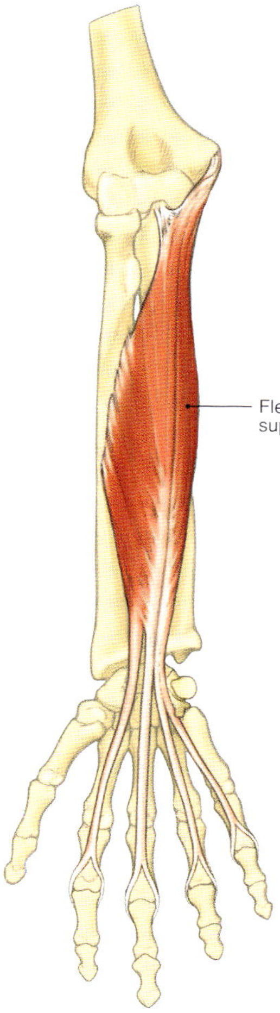

Fig. 354 Ventral muscles of the forearm; middle layer.

→ T 32

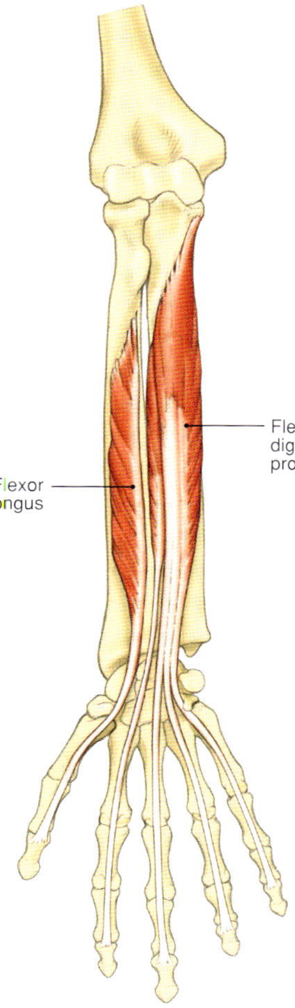

Fig. 355 Ventral muscles of the forearm; deep layer.

→ T 31, T32

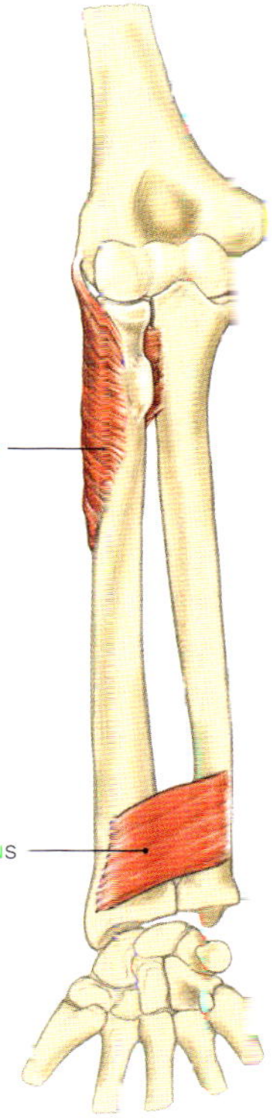

Fig. 356 Ventral muscles of the forearm deepest layer.

→ T 31, T 35

Muscles of the forearm

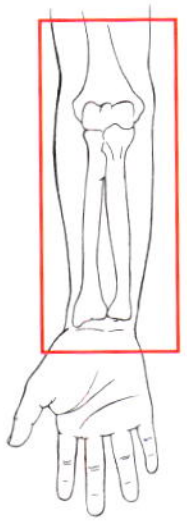

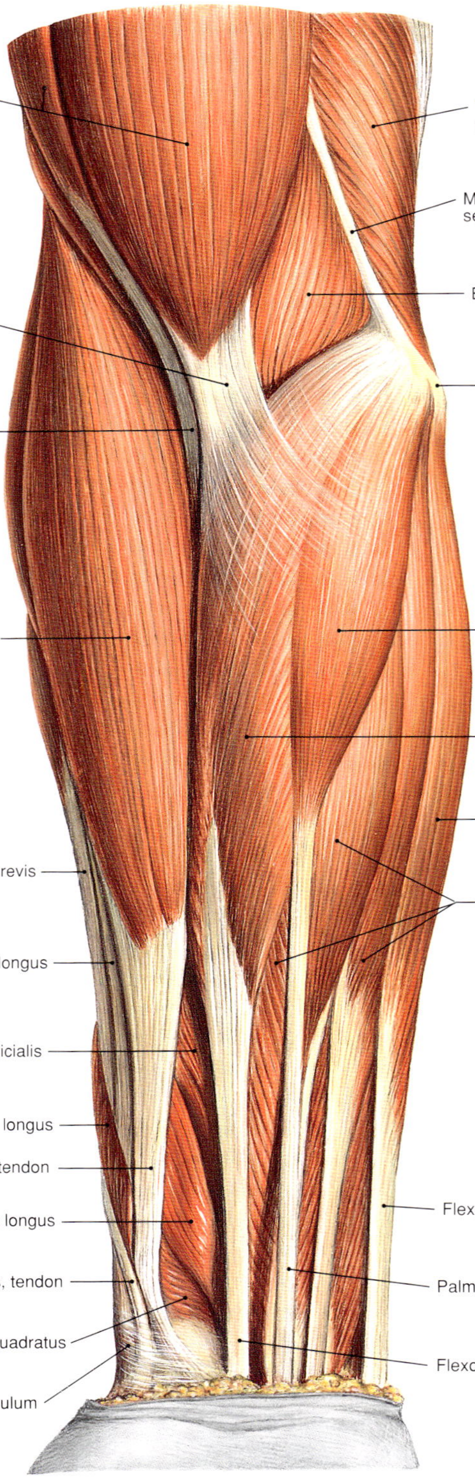

→ T 31

Fig. 357 Muscles of the forearm; flexor aspect, superficial layer.

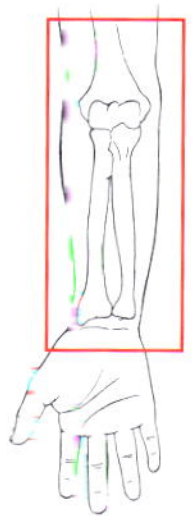

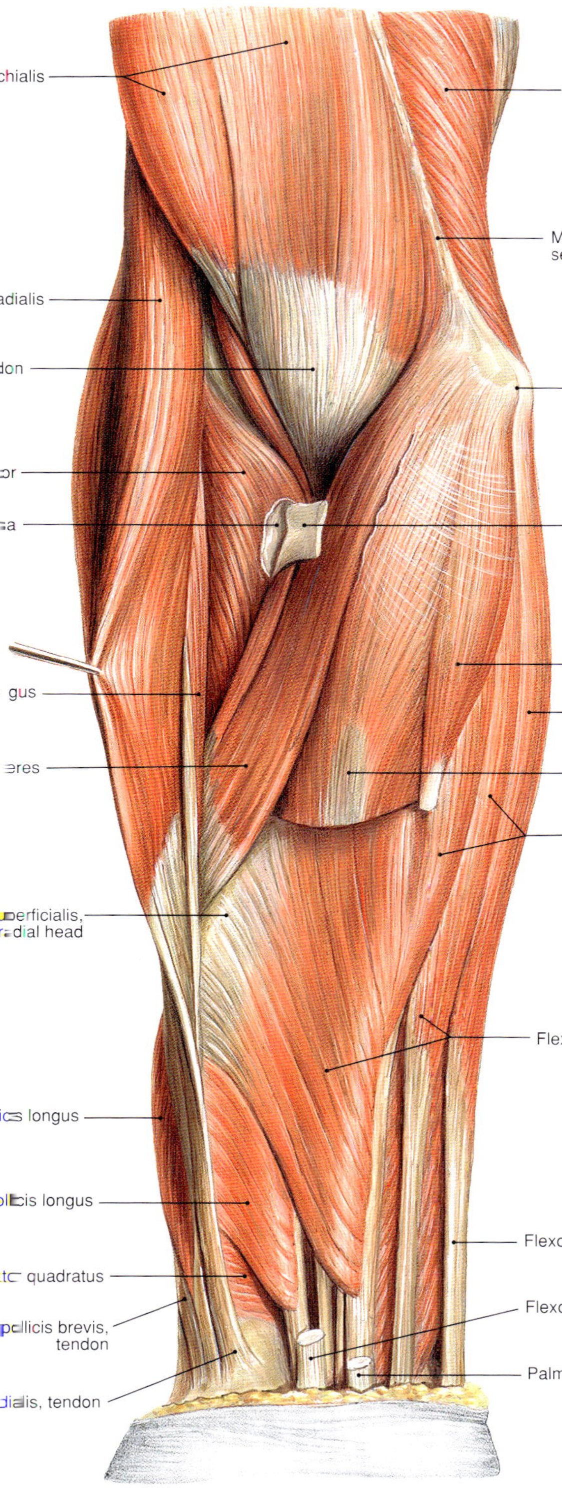

Fig. 358 Muscles of the forearm; flexor aspect, middle layer.

→ T 31

Muscles of the forearm

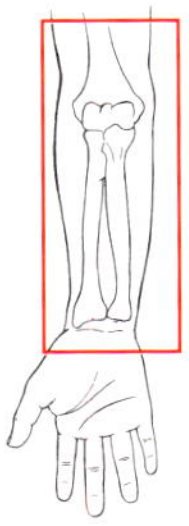

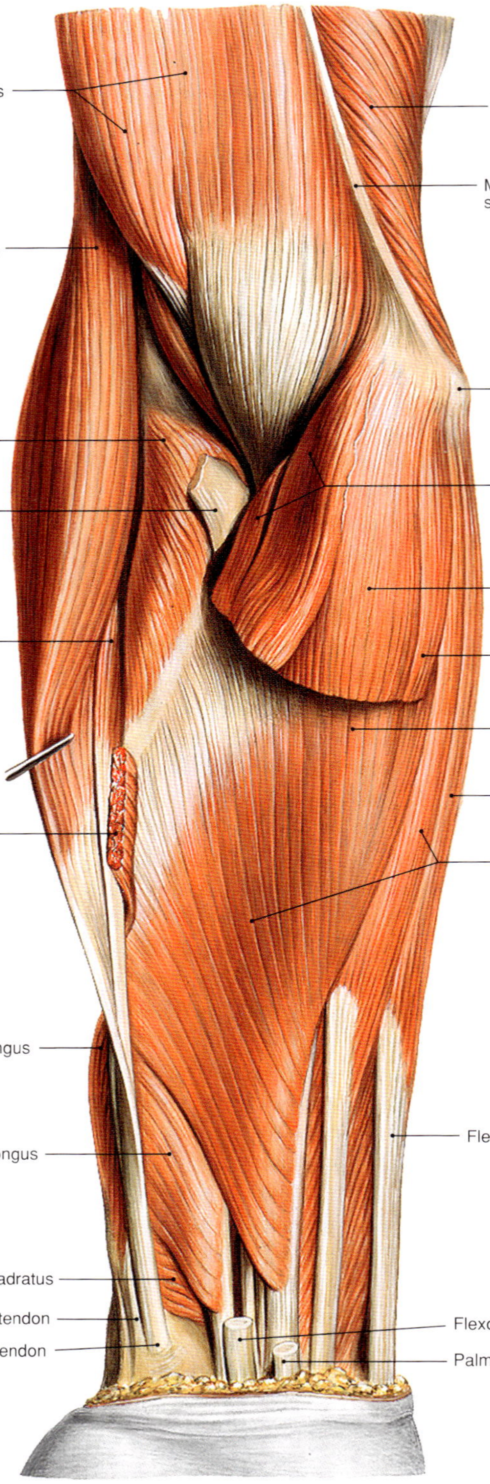

→ T 31, T 32

Fig. 359 Muscles of the forearm; flexor aspect, middle layer after section of the pronator teres muscle.

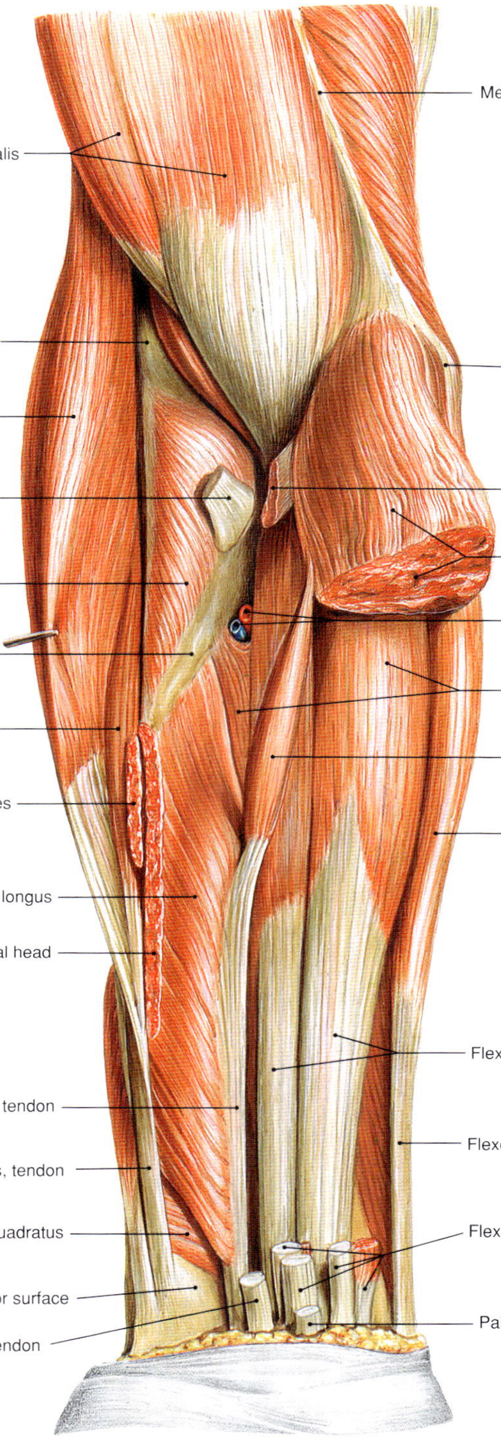

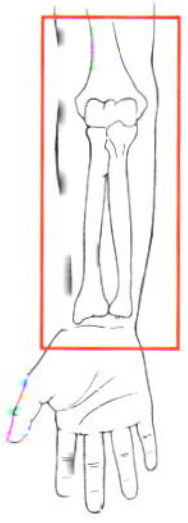

Fig. 360 Muscles of the forearm; flexor aspect, deep layer.

→ T 32

Origins and insertions of the dorsal muscles of the forearm

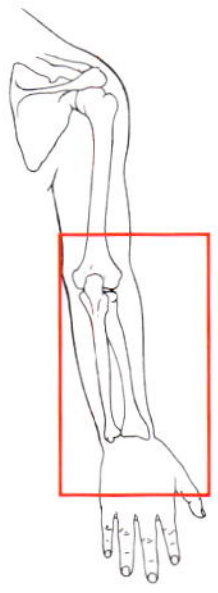

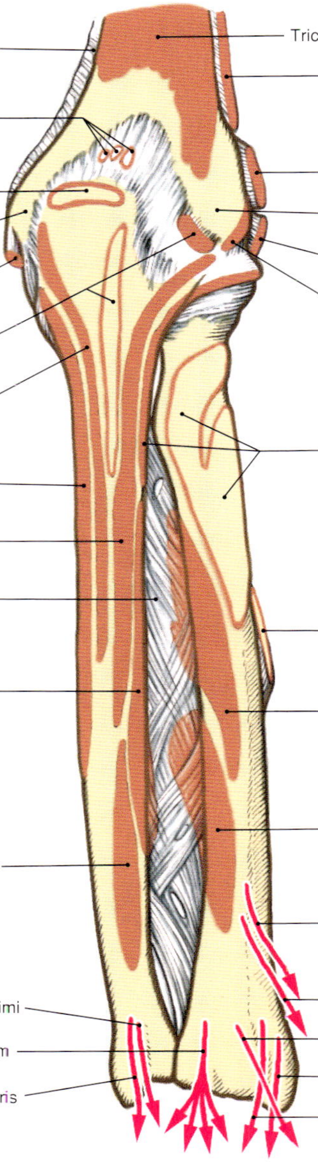

→ T 34, T 35

Fig. 361 Origins and insertions of the muscles at the radius, the ulna and the distal part of the humerus.

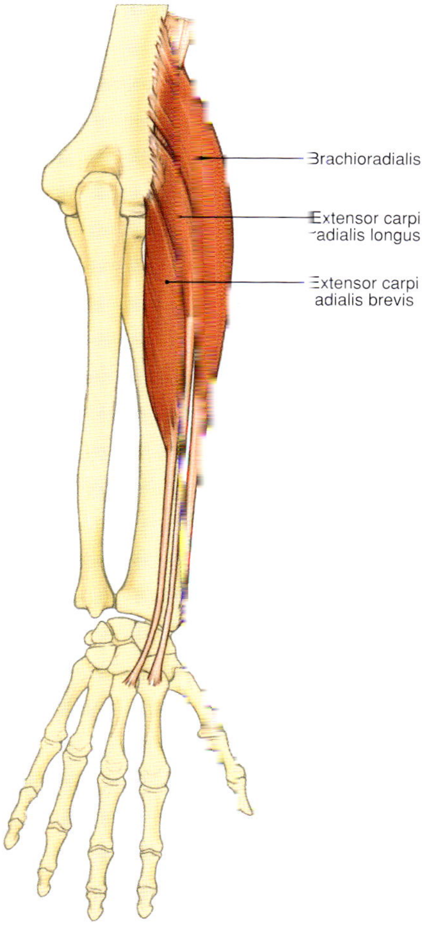

Fig. 362 Radial muscles of the forearm.

→ T 33

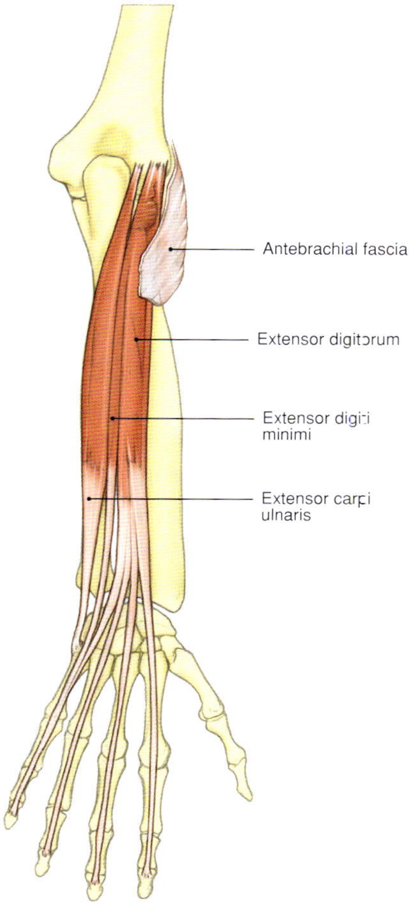

Fig. 363 Dorsal muscles of the forearm; superficial layer.

→ T 34

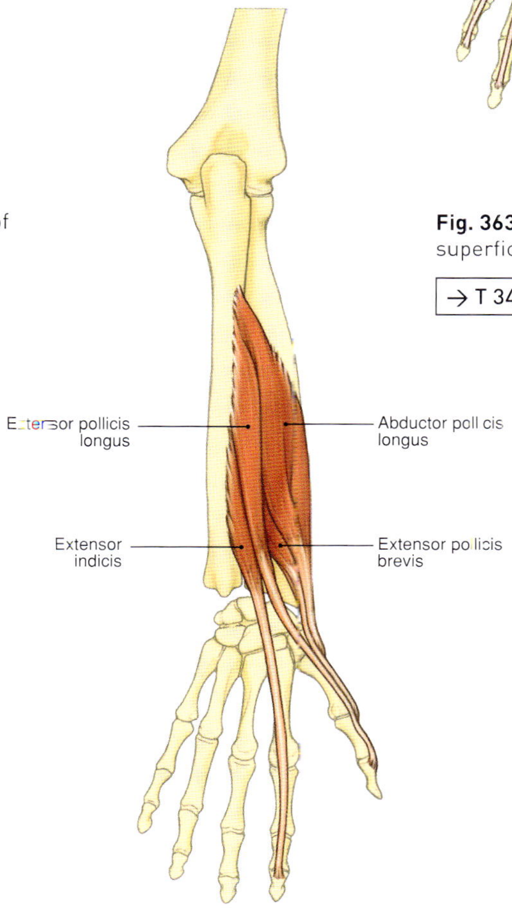

Fig. 364 Dorsal muscles of the forearm; middle layer.

→ T 35

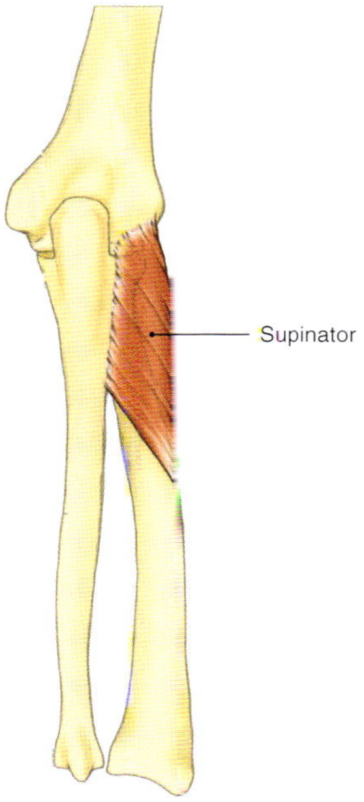

Fig. 365 Dorsal muscles of the forearm; deep layer.

→ T35

Muscles of the forearm

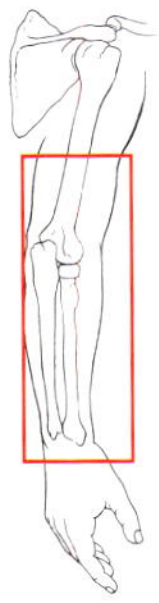

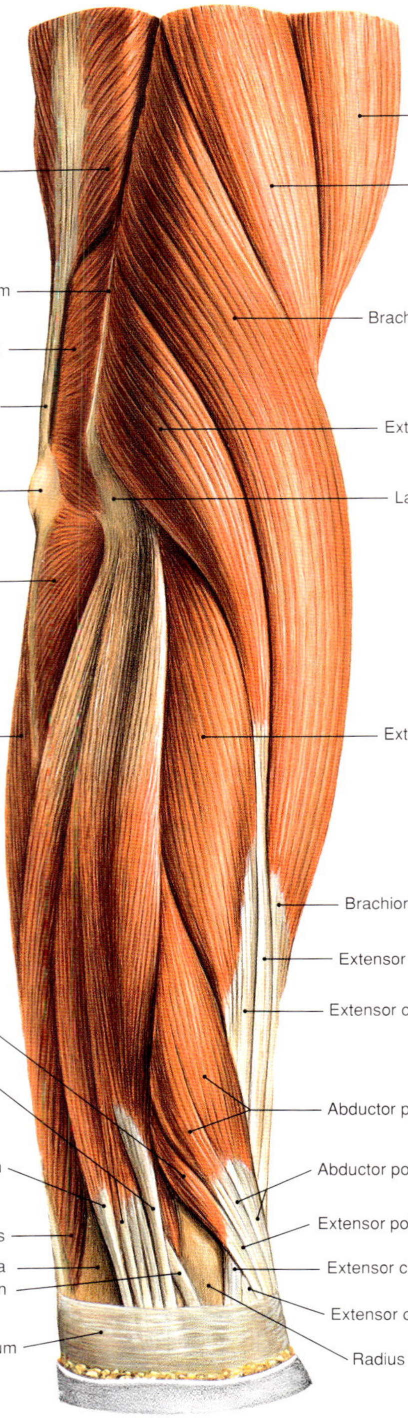

→ T 33

Fig. 366 Muscles of the forearm and the distal part of the arm; lateral view; intermediate position of the forearm between supination and pronation.

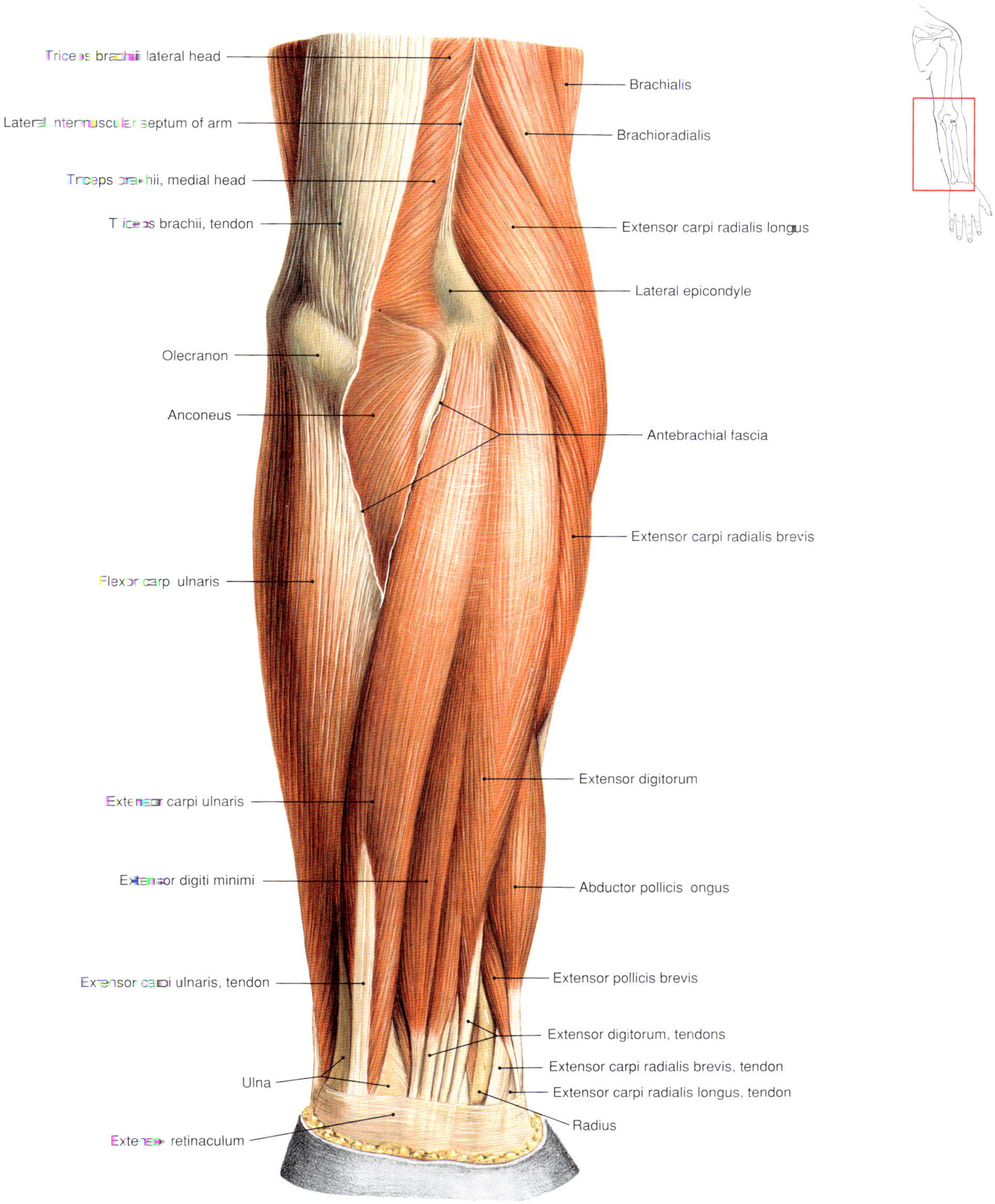

Fig. 367 Muscles of the forearm and the distal part of the arm; extensor aspect, superficial layer; intermediate position of the forearm between supination and pronation.

→ T 34

Muscles of the forearm

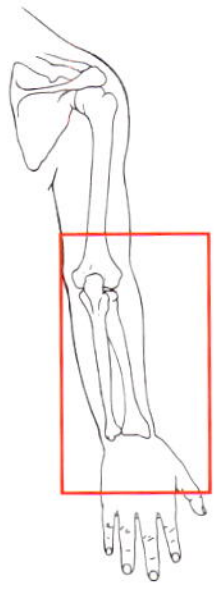

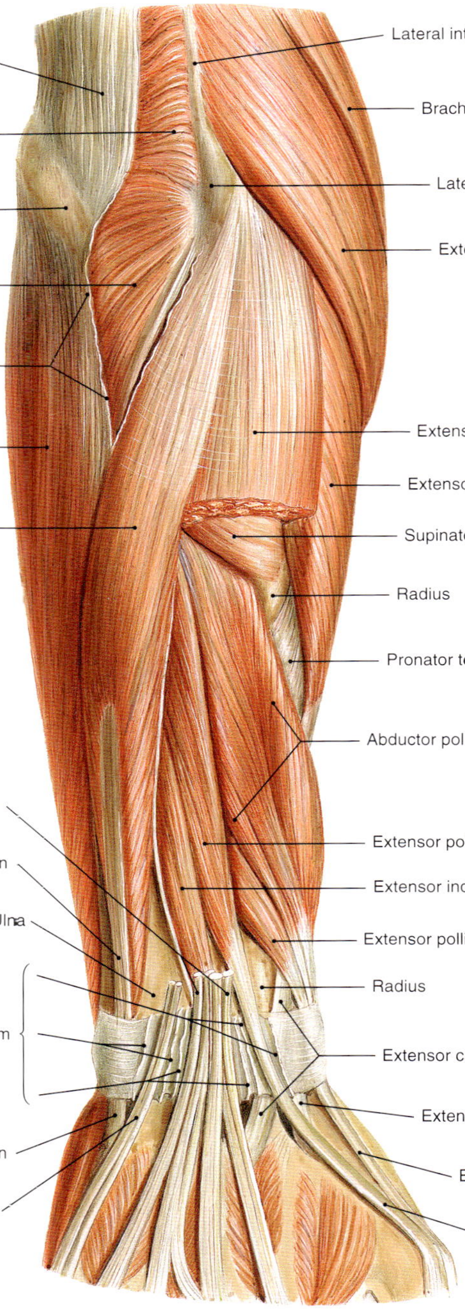

→ T 34, T 35

Fig. 368 Muscles of the forearm; extensor aspect, middle layer; intermediate position of the forearm between supination and pronation.

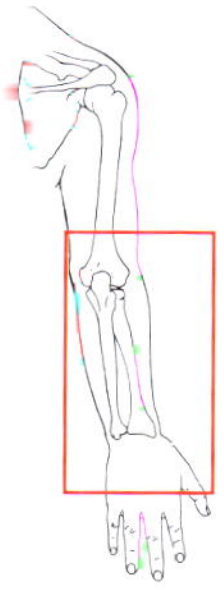

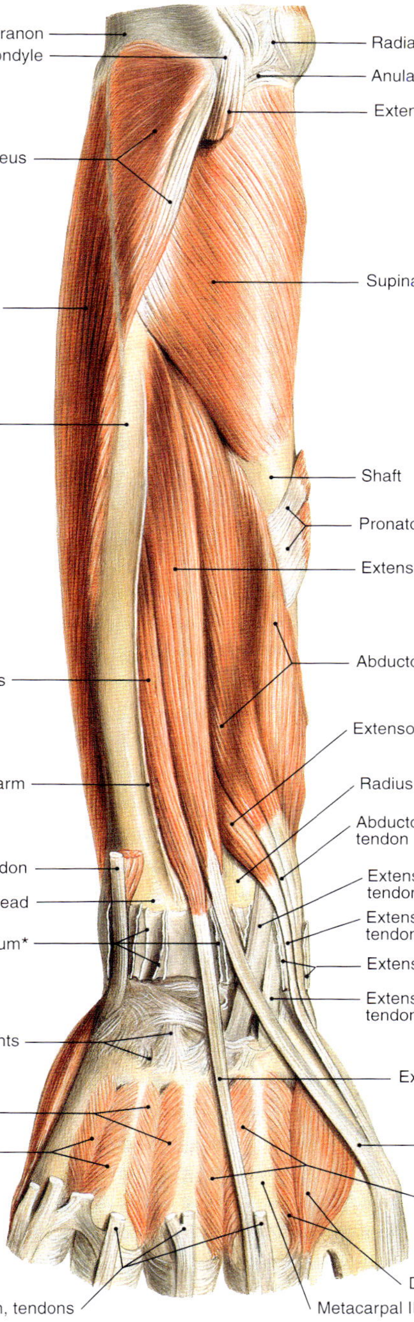

Fig. 369 Muscles of the forearm and the hand; extensor aspect, deep layer; intermediate position of the forearm between supination and pronation.

→ T 35

* The tendon compartments formed by the extensor retinaculum have been opened longitudinally.

Muscles of the forearm

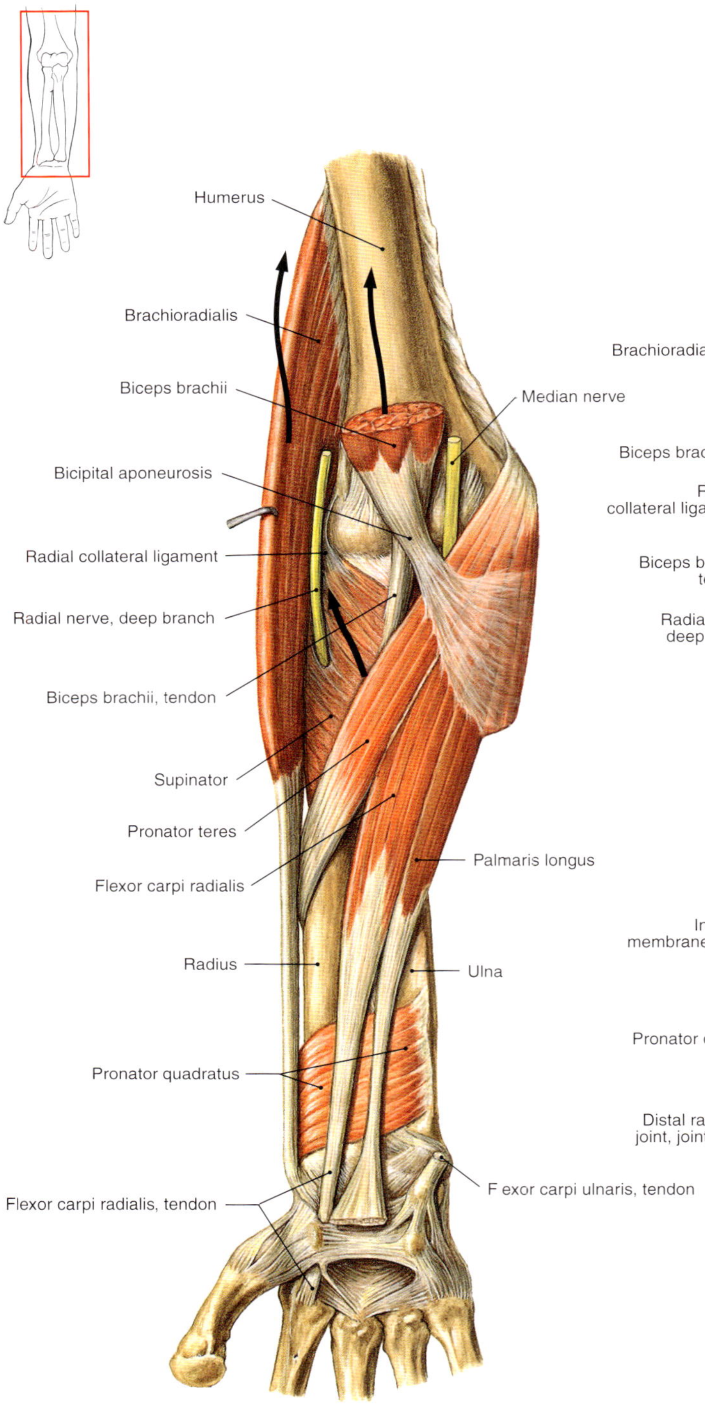

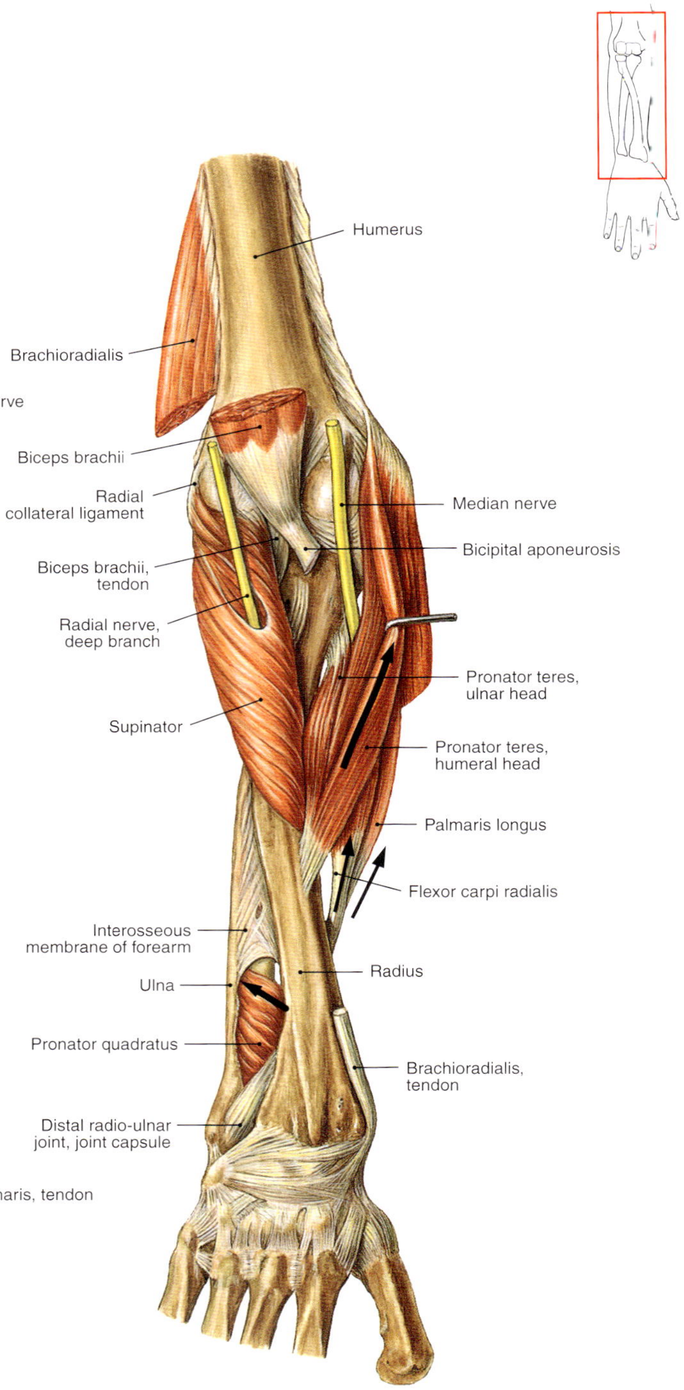

Fig. 370 Forearm in supination;
ventropalmar view.
Arrows indicate the direction of force generated by the main supinator muscles.

→ T 32, T 33, T 35

Fig. 371 Forearm in pronation;
ventral view of the elbow region, dorsal view of the dorsum of the hand.
Arrows indicate the direction of force generated by the main pronator muscles.

→ T 32, T 33, T 35

Origins and insertions of the muscles of the hand

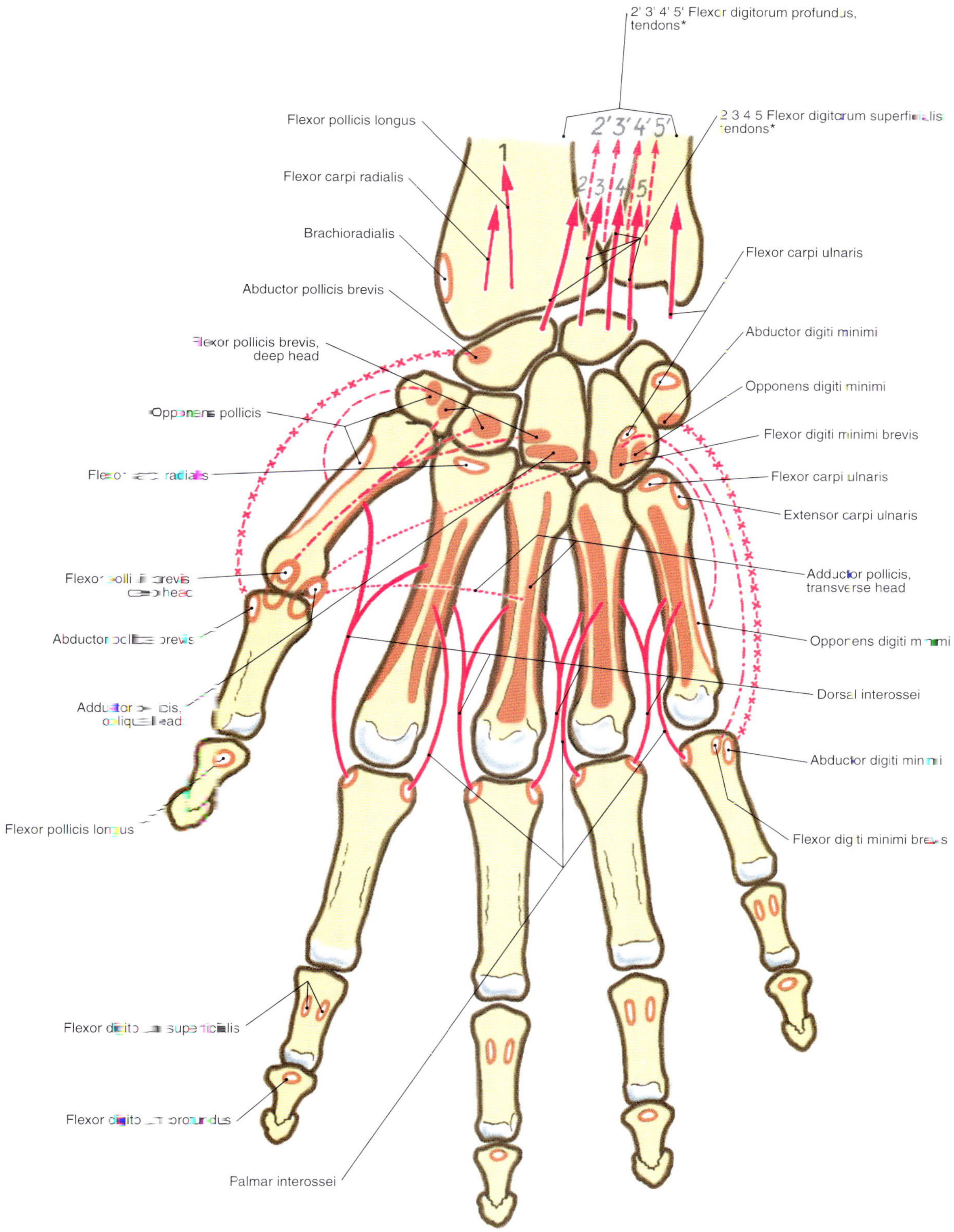

Fig. 372 Origins and insertions of the muscles of the hand at the bones of the hand.

→ T 35–T 38

* The flexors insert at the second to fifth digit.

Muscles of the hand

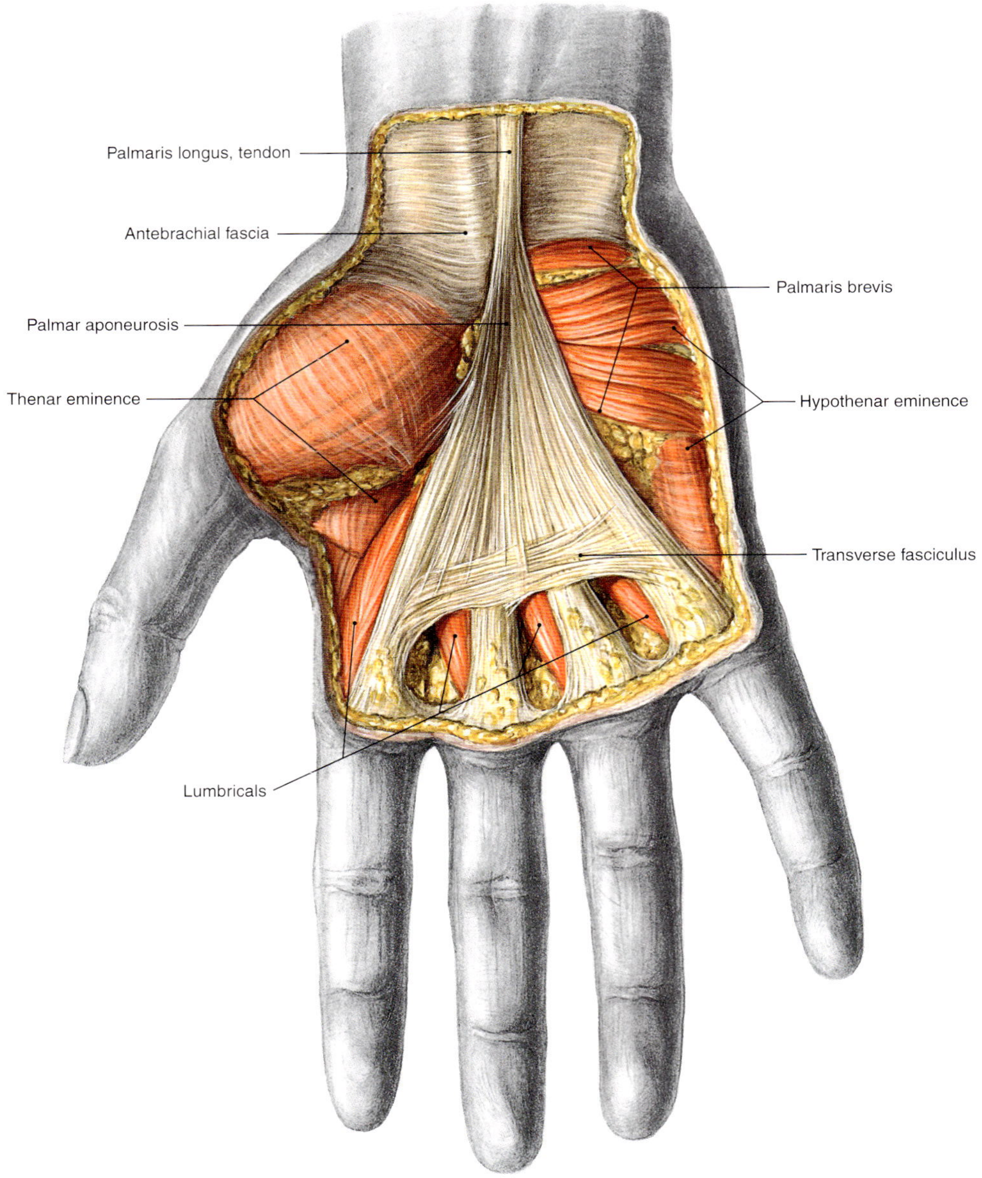

→ T 31, T 36–T 38

Fig. 373 Muscles of the palm; superficial layer.

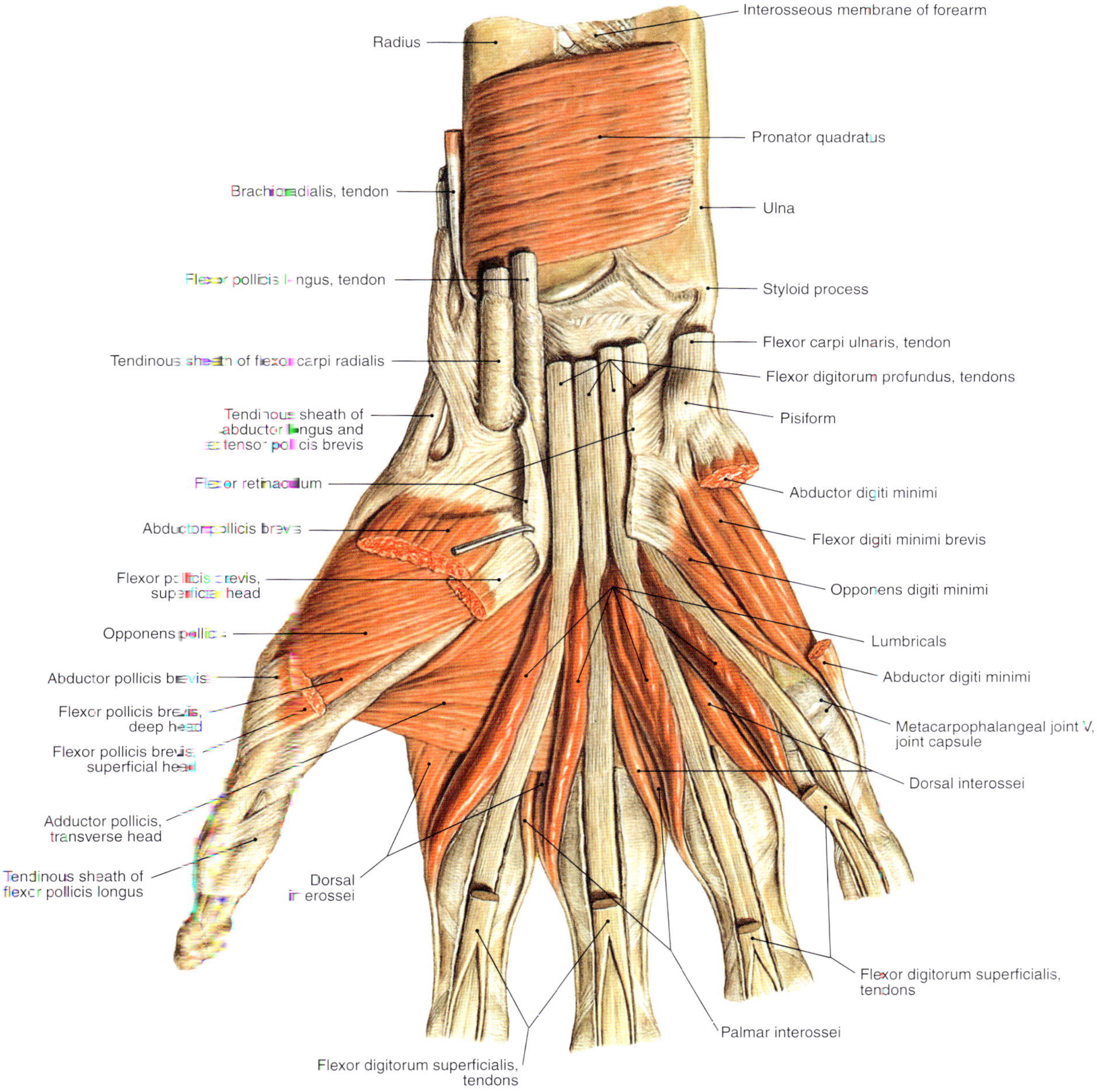

Fig. 374 Muscles of the palm; middle layer.

→ T 32, T 36–T 38

Tendon sheaths of the hand

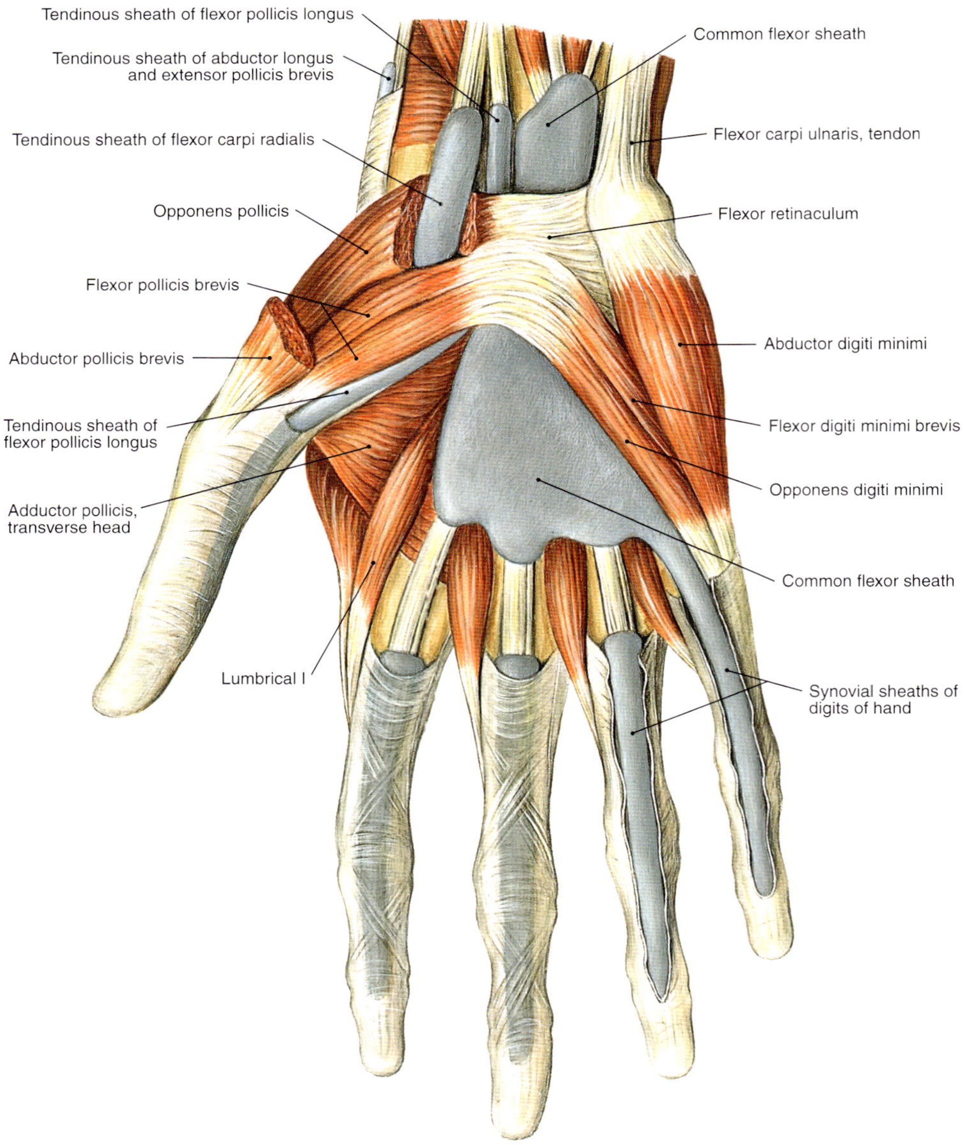

Fig. 375 Tendon sheaths of the hand.

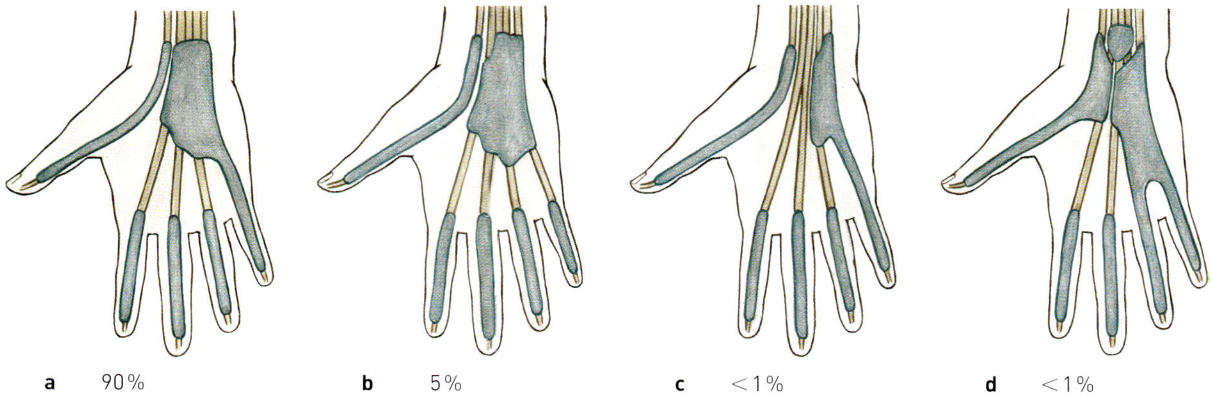

Fig. 376 a–d Frequent variations of the palmar tendon sheaths.

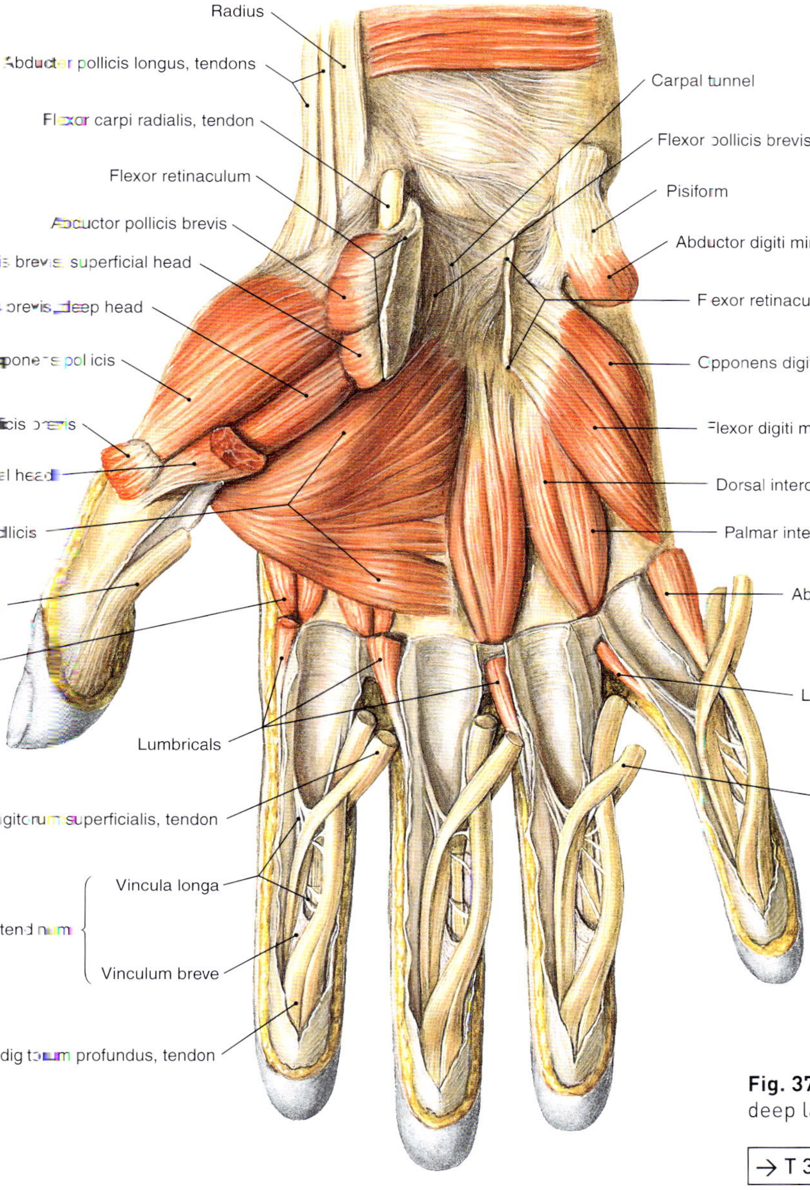

Fig. 377 Muscles of the palm; deep layer.

→ T 36–T 38

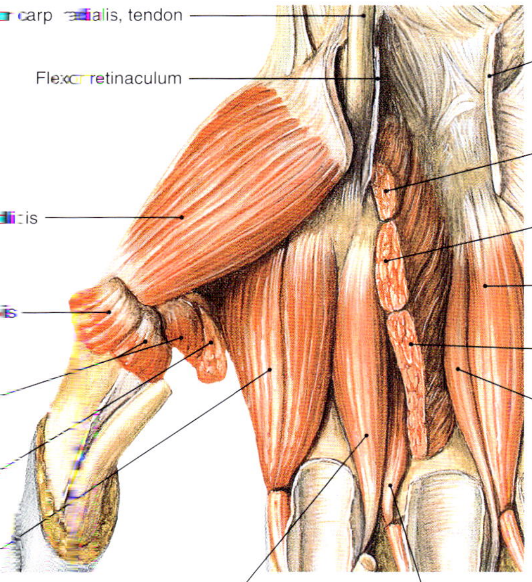

Fig. 378 Muscles of the palm; deepest layer.

→ T 36, T 37

Muscles of the hand

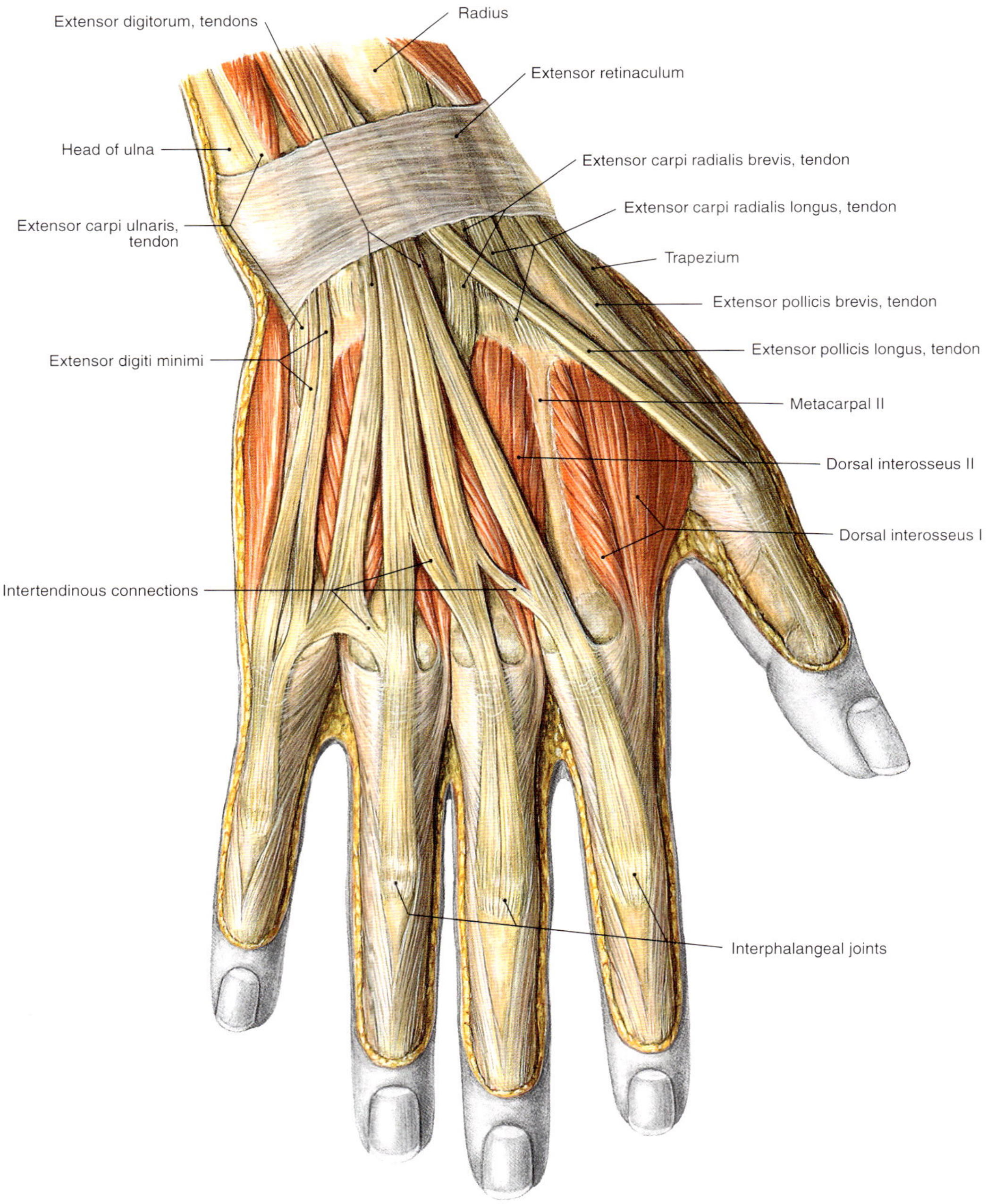

→ T 34, T 35, T 37

Fig. 379 Muscles of the dorsum of the hand.

Tendon sheaths of the hand

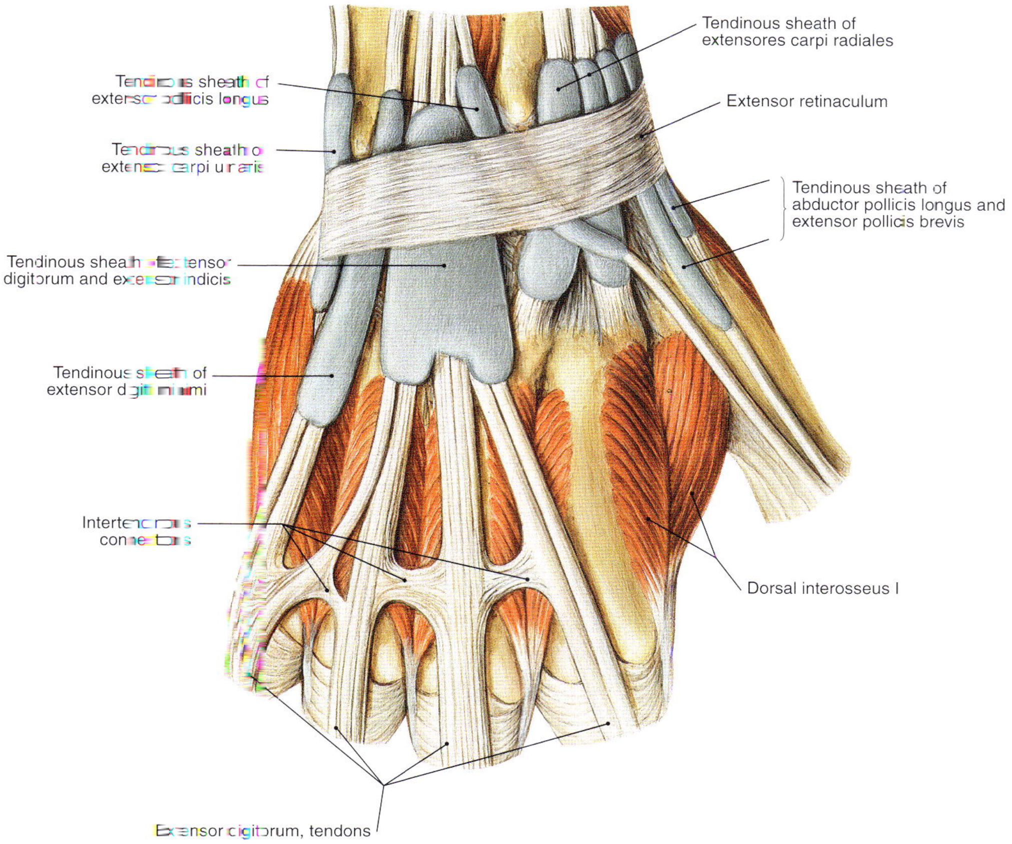

Fig. 380 Dorsal carpal tendon sheath.

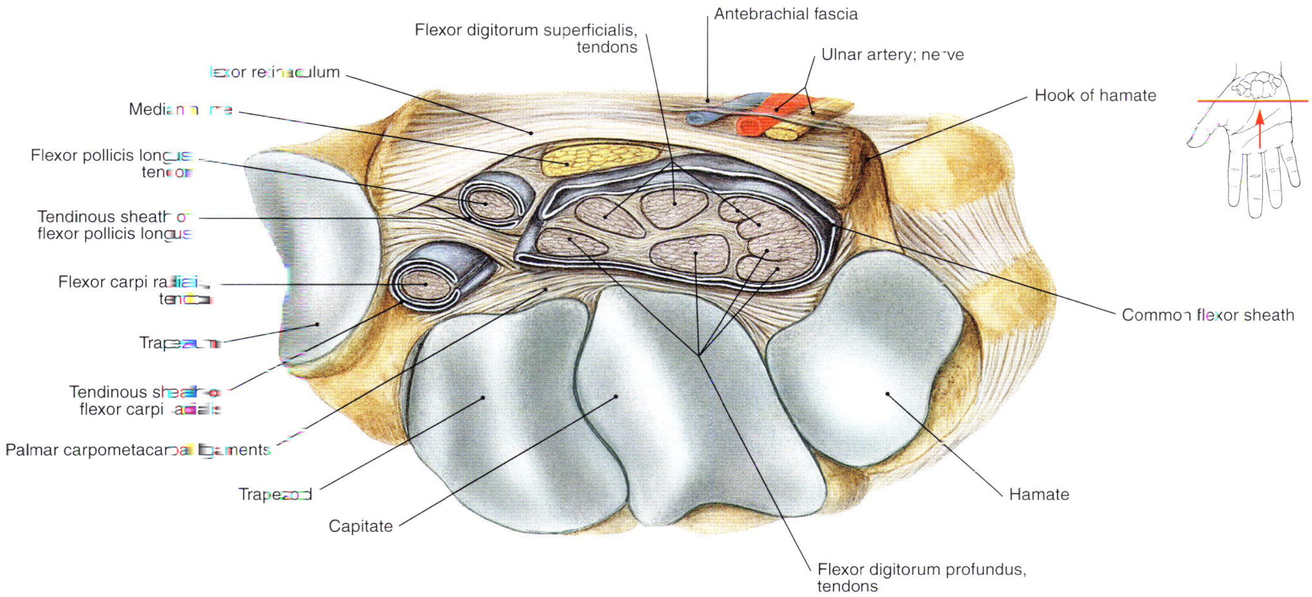

Fig. 381 Palmar carpal tendon sheaths; transverse section.

The compression of the median nerve in the carpal tunnel is known as "carpal tunnel syndrome".

Muscles of the hand

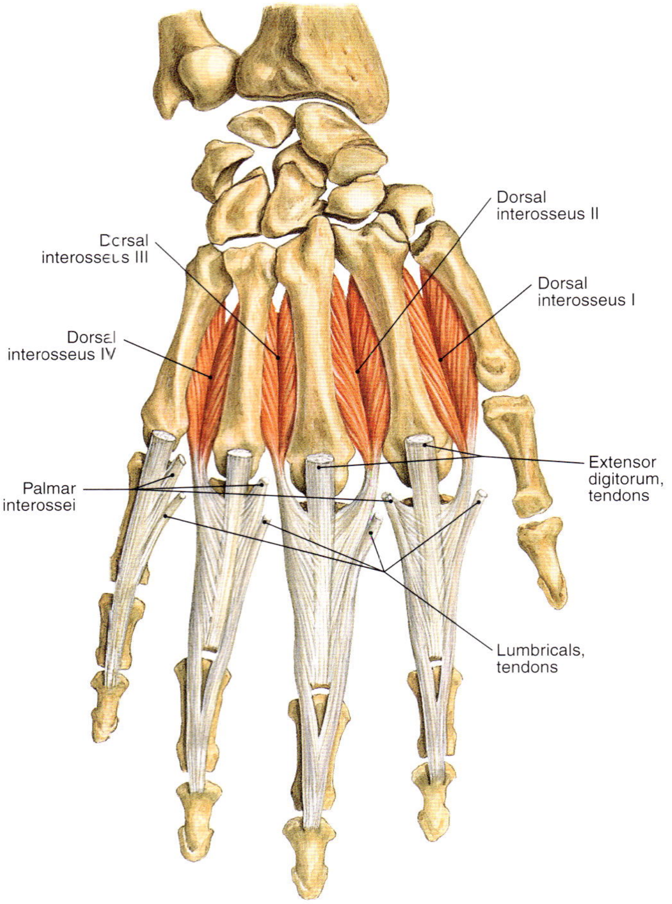

Fig. 382 Dorsal interosseous muscles; dorsal view.

→ T 37

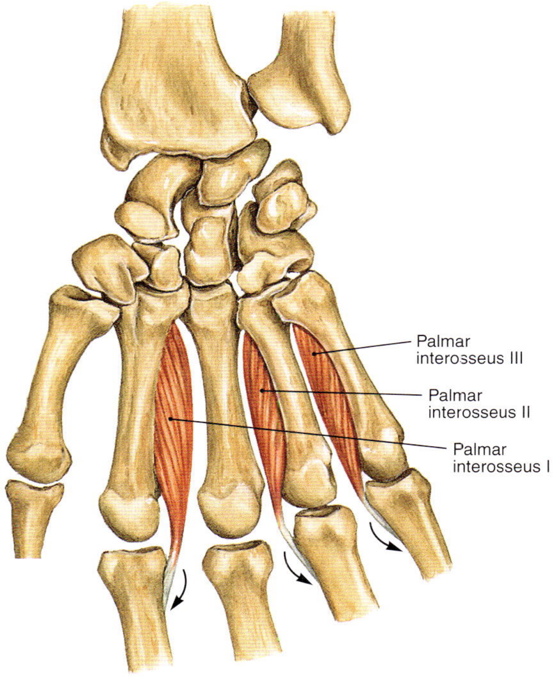

Fig. 383 Palmar interosseous muscles; palmar view.
The tendons of the interosseous and the lumbrical muscles radiate into the so-called dorsal aponeurosis of the fingers (arrows).

→ T 37

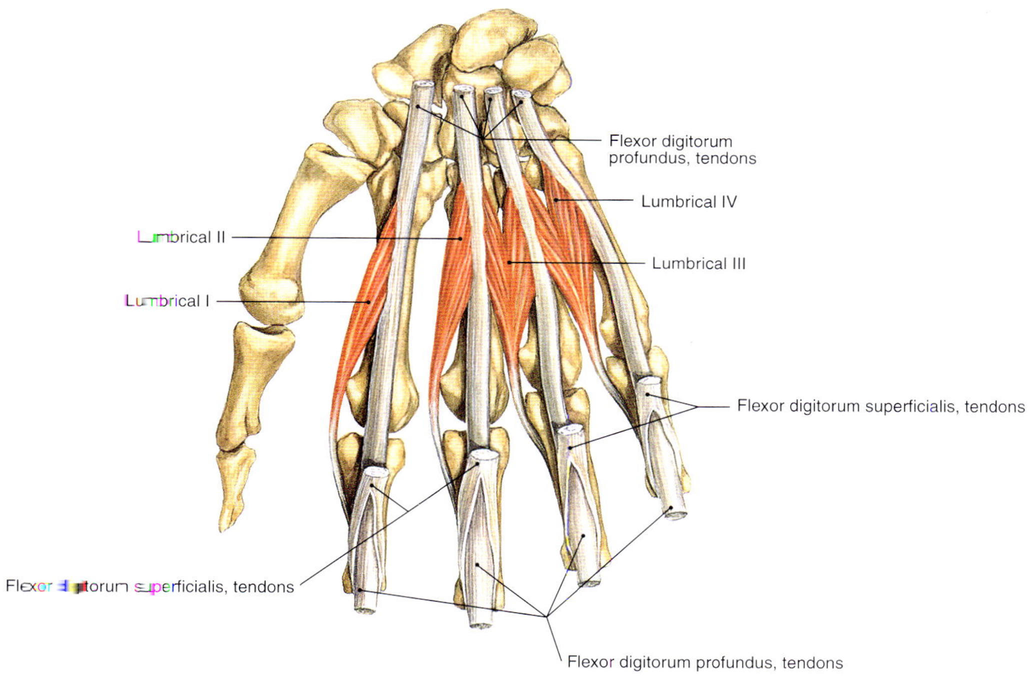

Fig. 384 Lumbrical muscles; palmar view.

→ T 37

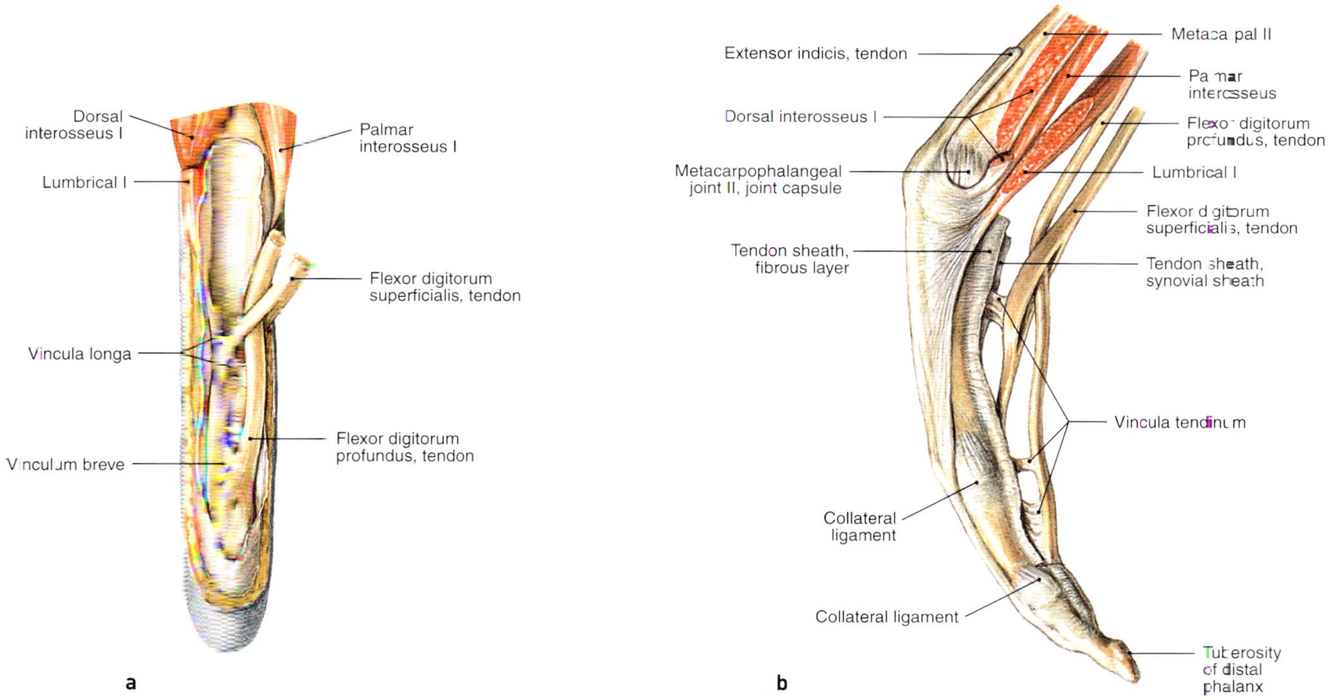

Fig. 385 a, b Tendon insertions at the index; the tendons of both flexors have been dissected from the tendon sheath.
a Palmar view
b Lateral view

Brachial plexus

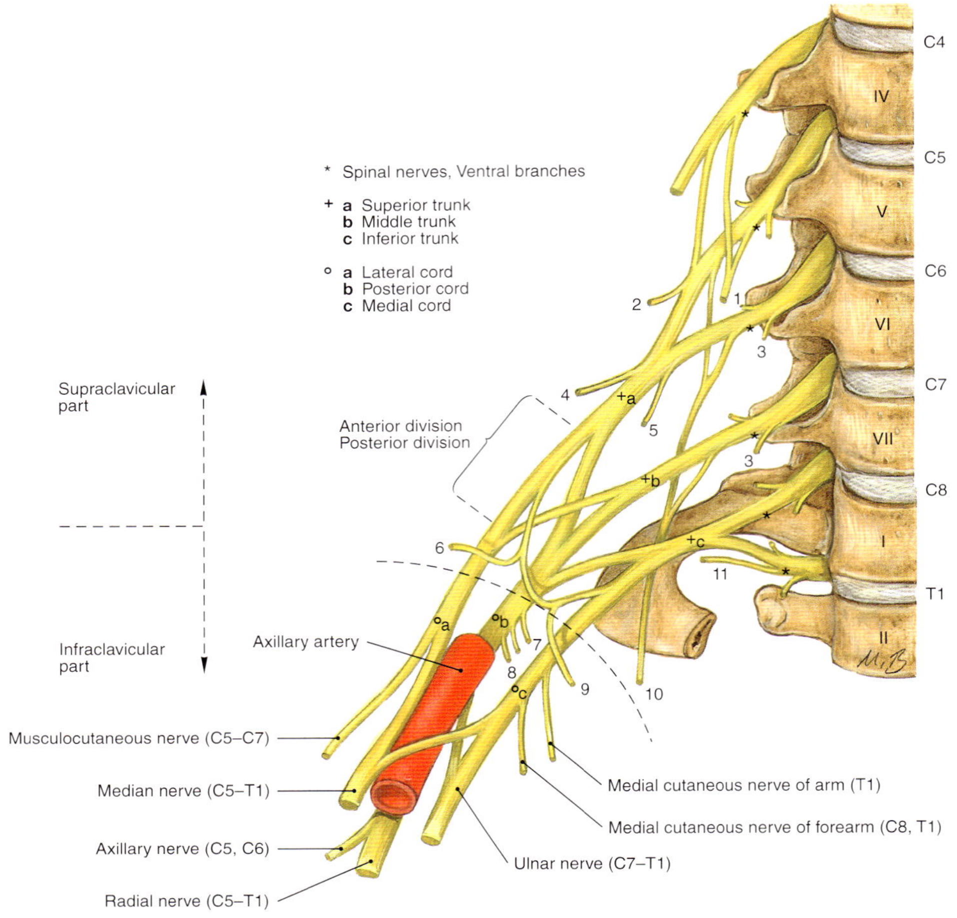

1 Phrenic nerve (Cervical plexus)
2 Dorsal scapular nerve (C5)
3 Muscular branches
4 Suprascapular nerve (C5, C6)
5 Subclavian nerve (C5, C6)
6 Lateral pectoral nerve (C5–C7)
7 Subscapular nerve (C5–C7)
8 Thoracodorsal nerve (C6–C8)
9 Medial pectoral nerve (C8, T1)
10 Long thoracic nerve (C5–C7)
11 Intercostal nerve (T1)

→ T 24, T 25

Fig. 386 Brachial plexus.

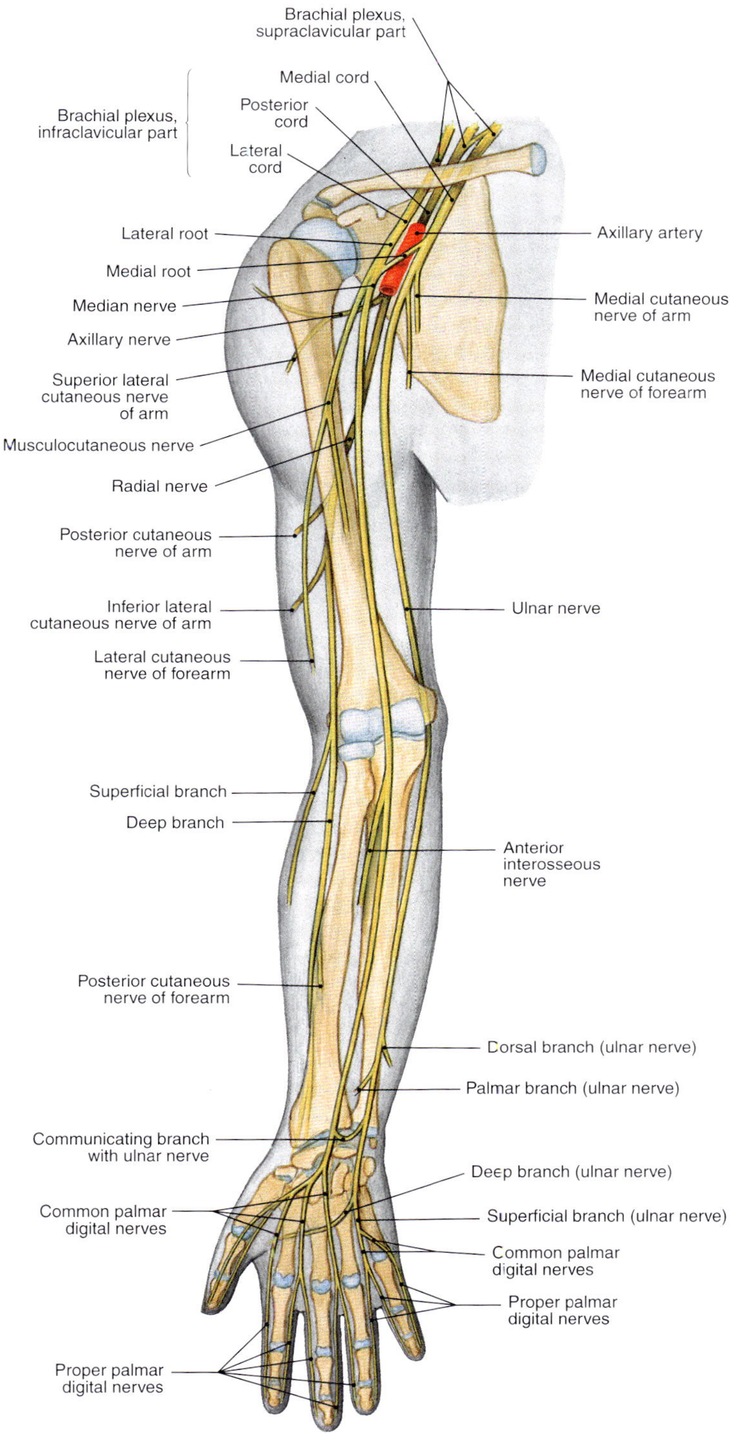

Fig. 387 Nerves of the upper limb; overview.

→ T 24, T 25

Cutaneous innervation

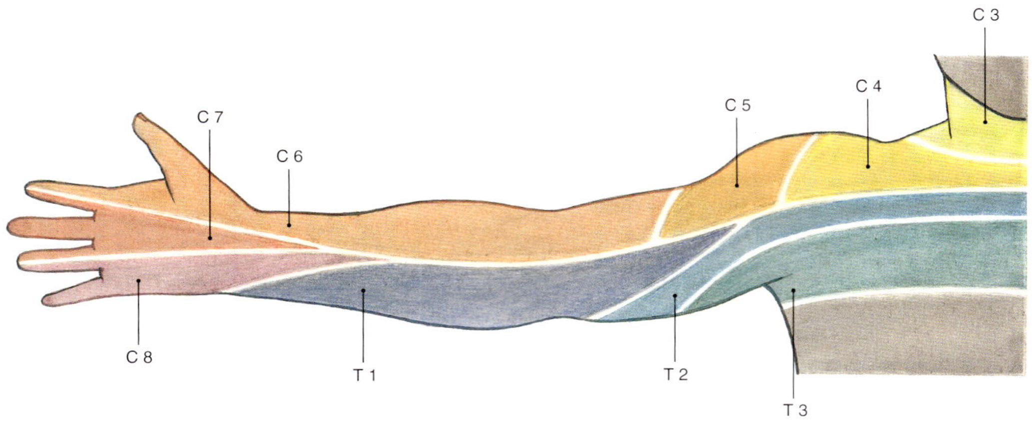

→ T 24

Fig. 388 Segmental cutaneous innervation (dermatomes) of the upper limb.

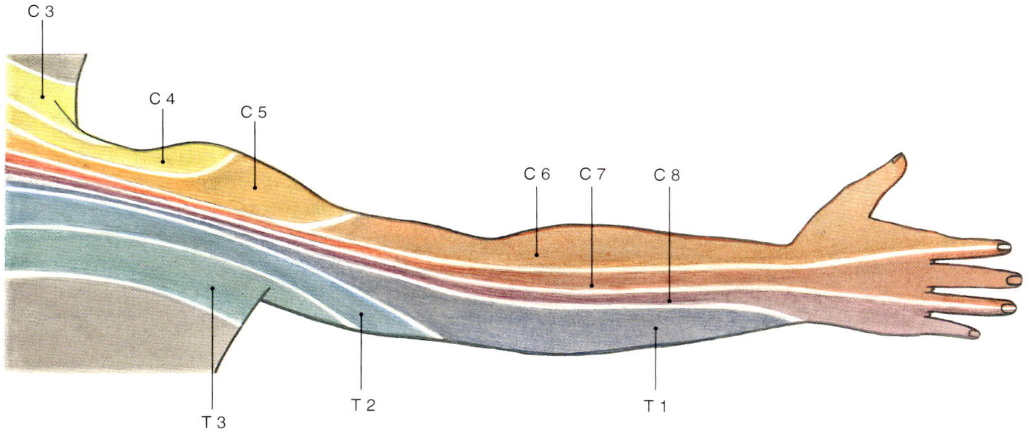

→ T 24

Fig. 389 Segmental cutaneous innervation (dermatomes) of the upper limb.

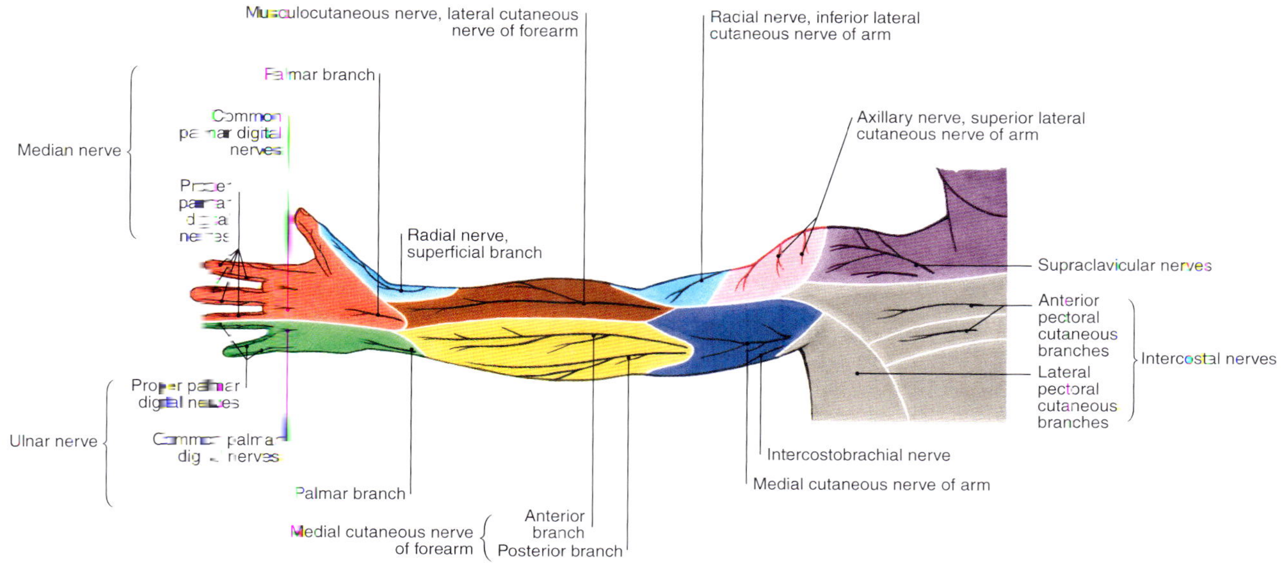

Fig. 390 Cutaneous nerves of the upper limb.

→ T 24

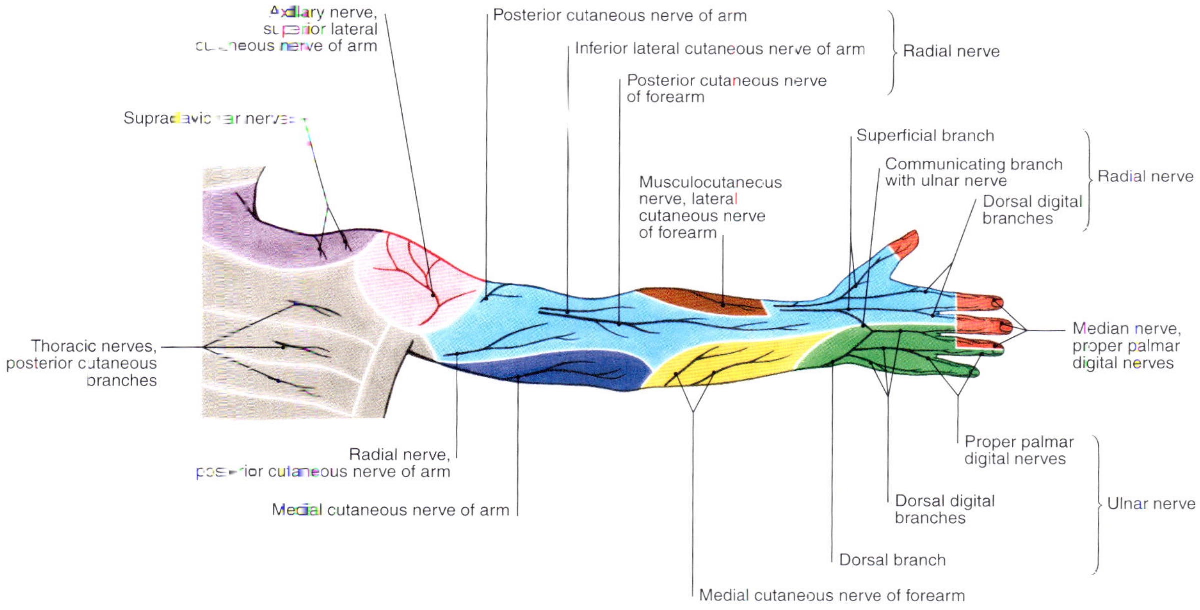

Fig. 391 Cutaneous nerves of the upper limb.

→ T 24

Musculocutaneous nerve

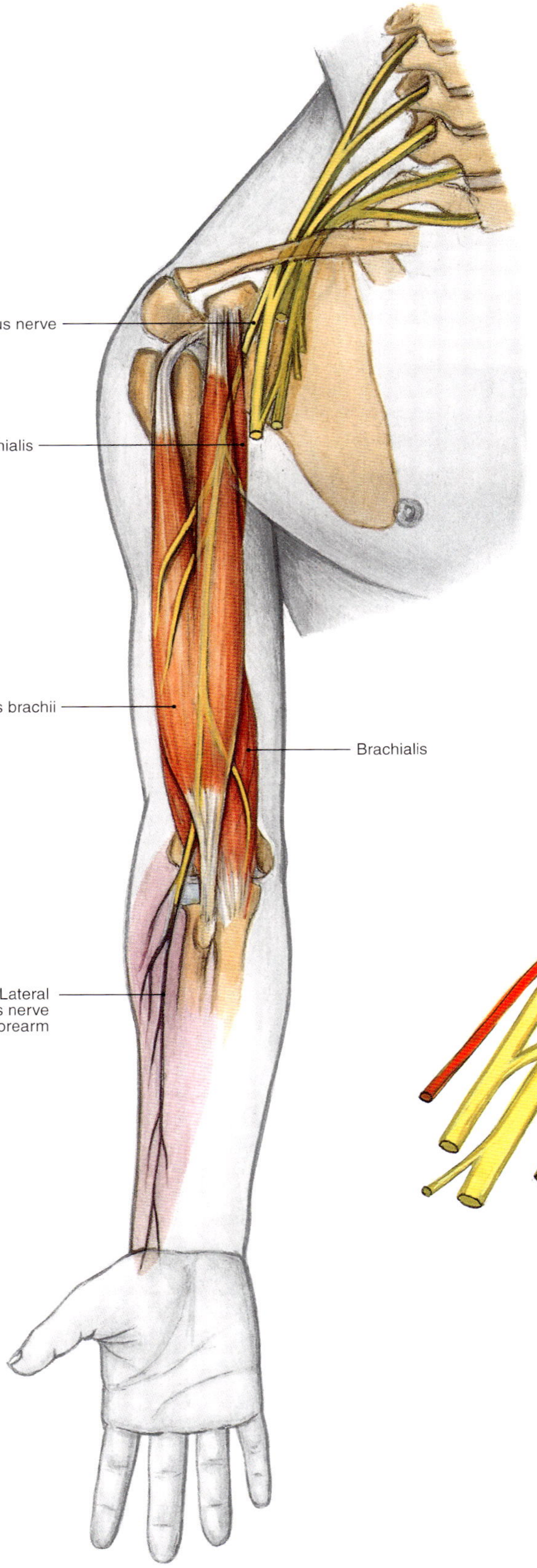

Fig. 392 Musculocutaneous nerve; supplying areas.
The skin branches and the cutaneous innervation are illustrated in blue.

→ 46, 386, T 24, T 25

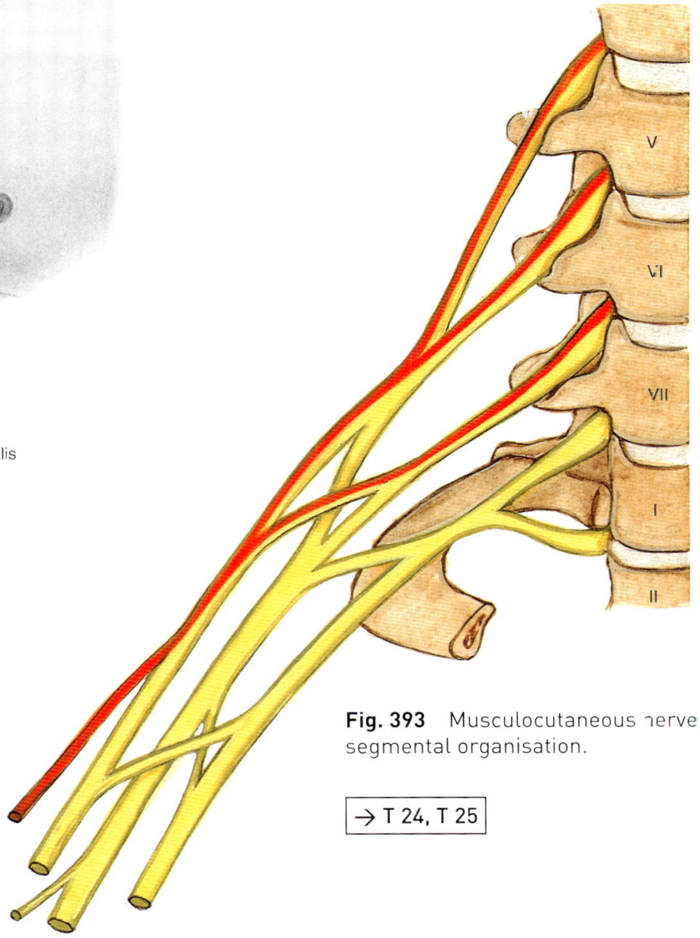

Fig. 393 Musculocutaneous nerve; segmental organisation.

→ T 24, T 25

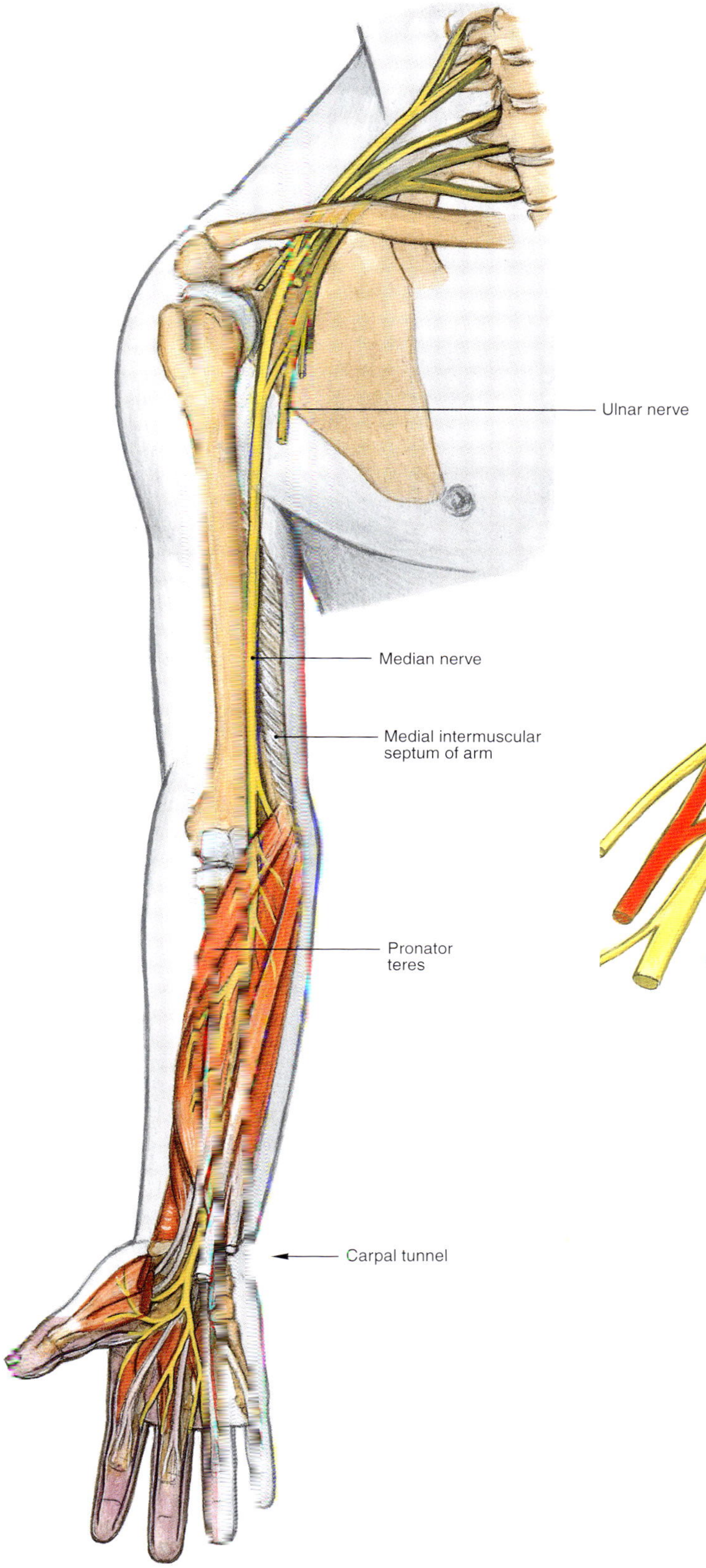

Fig. 394 Median nerve; supplying area

→ 46, 386, T 24, T 25

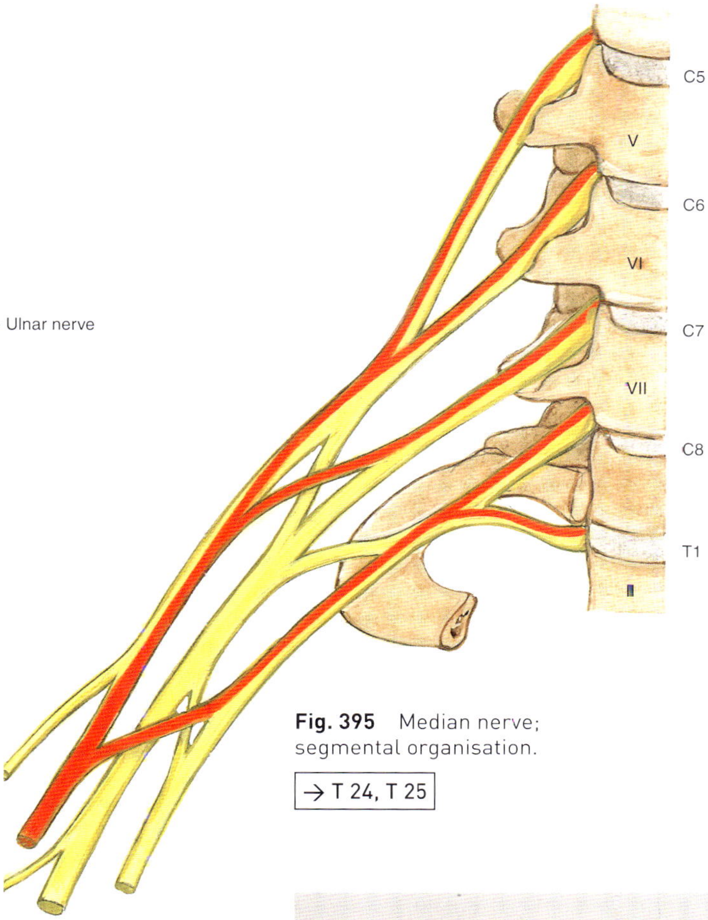

Fig. 395 Median nerve; segmental organisation.

→ T 24, T 25

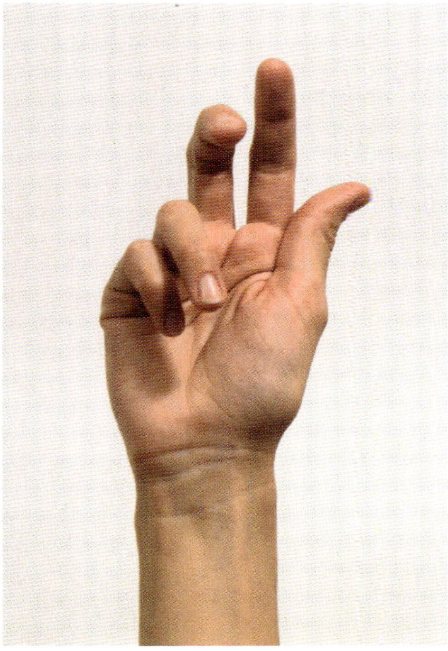

Fig. 396 Median nerve; proximal palsy: typical posture.

Ulnar nerve

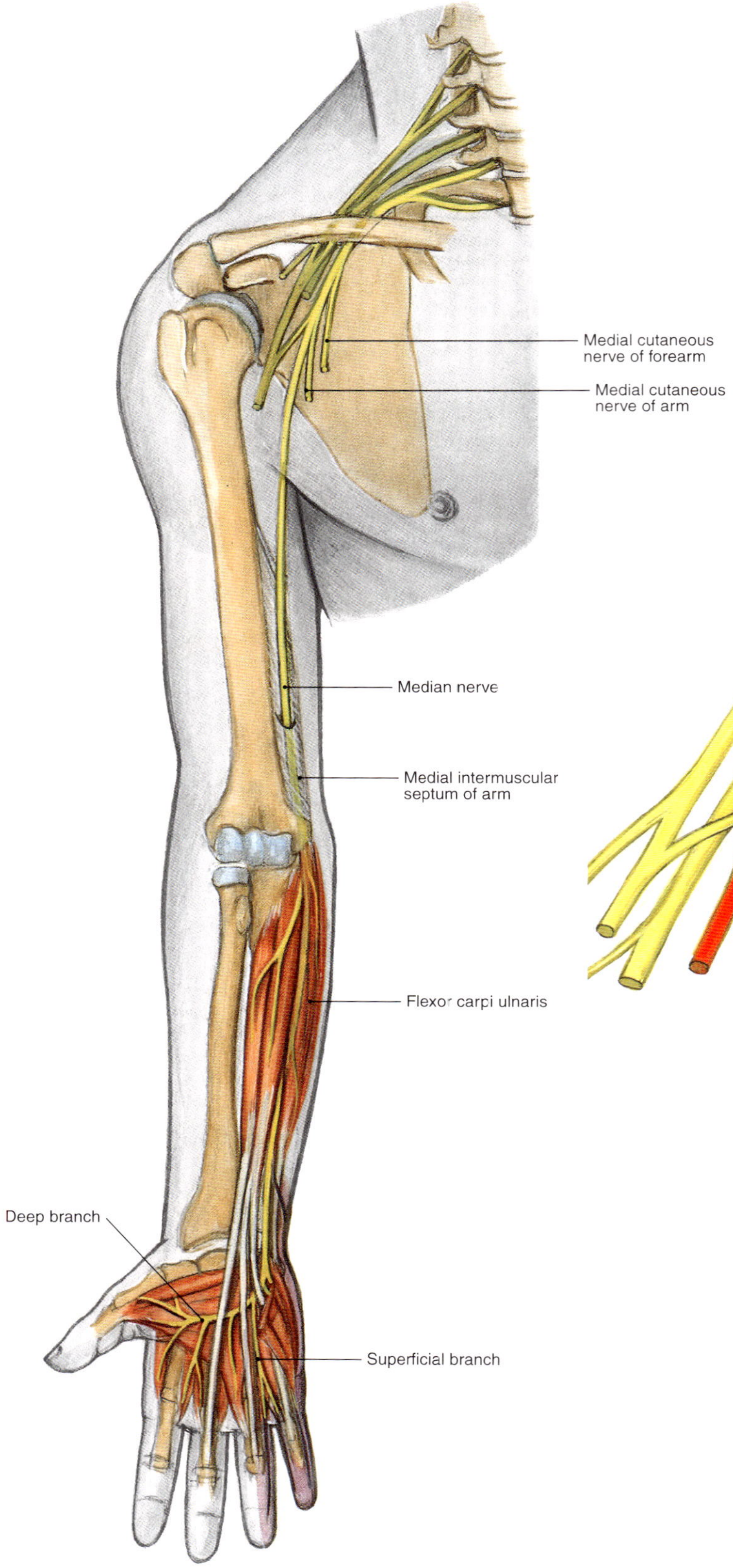

Fig. 397 Ulnar nerve; supplying areas.

→ 46, 386, T 24, T 25

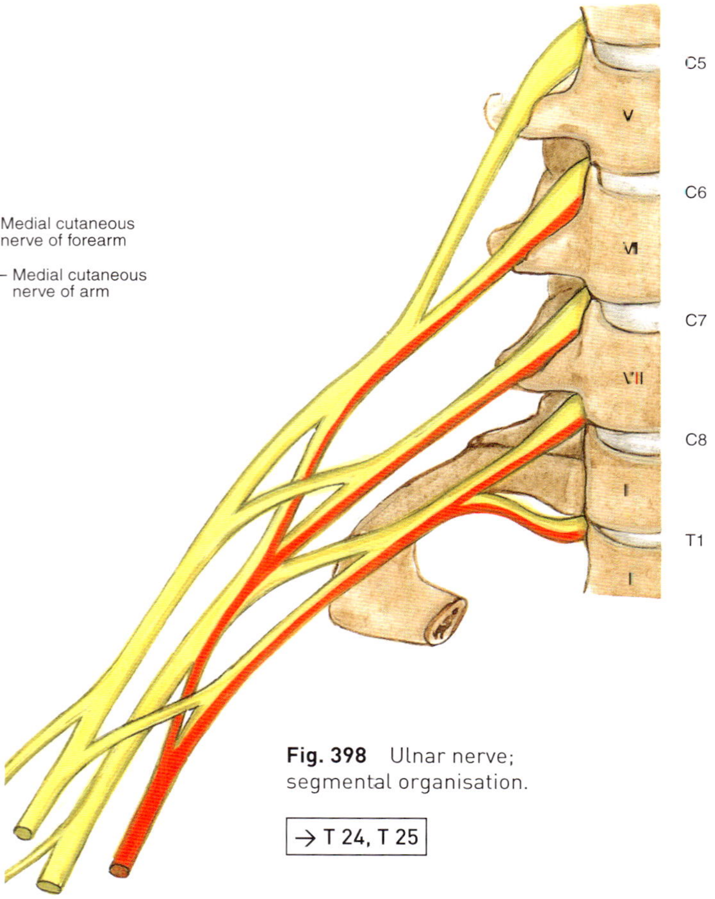

Fig. 398 Ulnar nerve; segmental organisation.

→ T 24, T 25

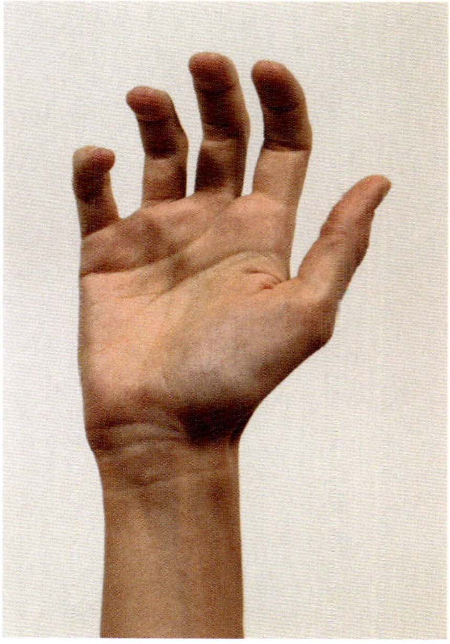

Fig. 399 Ulnar nerve; proximal palsy.

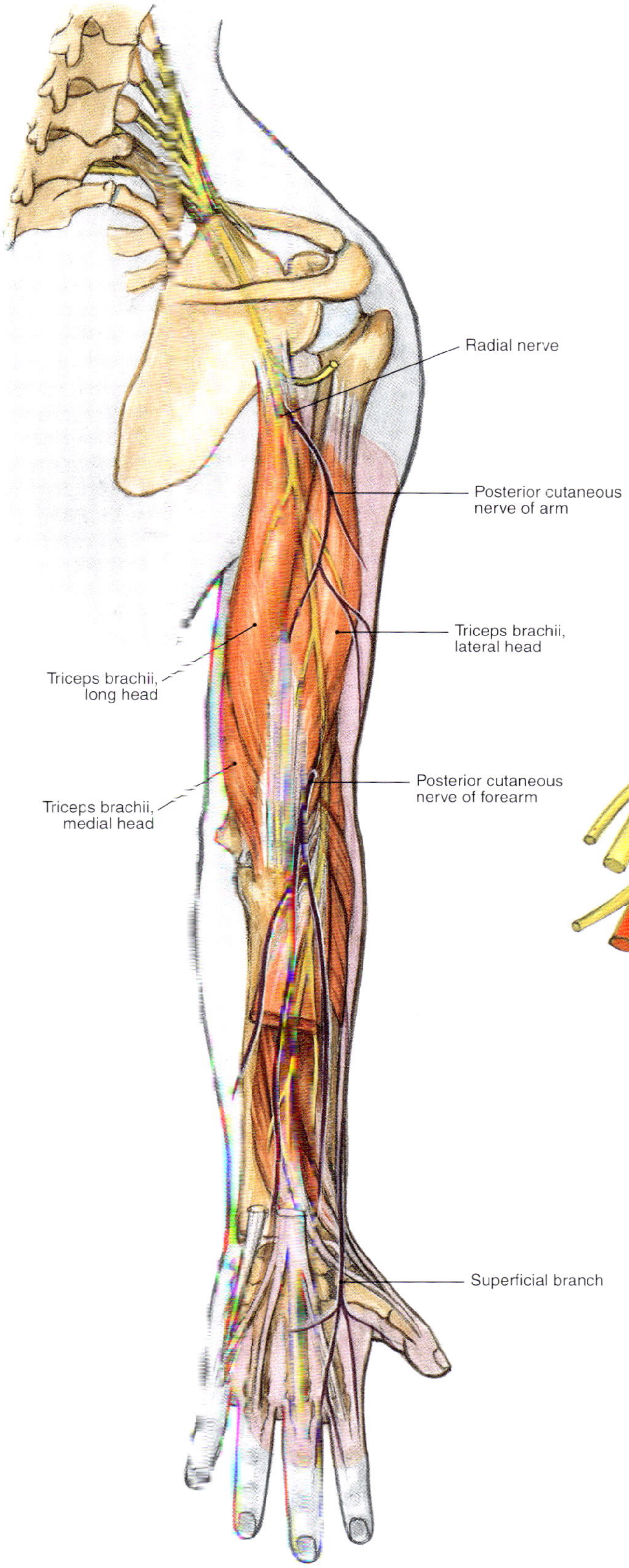

Fig. 400 Radial nerve supplying areas.

→ 46, 386, T 24, T 25

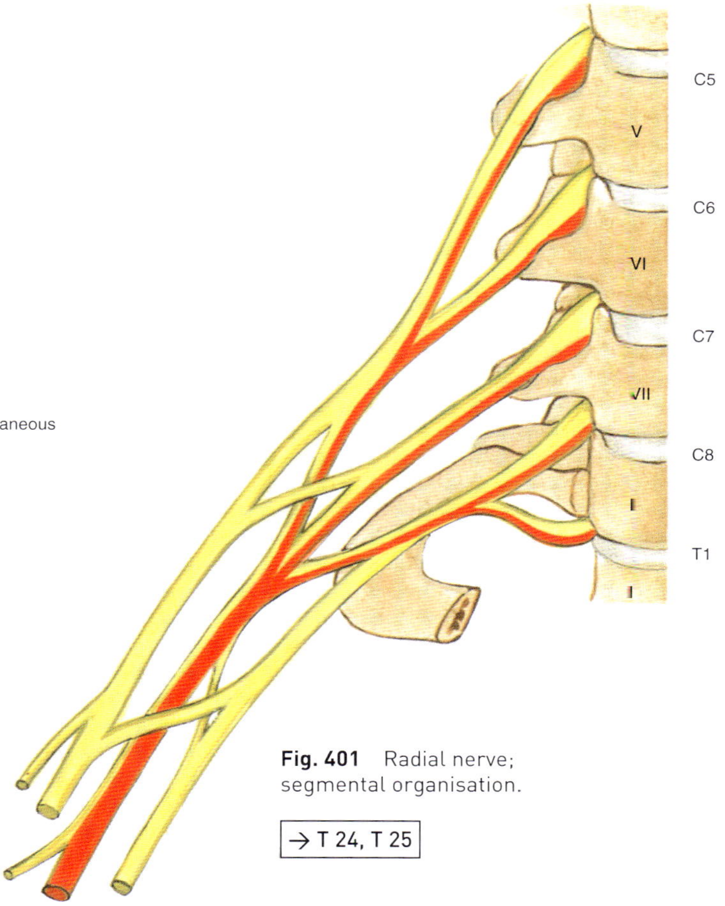

Fig. 401 Radial nerve; segmental organisation.

→ T 24, T 25

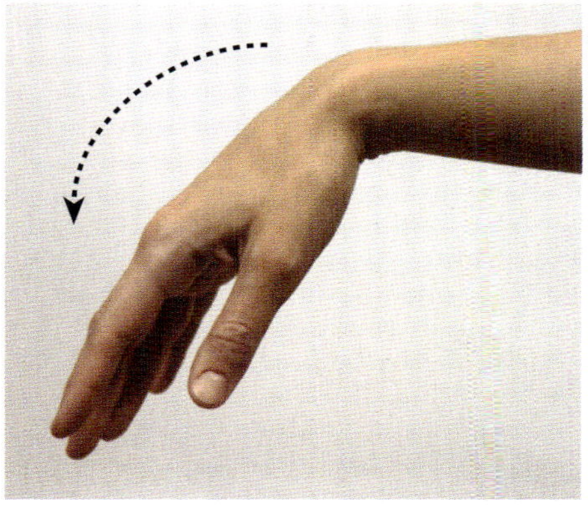

Fig. 402 Radial nerve; proximal palsy.

Axillary nerve

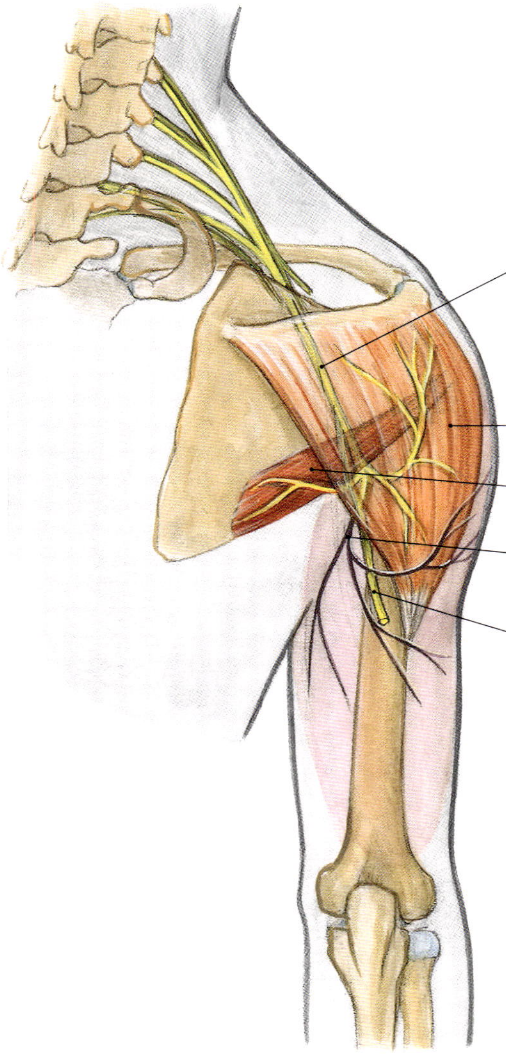

Fig. 403 Axillary nerve; supplying areas.
The axillary nerve passes to the dorsal side of the arm through the quadrangular space along with the posterior circumflex humeral artery.

→ 44, 386, T 24, T 25

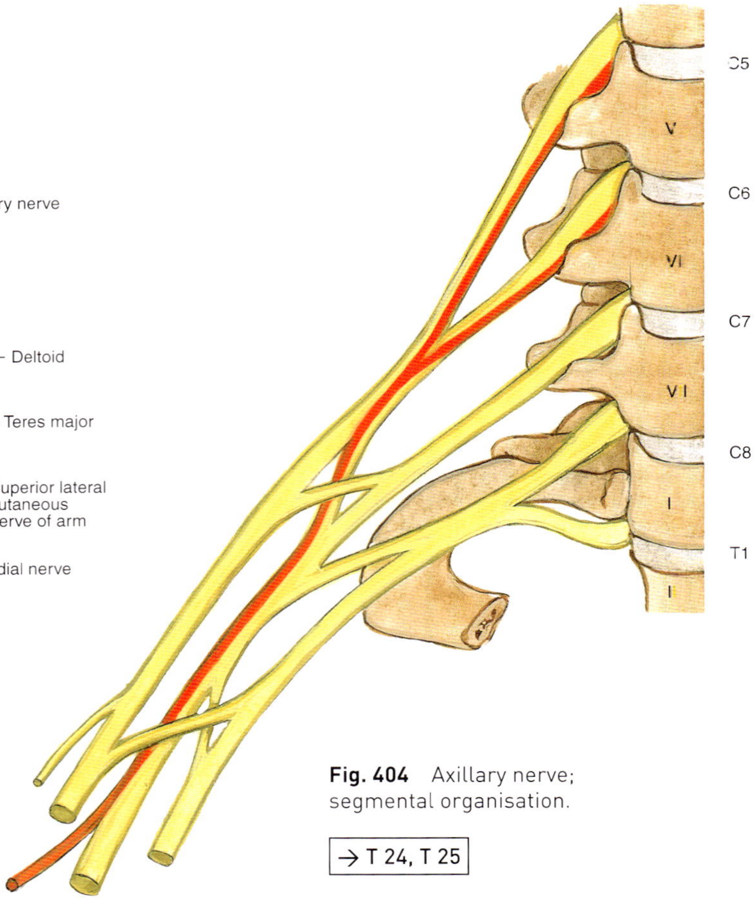

Fig. 404 Axillary nerve; segmental organisation.

→ T 24, T 25

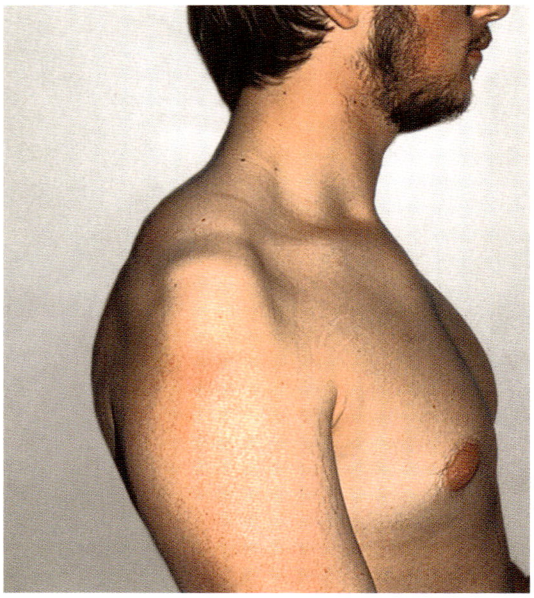

Fig. 405 Axillary nerve; palsy: deltoid muscle atrophy.

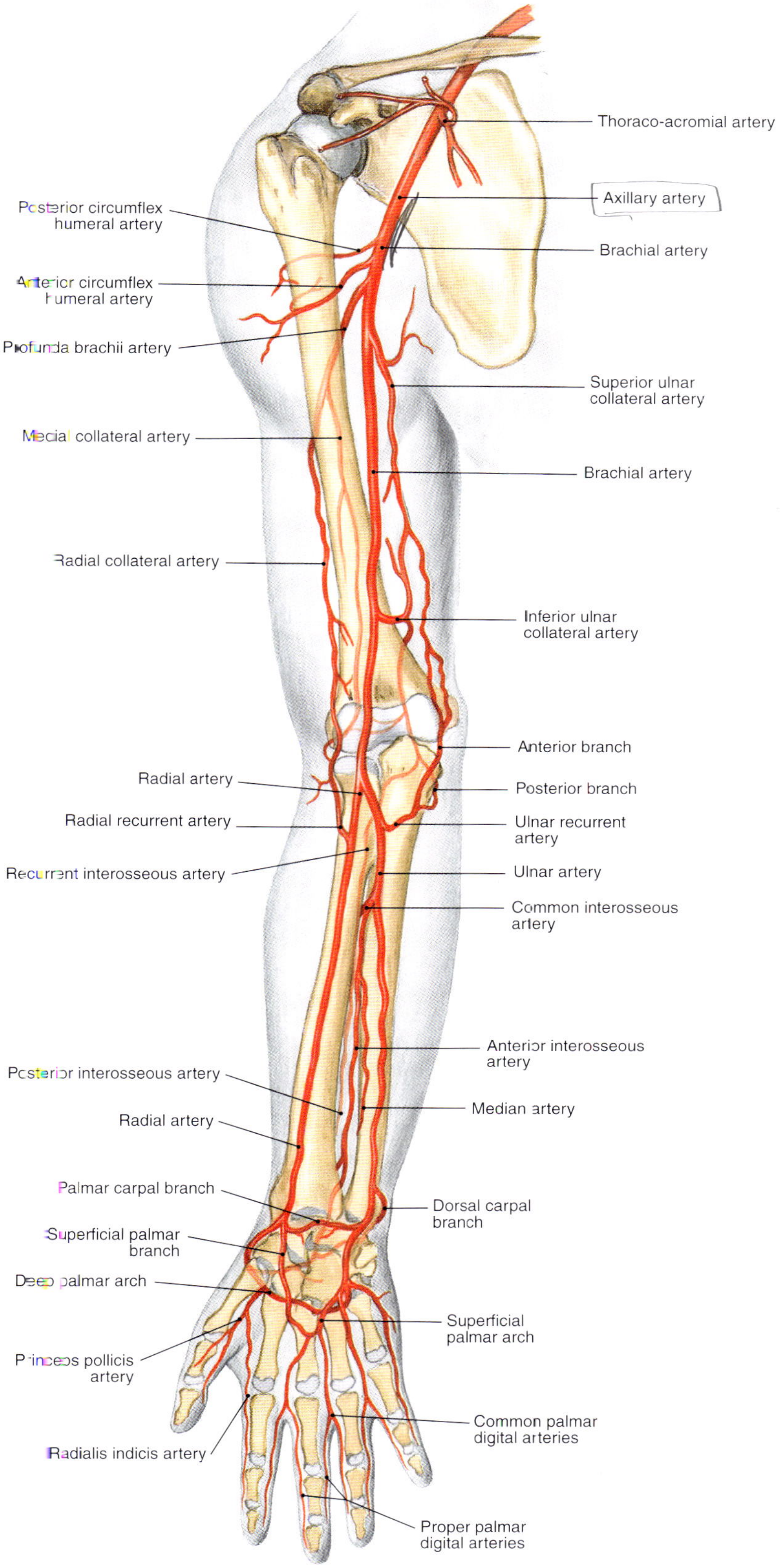

Fig. 406 Arteries of the upper limb; overview.
Arteries adjacent to the elbow joint form the cubital anastomosis.

→ 264

Lymphatics of the axilla

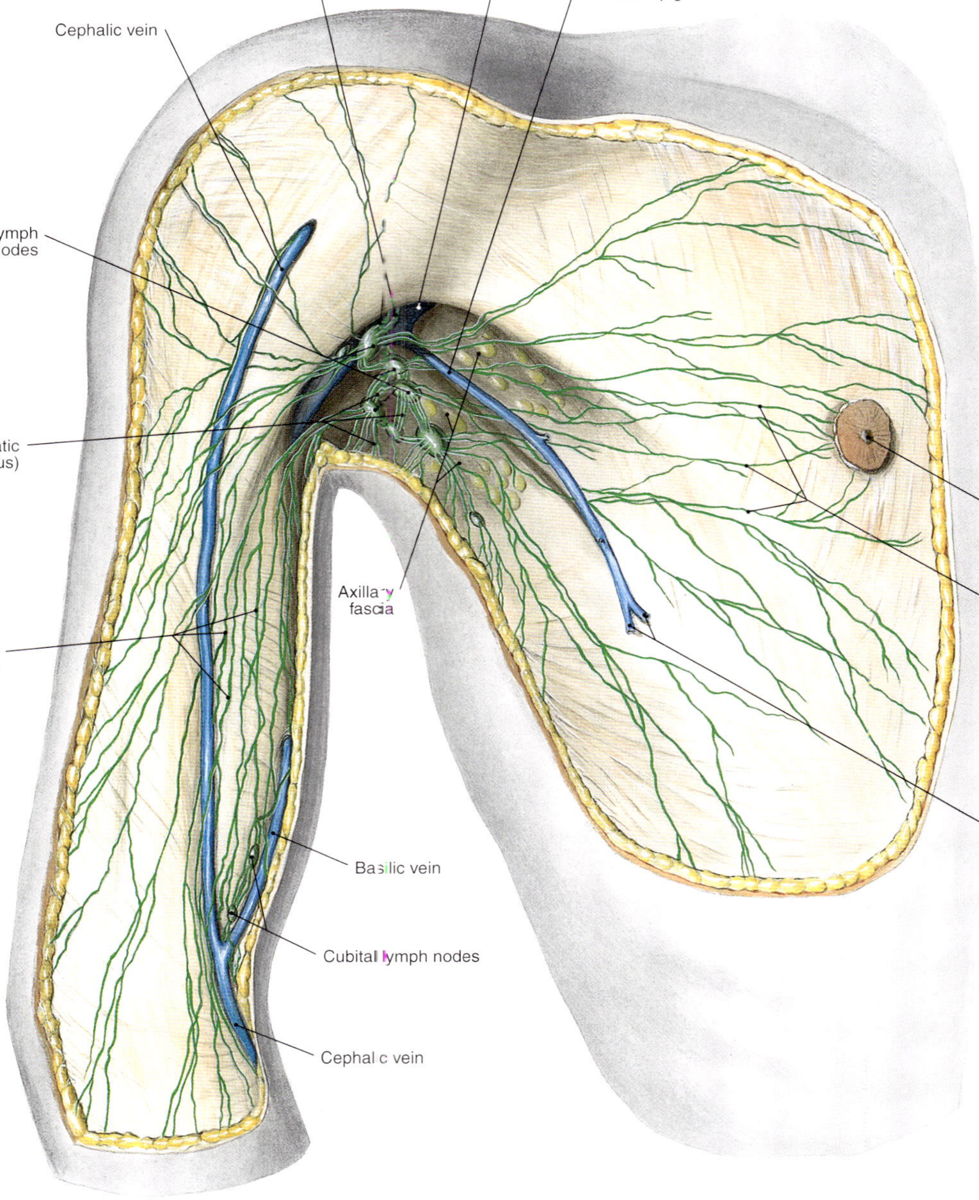

→ 42

408

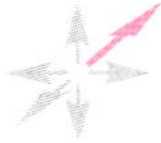

Fig. 407 Superficial lymphatics, lymph nodes and vein trunks in the regions of the arm, the lateral thoracic wall and the axilla.

Fascia of the chest, the shoulder and the axilla

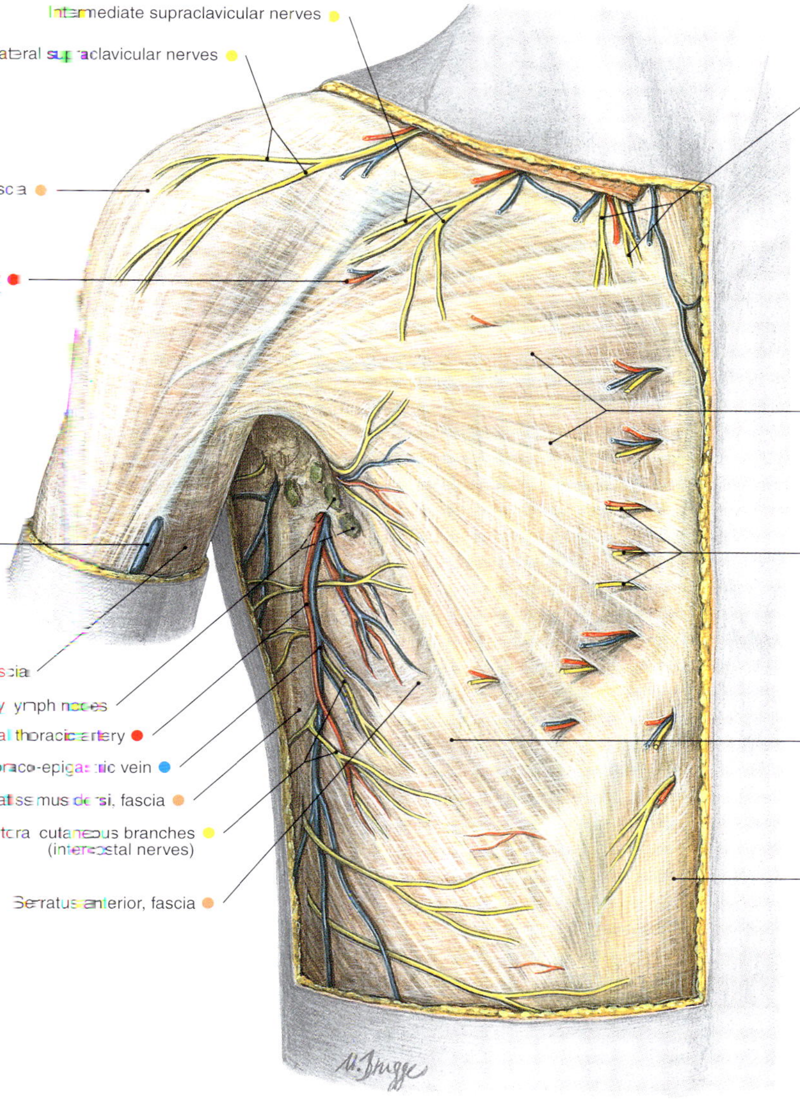

Fig. 408 Vessels and nerves in the regions of the upper arm as well as the shoulder, and the clavipectoral triangle.

253
409
407

Clavipectoral triangle

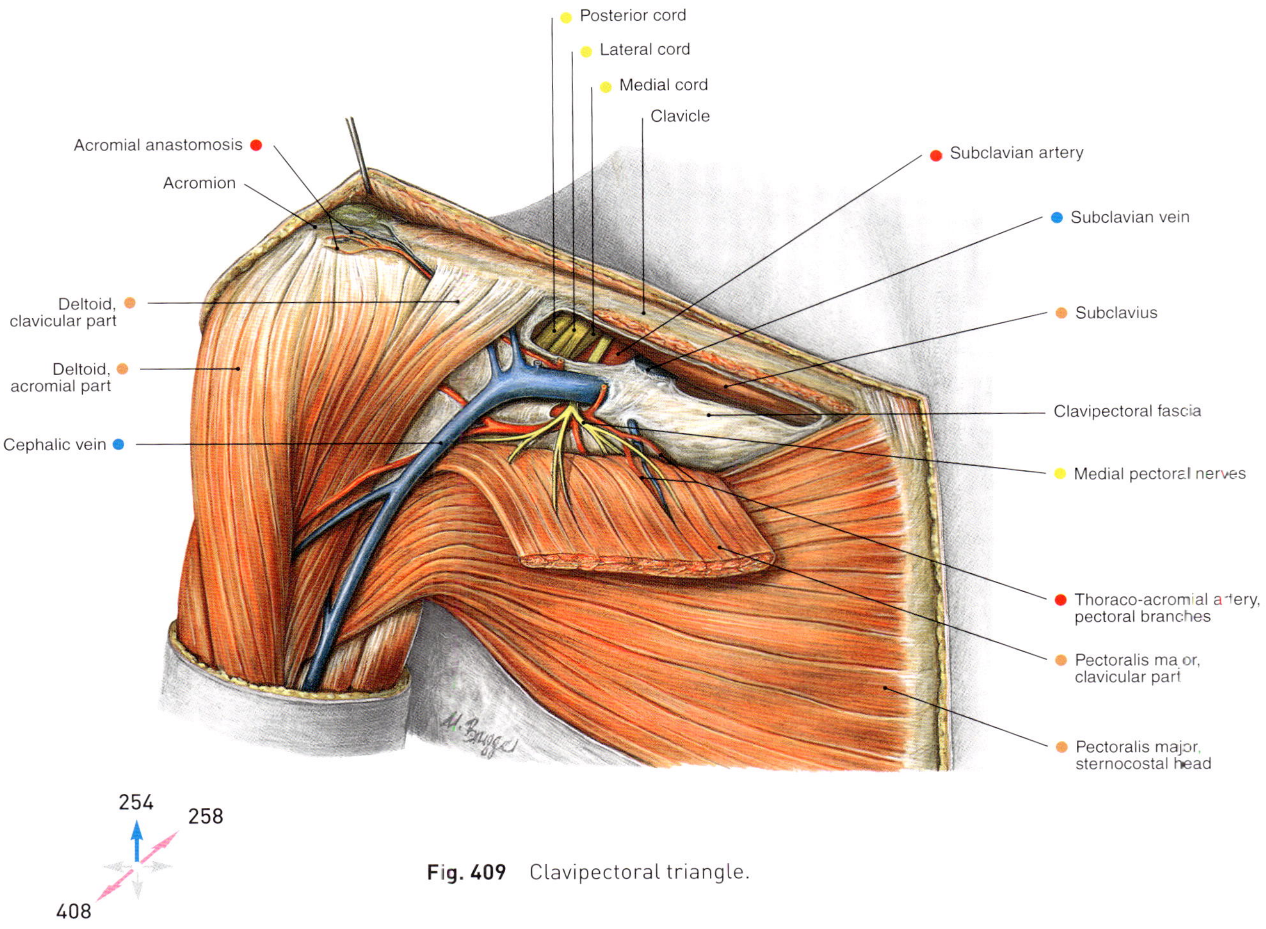

Fig. 409 Clavipectoral triangle.

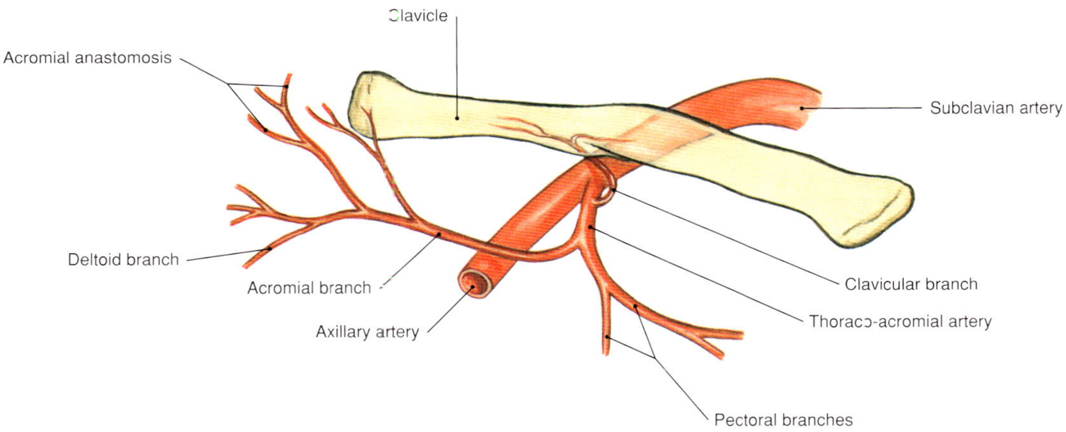

Fig. 410 Branching pattern of the thoraco-acromial artery.

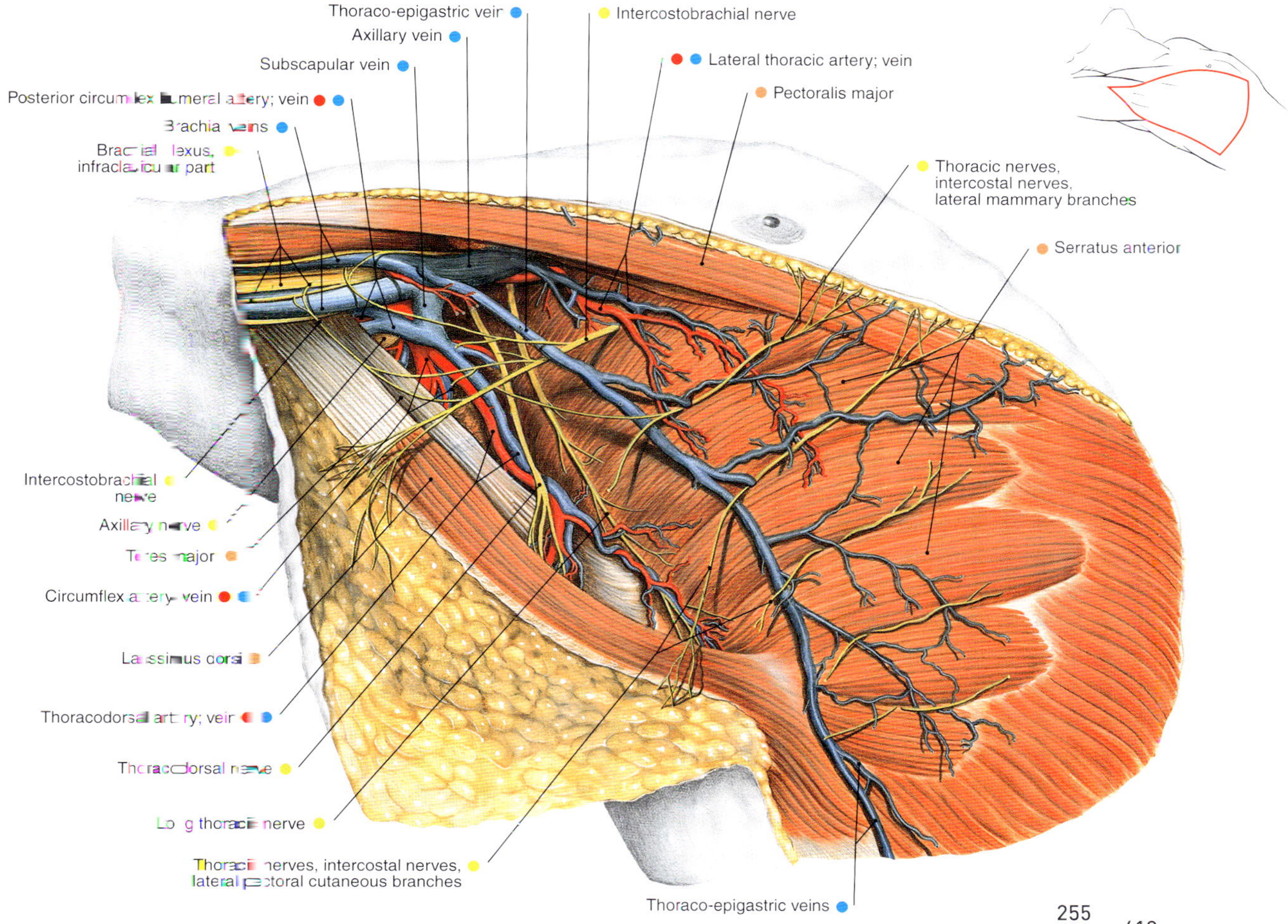

255
413
592
417
408

Fig. 411 Axillary fossa.

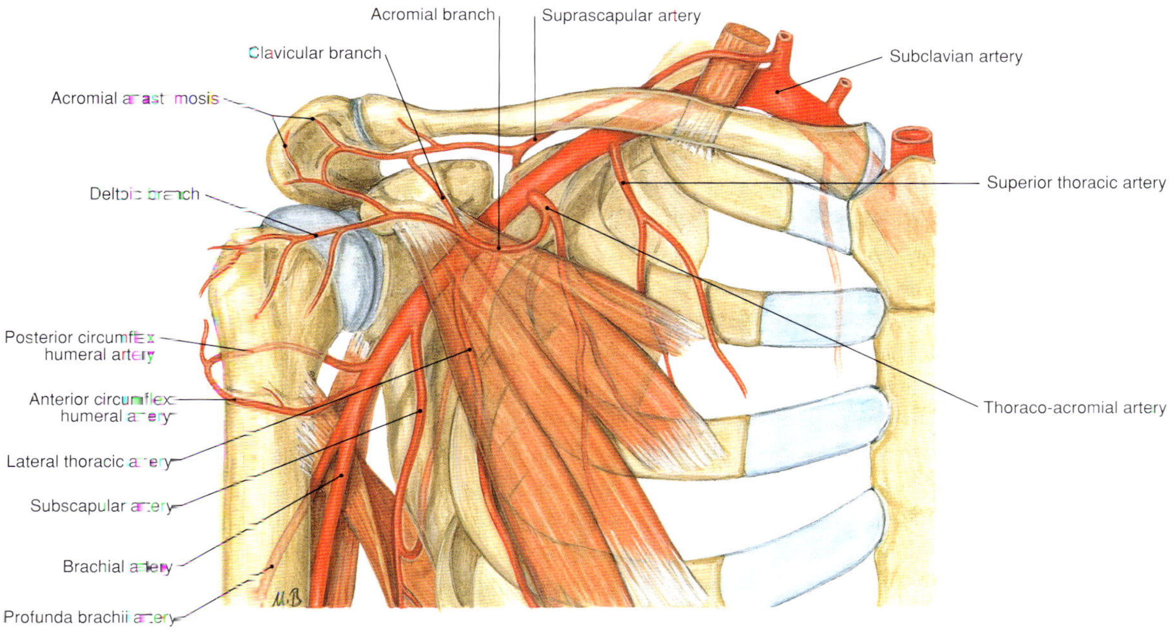

Fig. 412 Arteries of the shoulder region.

Neck and axillary fossa

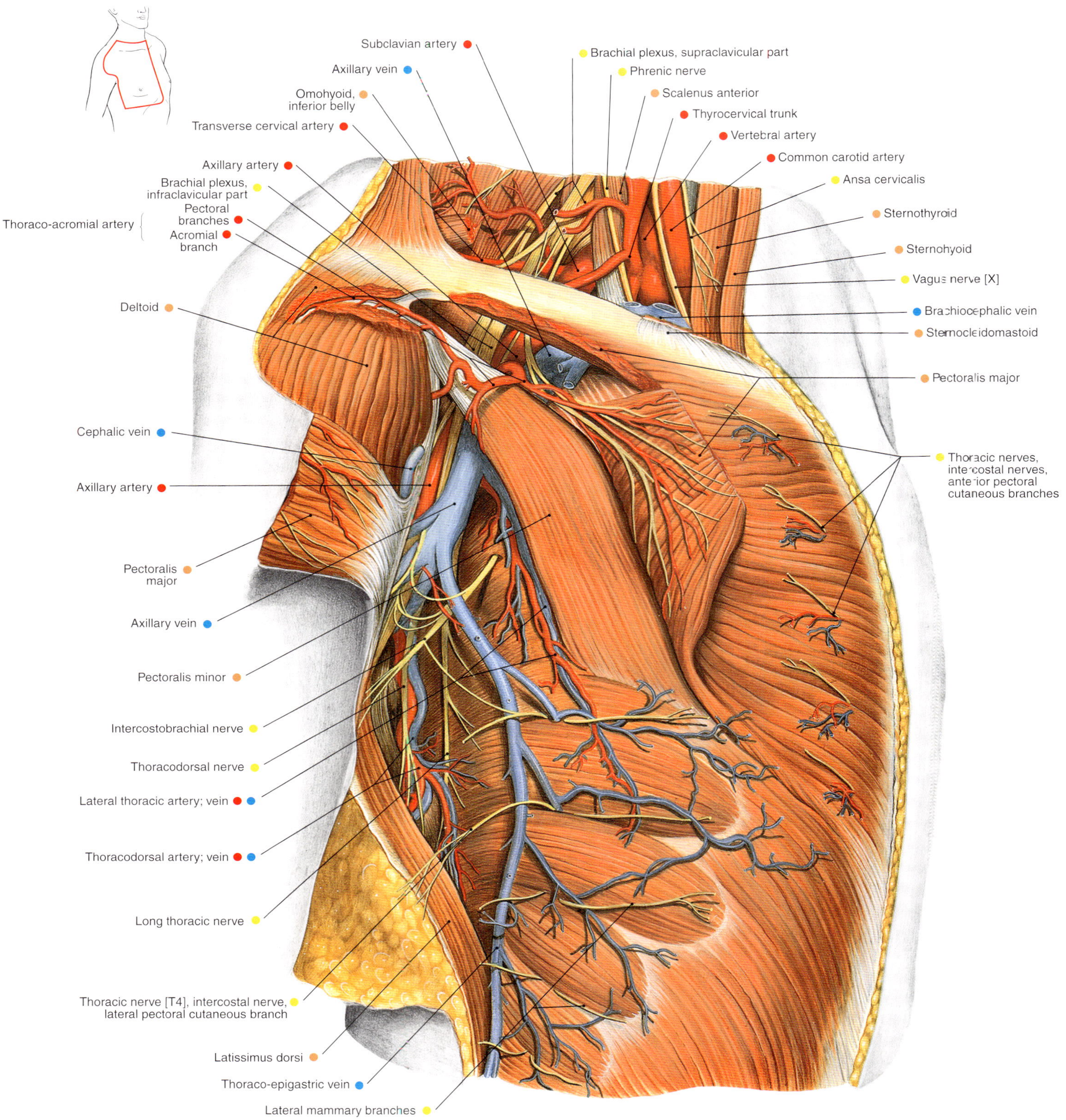

256
414
411
417

Fig. 413 Lateral thoracic wall; infraclavicular fossa and axillary fossa.

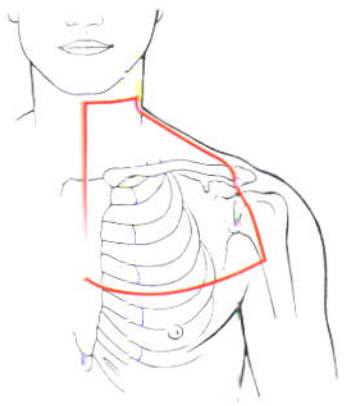

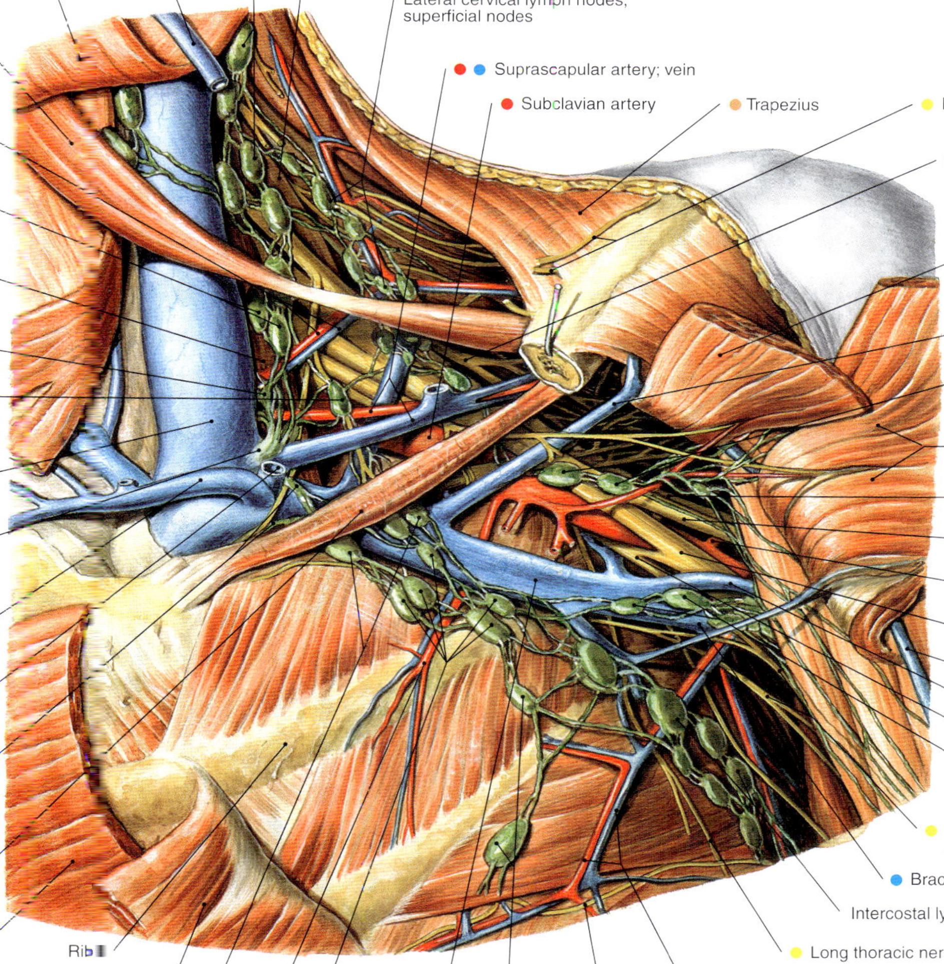

Fig. 414 Axillary fossa and deep cervical region; exemplary illustration of lymphatics and lymph nodes.

261
258
413
408
261
417

Vessels and nerves of the arm

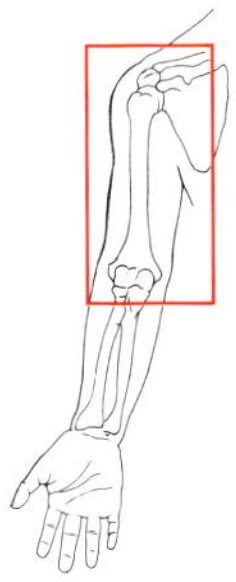

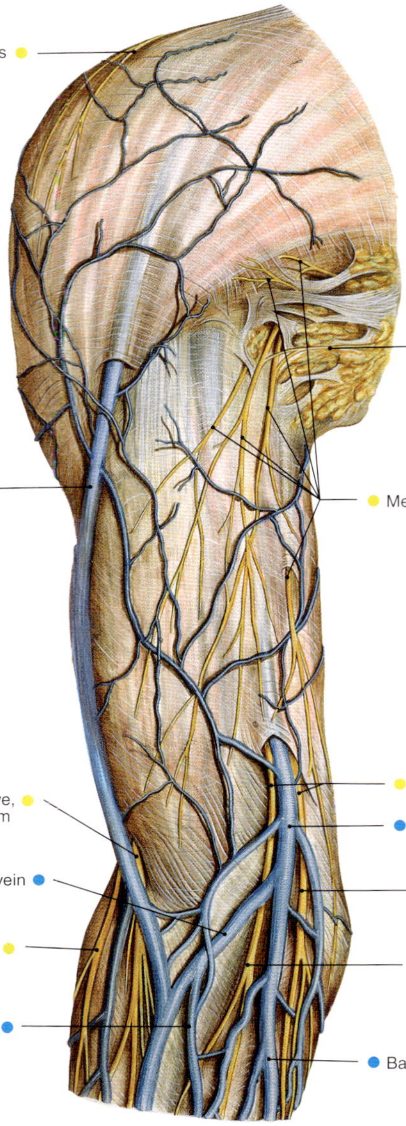

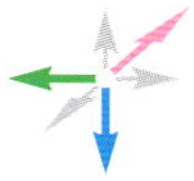
417
407
421

Fig. 415 Epifascial vessels and nerves of the shoulder, the anterior region of the arm and the anterior region of the elbow.

Vessels and nerves of the arm

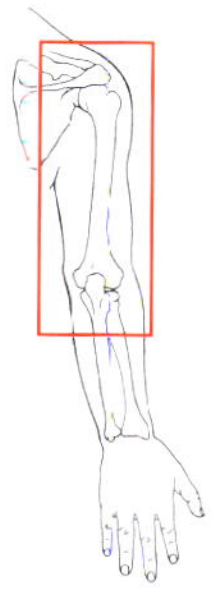

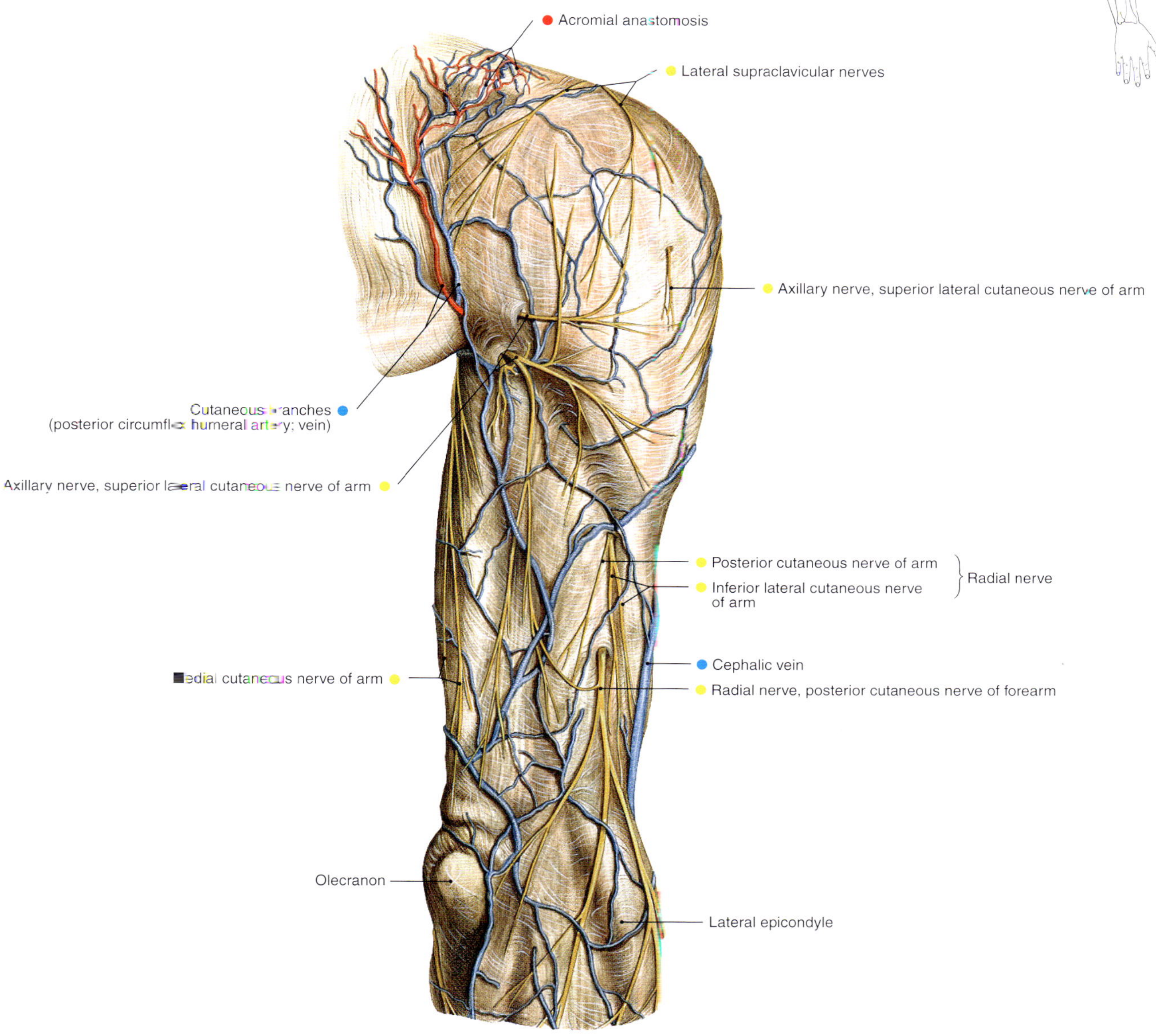

Fig. 416 Epifascial vessels and nerves of the shoulder, the posterior region of the arm and the posterior region of the elbow.

419
422

Vessels and nerves of the arm

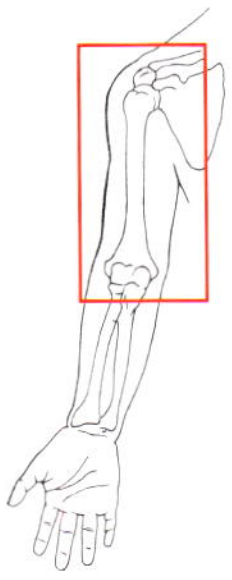

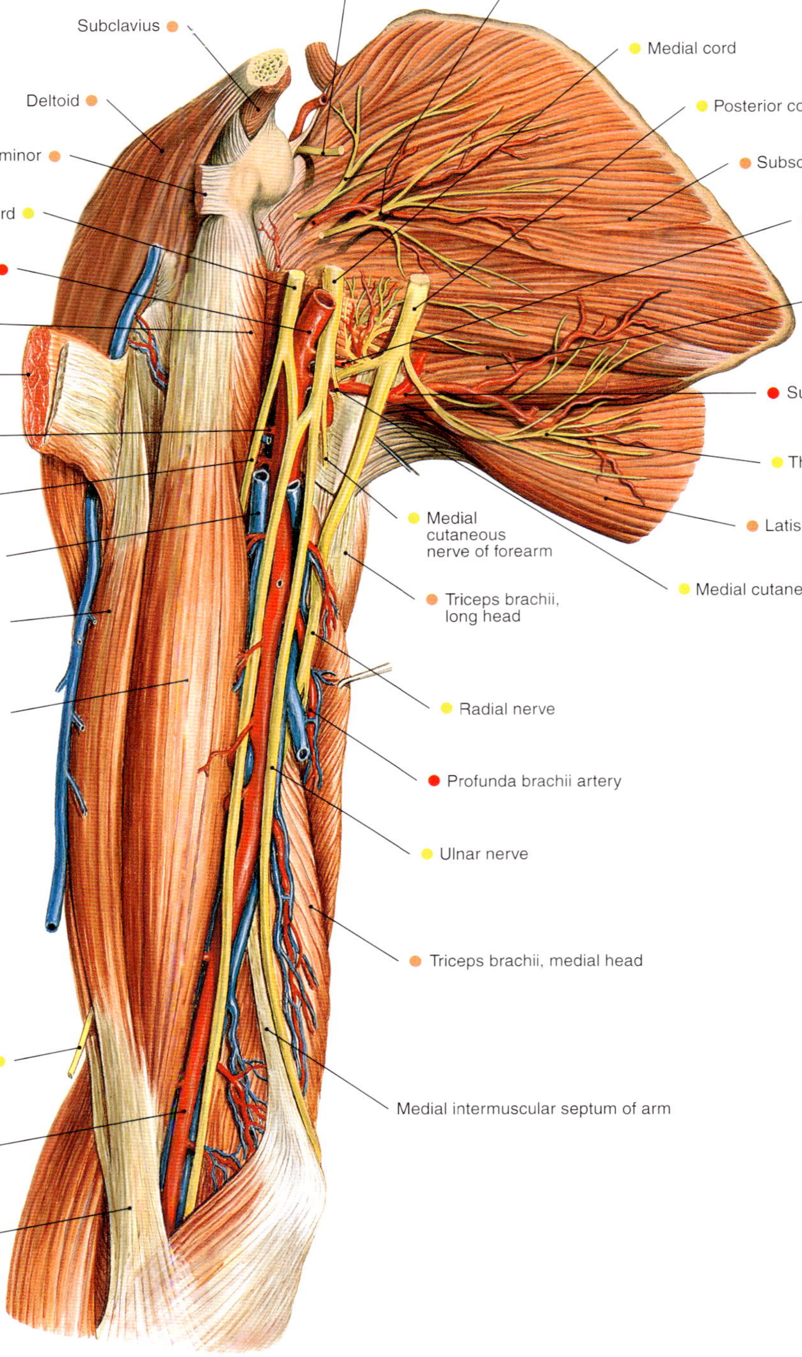

413
414
418
415
424

Fig. 417 Vessels and nerves of the anterior region of the arm.

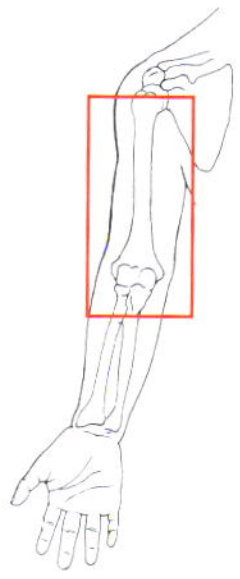

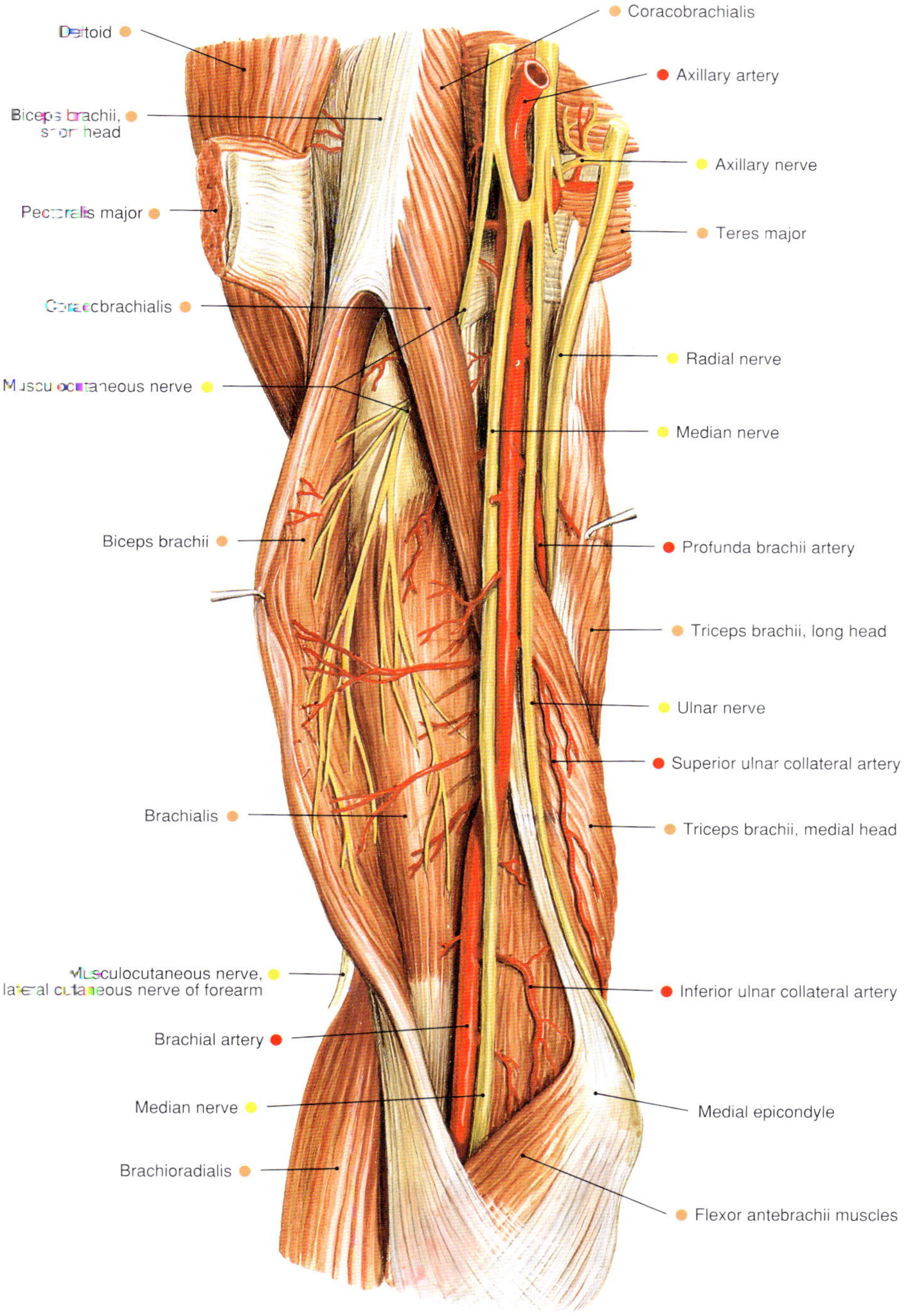

Fig. 418 Arteries and nerves of the anterior region of the arm.

414
413
417
425

Arteries and nerves of the arm

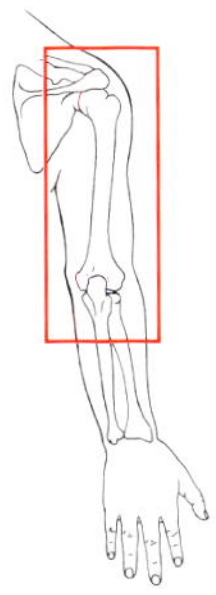

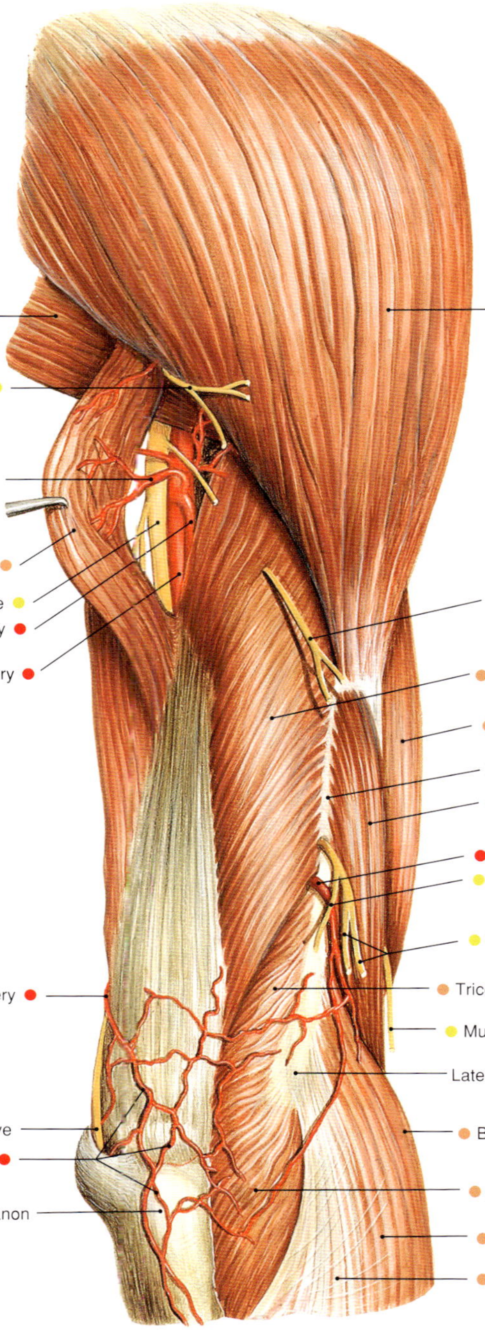

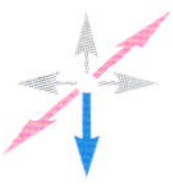

Fig. 419 Arteries and nerves of the posterior region of the arm.

Arteries and nerves of the arm

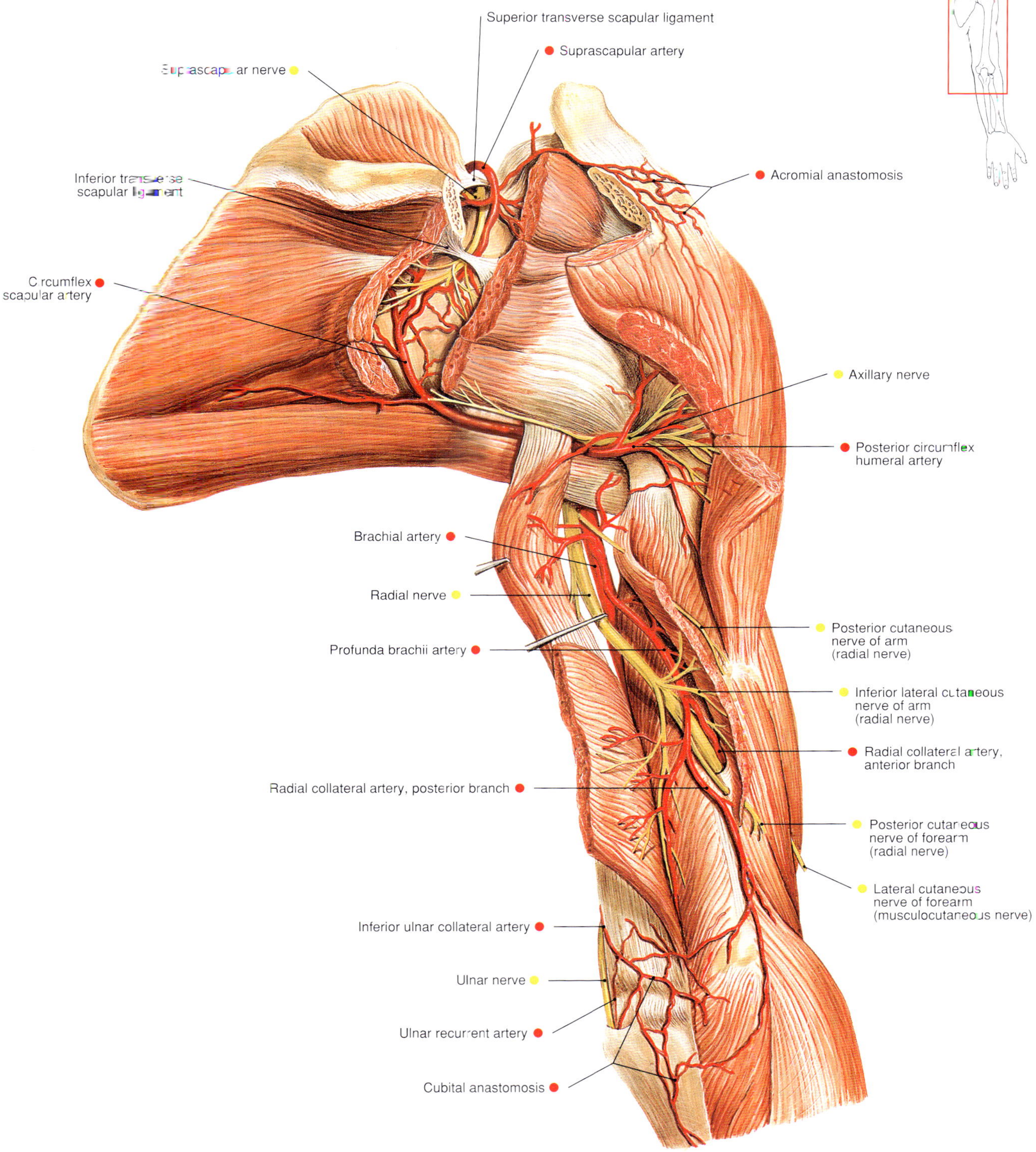

Fig. 420 Arteries and nerves of the scapular region and the posterior region of the arm.

419
430
431

Veins and nerves of the forearm

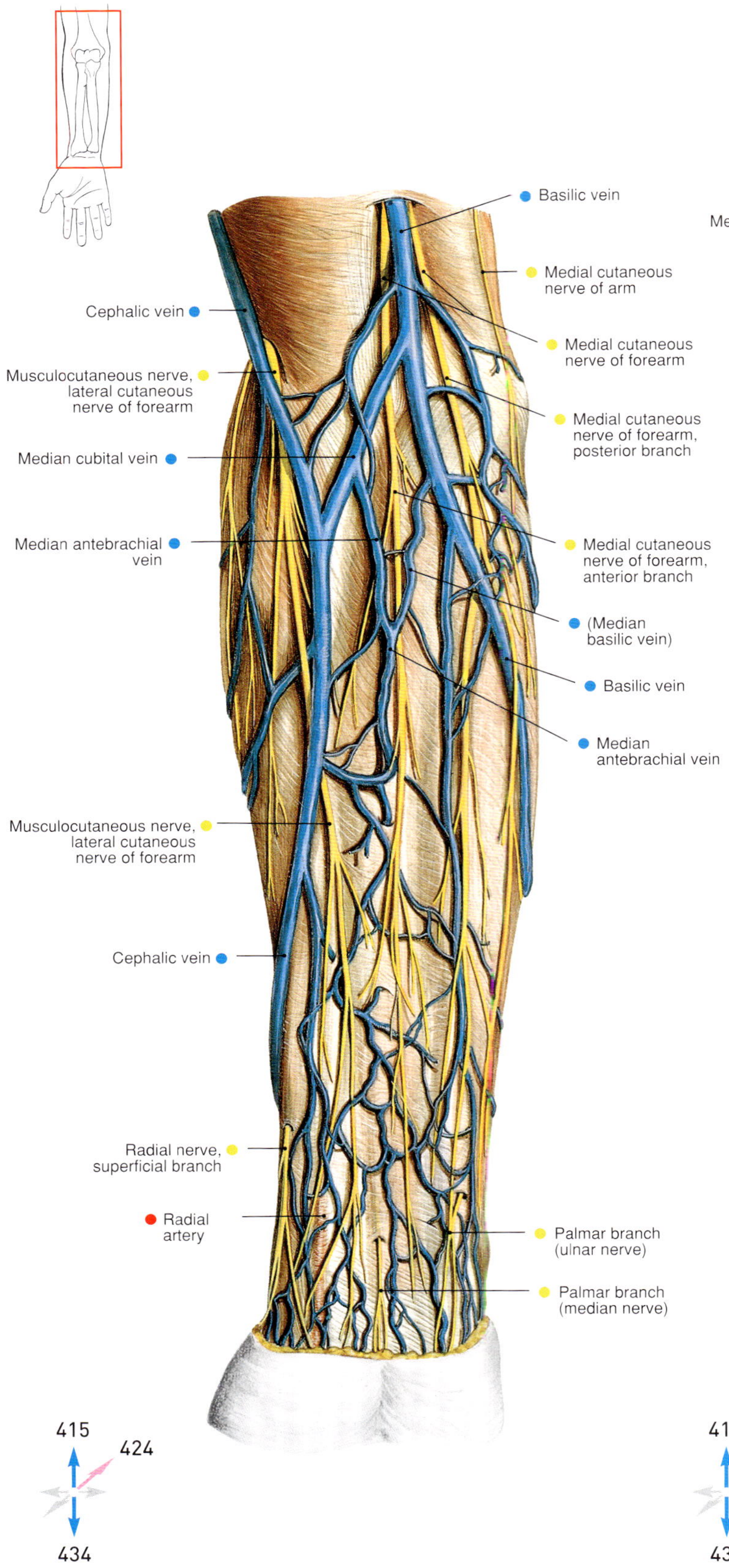

Fig. 421 Veins and nerves of the anterior region of the forearm; epifascial layer.

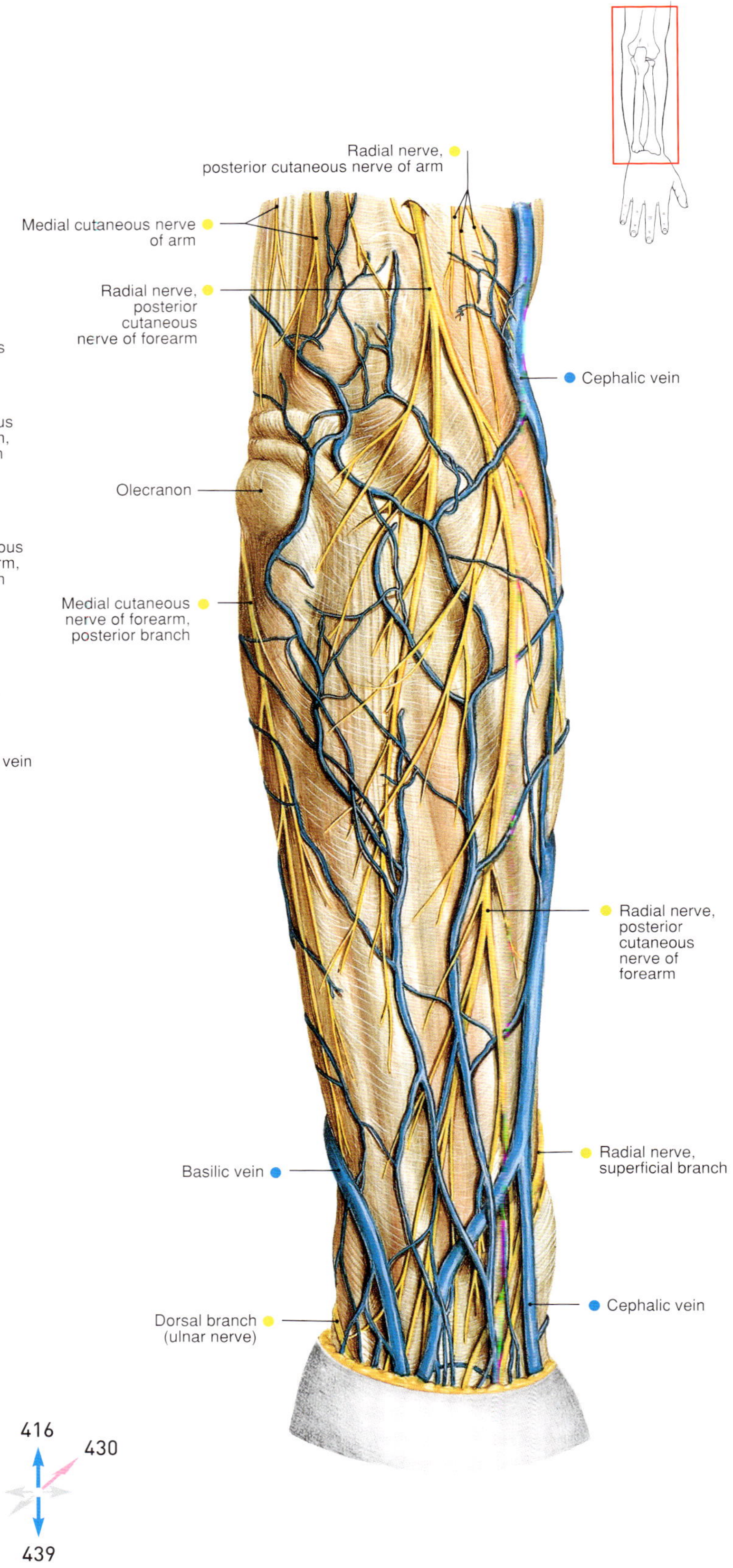

Fig. 422 Veins and nerves of the posterior region of the forearm; epifascial layer.

Veins of the cubital fossa

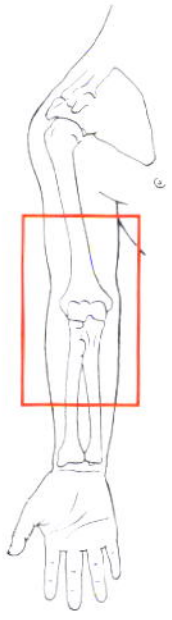

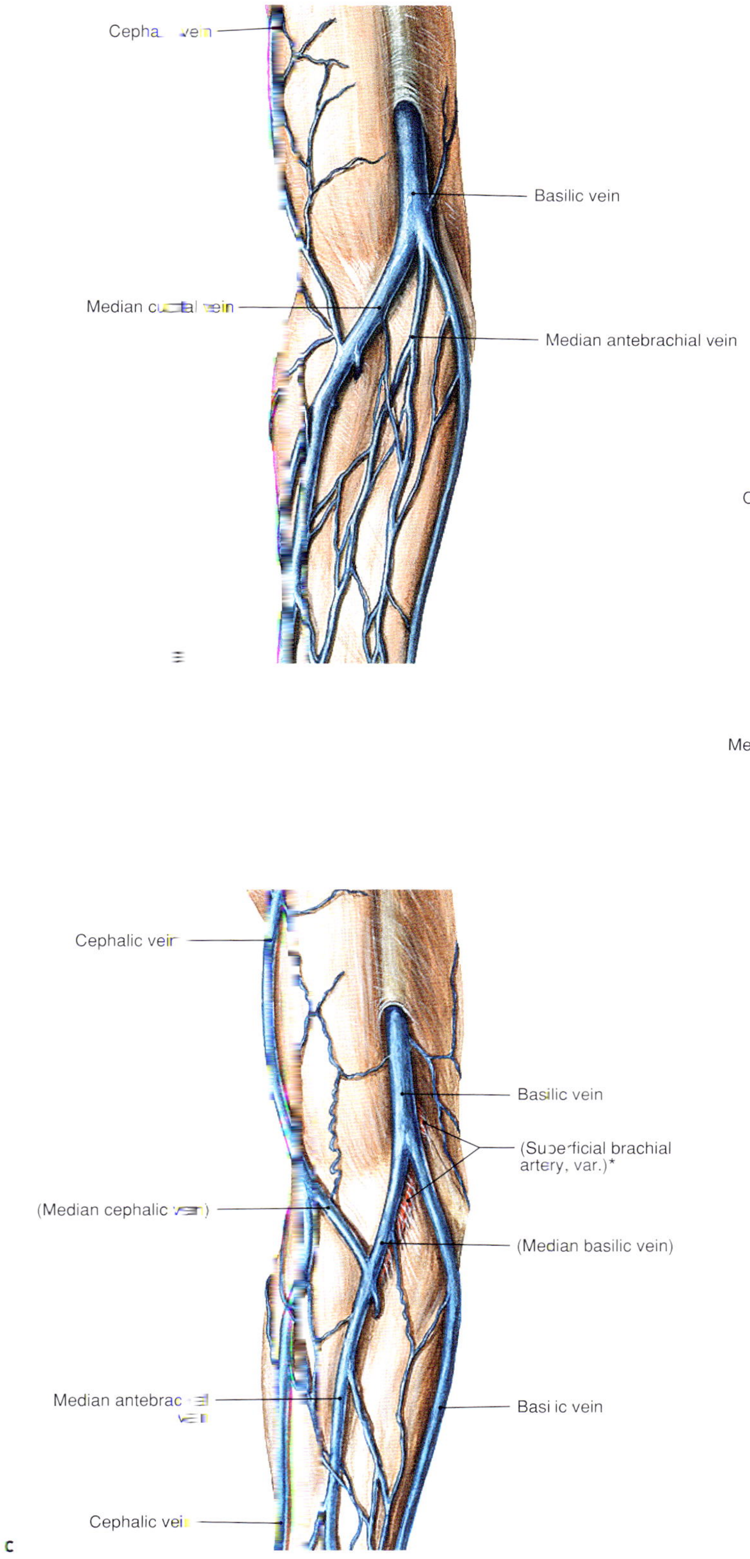

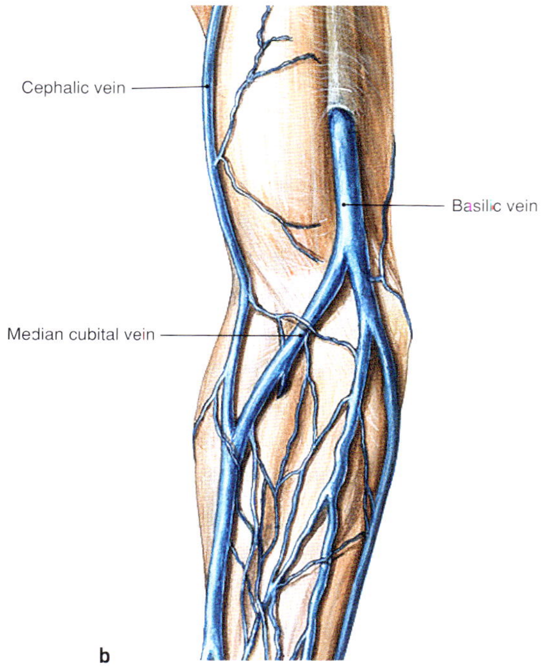

Fig. 423 a–c Variations in the epifascial veins of the cubital fossa.

* With regard to intravenous injections, this rare variation is particularly important, as a supposedly intravenous injection can mistakenly become intra-arterial.

Arteries and nerves of the arm

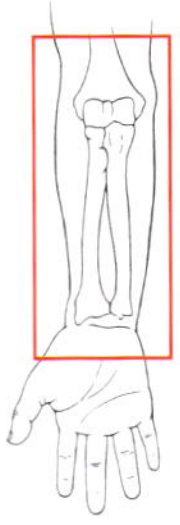

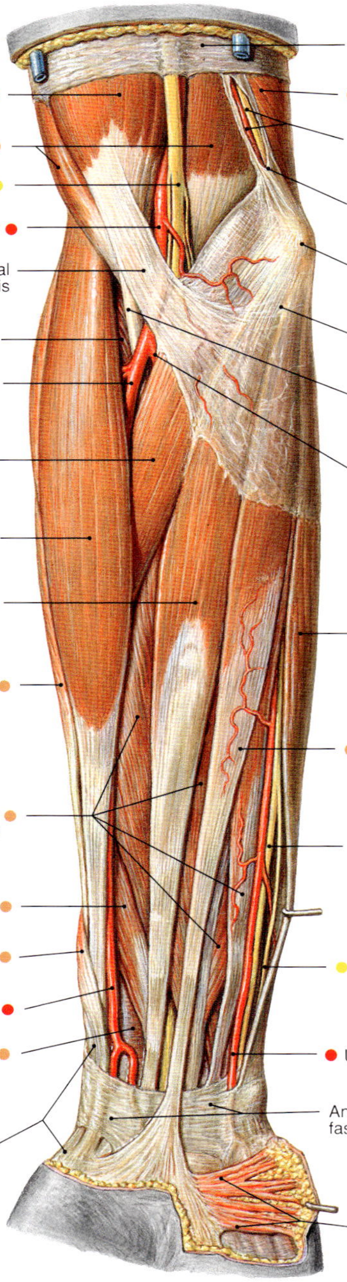

417 425 421 434

Fig. 424 Arteries and nerves of the anterior region of the forearm; subfascial layer.

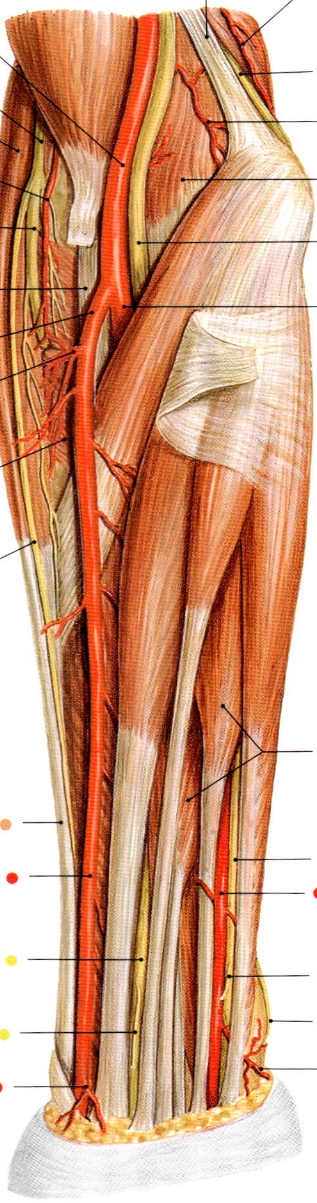

418 426 424 435

Fig. 425 Arteries and nerves of the anterior region of the forearm; course of the radial artery.

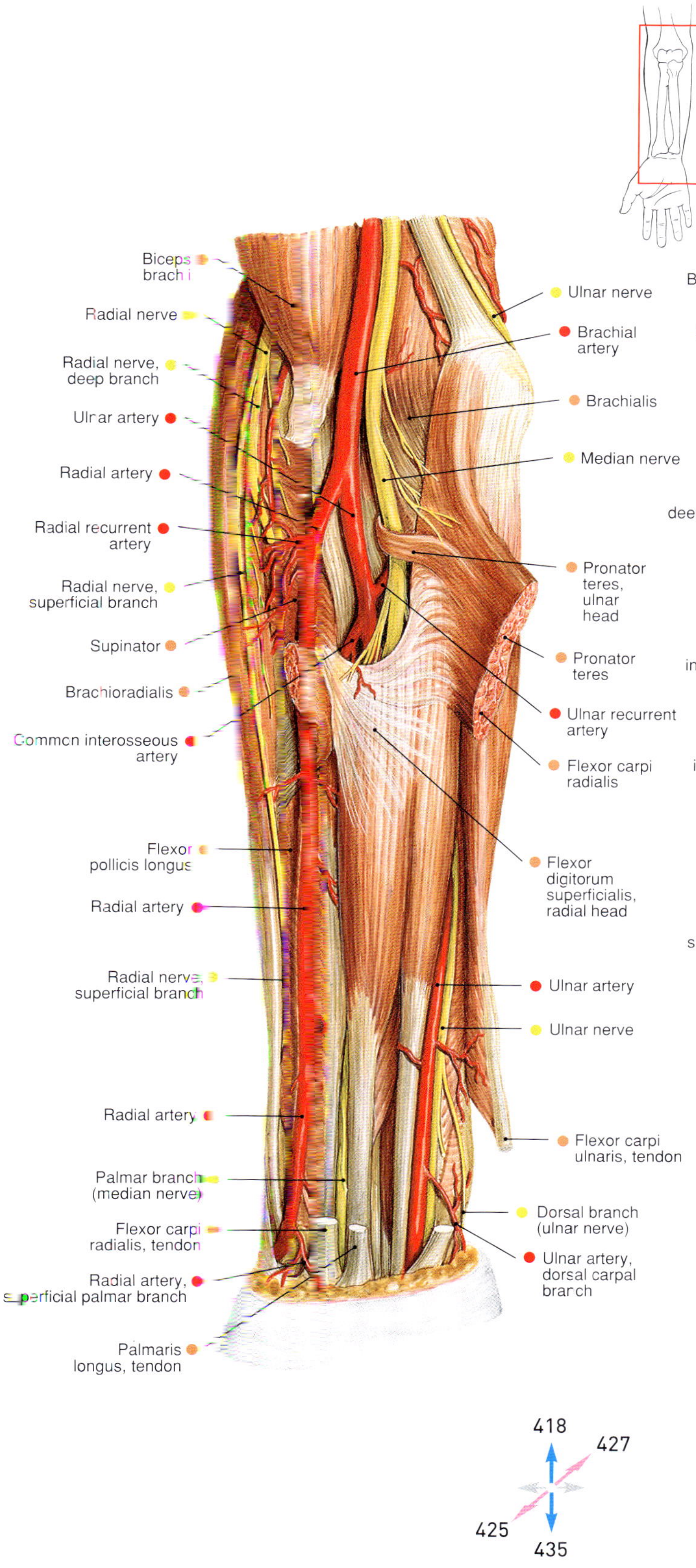

Fig. 426 Arteries and nerves of the anterior region of the forearm; deep layer.

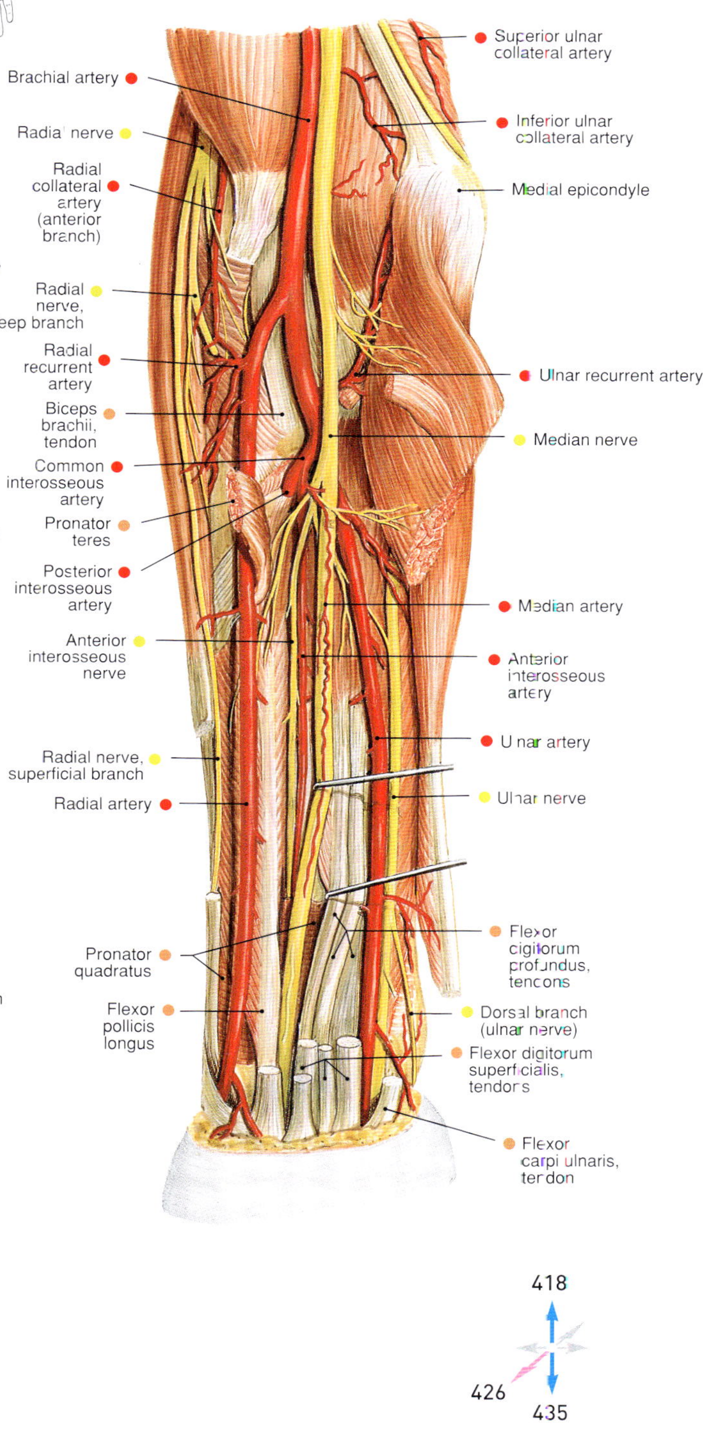

Fig. 427 Arteries and nerves of the anterior region of the forearm; deep layer after partial removal of the flexor digitorum superficialis muscle.

Arteries and nerves of the cubital fossa

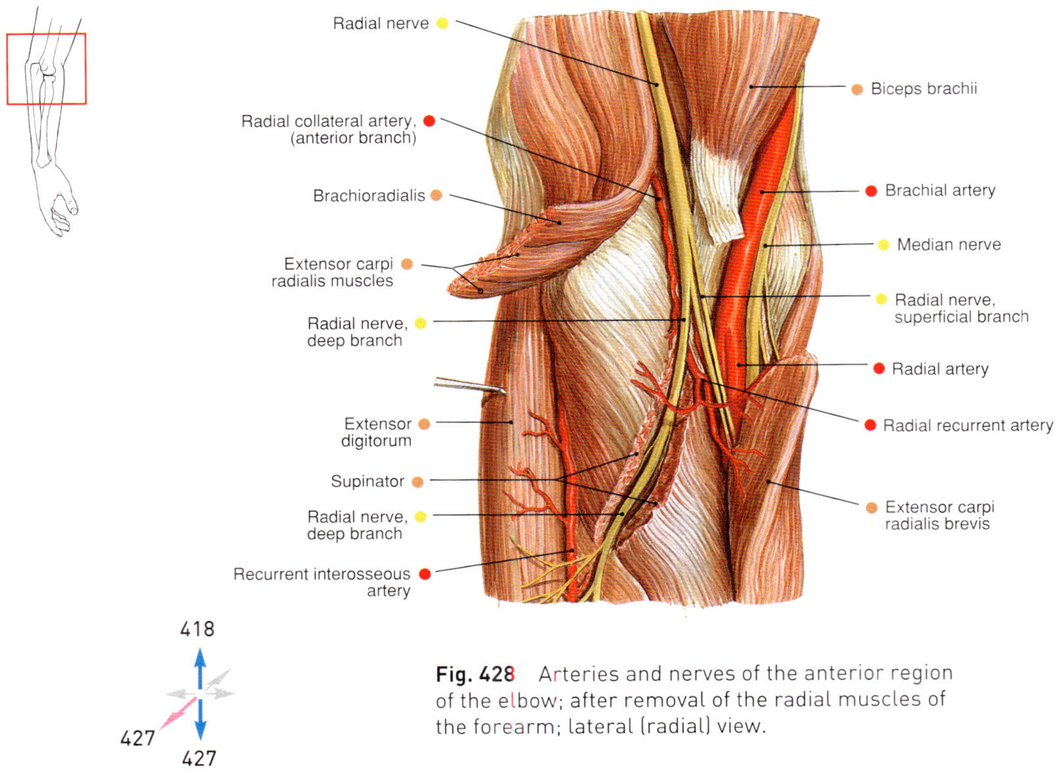

Fig. 428 Arteries and nerves of the anterior region of the elbow; after removal of the radial muscles of the forearm; lateral (radial) view.

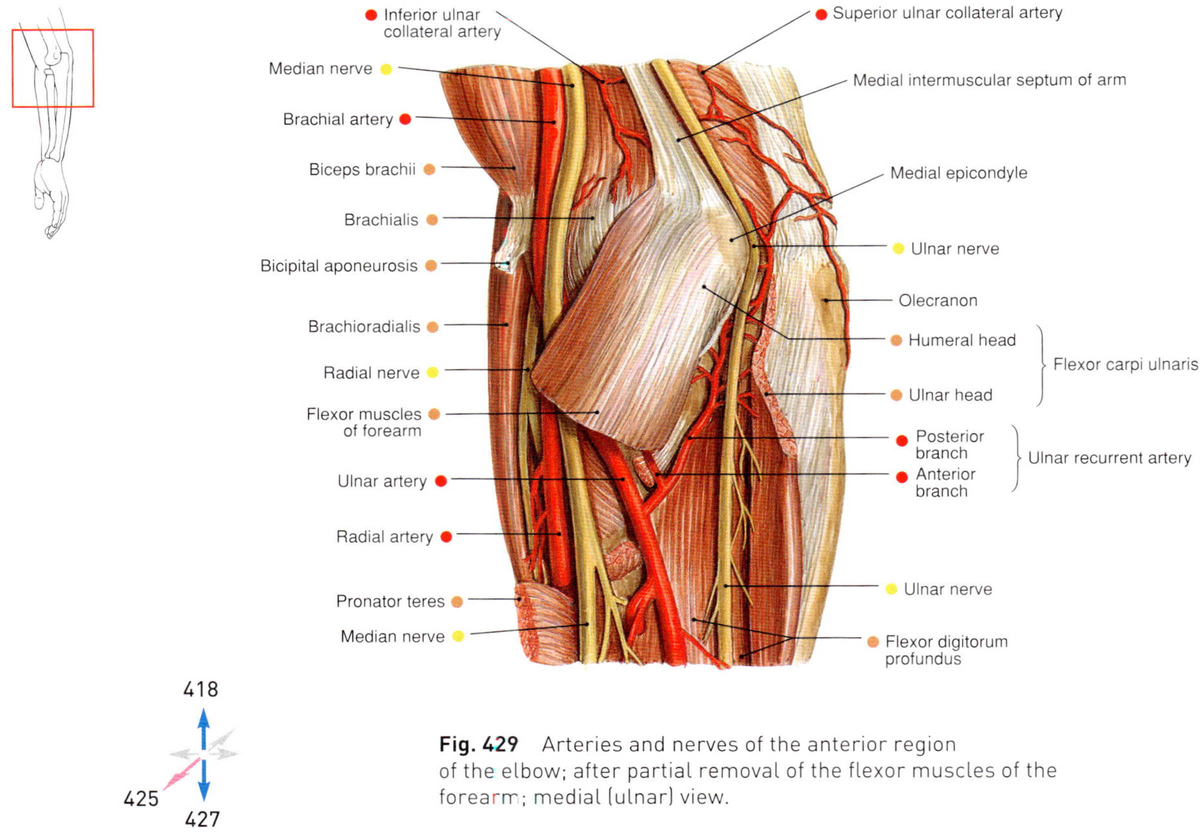

Fig. 429 Arteries and nerves of the anterior region of the elbow; after partial removal of the flexor muscles of the forearm; medial (ulnar) view.

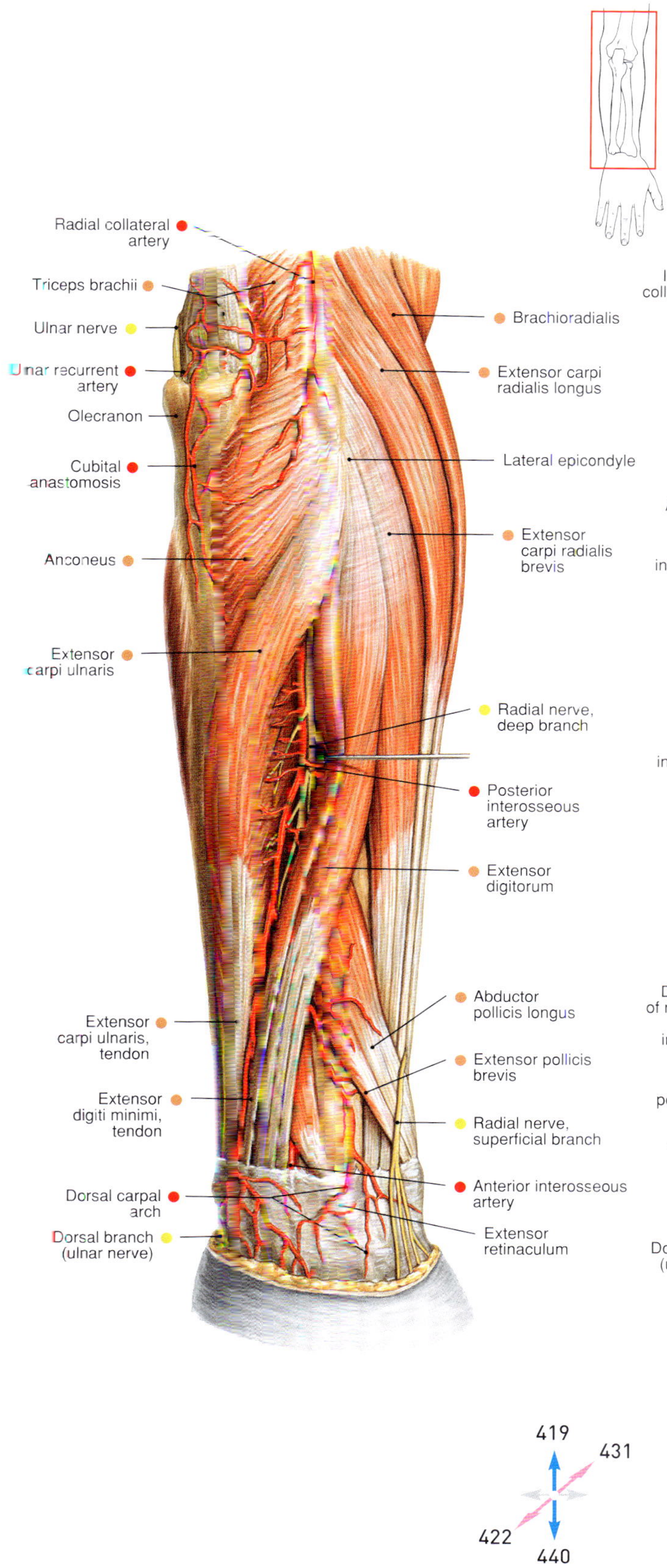

Fig. 430 Arteries and nerves of the posterior region of the forearm; superficial layer.

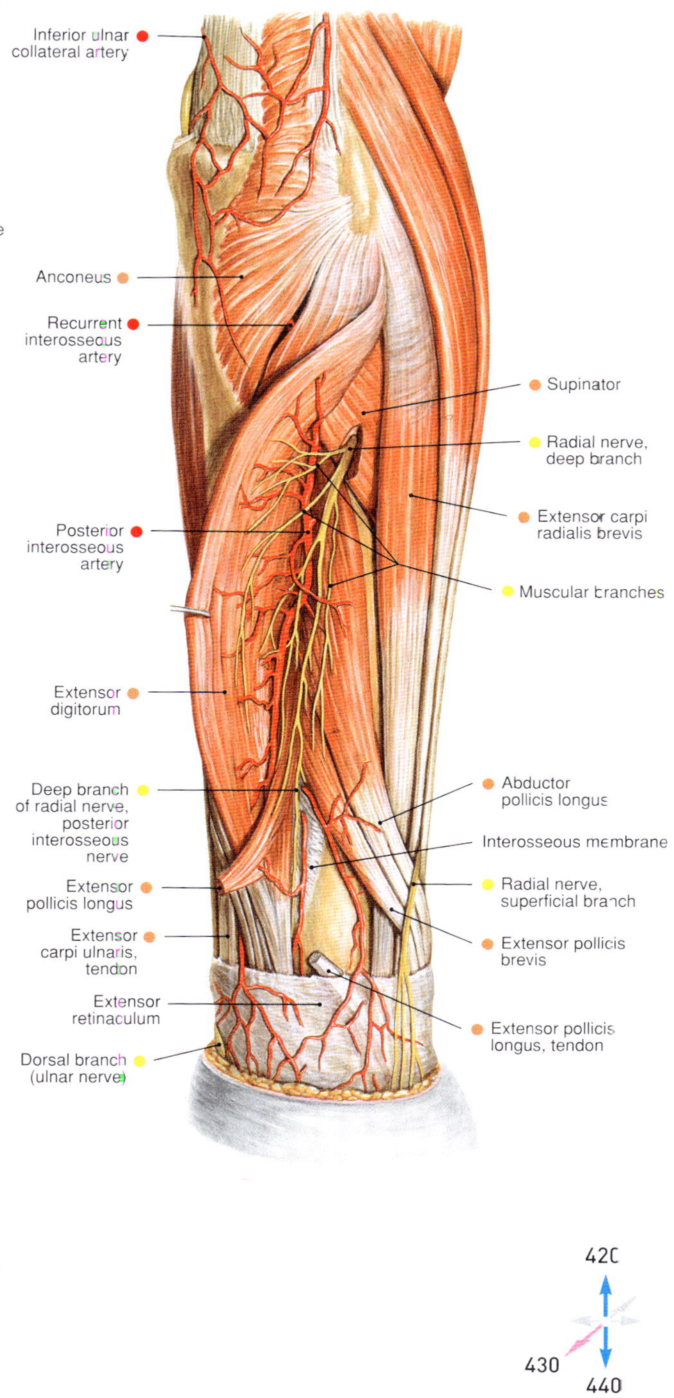

Fig. 431 Arteries and nerves of the posterior region of the forearm; deep layer.

Arteries of the hand

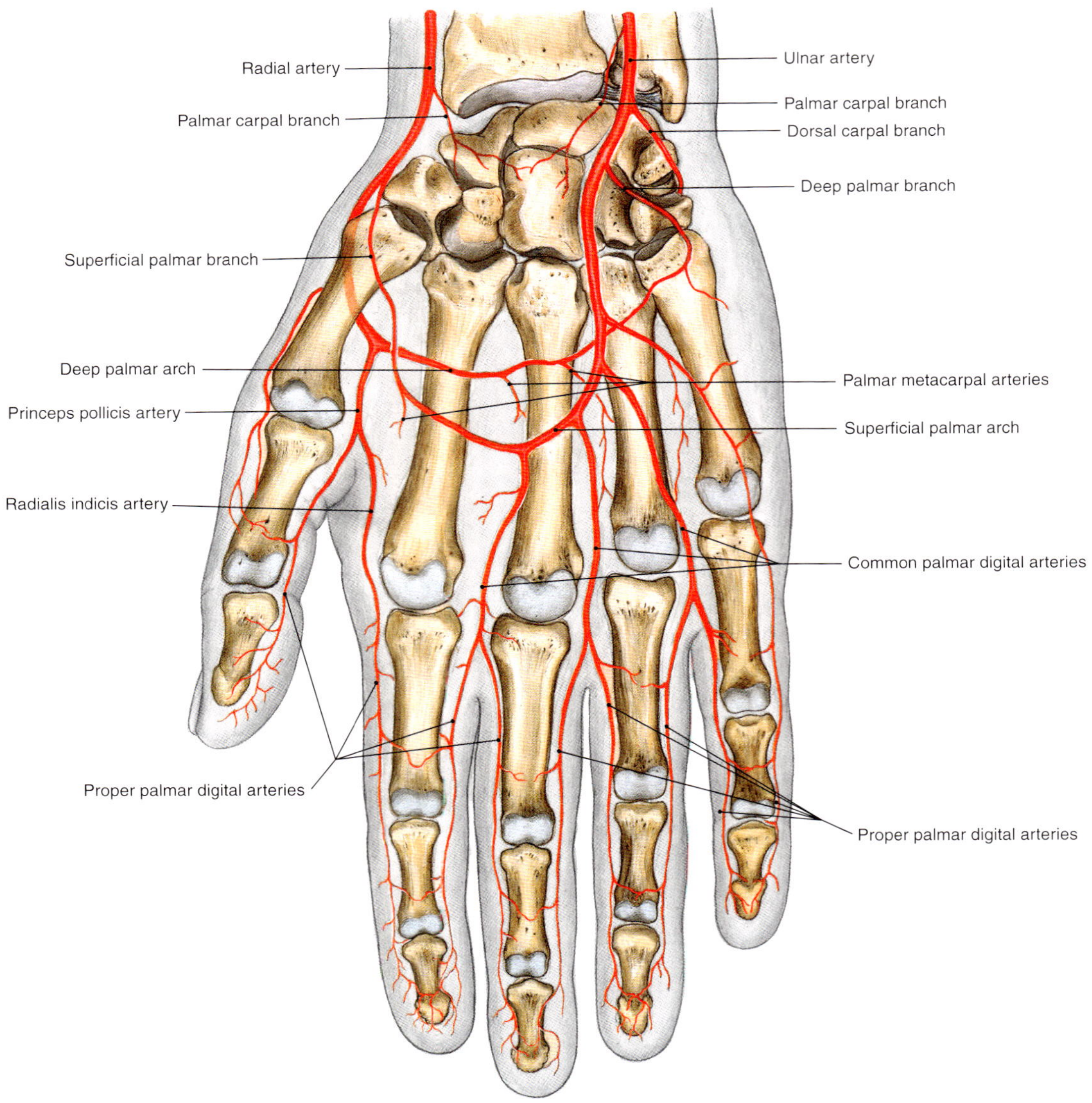

Fig. 432 Arteries of the palm; overview.

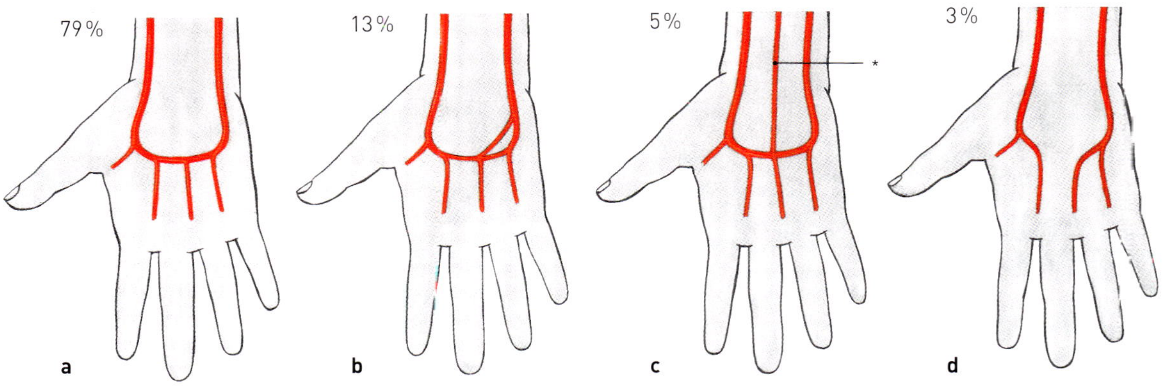

Fig. 433 a–d Variations of the deep palmar arch.

a "Textbook case", simple, closed arch

b Doubling of the ulnar part

c Anastomosis with the anterior interosseous artery (*)

d The radial artery supplies both radial fingers, whereas the ulnar artery supplies the three ulnar fingers.

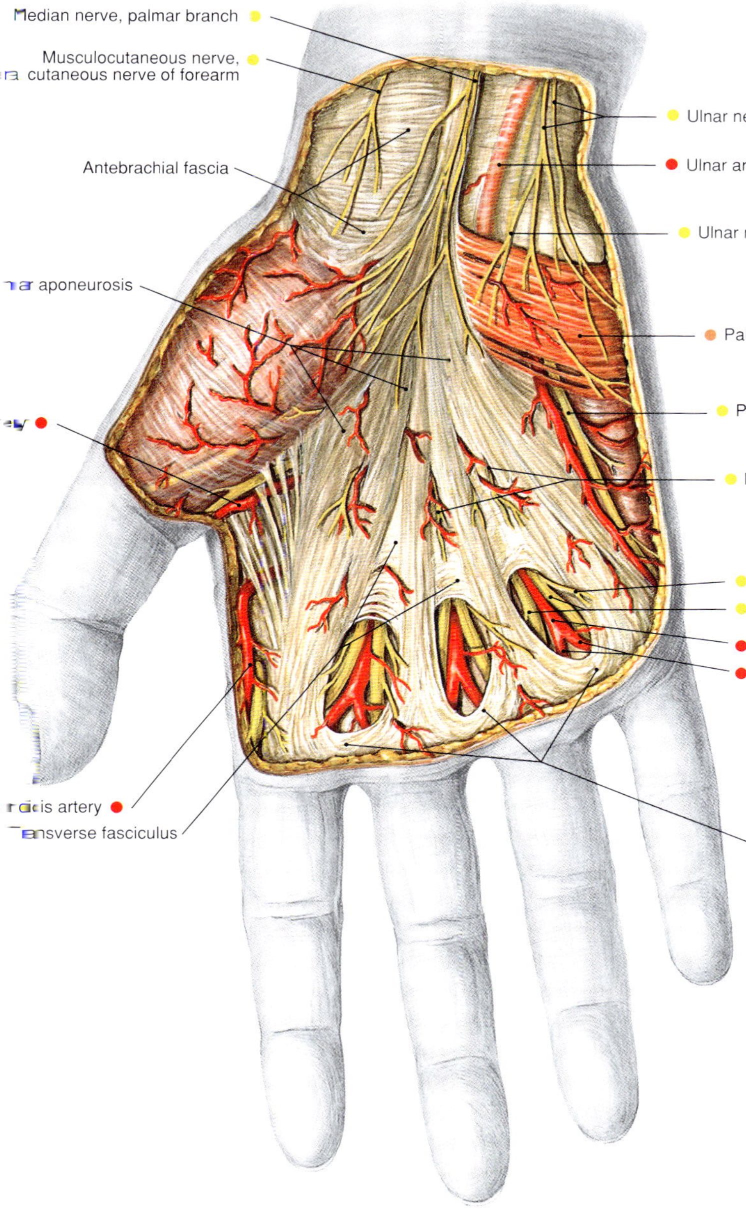

421
435

Fig. 434 Arteries and nerves of the palm; superficial layer.

Arteries and nerves of the hand

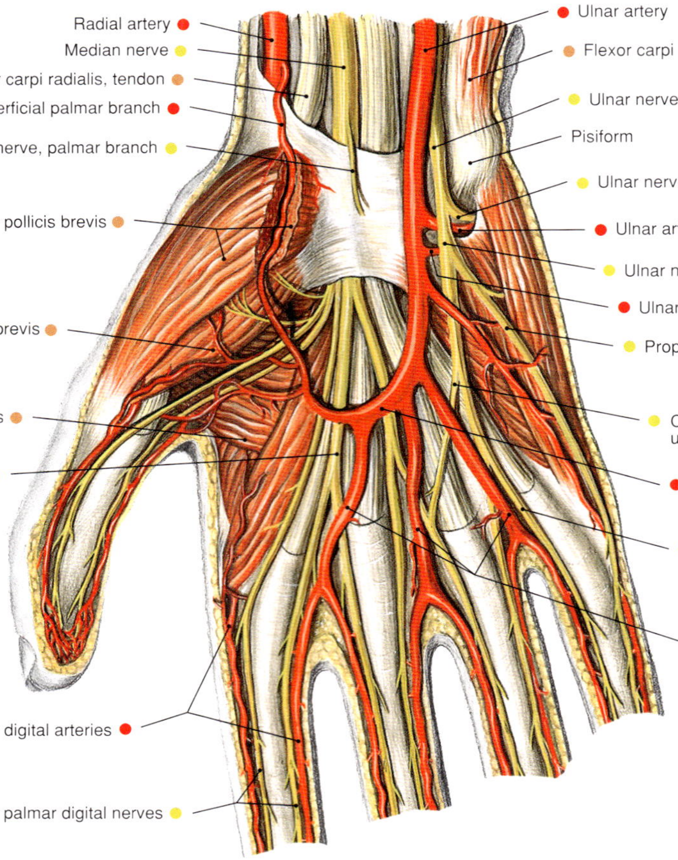

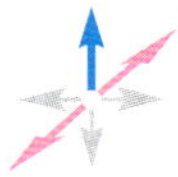

Fig. 435 Arteries and nerves of the palm; middle layer.

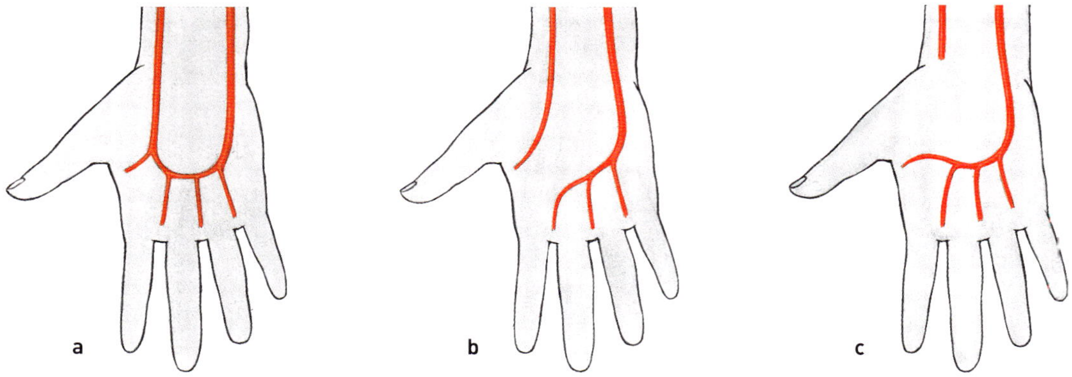

Fig. 436 a–c Variations of the superficial palmar arch.
a "Textbook case", closed arch
b The ulnar artery supplies the three ulnar fingers.
c All fingers are supplied by the ulnar artery.

Arteries and nerves of the hand

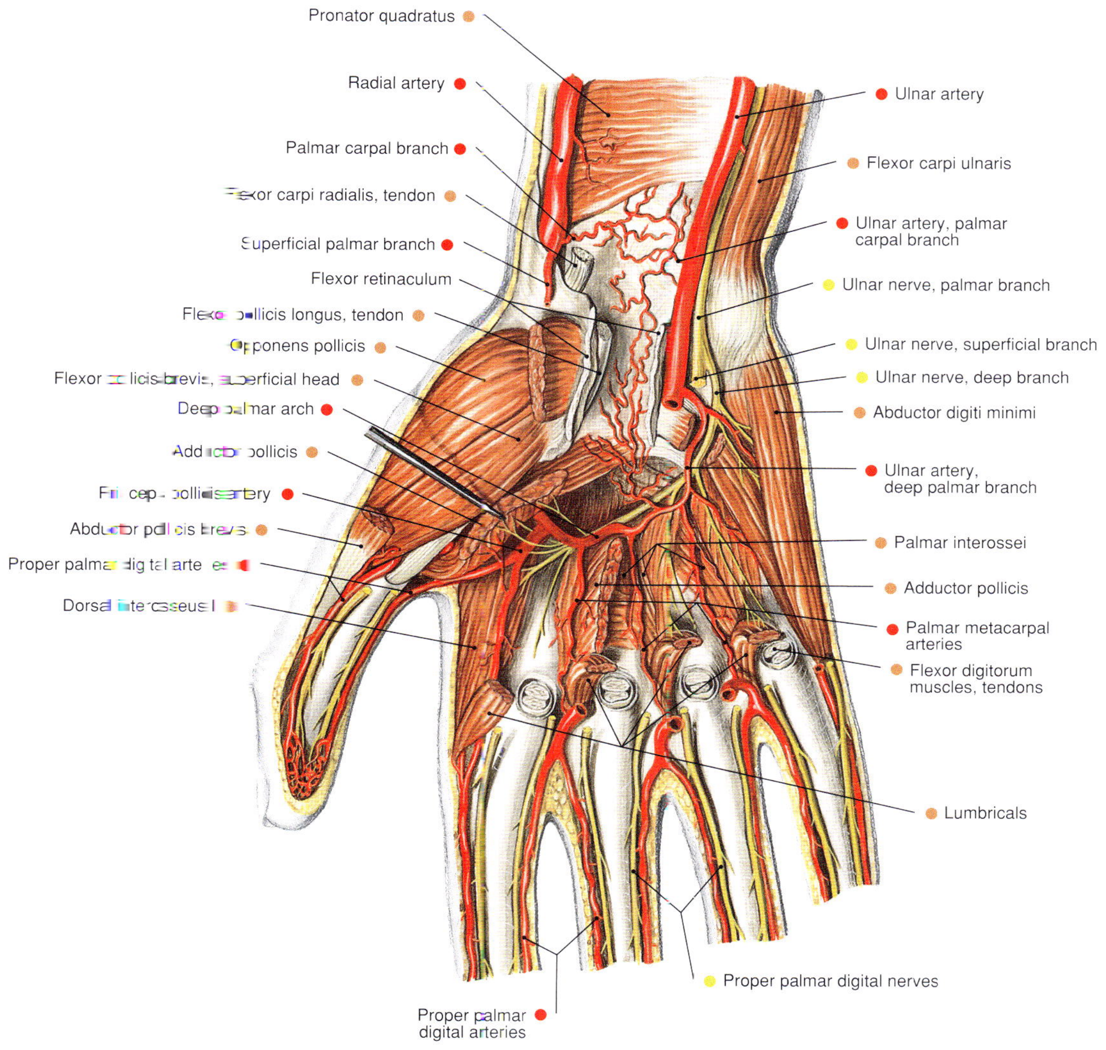

Fig. 437 Arteries and nerves of the palm; deep layer.

427
435

Arteries and nerves of the hand

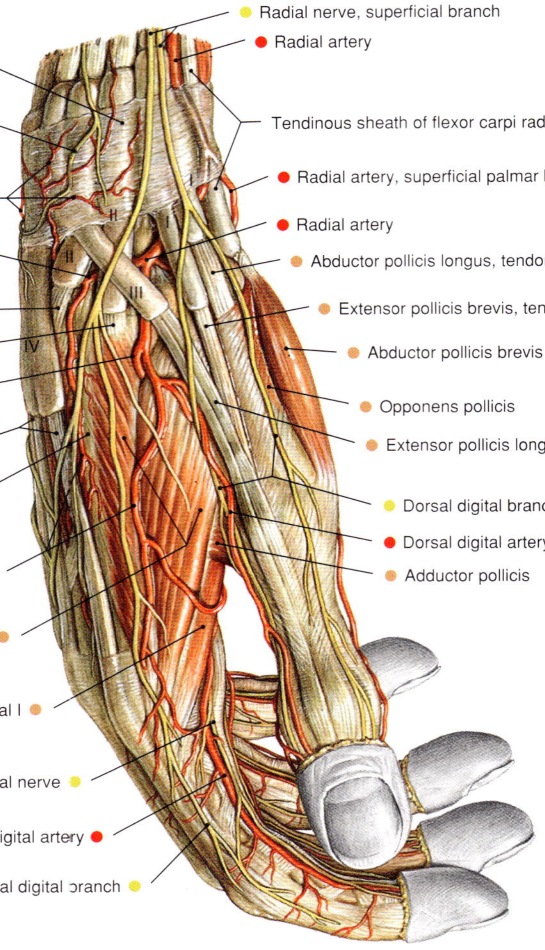

I–IV Tendinous sheath of extensores:
I Tendinous sheath of abductor longus and extensor pollicis brevis
II Tendinous sheath of extensores carpi radiales
III Tendinous sheath of extensor pollicis longus
IV Tendinous sheath of extensor digitorum and extensor indicis

430
440 434

Fig. 438 Arteries and nerves of the hand.

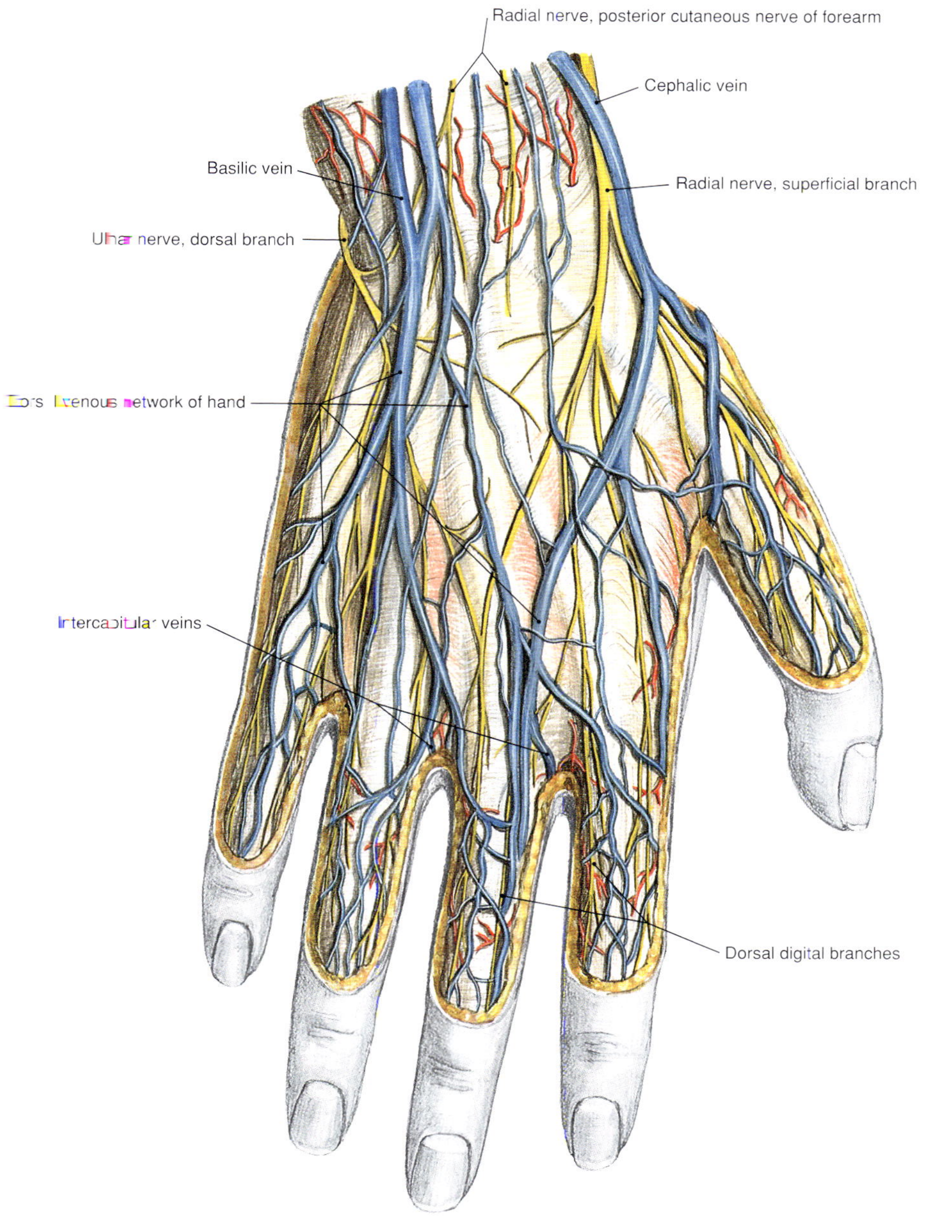

Fig. 439 Vessels and nerves of the dorsum of the hand; superficial layer.

422
440

Arteries and nerves of the hand

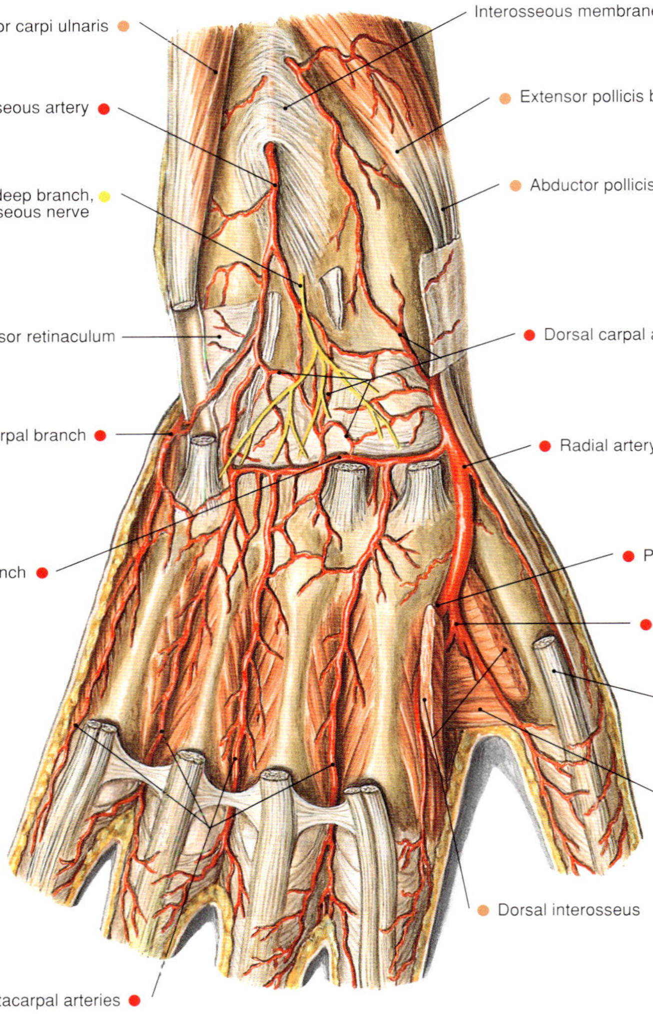

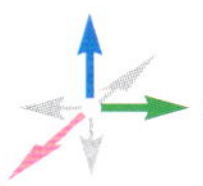

Fig. 440 Arteries and nerves of the dorsum of the hand; deep layer.

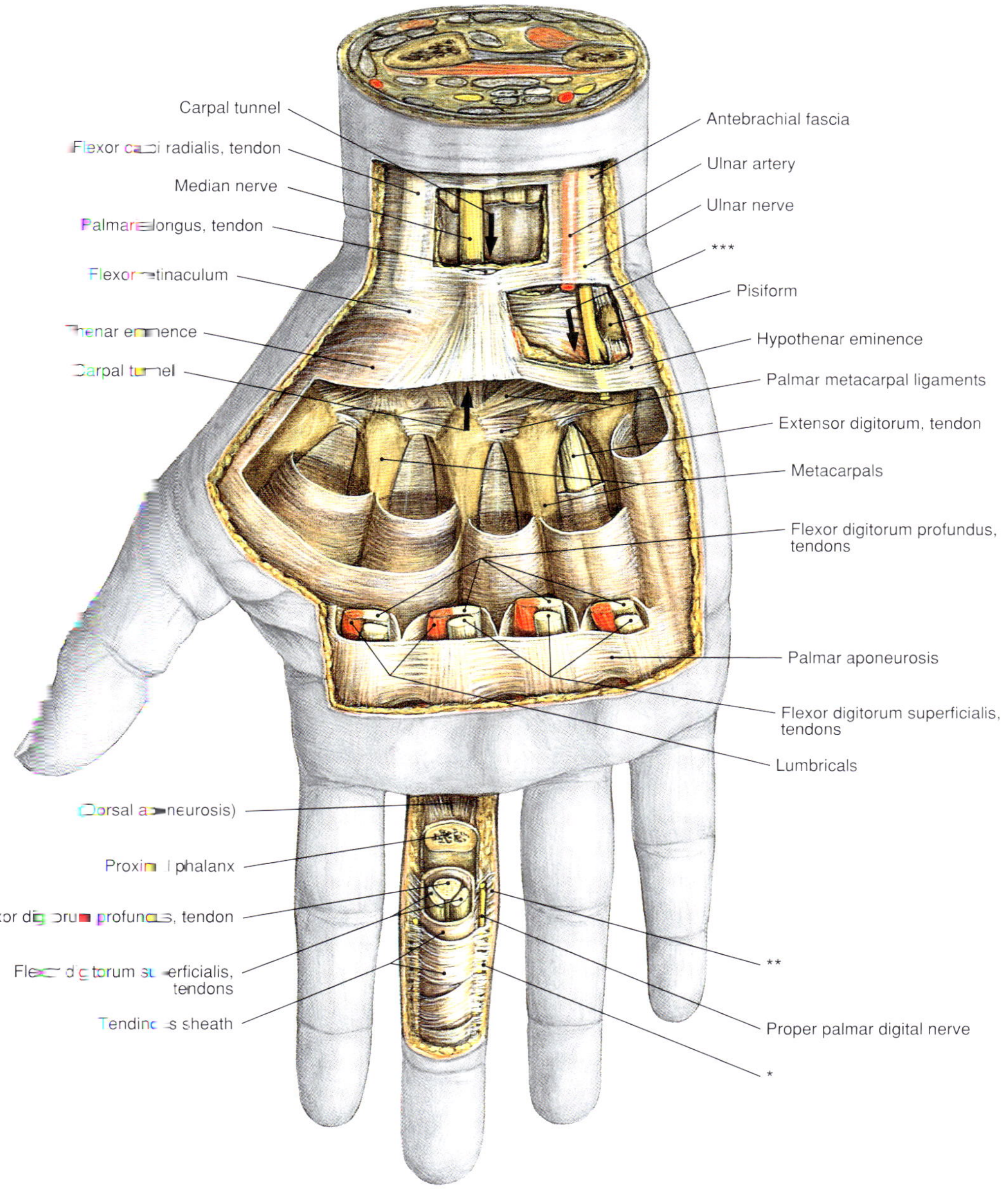

Fig. 441 Fascial compartments of the hand.

* Clinical term: ligament of GRAYSON
** Clinical term: ligament of CLELAND
*** Clinical term: ulnar canal (loge de GUYON)

Hand, sagittal section

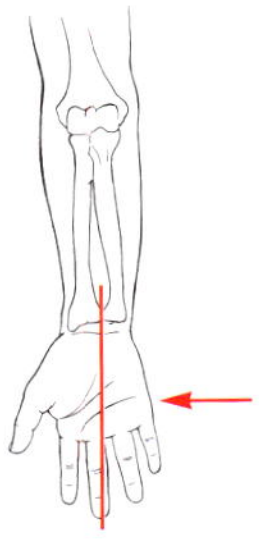

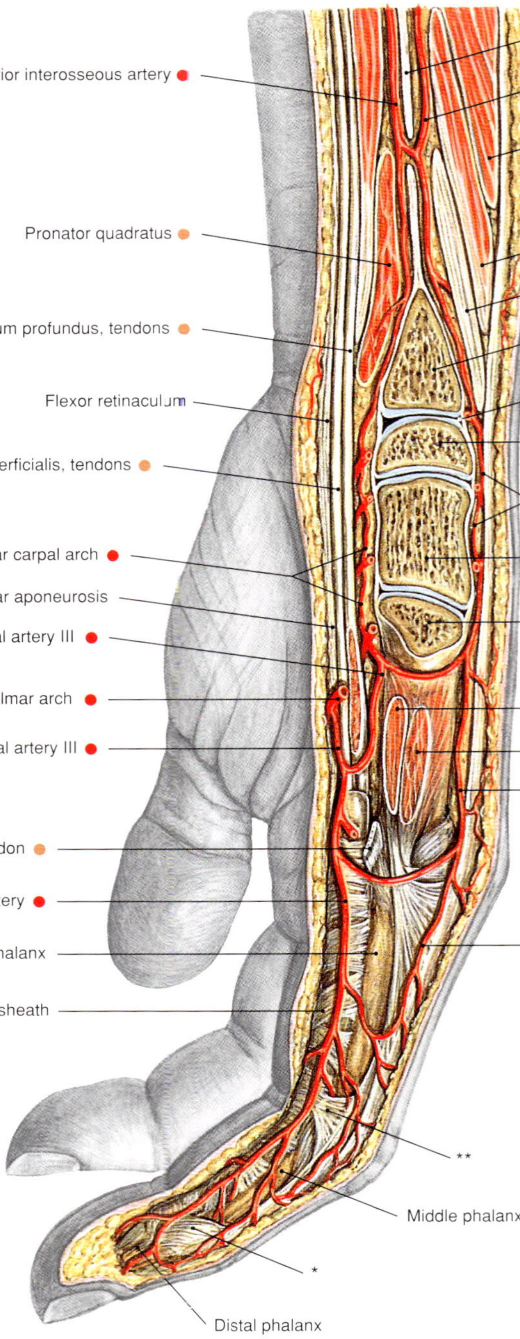

Fig. 442 Hand;
sagittal section at the level of the ulnar plane of the middle finger.

* Clinical term: ligament of CLELAND
** Clinical term: ligament of GRAYSON

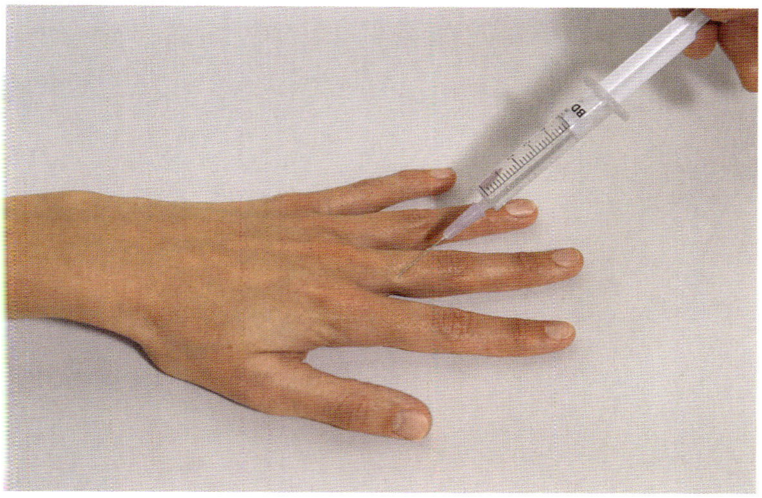

Fig. 443 Points of injection for regional conduction anaesthesia at the middle finger.

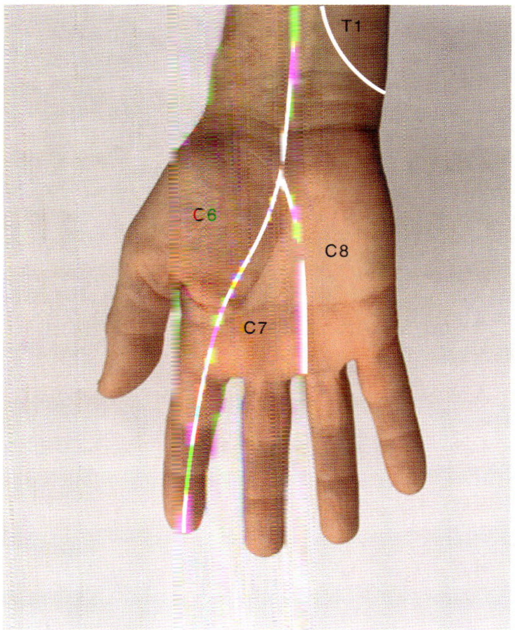

Fig. 444 Palm; segmental cutaneous innervation.

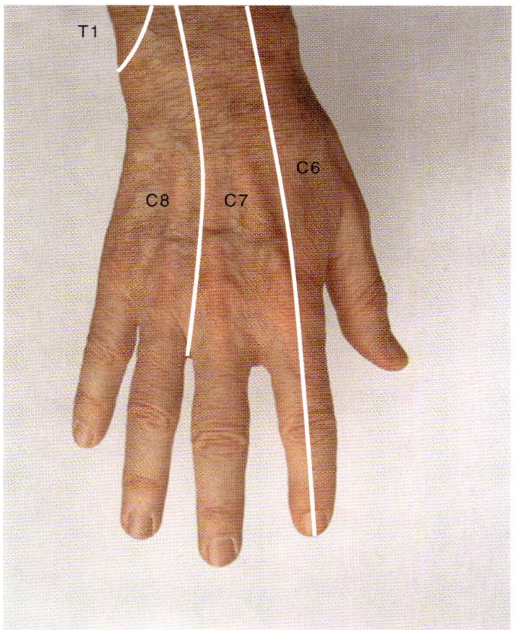

Fig. 445 Dorsum of the hand; segmental cutaneous innervation.

Arm, transverse sections

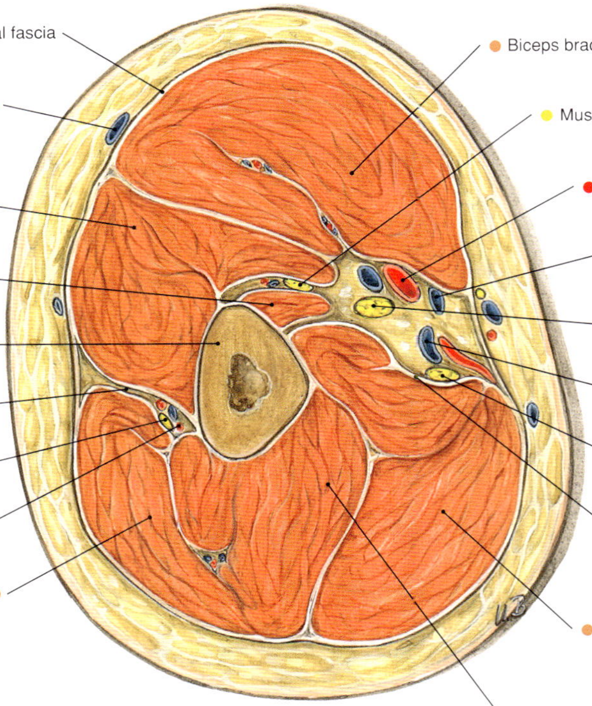

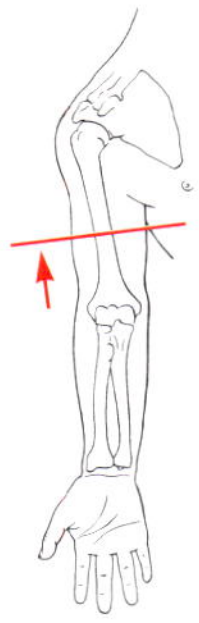

Fig. 446 Arm;
transverse section.

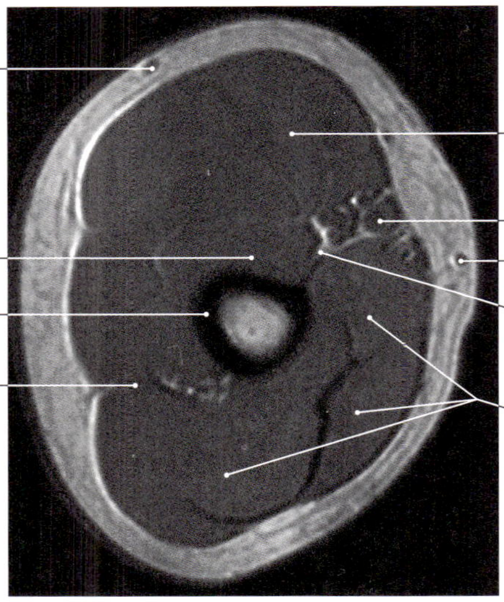

Fig. 447 Arm;
magnetic resonance tomographic image (MRI);
cross-section at the level of the middle of the arm;
distal view.

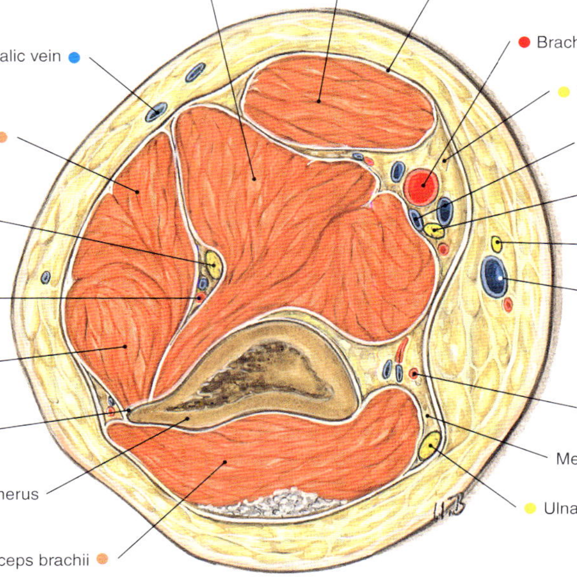

Fig. 448 Arm;
transverse section through the lower third of the arm.

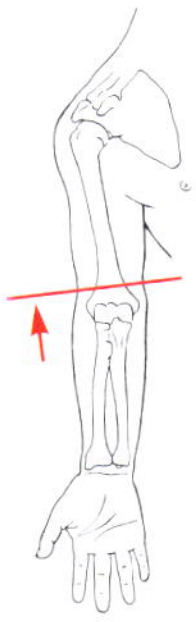

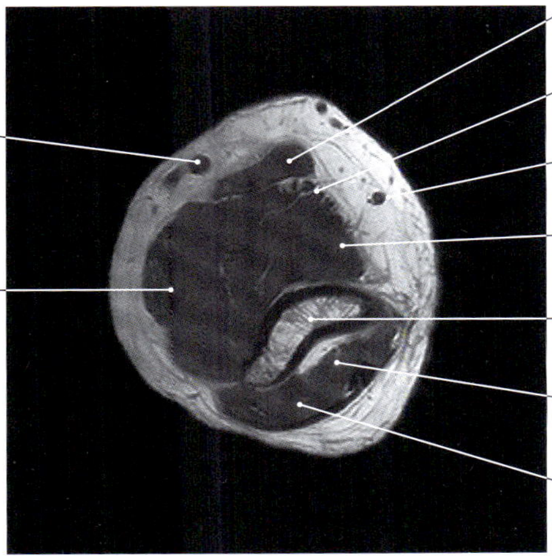

Fig. 449 Arm;
magnetic resonance tomographic image (MRI);
cross-section at the level of the lower third of the arm;
distal view.

Forearm, transverse sections

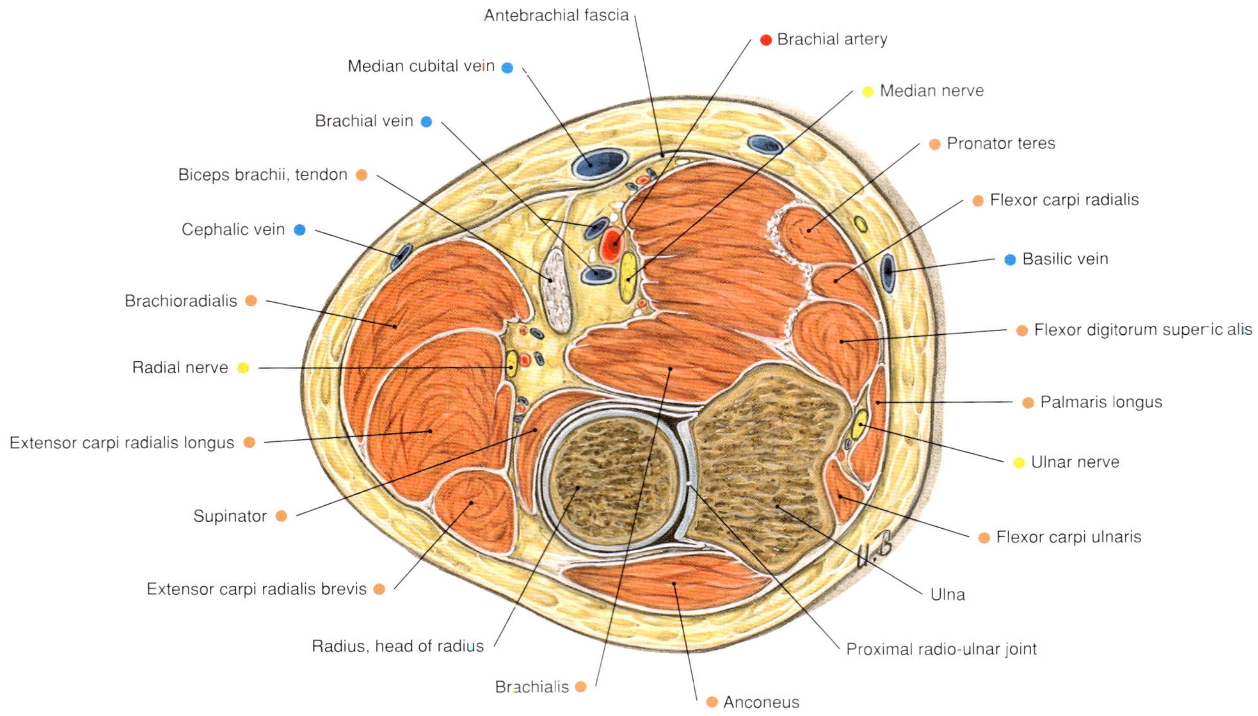

Fig. 450 Forearm;
transverse section at the level of the proximal radio-ulnar joint.

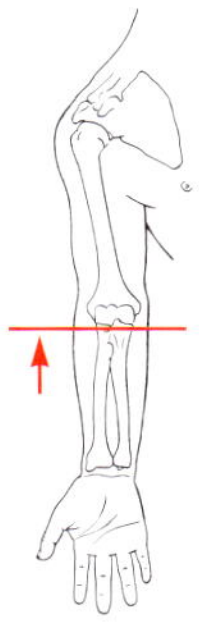

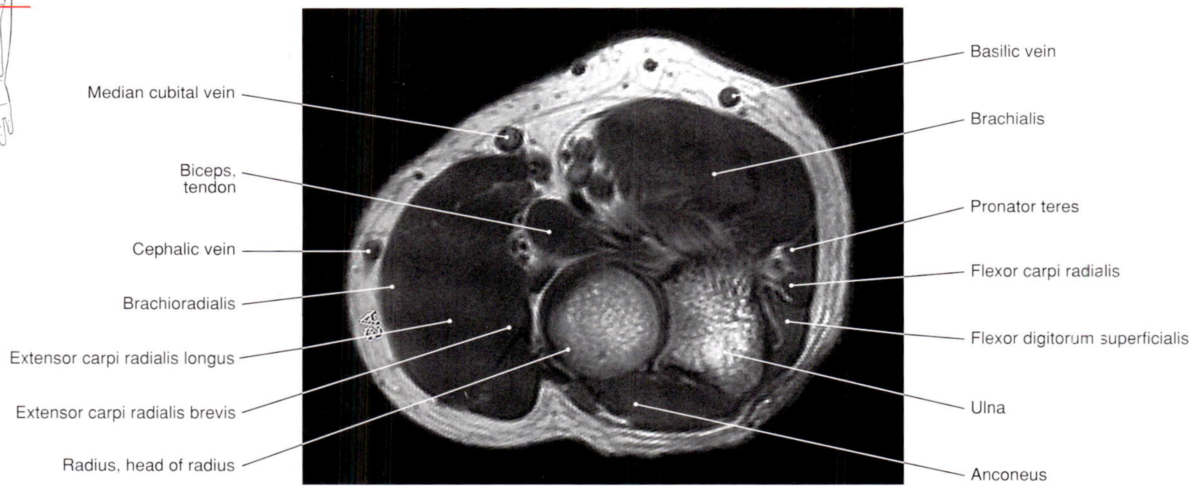

Fig. 451 Forearm;
magnetic resonance tomographic image (MRI);
cross-section at the level of the elbow joint;
distal view.

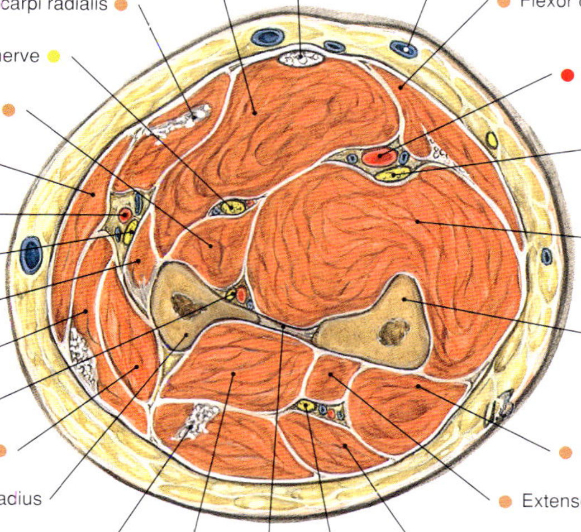

Fig. 452 Forearm;
transverse section through the lower third of the forearm.

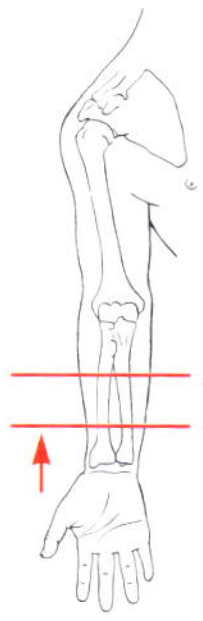

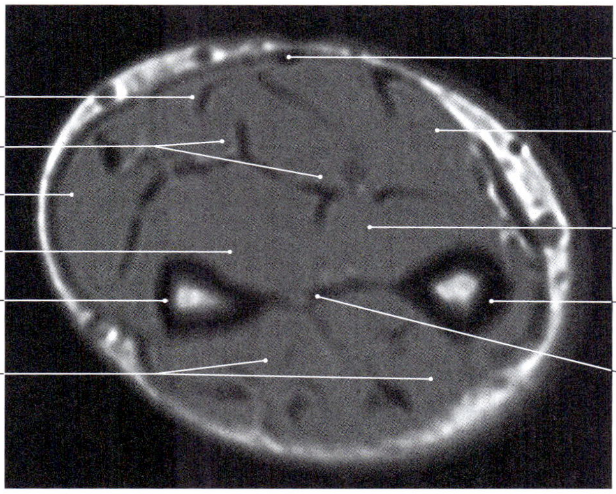

Fig. 453 Forearm;
magnetic resonance tomographic image (MRI);
cross-section at the level of the middle of the forearm;
distal view.

Forearm, transverse sections

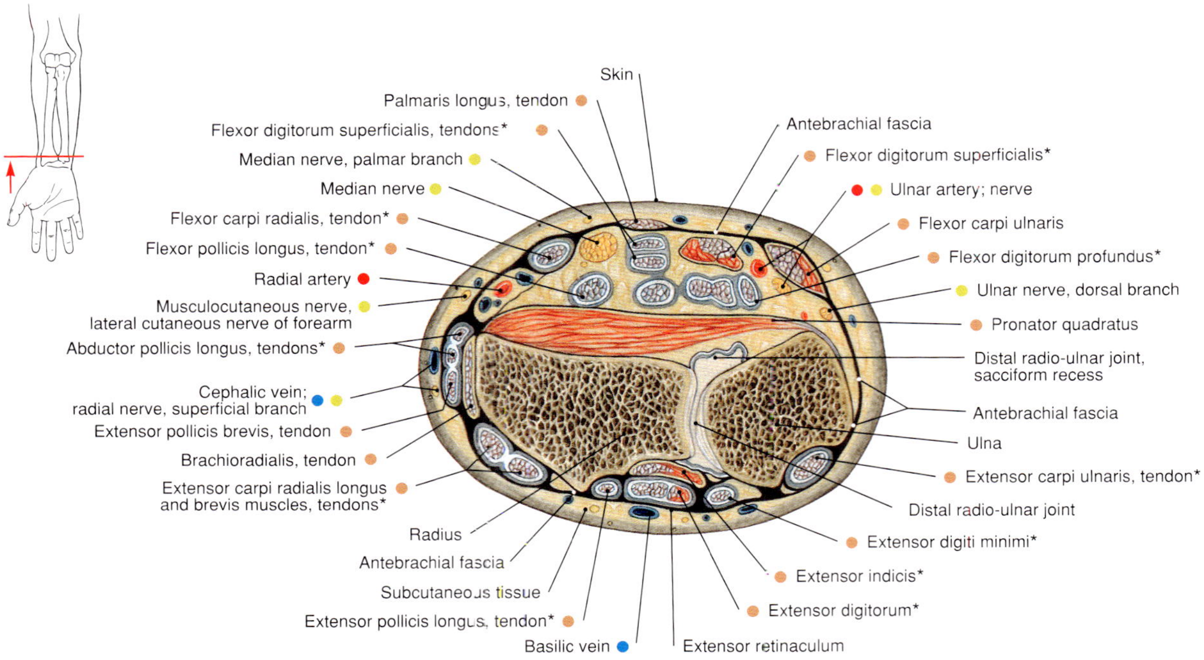

Fig. 454 Forearm;
transverse section at the level of the distal radio-ulnar joint.
At this level the muscle tendons marked with * run within tendon sheaths.

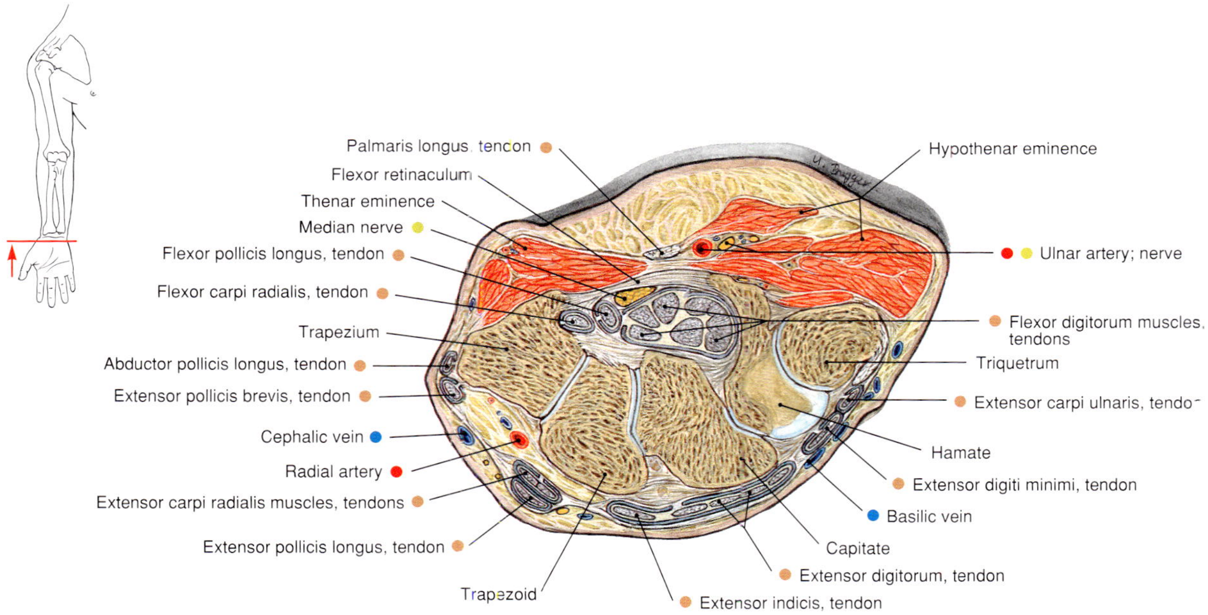

Fig. 455 Wrist;
transverse section at the level of the hook of the hamate bone.

* Carpal tunnel
** ulnar canal (loge de GUYON)

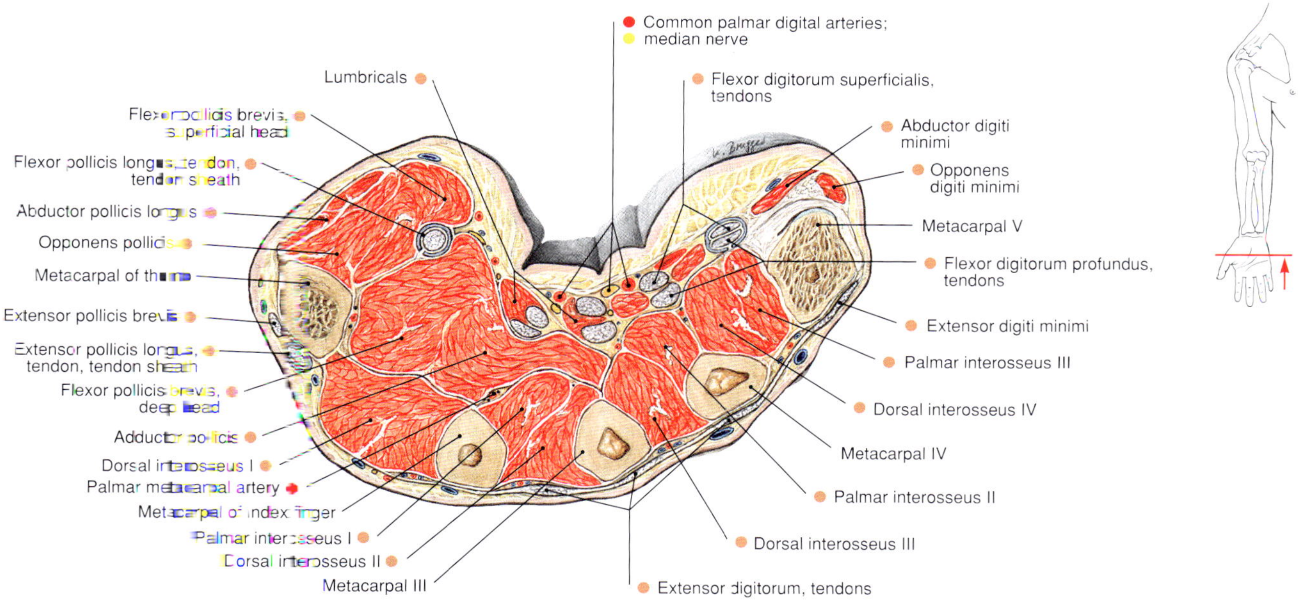

Fig. 456 Metacarpus; transverse section at the level of the third metacarpal bone.

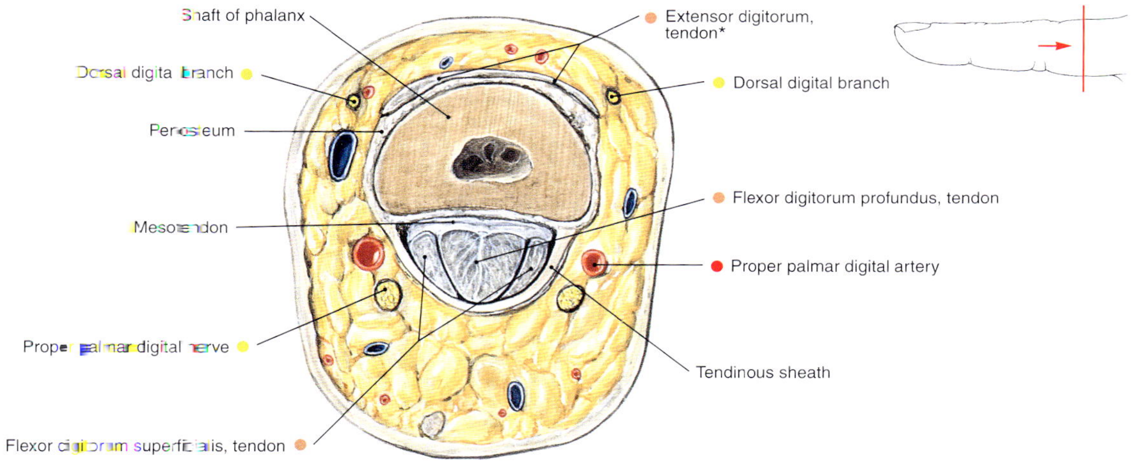

Fig. 457 Middle finger; transverse section through the shaft of the proximal phalanx.

* So-called dorsal aponeurosis into which the branching tendon of the extensor digitorum muscle, as well as the tendons of the interosseous and lumbrical muscles radiate

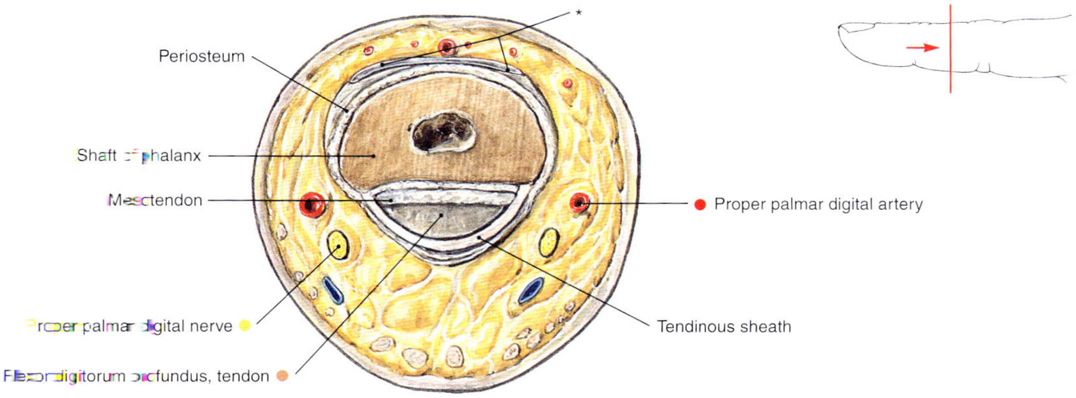

Fig. 458 Middle finger; transverse section through the shaft of the middle phalanx.

* So-called dorsal aponeurosis

Regions

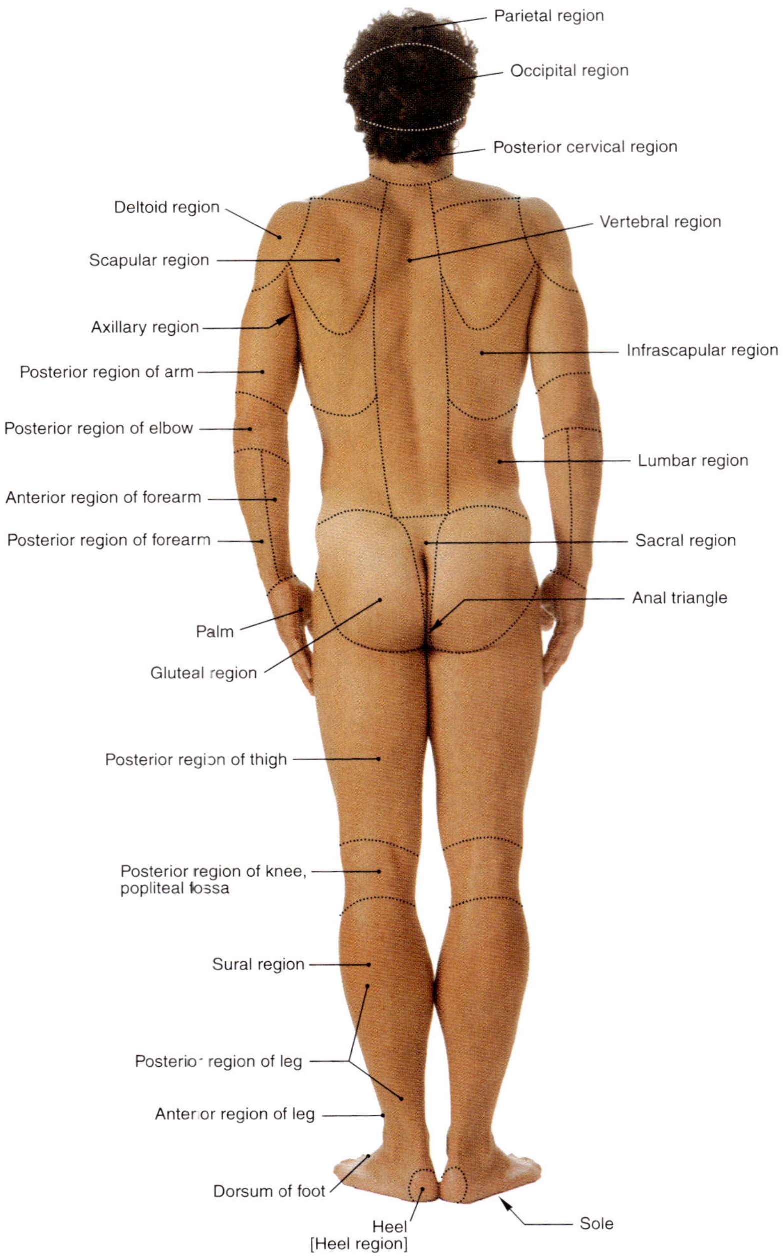

Fig. 459 Regions of the human body.

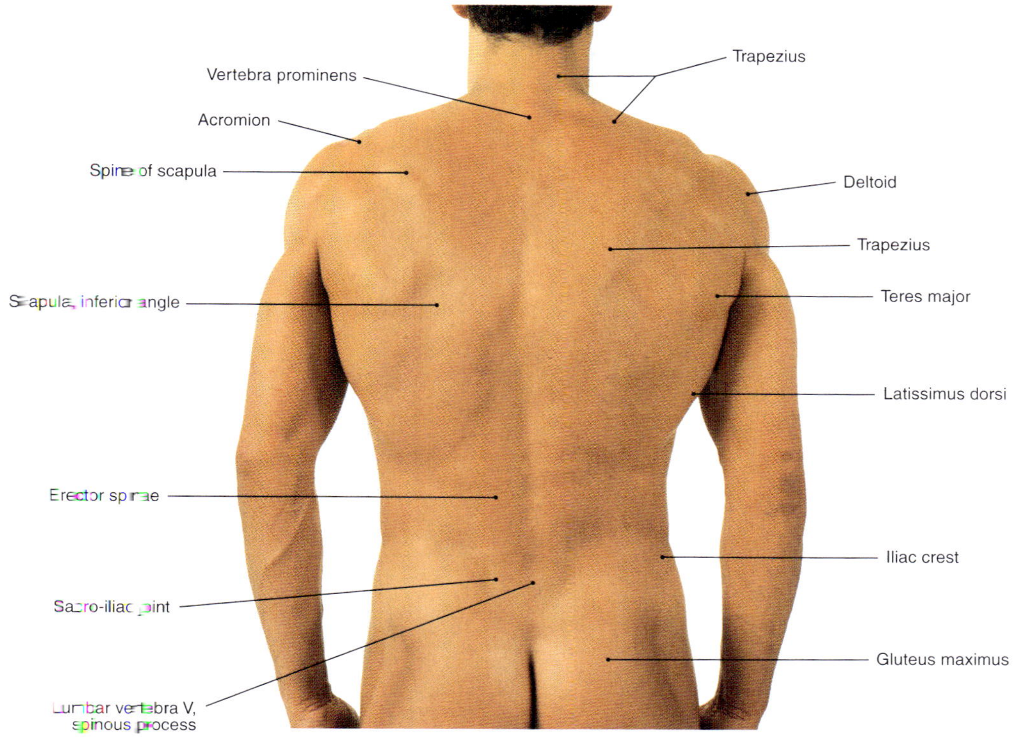

Fig. 460 Back; surface anatomy.

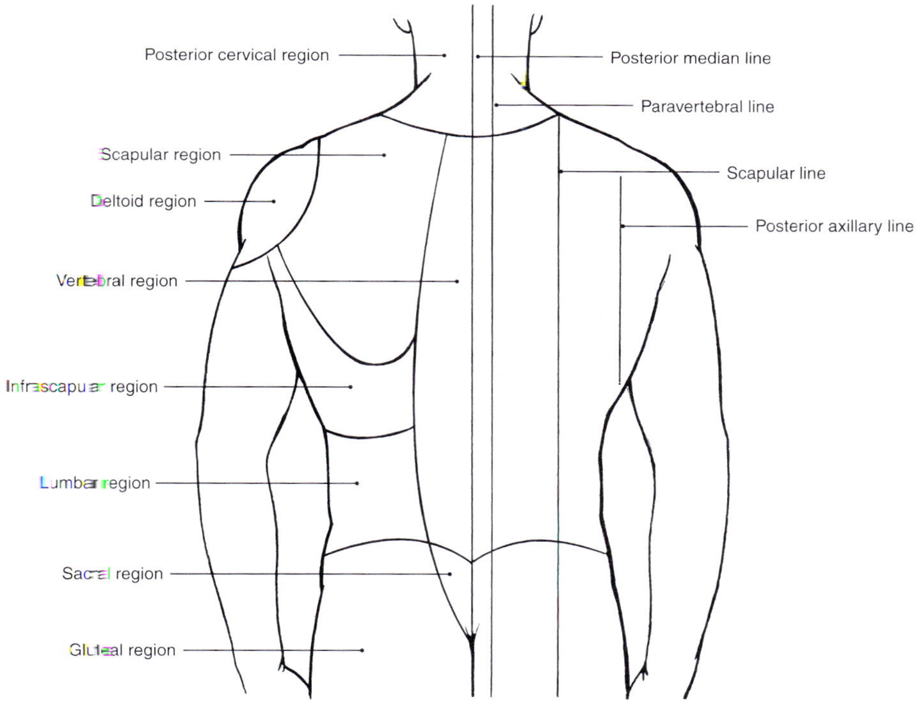

Fig. 461 Regions and orientation lines of the back.

Skeleton of the trunk

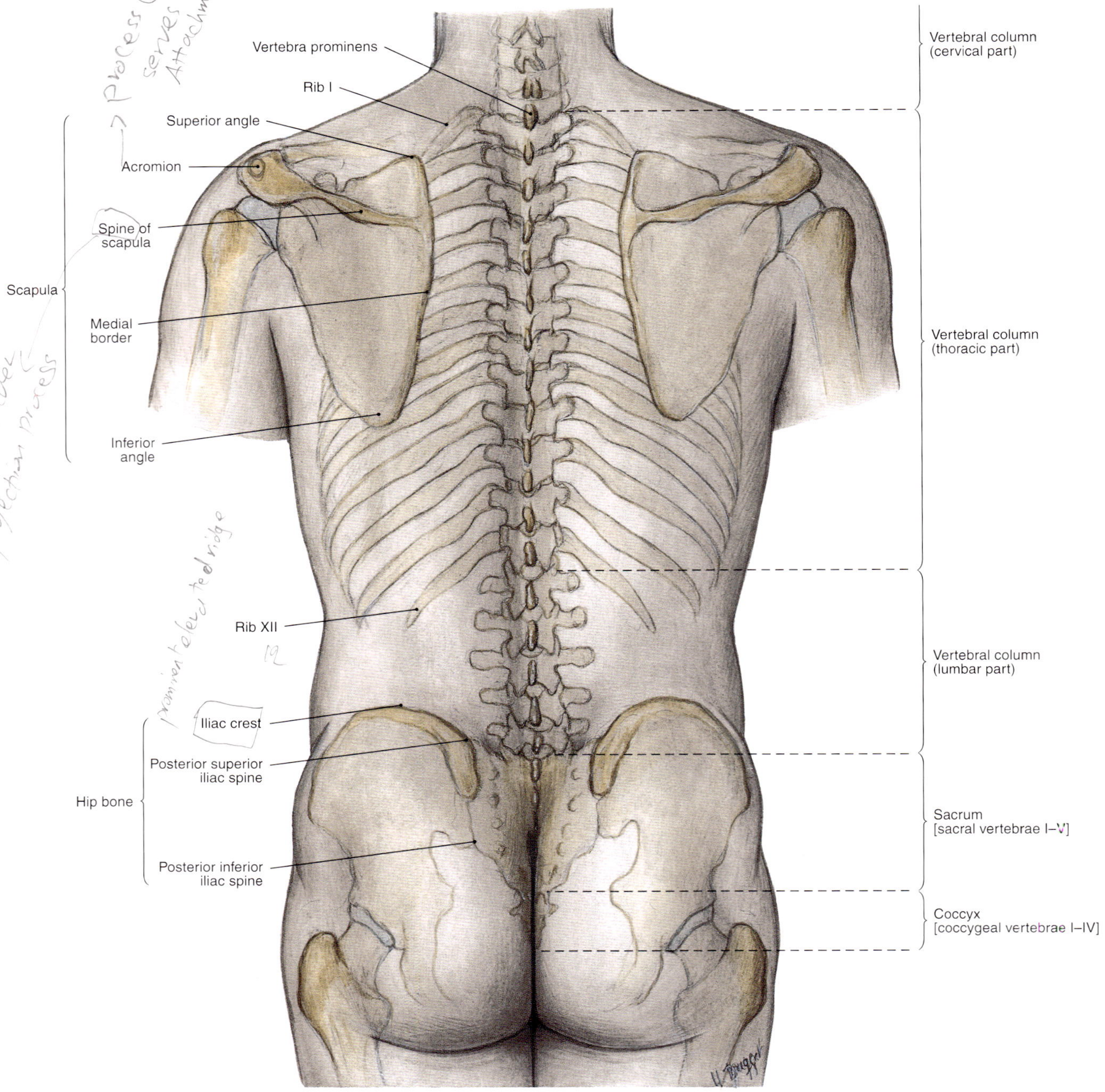

Fig. 462 Skeletal system of the trunk.

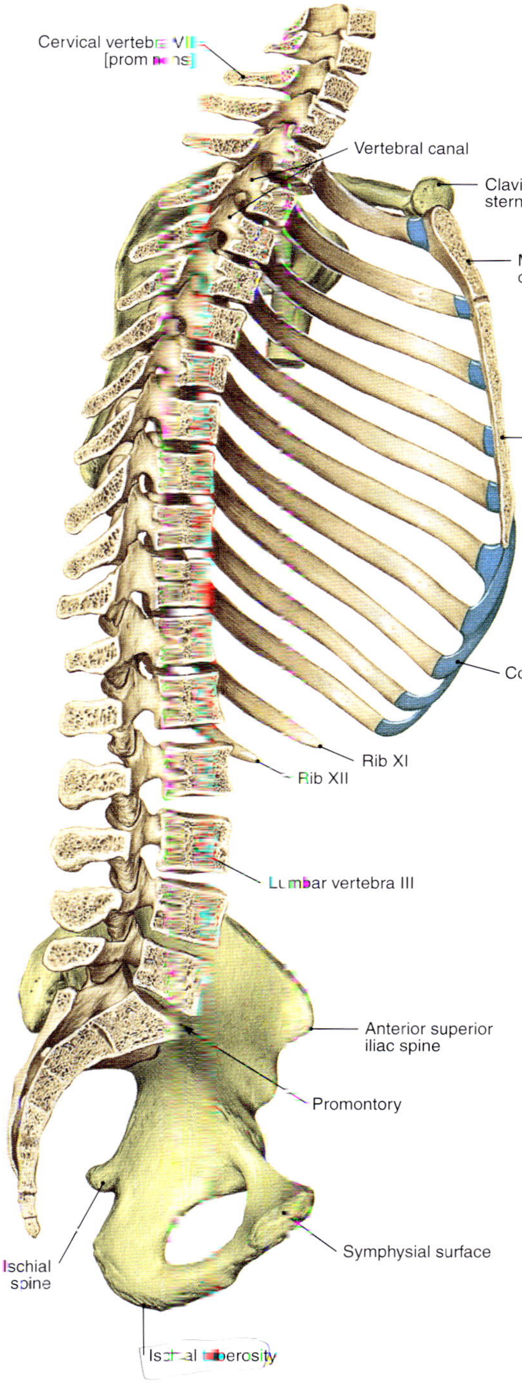

Fig. 463 Vertebral column; pectoral girdle and pelvic girdle; median section through the vertebral column; medial view.

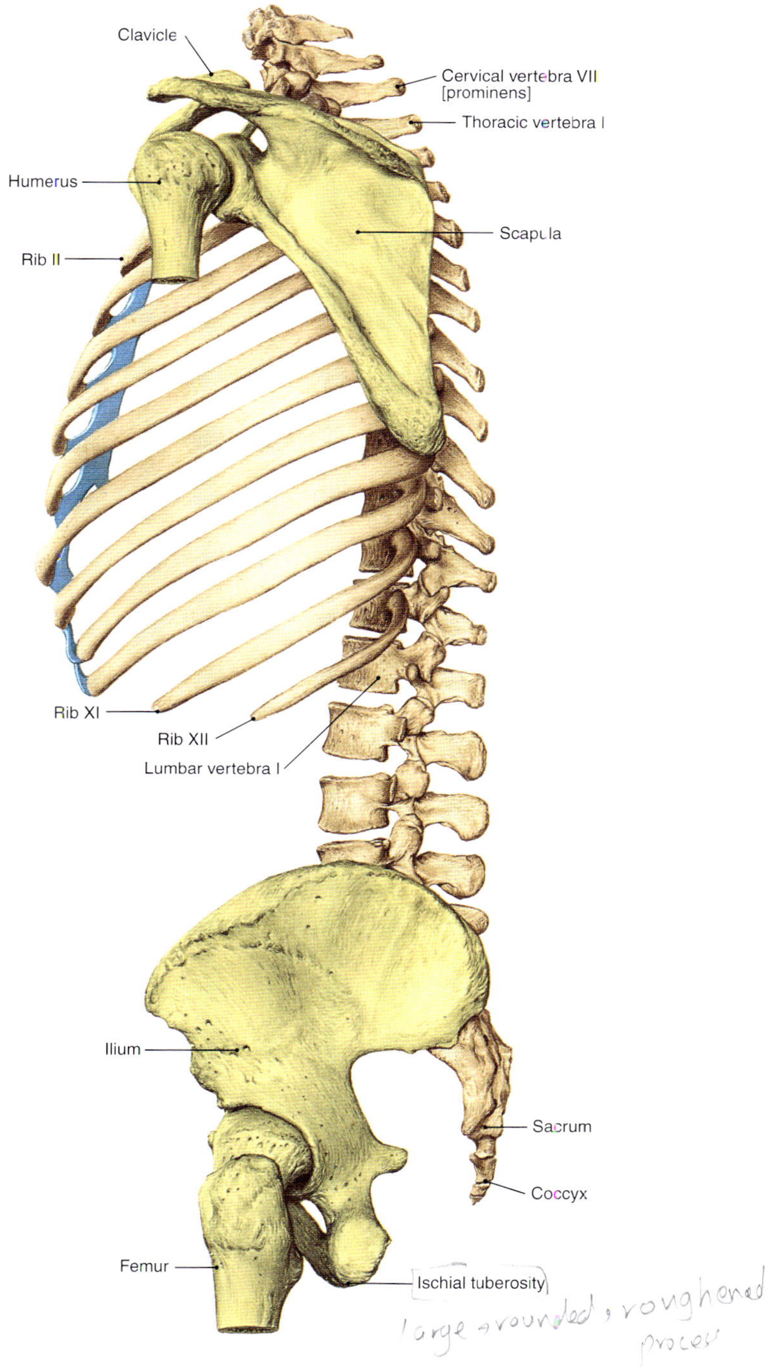

Fig. 464 Vertebral column; pectoral girdle and pelvic girdle; median section through the vertebral column; viewed from the left.

Vertebral column

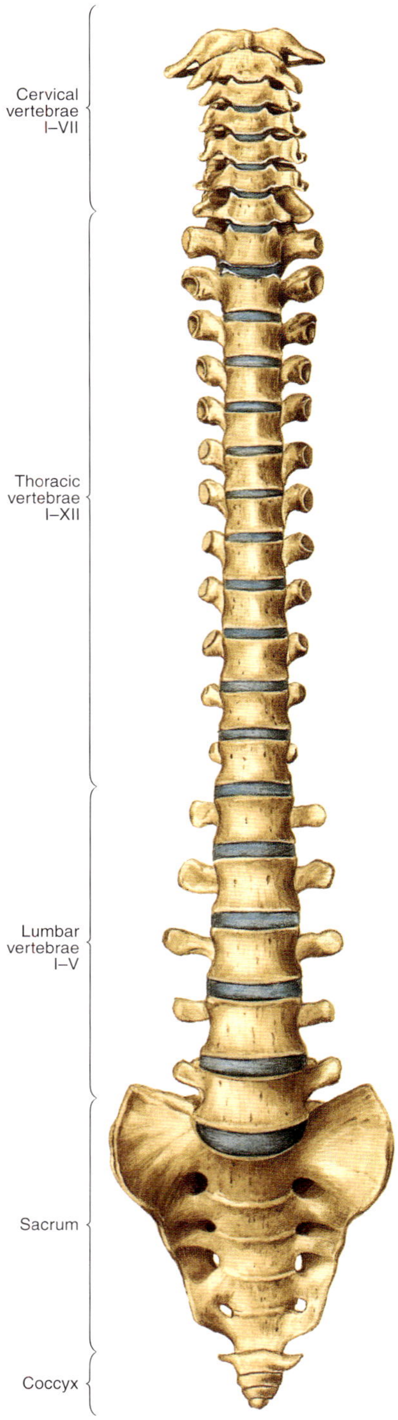

Fig. 465 Vertebral column; ventral view.

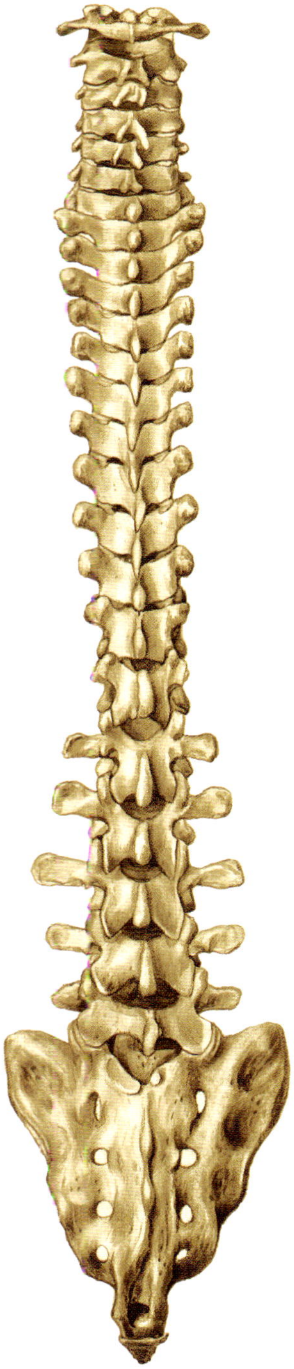

Fig. 466 Vertebral column; dorsal view.

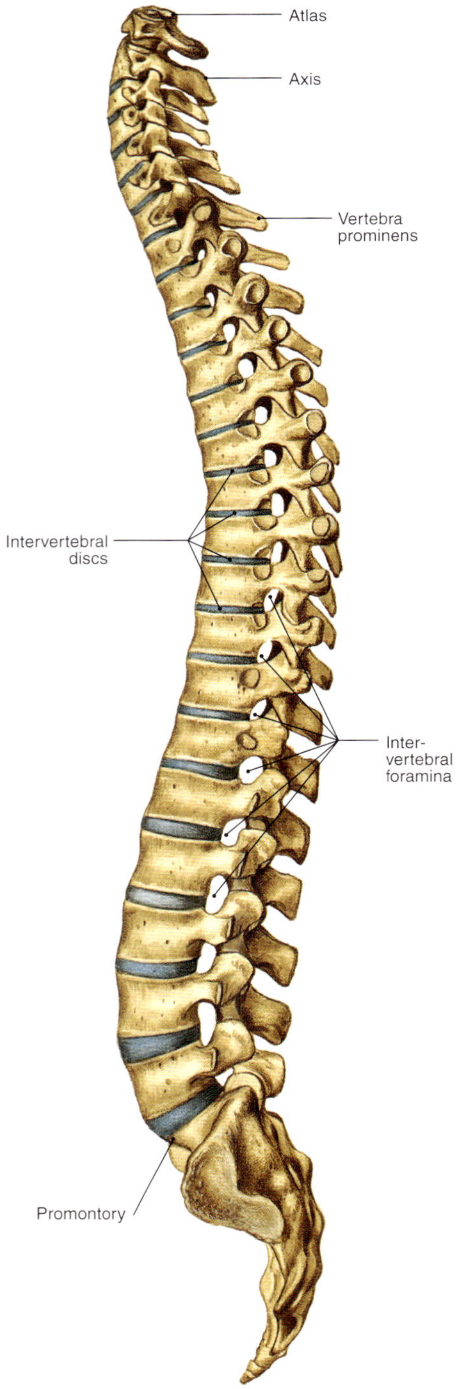

Fig. 467 Vertebral column; viewed from the left.

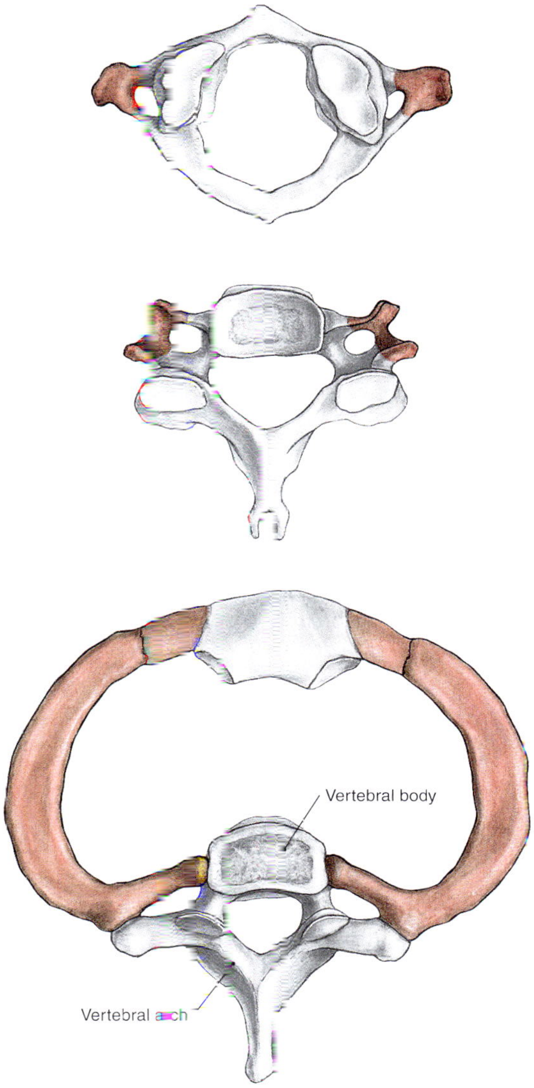

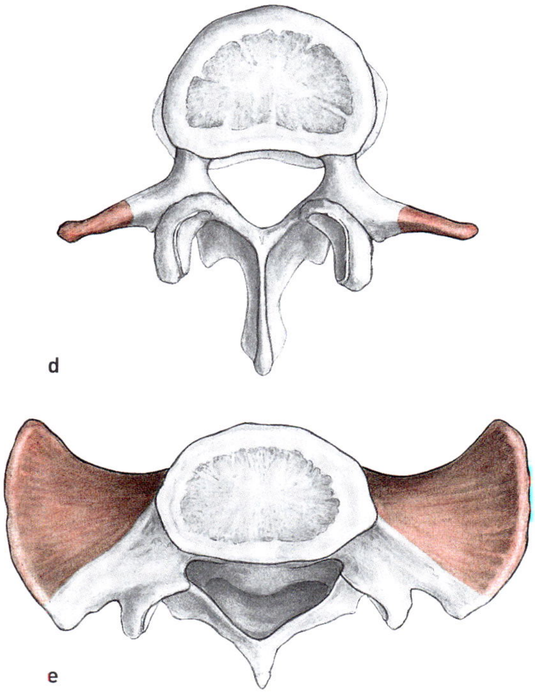

Fig. 468 a–e Regional characteristics of the vertebrae.
Only in the thoracic region of the vertebral column do the lateral parts (labelled in red) remain separated and form ribs.

a First cervical vertebra, atlas
b Fourth cervical vertebra
c First thoracic vertebra with corresponding ribs and sternum
d Third lumbar vertebra
e Sacrum

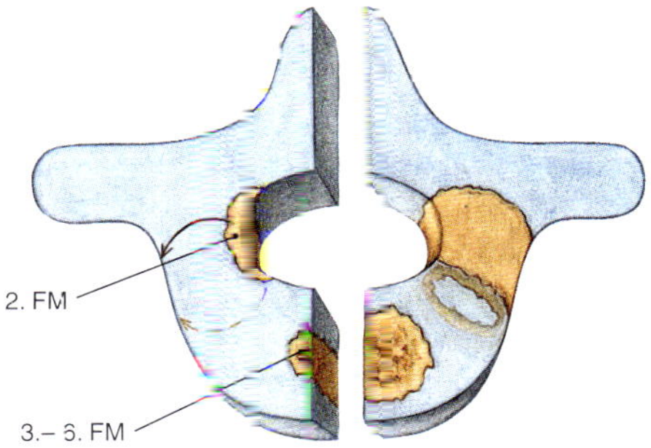

Fig. 469 Vertebral development.
Demonstration of the appearance of primary ossification centres in a lumbar vertebra (pedicle: second foetal month; corpus: third to sixth foetal month).
Synostosis of the ossification centres of the vertebral arch with those of the corpus occurs between the third and the sixth year of life.

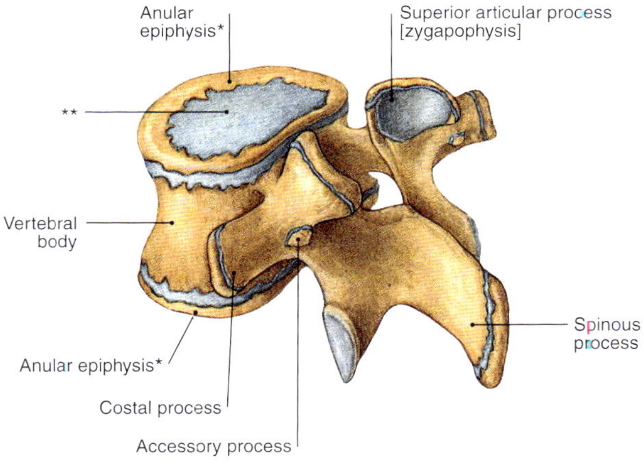

Fig. 470 Vertebral development.
Circular ossification centres (= rims*) appear in the epiphyses of the vertebrae during the eighth year of life and fuse with the vertebral bodies until the eighteenth year of life.
The central portions of the epiphyses remain as hyaline cartilaginous laminae ** throughout life.
Secondary ossification centres (apophyses) develop at the processes.

Atlas and axis

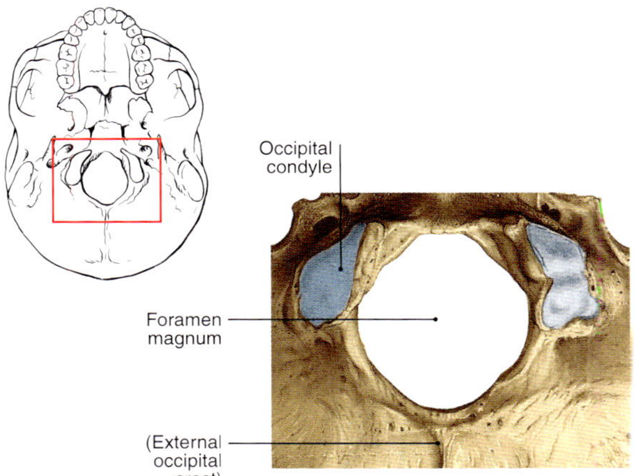

Fig. 471 Occipital bone;
section illustrating the foramen magnum and the articular surfaces of the atlanto-occipital joint;
inferior view.

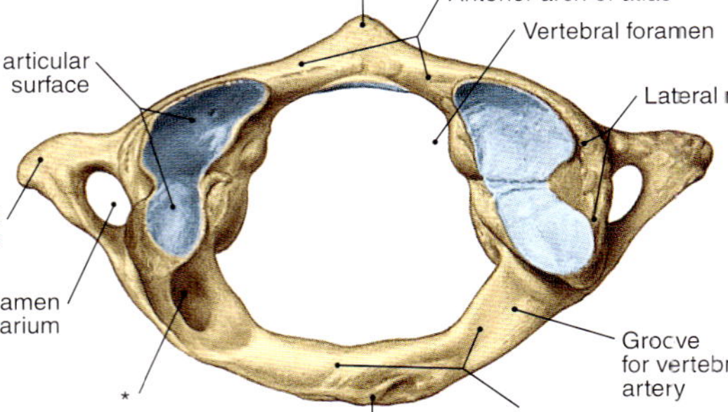

Fig. 472 First cervical vertebra, atlas;
superior view.
The superior articular surfaces of the atlas are frequently divided.

* Canal for vertebral artery as a variation

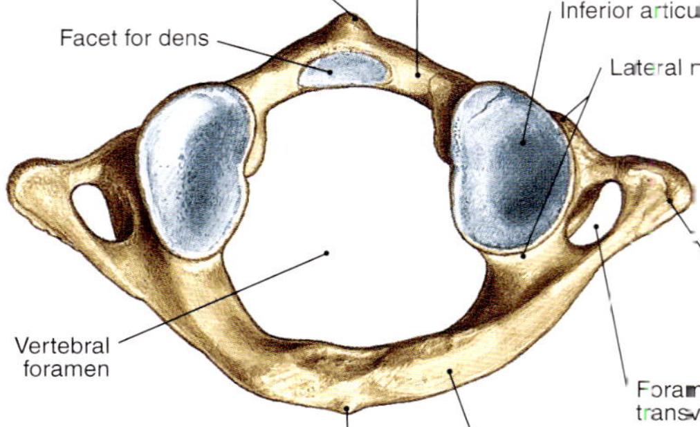

Fig. 473 First cervical vertebra, atlas;
inferior view.

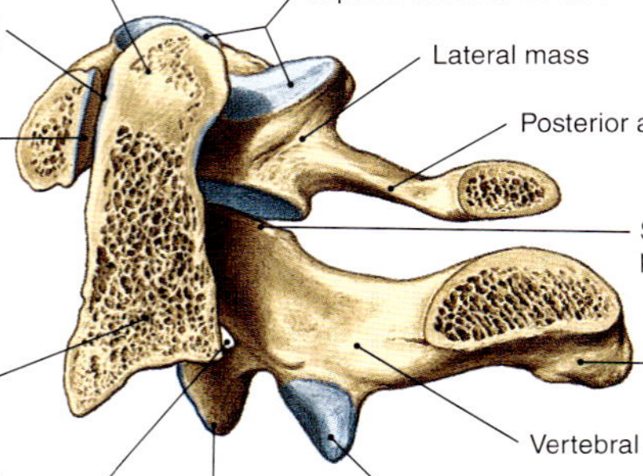

Fig. 474 First and second cervical vertebrae, atlas and axis;
median section.

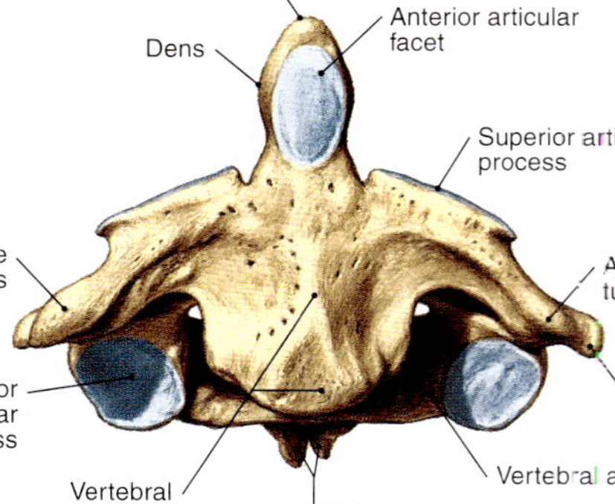

Fig. 475 Second cervical vertebra, axis;
ventral view.

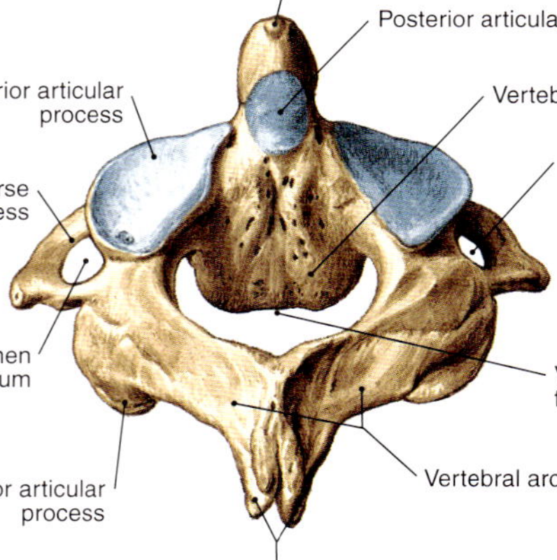

Fig. 476 Second cervical vertebra, axis;
dorsosuperior view.

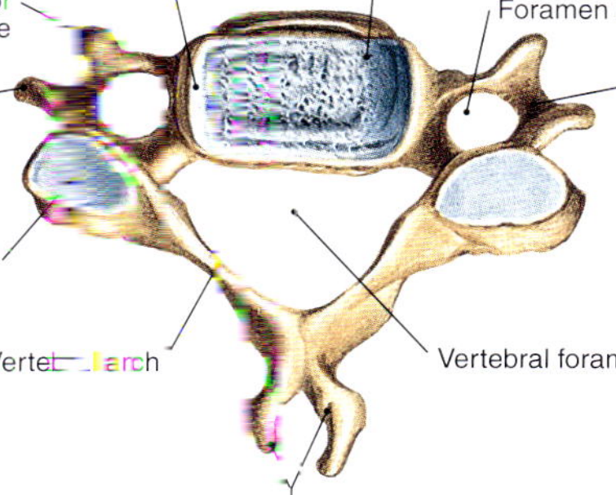

Fig. 477 Fifth cervical vertebra; superior view.
The tips of the spinous processes of the cervical vertebrae II–VI are frequently divided.

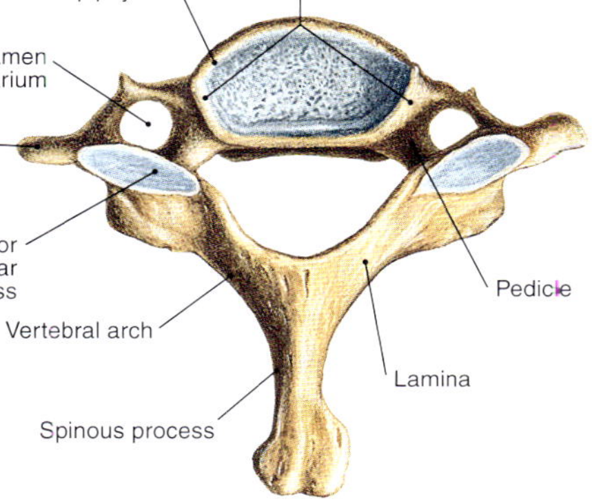

Fig. 478 Seventh cervical vertebra; superior view.
In general the seventh cervical vertebra can be easily identified by its protruding spinous process and is referred to as vertebra prominens. In fact, the spinous process of the first thoracic vertebra often protrudes even further.

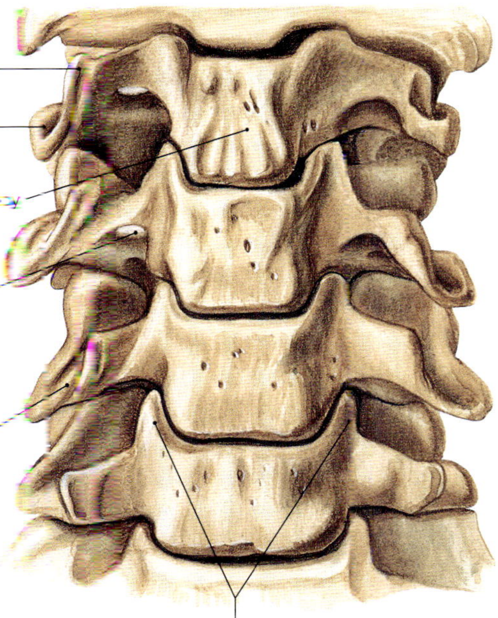

Fig. 479 Second to seventh cervical vertebrae; ventral view.

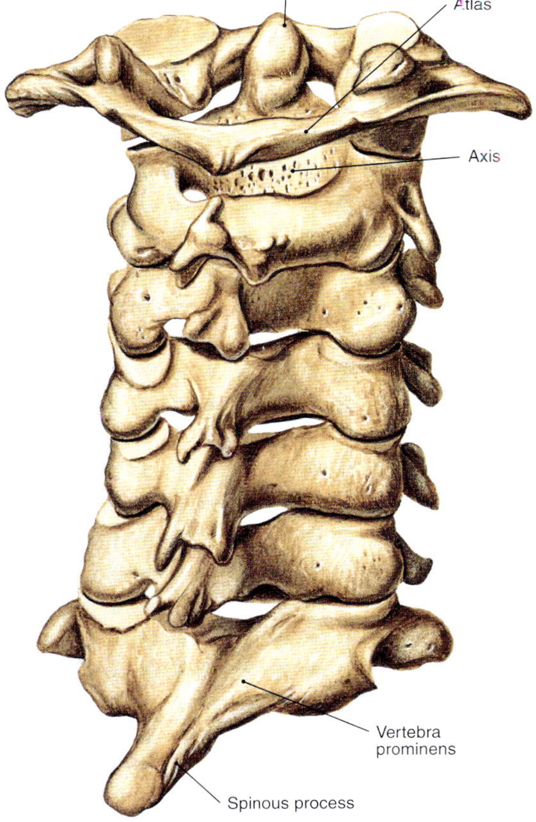

Fig. 480 First to seventh cervical vertebrae; dorsolateral view.

Thoracic and lumbar vertebrae

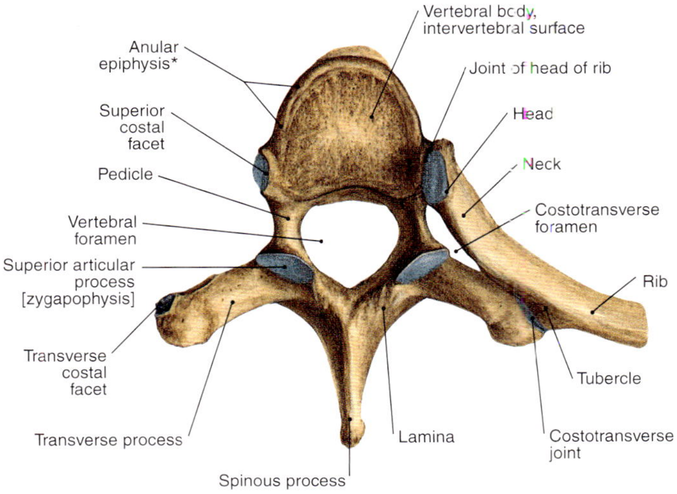

Fig. 481 Vertebra; typical structural features exemplified by the fifth thoracic vertebra; superior view.

* Also: rim of vertebral body

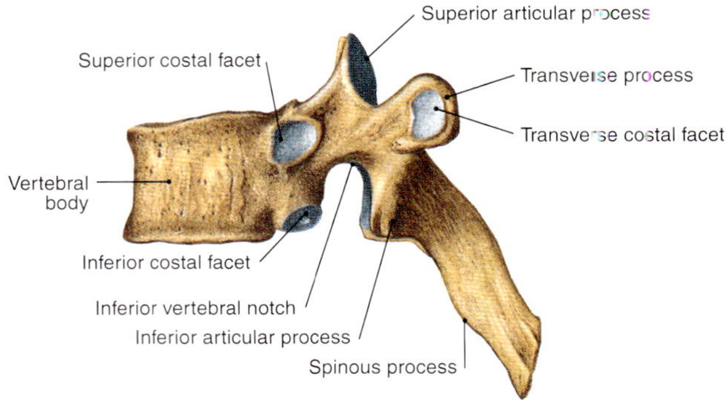

Fig. 482 Sixth thoracic vertebra; viewed from the left.

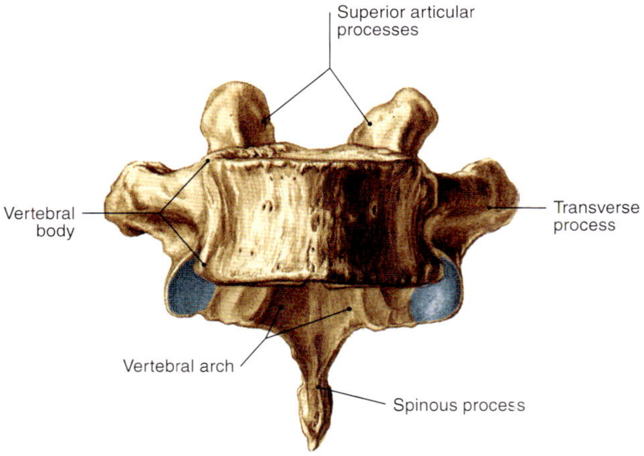

Fig. 483 Tenth thoracic vertebra; ventral view.

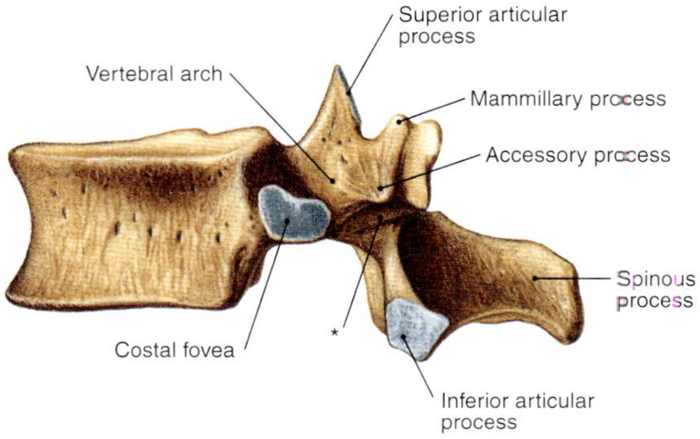

Fig. 484 Twelfth thoracic vertebra; viewed from the left.

* Region of the vertebral arch between the superior and inferior articular processes („isthmus" = interarticular portion)

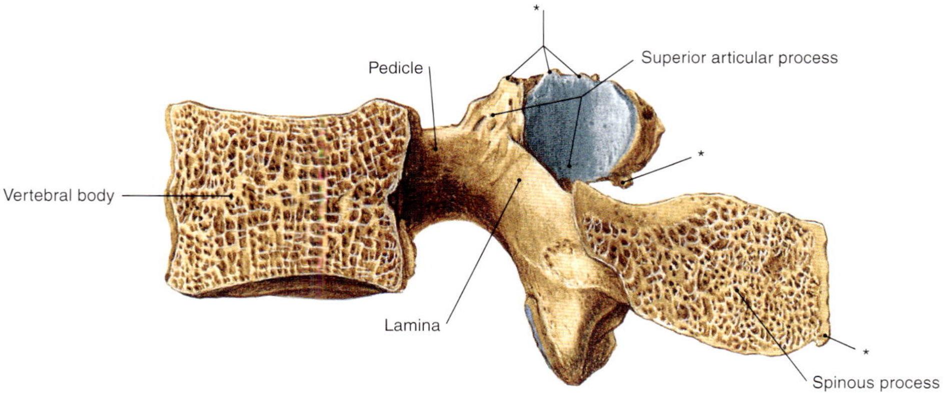

Fig. 485 Third lumbar vertebra; median section; specimen of an older individual.

* Ossification of the ligamentous insertions

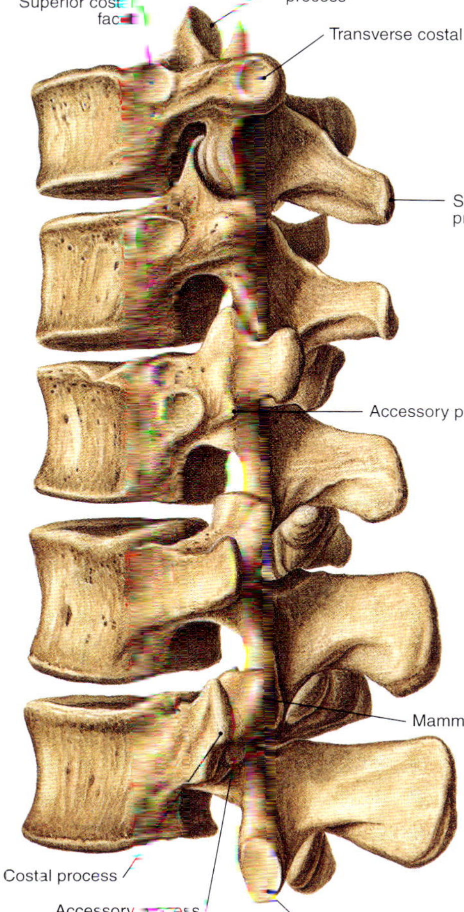

Fig. 486 Tenth to twelfth thoracic vertebrae and first to second lumbar vertebrae; dorsal view from the left.

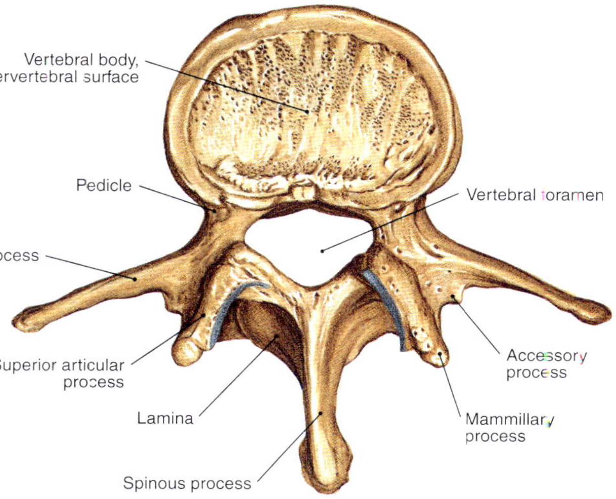

Fig. 487 Fourth lumbar vertebra; superior view.

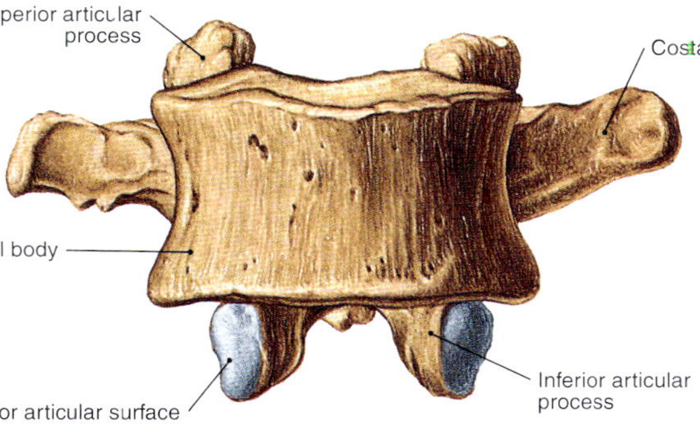

Fig. 488 Fourth lumbar vertebra; ventral view.

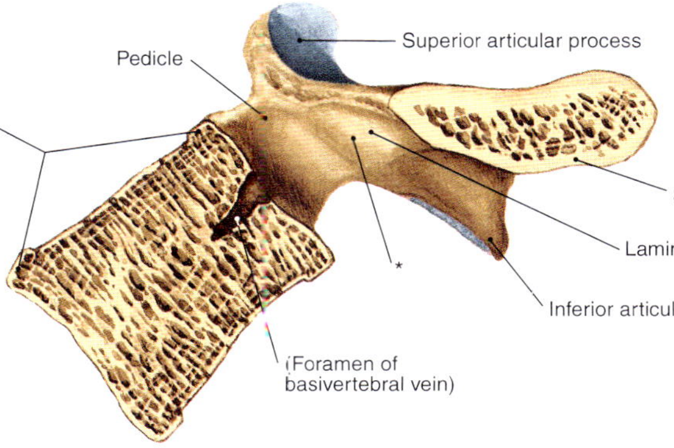

Fig. 489 Fifth lumbar vertebra; median section.
Note the characteristic wedge-shape of the body of the fifth lumbar vertebra.

* Region of the vertebral arch between the superior and inferior articular process. Here in the fifth and less frequently in the fourth lumbar vertebra a cleft, bridged by connective tissue (spondylolysis) can be formed. This is probably caused by local bending stress. As a consequence, the superior vertebra may slip (olisthesis) onto the inferior vertebra (spondylolisthesis).

Sacrum

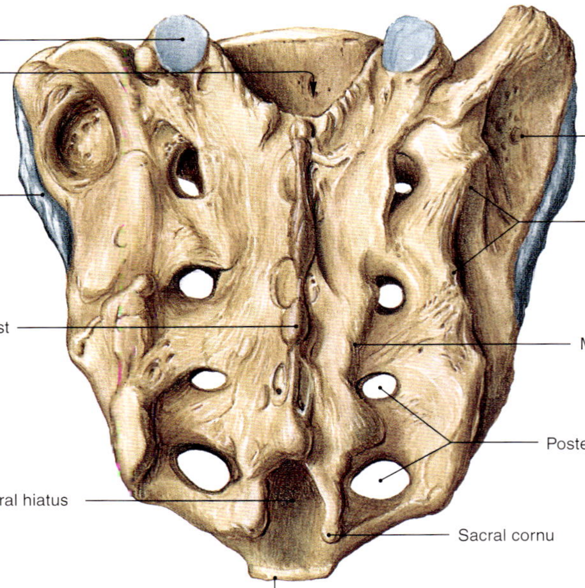

Fig. 490 Sacrum; dorsal view.

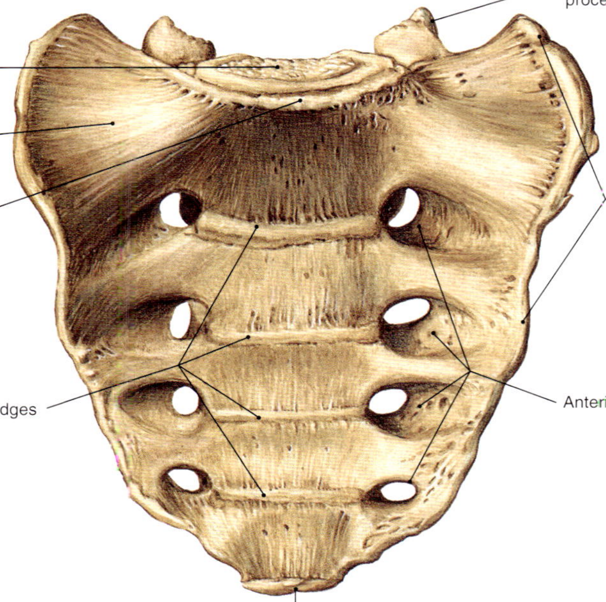

Fig. 491 Sacrum; ventroinferior view.

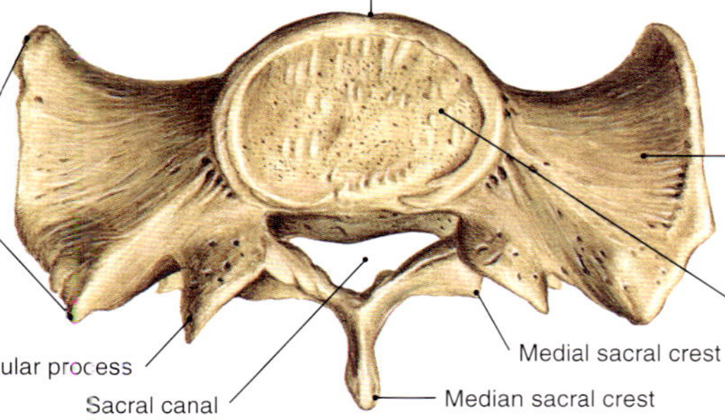

Fig. 492 Sacrum; the bone has been sectioned at the level of the second sacral vertebra; superior view.

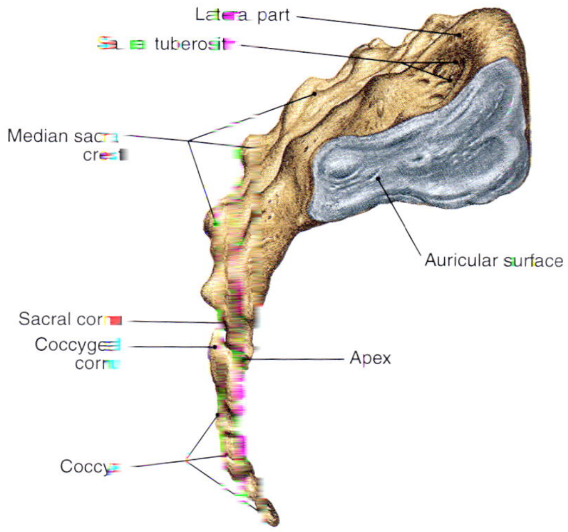

Fig. 493 Sacrum;
viewed from the right.

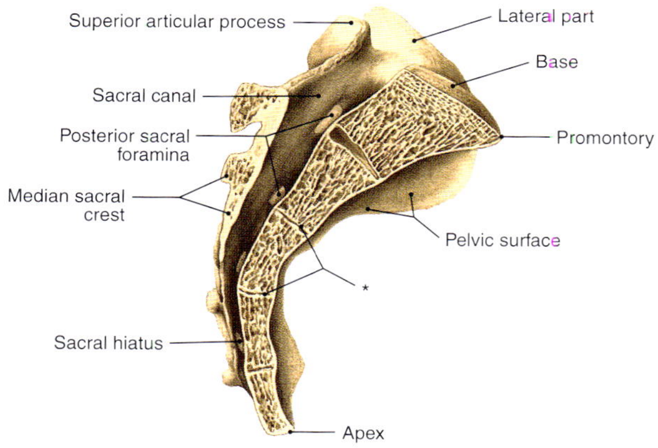

Fig. 494 Sacrum;
median section.

* Remnants of intervertebral disc tissue persist even in the adult.

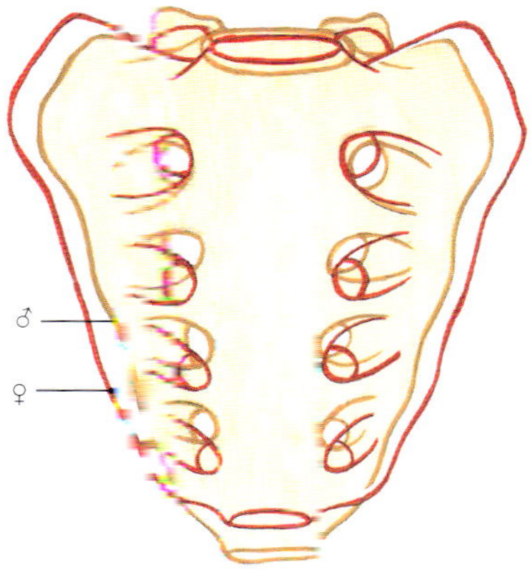

Fig. 495 Sacrum;
gender differences.

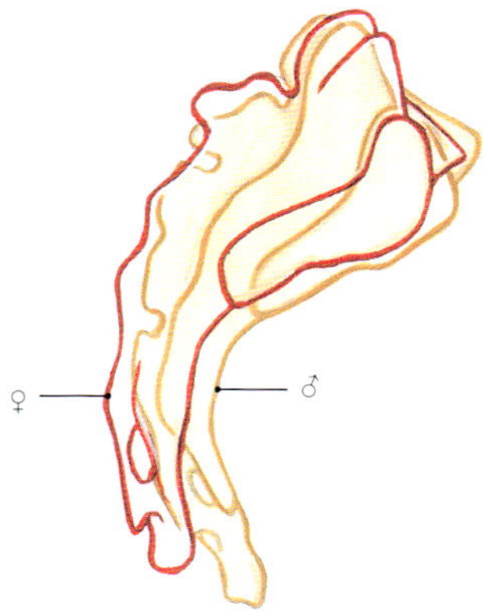

Fig. 496 Sacrum;
gender differences.

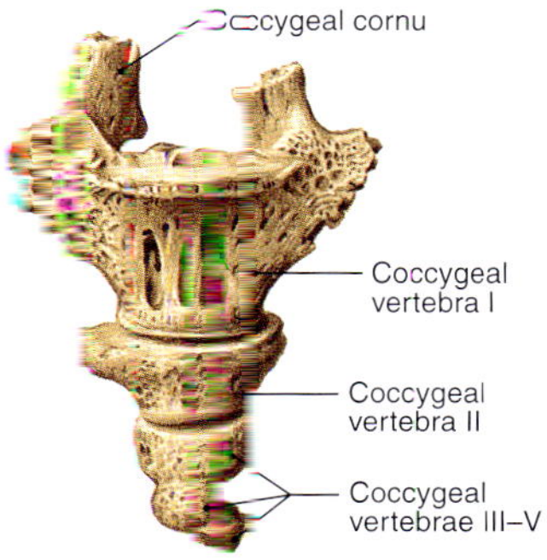

Fig. 497 Coccyx;
ventrosuperior view.

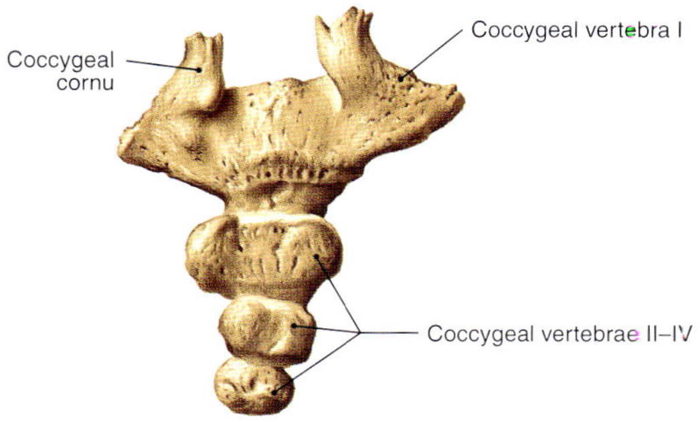

Fig. 498 Coccyx;
dorsoinferior view.

Cervical part of the vertebral column, radiography

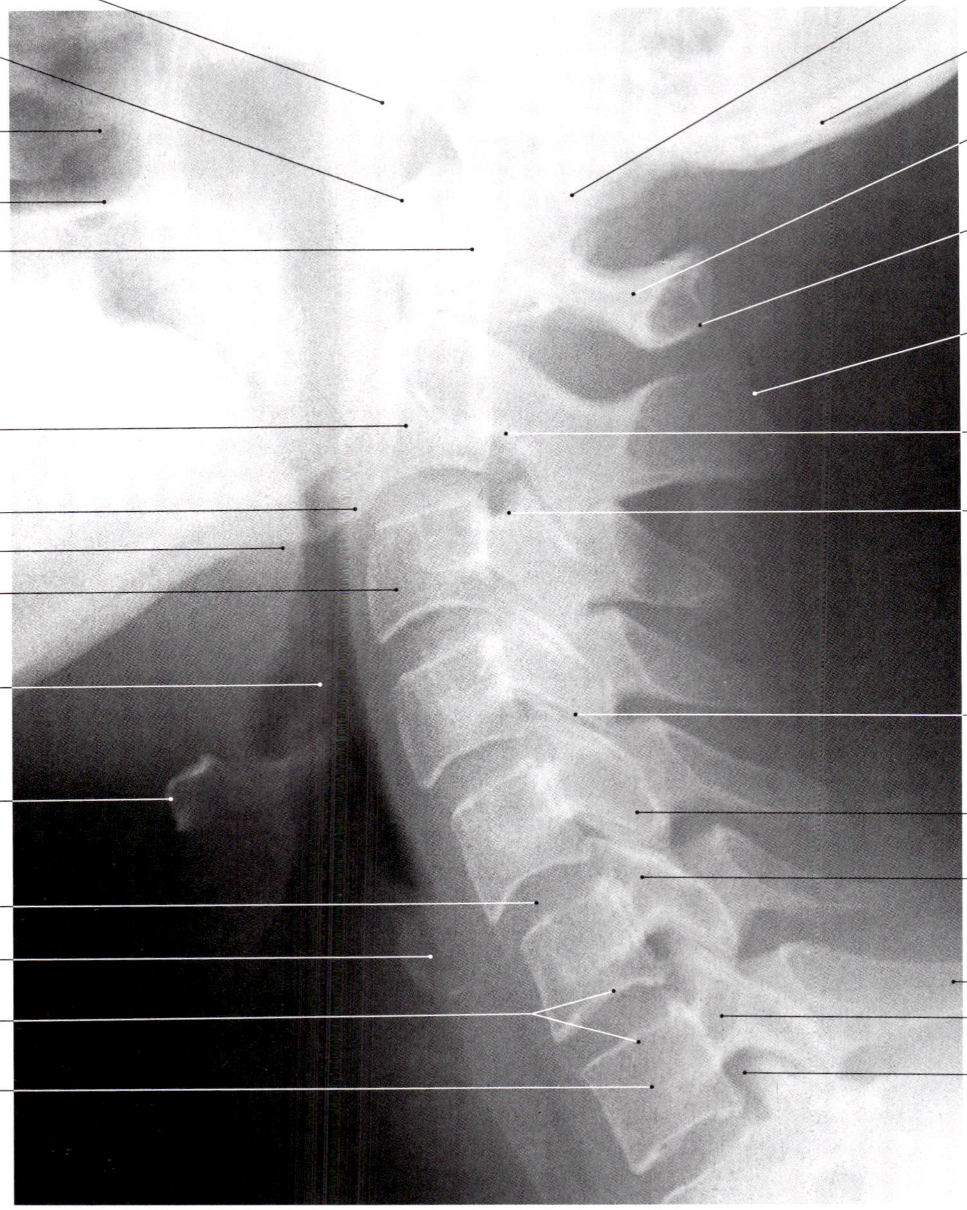

Fig. 499 Cervical vertebrae;
lateral radiograph of the cervical part of the vertebral column;
upright position; the central beam is directed
onto the third cervical vertebra;
shoulders are pulled downwards.

Cervical part of the vertebral column, radiography

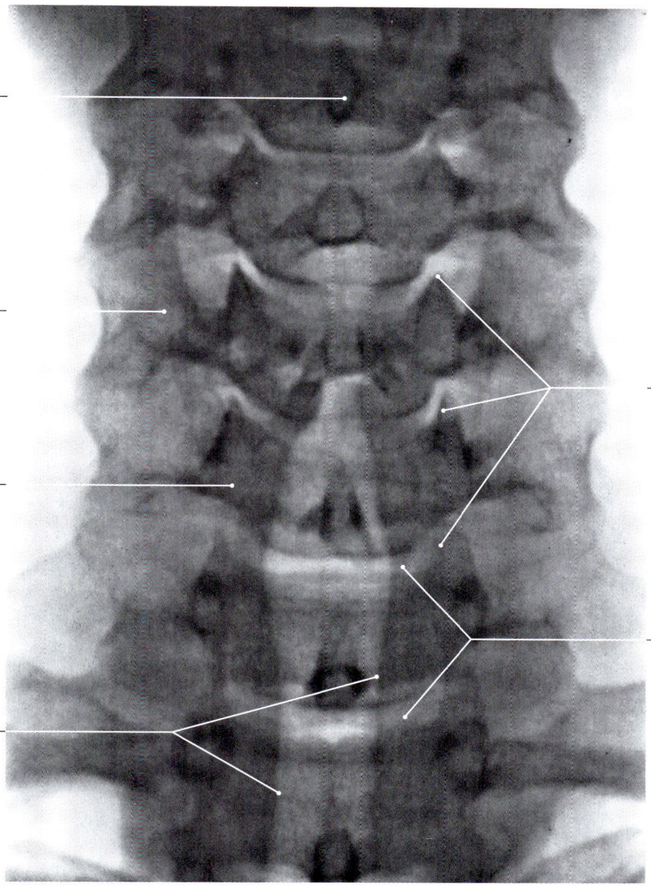

Fig. 500 Cervical vertebrae;
AP-radiograph of the cervical part of the vertebral column; upright position; the central beam is directed onto the third cervical vertebra.

* Intervertebral disc spaces

Thoracic part of the vertebral column, radiography

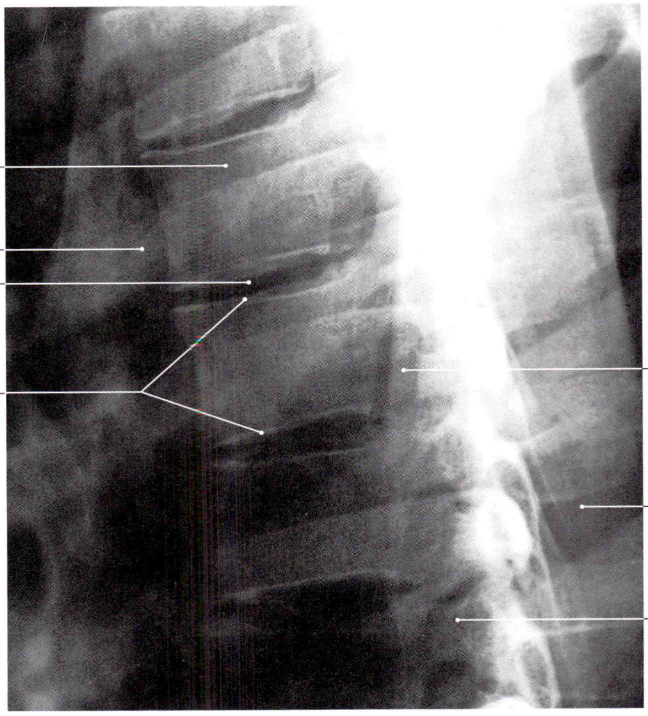

Fig. 501 Thoracic vertebrae;
lateral radiograph of the thoracic part of the vertebral column;
upright position with the thorax in inspiration;
the central beam is directed onto the sixth thoracic vertebra.

* Intervertebral disc space
** Clinical term: end-plates

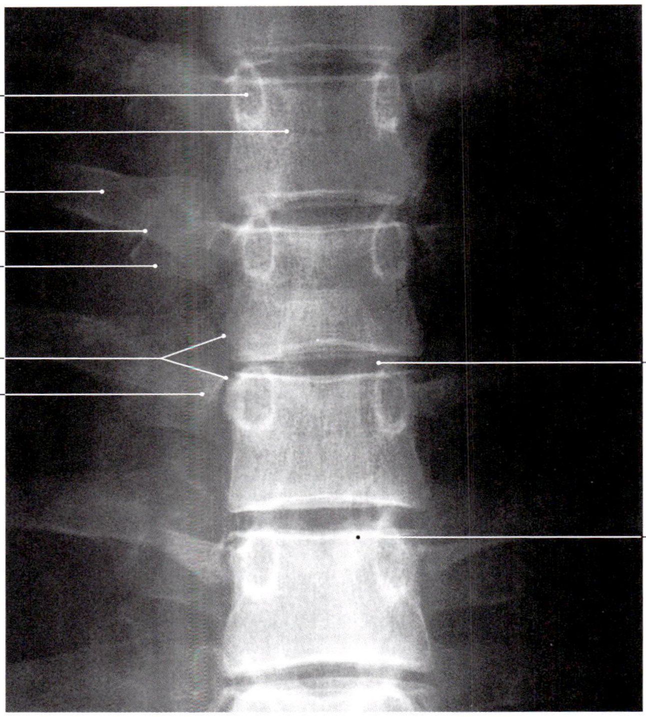

Fig. 502 Thoracic vertebrae;
AP-radiograph of the thoracic part of the vertebral column;
upright position with the thorax in inspiration;
the central beam is directed onto the sixth thoracic vertebra.

* Intervertebral disc space

Lumbar part of the vertebral column, radiography

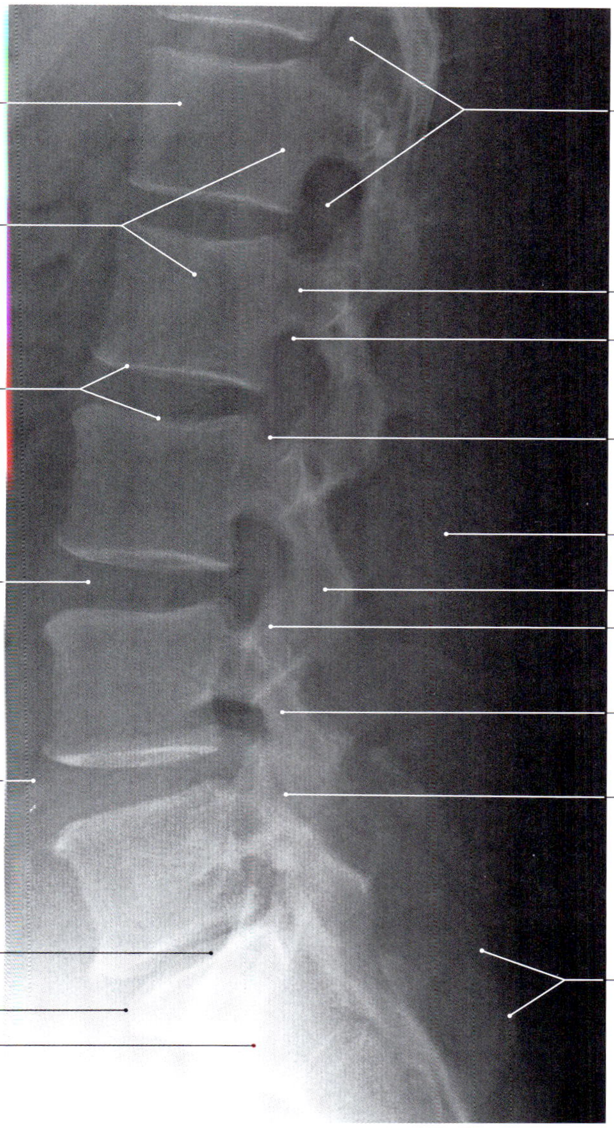

Fig. 503 Lumbar vertebrae;
lateral radiograph of the lumbar part of the vertebral column;
upright position;
the central beam is directed onto the second lumbar vertebra.
In this case, the anterior edges of the lower lumbar vertebrae are oblique due to pathological alterations.

* Intervertebral disc space
** Region of the vertebral arch between the superior and inferior articular processes („isthmus" = interarticular portion)
*** The marks indicate the position of the twelfth rib, which is poorly visible in this copy of the radiograph.

Lumbar part of the vertebral column, radiography

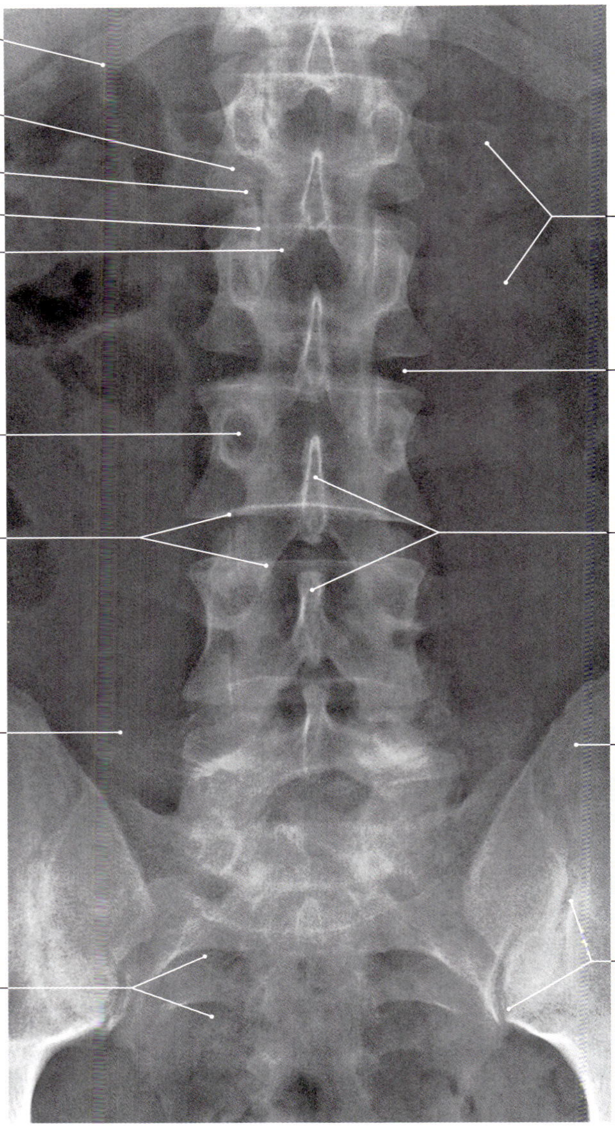

Fig. 504 Lumbar vertebrae;
AP-radiograph of the lumbar part of the vertebral column and the sacrum;
upright position; the central beam is directed onto the second lumbar vertebra.

* Intervertebral disc space

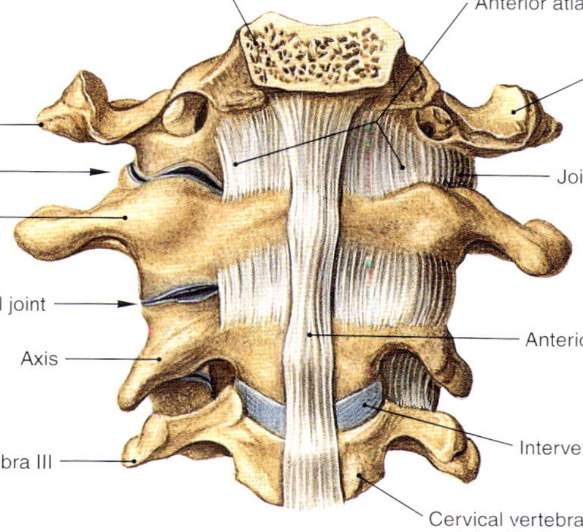

Fig. 505 Craniocervical junctions and the upper cervical part of the vertebral column; ventral view.

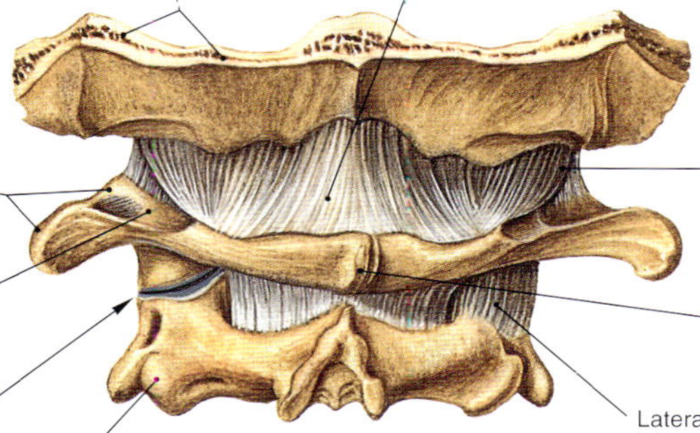

Fig. 506 Craniocervical junctions; dorsal view.

Craniocervical junctions

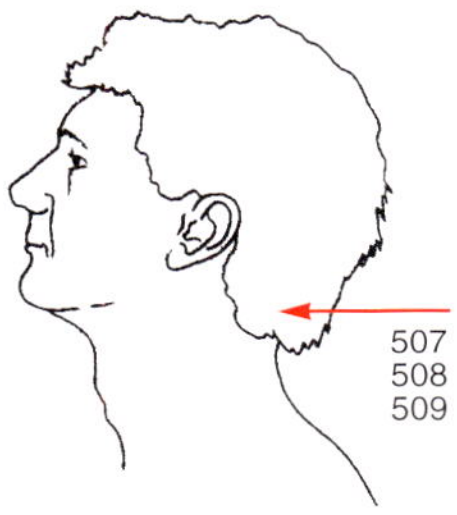

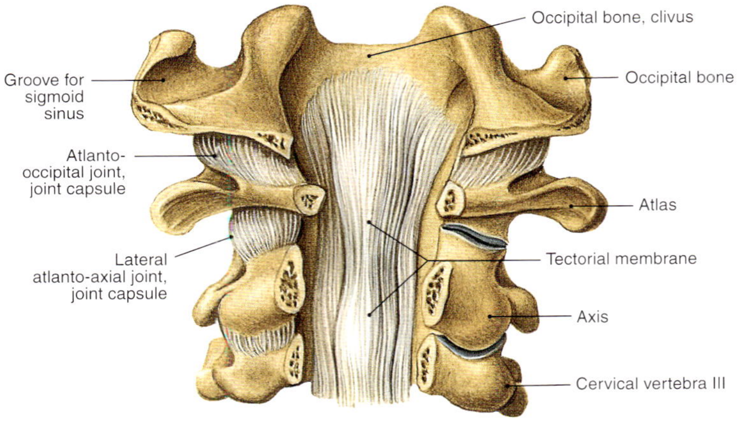

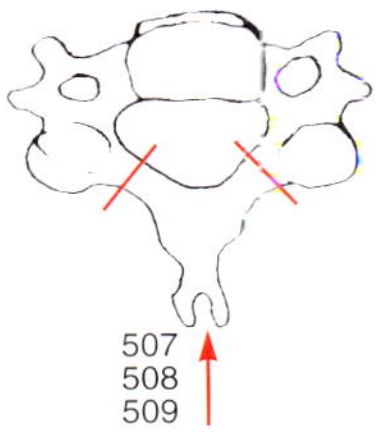

Fig. 507 Craniocervical junctions, deep ligaments; dorsal view.

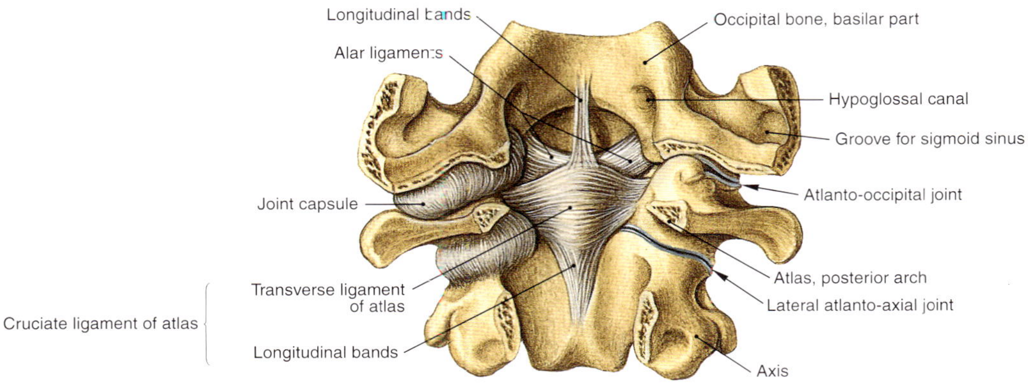

Fig. 508 Craniocervical junctions, deep ligaments; dorsal view.

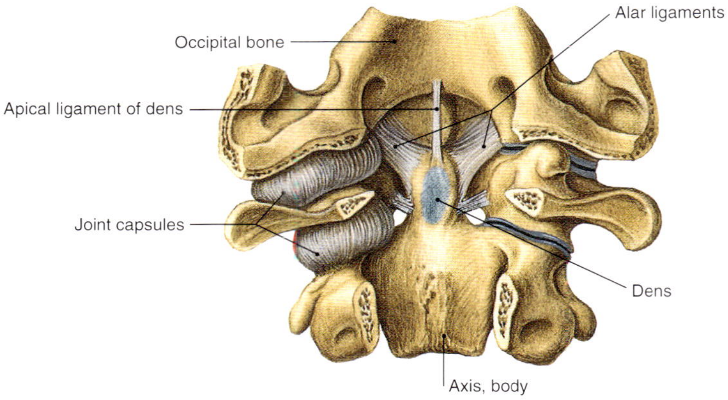

Fig. 509 Craniocervical junctions, deep ligaments; dorsal view.
The alar ligaments frequently extend to the lateral masses of the atlas.

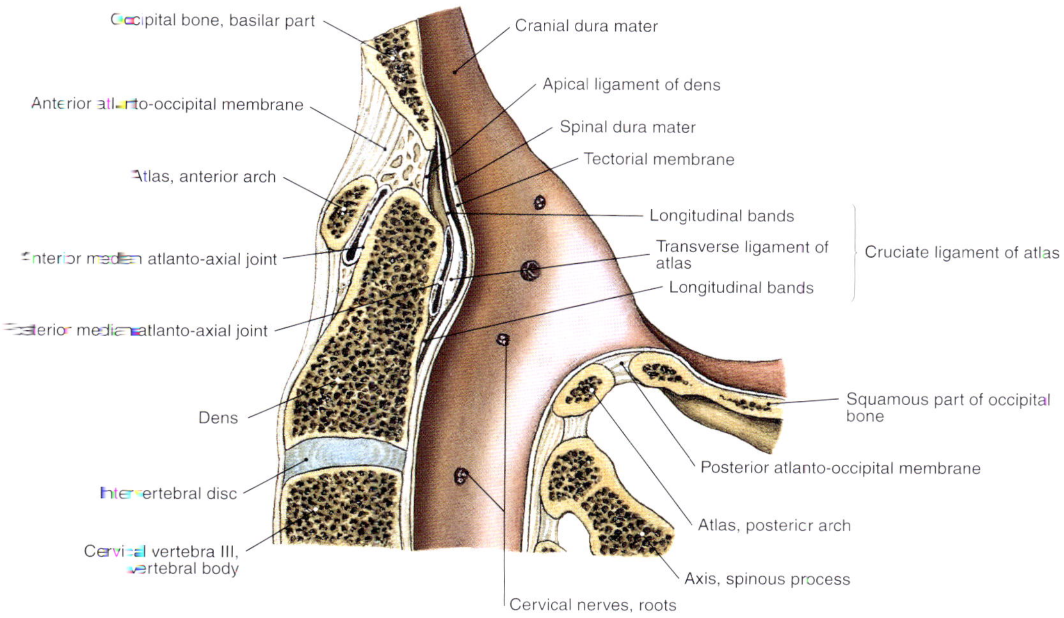

Fig. 510 Craniocervical junctions; median section.

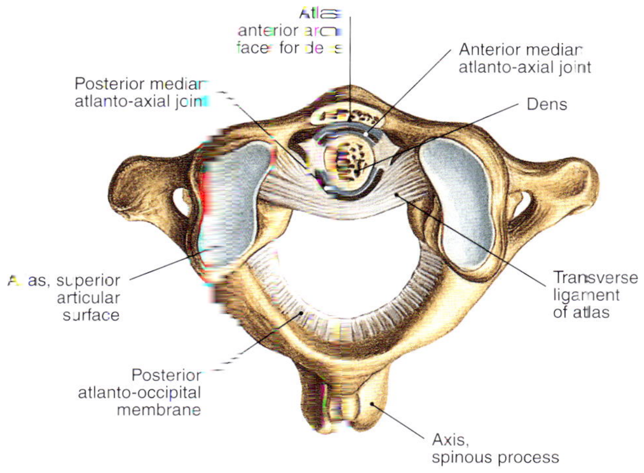

Fig. 511 Craniocervical junctions; superior view.

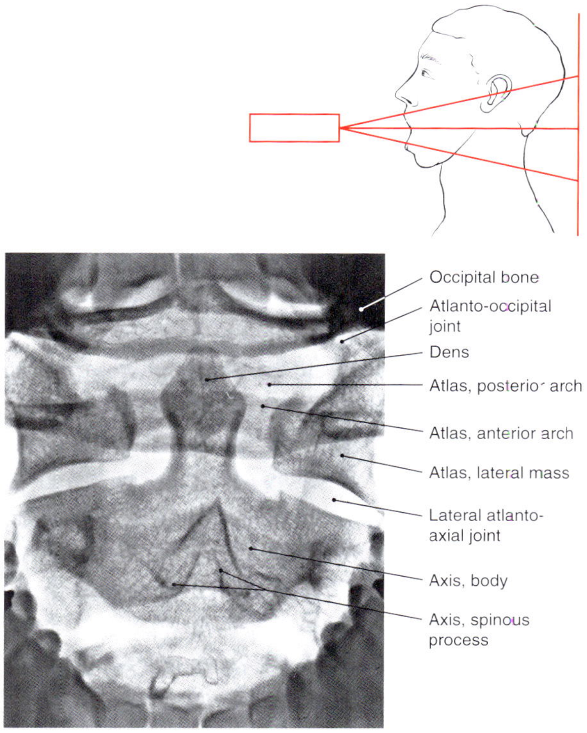

Fig. 512 Craniocervical junctions; AP-radiograph.

Ligaments of the vertebral column

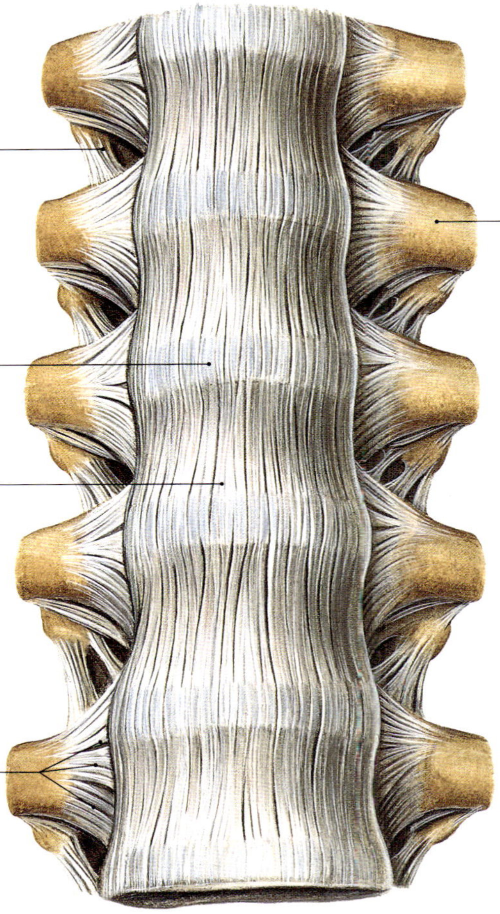

Fig. 513 Ligaments of the vertebral column; exemplified by the lower thoracic part of the vertebral column; ventral view.

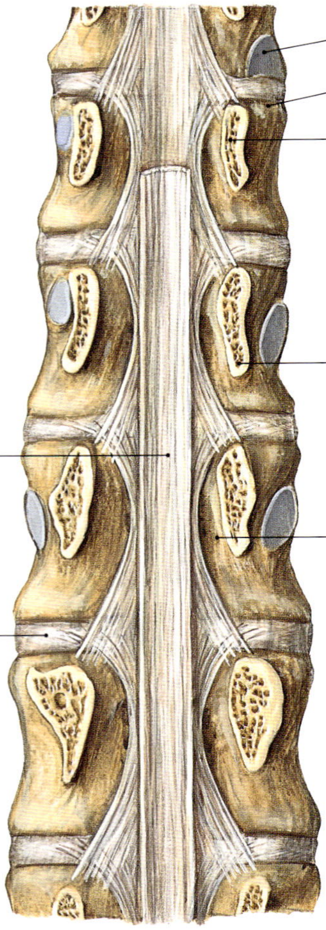

Fig. 514 Ligaments of the vertebral column; exemplified by the lower thoracic and the upper lumbar part of the vertebral column; dorsal view.

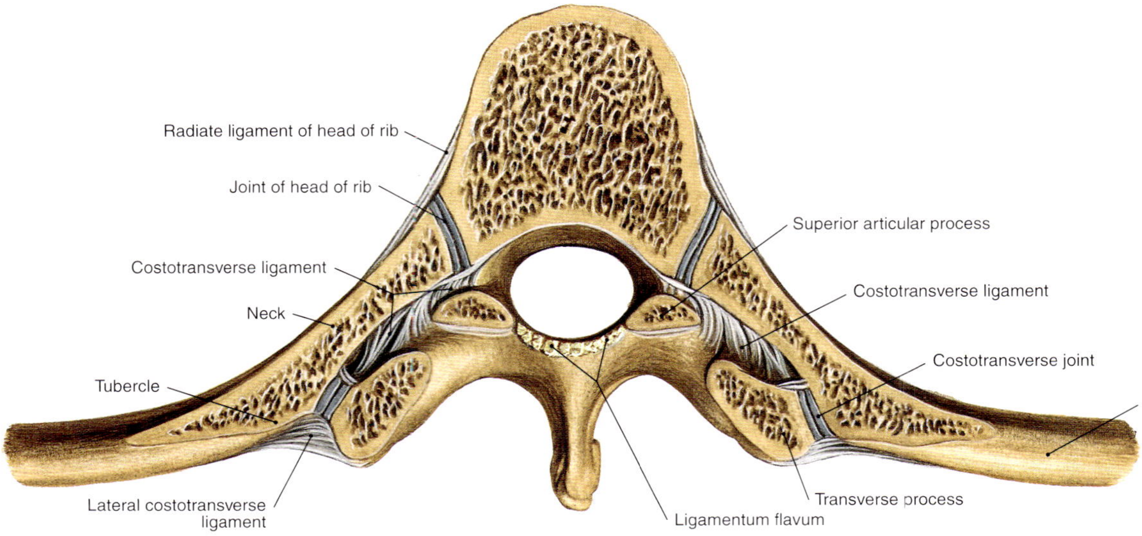

Fig. 515 Costovertebral joints; cross-section at the level of the lower part of the joint at a head of a rib; superior view.

Ligaments of the vertebral column

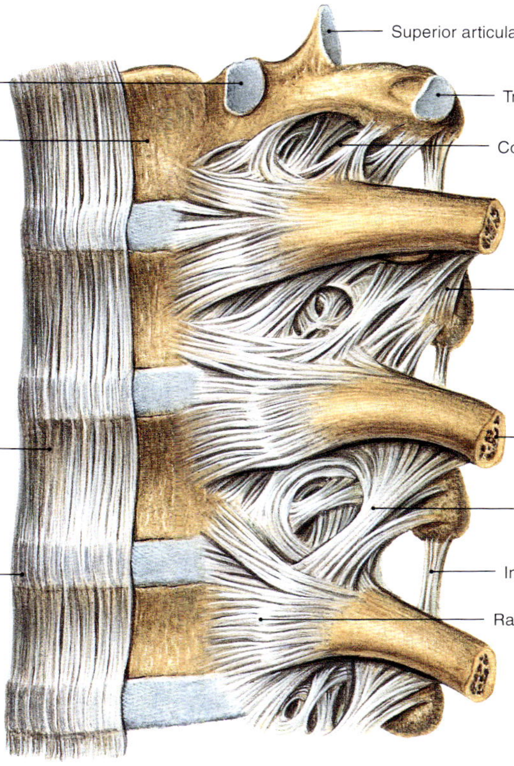

Fig. 516 Ligaments of the vertebral column and the costovertebral joints;
lateral parts of the anterior longitudinal ligament have been removed;
viewed from the left.

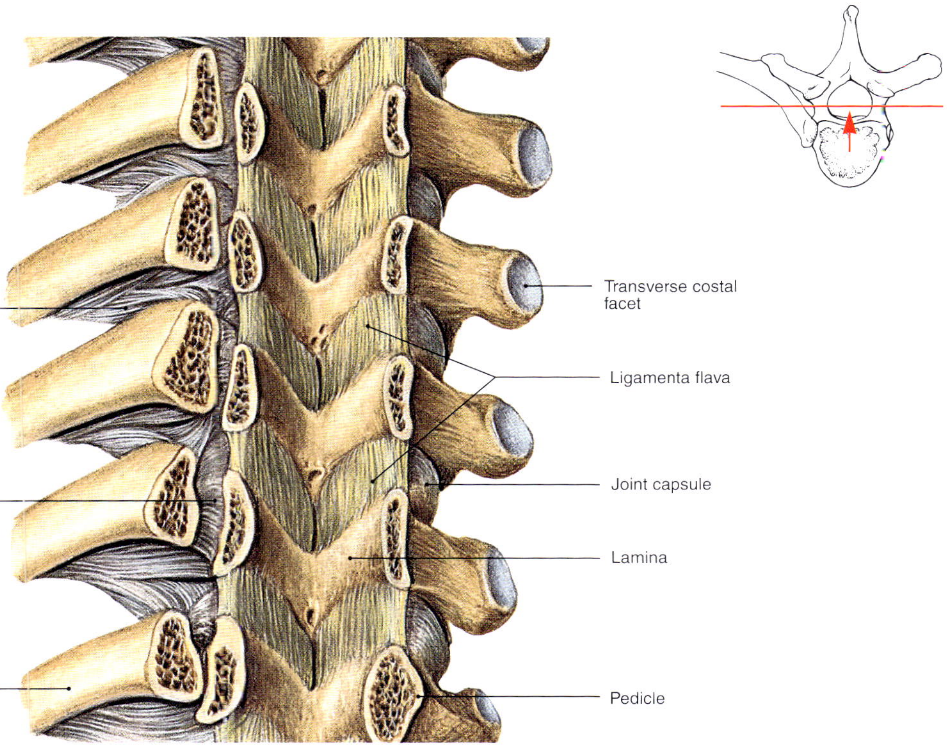

Fig. 517 Junctions between the vertebral arches;
ventral view.

Costovertebral joints

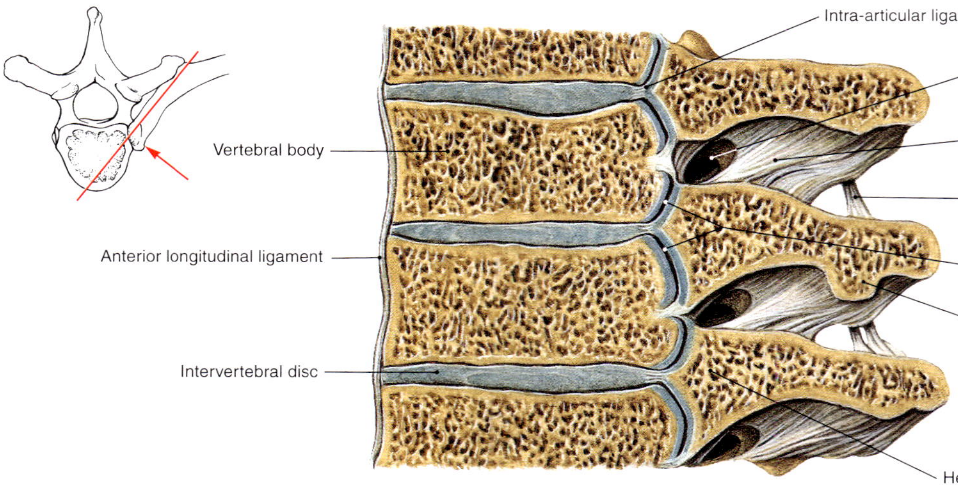

Fig. 518 Costovertebral joints; ventral view from the left.

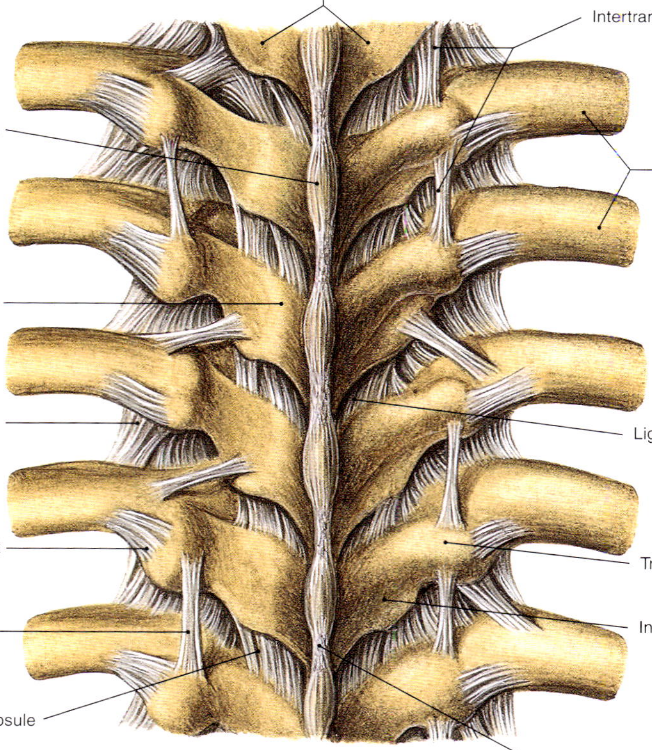

Fig. 519 Ligaments of the vertebral arches and the costovertebral joints; dorsal view.

* The median portion of the thoracolumbar fascia is referred to as supraspinous ligament.

Ligaments of the lumbar part of the vertebral column

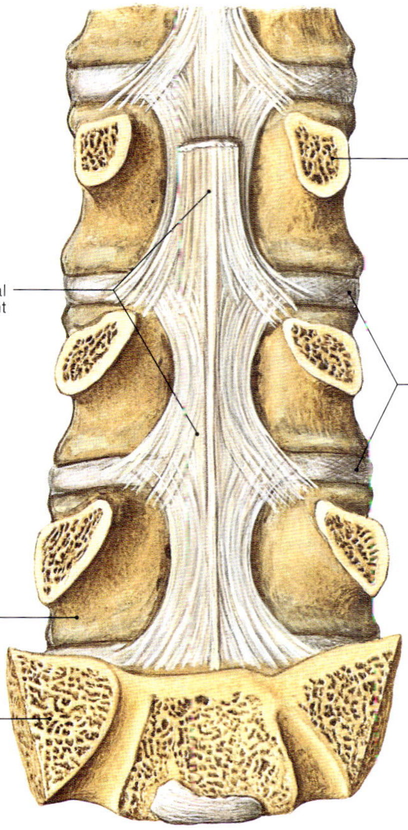

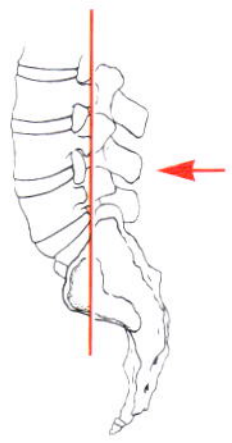

Fig. 520 Ligaments of the lumbar part of the vertebral column.

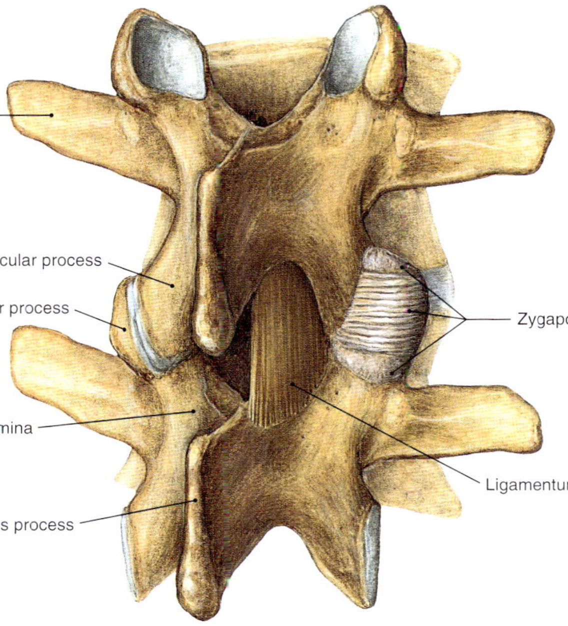

Fig. 521 Vertebral joints of the lumbar part of the vertebral column; dorsal view from the right.

Reinforcement of the interarticular joints by strong and transverse fibres (transverse ligaments) is restricted to the lumbar part of the vertebral column.

Intervertrebal discs

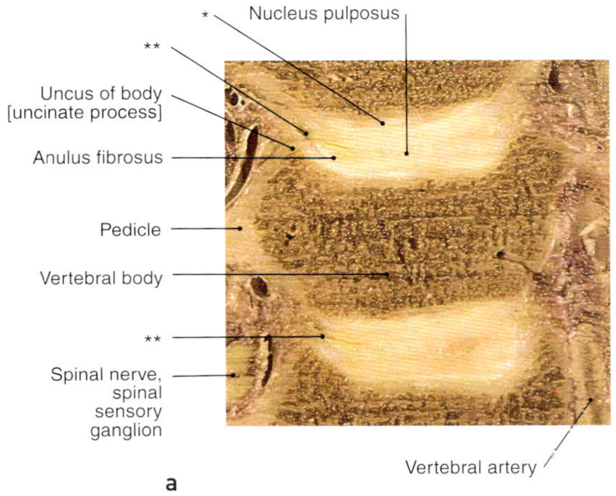

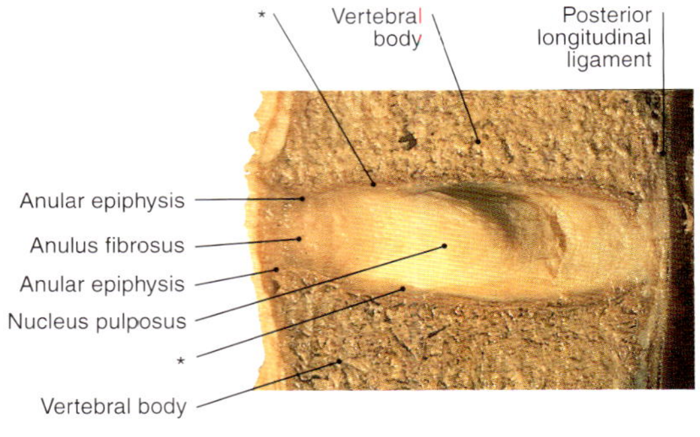

Fig. 522 a, b Intervertebral discs
a Cervical intervertebral discs; frontal section
b Lumbar intervertebral disc;
median section

* Hyaline cartilaginous covering of the end-plates of the vertebral bodies reflecting the non-ossified portion of the epiphyses

** In the first decade of life, so-called uncovertebral clefts develop in the lateral zones of the cervical intervertebral discs, which can progress further towards the middle in the following decades.

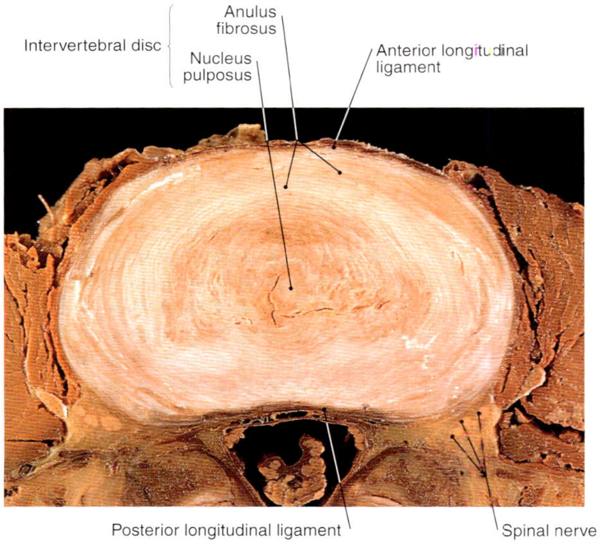

Fig. 523 Lumbar intervertebral disc; superior view.

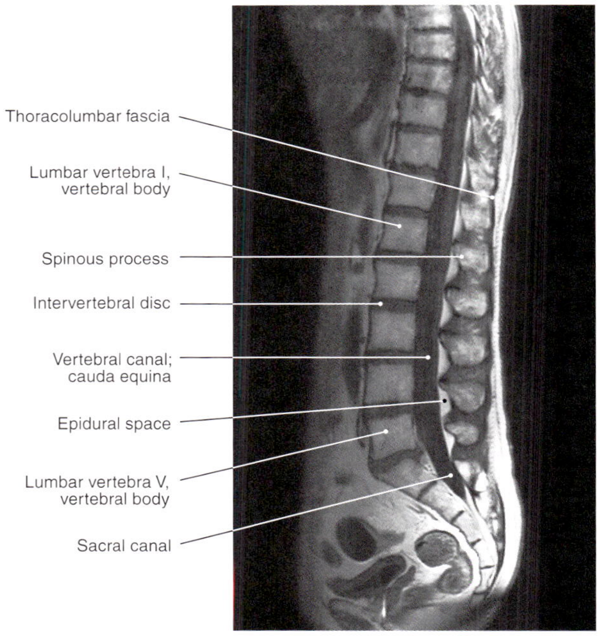

Fig. 524 Lumbar parts of the vertebral column; magnetic resonance tomographic image (MRI); median section.

Motion segments

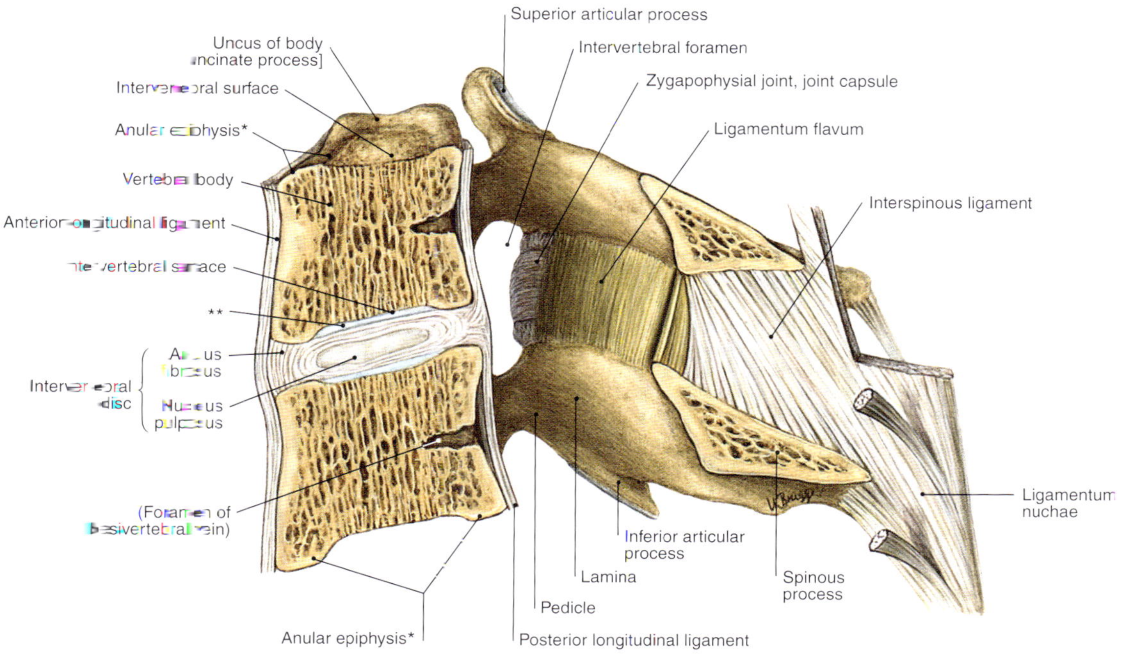

Fig. 525 Cervical motion segment; schematic median section.

* Also: rim of vertebral body
** Hyaline cartilaginous covering of the end-plate of the vertebral body reflecting the non-ossified portion of the epiphysis

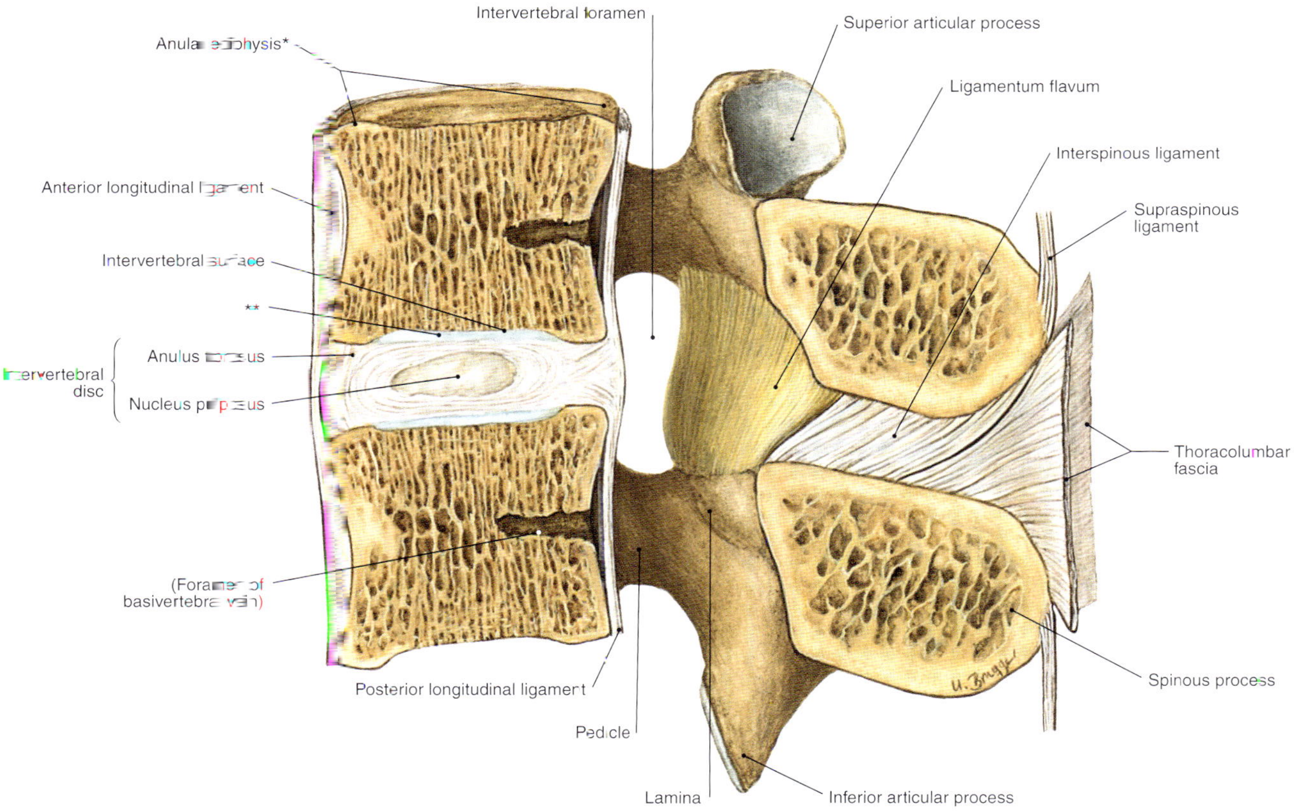

Fig. 526 Lumbar motion segment; schematic median section.

* Also: rim of vertebral body
** Hyaline cartilaginous covering of the end-plate of the vertebral body reflecting the non-ossified portion of the epiphysis

Superficial muscles of the back

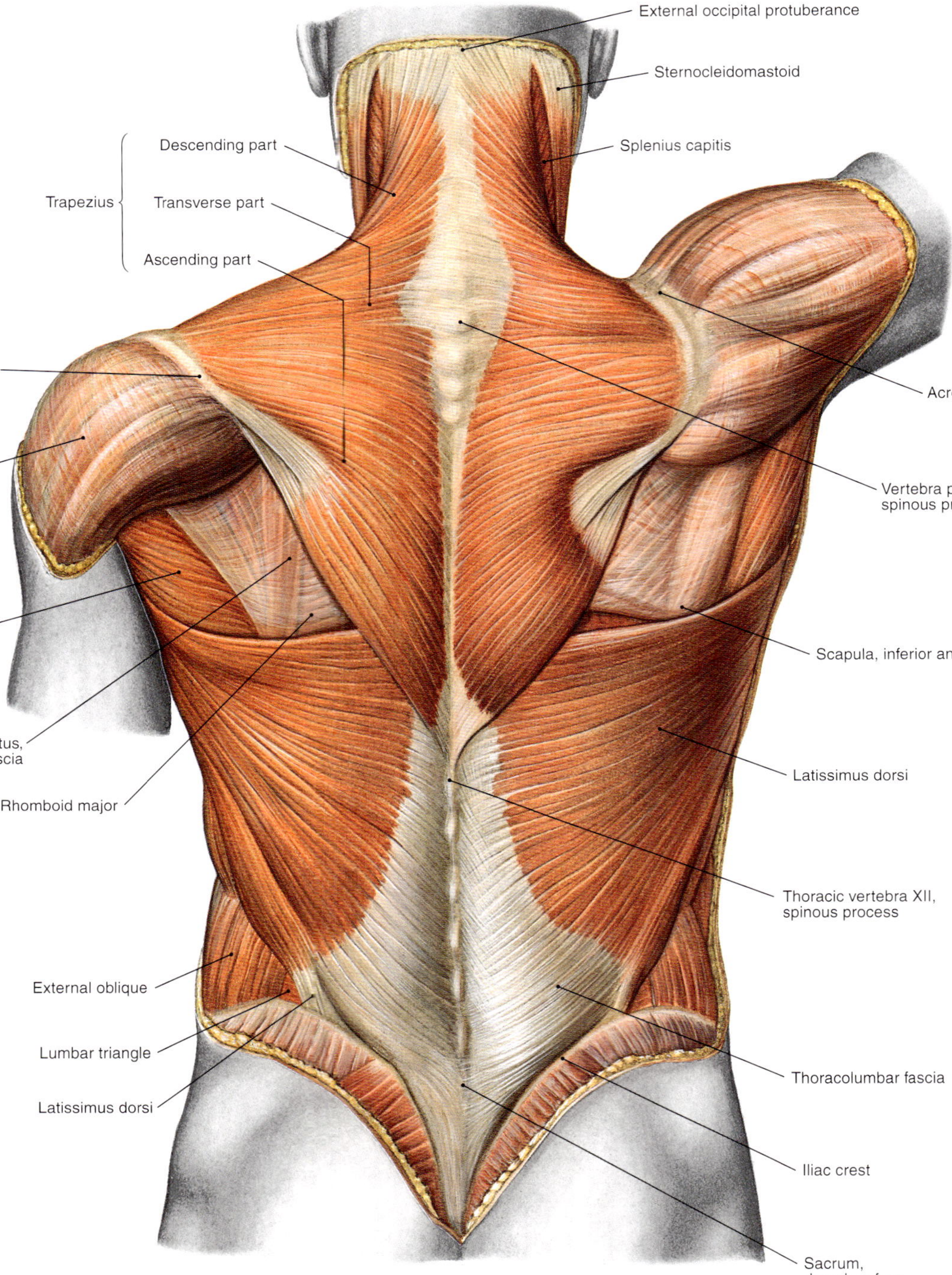

→ T 17, T 18

Fig. 527 Muscles of the back;
superficial layer of the trunk-arm and trunk-shoulder girdle muscles.

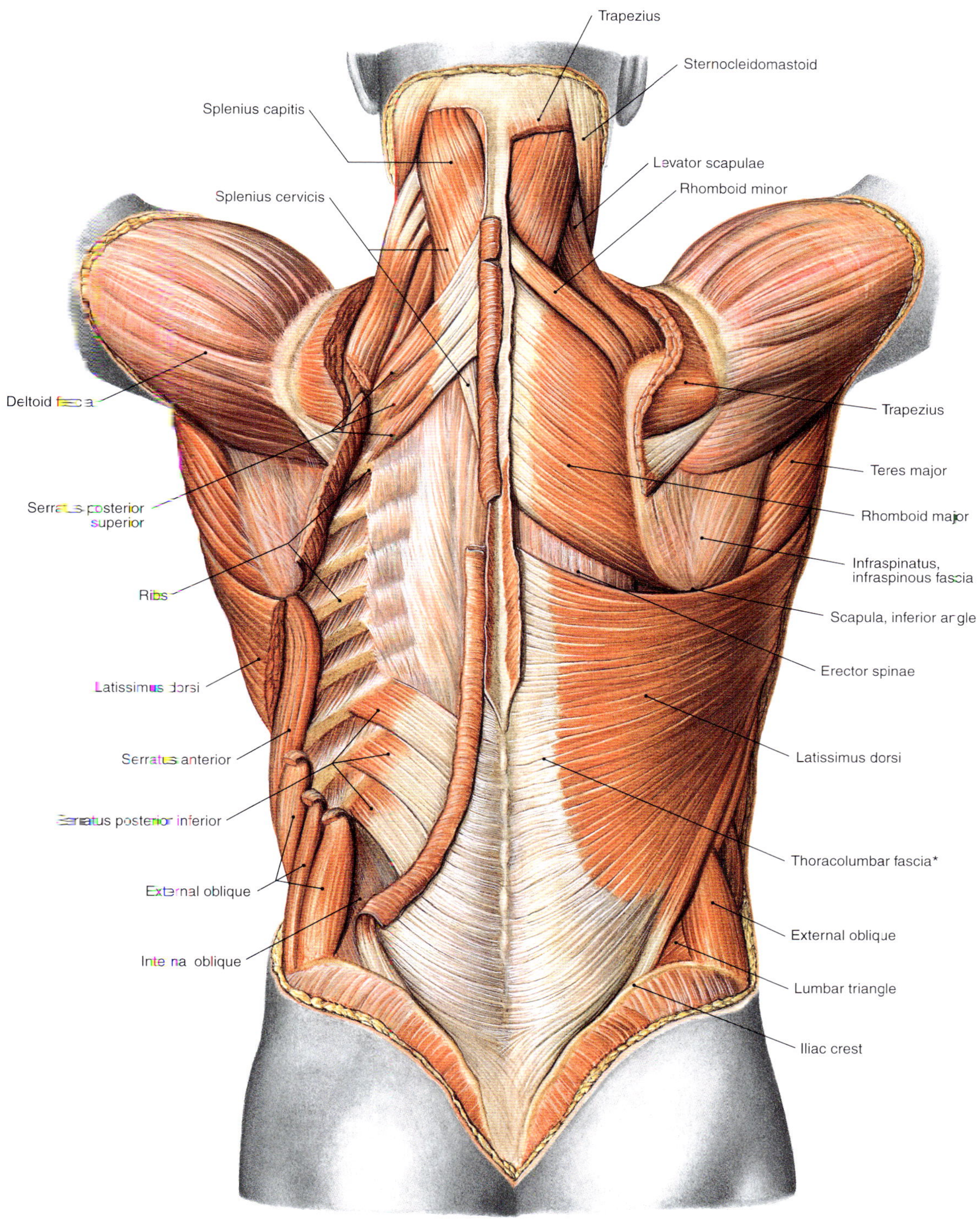

Fig. 528 Muscles of the back;
deep layer of the trunk-arm and trunk-shoulder girdle muscles.

* The so-called thoracolumbar fascia forms a dense aponeurosis.

→ T 17–T 19

Deep muscles of the back

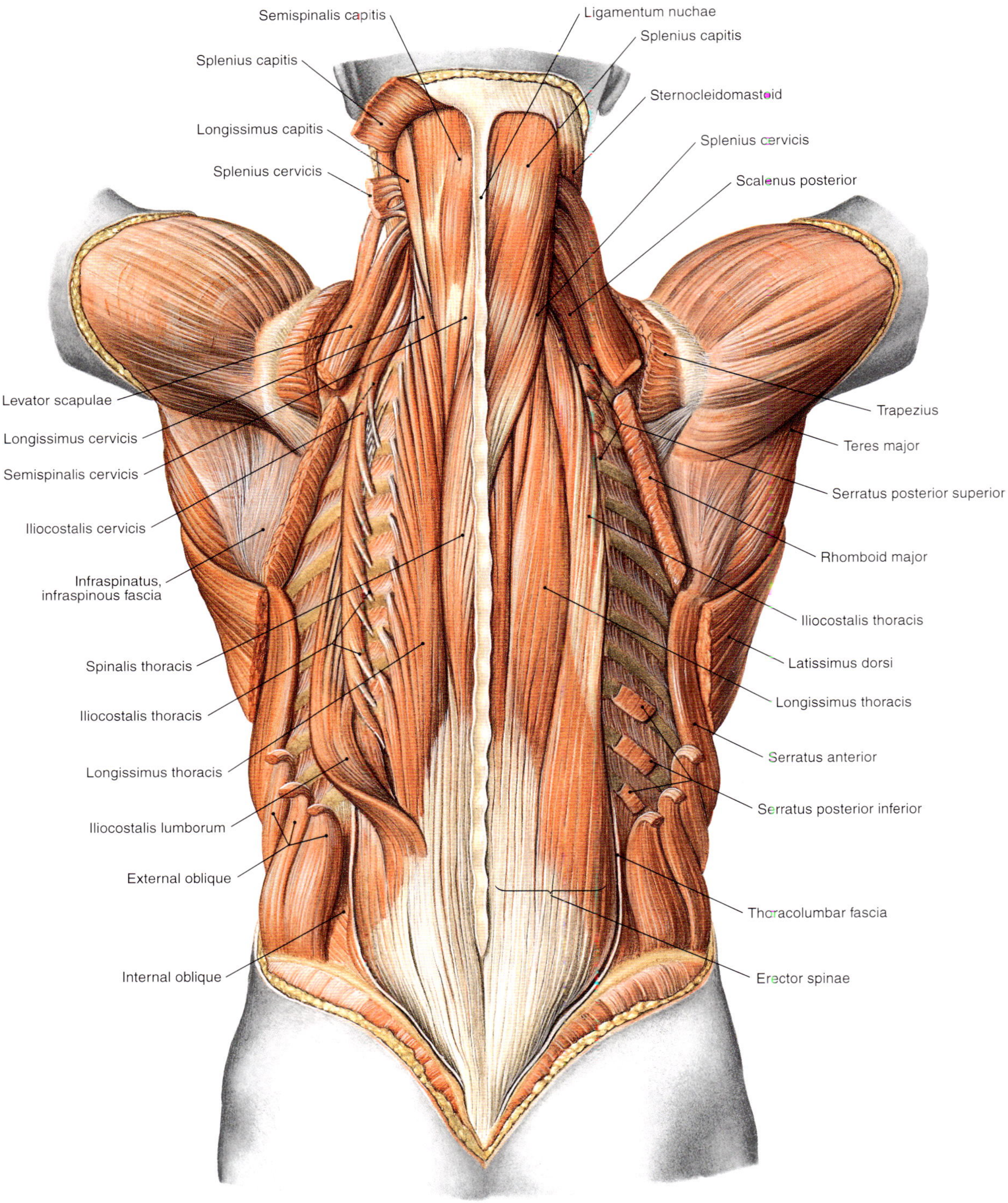

→ T 20 a, b

Fig. 529 Muscles of the back;
superficial layer of the deep (autochthonous) muscles.

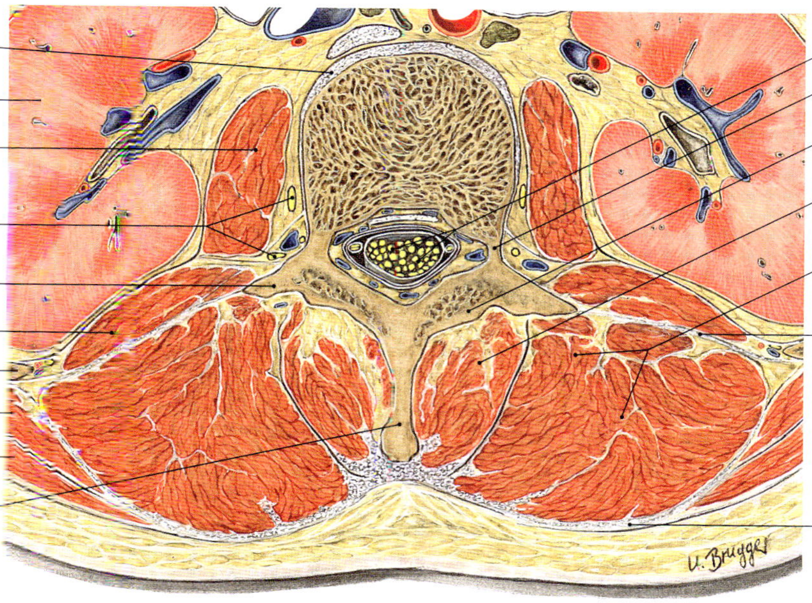

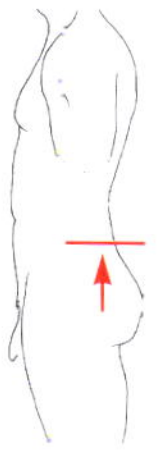

Fig. 530 Muscles of the back; cross-section at the level of the second lumbar vertebra; inferior view.

The deep (autochthonous) muscles of the back lie within an osteofibrous tube formed by dorsal parts of the vertebrae and the surrounding aponeurotic thoracolumbar fascia. The muscles are divided into a lateral * and a medial ** tract.

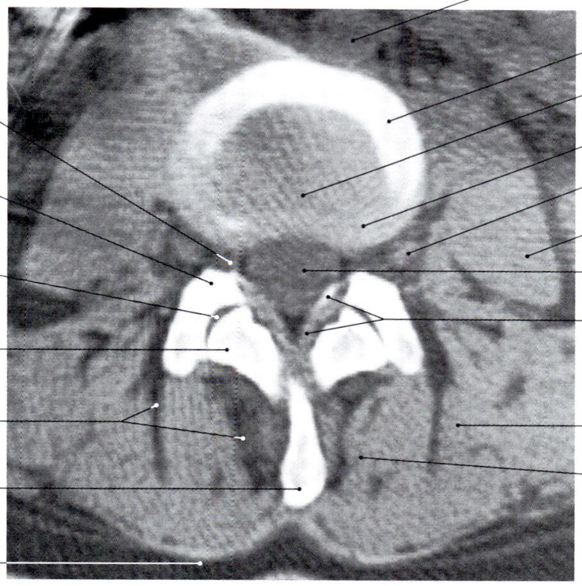

Fig. 531 Muscles of the back; computed tomographic cross-section (CT) at the level of the intervertebral disc between the third and the fourth lumbar vertebra; inferior view.

* Calcification or ossification frequently occurs at the sites of insertion of the ligamenta flava, even in younger individuals.

** Adipose tissue deposits

Deep muscles of the back

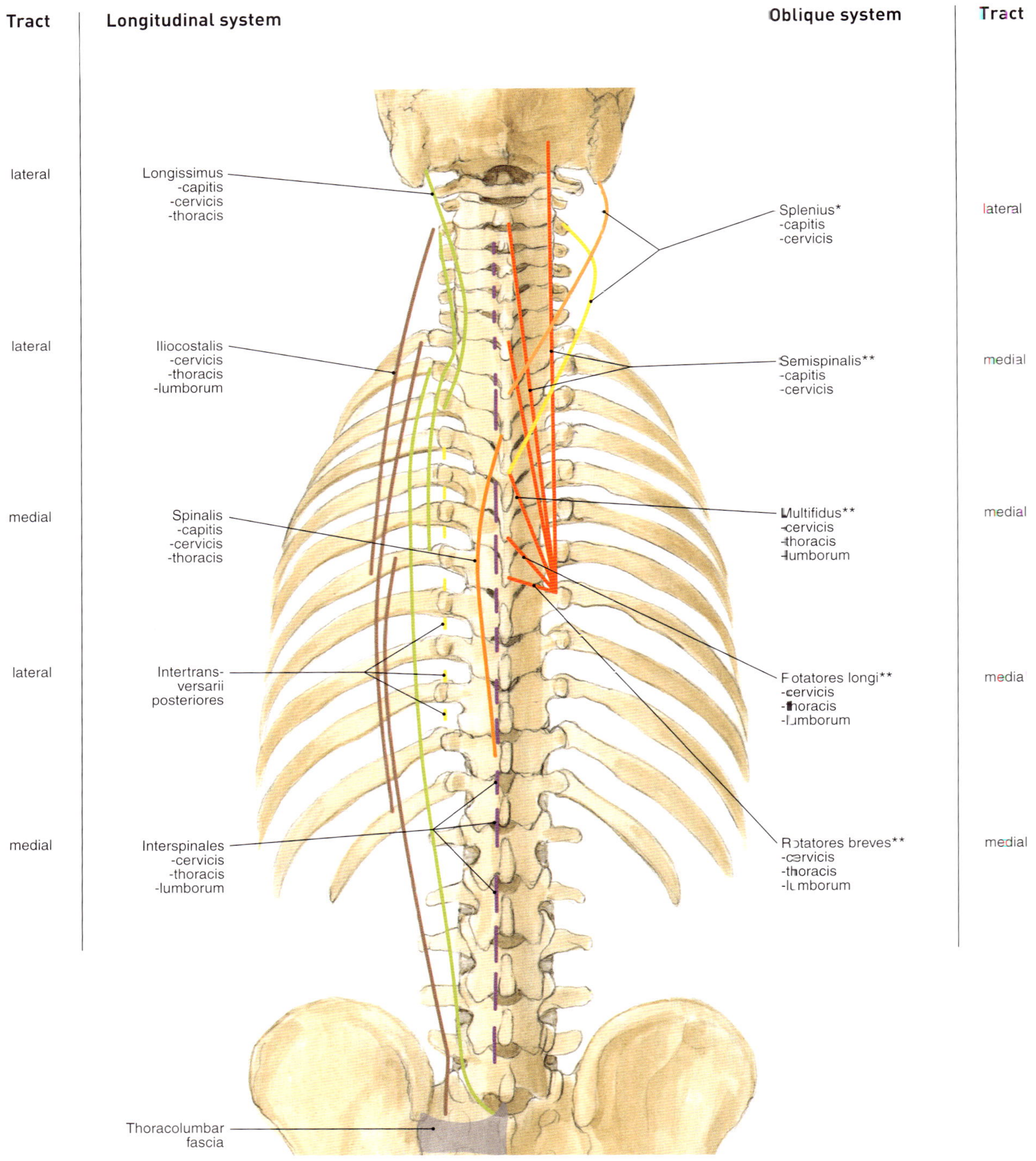

Fig. 532 Deep (autochthonous) muscles of the back; diagram of the different groups of muscles.
The deep (autochthonous) muscles of the back can be divided into a longitudinal and an oblique system, as well as into a medial and a lateral tract.

* Spinotransverse
** Transversospinal

Deep muscles of the back

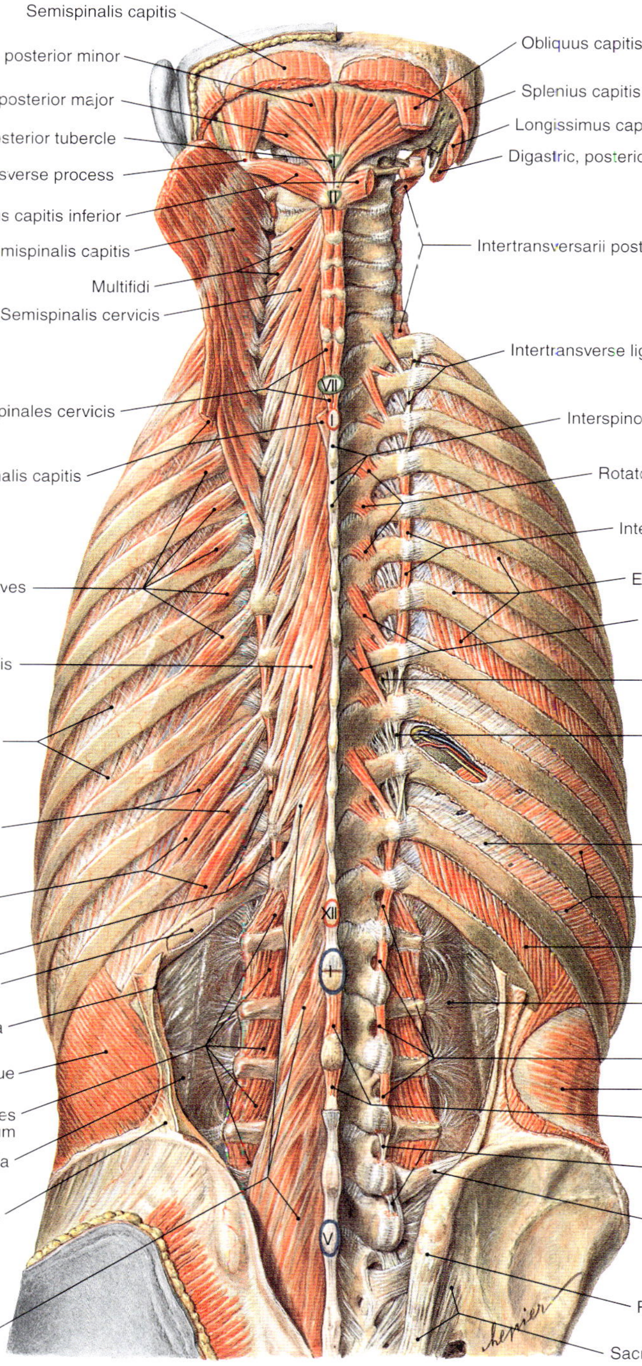

Fig. 533 Muscles of the back and suboccipital muscles.

→ T 20 b, c

Deep muscles of the back

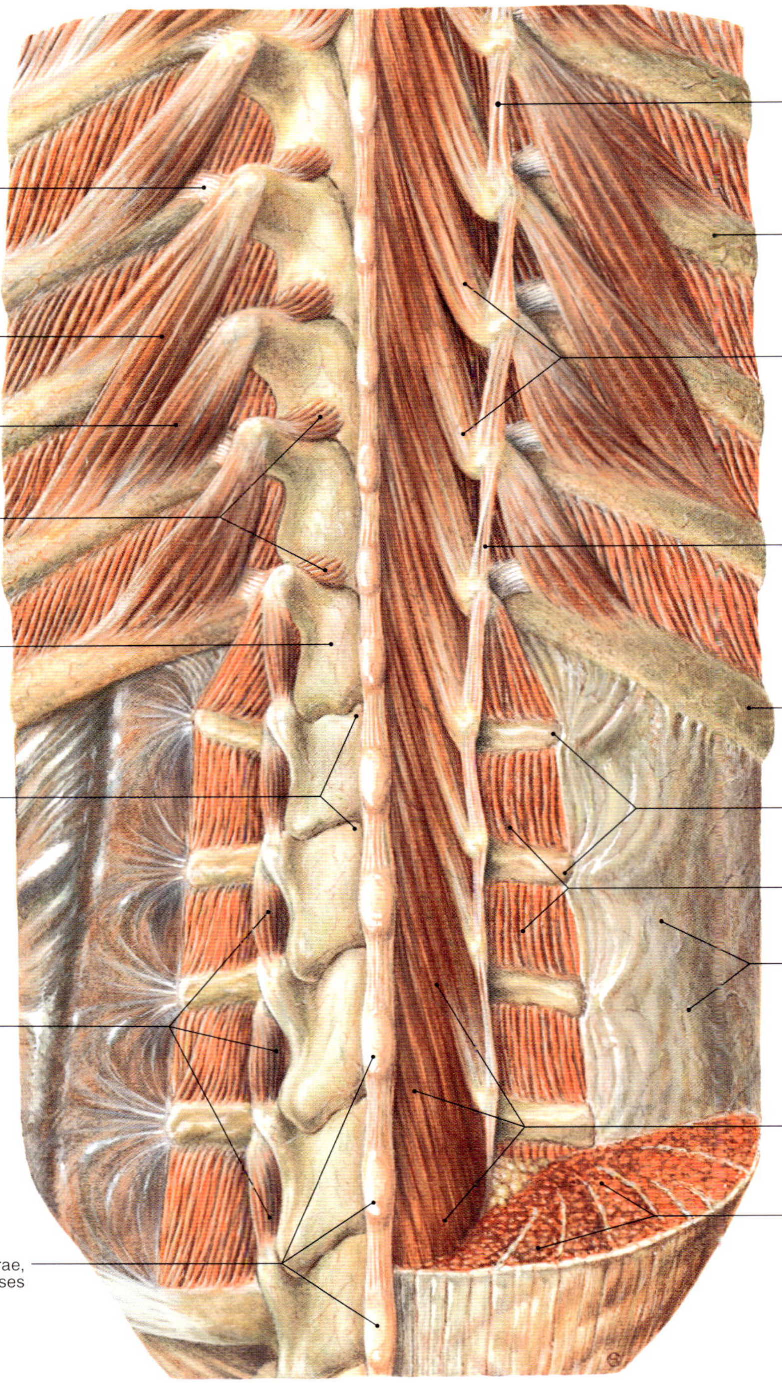

→ T 20 a, b

Fig. 534 Muscles of the back;
deepest layer in the region of the lower thoracic and the lumbar part of the vertebral column.

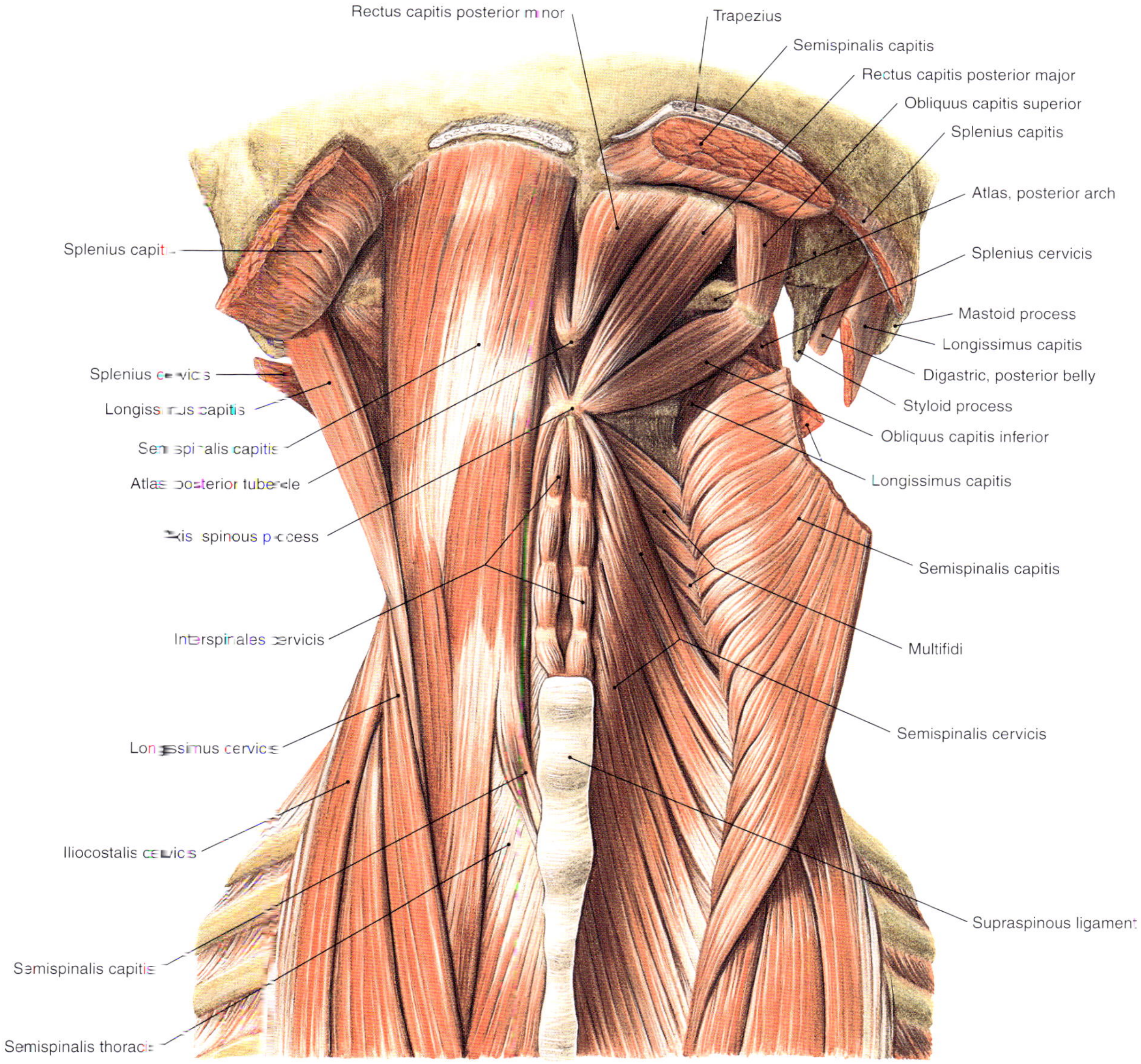

Fig. 535 Muscles of the back and suboccipital muscles.

→ T 20 b, c

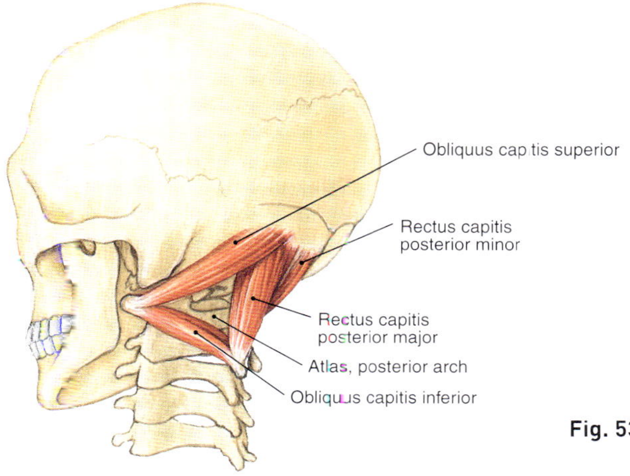

Fig. 536 Suboccipital muscles.

→ T 20 c

Suboccipital muscles

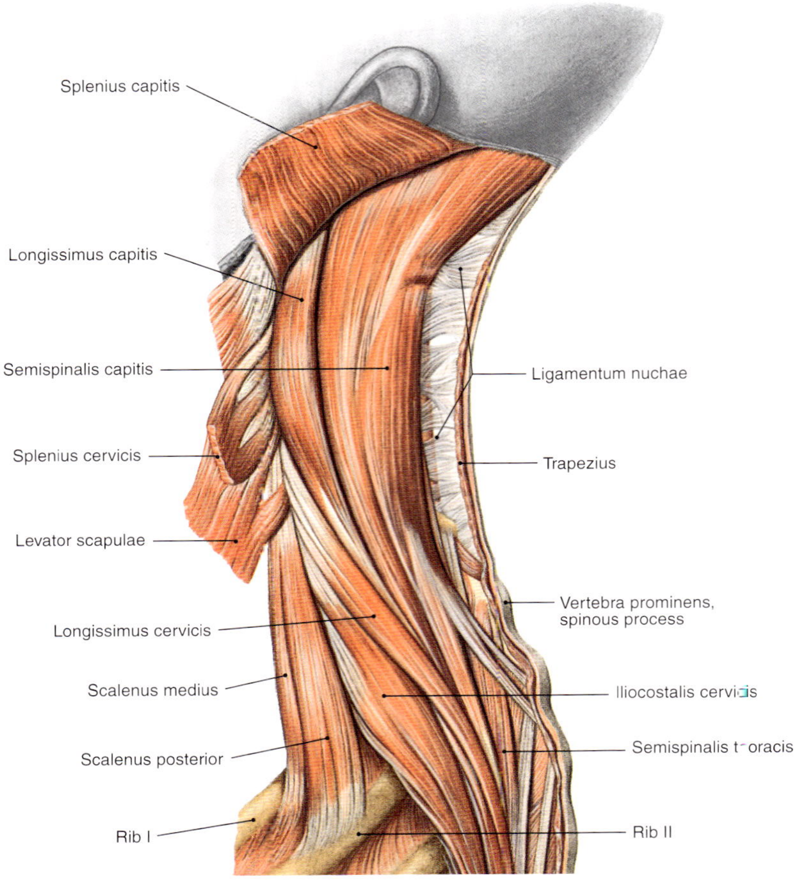

→ T 20 a, b

Fig. 537 Muscles of the back and muscles of the neck.

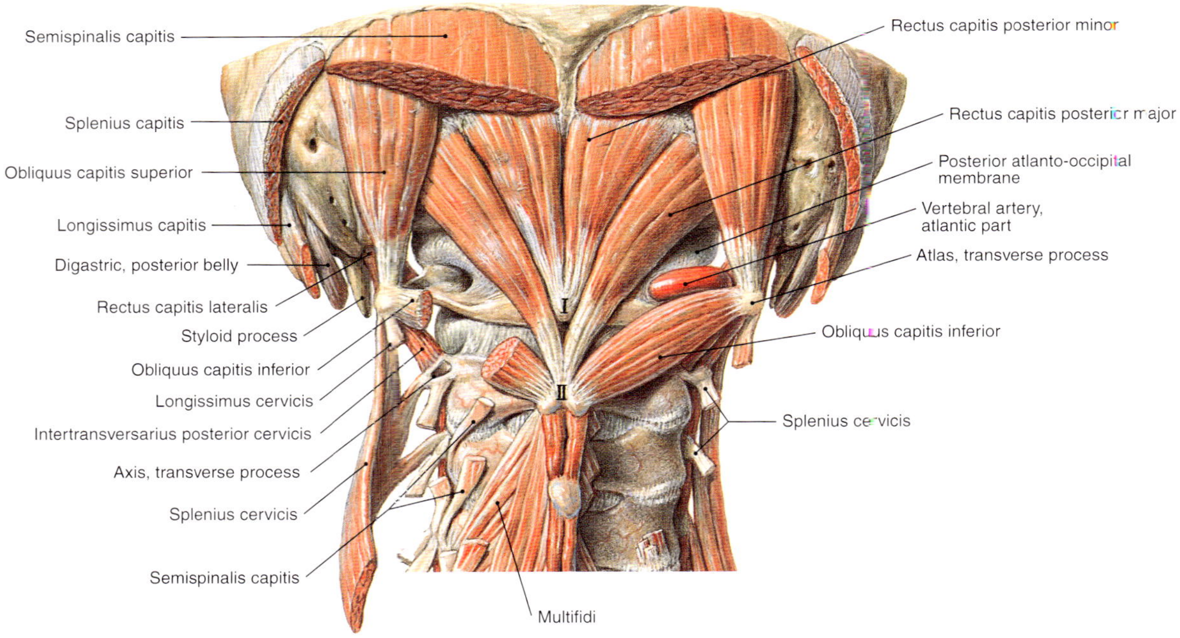

→ T 20 c

Fig. 538 Suboccipital muscles.

I = Posterior tubercle of the atlas
II = Spinous process of the axis

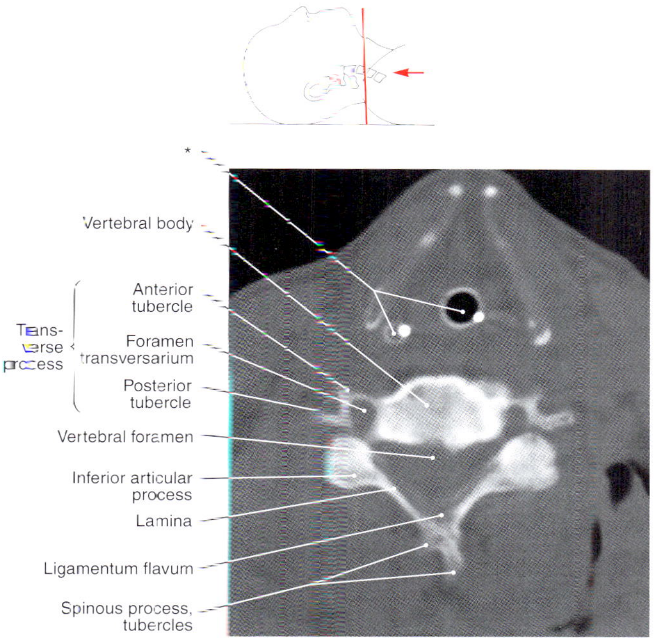

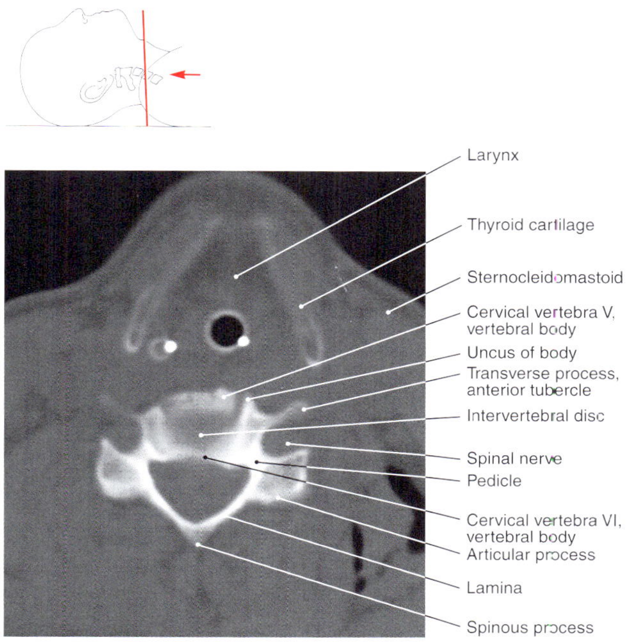

Fig. 539 Cervical part of the vertebral column; computed tomographic cross-section (CT) at the level of the intervertebral disc between the fourth and the fifth cervical vertebra

* Endotracheal tube and endoscope

Fig. 540 Cervical part of the vertebral column; computed tomographic cross-section (CT) at the level of the fifth and the sixth cervical vertebra.

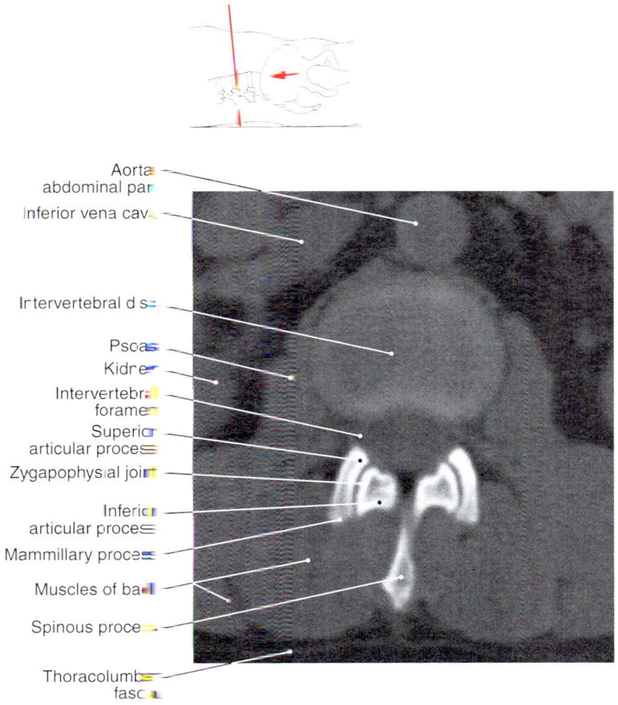

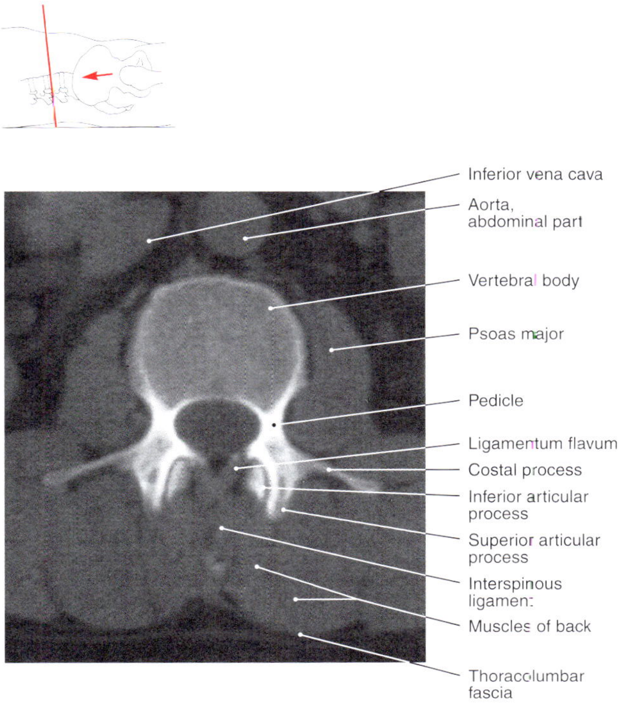

Fig. 541 Lumbar part of the vertebral column; computed tomographic cross-section (CT) at the level of the intervertebral disc between the second and the third lumbar vertebra.

Fig. 542 Lumbar part of the vertebral column; computed tomographic cross-section (CT) at the level of the pedicles of the third lumbar vertebra.

Cutaneous innervation

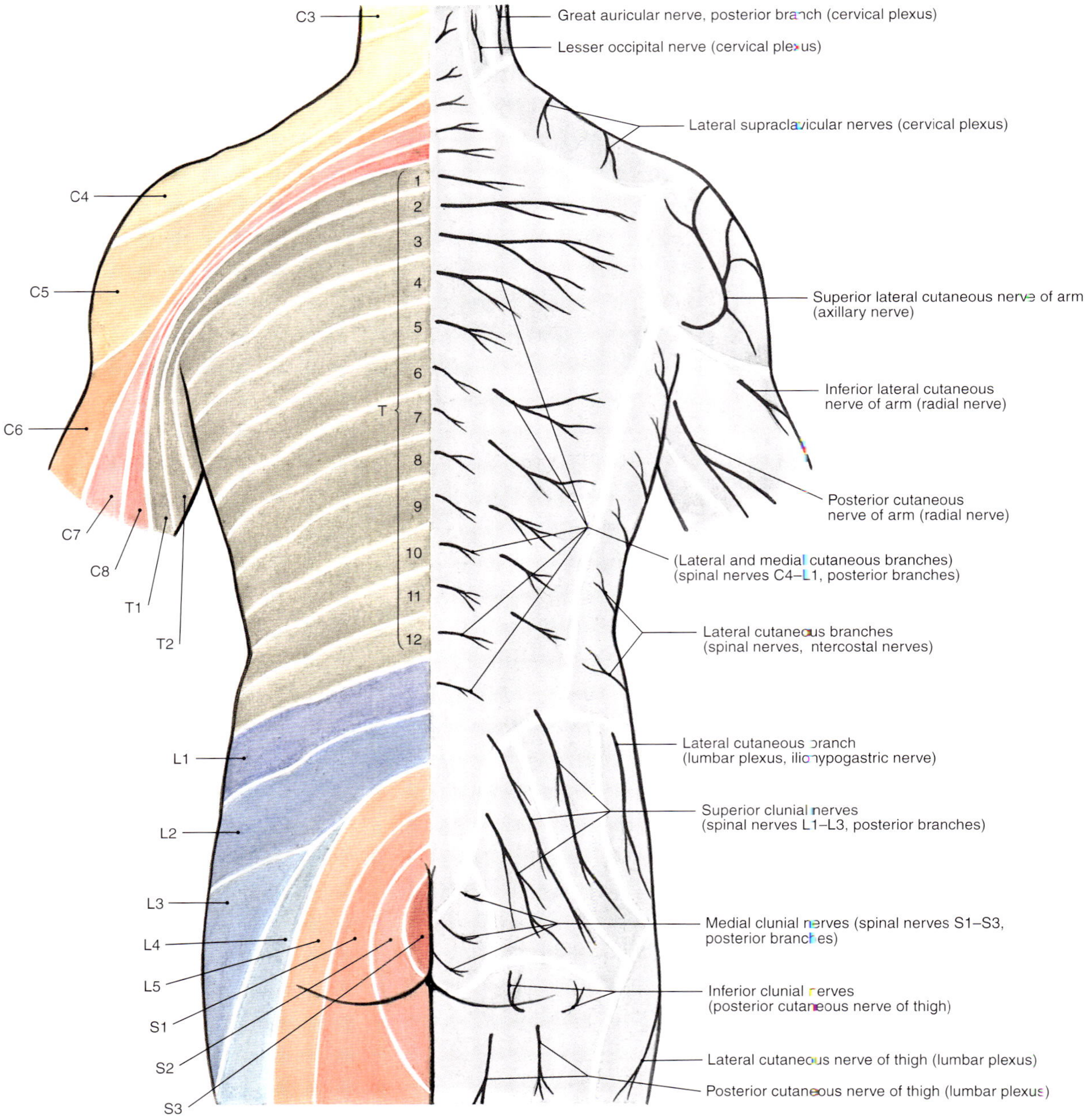

Fig. 543 Segmental cutaneous innervation (dermatomes) and cutaneous nerves of the back.

Vessels and nerves of the back

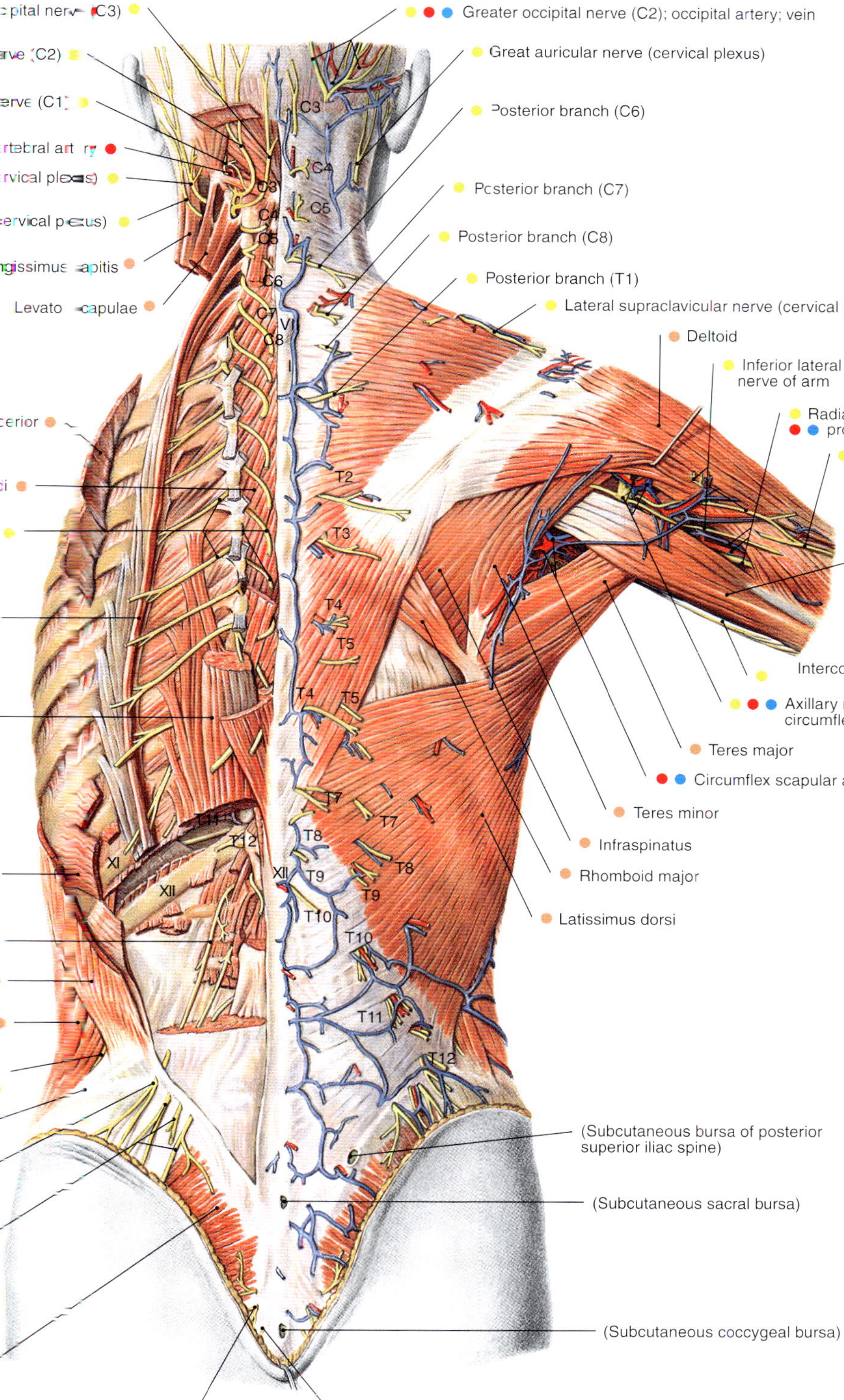

545
546

Fig. 544 Vessels and nerves of the back.
* Vessels and nerves of the triangular space
** Vessels and nerves of the quadrangular space

Vessels and nerves of the posterior cervical region

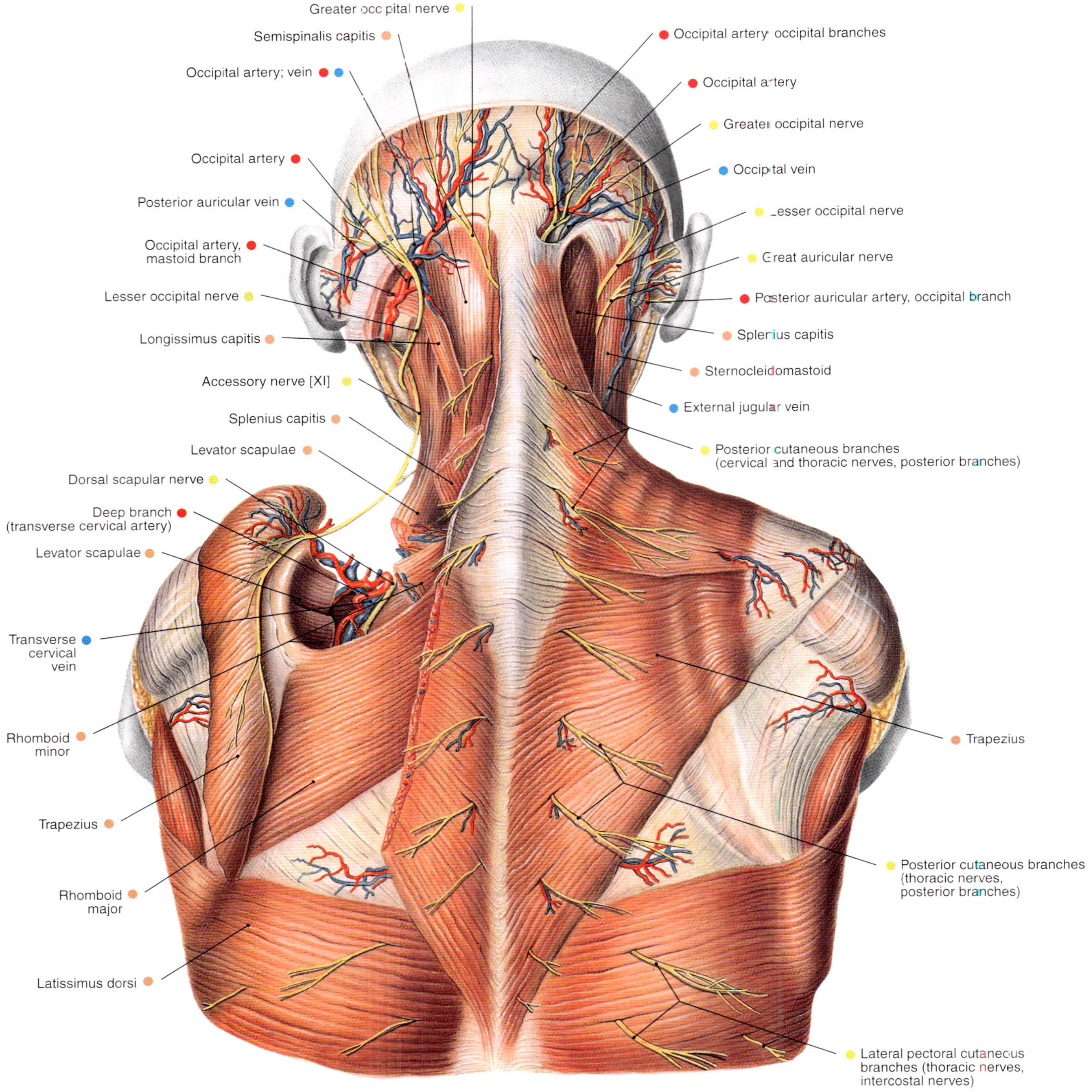

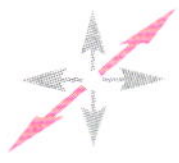

Fig. 545 Vessels and nerves of the occipital region, the posterior cervical region and the upper back.

Vessels and nerves of the posterior cervical region

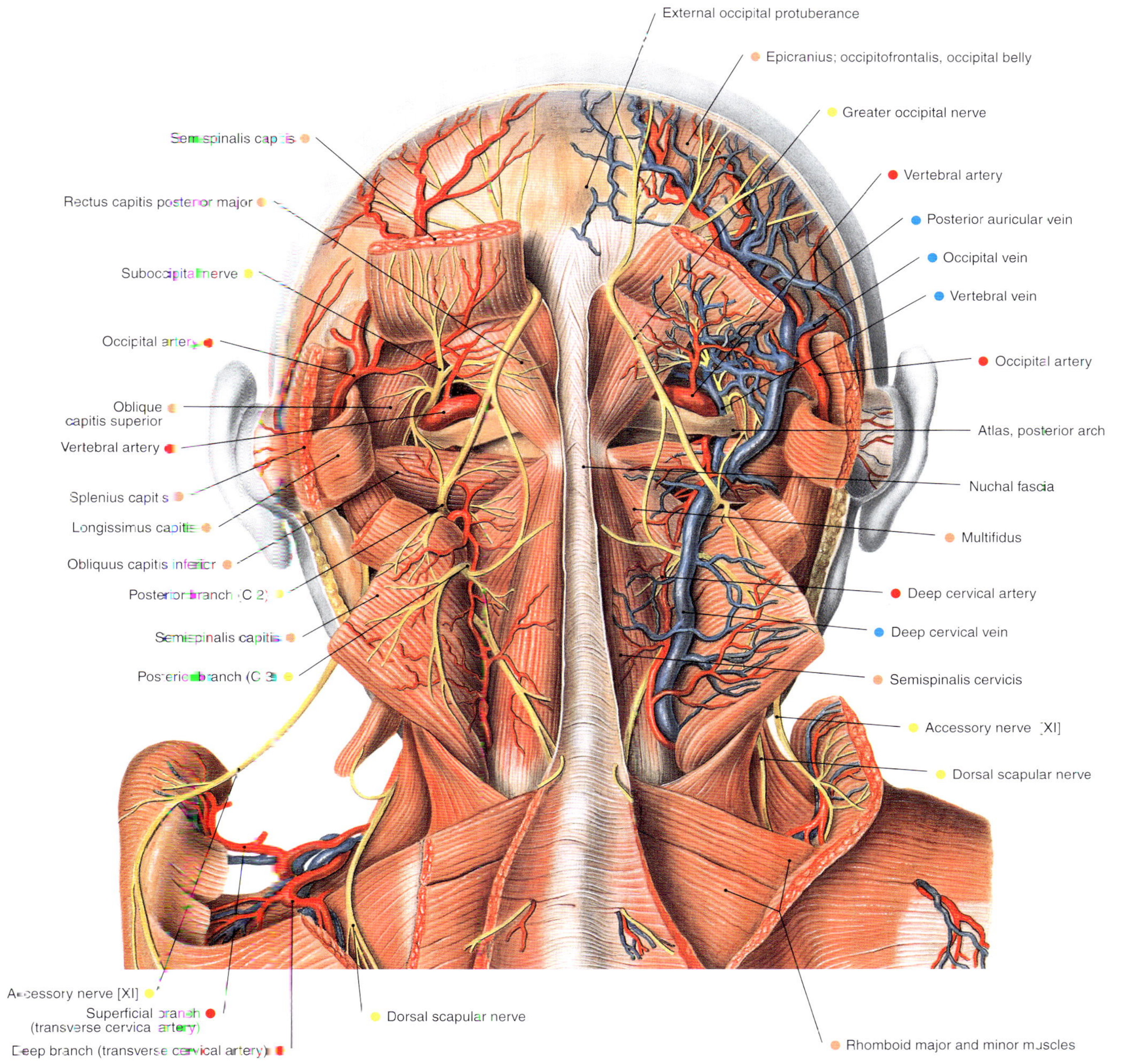

Fig. 546 Vessels and nerves of the occipital region and the posterior cervical region.

547
545

Cervical part of the vertebral canal

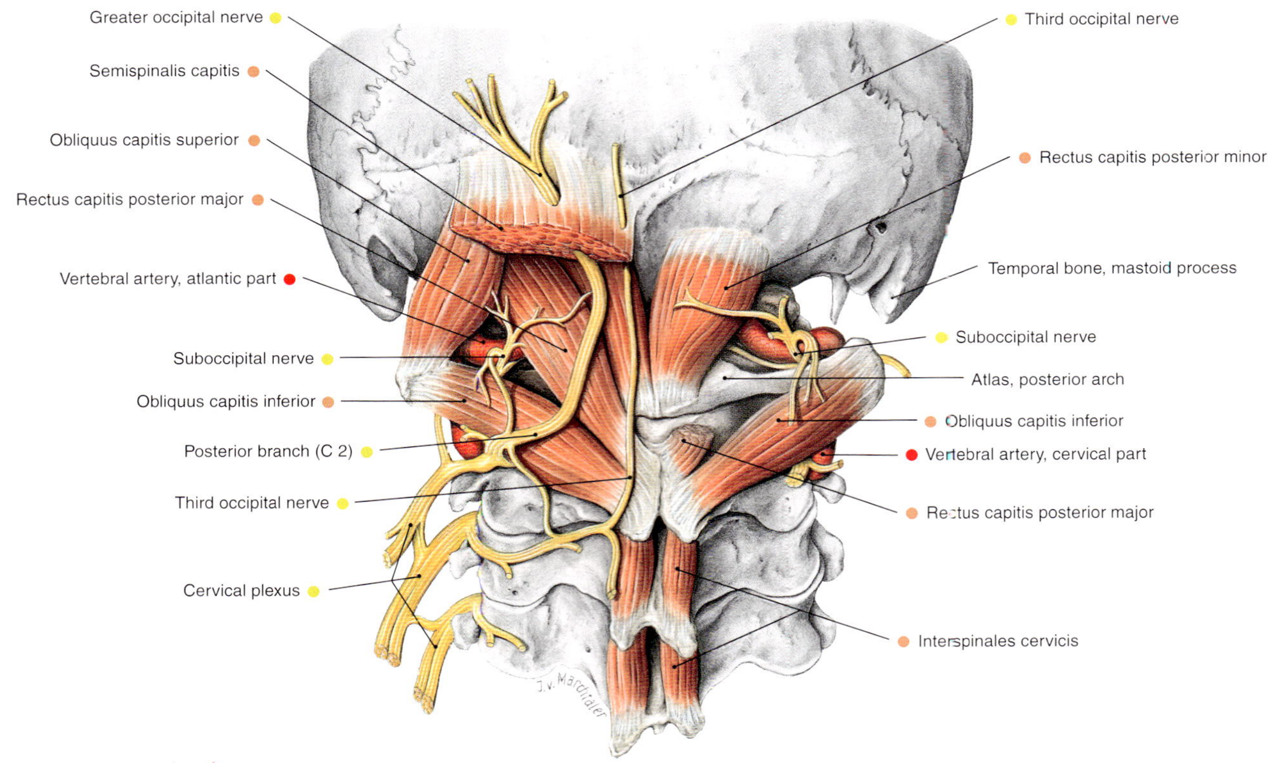

546

Fig. 547 Nerves of the posterior cervical region and the vertebral artery.

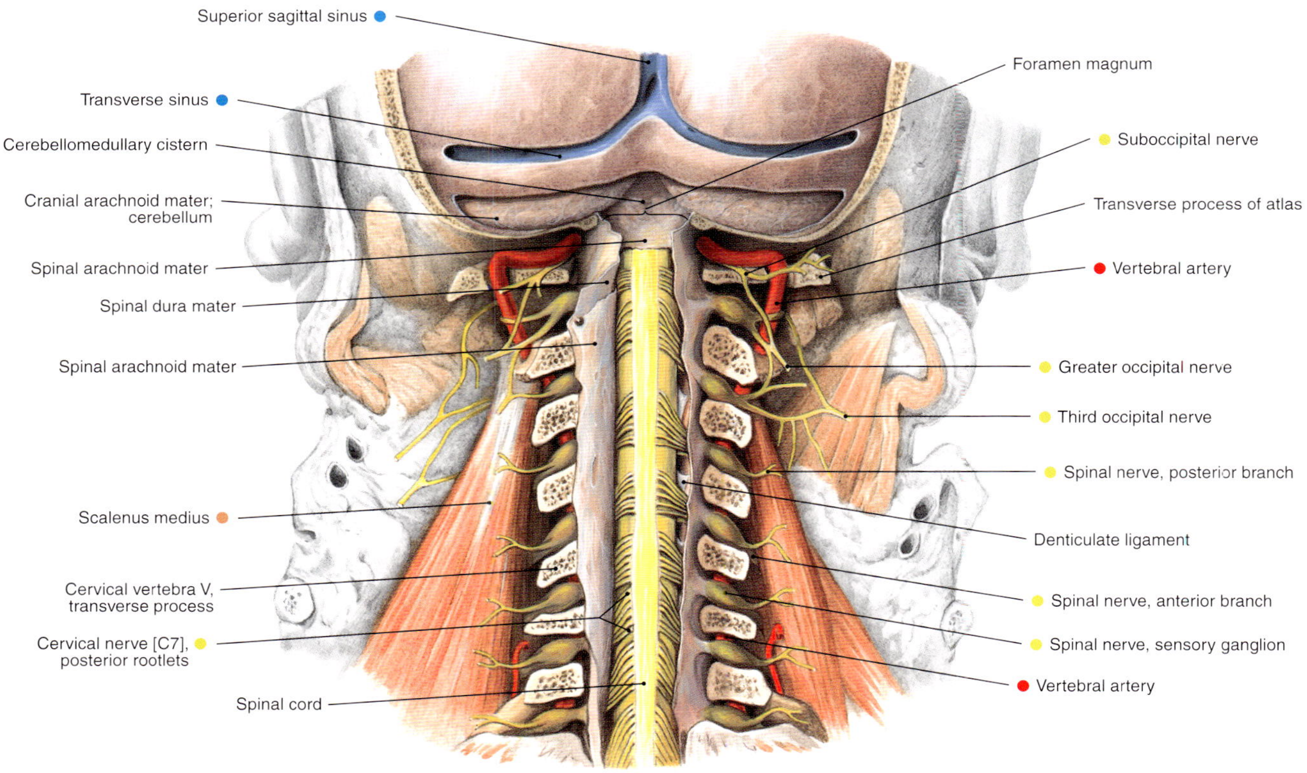

Fig. 548 Vessels and nerves of the deep posterior cervical region and the content of the vertebral canal.

Lumbar part of the vertebral canal

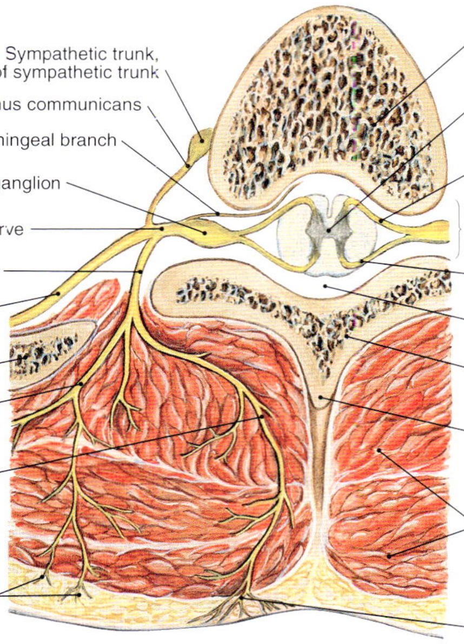

Fig. 549 Spinal nerve; in the thoracic region.

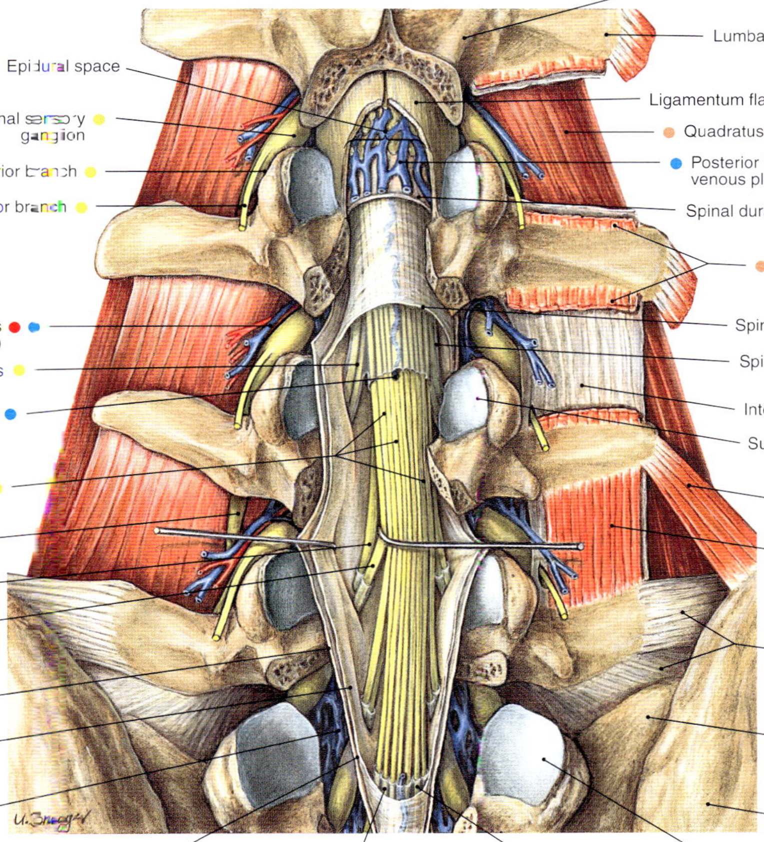

Fig. 550 Vessels and nerves of the lumbar part of the vertebral canal.

Veins and nerves of the lumbar part of the vertebral column

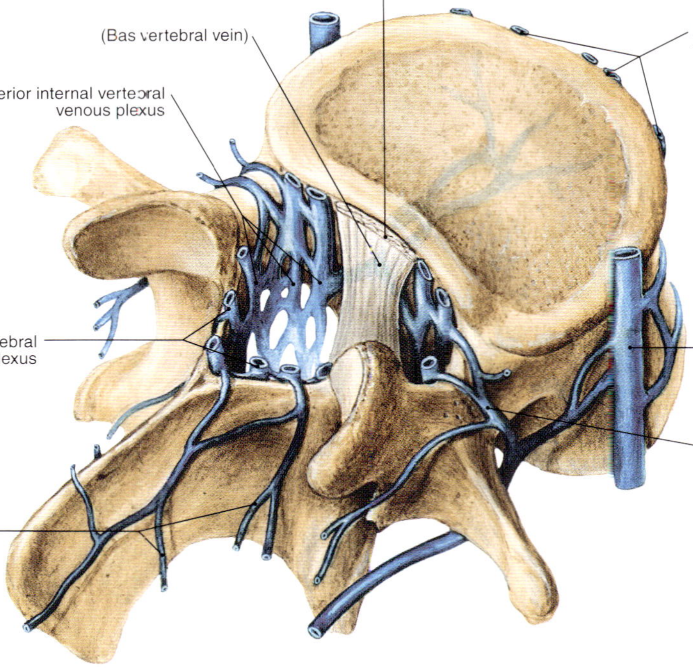

Fig. 551 Veins of the vertebral canal; venous plexus.

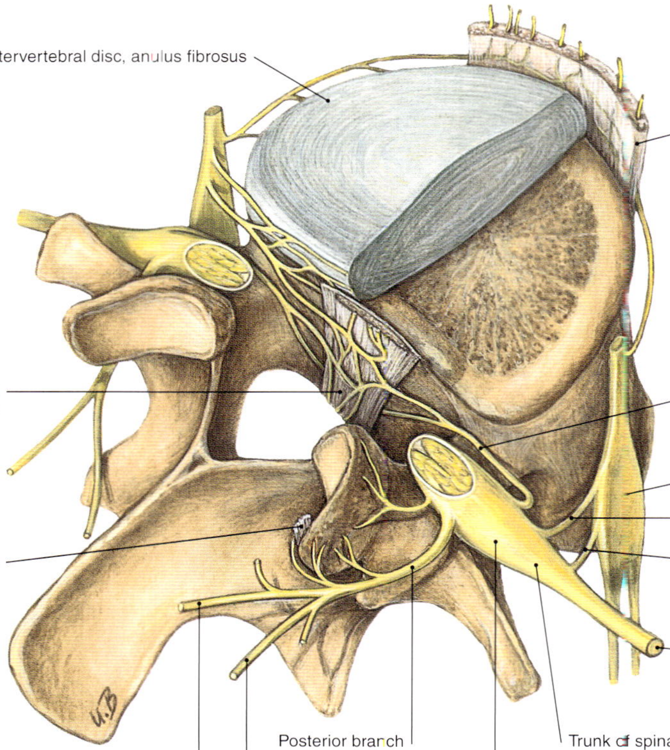

Fig. 552 Nerves of the vertebral column; somatic and autonomous innervation.

Vessels and nerves of the vertebral canal

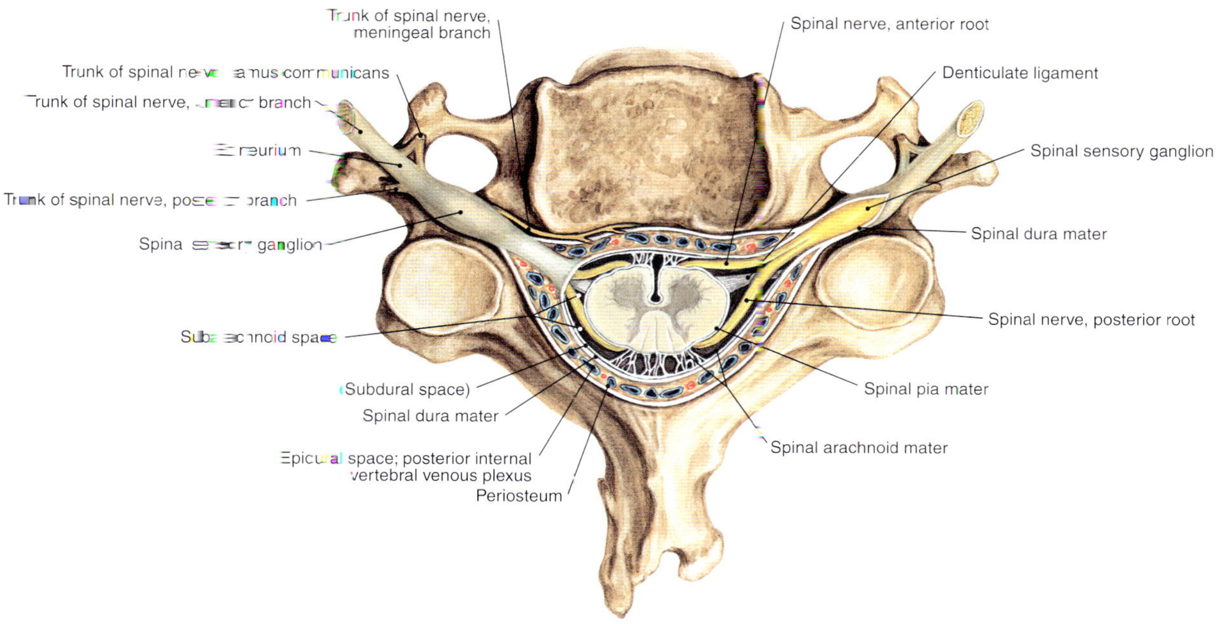

Fig. 553 Content of the vertebral canal; cross-section at the level of the fifth cervical vertebra.

→ 1304 ff

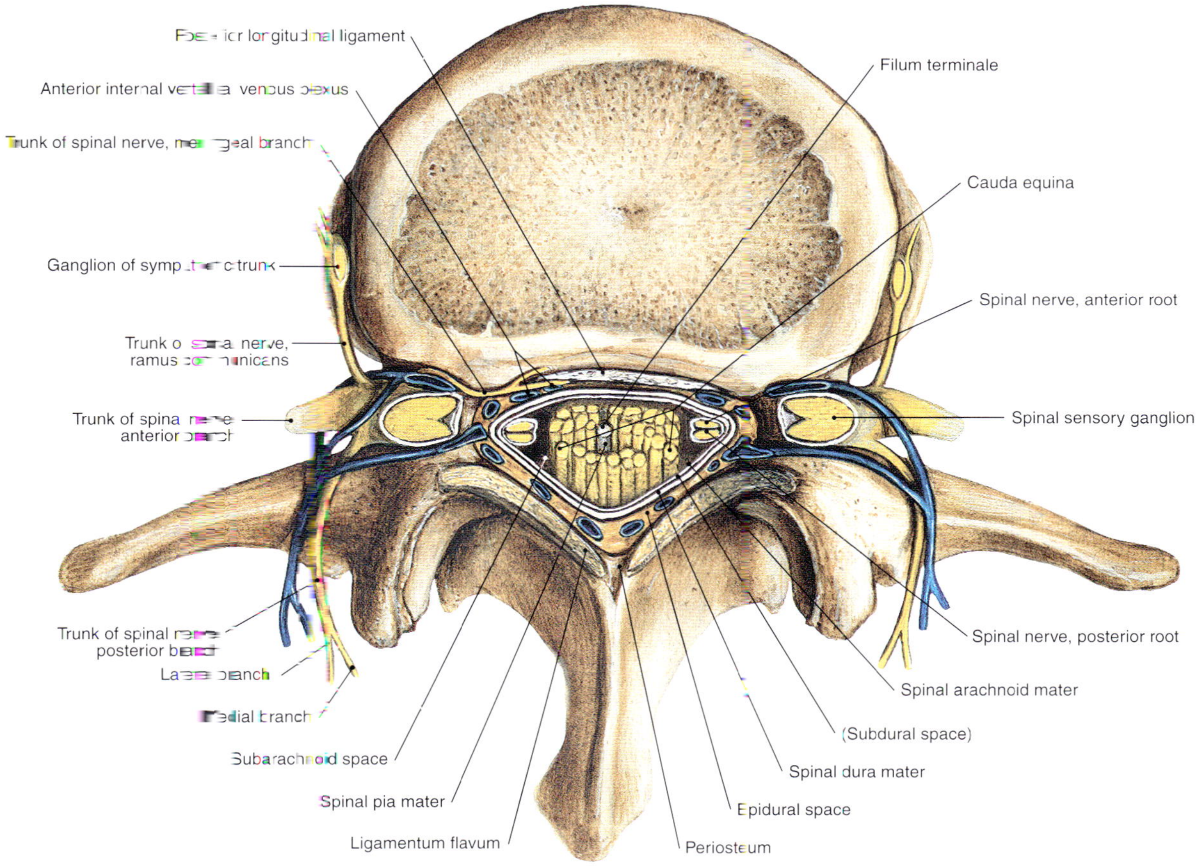

Fig. 554 Content of the vertebral canal; cross-section at the level of the third lumbar vertebra.

→ 1304 ff

Lumbar and sacral puncture

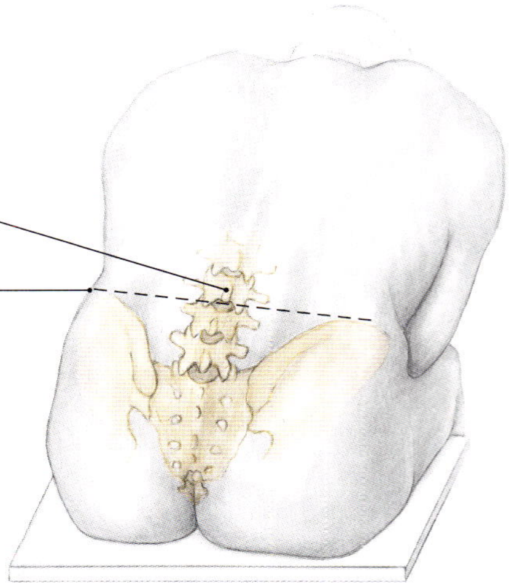

Fig. 555 Lumbar puncture to obtain cerebrospinal fluid or for lumbal anaesthesia; position of the patient.

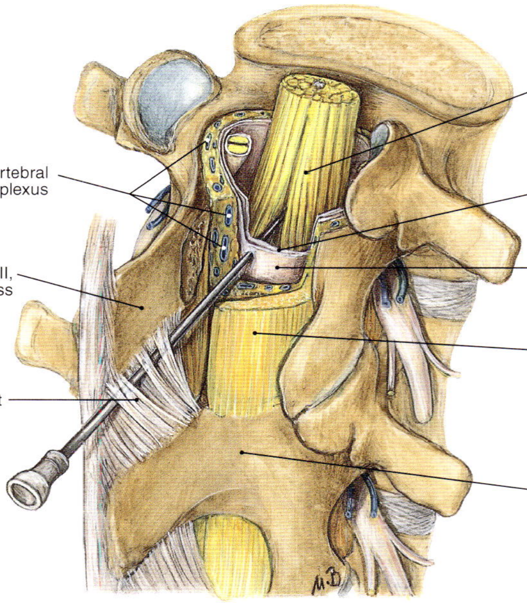

→ 550

Fig. 556 Lumbar puncture; guidance of the puncture needle.

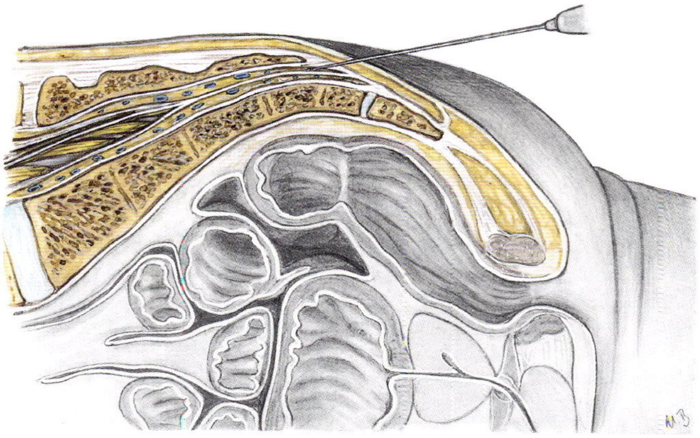

Fig. 557 Sacral puncture; guidance of the puncture needle.

Vessels and nerves of the vertebral canal

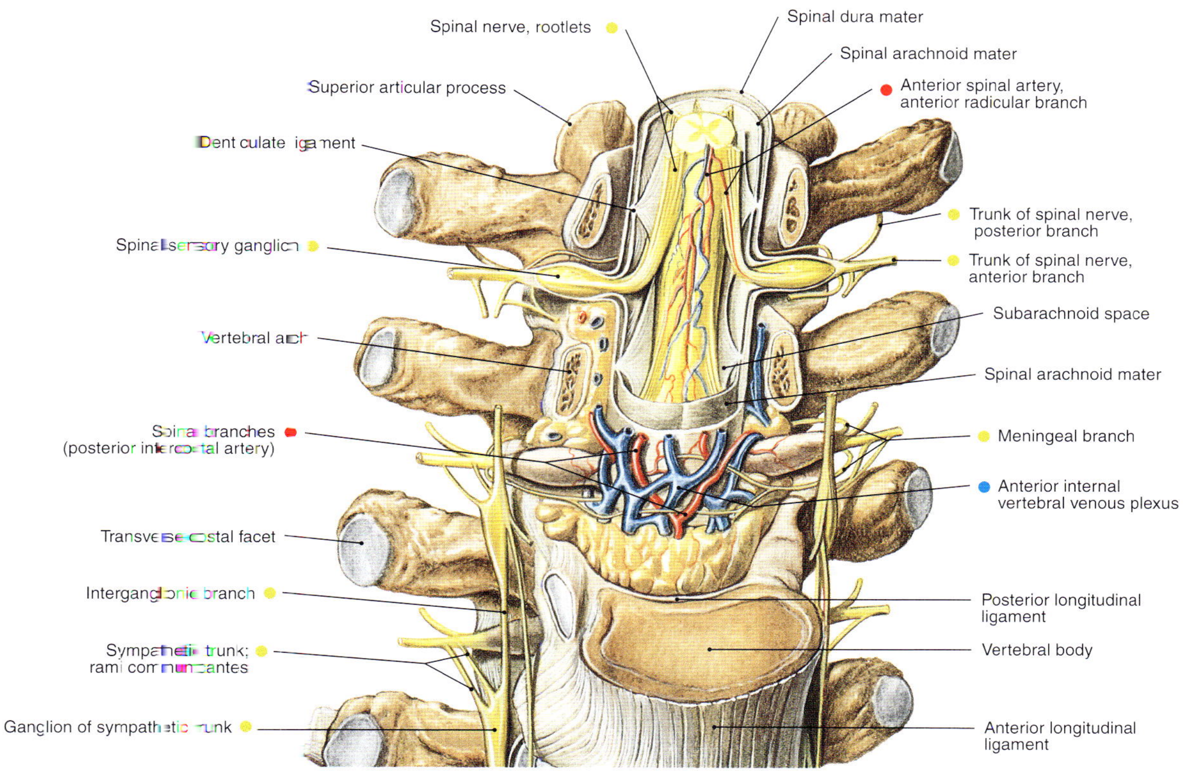

Fig. 558 Content of the vertebral canal; thoracic portion after stepwise exposure; ventral view.

→ 1304 ff

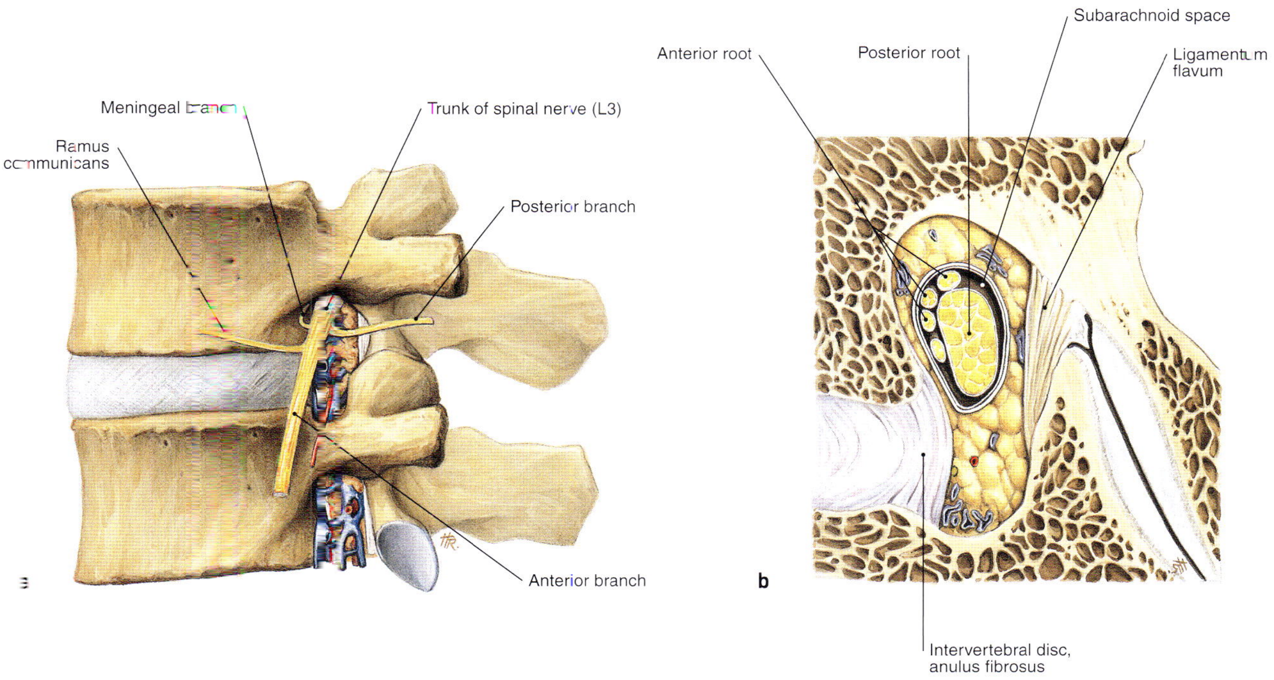

Fig. 559 a, b Intervertebral foramina; lumbar part of the vertebral column.

a Viewed from the left
b Sagittal section

Surface anatomy

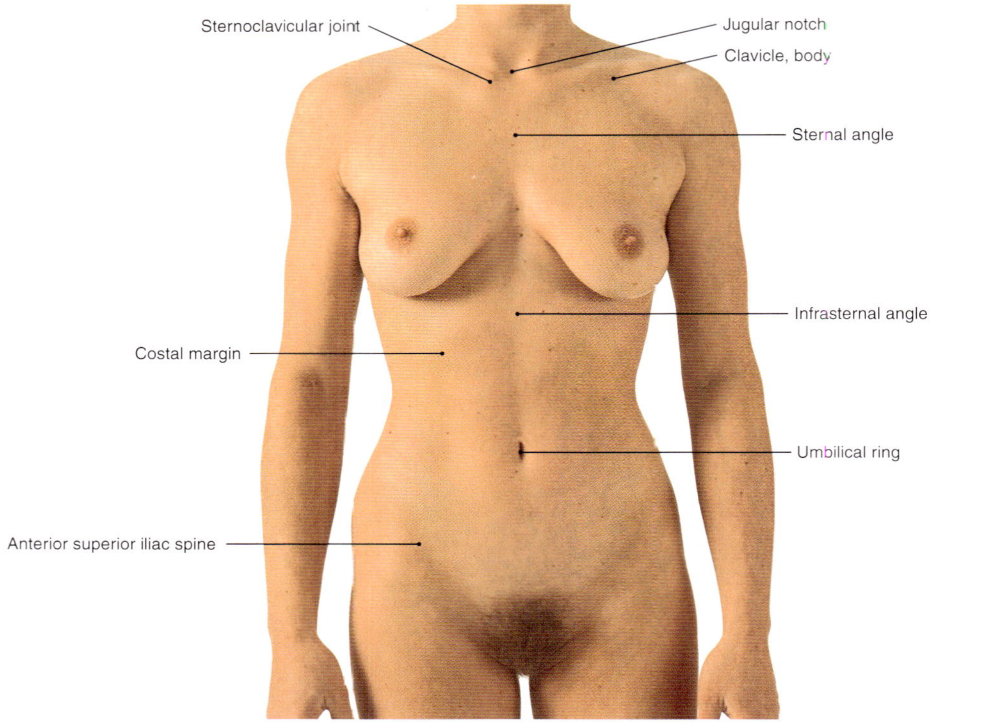

Fig. 560 Surface anatomy of the thoracic and abdominal wall of a young woman.

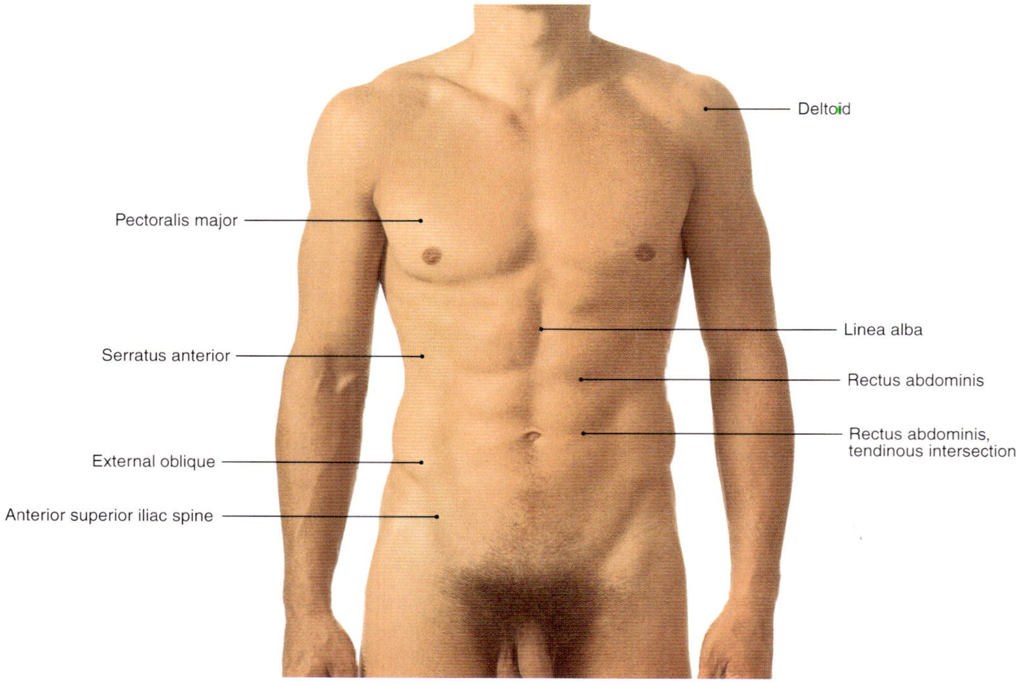

Fig. 561 Surface anatomy of the thoracic and abdominal wall of a young man.

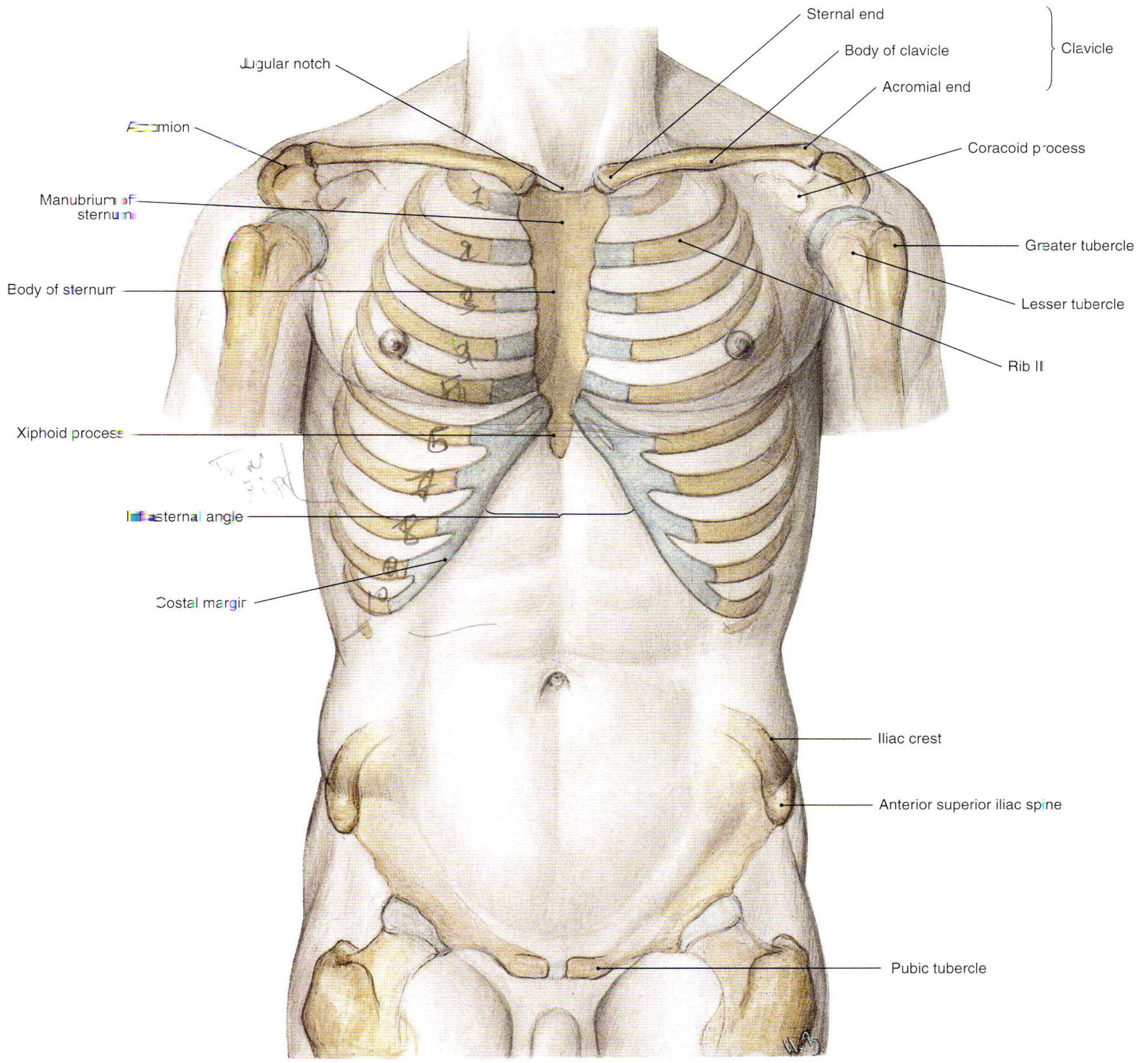

Fig. 562 Projection of the skeleton onto the thoracic and abdominal wall.

Skeleton of the trunk

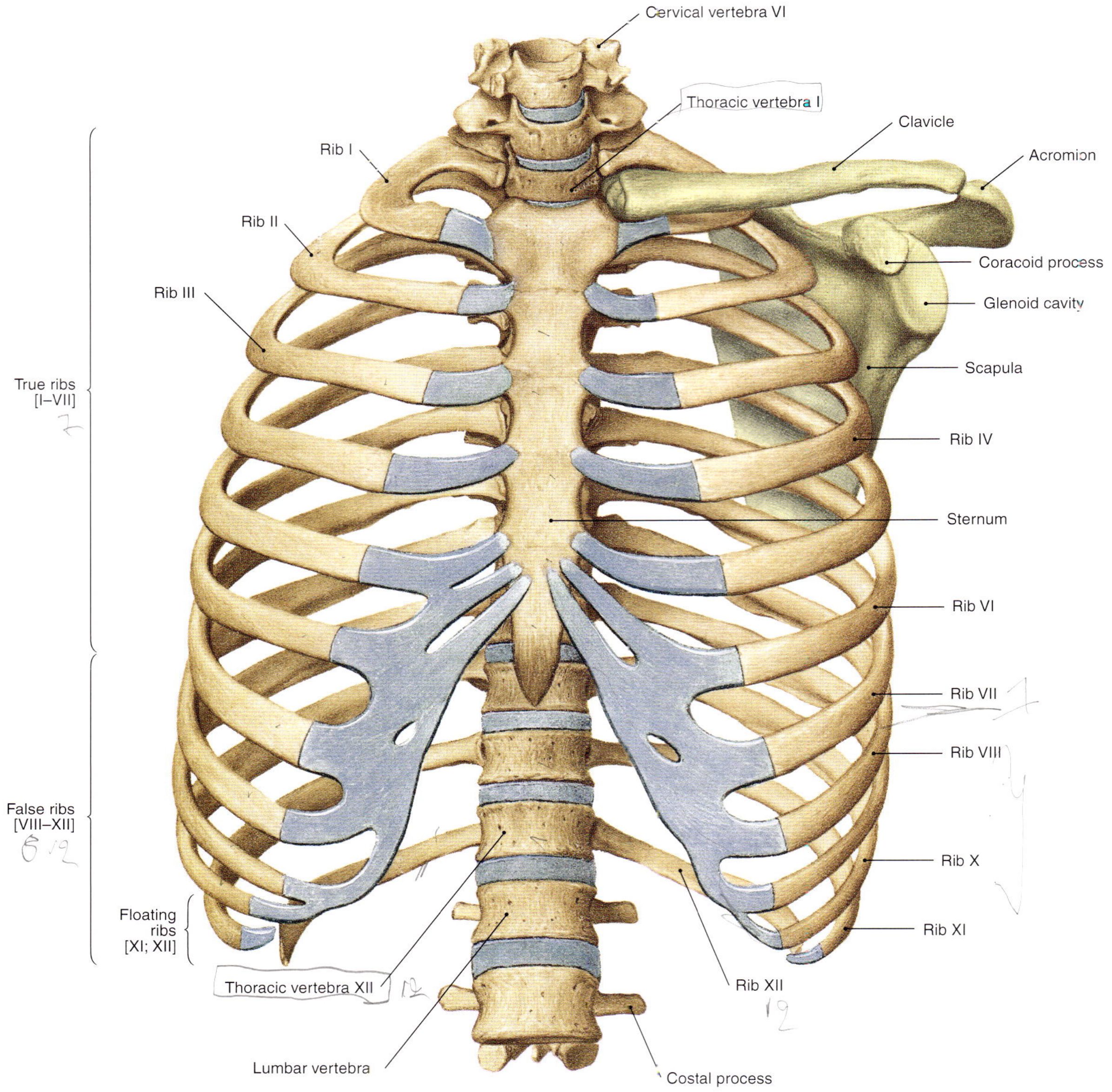

Fig. 563 Thoracic cage and left shoulder girdle.

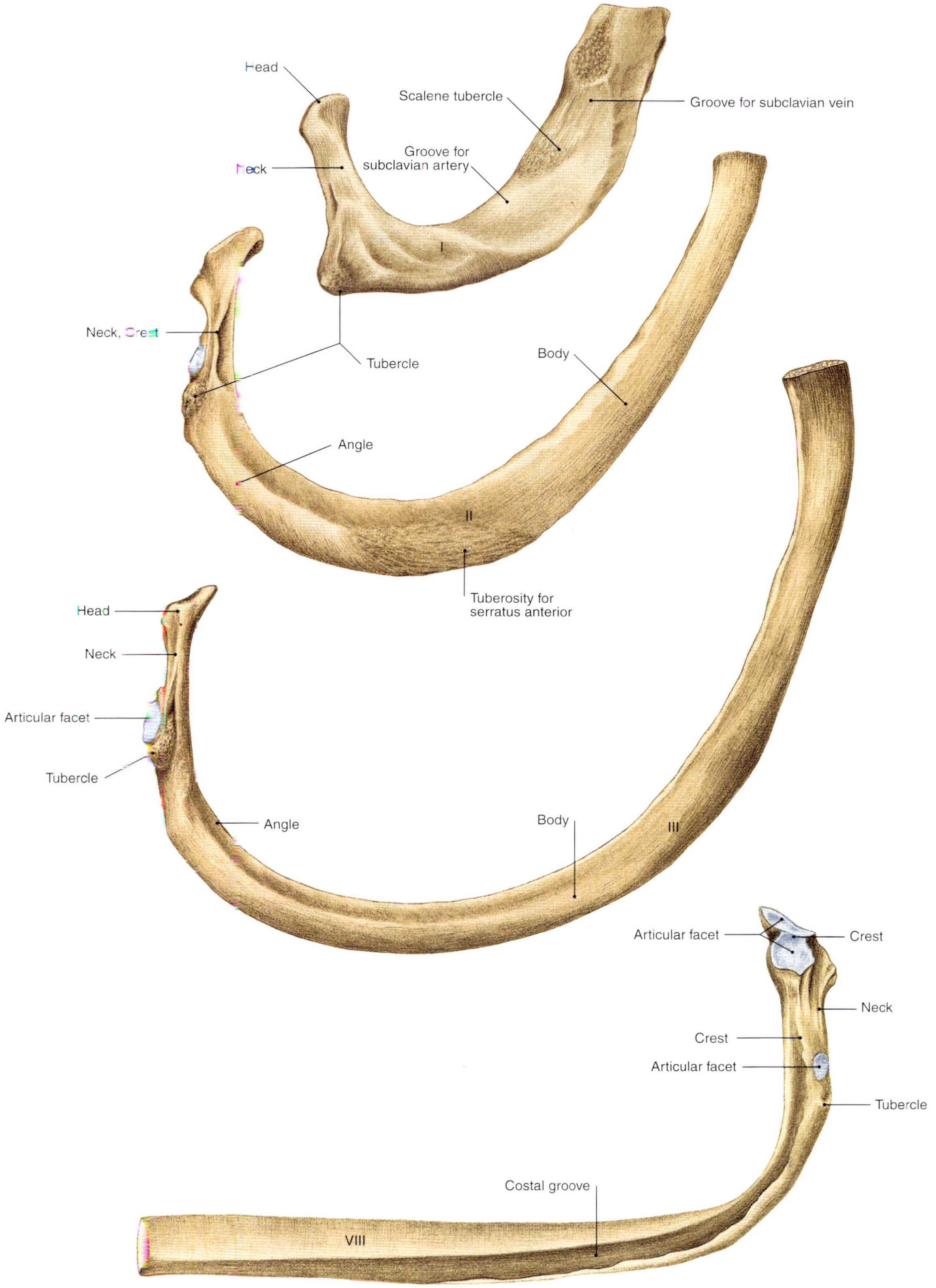

Fig. 564 Ribs;
I.–III. rib, superior view;
VIII. rib, inferior view.

Sternum is made of 3 individual parts
* The most superior part is the manubrium
* The inferior to the manubrium is body of the sternum
* The most inferior portion of sternum is xiphoid process.

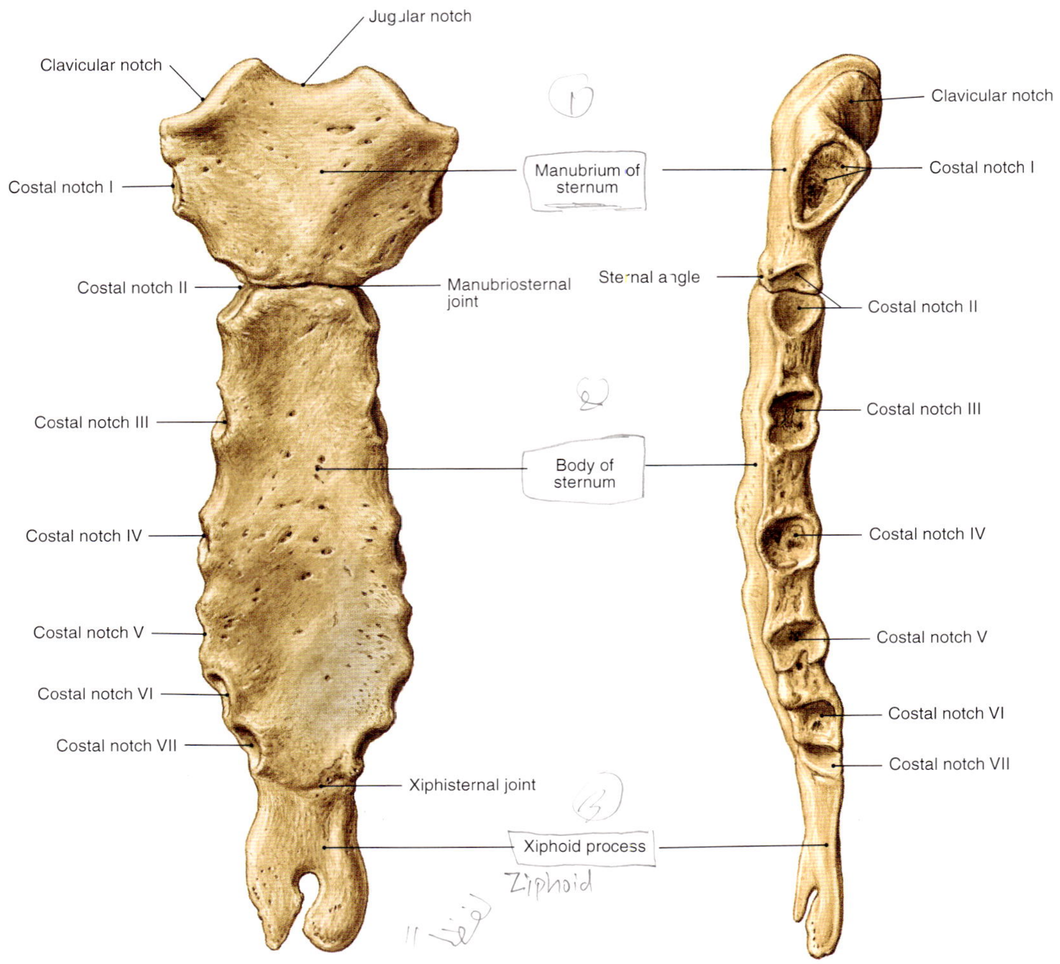

Fig. 565 Sternum.

Fig. 566 Sternum.

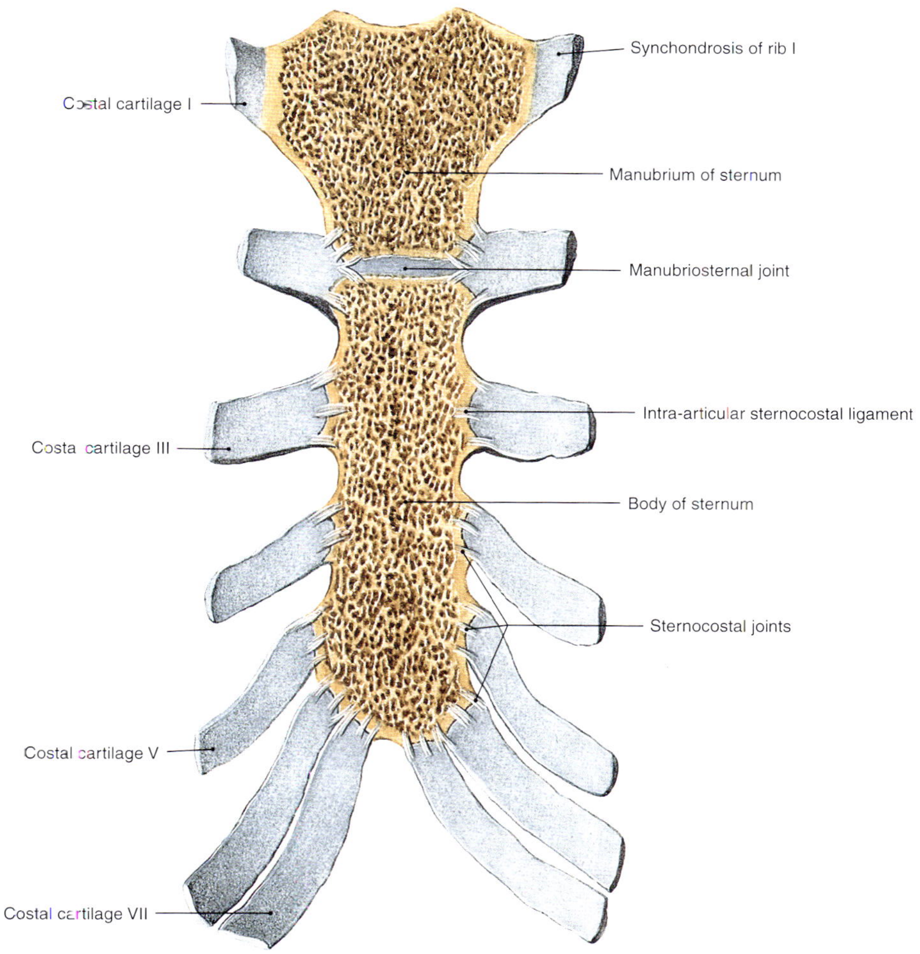

Fig. 567 Sternum and costal cartilages; section.

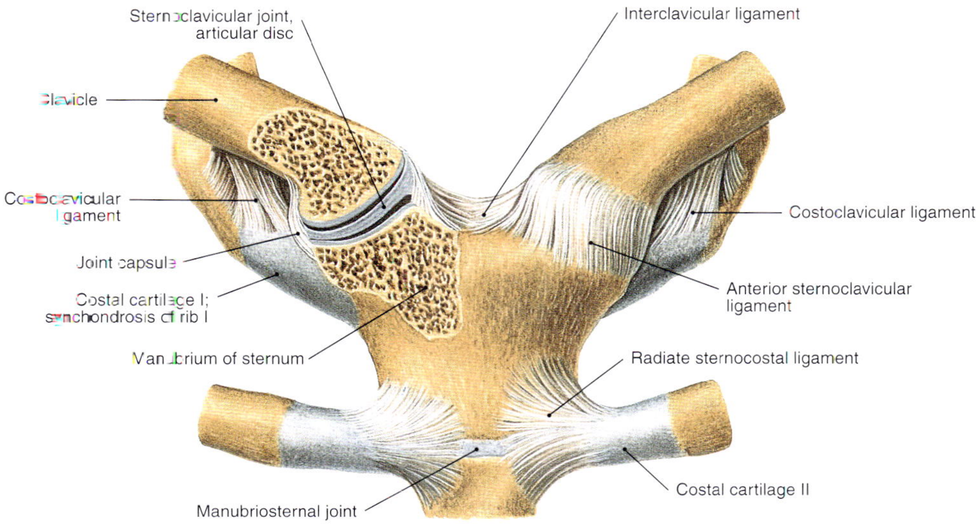

Fig. 568 Sternoclavicular joint.

Muscles of the thoracic and the abdominal wall

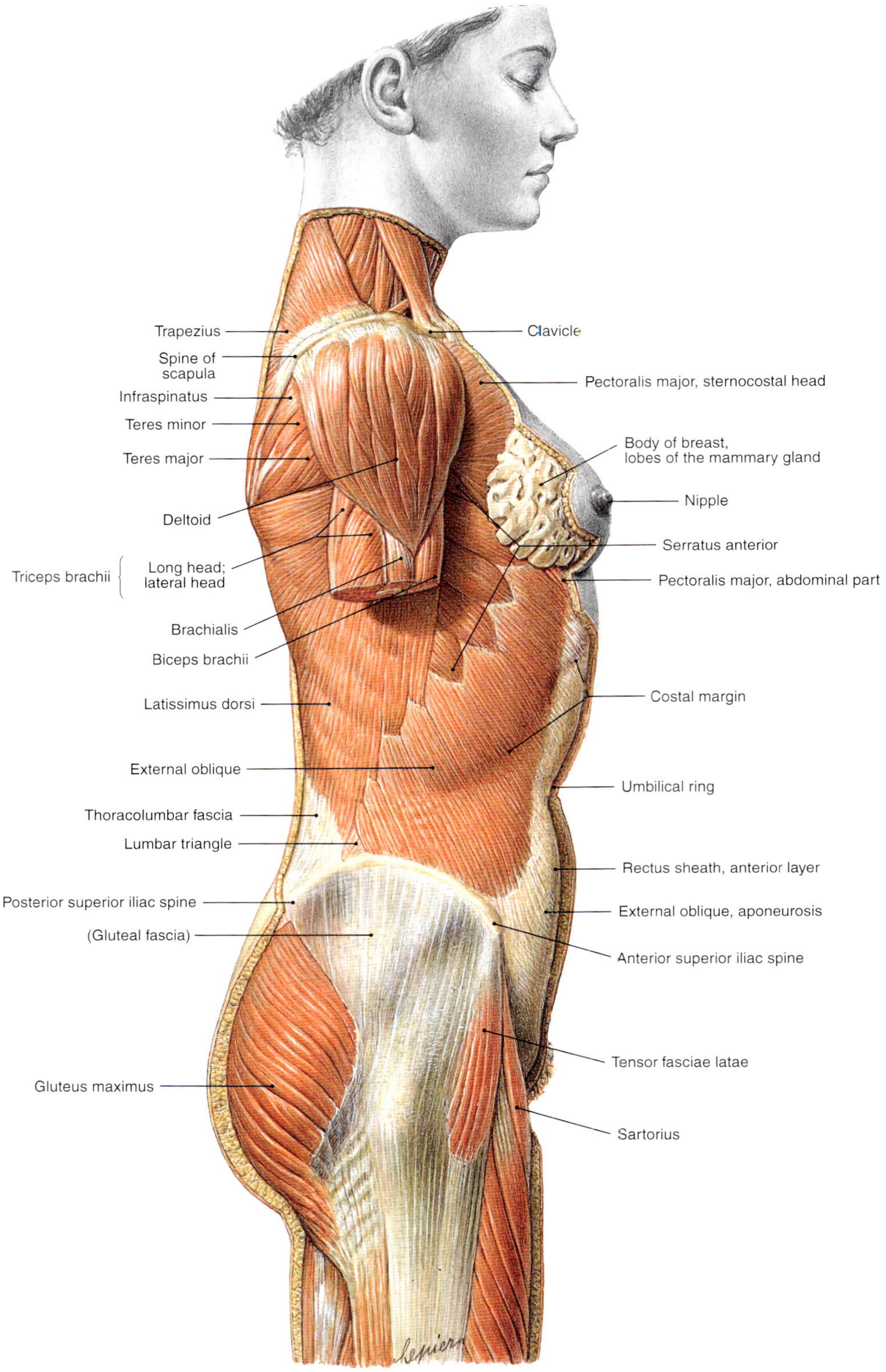

→ T 15, T 17, T 18, T 26

Fig. 569 Muscles of the thoracic and the abdominal wall.

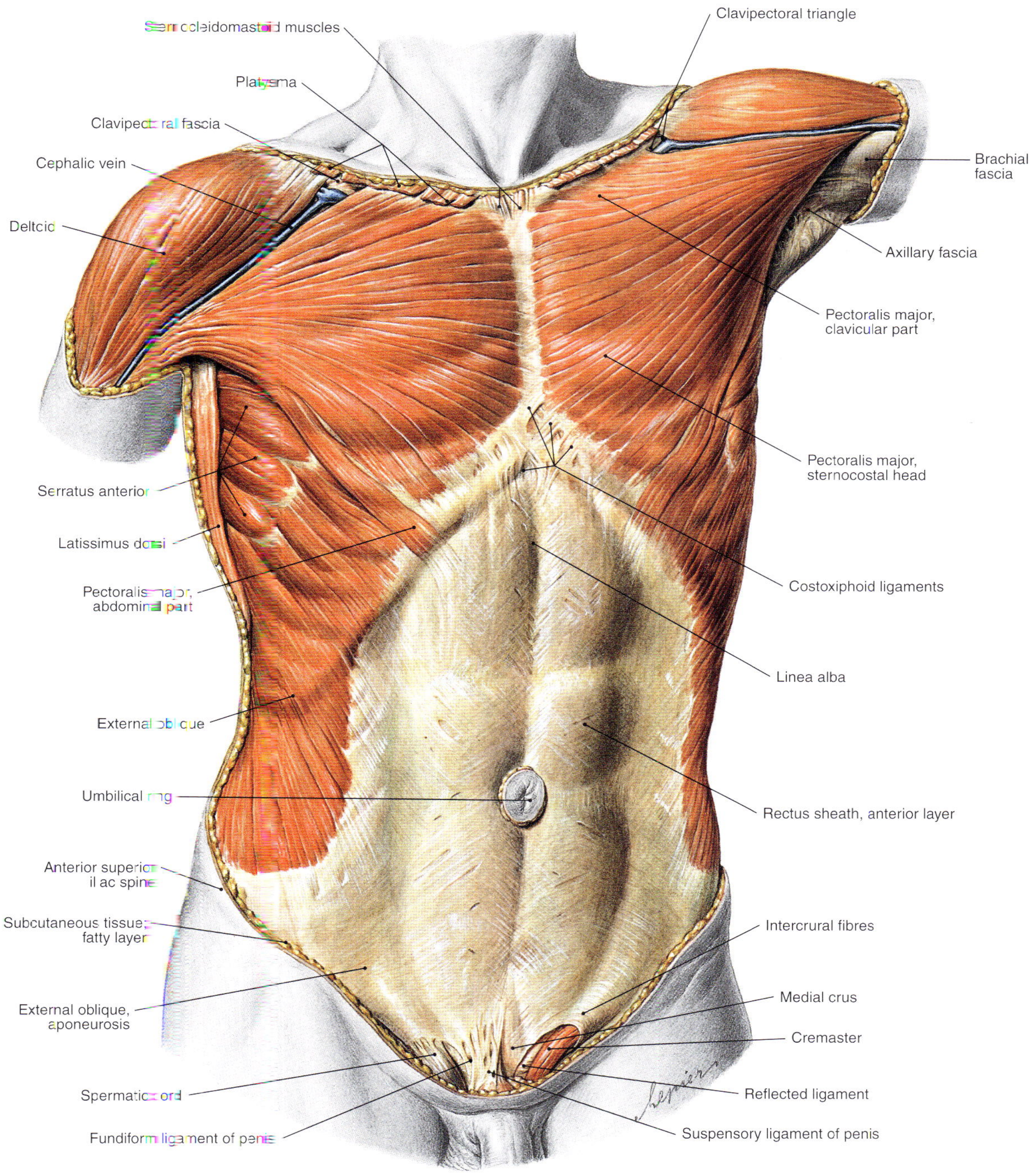

Fig. 570 Muscles of the thoracic and the abdominal wall; superficial layer.

→ T 15, T 17, T 18, T 26

Muscles of the thoracic and the abdominal wall

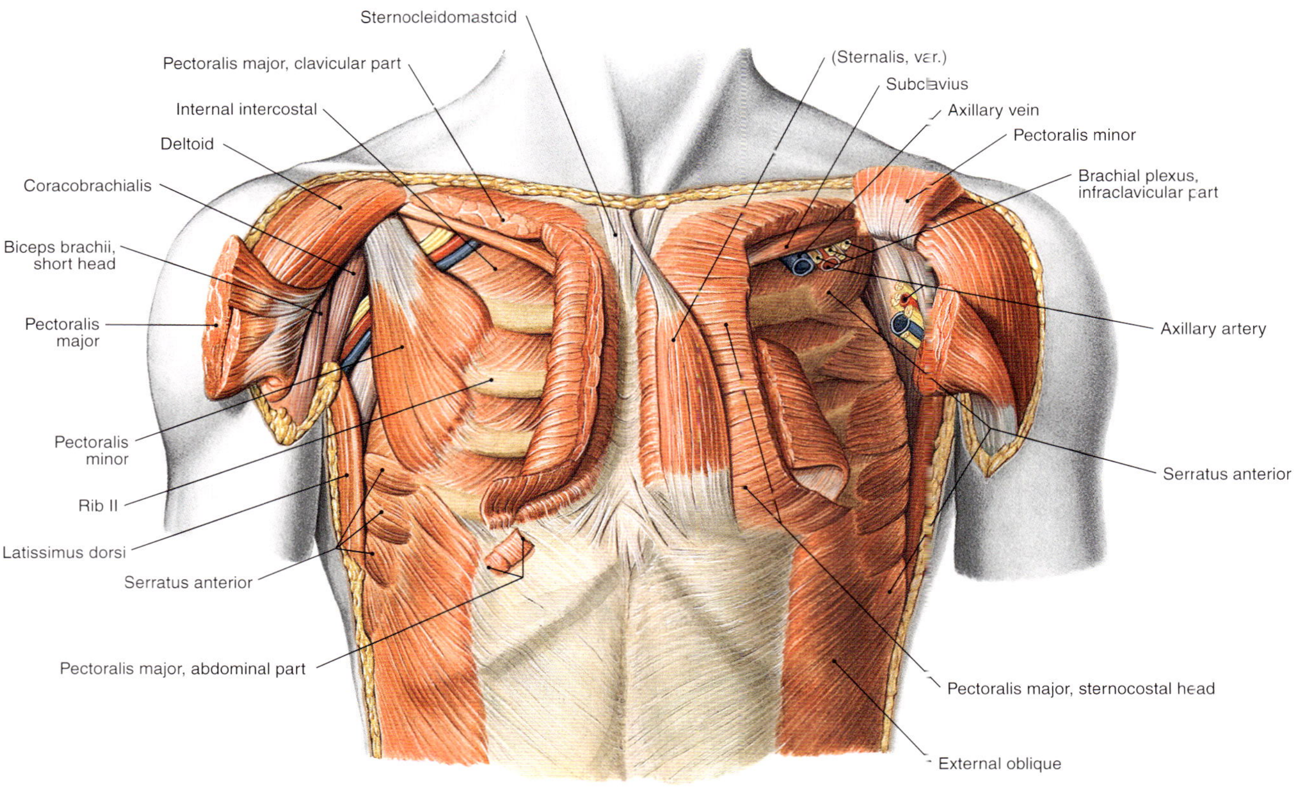

→ T 13, T 15, T 26

Fig. 571 Muscles of the thoracic wall.

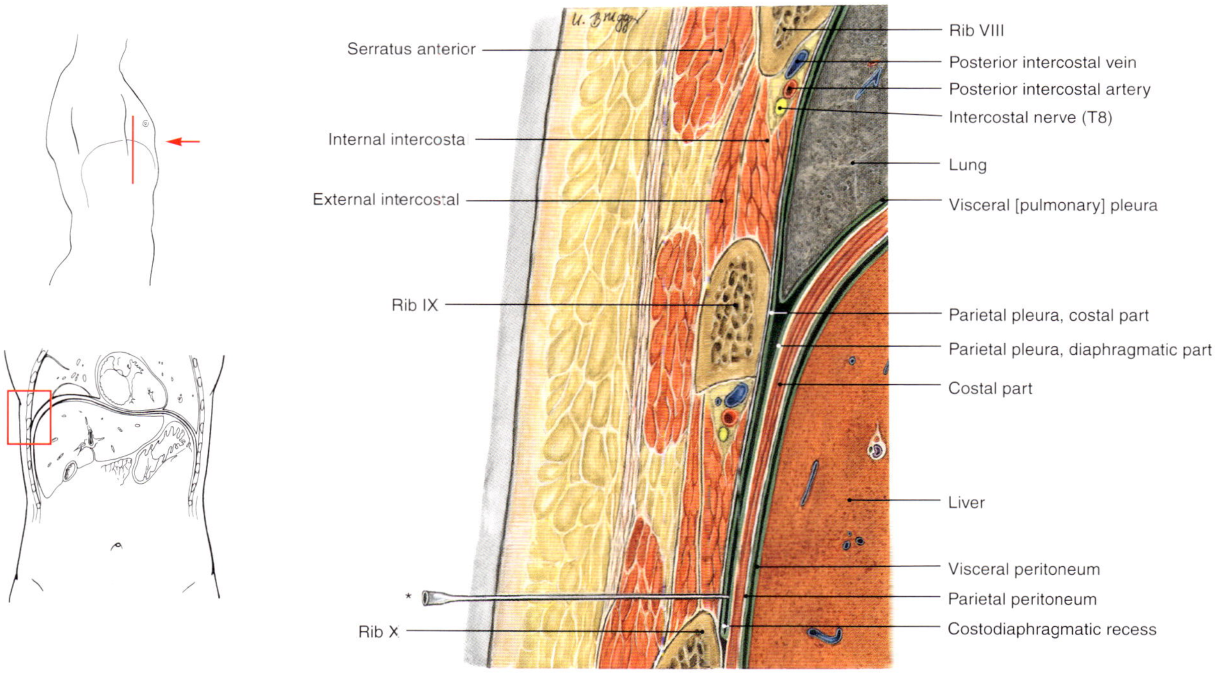

→ T 13

Fig. 572 Muscles of the thoracic wall; frontal section.

* Position of the needle for puncture of the pleural cavity (pleurocentesis)

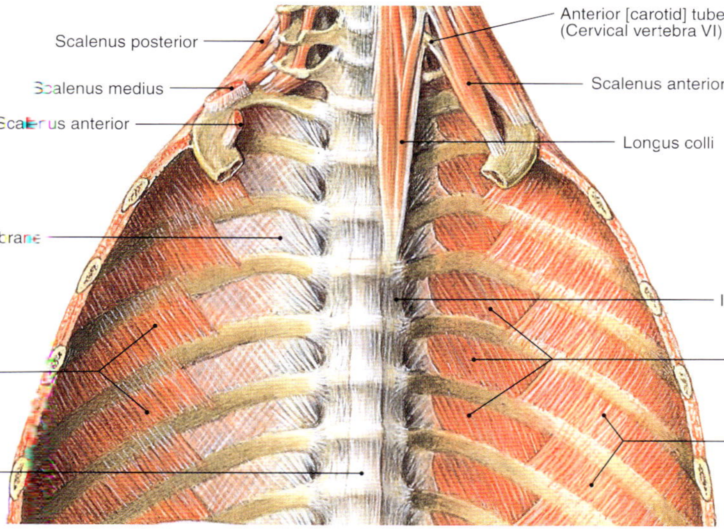

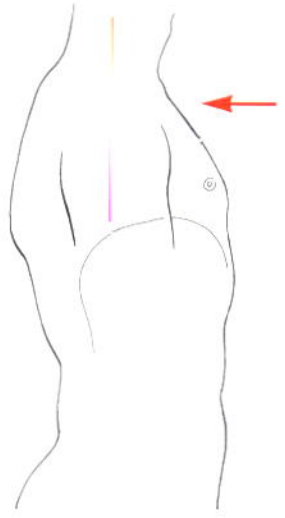

Fig. 573 Thoracic cage; posterior wall.

→ T 11–T 13

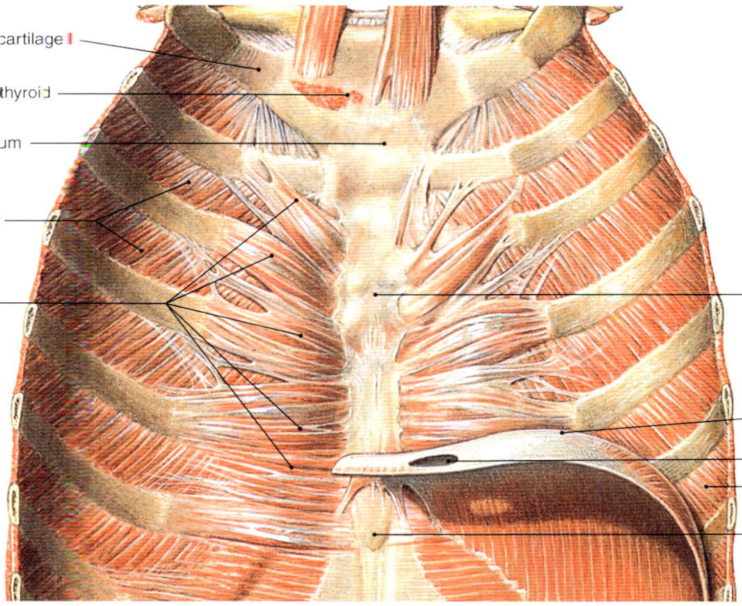

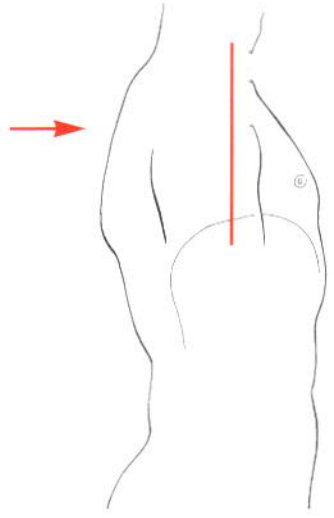

Fig. 574 Thoracic cage; anterior wall.

→ T 13

Abdominal muscles

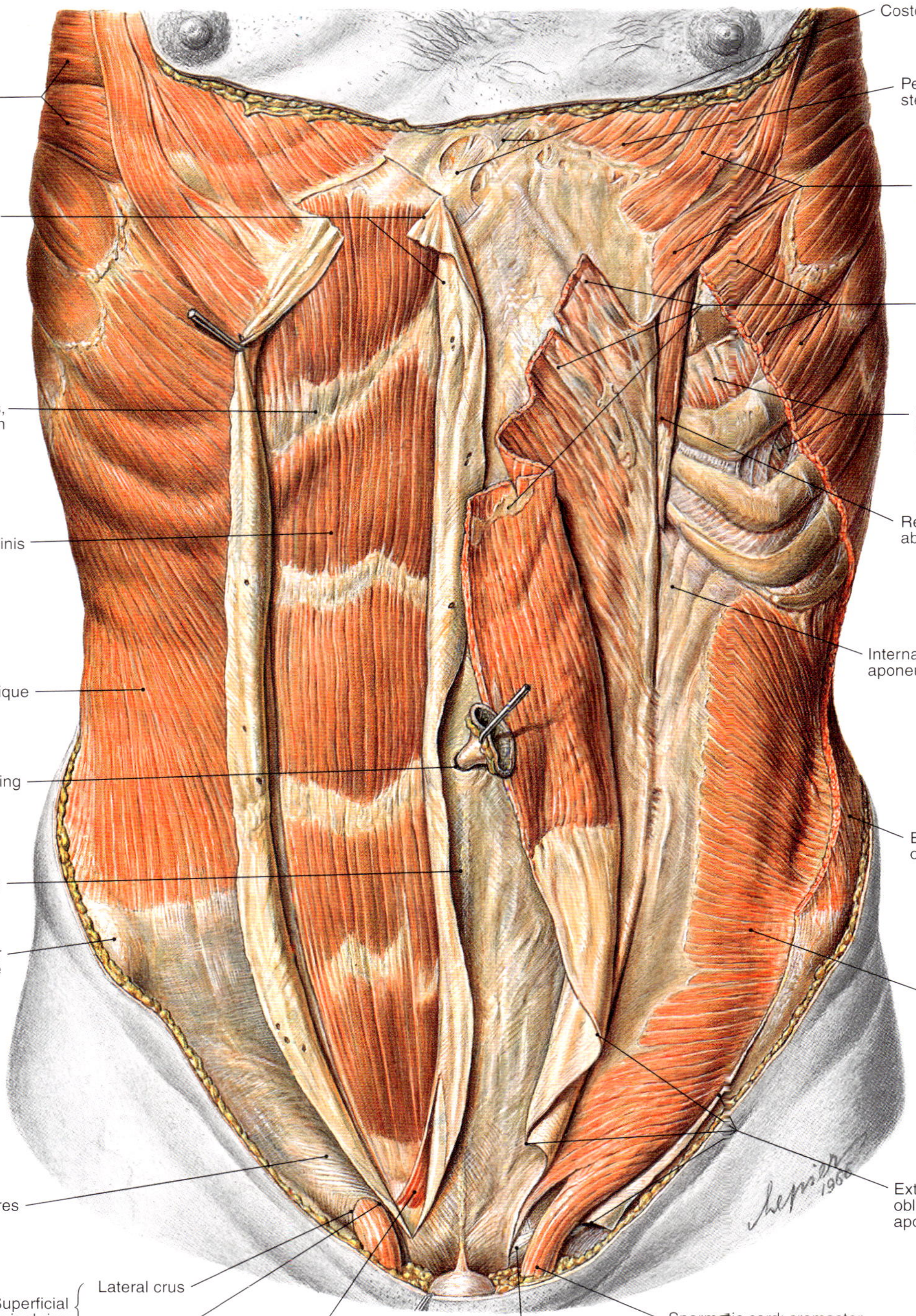

→ T 13–T 15, T 17, T 26

Fig. 575 Muscles of the abdominal wall; superficial and middle layer.

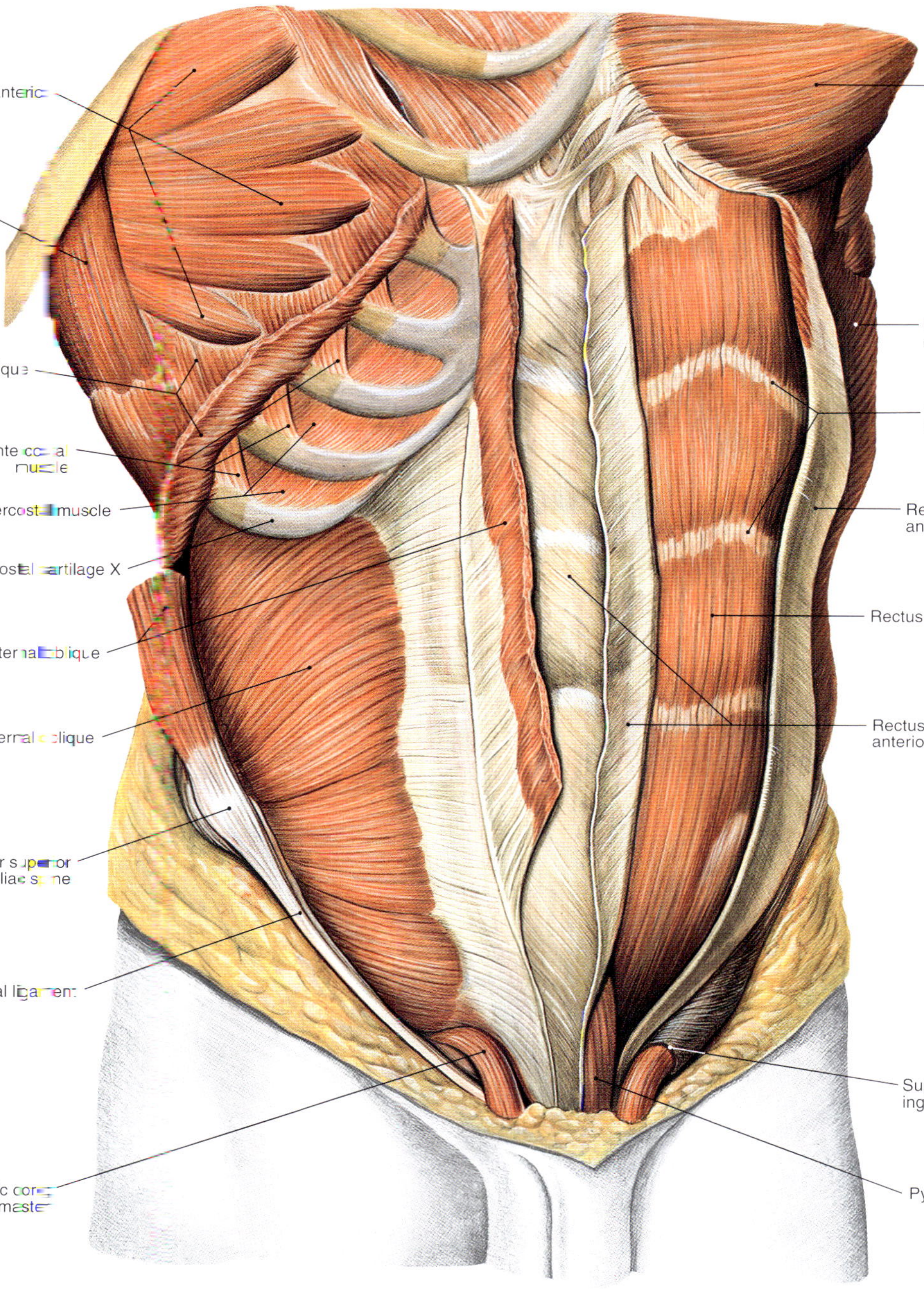

Fig. 576 Muscles of the abdominal wall; middle layer.

→ T 13–T 15, T 17

Abdominal muscles

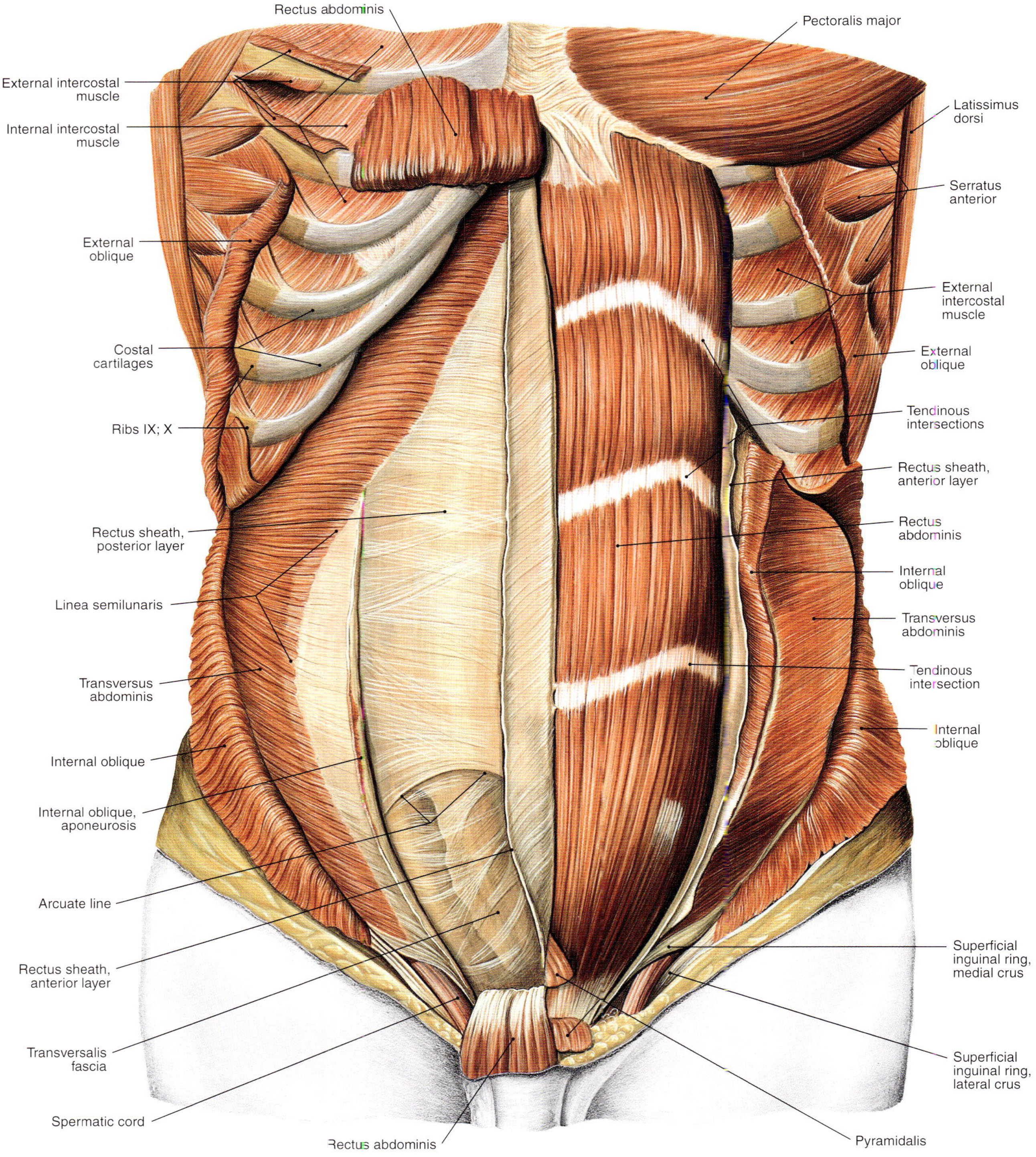

→ T 13–T 15

Fig. 577 Muscles of the abdominal wall; deep layer.

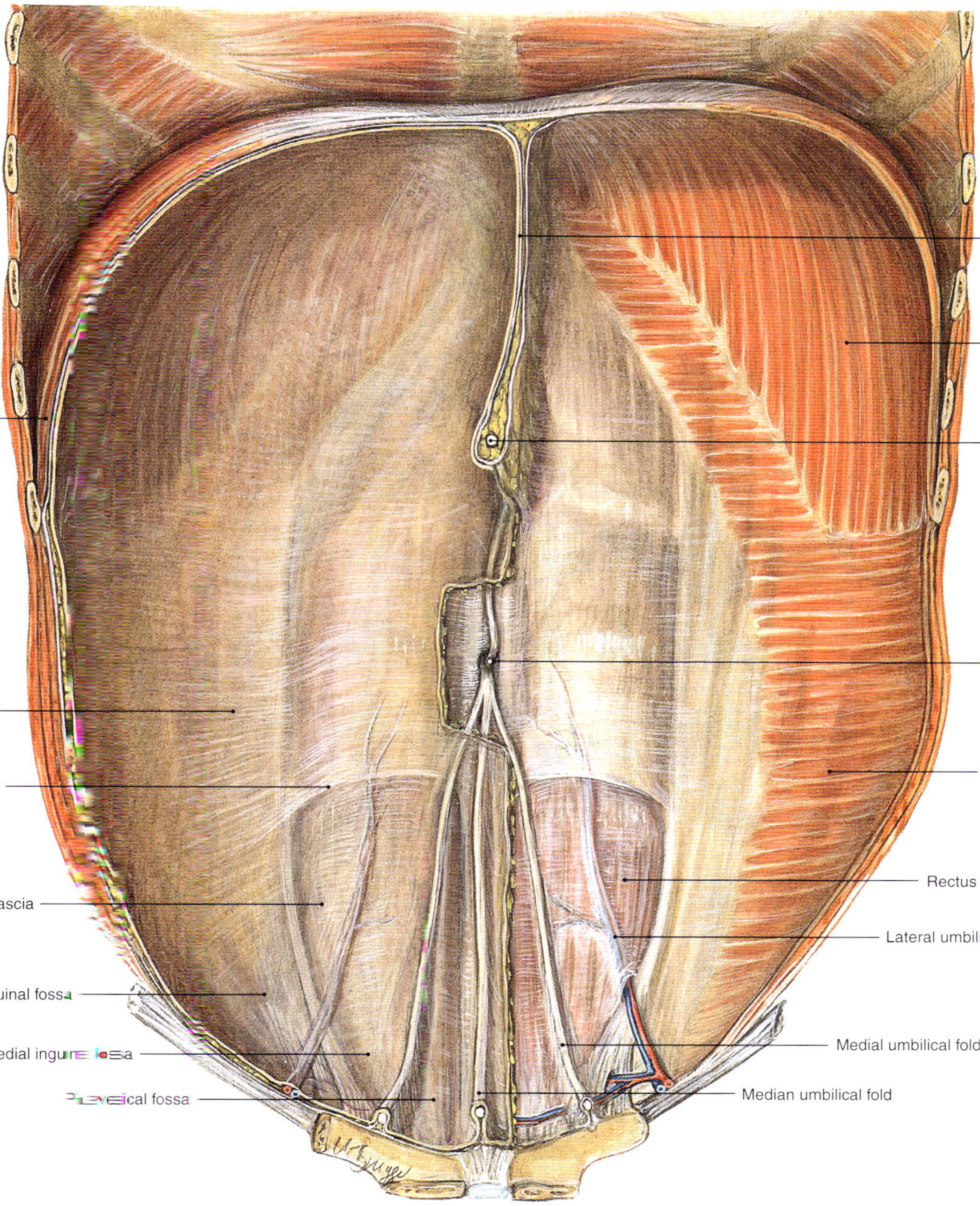

Fig. 578 Internal surface of the anterior abdominal wall.

→ T 14, T 15, T 21

Inguinal canal

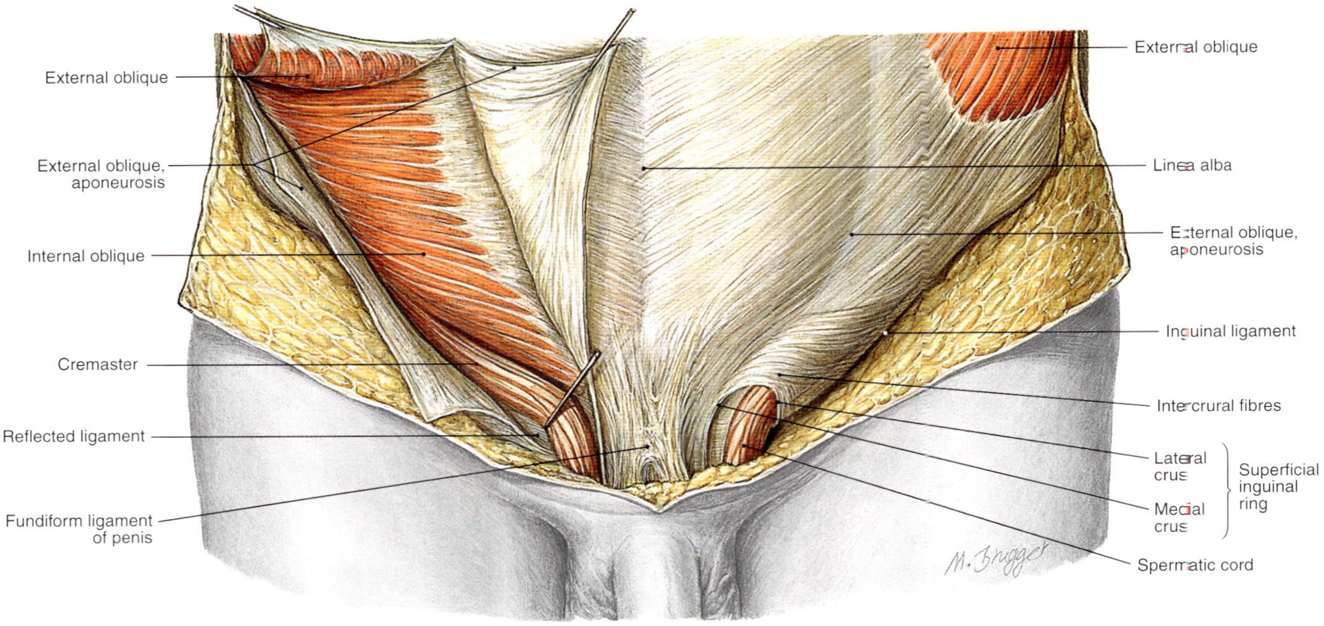

Fig. 579 Superficial inguinal ring.

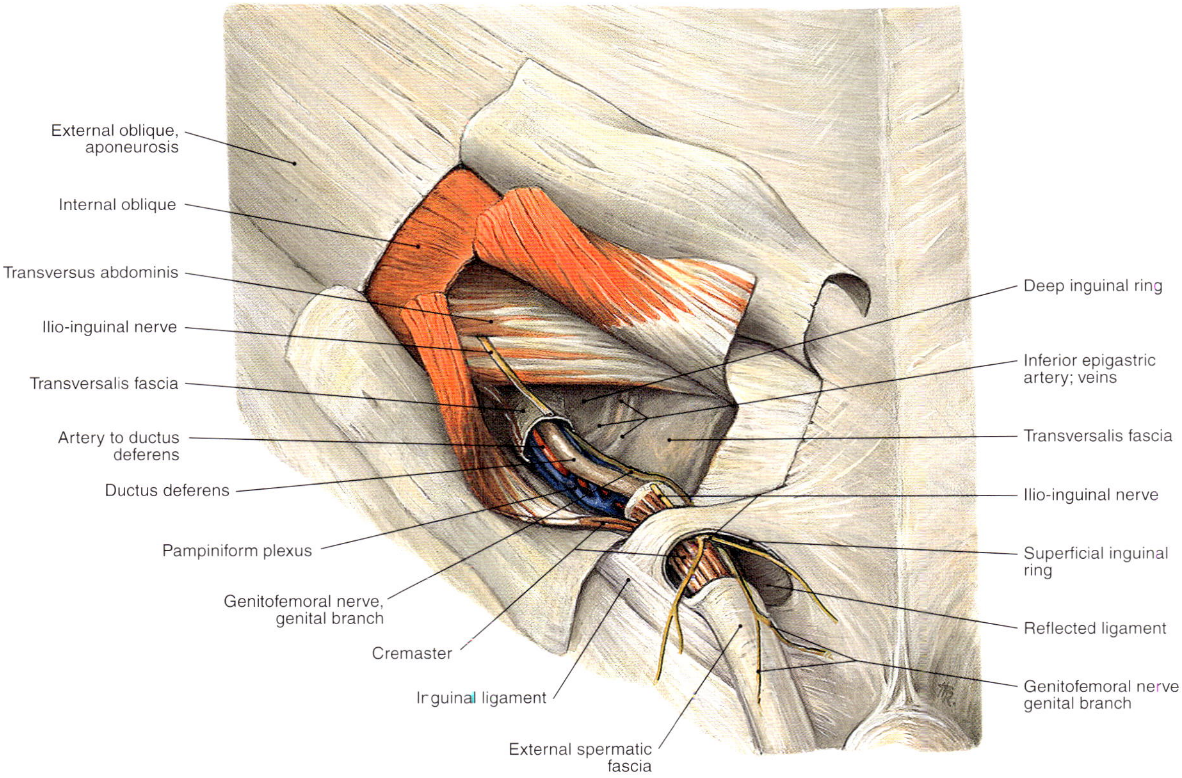

Fig. 580 Walls of the inguinal canal.

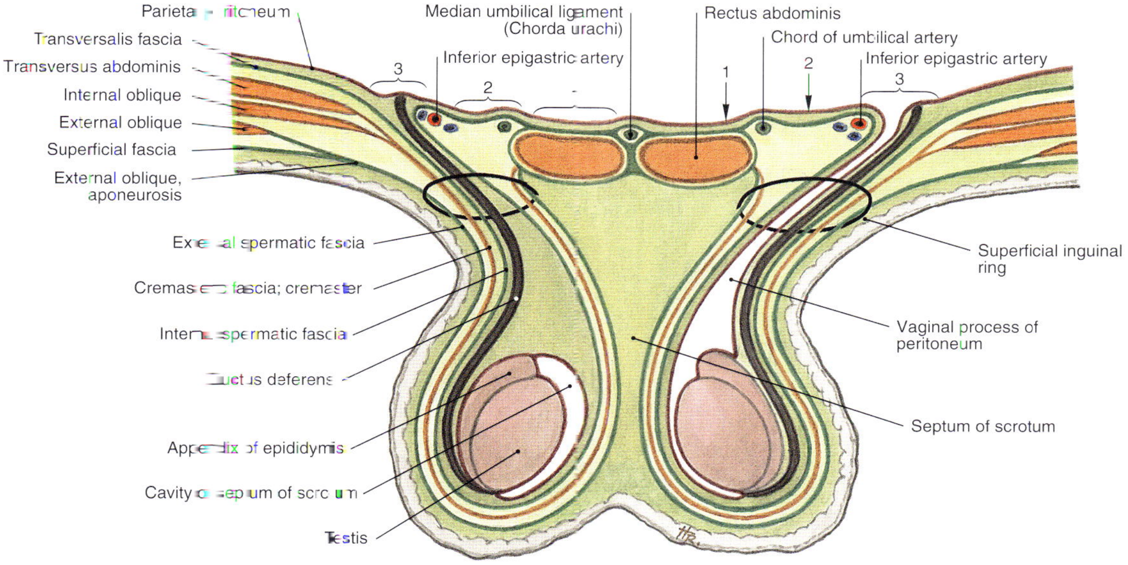

Fig. 581 Diagram of the inguinal canal.
The inguinal canal, the spermatic cord and the scrotum are illustrated in the same plane for didactical reasons.

1 Supravesical fossa
2 Medial inguinal fossa
3 Lateral inguinal fossa

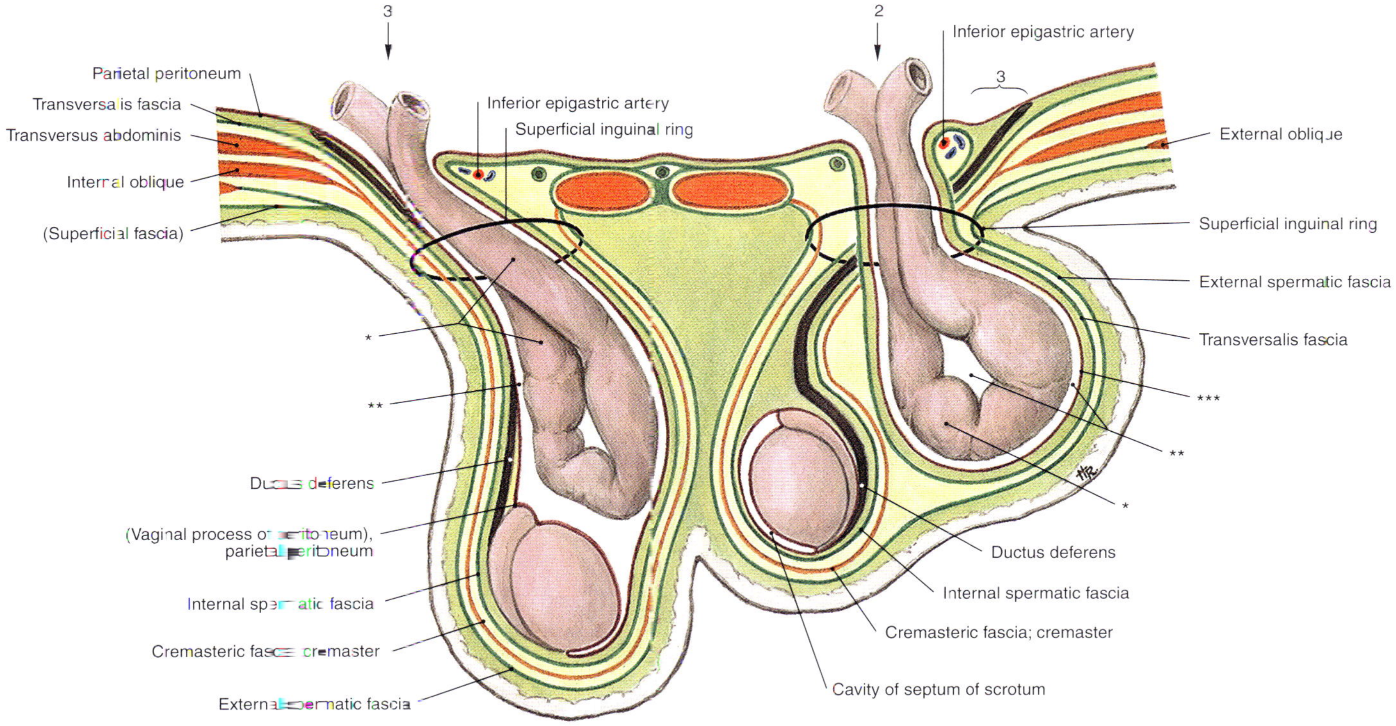

Fig. 582 Diagram of inguinal hernias;
left side: lateral, indirect hernia;
right side: medial, direct hernia.

* Hernial sac with an intestinal loop
** Peritoneal space
*** Newly formed peritoneal hernial sac

Diaphragm and posterior abdominal wall

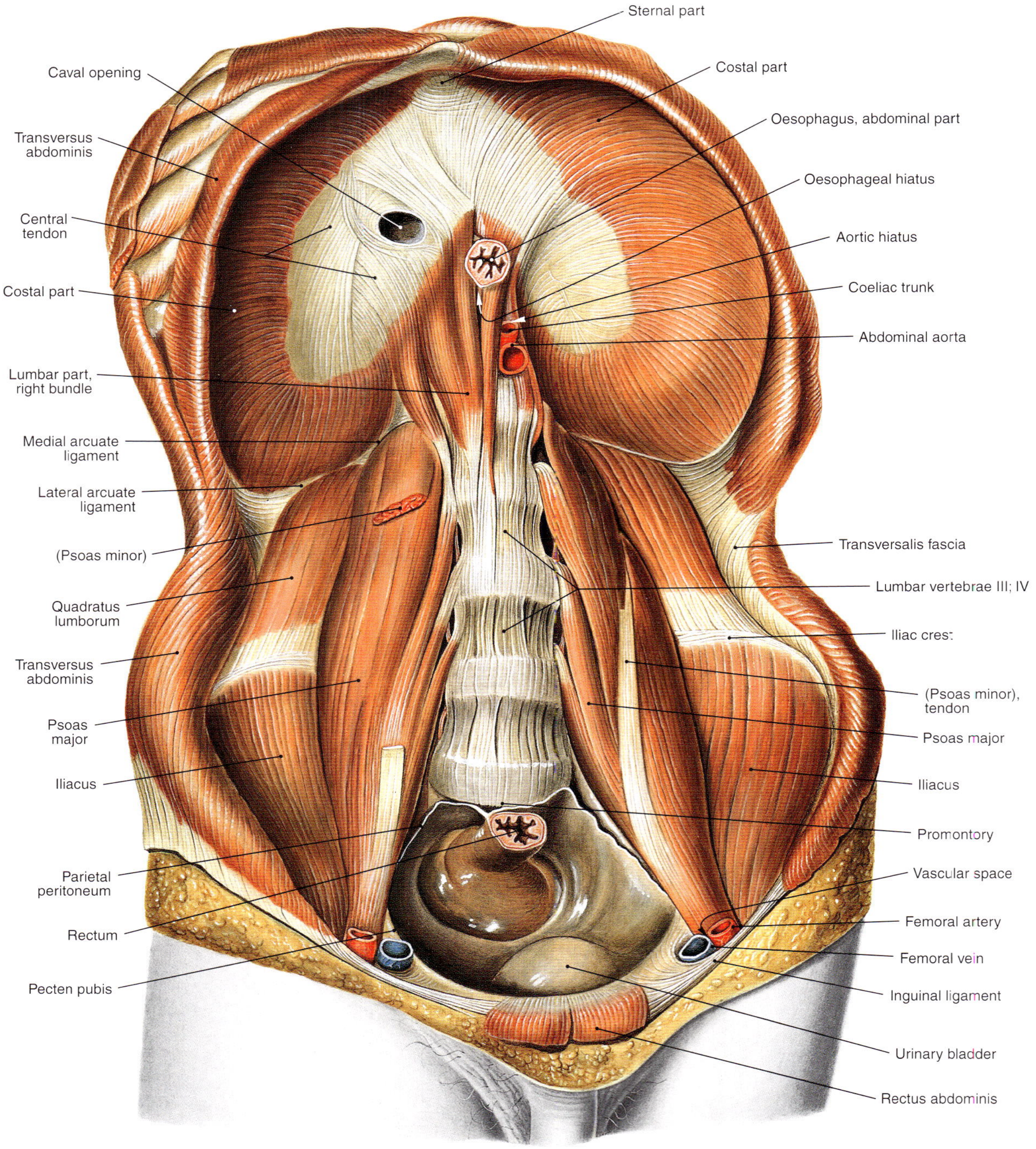

→ T 15, T 16, T 21, T 42

Fig. 583 Diaphragm and muscles of the abdominal wall.

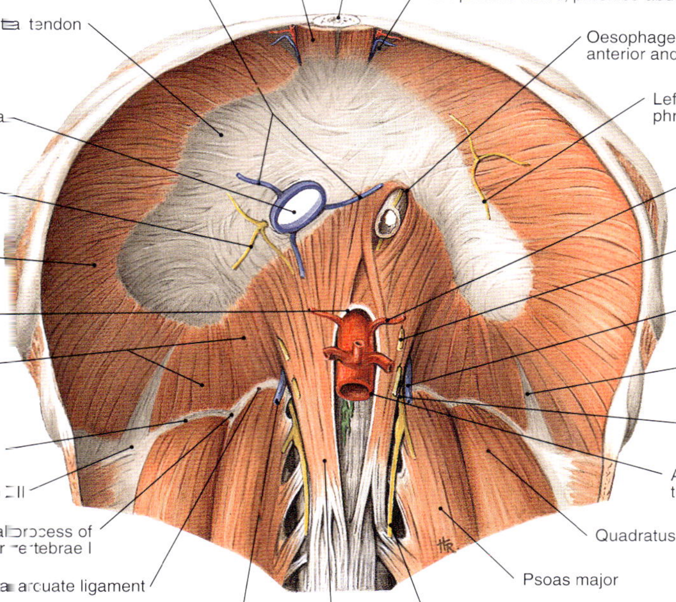

Fig. 584 Diaphragm.

→ T 21

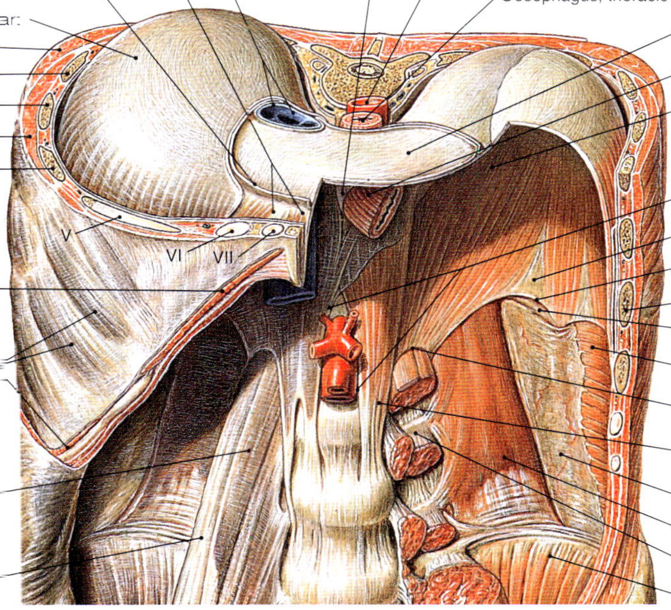

Fig. 585 Diaphragm with apertures and muscles of the posterior abdominal wall.

→ T 21

* Clinical term: BOCHDALEK's triangle
** Psoas arcade

Breast

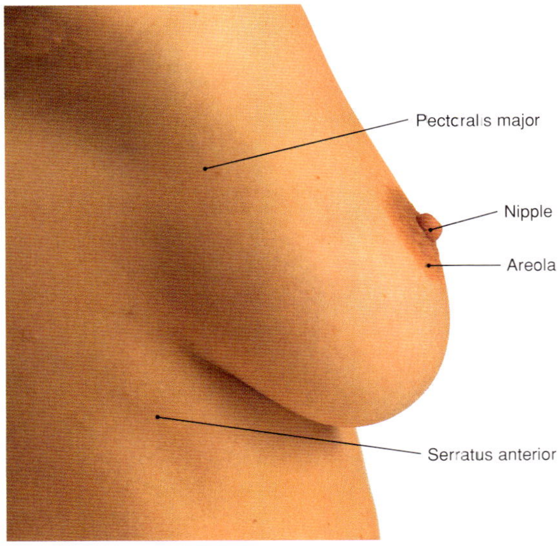

Fig. 586 Breast.

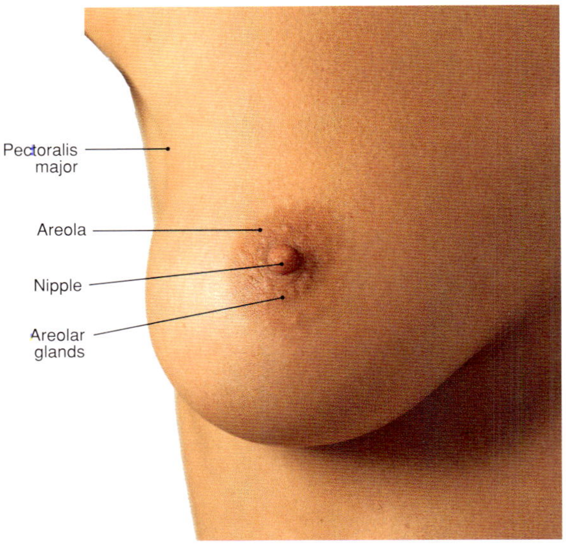

Fig. 587 Breast.

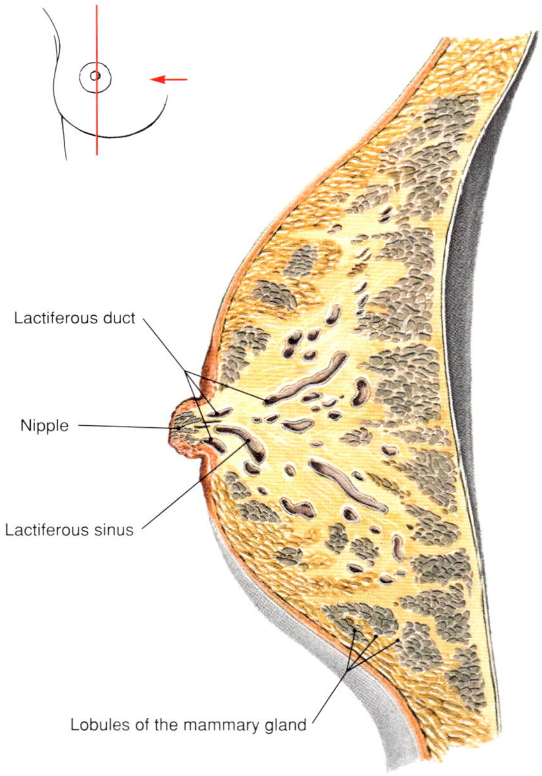

Fig. 588 Breast of a pregnant woman.

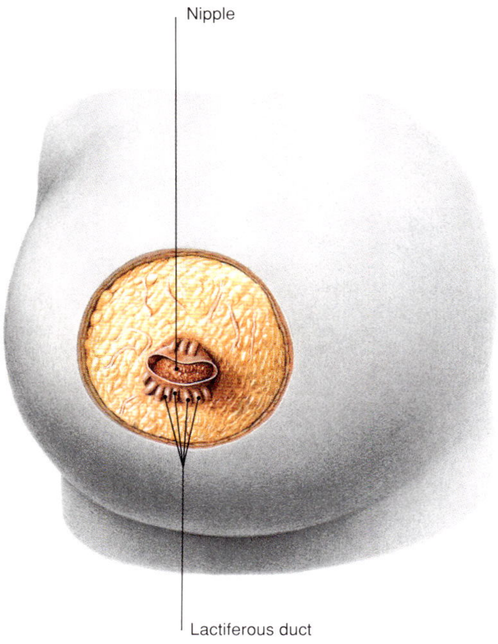

Fig. 589 Breast of a pregnant woman.

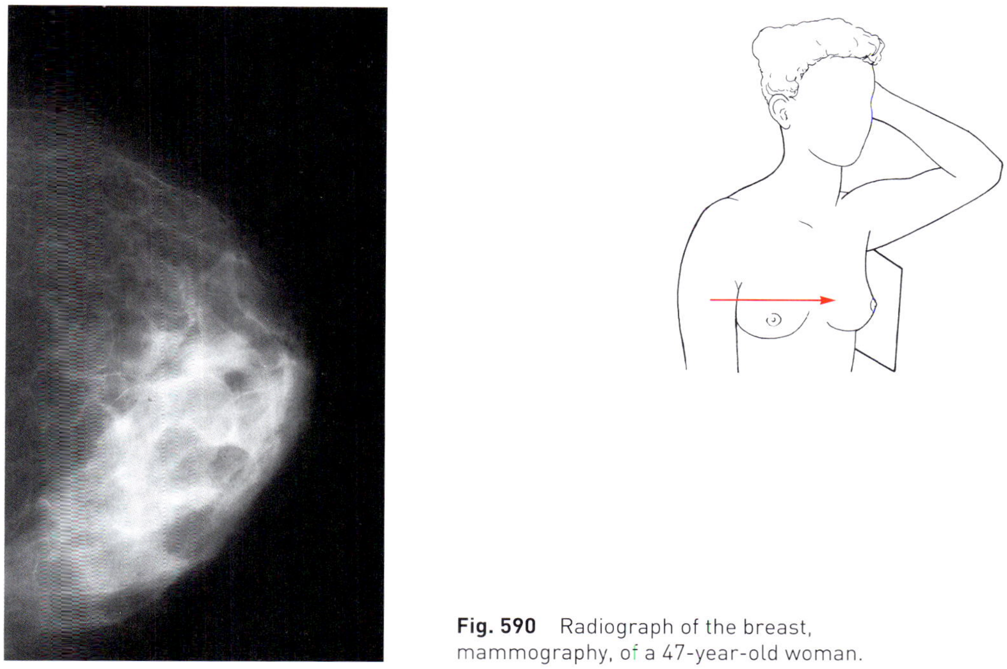

Fig. 590 Radiograph of the breast, mammography, of a 47-year-old woman.

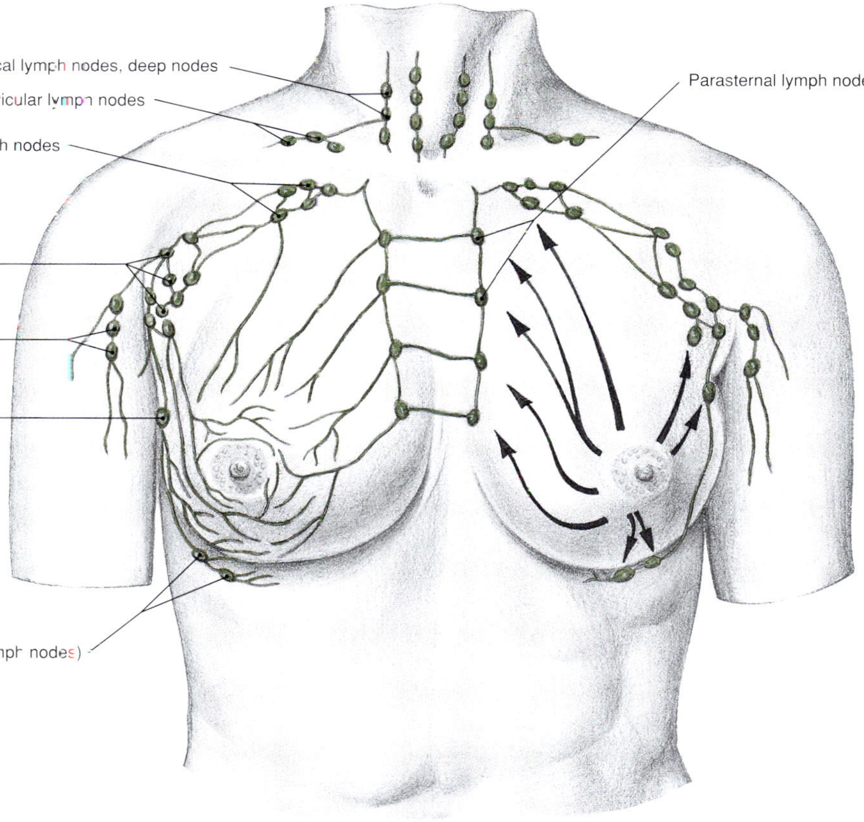

Fig. 591 Lymphatic drainage of the breast and location of the regional lymph nodes.

Vessels and nerves of the wall of the trunk

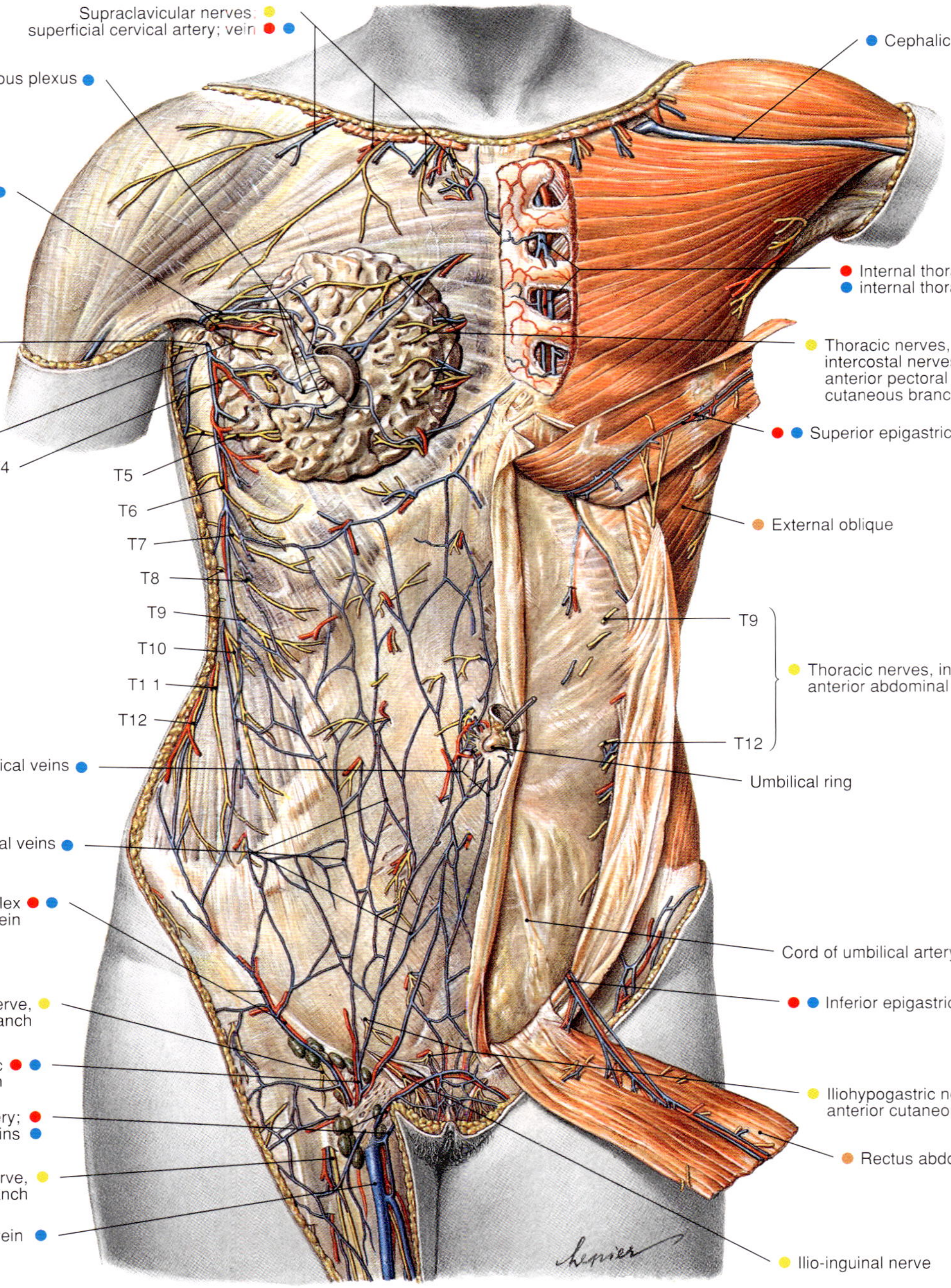

Fig. 592 Vessels and nerves of the thoracic and the abdominal wall.

* Clinical term: internal mammary artery

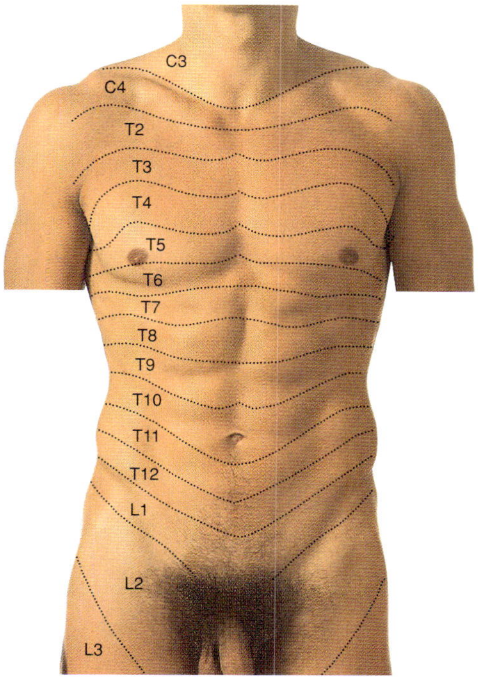

Fig. 593 Segmental sensory innervation of the anterior thoracic and abdominal wall (dermatomes).

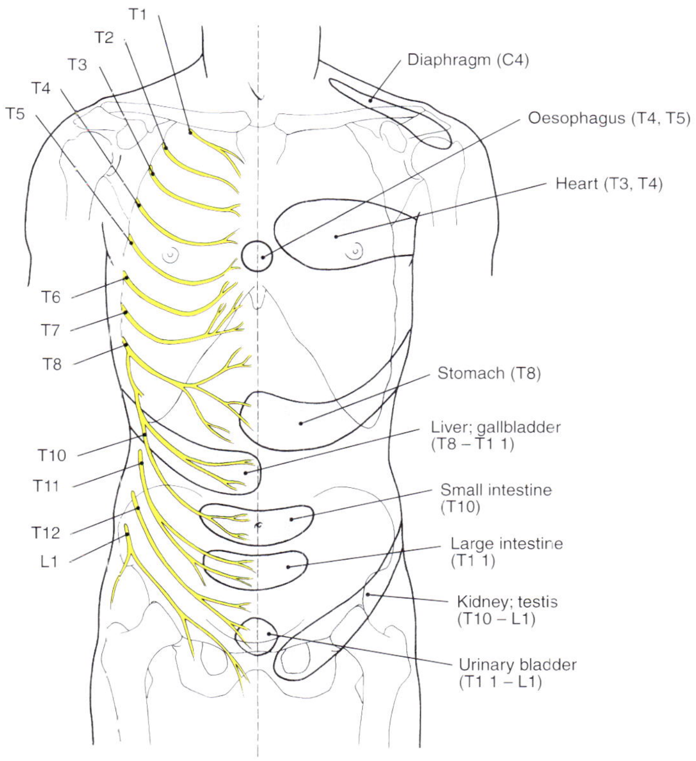

Fig. 594 Segmental sensory innervation of the anterior thoracic and abdominal wall.
Regions to which pain from diseased viscera (zones of HEAD) is referred to are indicated in grey.

Lumbosacral plexus

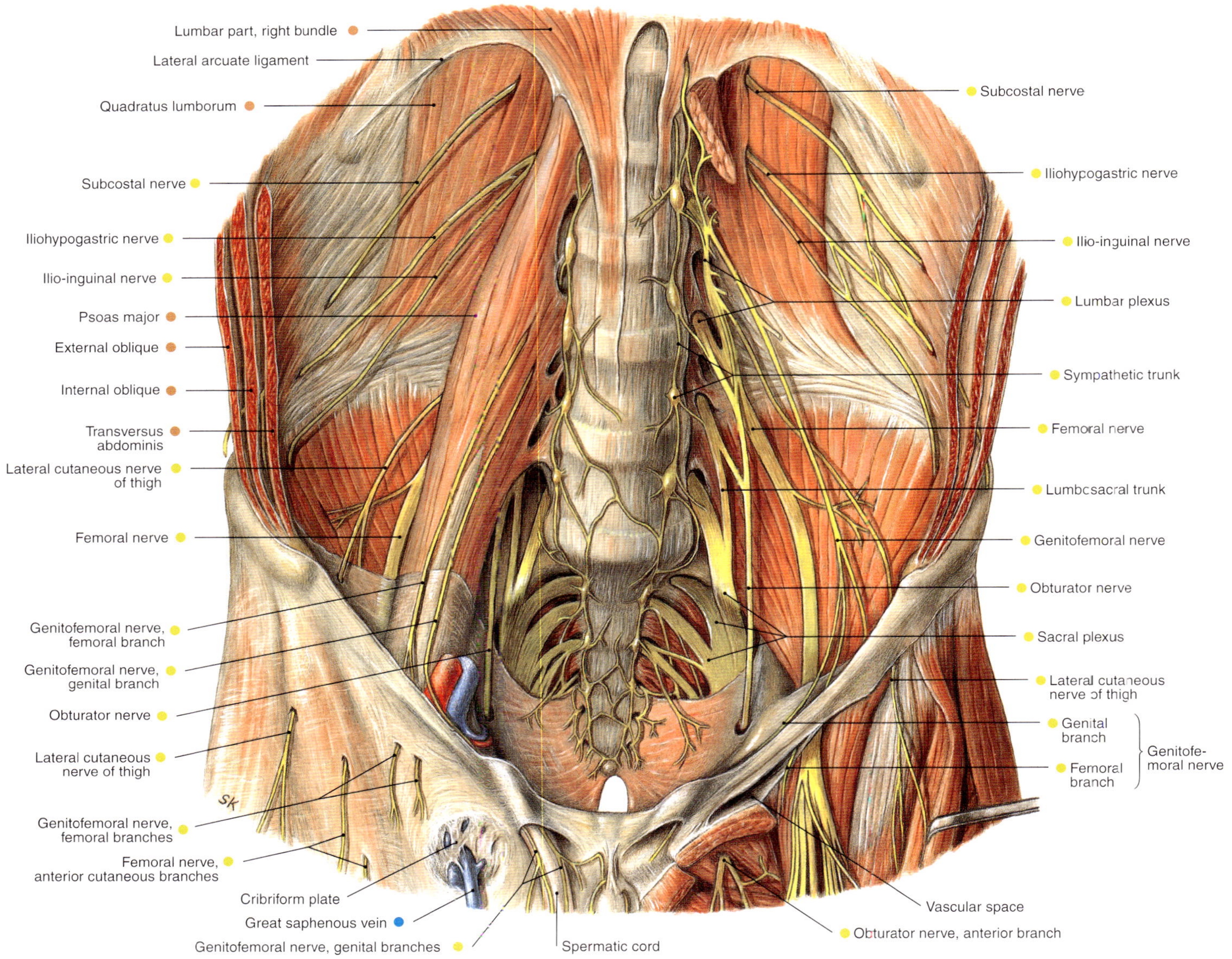

Fig. 595 Lumbosacral plexus.

→ 47, 1102, T 40

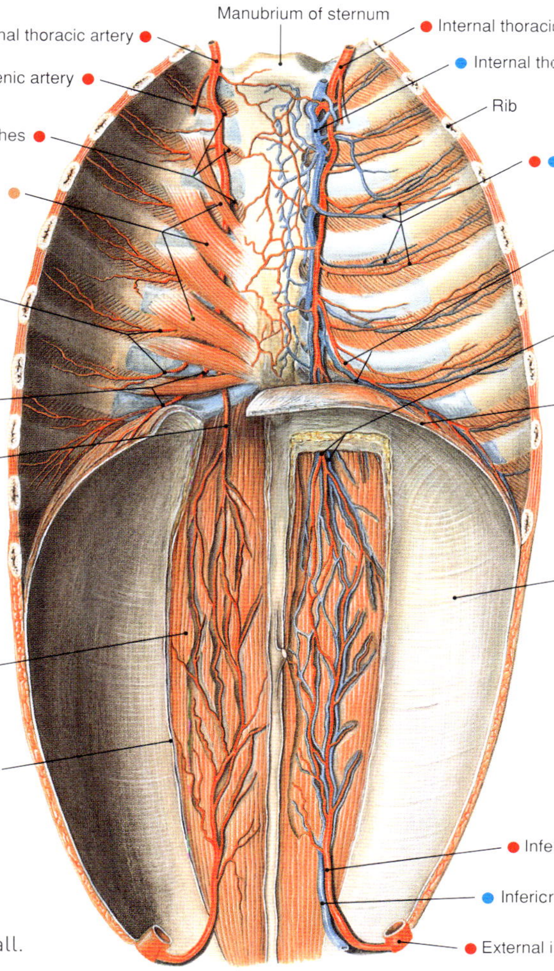

Fig. 596 Vessels of the anterior thoracic and abdominal wall.

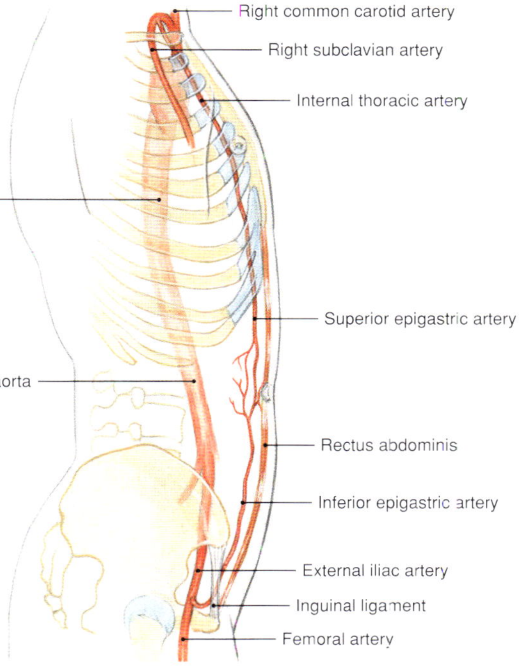

Fig. 597 Diagram of the collateral circulation via the internal thoracic artery, the superior epigastric artery and the inferior epigastric artery, in the case of aortic occlusion; viewed from the right.

Abdominal wall of neonate

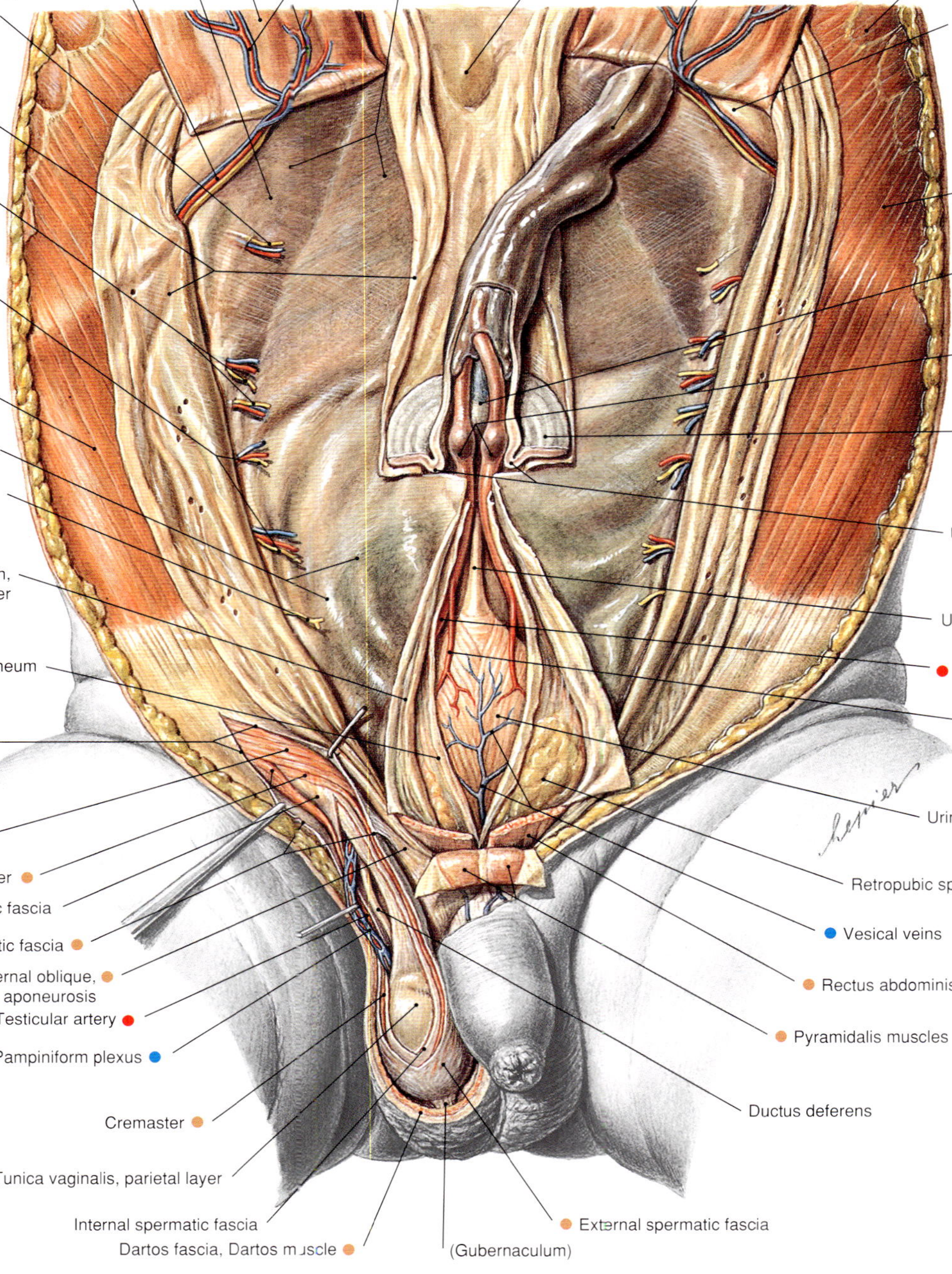

Fig. 598 Anterior abdominal wall of a neonate.

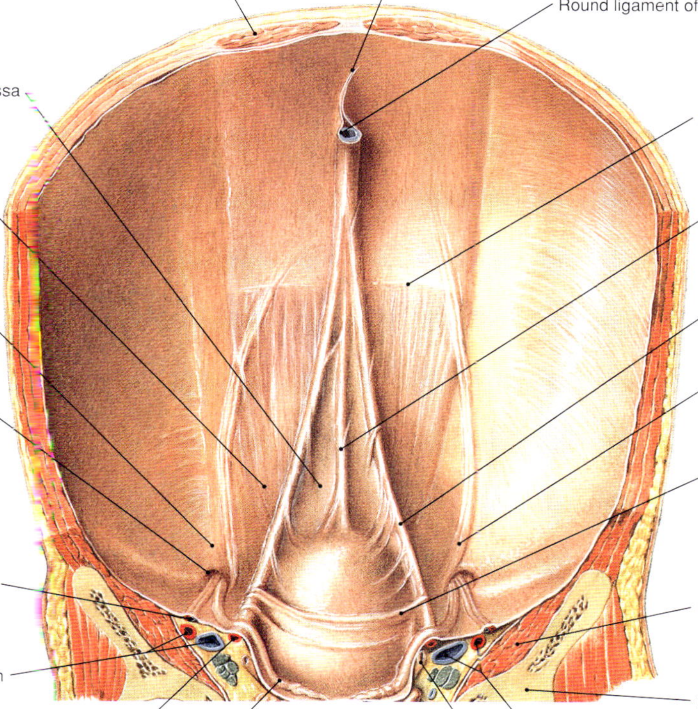

Fig. 599 Anterior abdominal wall of a neonate.

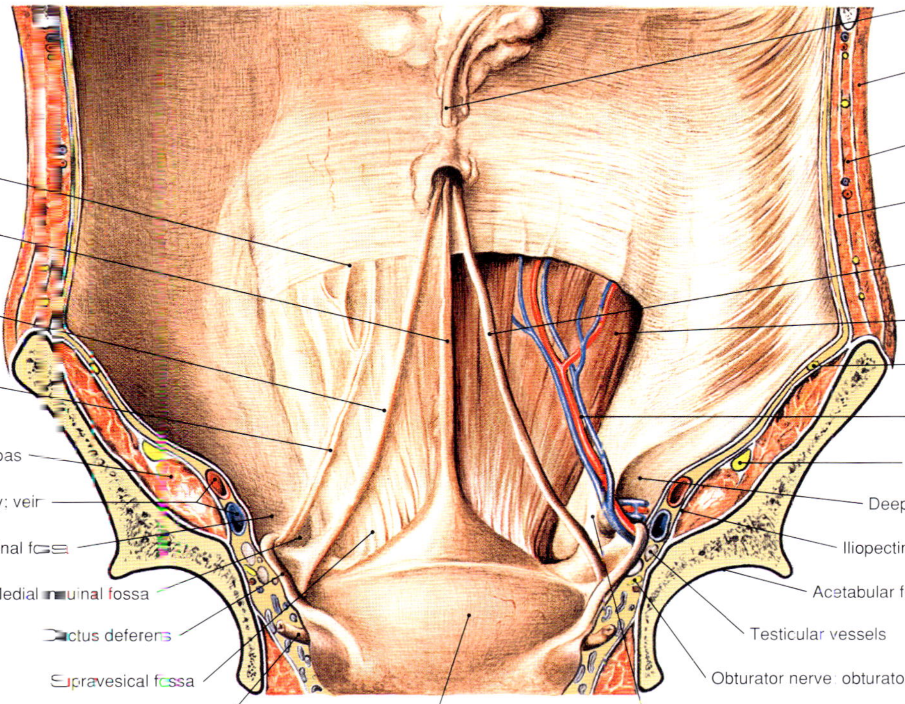

Fig. 600 Anterior abdominal wall, internal aspect.

Abdominal wall, sections

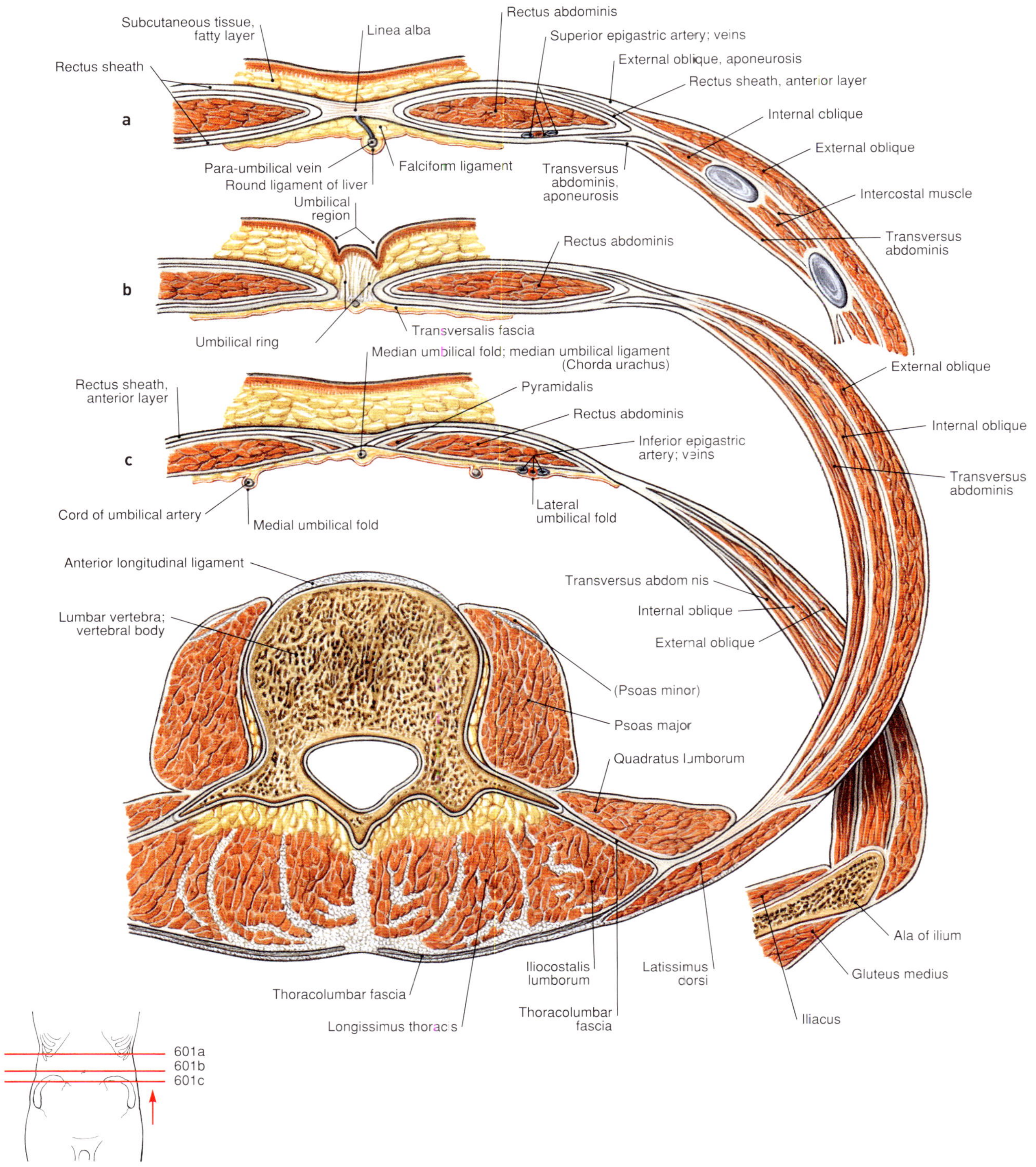

→ T 14–T 16, T 20a, b, T 42

Fig. 601 a–c Muscles of the abdominal wall; horizontal section.

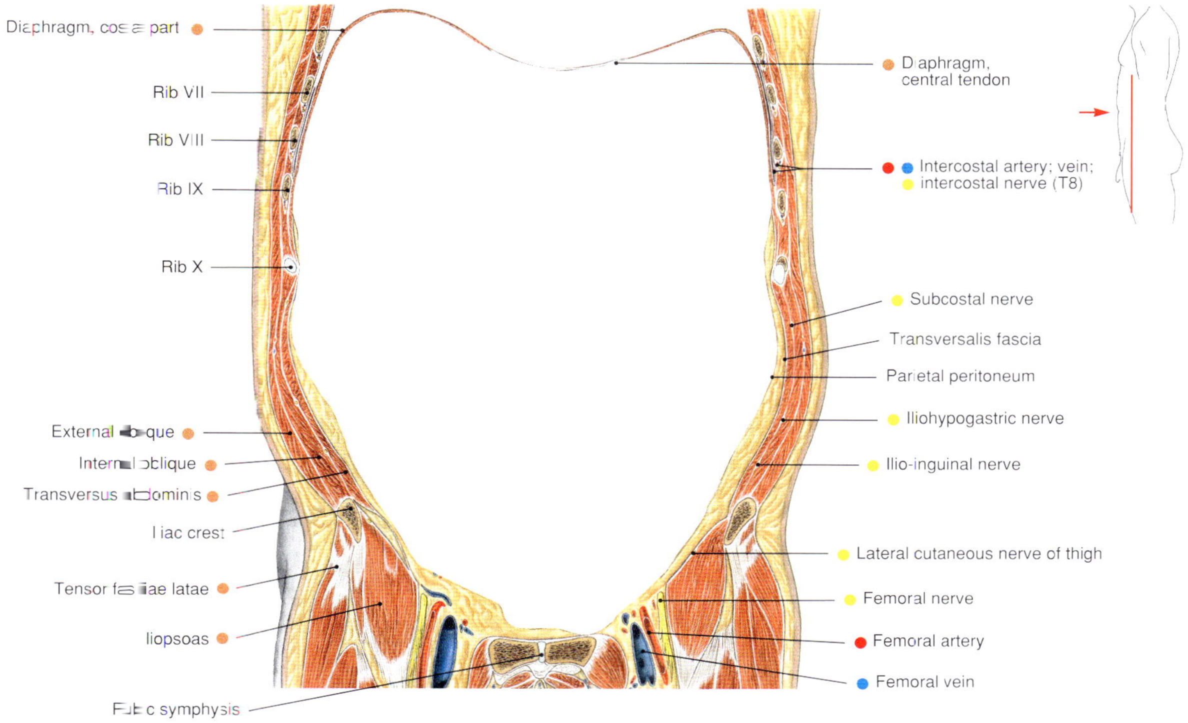

Fig. 602 Muscles of the abdominal wall; frontal section.

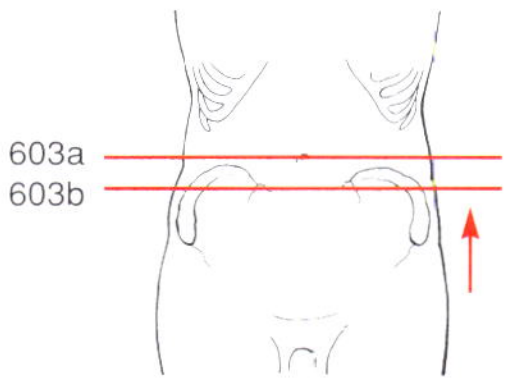

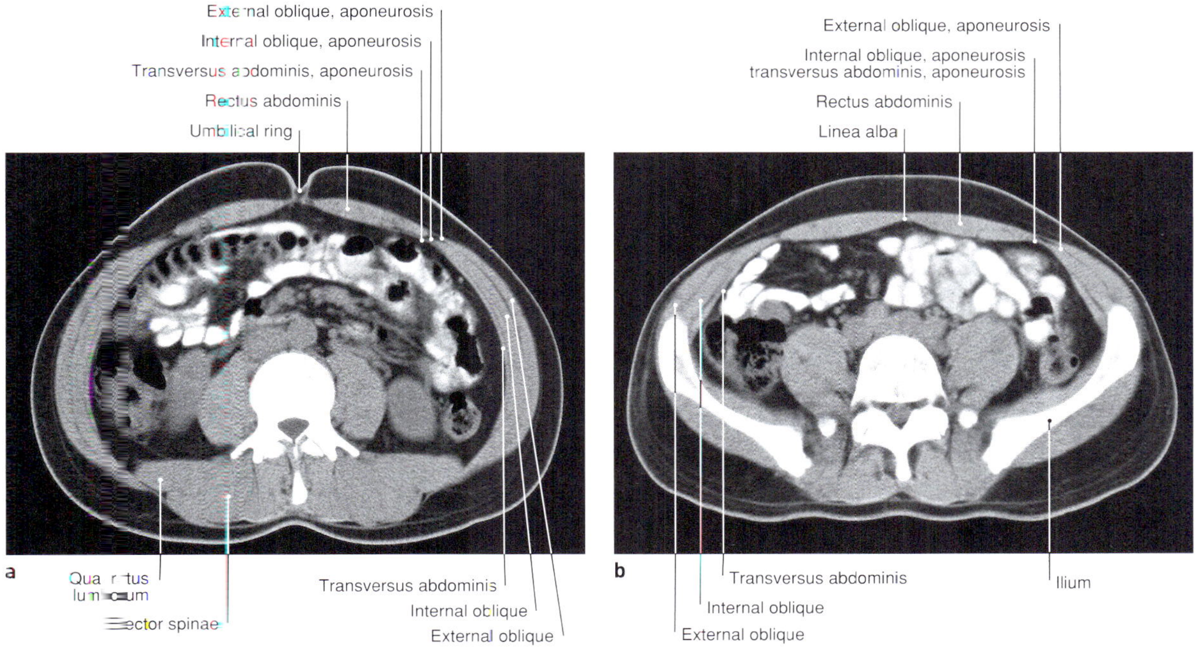

Fig. 603 a, b Muscles of the abdominal wall; computed tomographic cross-sections (CT).

Heart

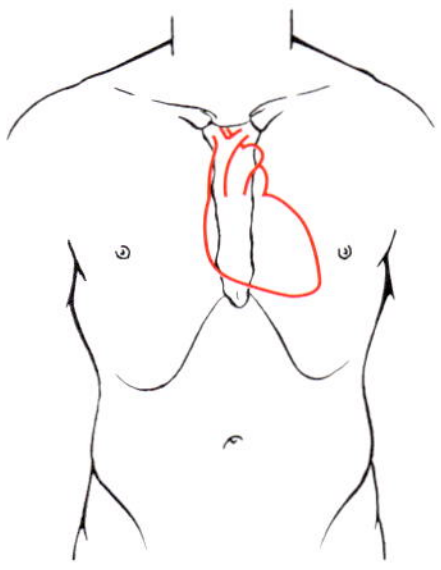

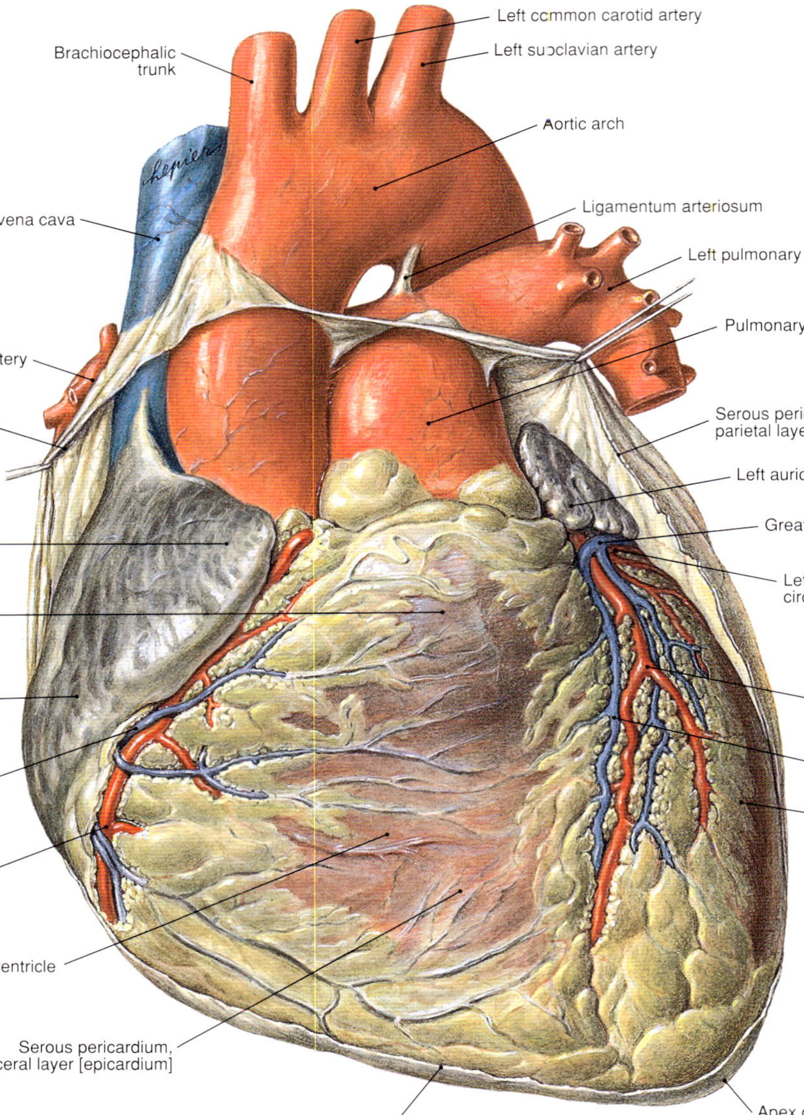

Fig. 604 Heart.

Fibrous pericardium	}	Pericardium
Serous pericardium		
Parietal layer		
Visceral layer	=	Epicardium

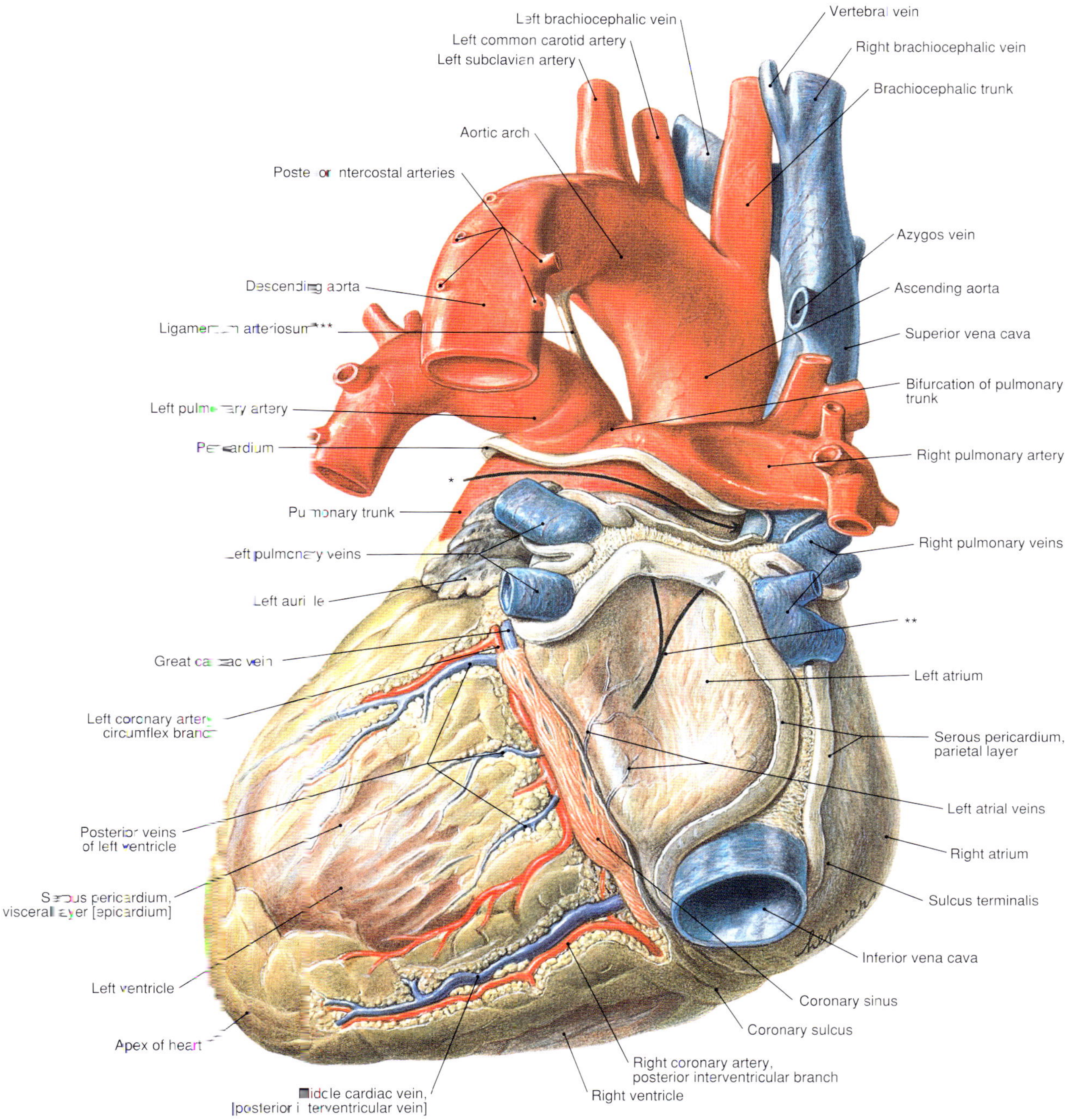

Fig. 605 Heart and great vessels; dorsal view.

* Arrow in the transverse pericardial sinus
** Double arrows in the oblique pericardial sinus
*** Remnants of the foetal ductus arteriosus (BOTALLO's ligament)

Myocardium

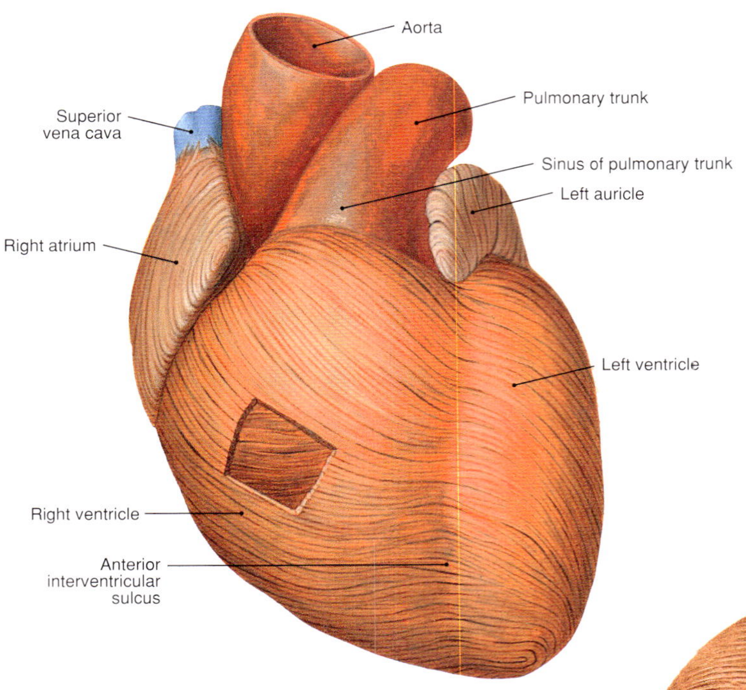

Fig. 606 Myocardium; ventral view.

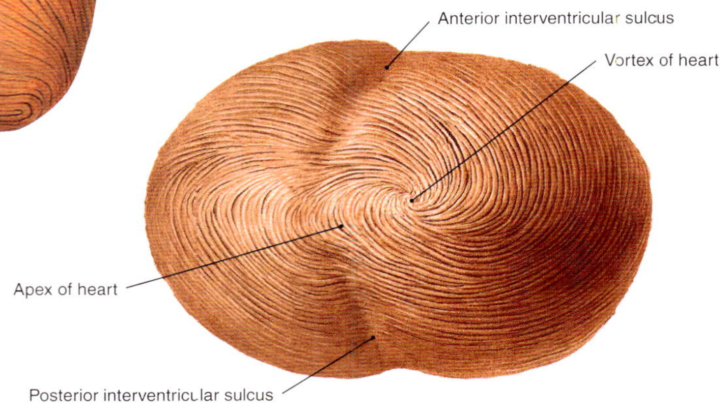

Fig. 607 Myocardium; viewed from the apex of the heart.

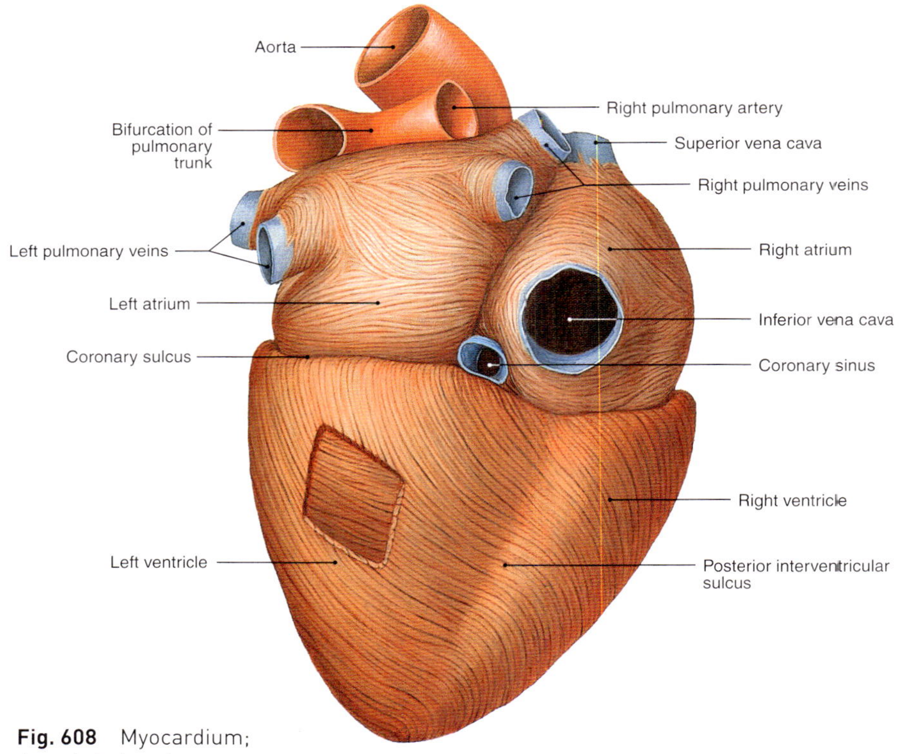

Fig. 608 Myocardium; dorsoinferior view.

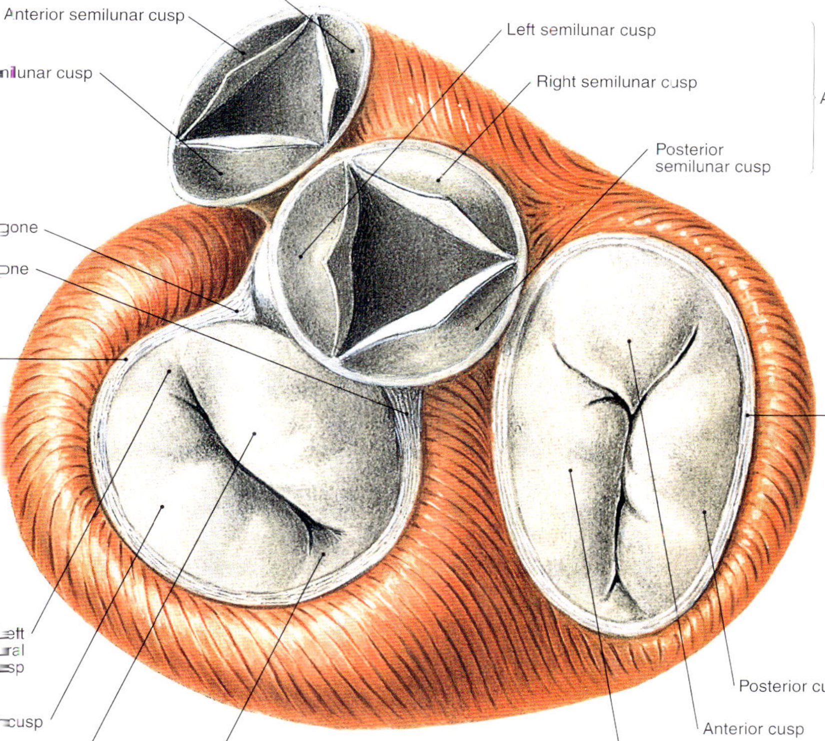

Fig. 609 Valves of the heart; superior view.

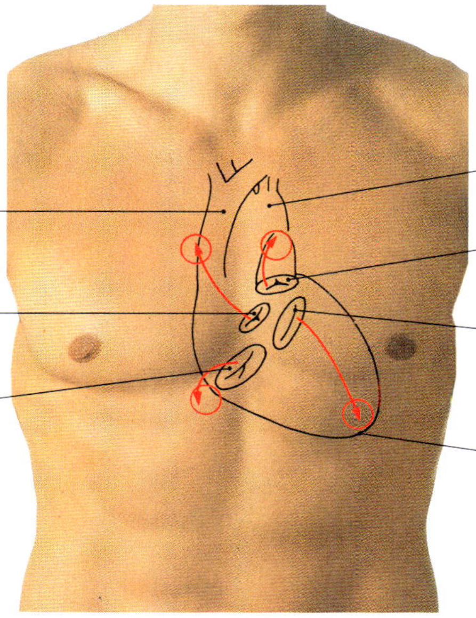

Fig. 610 Contour of the heart, valves of the heart, and points of auscultation projected onto the anterior thoracic wall (circles). The heart sounds and (where applicable) the heart murmurs are spreading in the direction of the arrows.

Internal spaces of the heart

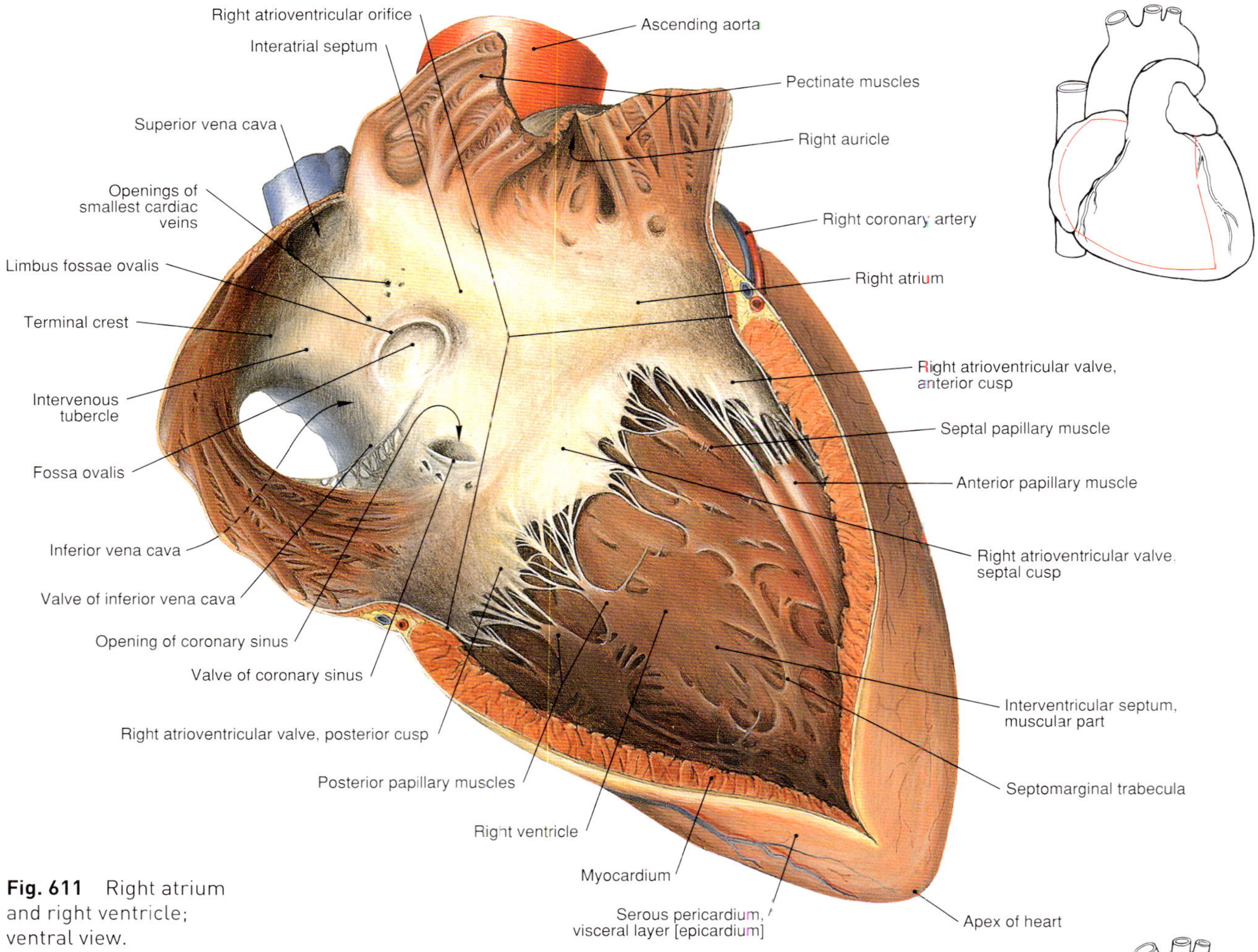

Fig. 611 Right atrium and right ventricle; ventral view.

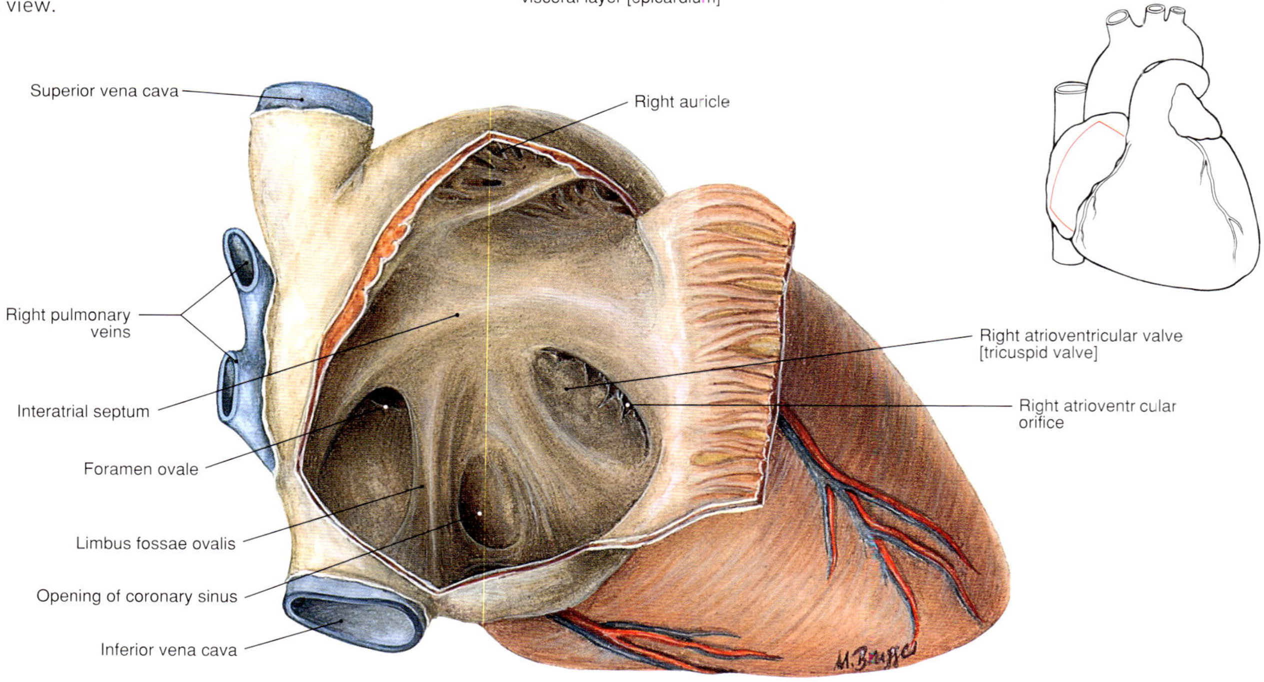

Fig. 612 Right atrium of a neonate; ventral view from the right.

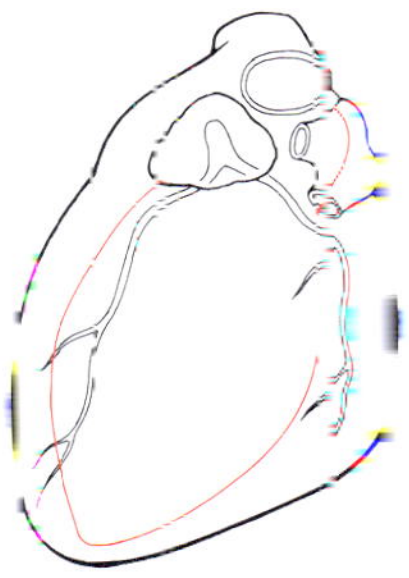
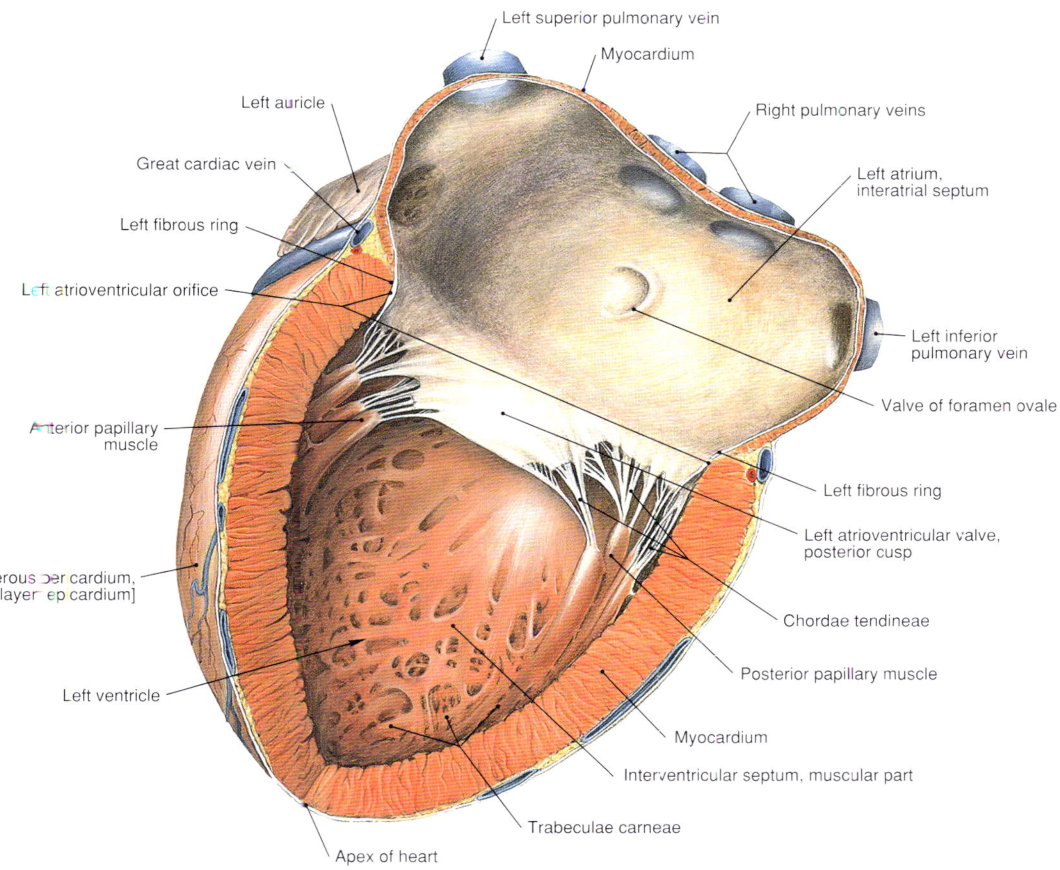

Fig. 613 Left atrium and left ventricle; lateral view.

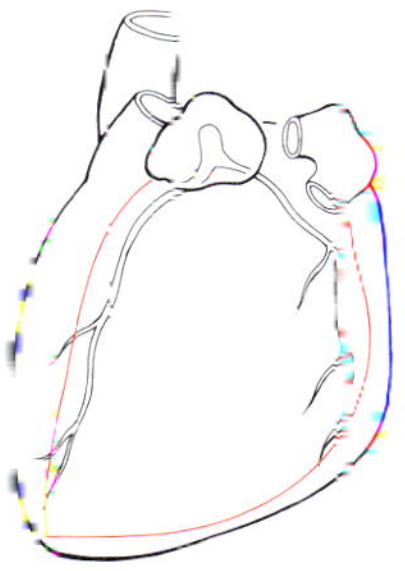
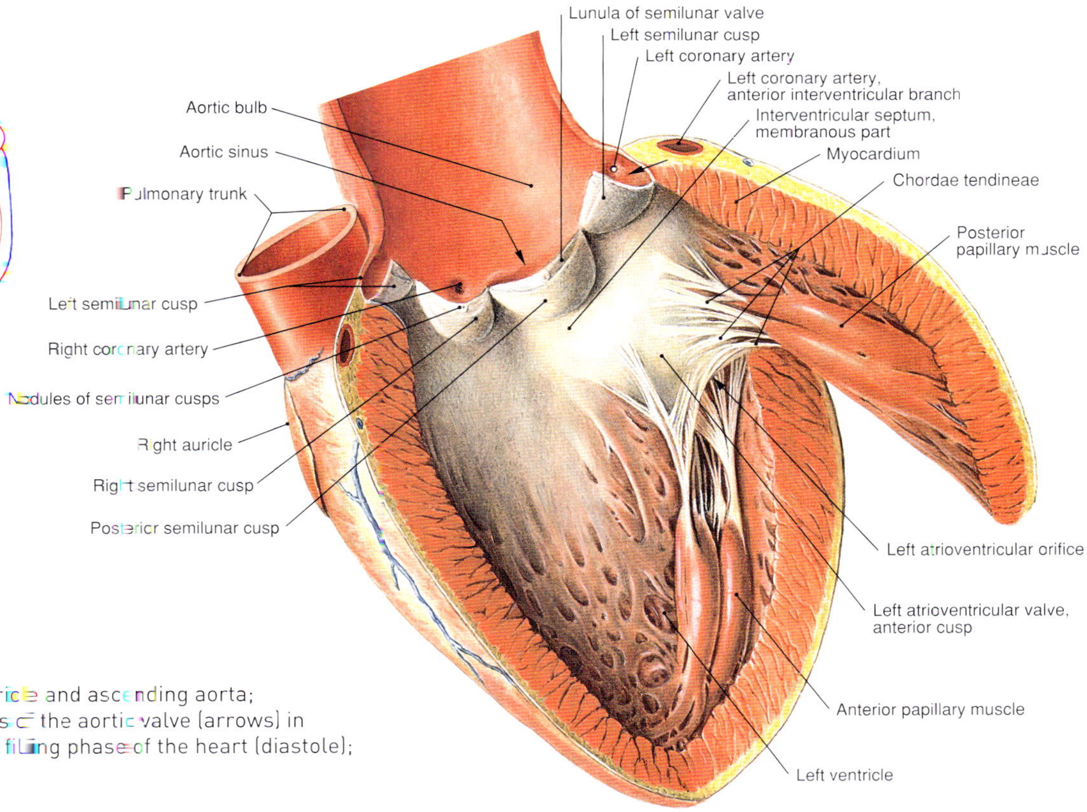

Fig. 614 Left ventricle and ascending aorta; position of the cusps of the aortic valve (arrows) in their position at the filling phase of the heart (diastole); lateral view.

Internal spaces of the heart

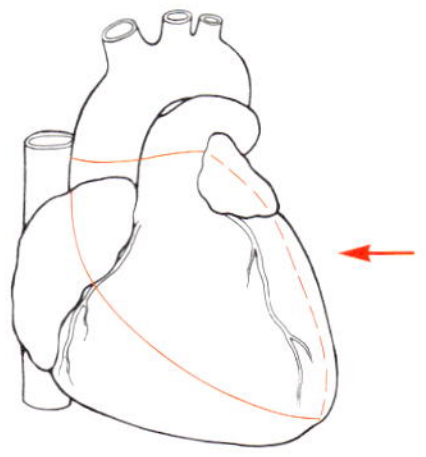

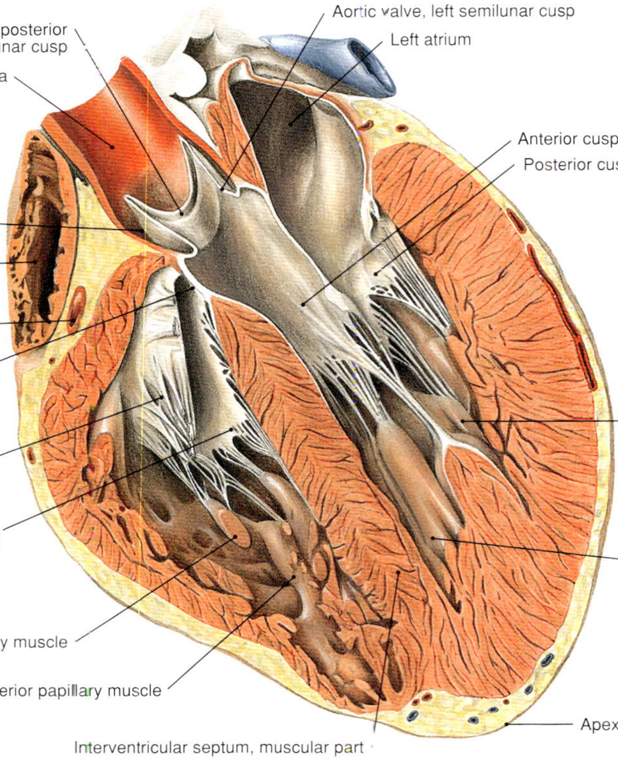

Fig. 615 Left and right ventricle.

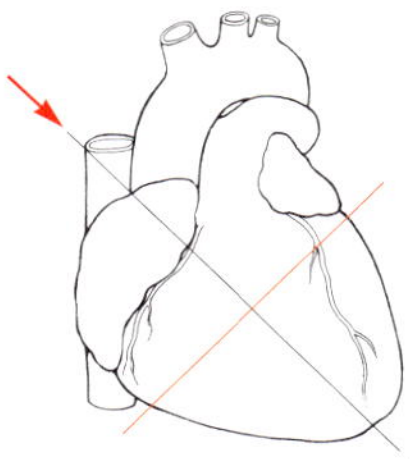

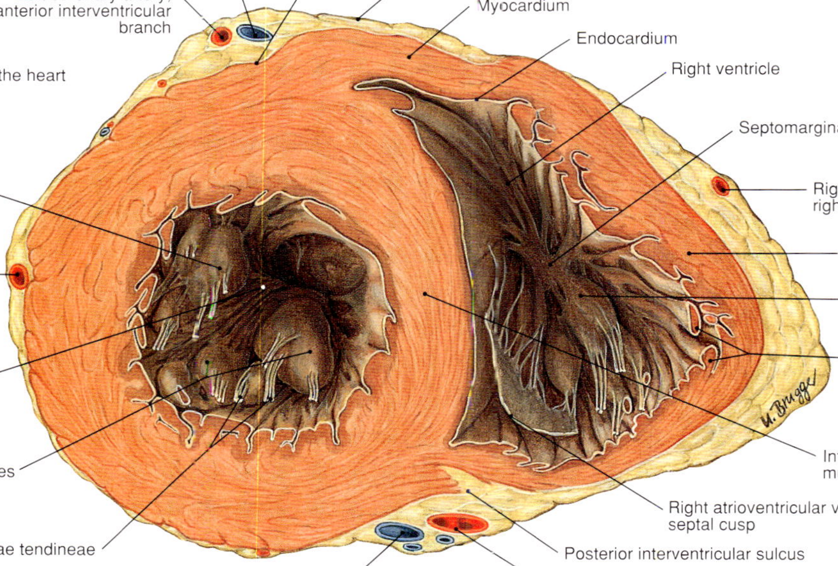

Fig. 616 Left and right ventricle; superior view.

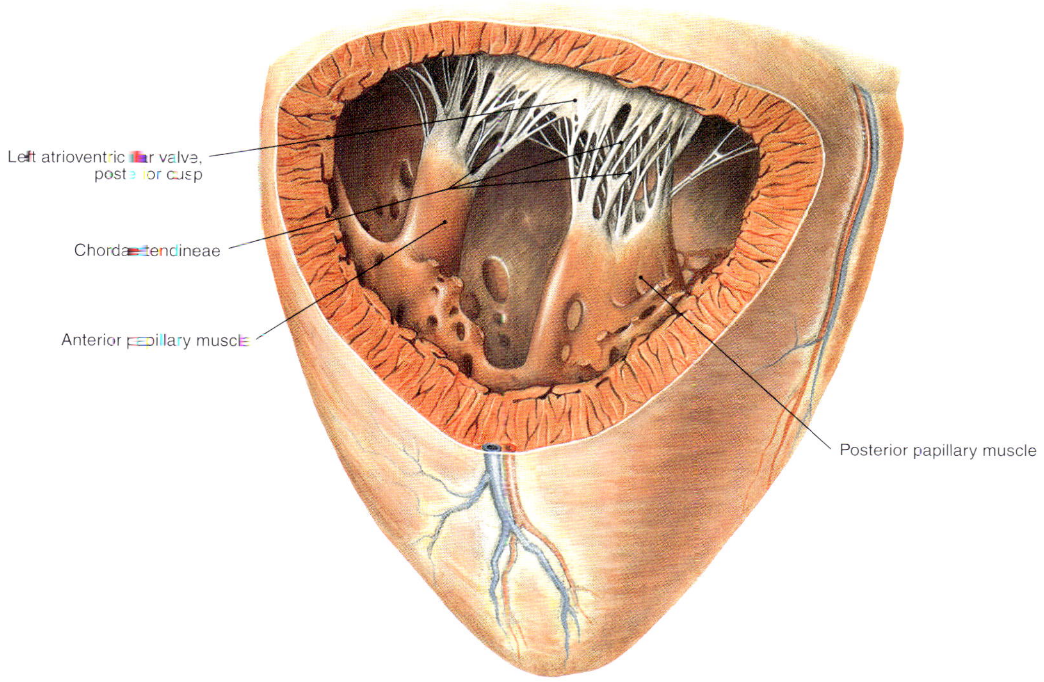

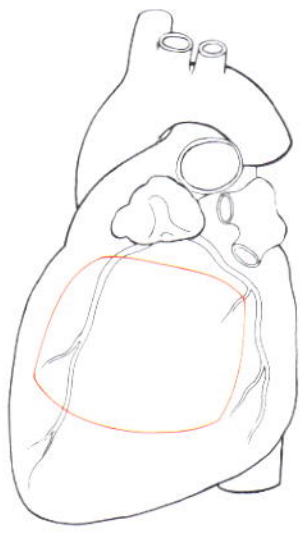

Fig. 617 Left ventricle; ventrosuperior view from the left.

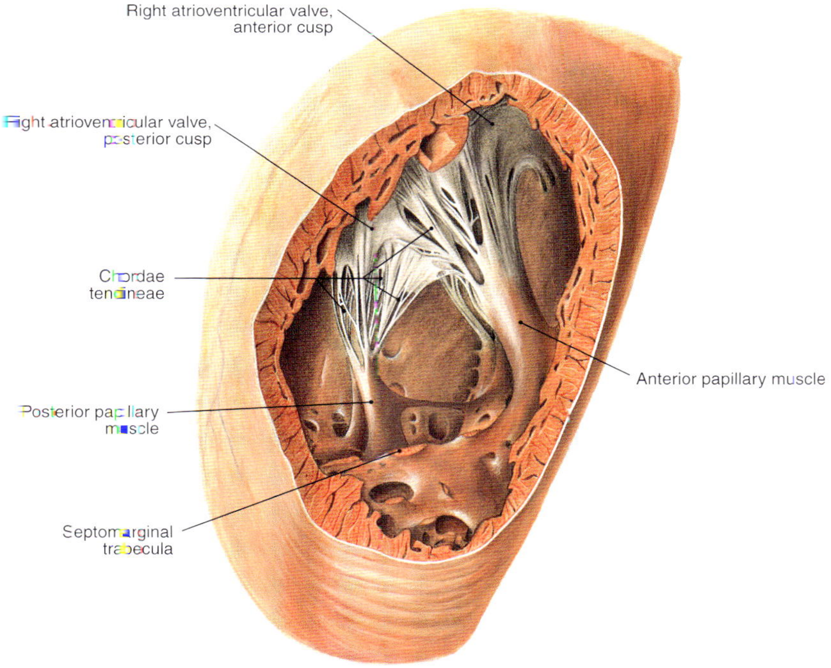

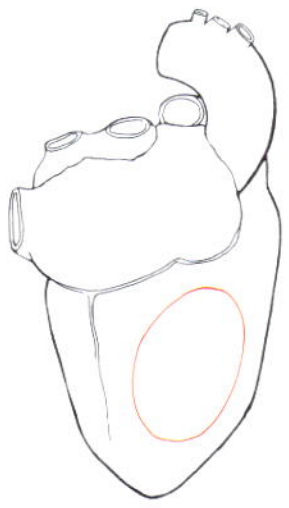

Fig. 618 Right ventricle; dorsal view.

Conducting system

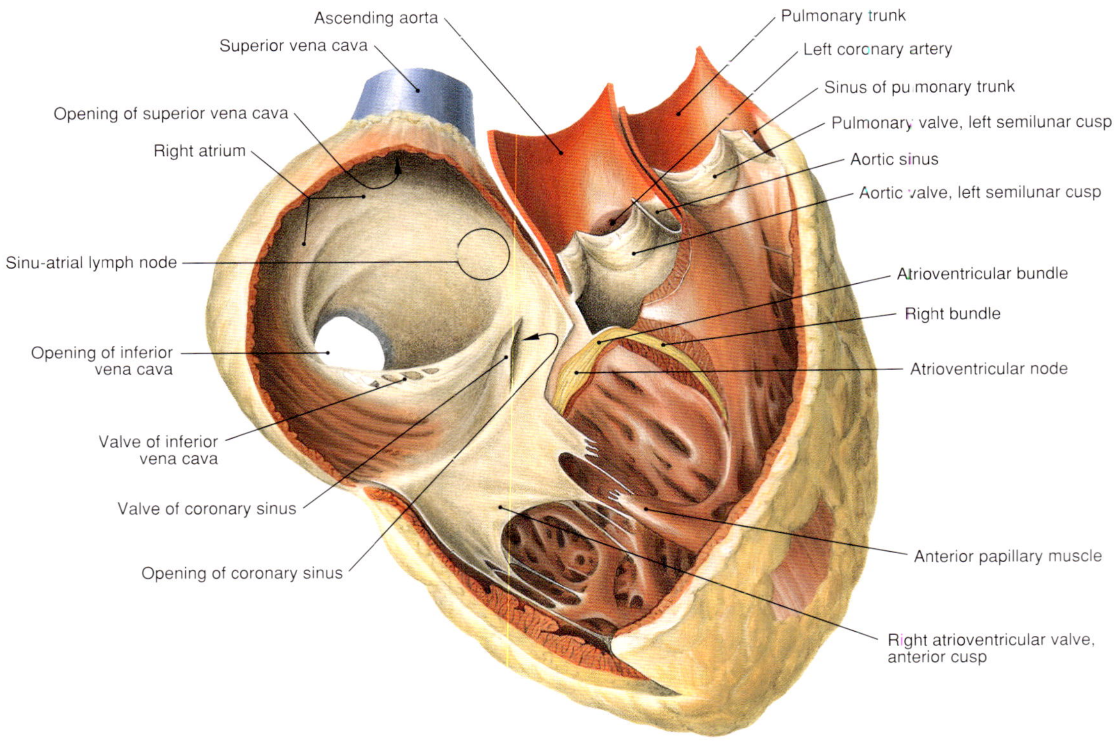

Fig. 619 Right atrium and right ventricle; conducting system highlighted in yellow; ventral view.

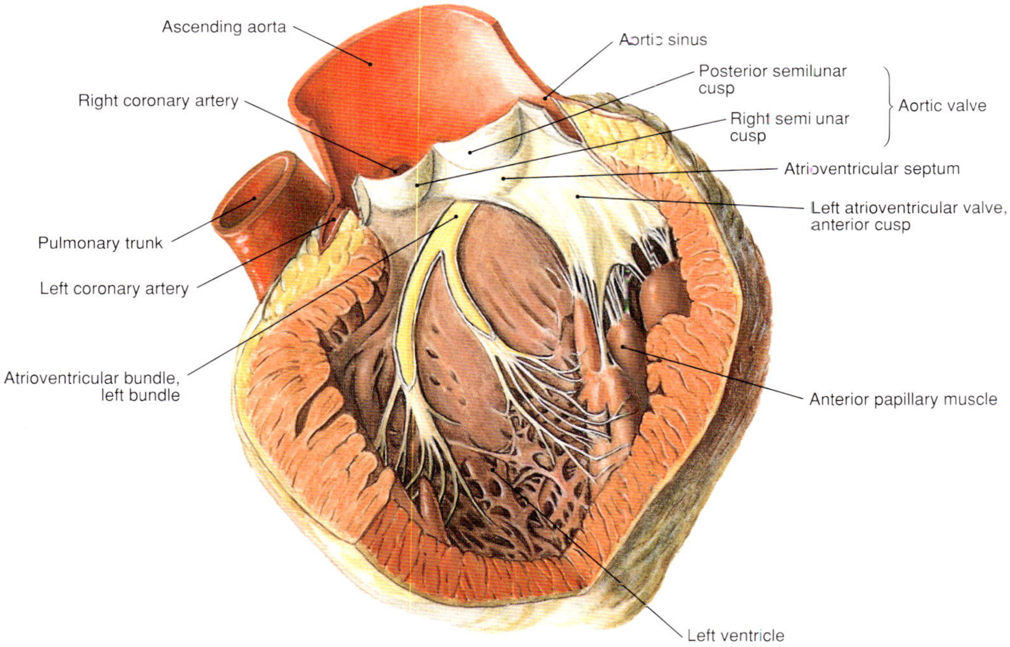

Fig. 620 Left ventricle; conducting system highlighted in yellow; ventral view from the left.

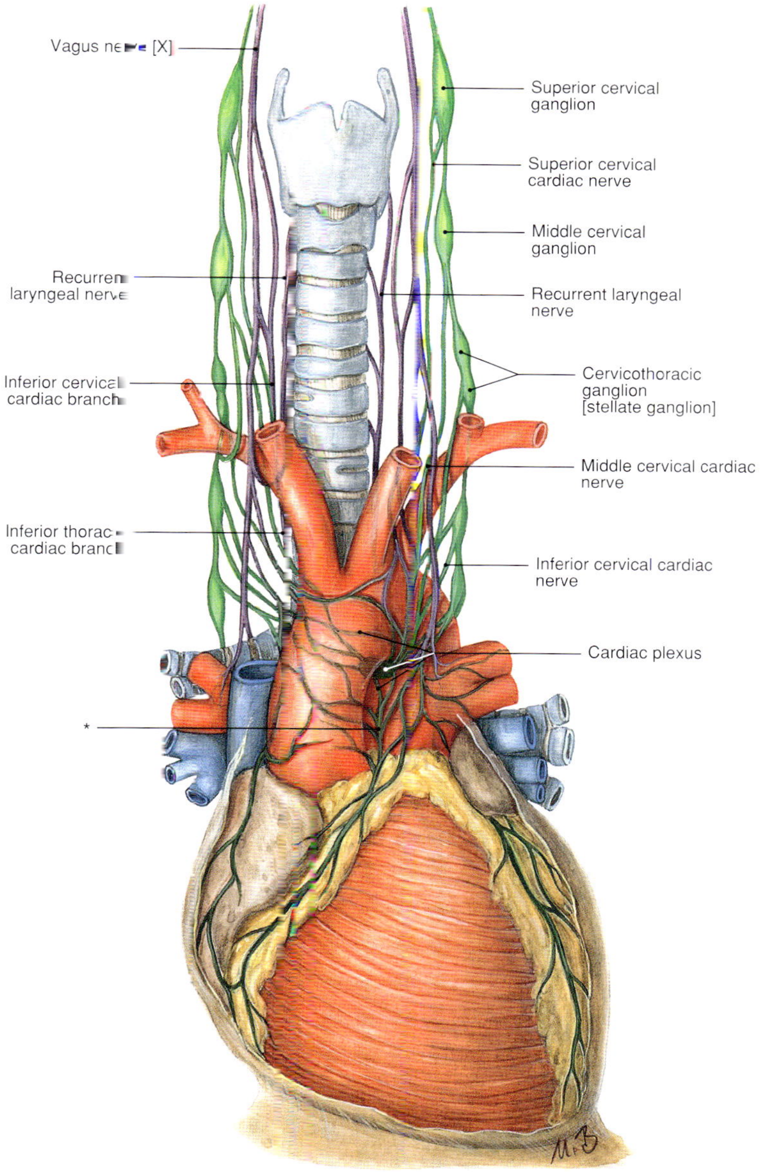

Fig. 621 Innervation of the heart, diagram; sympathetic trunk: green; vagus nerve: purple.

* The branches beyond the cardiac plexus contain sympathetic and vagal fibres.

→ 688

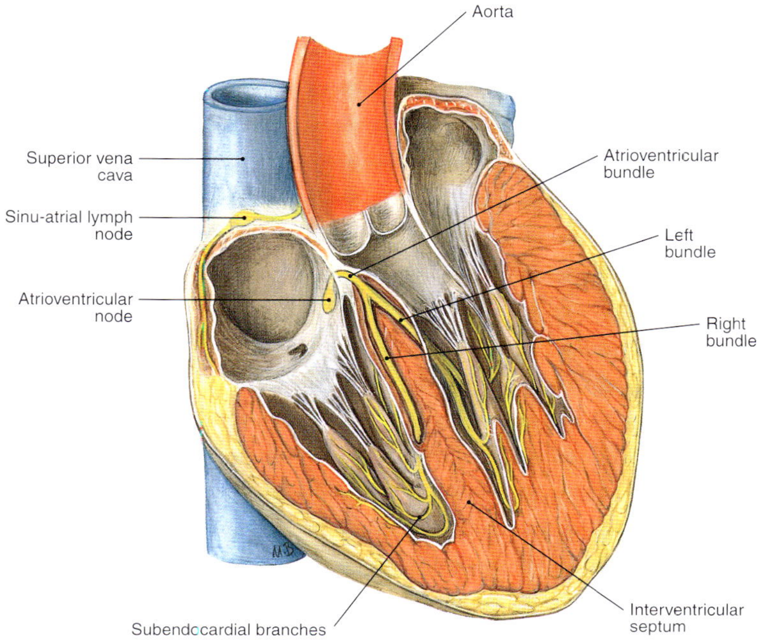

Fig. 622 Conducting system of heart; section at the plane of the axis of the heart.

Coronary arteries

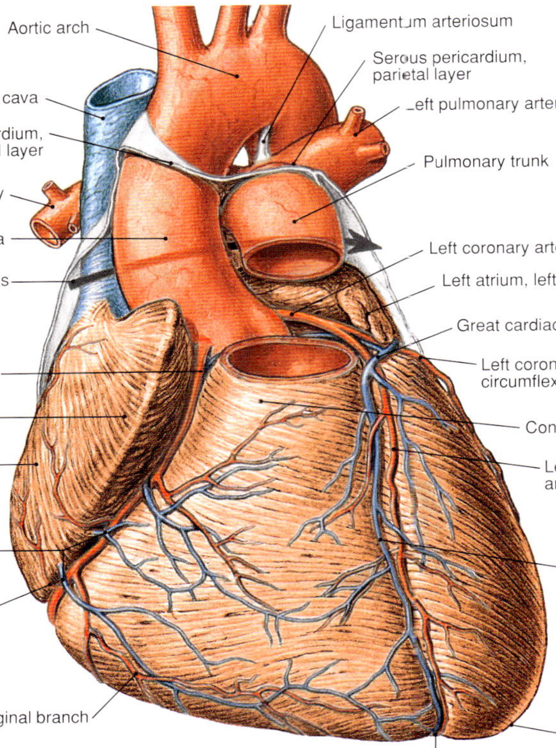

Fig. 623 Coronary arteries; ventral view.
Arrow in the transverse pericardial sinus

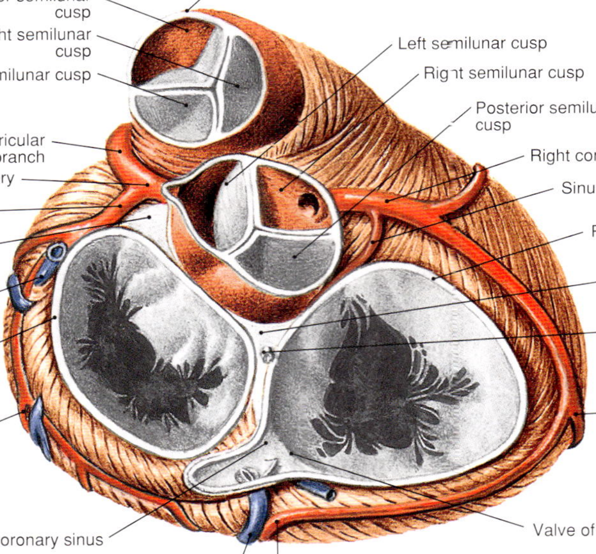

Fig. 624 Coronary arteries; superior view.

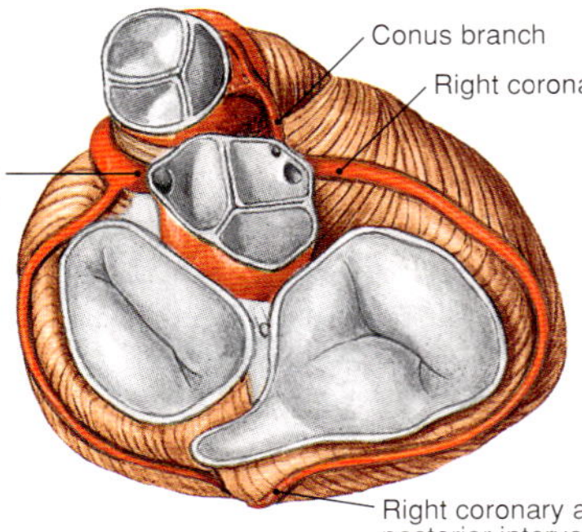

Fig. 625 Variability of the coronary arteries. The conus arteriosus branch arises from the aorta as an independent artery (~37%).

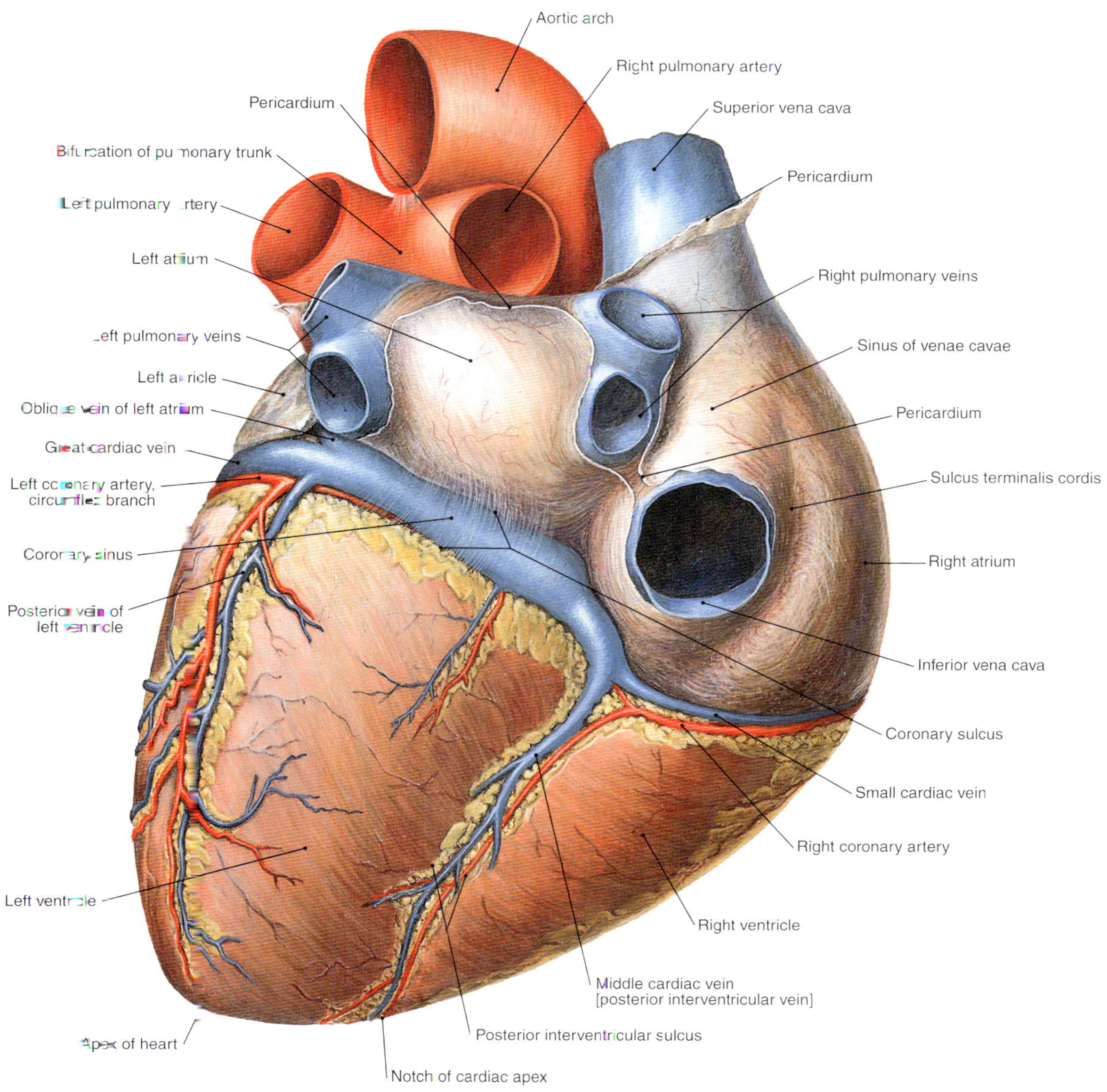

Fig. 626 Veins of the heart.

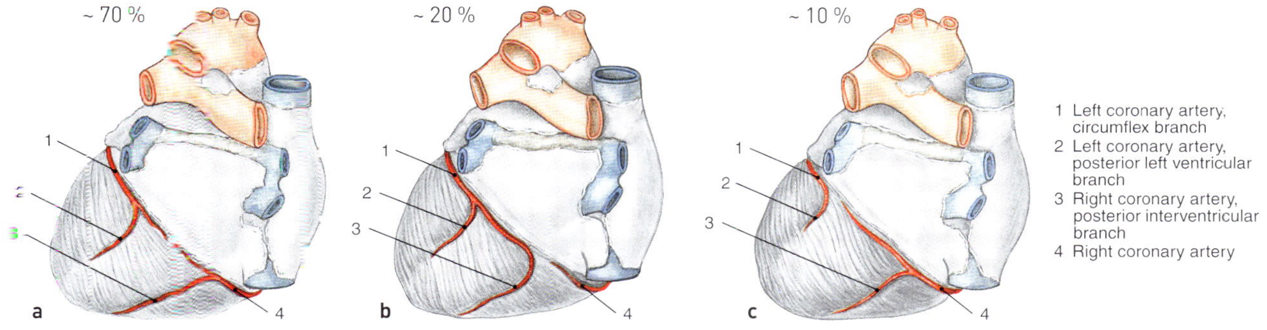

Fig. 627 a–c Variations in the arterial supply of the posterior aspect of the heart; dorsal view.

a Balanced coronary artery supply
b Dominant left coronary artery supply
c Dominant right coronary artery supply

Coronary arteries, variability of supply

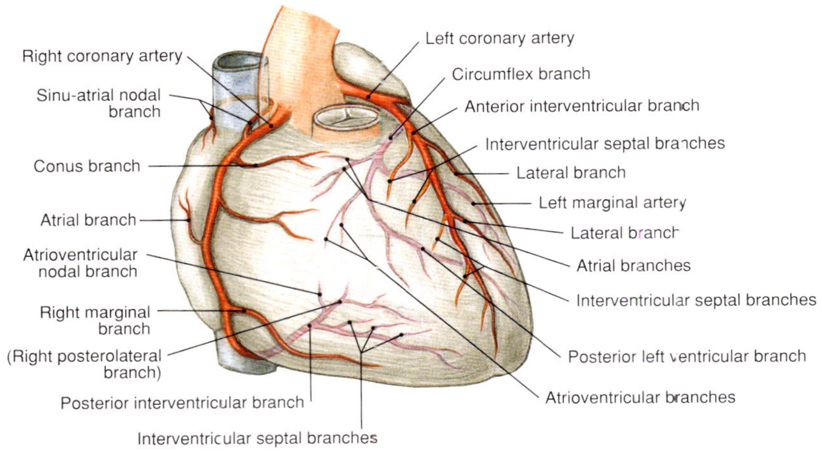

Fig. 628 Coronary arteries;
posterior arterial branches are shown in a lighter colour;
the posterior interventricular branch arises from the right coronary artery (balanced coronary artery supply);
ventral view.

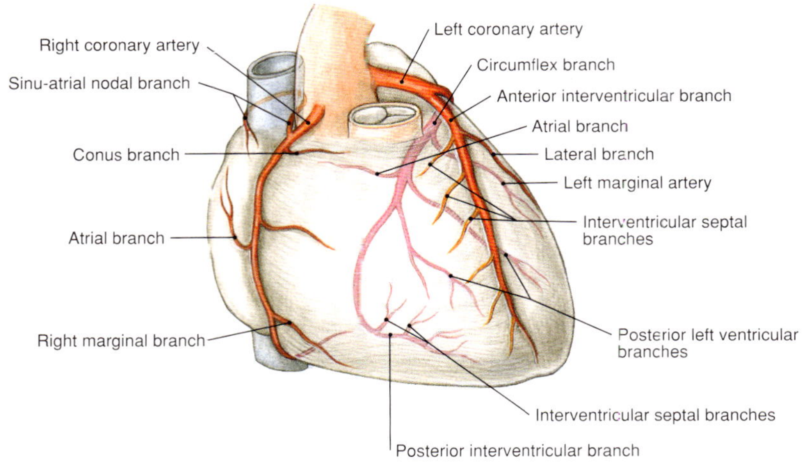

Fig. 629 Coronary arteries;
the posterior interventricular branch arises from the left coronary artery (dominant left coronary artery supply);
ventral view.

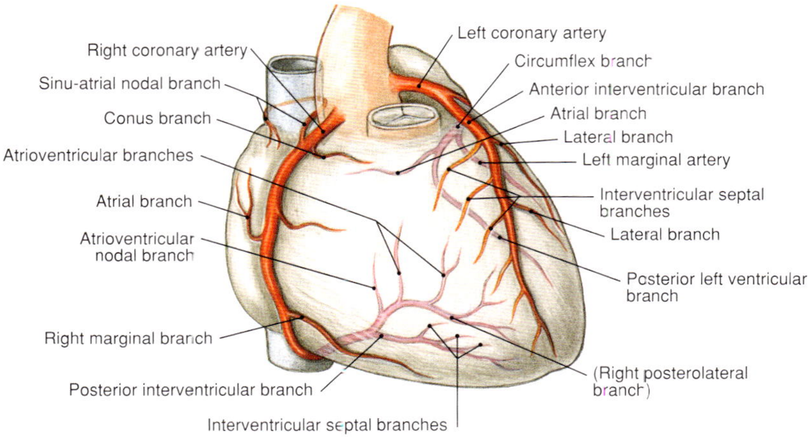

Fig. 630 Coronary arteries;
the posterior wall of the ventricles is mainly supplied by branches of the right coronary artery (dominant right coronary artery supply);
ventral view.

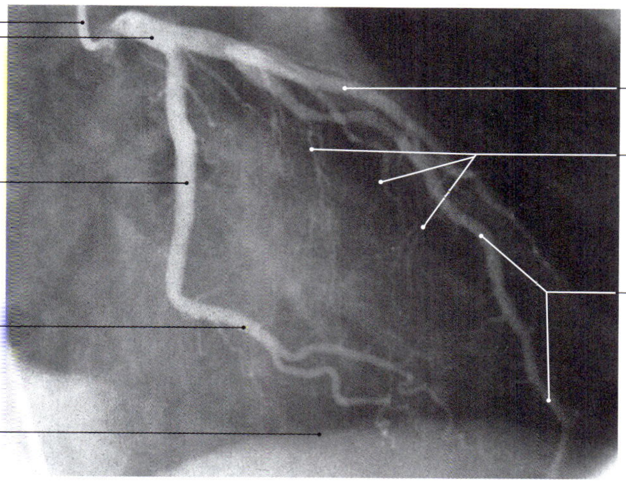

Fig. 631 Left coronary artery; coronary angiography; the beam is directed obliquely from right anterior to left posterior (RAO).

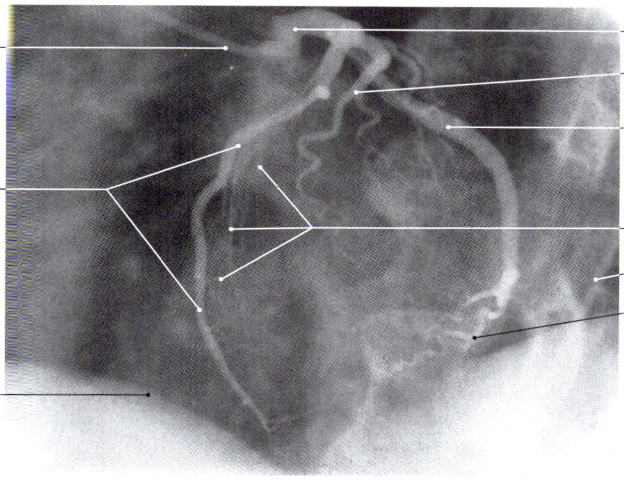

Fig. 632 Left coronary artery; coronary angiography; the beam is directed obliquely from left anterior to right posterior (LAO).

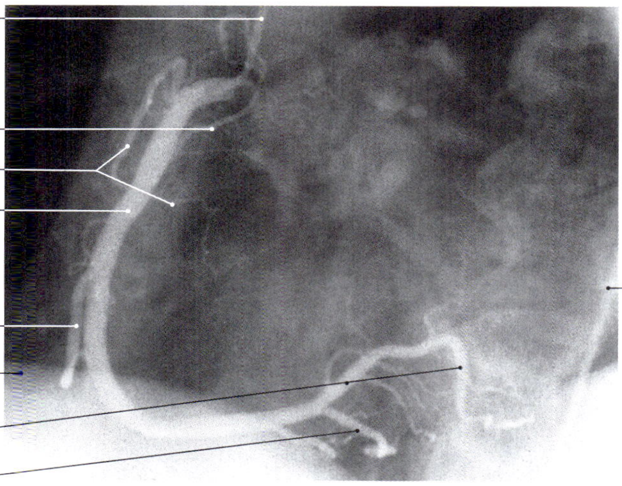

Fig. 633 Right coronary artery; coronary angiography; the beam is directed obliquely from left anterior to right posterior (LAO).

Heart situs

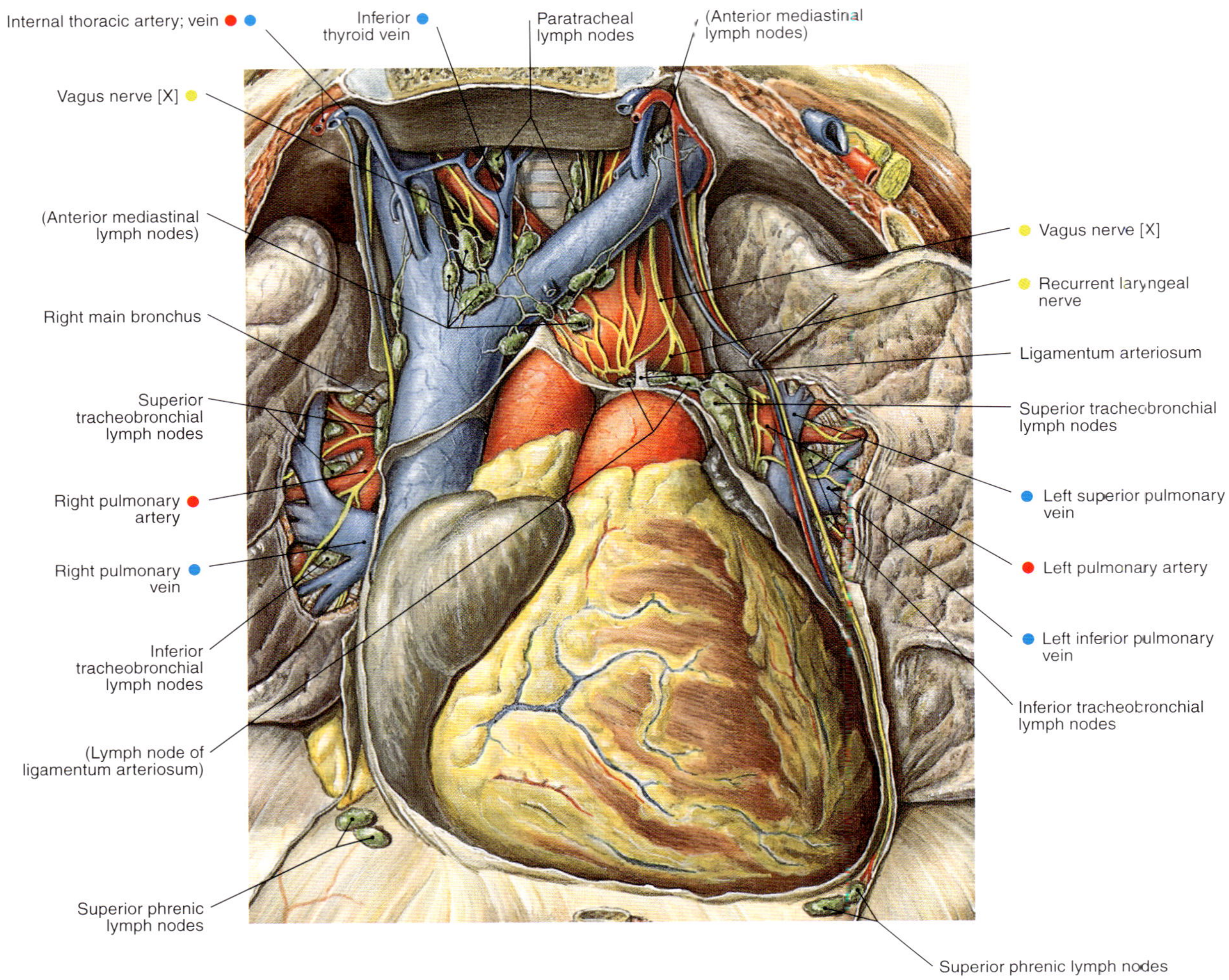

Fig. 634 Position of the heart in the thorax.

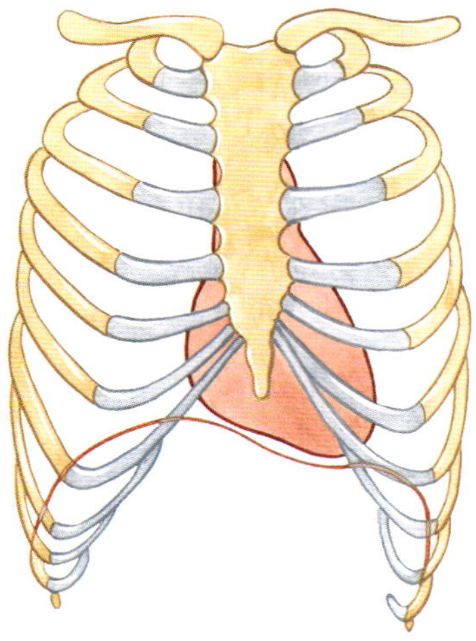

Fig. 635 Position of the heart; inspiration.

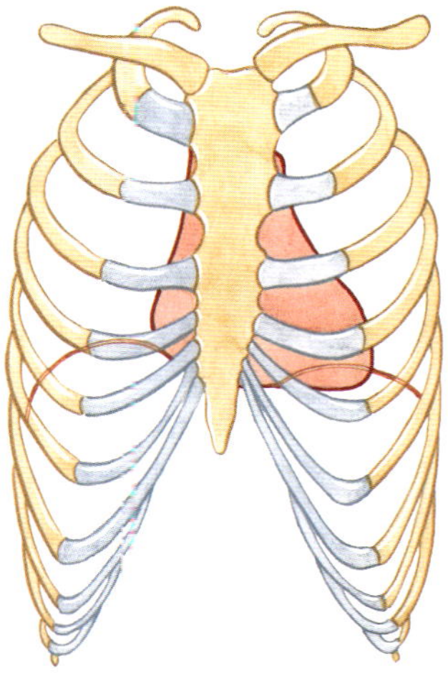

Fig. 636 Position of the heart; expiration.

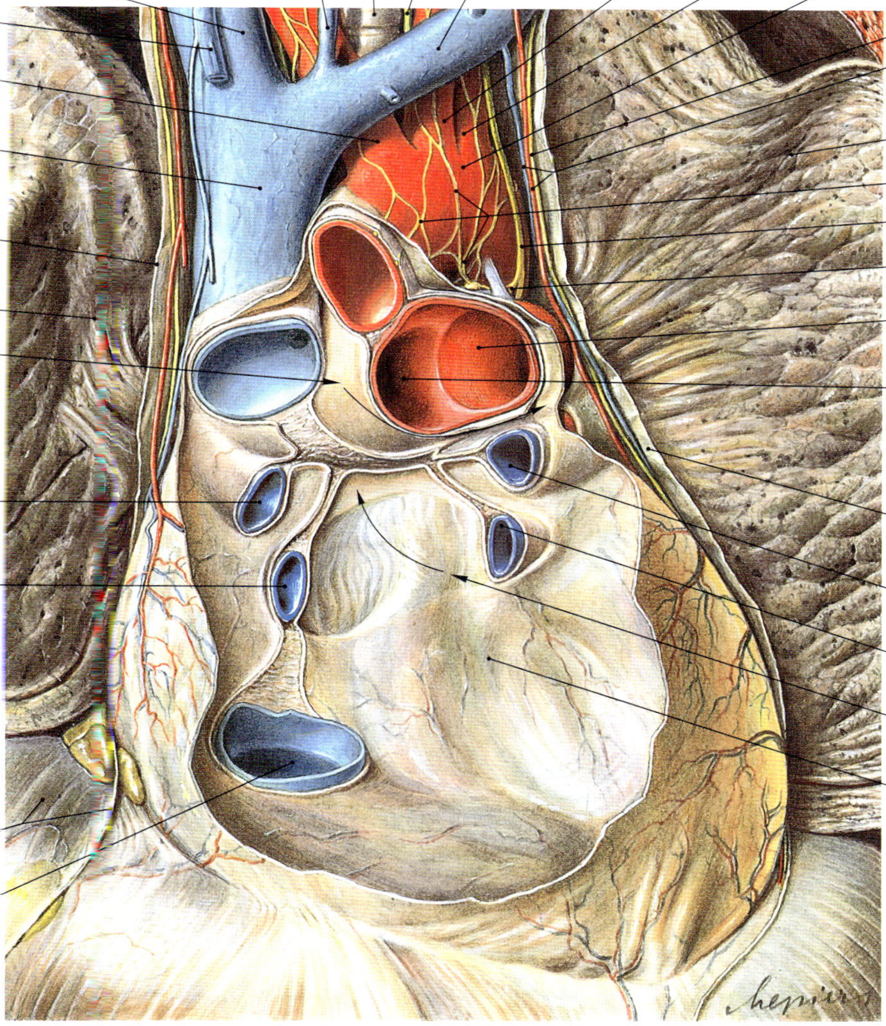

Fig. 637 Pericardium.

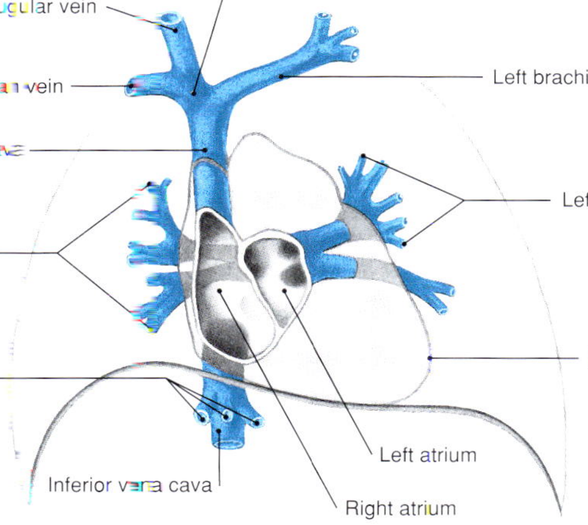

Fig. 638 Openings of the large veins into the heart; ventral view.

Trachea and bronchi

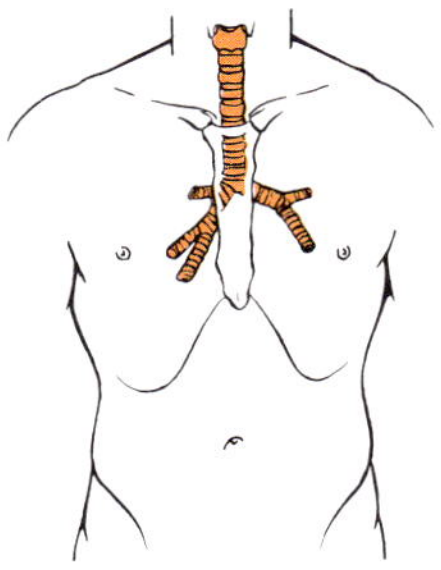

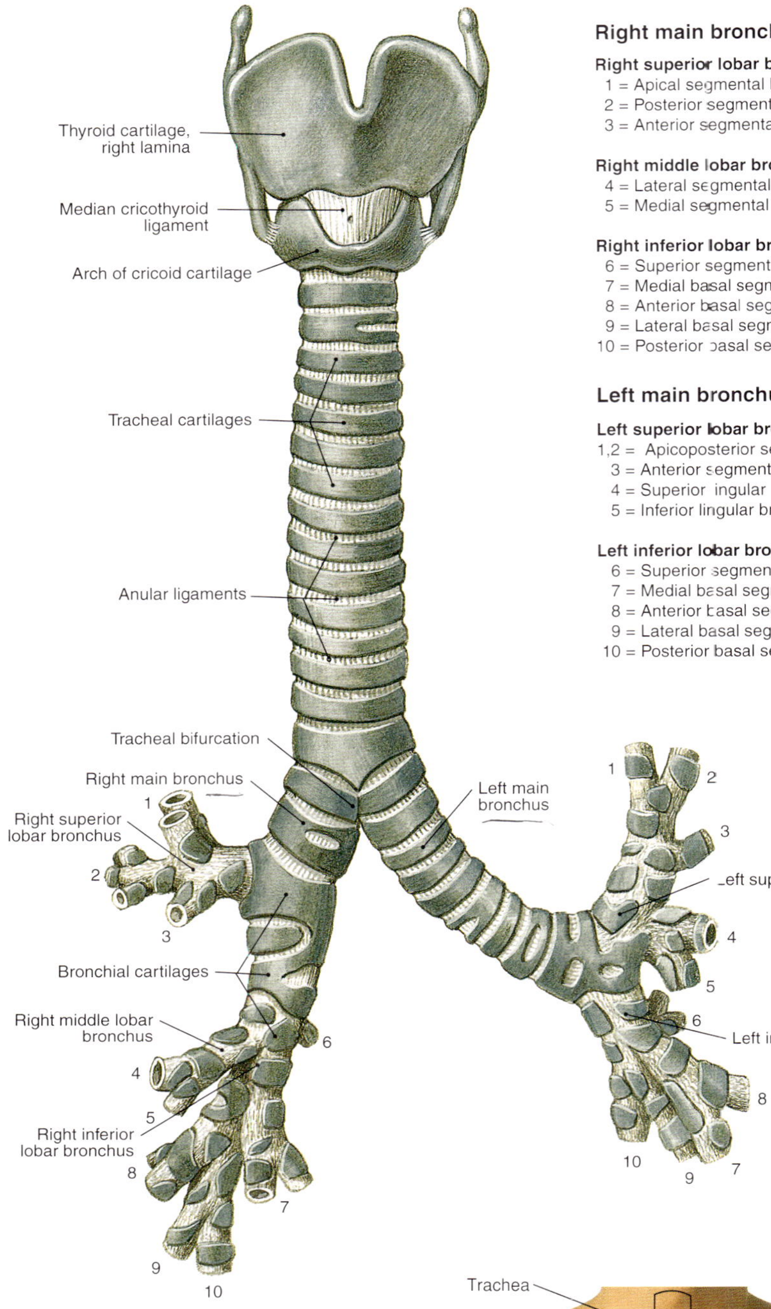

Right main bronchus

Right superior lobar bronchus
1 = Apical segmental bronchus [B I]
2 = Posterior segmental bronchus [B II]
3 = Anterior segmental bronchus [B III]

Right middle lobar bronchus
4 = Lateral segmental bronchus [B IV]
5 = Medial segmental bronchus [B V]

Right inferior lobar bronchus
6 = Superior segmental bronchus [B VI]
7 = Medial basal segmental bronchus [B VII] [B VII]
8 = Anterior basal segmental bronchus [B VIII]
9 = Lateral basal segmental bronchus [B IX]
10 = Posterior basal segmental bronchus [B X]

Left main bronchus

Left superior lobar bronchus
1,2 = Apicoposterior segmental bronchus [B I + II]
3 = Anterior segmental bronchus [B III]
4 = Superior lingular bronchus [B IV]
5 = Inferior lingular bronchus [B V]

Left inferior lobar bronchus
6 = Superior segmental bronchus [B VI]
7 = Medial basal segmental bronchus [B VII] [B VII]
8 = Anterior basal segmental bronchus [B VIII]
9 = Lateral basal segmental bronchus [B IX]
10 = Posterior basal segmental bronchus [B X]

Fig. 639 Larynx; trachea and bronchi.

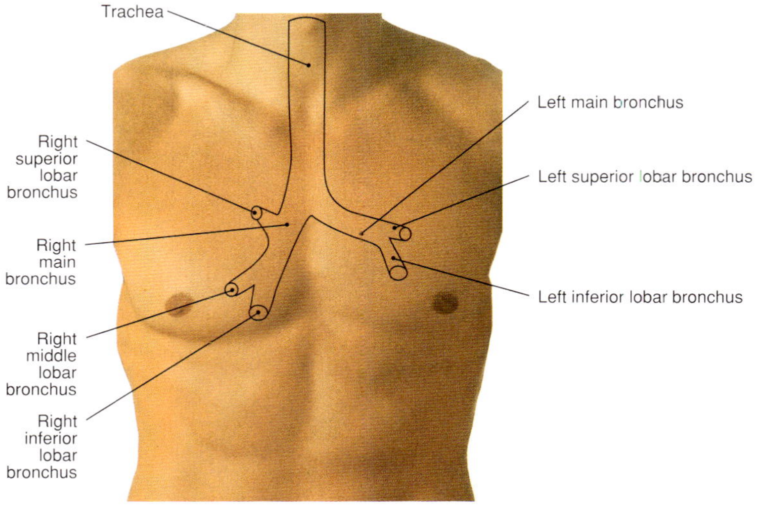

Fig. 640 Projection of the trachea and the bronchi onto the anterior thoracic wall.

* Connect the upper RT with the lower RT
* 9–15 cm in length
* located in front the esophagus and behind the thyroid gland in the neck
– considered to be in the superior and middle mediastinum.
* it's made up of 16–20 incomplete hyaline cartilagenous rings that open posteriorly.

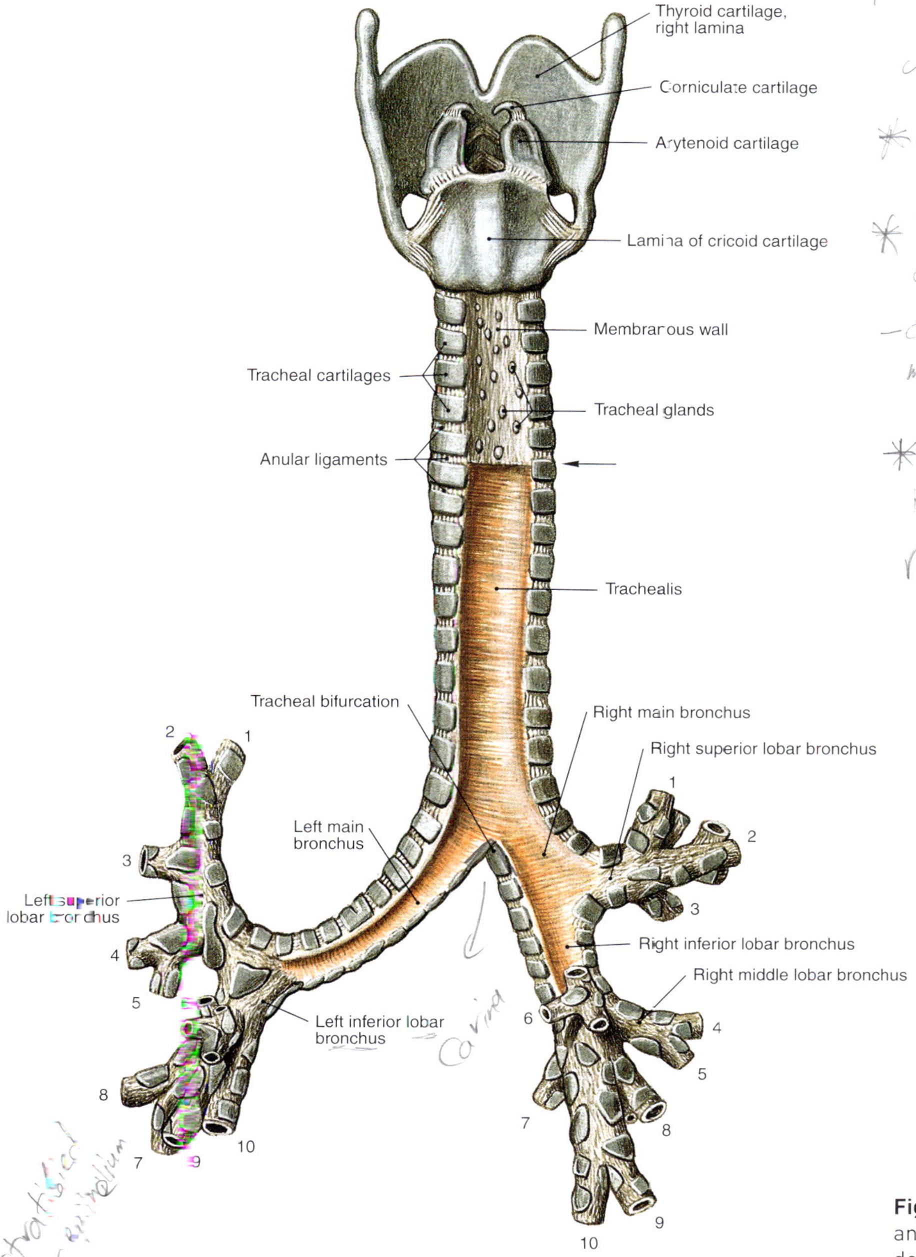

Fig. 641 Larynx; trachea and bronchi; dorsal view.

Ciliated pseudostratified columnar epithelium

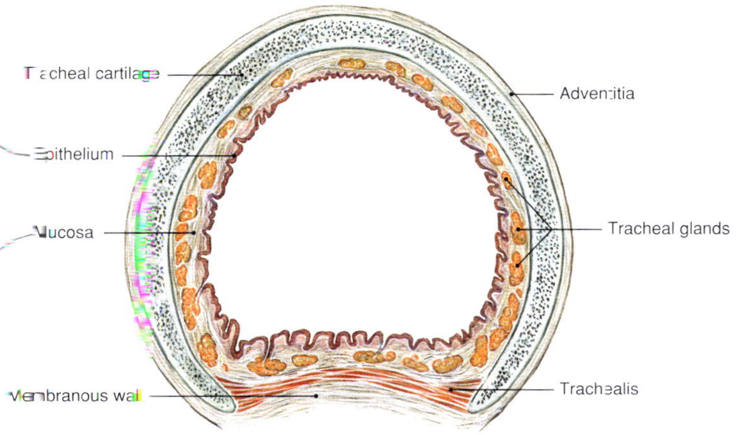

Secreting goblet cells

Fig. 642 Trachea; cross-section; microscopic enlargement at low magnification.

Segmental bronchi

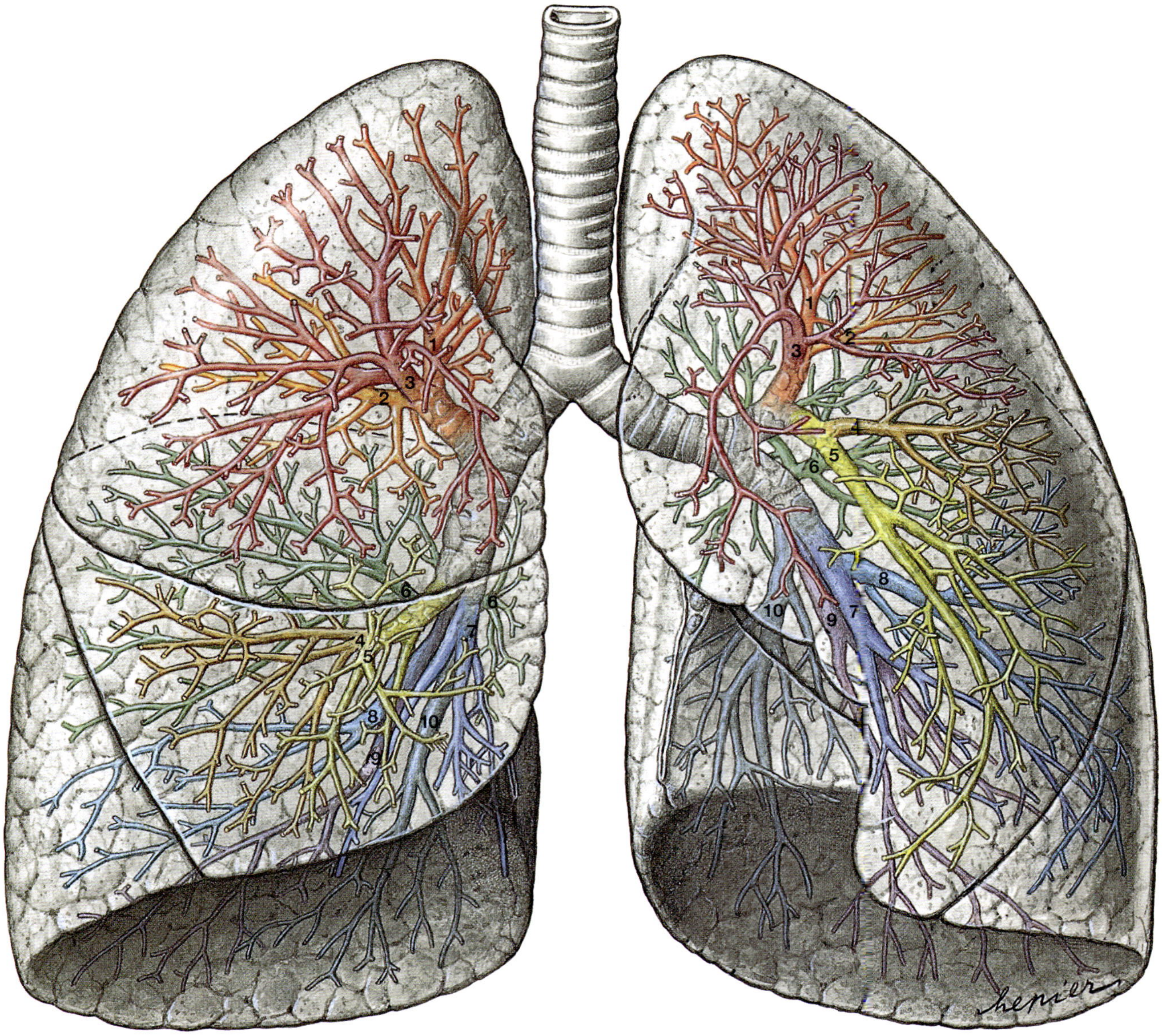

Fig. 643 Bronchi;
the lobar and the segmental bronchi have been projected onto the lungs and are illustrated with different colours; ventral view.
Numbers indicate the segmental bronchi (see p. 348).

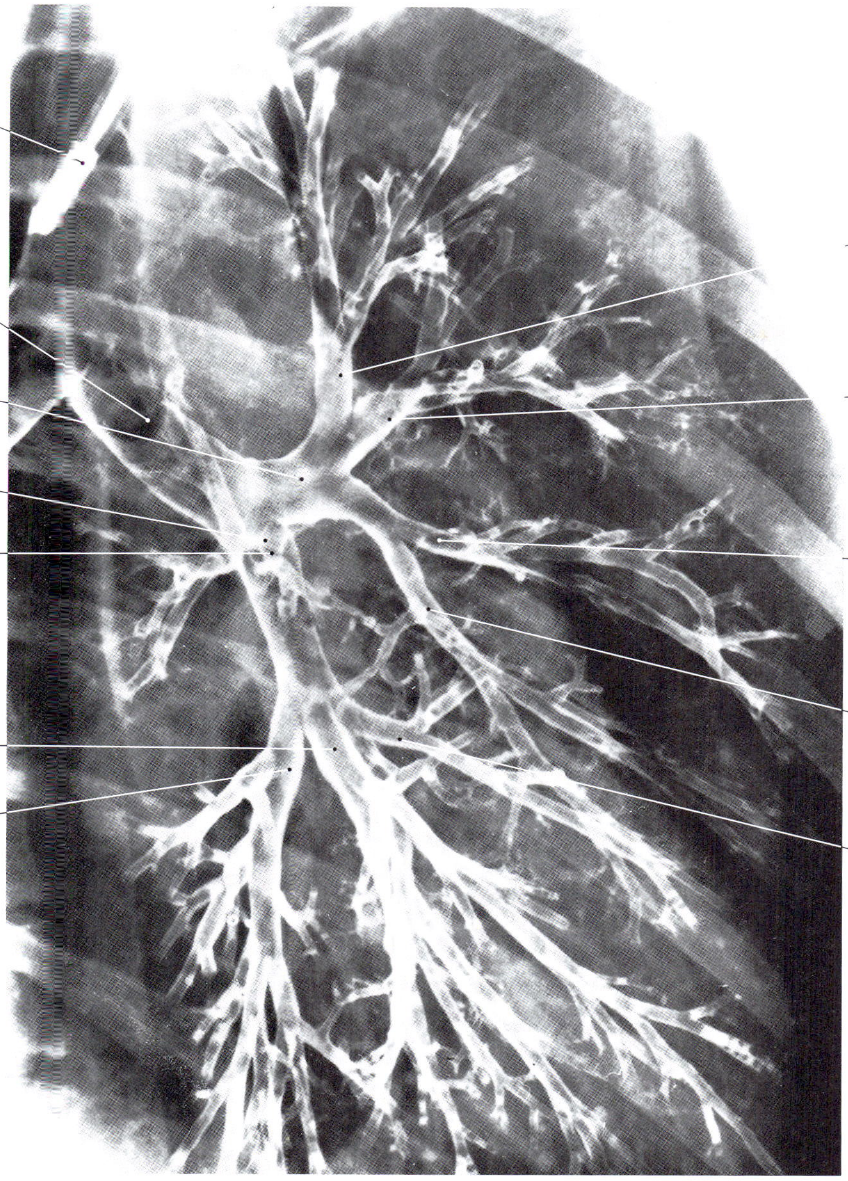

Fig. 644 Bronchi;
AP-radiograph; bronchography of the left lung.

* Bronchography catheter in the trachea

Lungs

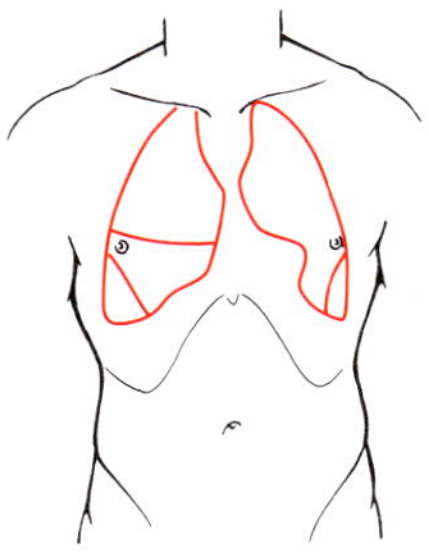

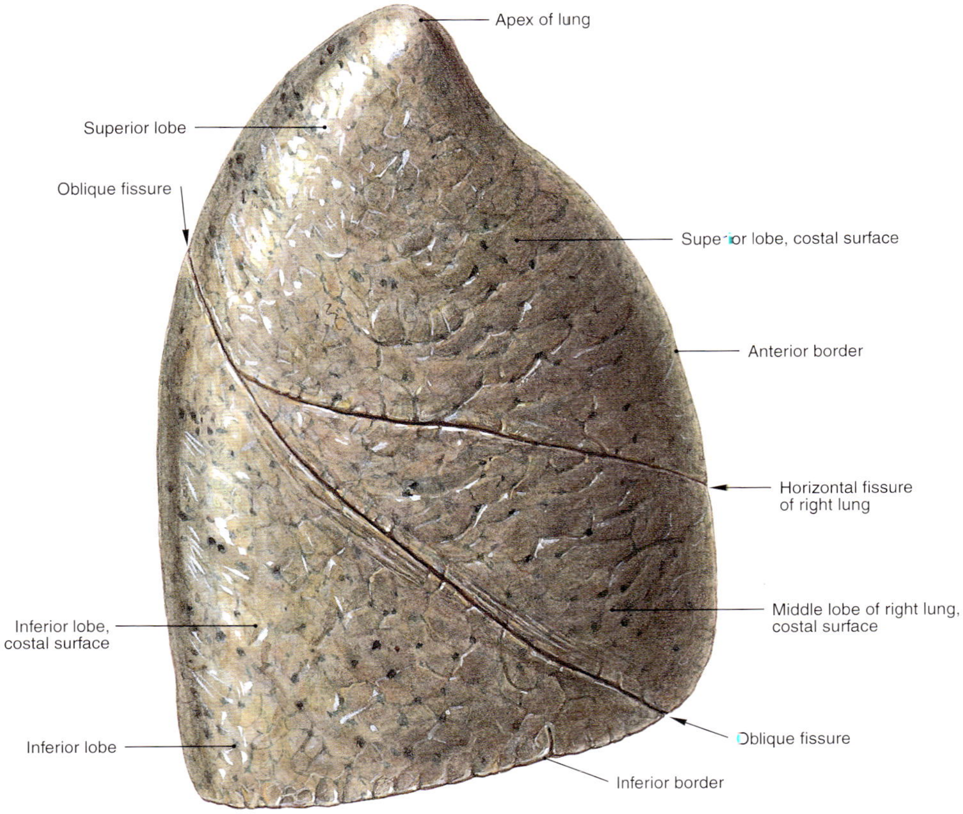

Fig. 645 Right lung; lateral view.

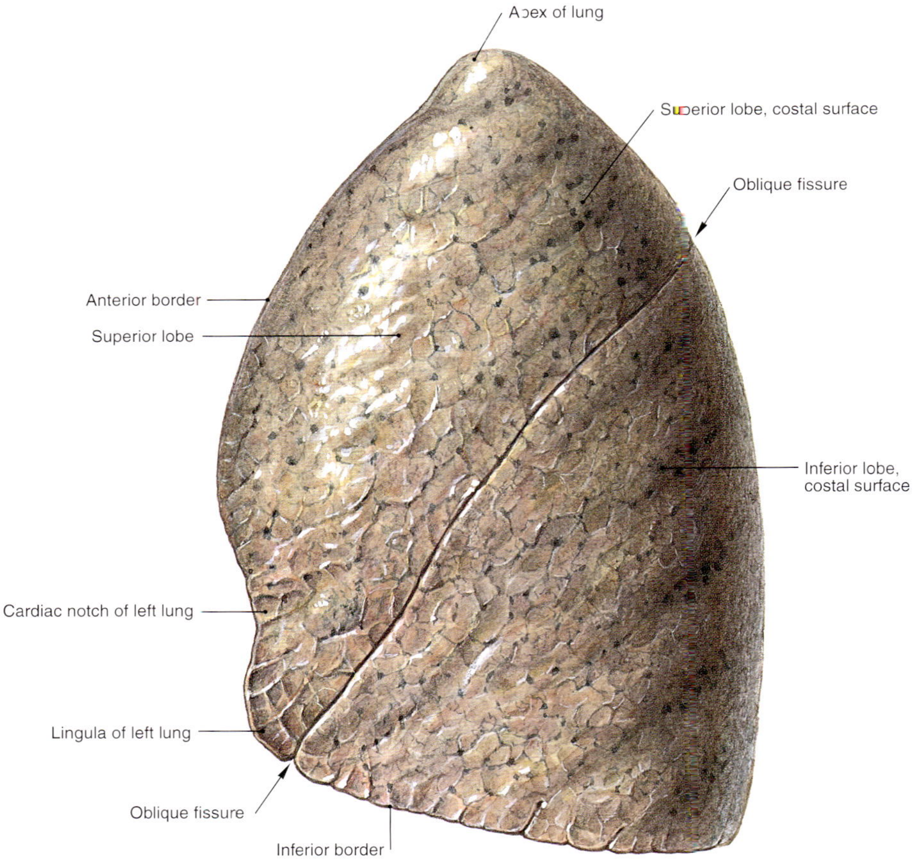

Fig. 646 Left lung; lateral view.

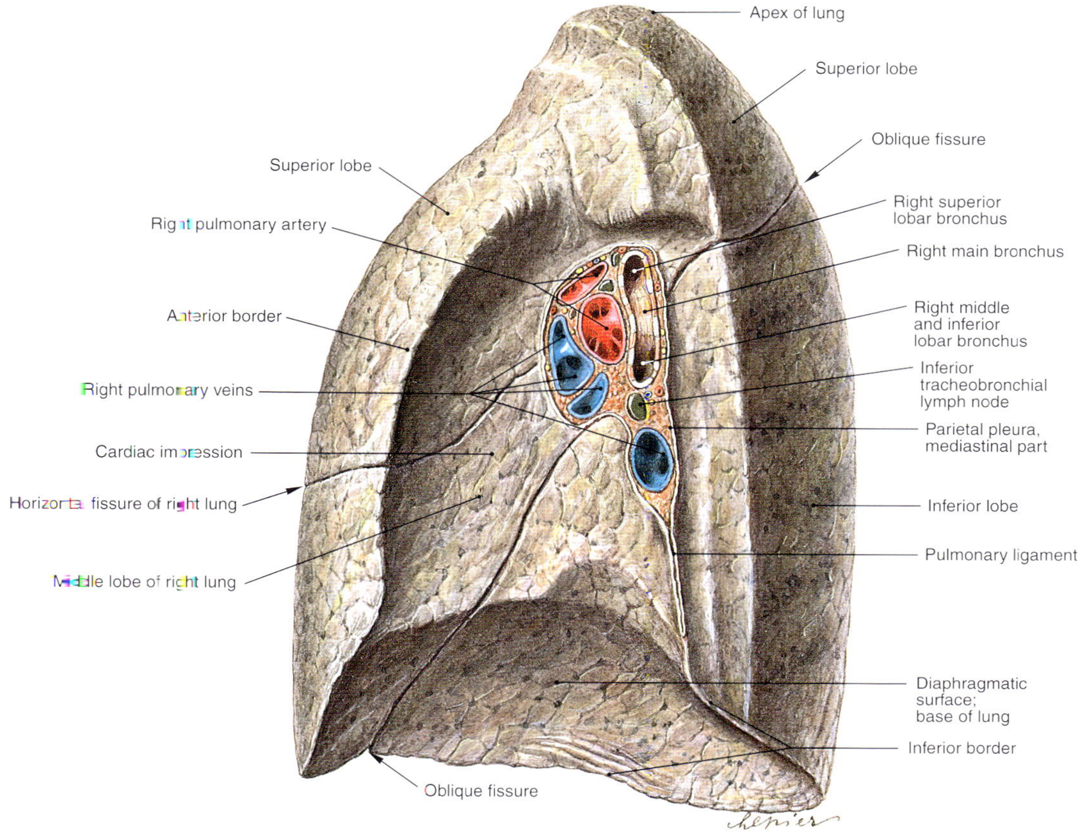

Fig. 647 Right lung;
sagittal section at the plane of the hilum of the lung;
medial view.

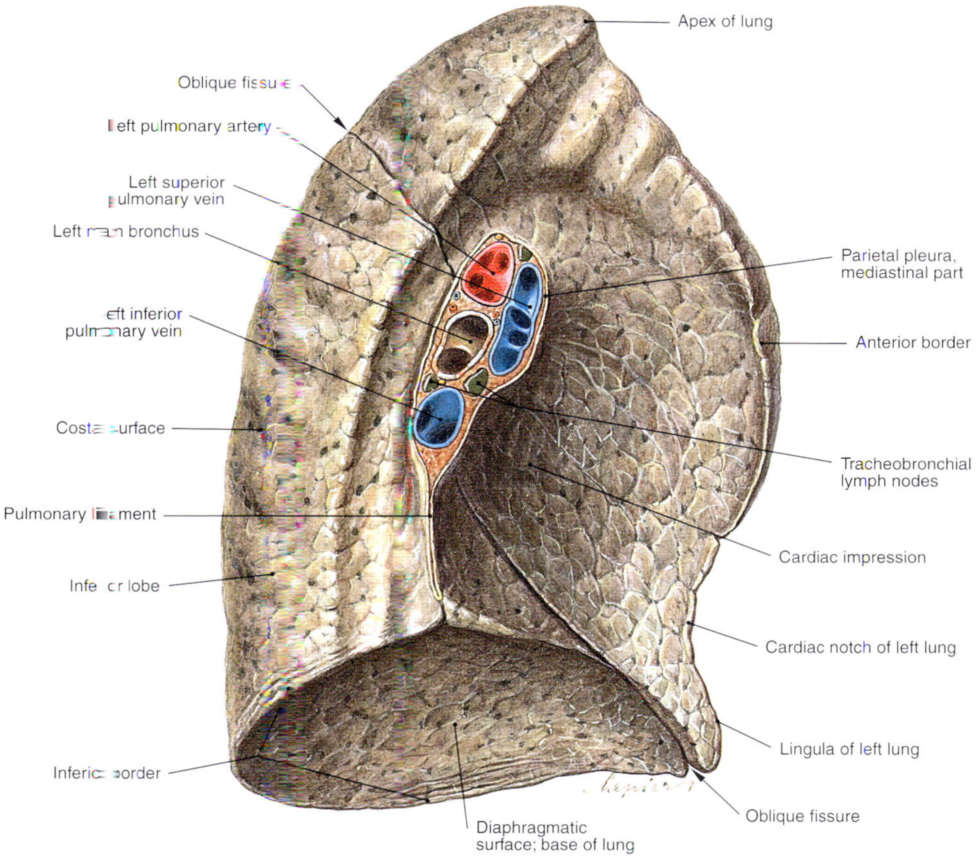

Fig. 648 Left lung;
sagittal section at the plane of the hilum of the lung;
medial view.

Bronchopulmonary segments

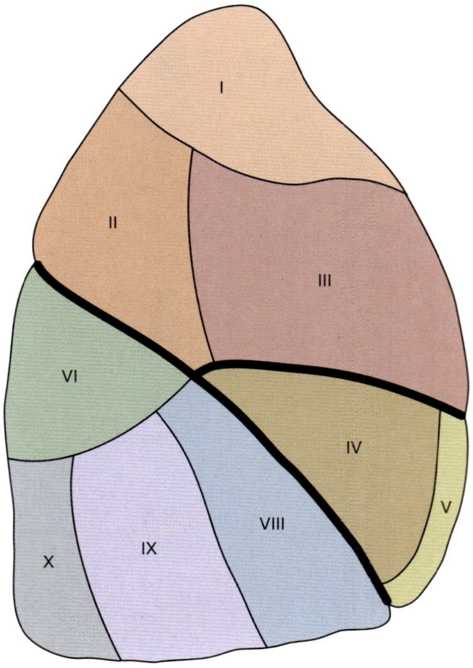

Right lung

Right lung, superior lobe

- Apical segment [S I]
- Posterior segment [S II]
- Anterior segment [S III]

Right lung, median lobe

- Lateral segment [S IV]
- Medial segment [S V]

Right lung, inferior lobe

- Superior segment [S VI]
- Medial basal [cardiac] segment [S VII]
- Anterior basal segment [S VIII]
- Lateral basal segment [S IX]
- Posterior basal segment [S X]

Fig. 649 Right lung; bronchopulmonary segments; lateral view

Left lung

Left lung, superior lobe

- Apicoposterior segment [S I + II]
- Anterior segment [S III]
- Superior lingular segment [S IV]
- Inferior lingular segment [S V]

Left lung, inferior lobe

- Superior segment [S VI]
- Medial basal [cardiac] segment [S VII]*
- Anterior basal segment [S VIII]
- Lateral basal segment [S IX]
- Posterior basal segment [S X]

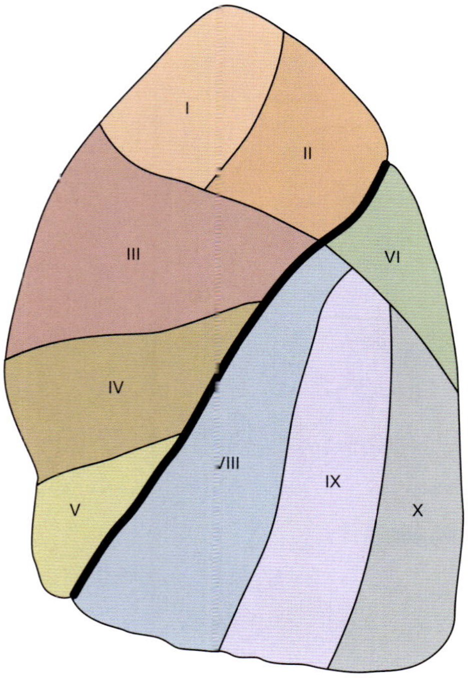

Fig. 650 Left lung; bronchopulmonary segments; lateral view.

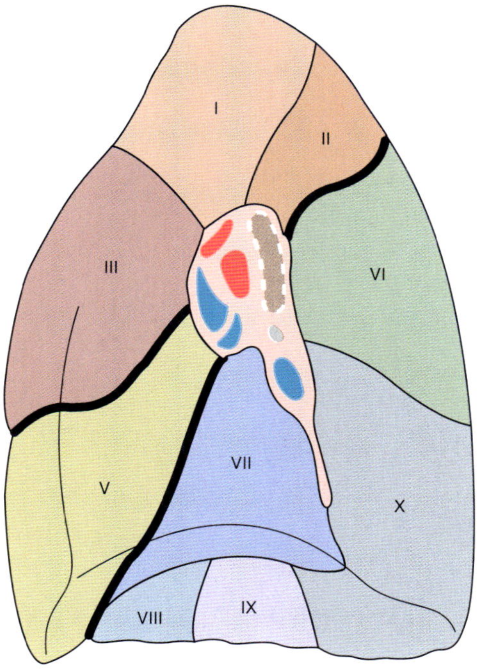

Fig. 65 Right lung; bronchopulmonary segments; medial view.

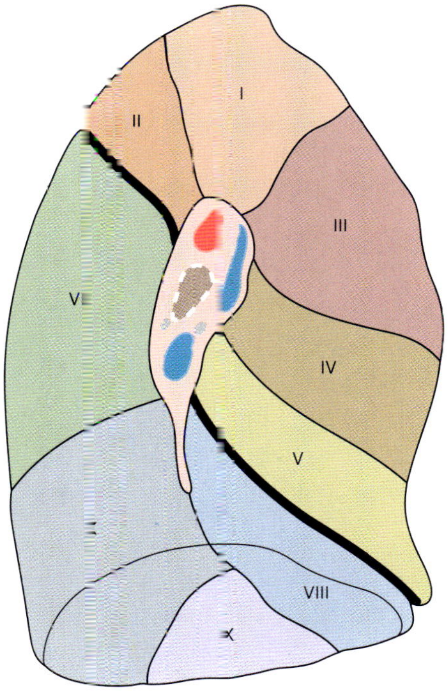

Fig. 652 Left lung; bronchopulmonary segments; medial view.

Lungs, structure

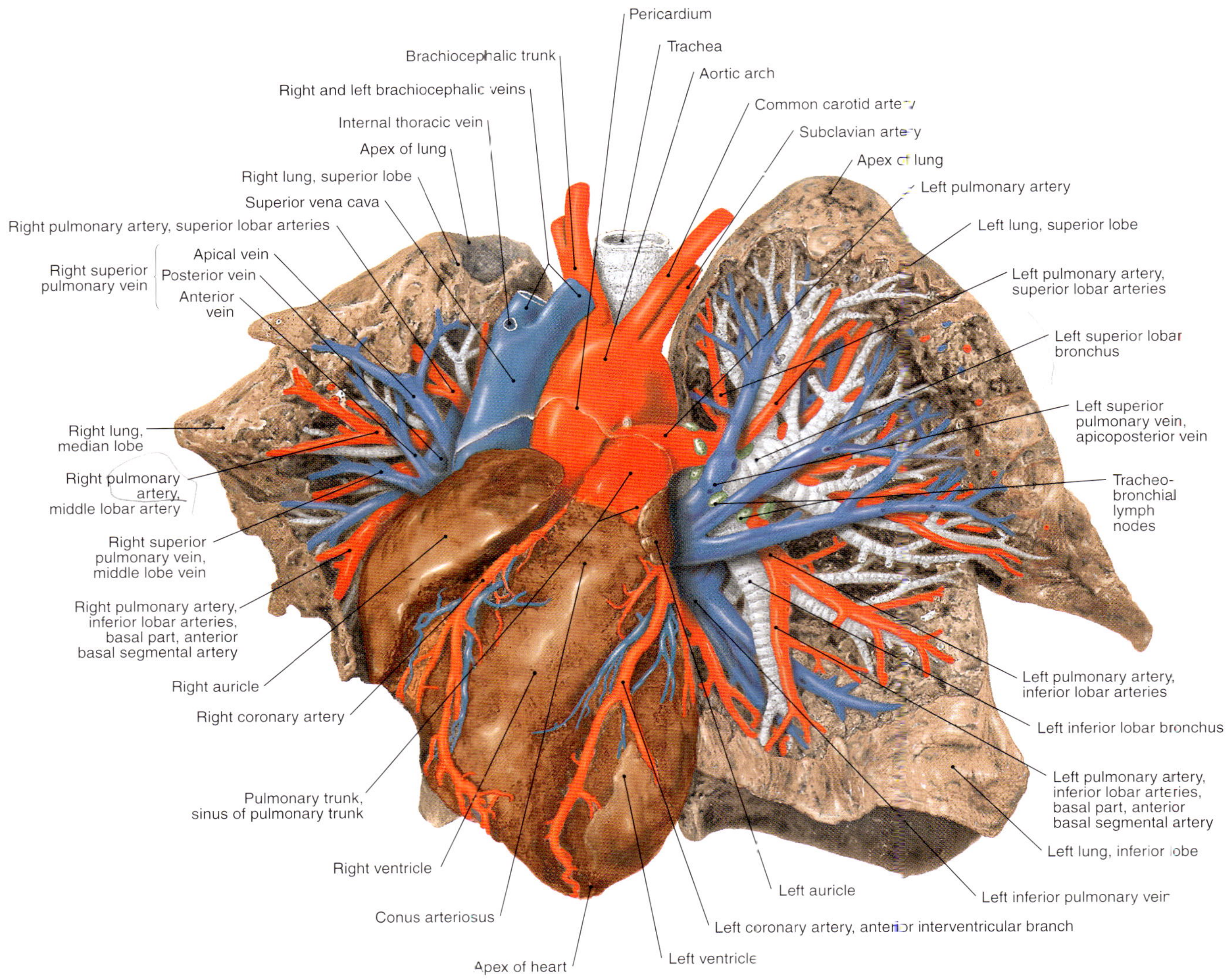

Fig. 653 Lungs and heart;
the arteries, the veins and the bronchi have been dissected up to the external surface of the lungs.

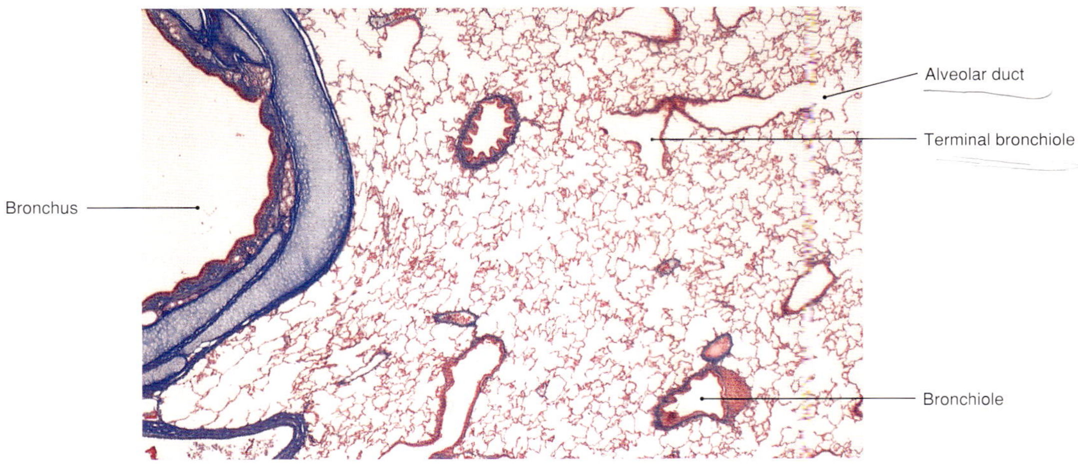

Fig. 654 Lung;
overview of the lung structure;
microscopic enlargement at low magnification.

Vessels of the lungs and bronchi

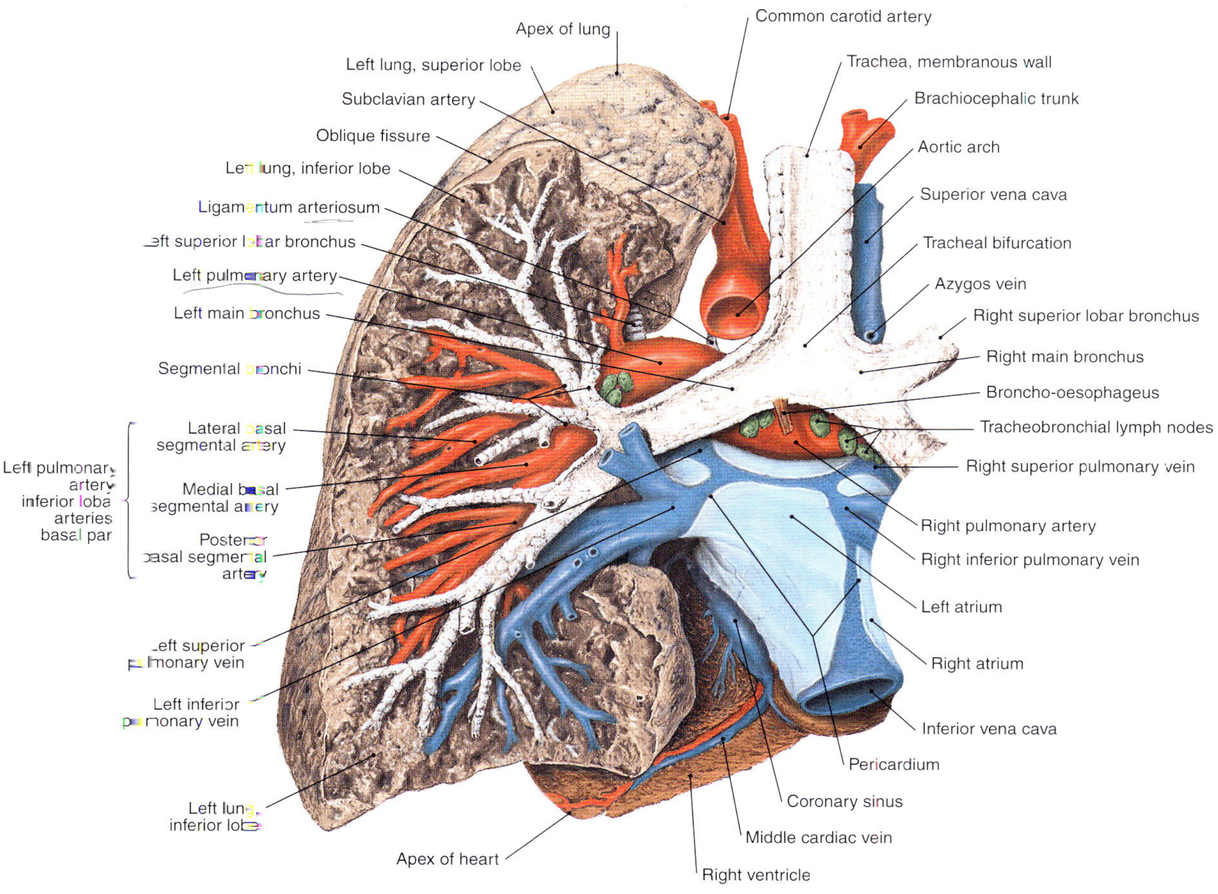

Fig. 655 Vessels of the left lung; dorsal view.

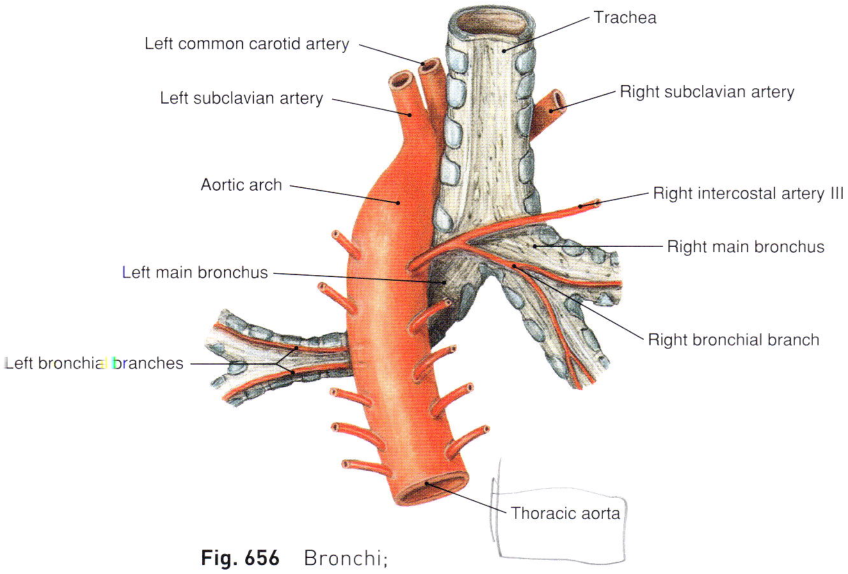

Fig. 656 Bronchi; arterial supply.

Vessels of the lung, radiography

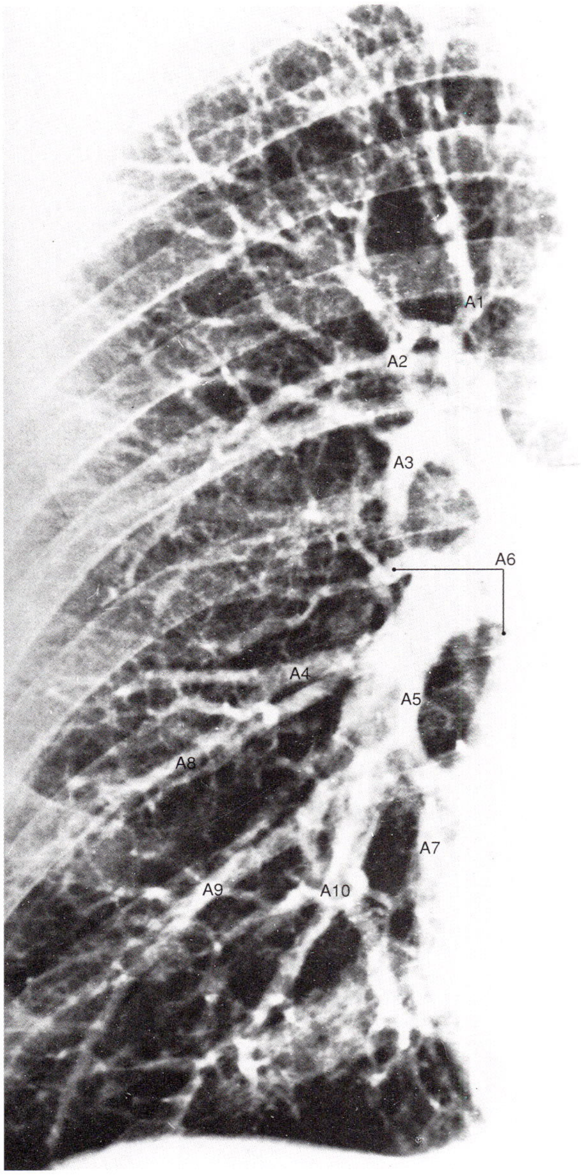

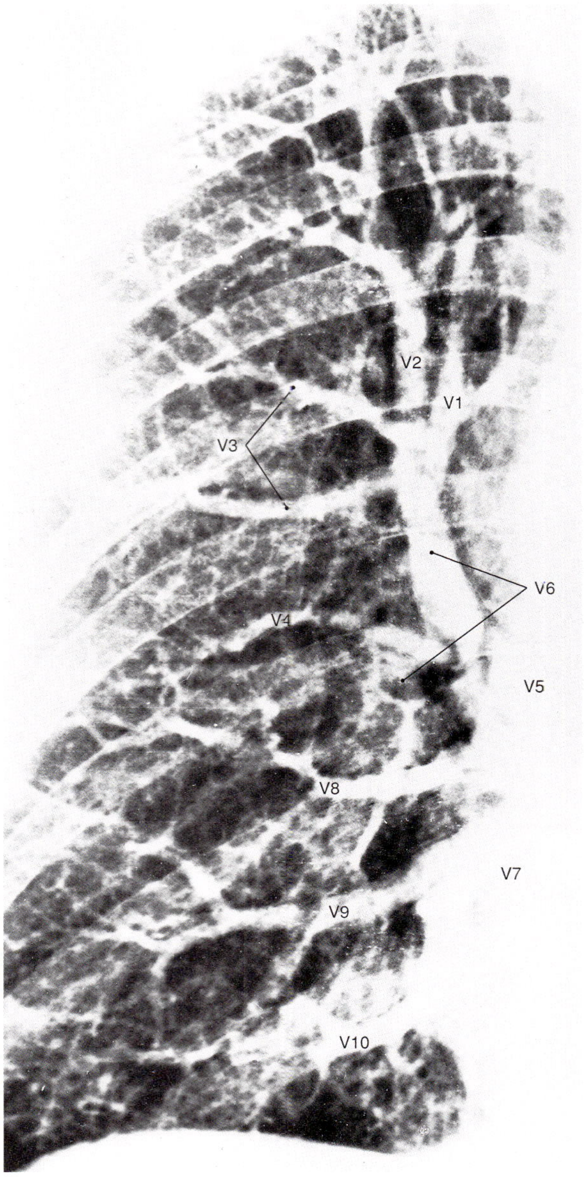

Fig. 657 Arteries of the right lung;
AP-radiograph (pulmonary angiography); after injection of a contrast medium into the right ventricle;
ventral view.
The numbers designate the segmental arteries (compare p. 354).

Fig. 658 Veins of the right lung;
AP-radiograph (return via pulmonary veins of the contrast medium injected into the right ventricle);
ventral view.
Numbers indicate the segmental veins (compare p. 354).

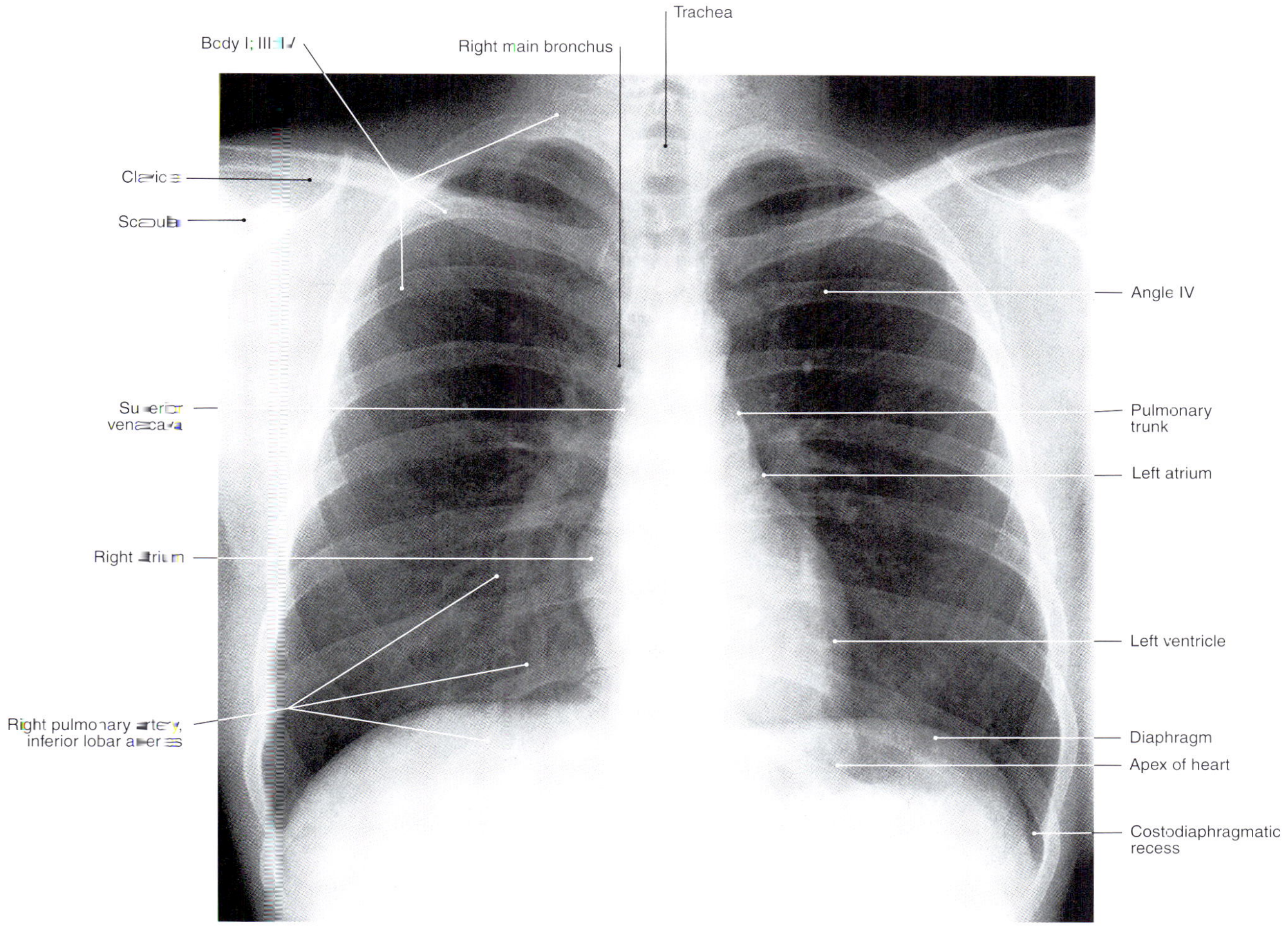

Fig. 659 Thoracic cage and thoracic viscera; PA-radiograph of a 27-year-old male (thorax radiograph).

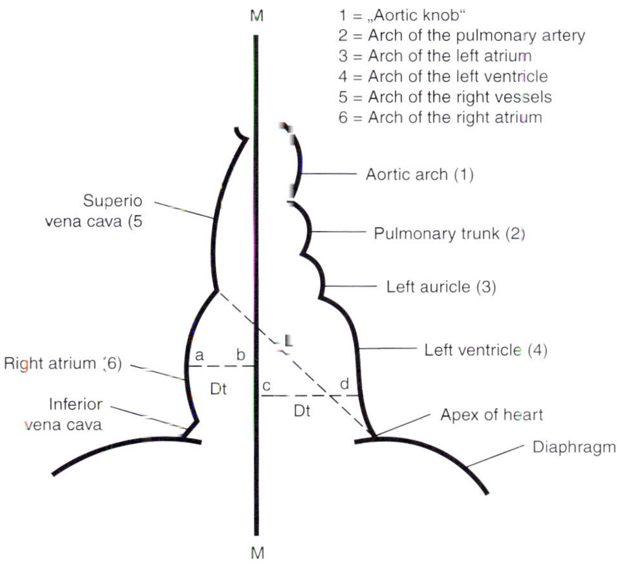

Fig. 660 Outline of the heart shadow in the radiograph;
Dt = Transverse diameter,
ab + cd = 13–14 cm
L = Longitudinal axis of the heart (from the superior border of the right atrial contour to the apex of the heart) = 15–16 cm
M = Median plane of the body

Bronchoscopy

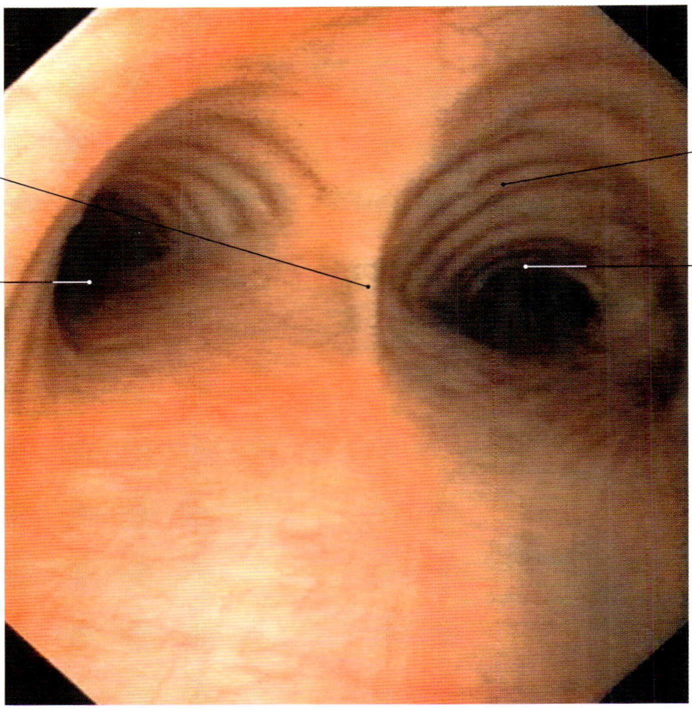

Fig. 661 Bronchi;
bronchoscopy of a healthy individual displaying the tracheal bifurcation and the carina of trachea.

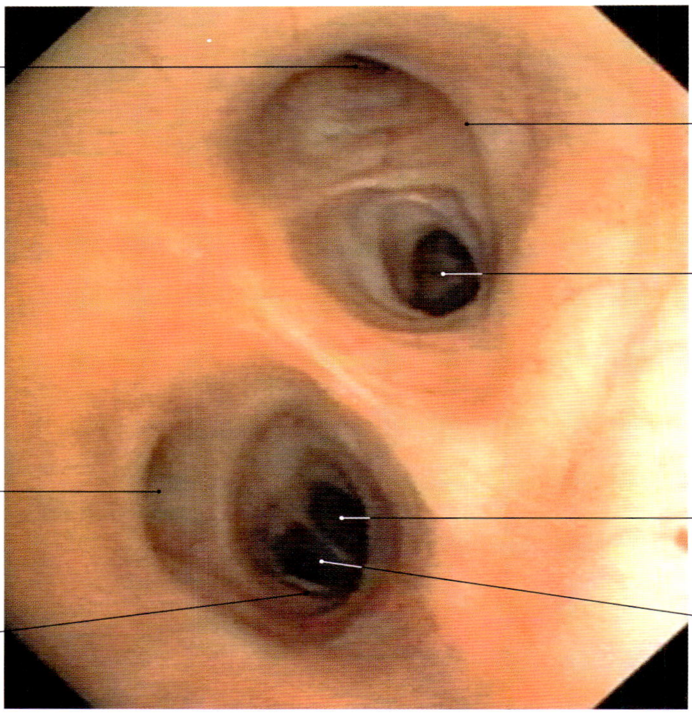

Fig. 662 Bronchi;
bronchoscopic view of the left segmental bronchi.

Lungs, surface projections

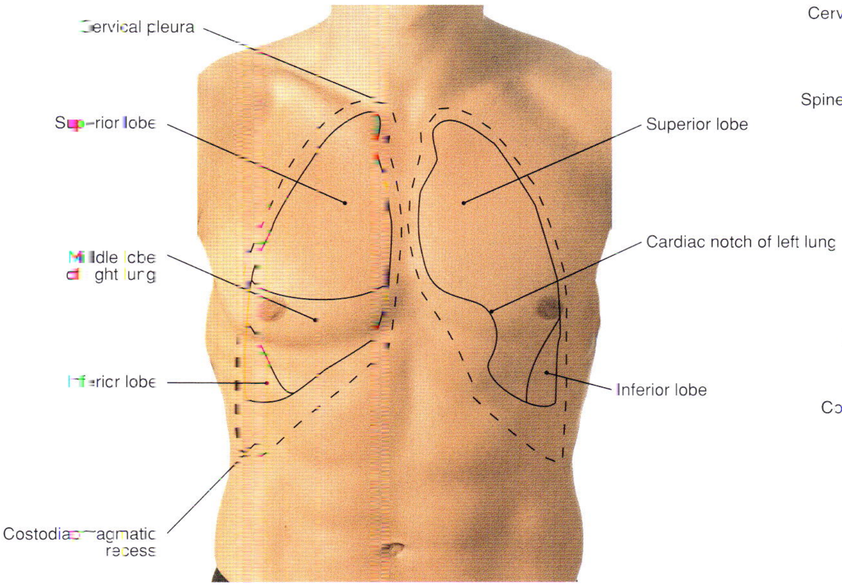

Fig. 663 Projection of the pulmonary and the pleural borders onto the anterior thoracic wall.

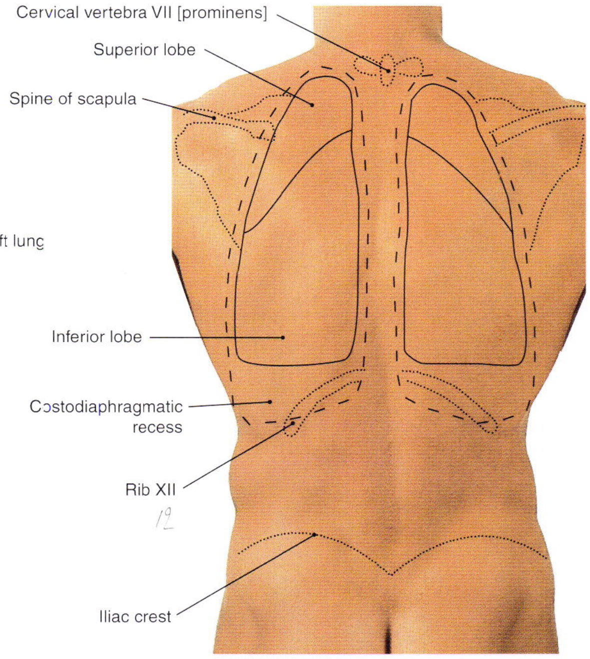

Fig. 664 Projection of the pulmonary and the pleural borders onto the posterior thoracic wall.

Borders of the lungs – line
Borders of the pleura – dashed line

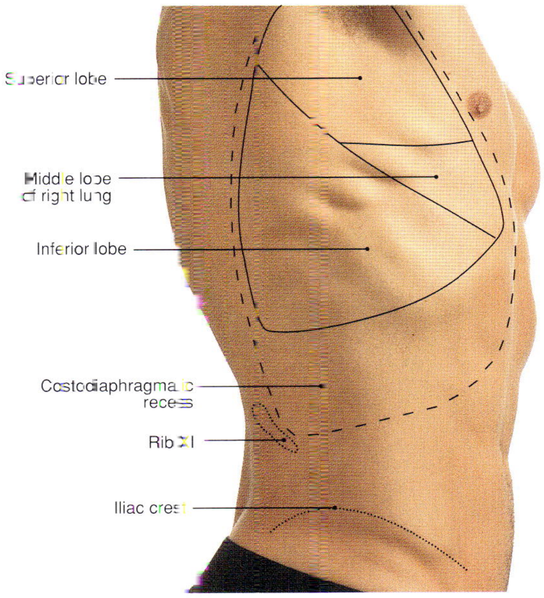

Fig. 665 Projection of the pulmonary and the pleural borders onto the lateral thoracic wall.

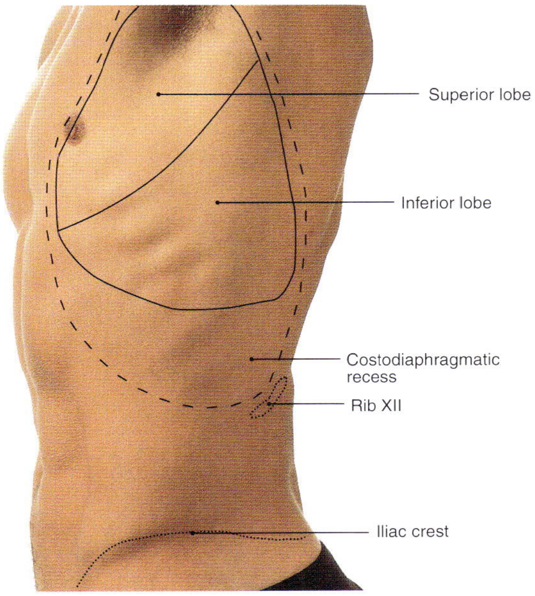

Fig. 666 Projection of the pulmonary and the pleural borders onto the lateral thoracic wall.

Oesophagus

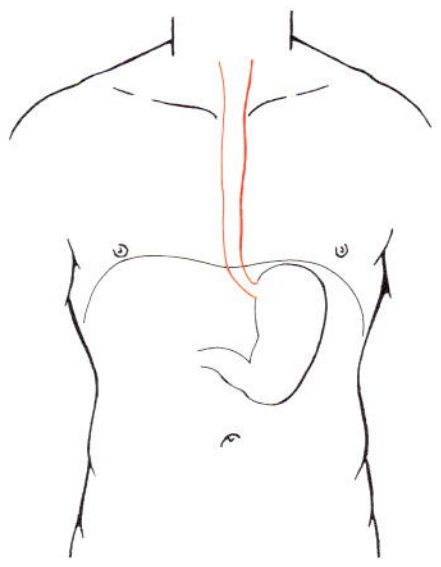

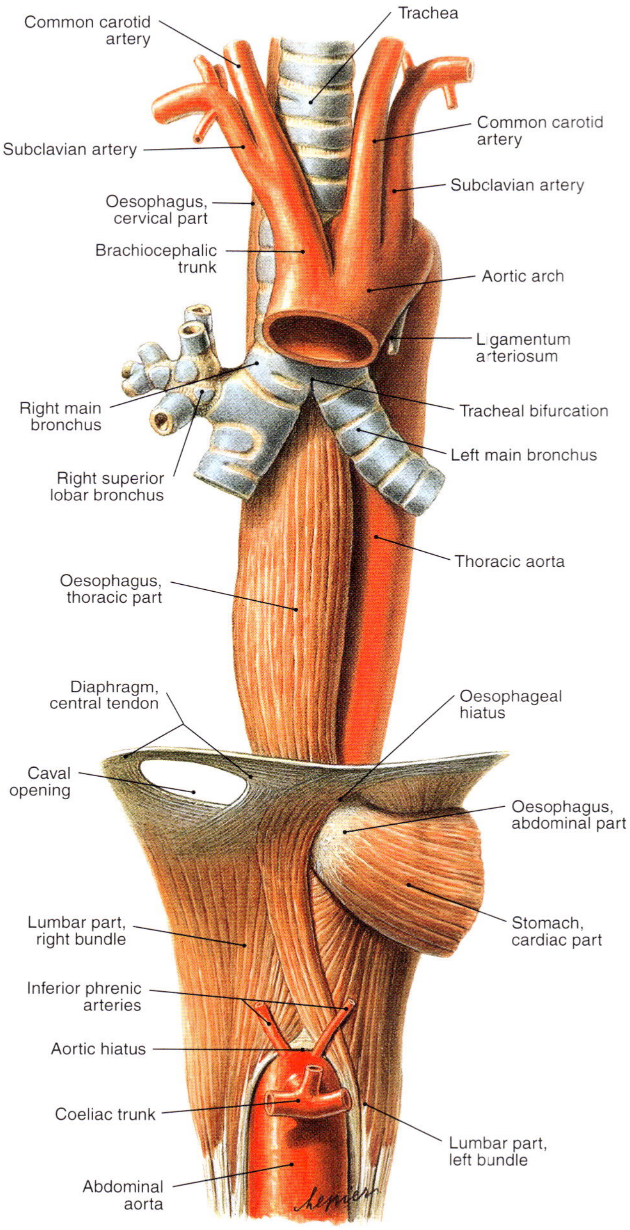

Fig. 667 Oesophagus; trachea and the thoracic aorta; ventral view.

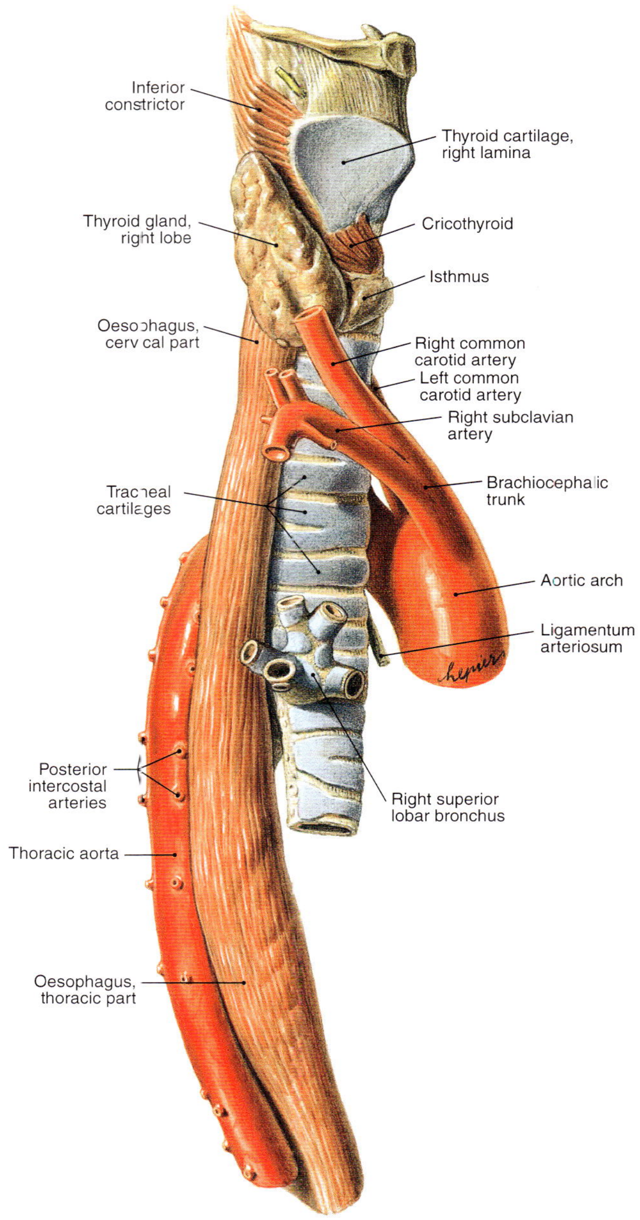

Fig. 668 Oesophagus; trachea and the thoracic aorta; viewed from the right.

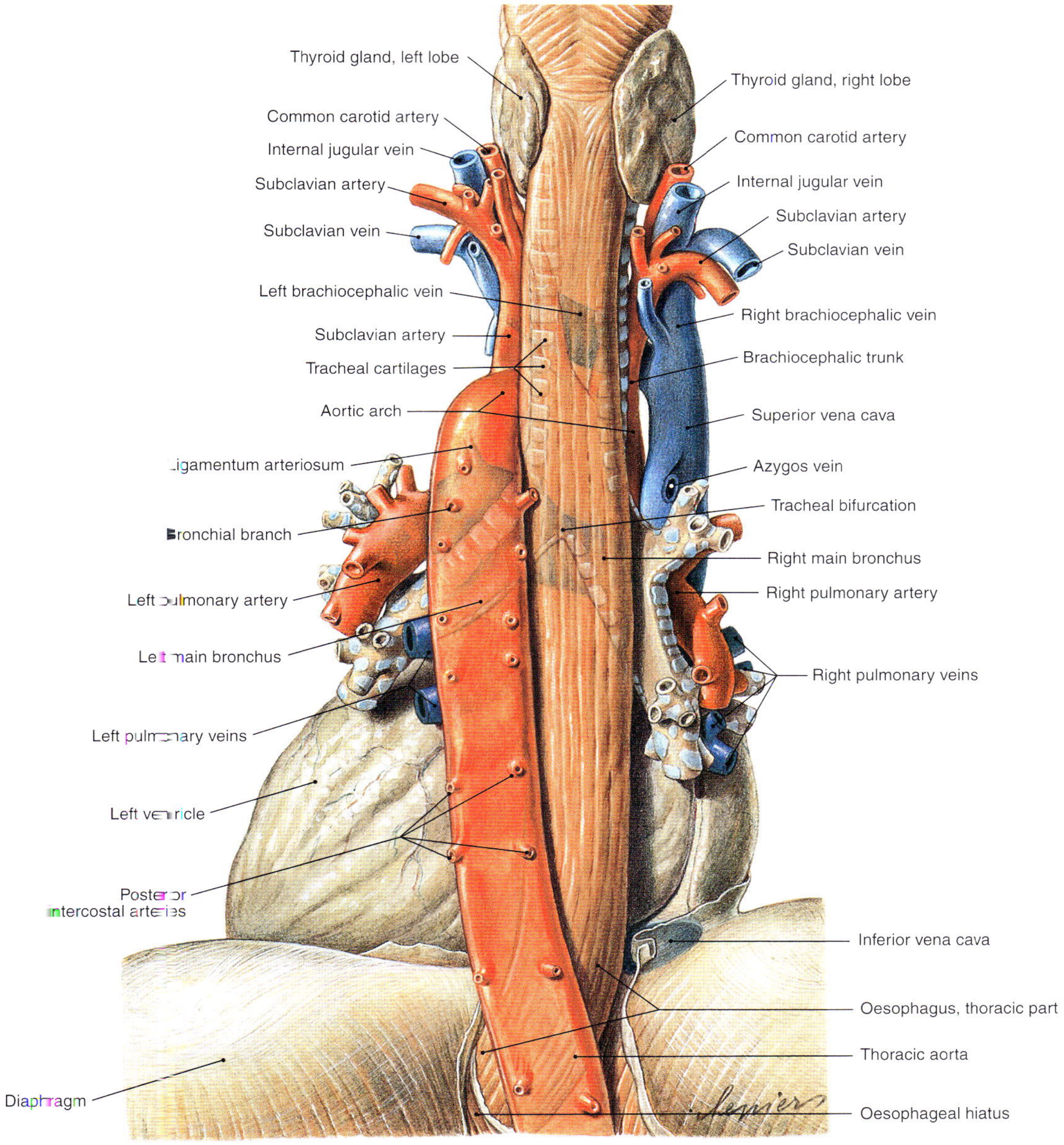

Fig. 669 Oesophagus and the thoracic aorta; dorsal view.

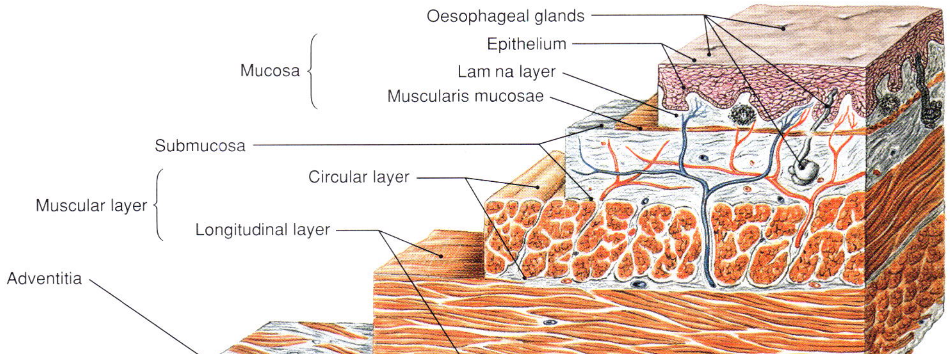

Fig. 670 Oesophagus; microscopic enlargement at low magnification.

Vessels of the oesophagus

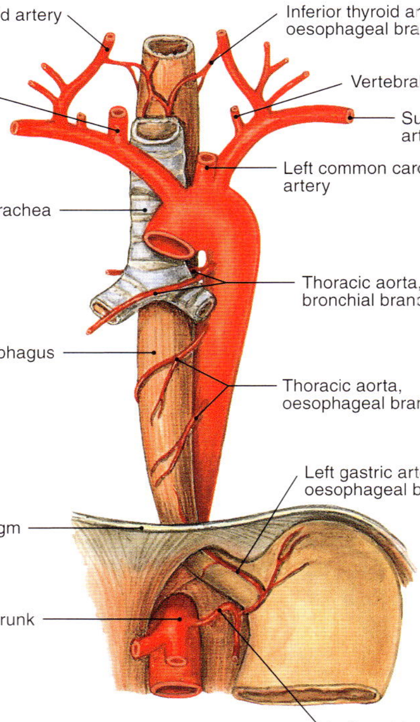

Fig. 671 Oesophagus; supplying arteries; ventral view.

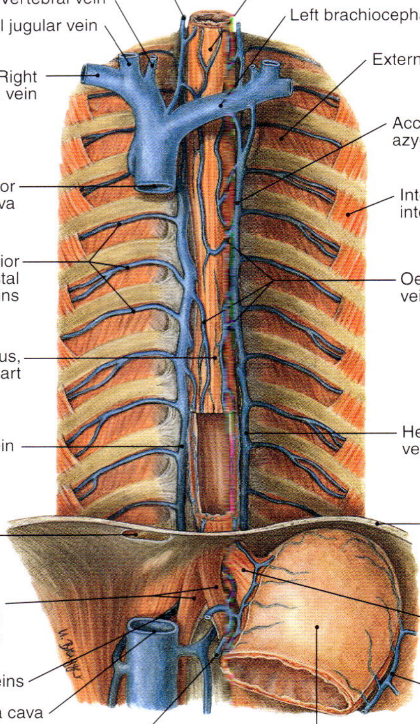

Fig. 672 Veins of the oesophagus.

→ 809, 810

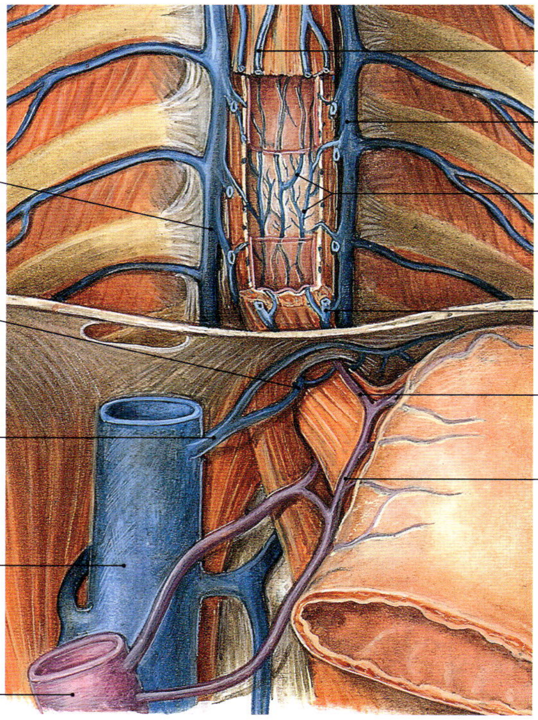

→ 810

Fig. 673 Veins of the oesophagus; magnification of Fig. 672; demonstration of anastomoses between branches of the hepatic portal vein and the superior vena cava.

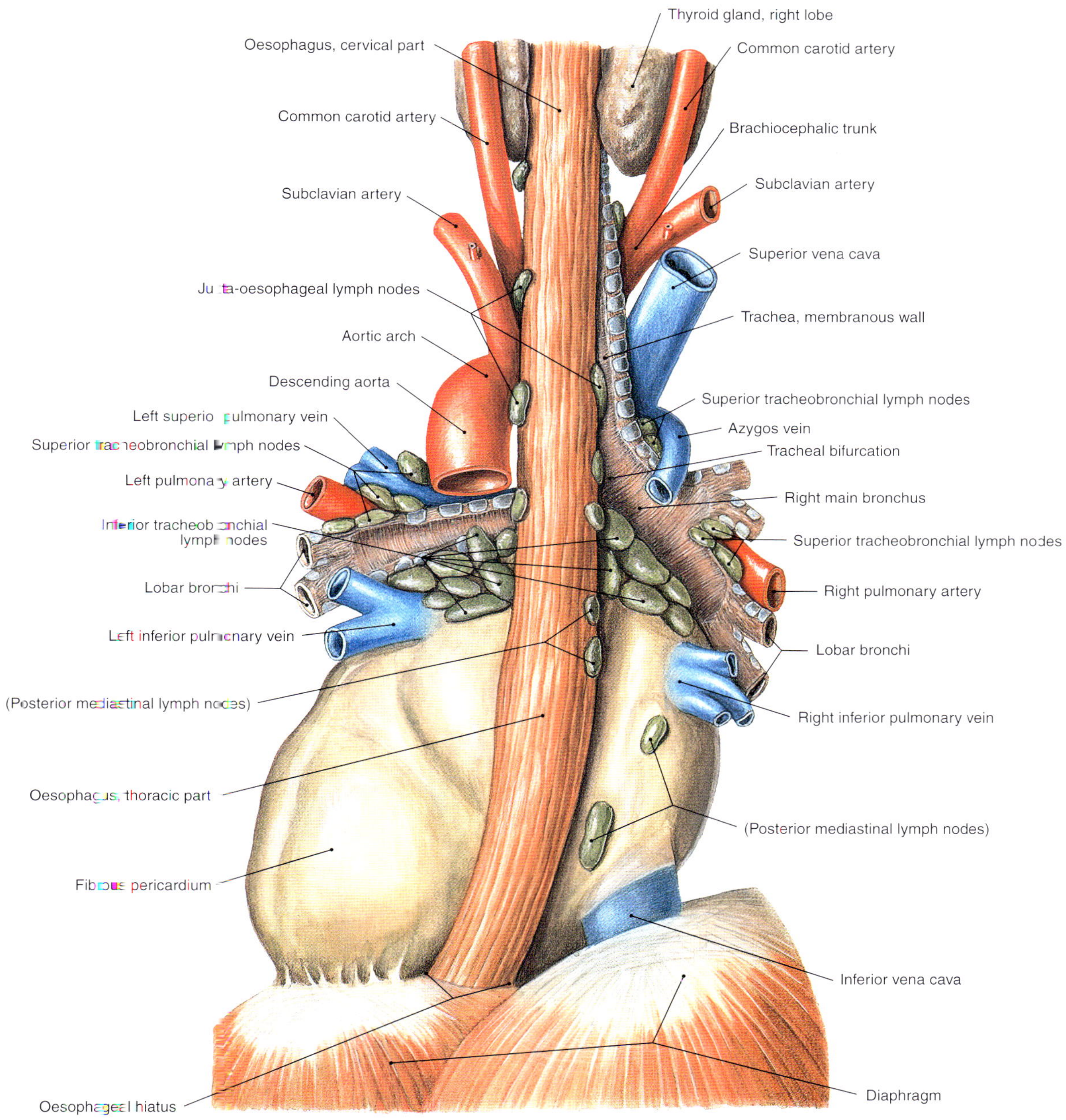

Fig. 674 Thoracic lymph nodes; dorsal view.

Oesophagus, radiography and oesophagoscopy

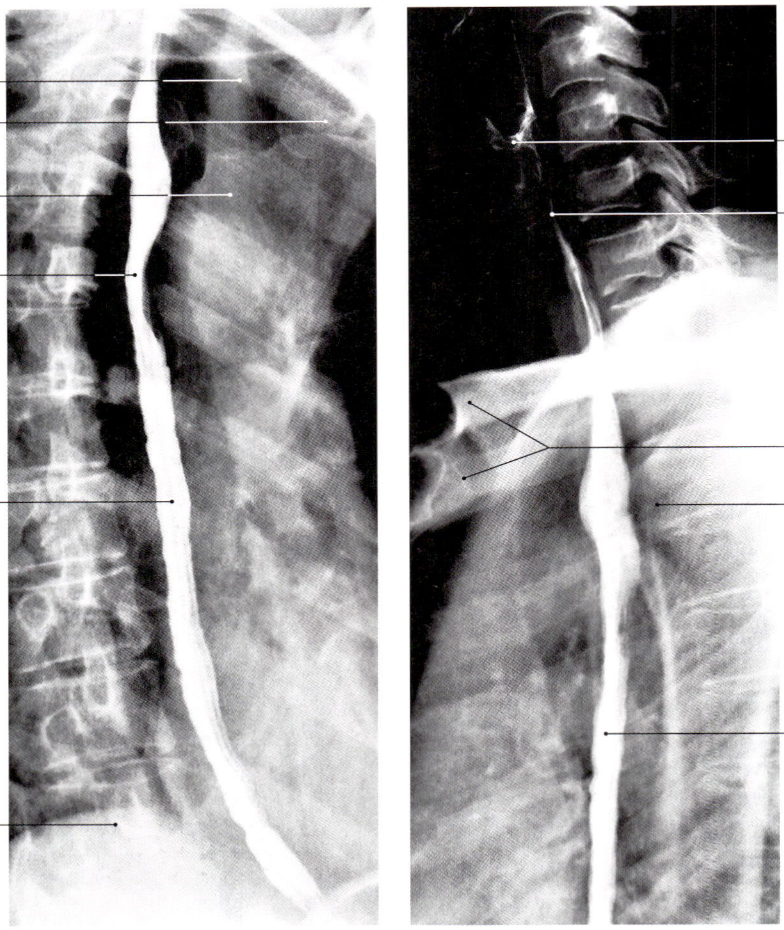

Fig. 675 a, b Oesophagus;
radiograph after swallowing of a contrast medium.
a Right anterior oblique position, oblique diameter I (beam directed from left anterior to right posterior)
b Left anterior oblique position, oblique diameter II (beam directed from right anterior to left posterior)

* Oesophageal constriction caused by the aortic arch
** Retrocardial portion of the oesophagus
*** Oesophageal constriction at the junction of the pharynx with the oesophagus

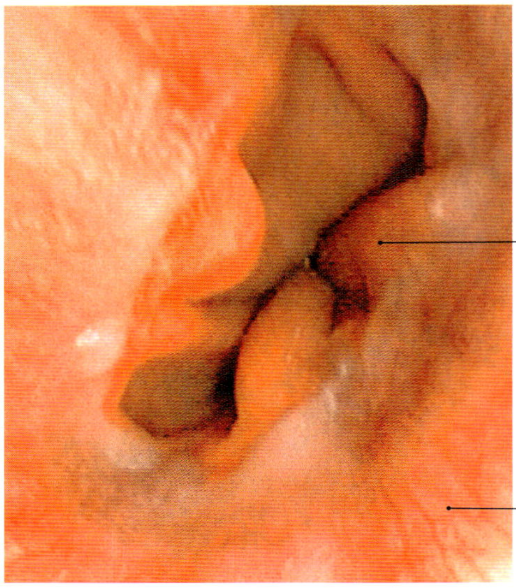

Fig. 676 Oesophagus;
oesophagoscopy (technical details see Fig. 718);
superior view.

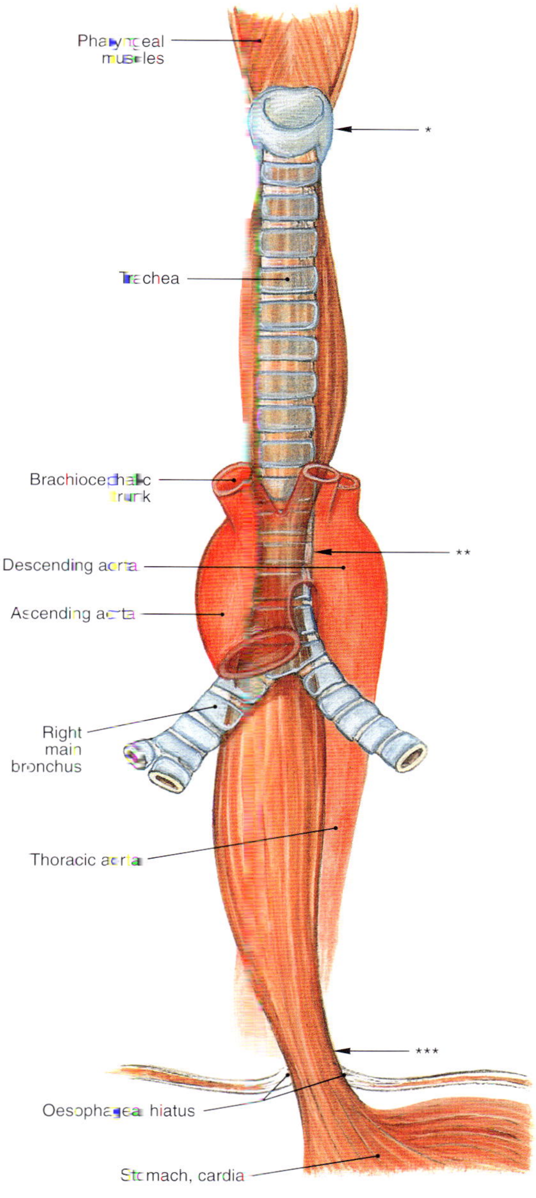

Fig. 677 Oesophagus; constrictions.

* Upper oesophageal sphincter
** Narrowing caused by the aortic arch
*** Diaphragmatic constriction

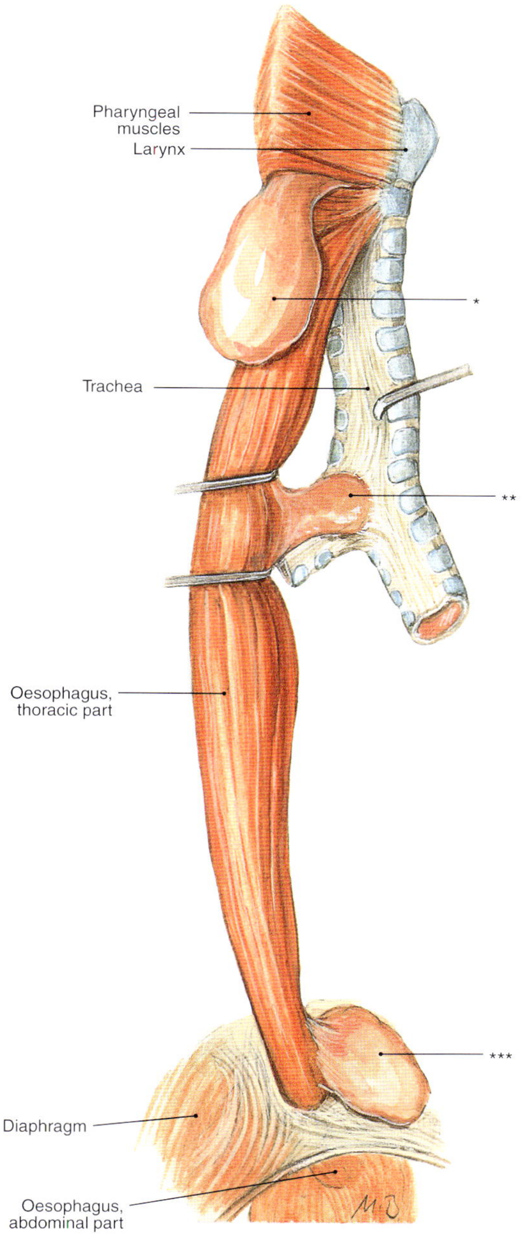

Fig. 678 Oesophagus; typical location and frequency of diverticula.

* Cervical diverticulum (ZENKER's diverticulum), (~70%)
** Mid-oesophageal diverticulum (~22%)
*** Epiphrenic diverticulum (~8%)

Thymus

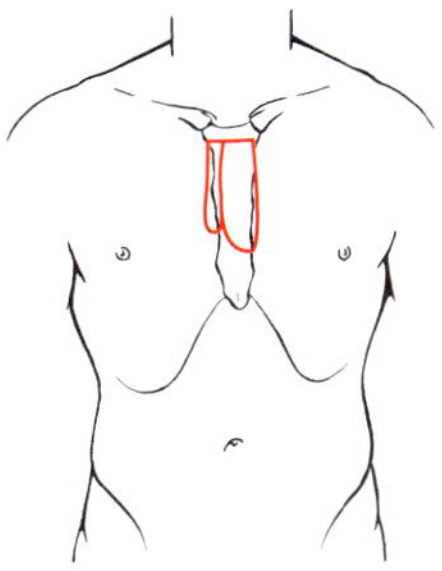

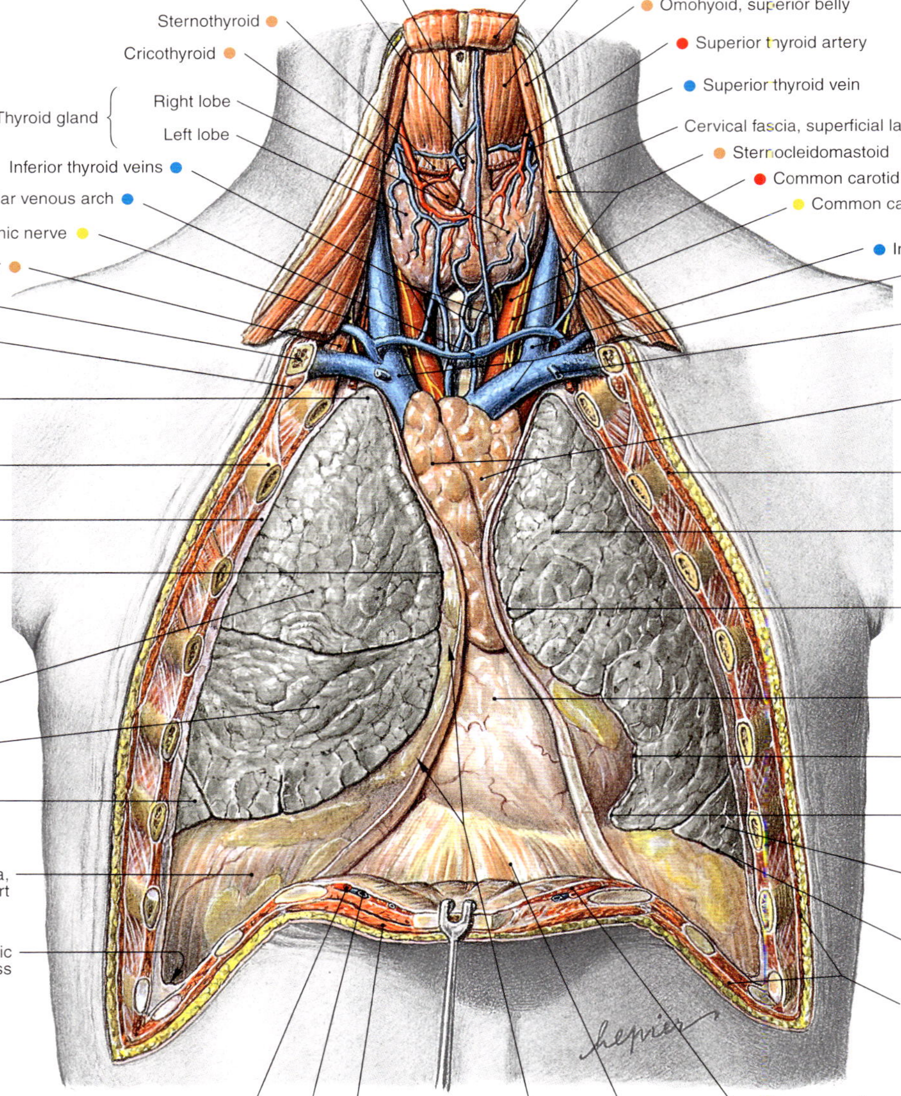

→ 781

Fig. 679 Thymus; pericardium and lungs of an adolescent.
Note the size of the adolescent thymus. In older individuals, the thymic tissue is almost entirely replaced by adipose tissue

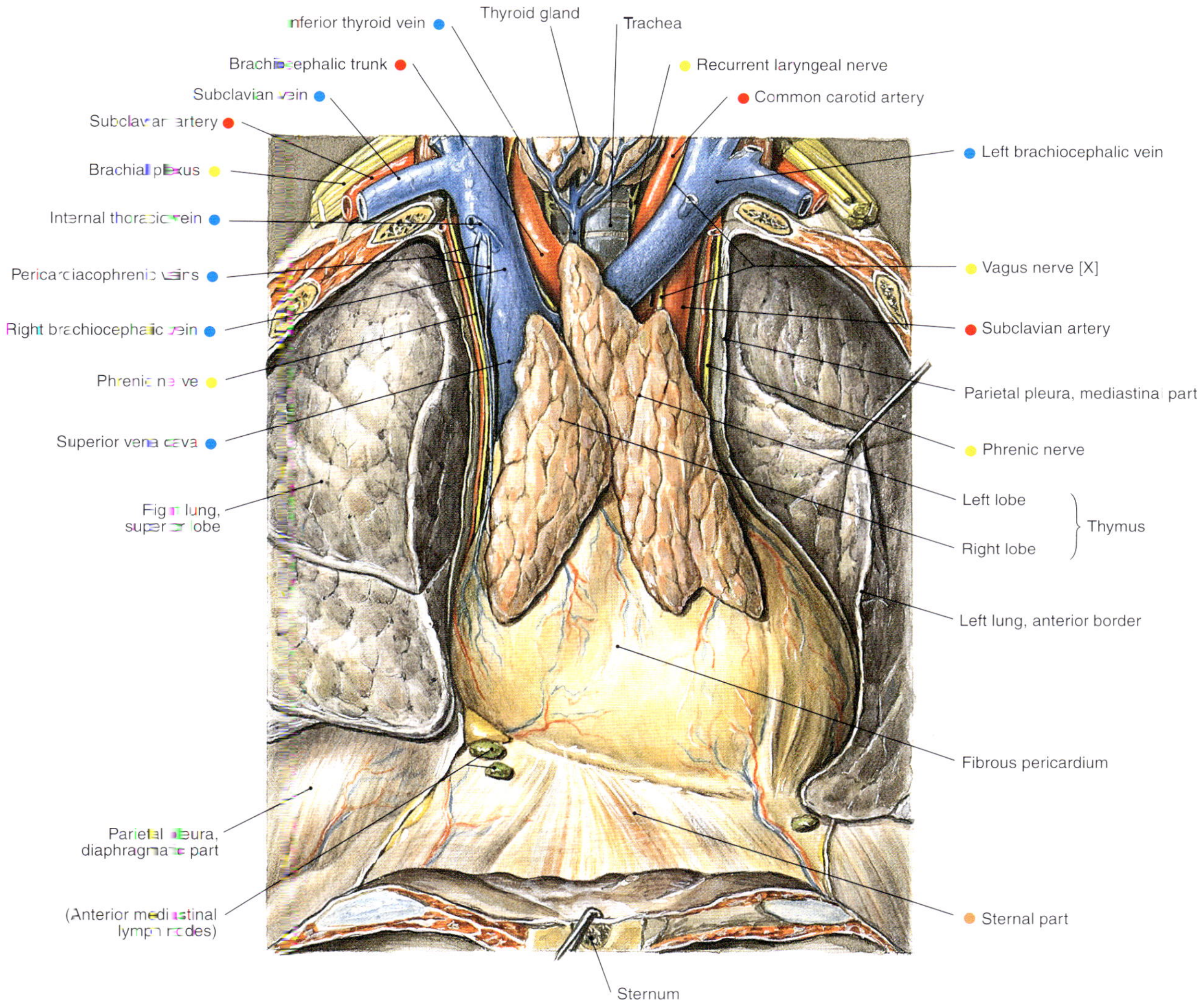

Fig. 680 Thymus of an adolescent.

→ 781

Pleural cavity

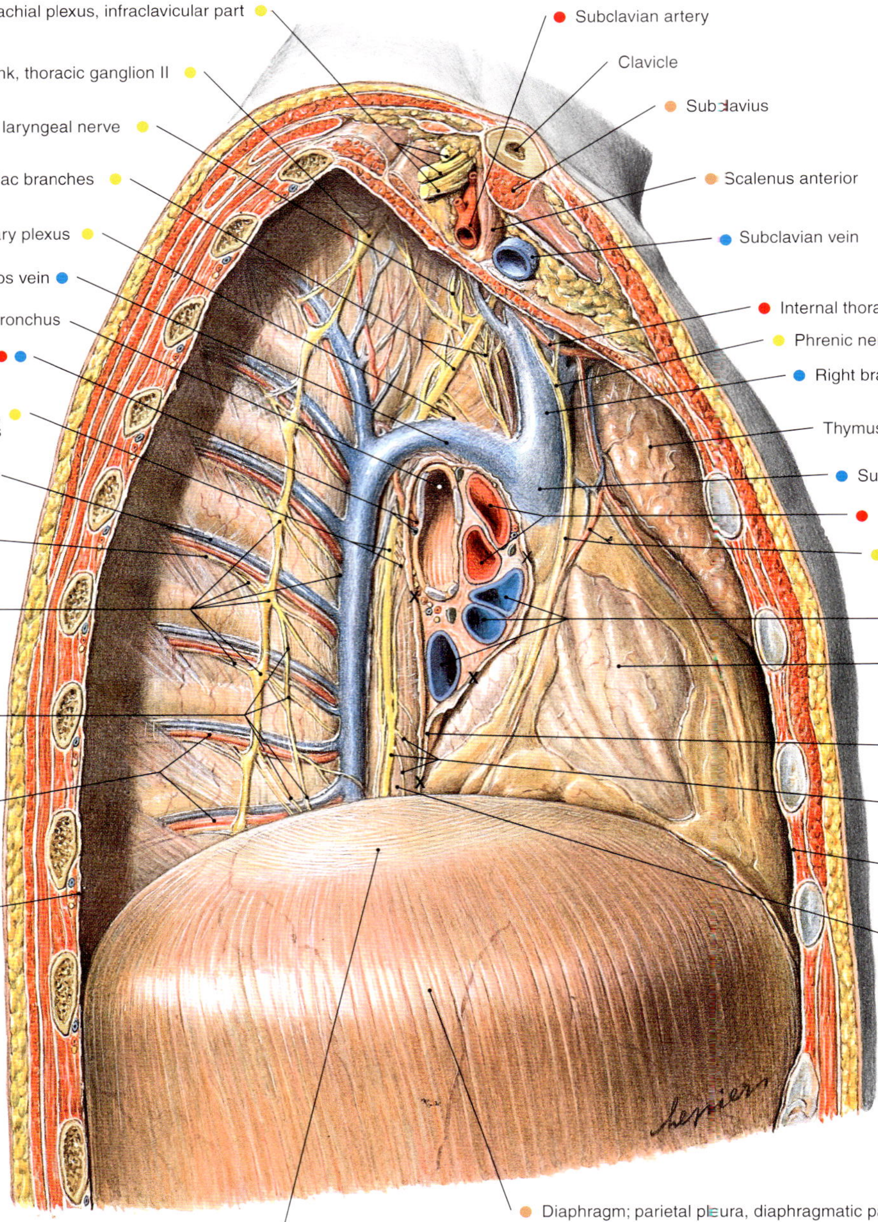

Fig. 681 Pleural cavity and mediastinum of an adolescent; lateral thoracic wall and right lung have been removed; viewed from the right.
The x indicate the areas at the root of the lung and the pulmonary ligament, respectively, where the visceral pleura folds back into the parietal pleura.

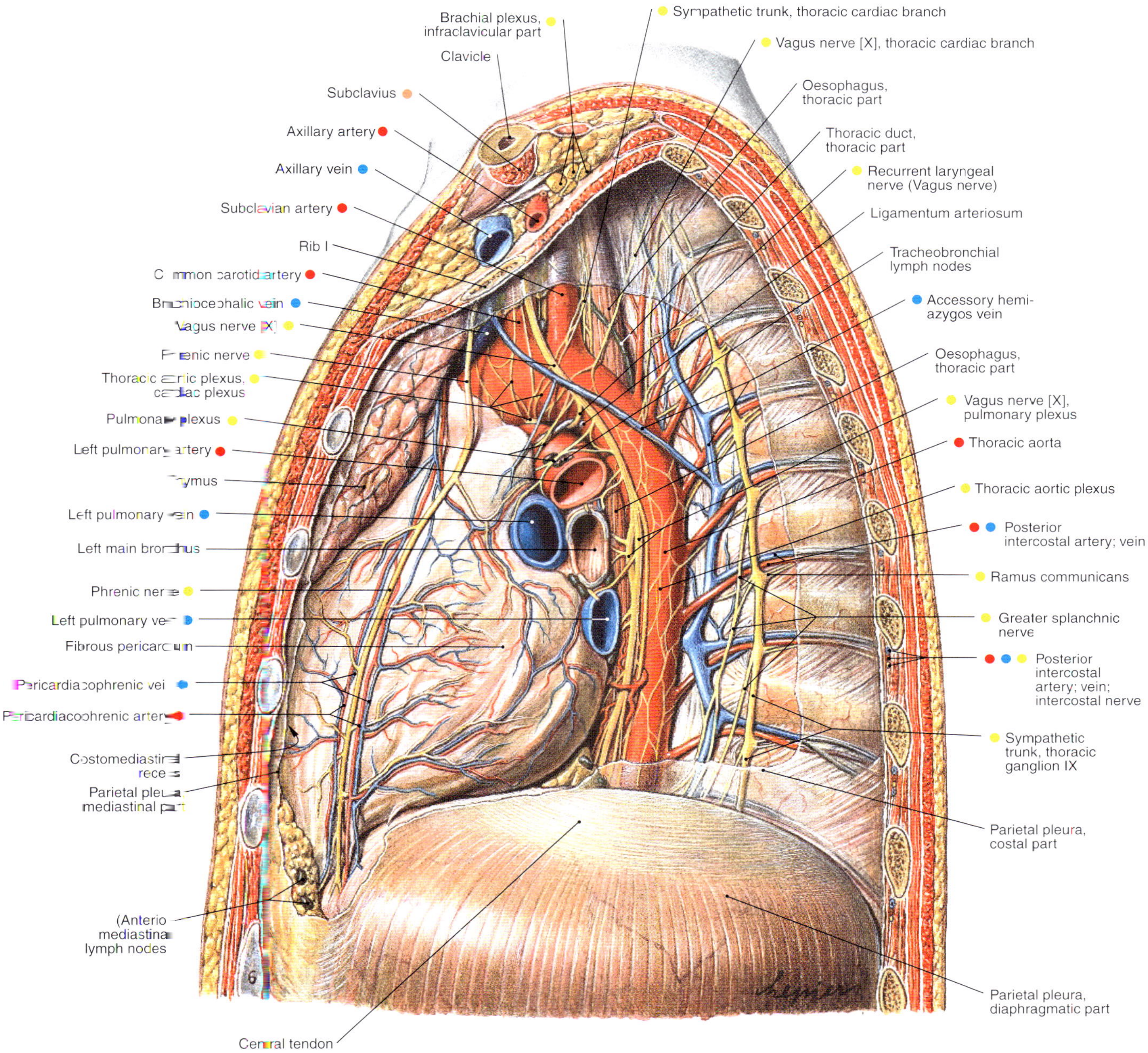

Fig. 682 Pleural cavity and mediastinum of an adolescent; viewed from the left.
In older individuals, the thymic tissue is almost entirely replaced by adipose tissue.

Aortic arch

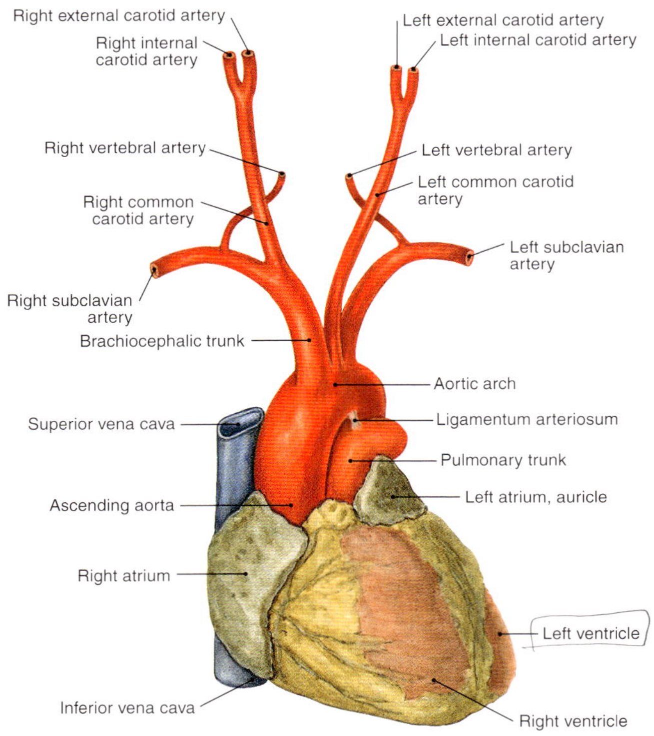

Fig. 683 Heart and aortic arch with the origins of the major arteries; ventral view.

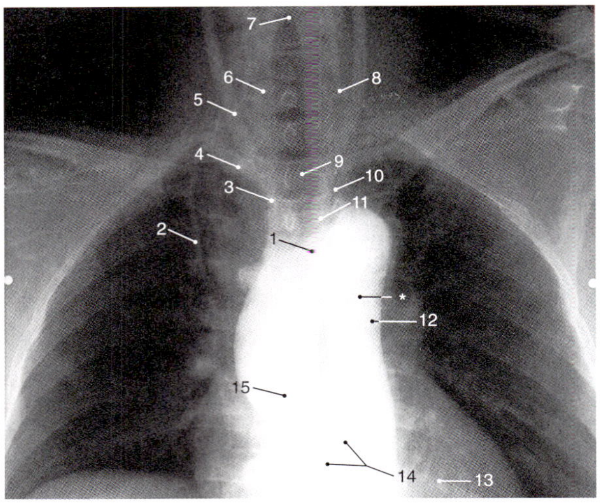

1 Aortic arch
2 Internal thoracic artery
3 Brachiocephalic trunk
4 Right subclavian artery
5 Right common carotid artery
6 Right vertebral artery
7 Rima glottidis
8 Left vertebral artery
9 Trachea
10 Left subclavian artery
11 Left common carotid artery
12 Descending aorta
13 Heart
14 Aortic valve
15 Ascending aorta

Fig. 684 Aortic arch and branches; AP-radiograph after injection of a contrast medium into the aortic bulb; ventral view.

* Catheter

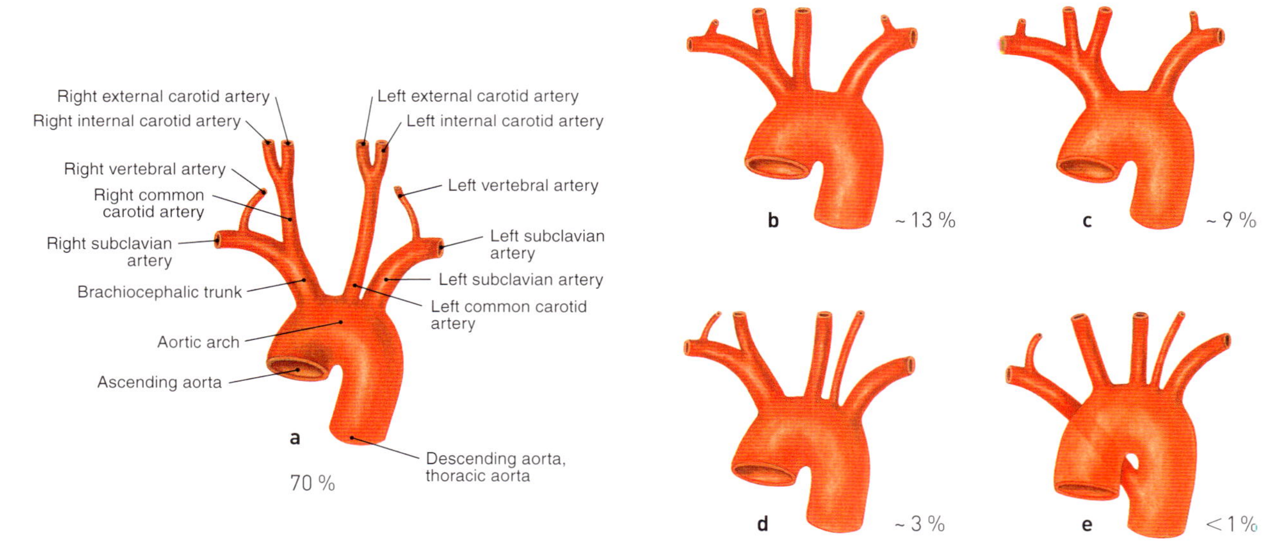

Fig. 685 a–e Variability of the origin of the major arteries from the aortic arch.

a "Textbook case"
b Common origin of the brachiocephalic trunk and the left common carotid artery
c Common trunk for the brachiocephalic trunk and the left common carotid artery
d Left vertebral artery branching off the aortic arch independently
e Right subclavian artery as the ultimate branch of the aortic arch
This abnormal artery frequently passes behind the oesophagus to the right, which can result in swallowing difficulties (Dysphagia lusoria).

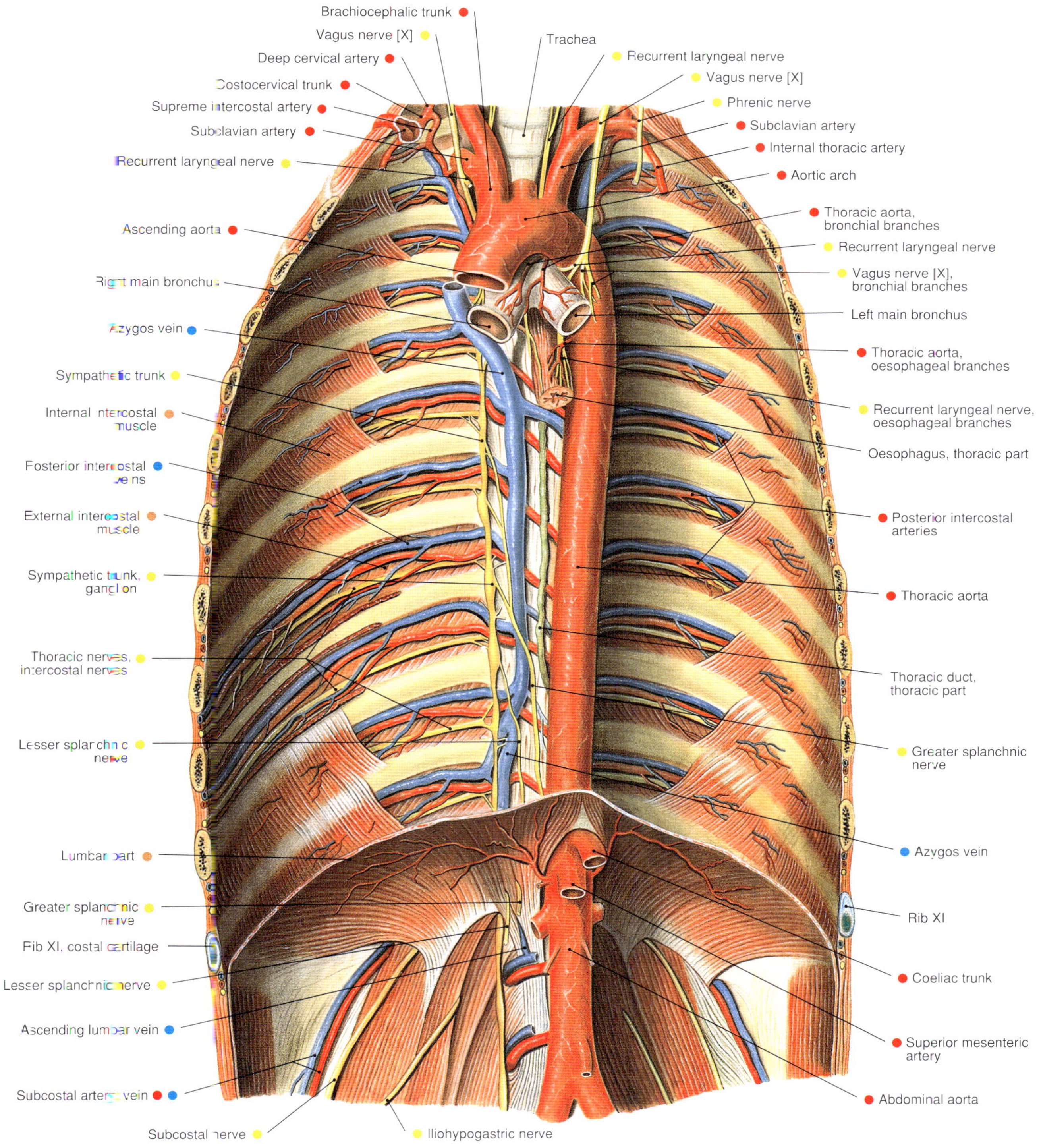

Fig. 686 Thoracic and abdominal aorta.

Posterior mediastinum

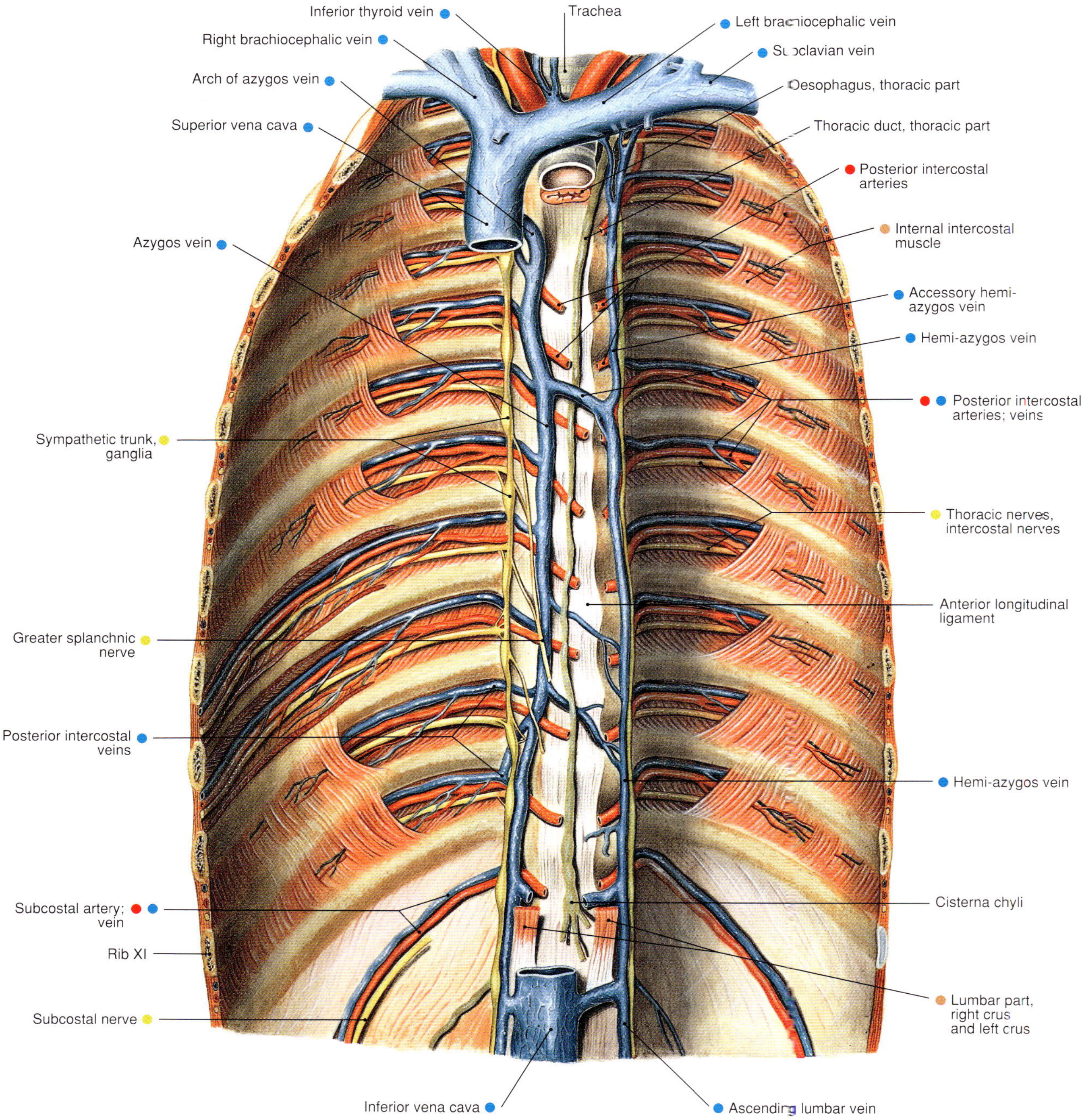

Fig. 687 Vessels and nerves of the posterior mediastinum.

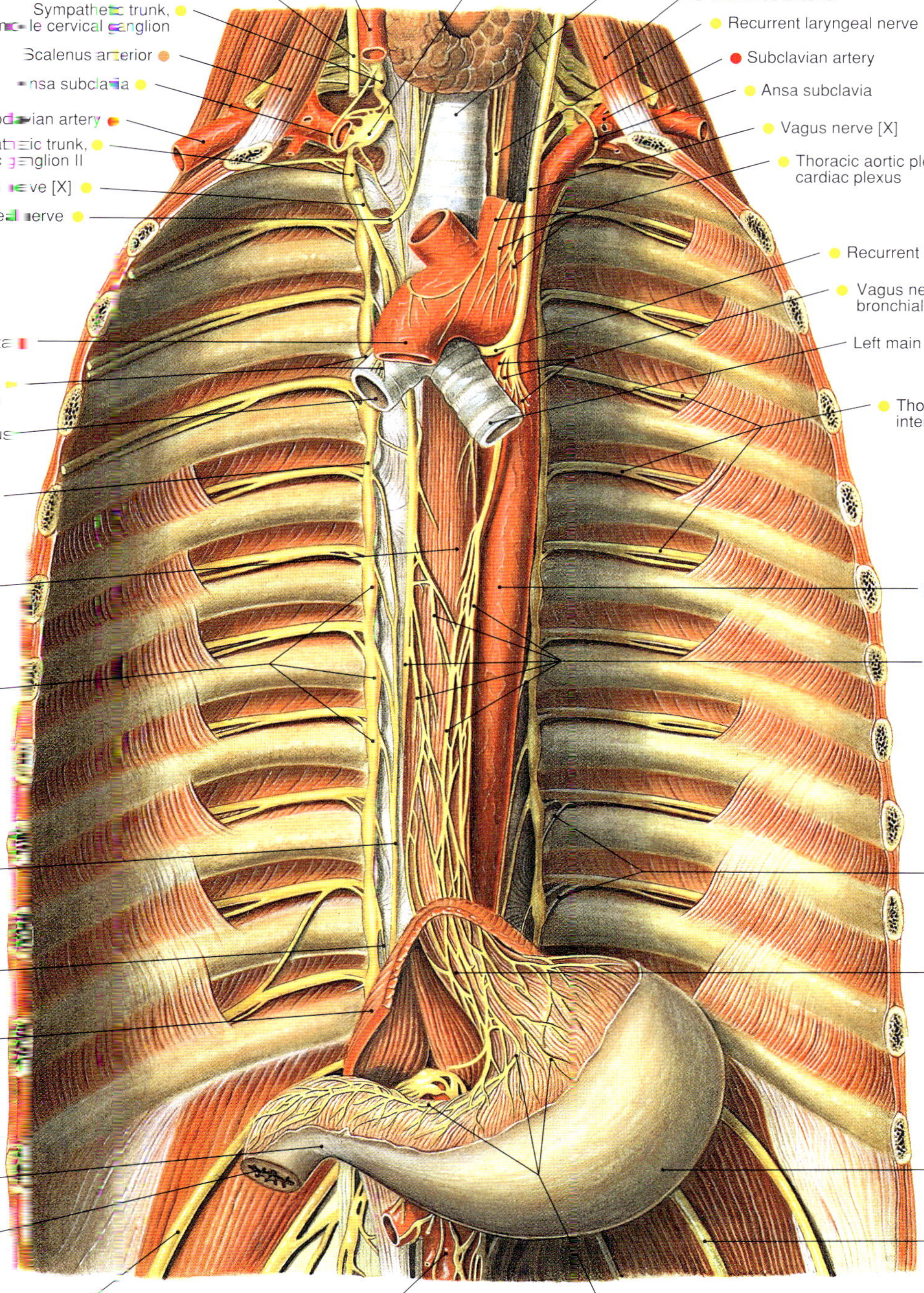

Fig. 688 Autonomous nervous system of the thoracic cavity.

→ 49, 50

Phrenic nerve

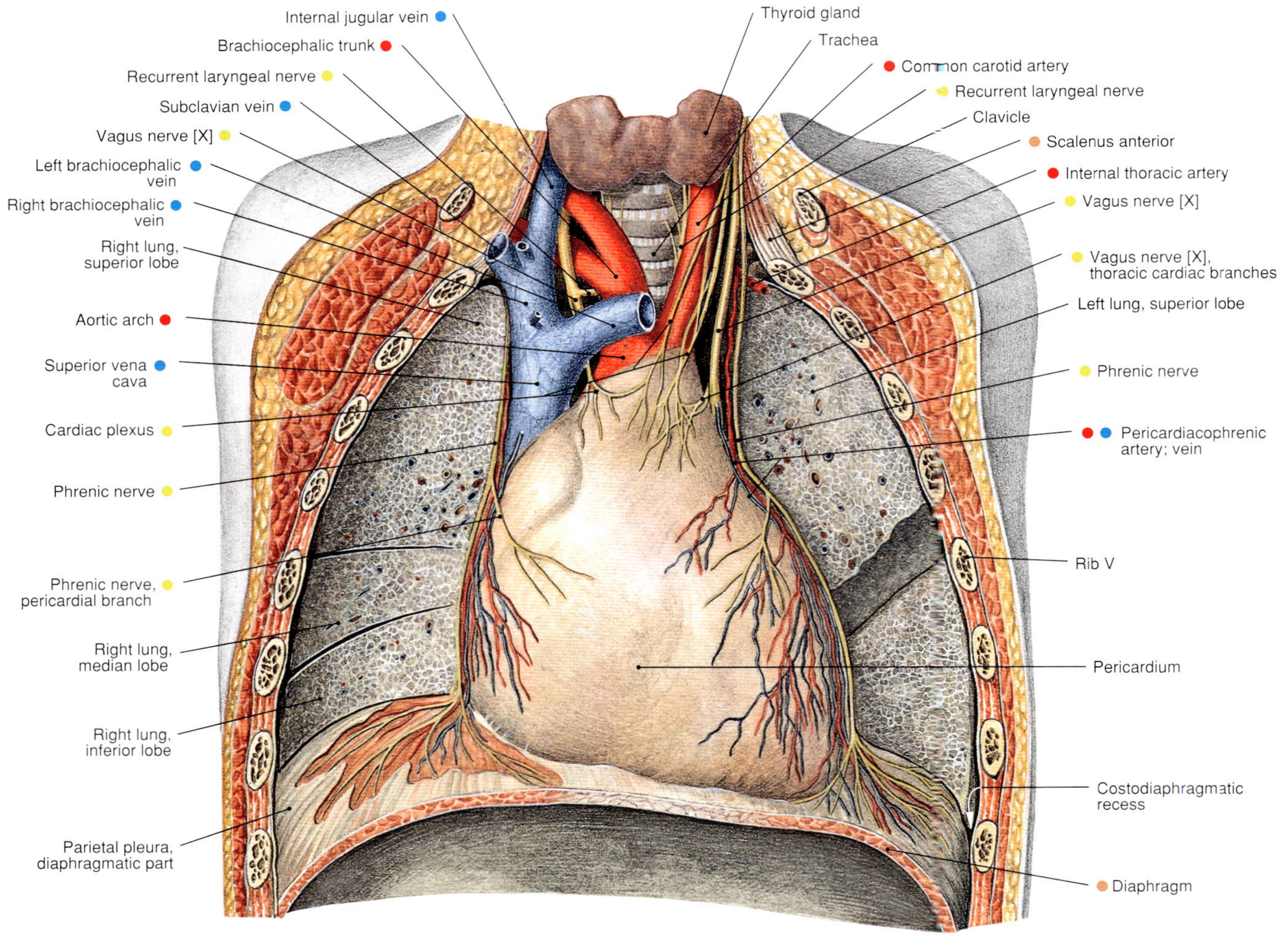

Fig. 689 Thoracic viscera of an adult; the anterior thoracic wall has been removed, and the right and the left lung have been sectioned in the frontal plane; ventral view.

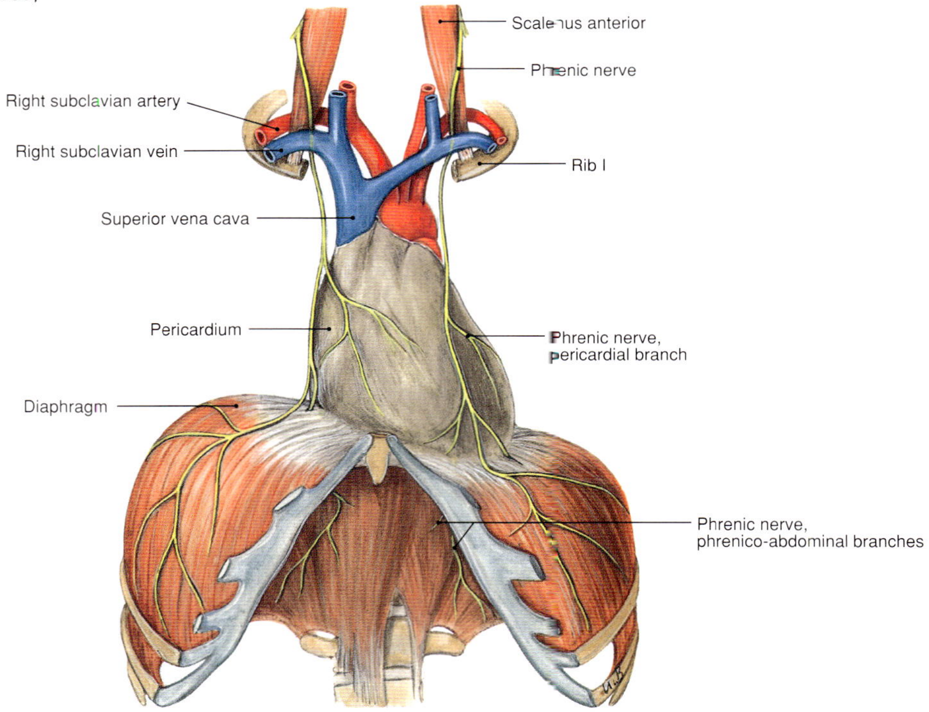

Fig. 690 Course of the phrenic nerve.

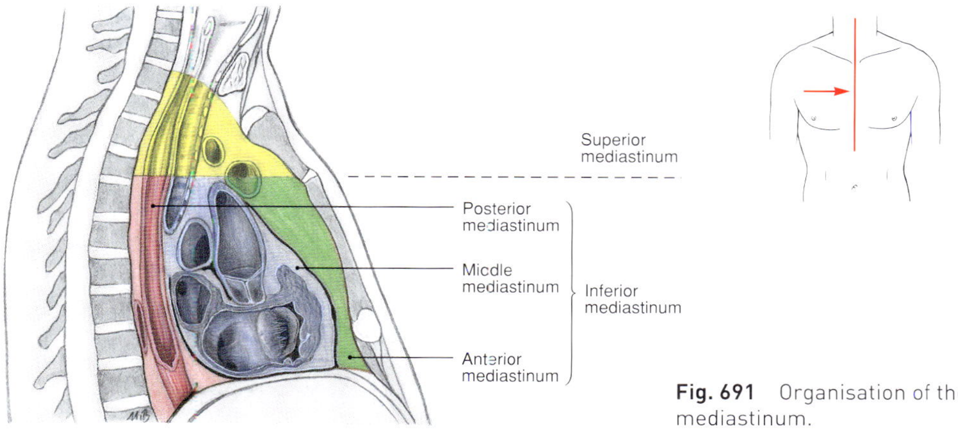

Fig. 691 Organisation of the mediastinum.

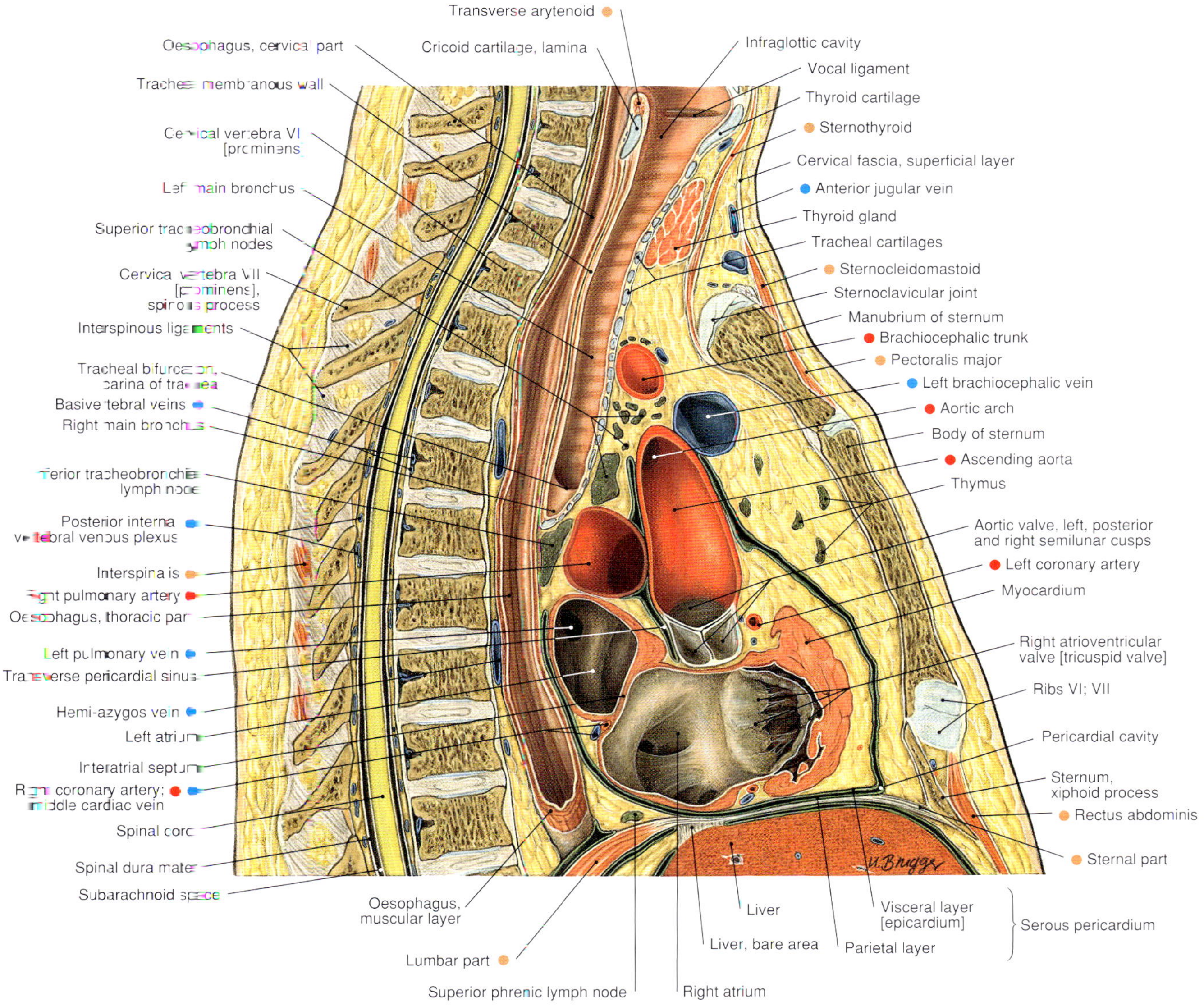

Fig. 692 Thoracic cavity and mediastinum; median sagittal section through the neck and the thorax; lateral view from the right.

Thorax, frontal sections

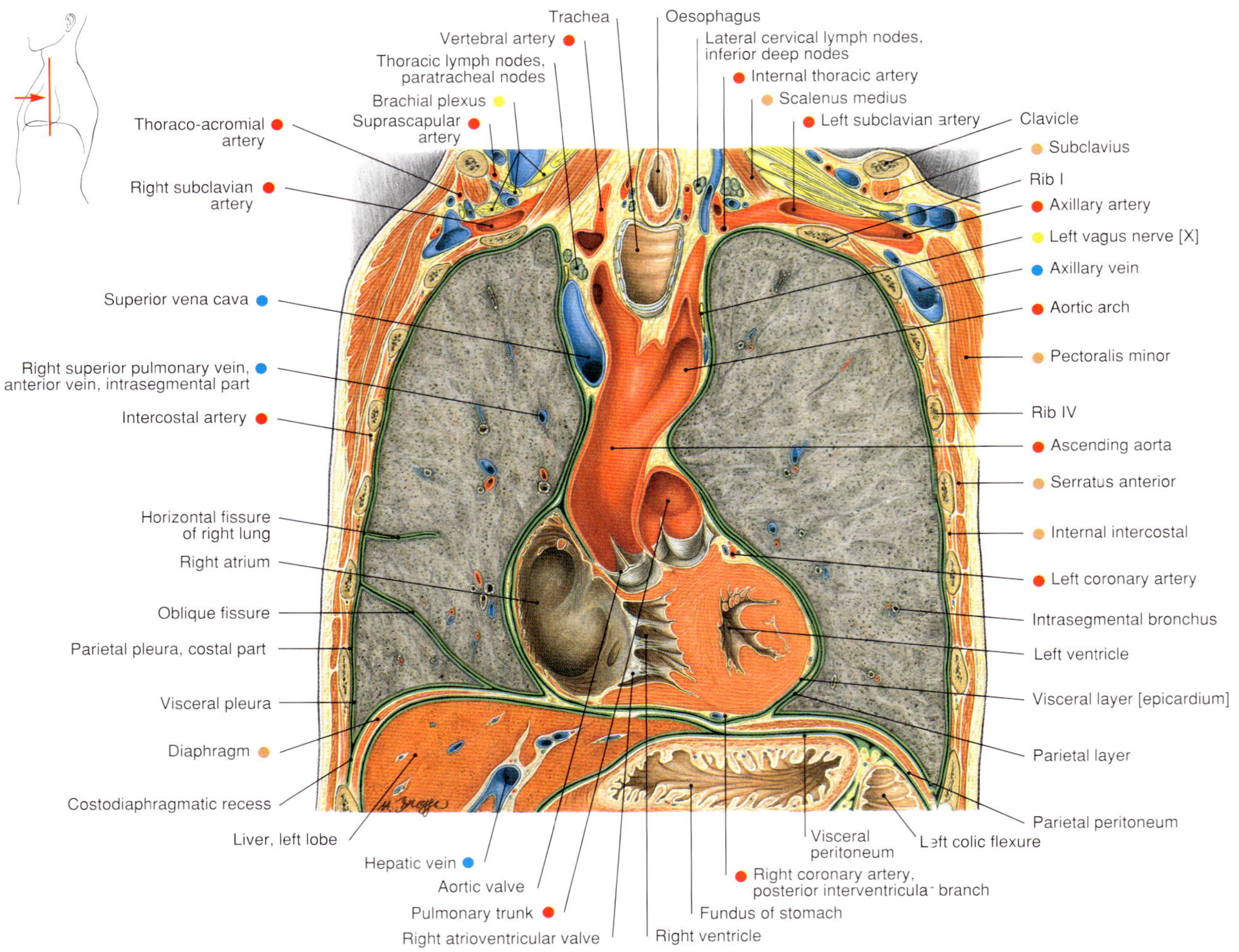

Fig. 693 Thoracic cavity.

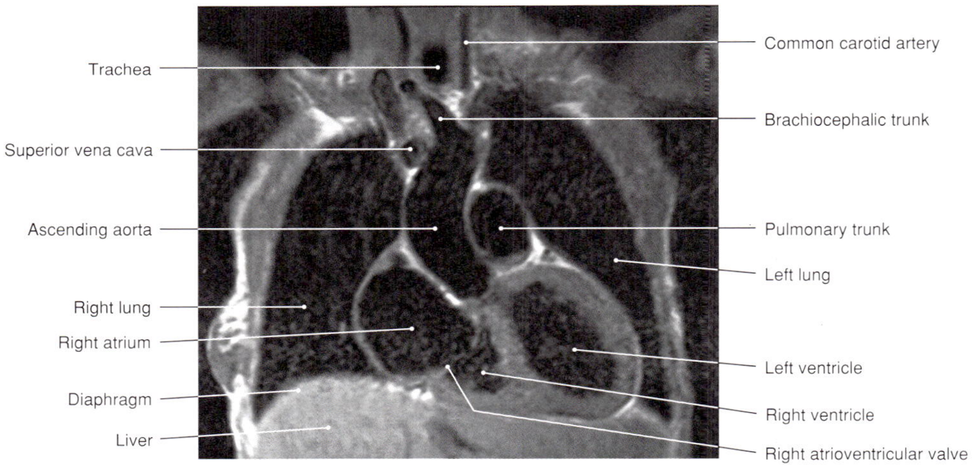

Fig. 694 Thoracic cavity;
magnetic resonance tomographic image (MRI);
frontal section at the level of the superior vena cava;
ventral view.

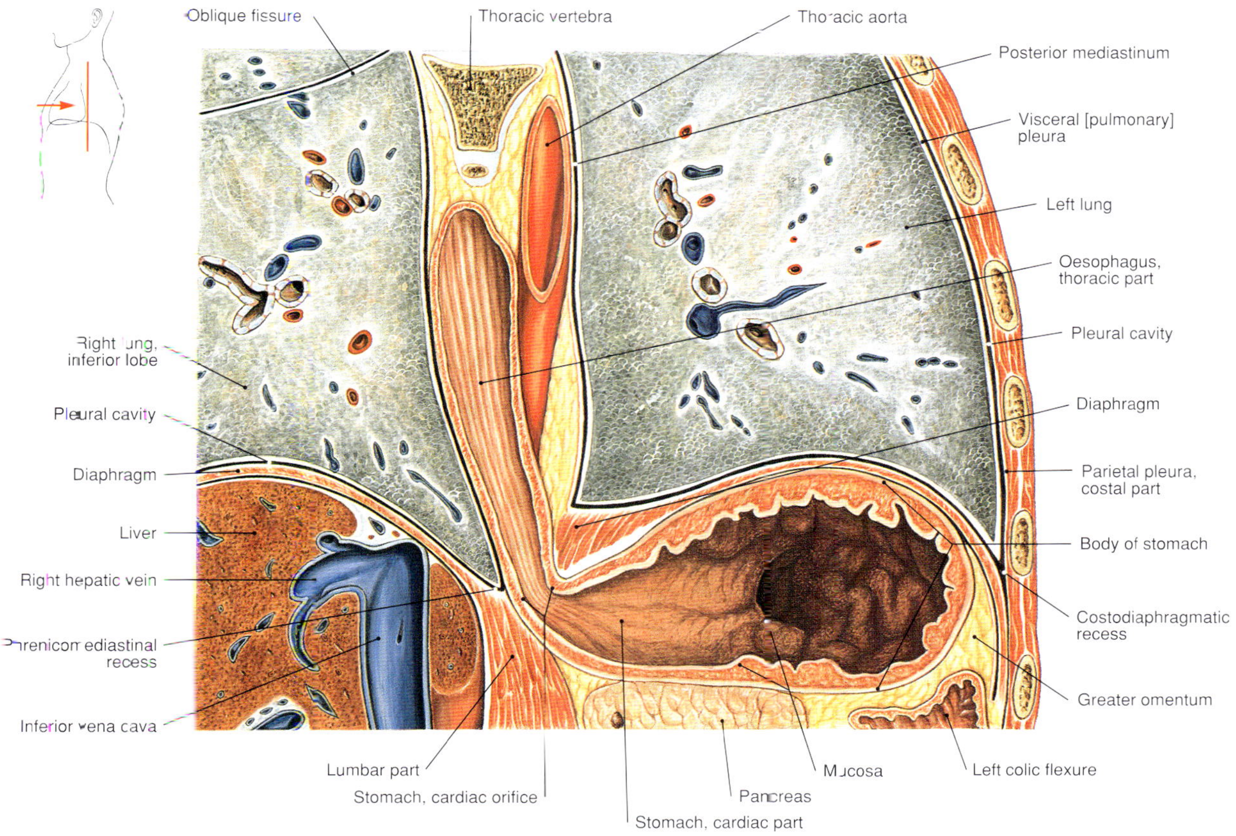

Fig. 695 Diaphragm and oesophagus with its transition into the stomach;
frontal section through the lower part of the thoracic cavity and the upper part of the abdominal cavity.

→ 919

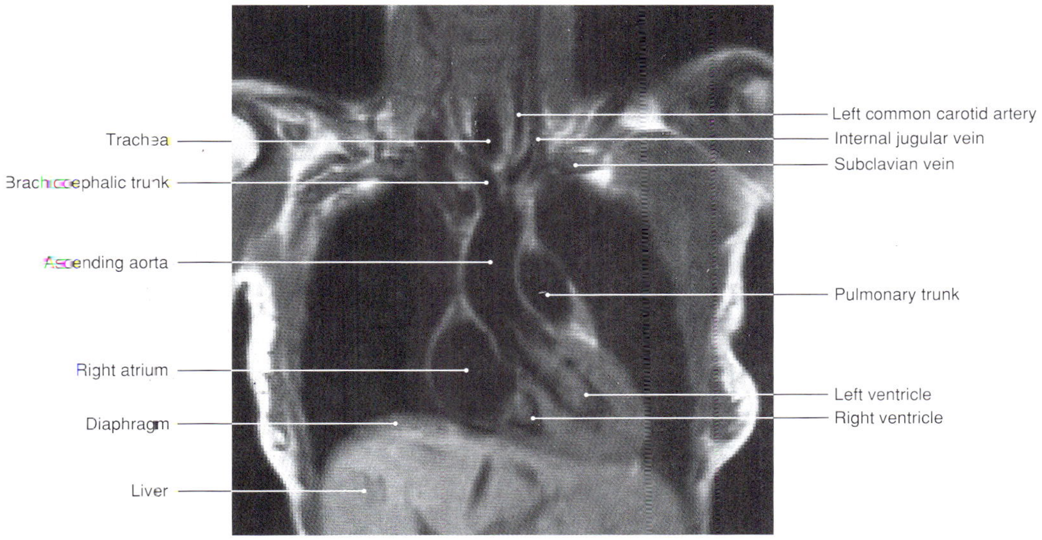

Fig. 696 Thoracic cavity;
magnetic resonance tomographic image (MRI);
frontal section at the level of the aortic valve;
ventral view.

Thorax, frontal sections

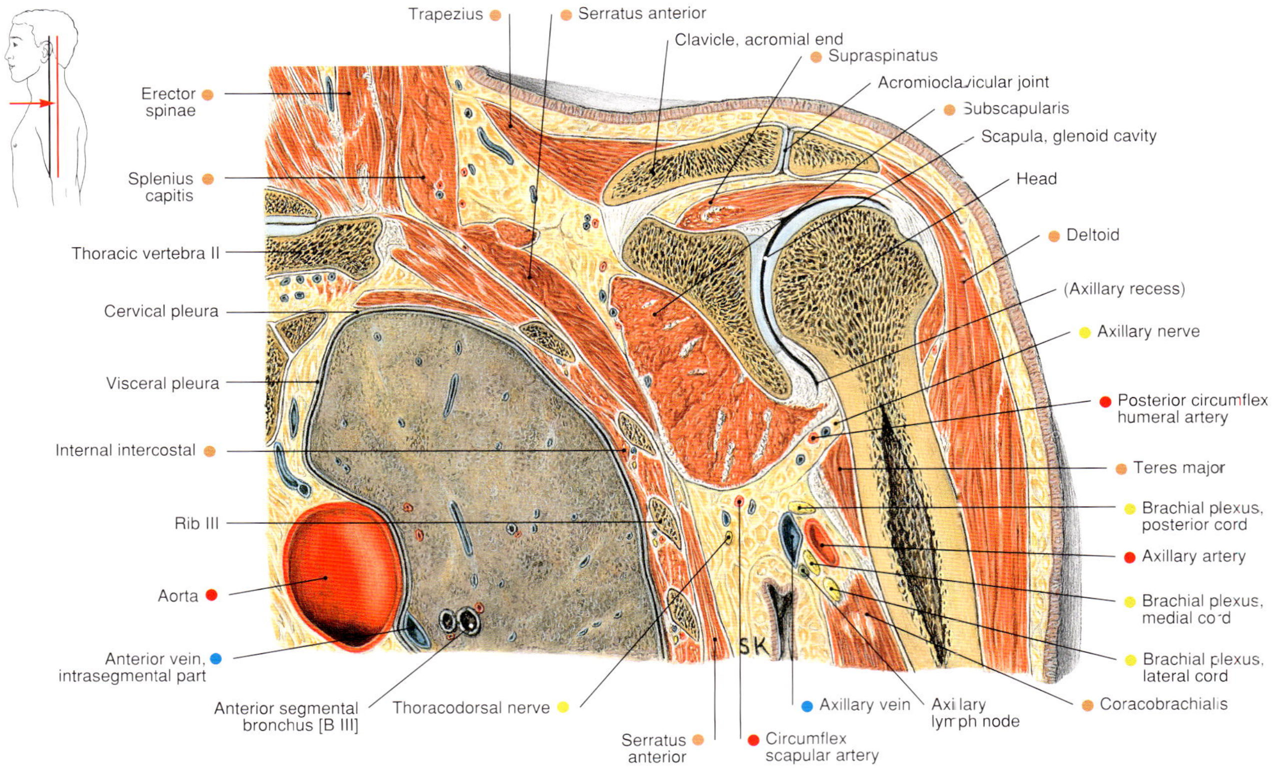

Fig. 697 Thoracic cavity; axilla and shoulder joint.

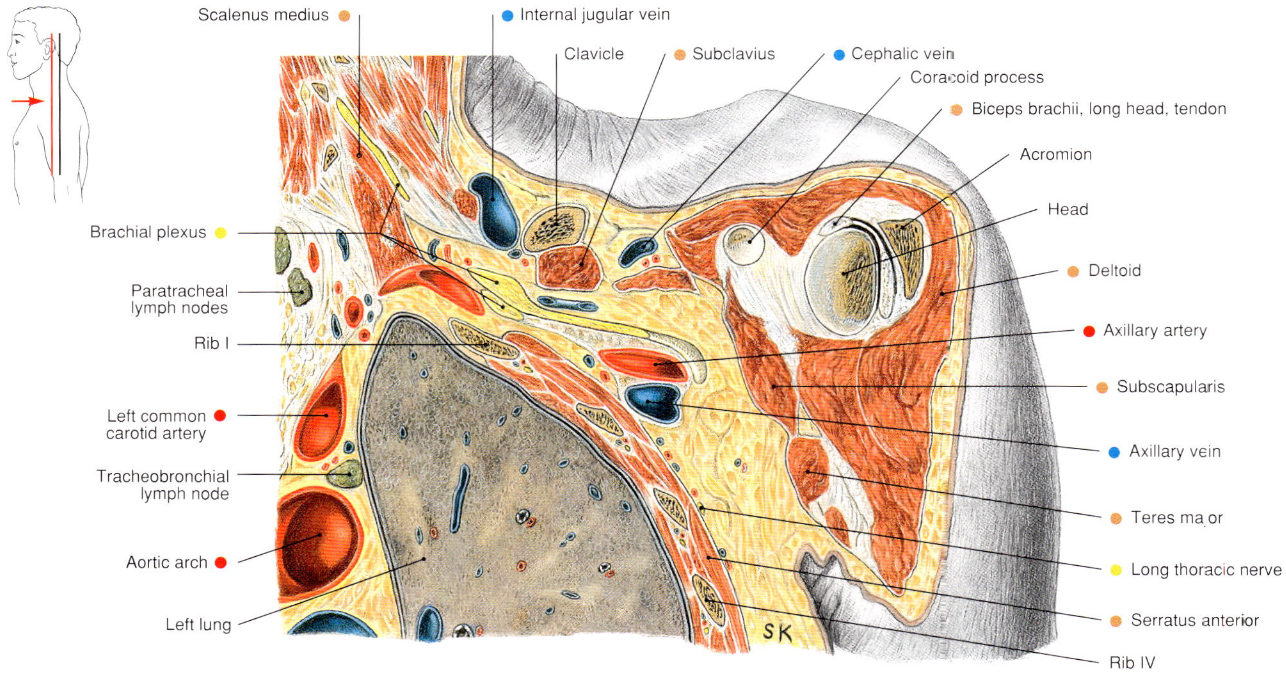

Fig. 698 Thoracic cavity; axilla and shoulder joint.

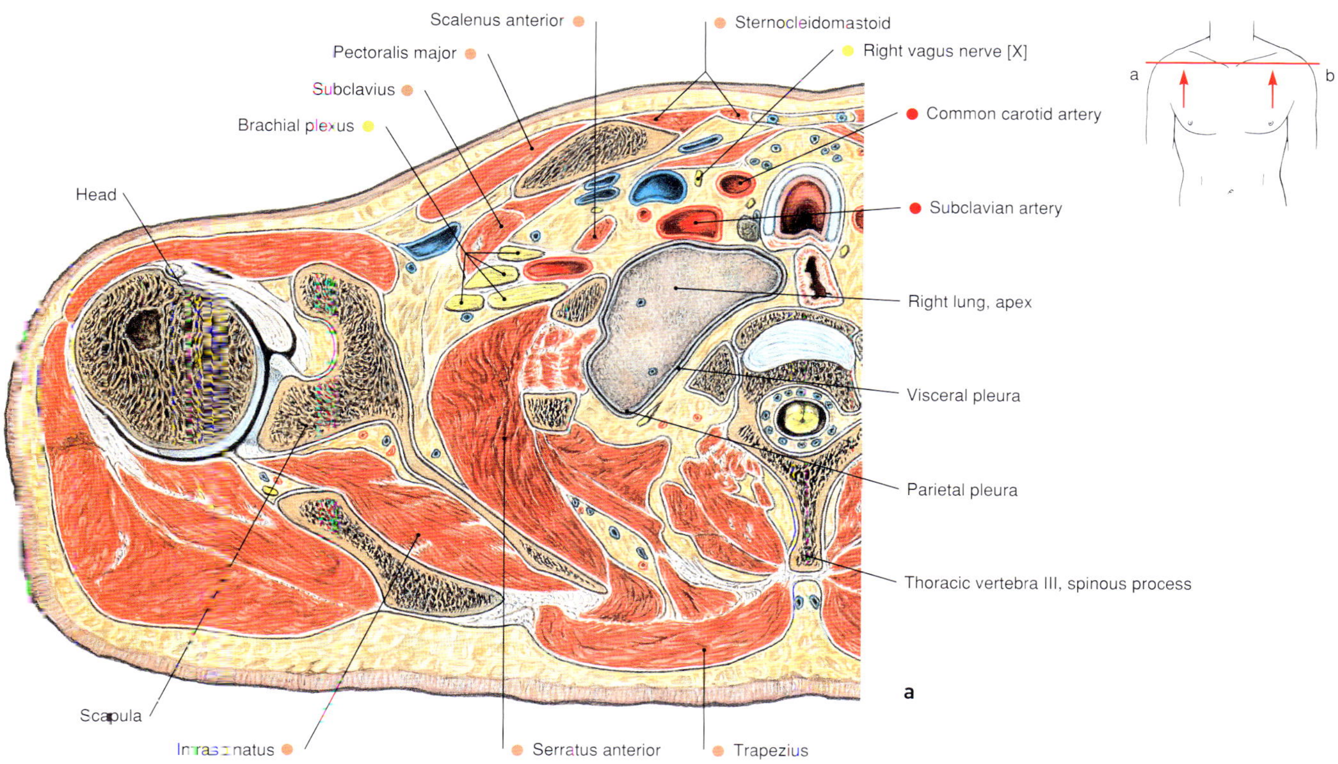

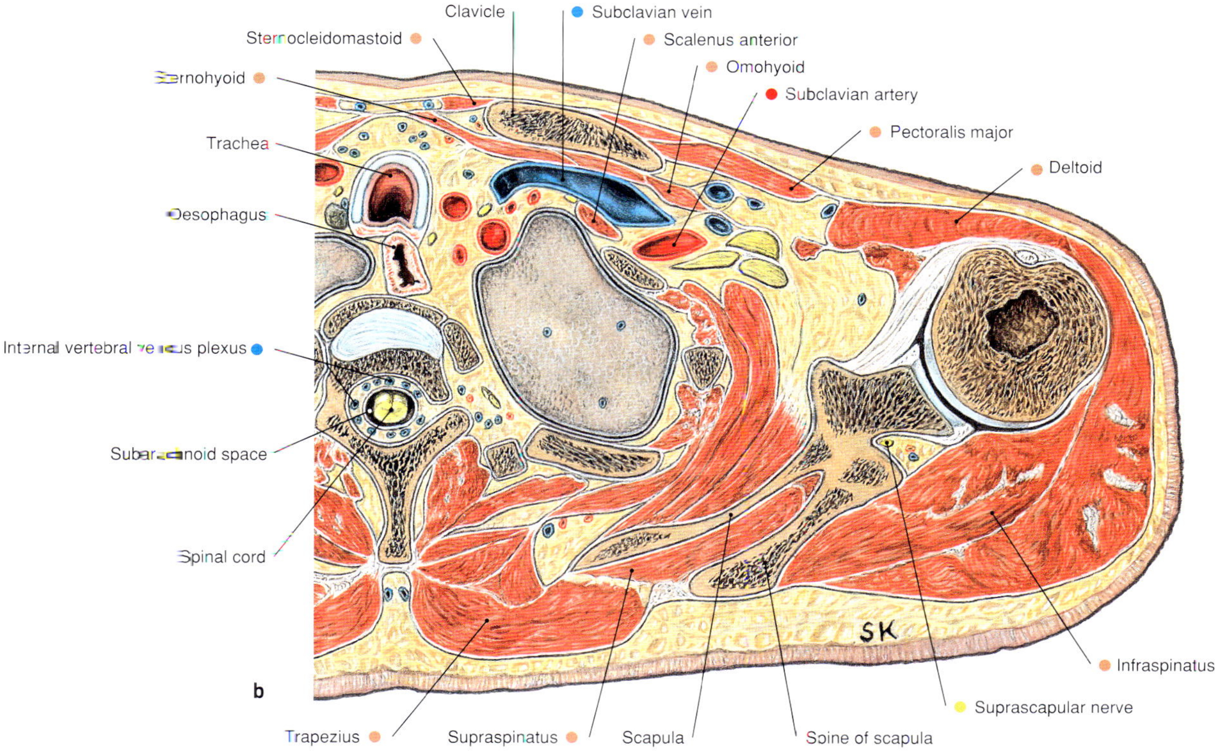

Fig. 499 a, b Thoracic cavity; axilla and shoulder joint.

a Right part of the body
b Left part of the body

→ 294

Thorax, transverse sections

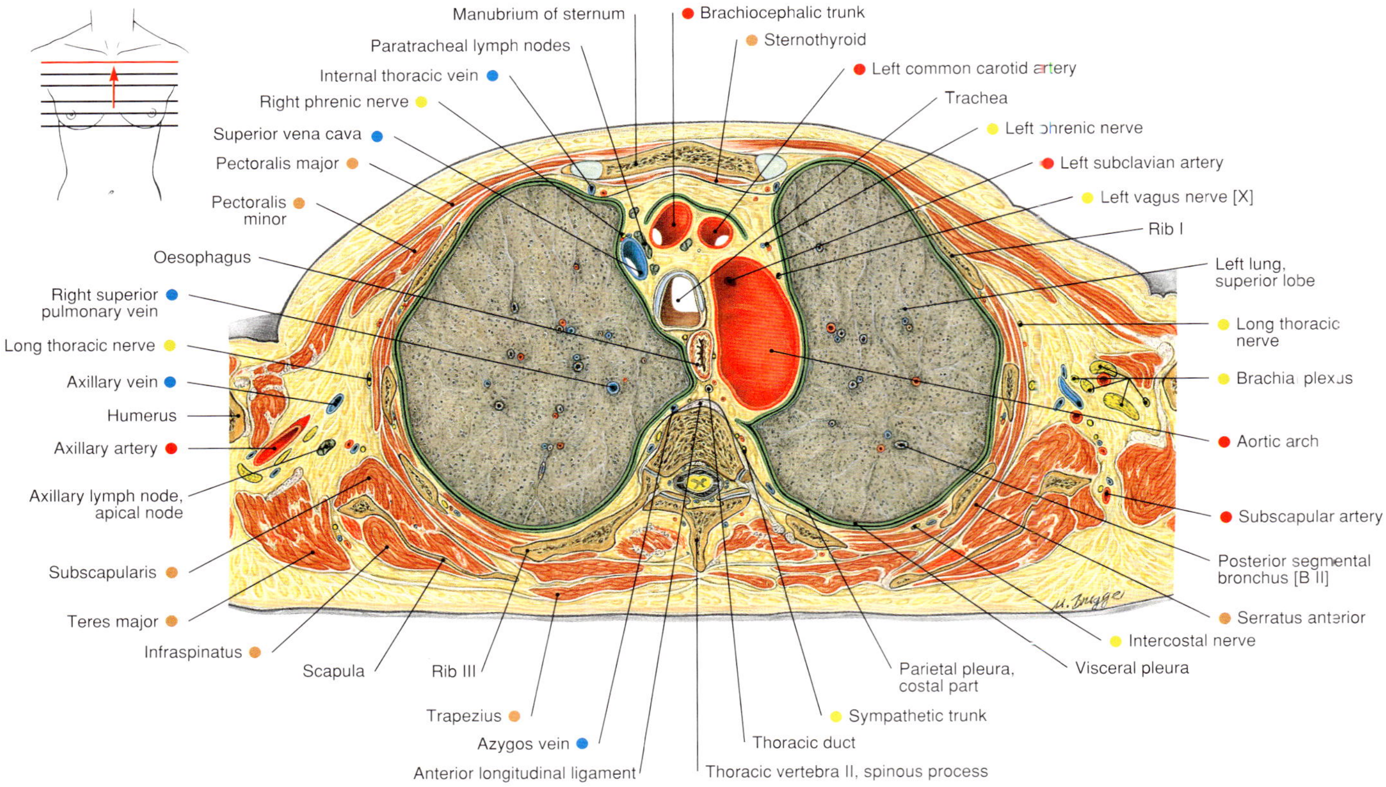

Fig. 700 Thoracic cavity.

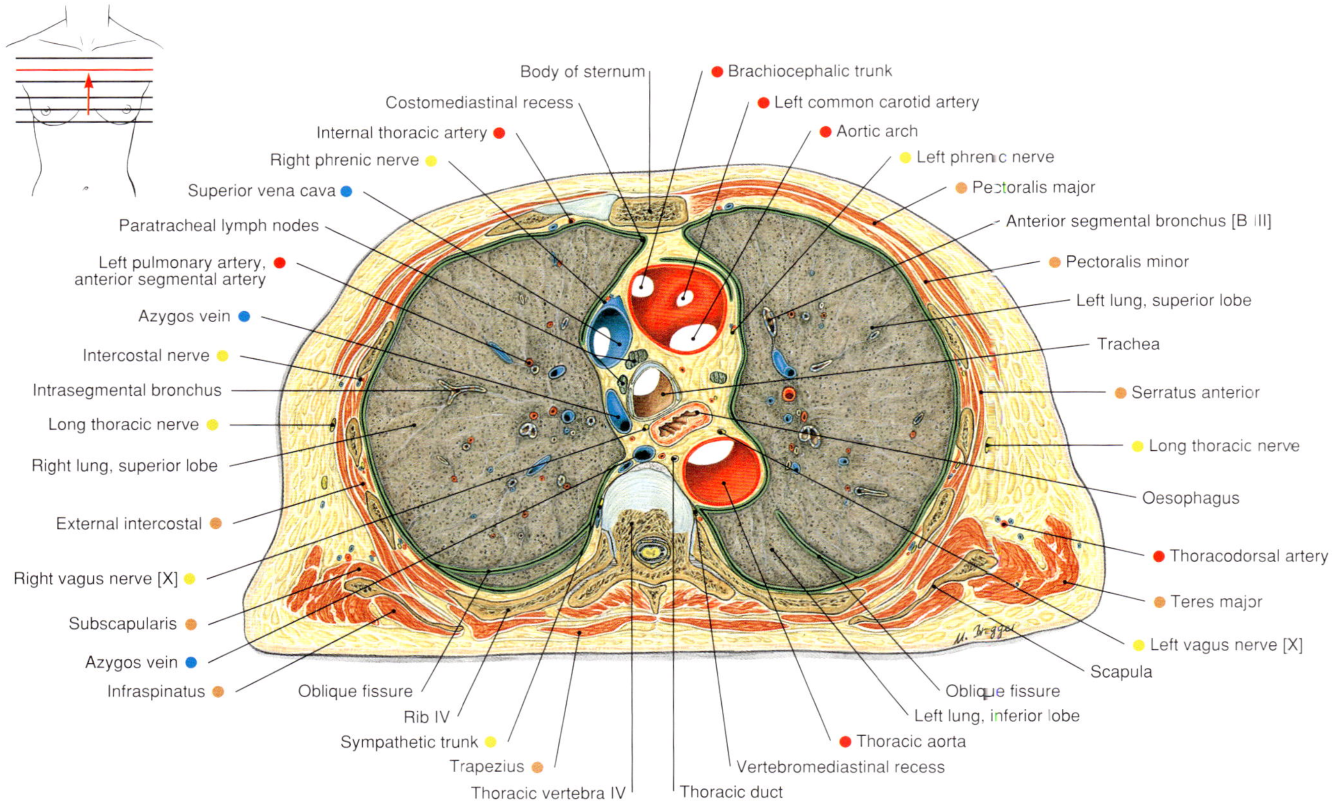

Fig. 701 Thoracic cavity.

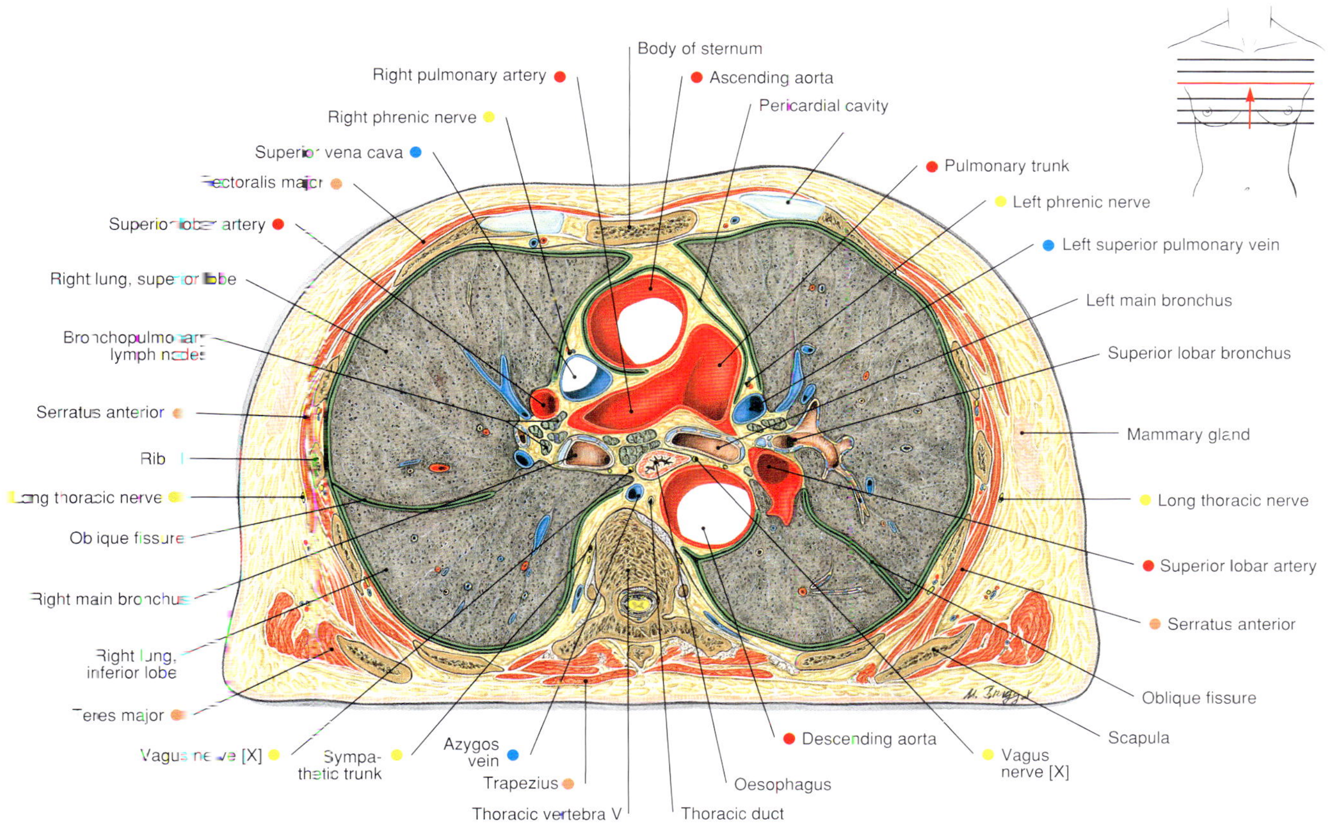

Fig. 702 Thoracic cavity.

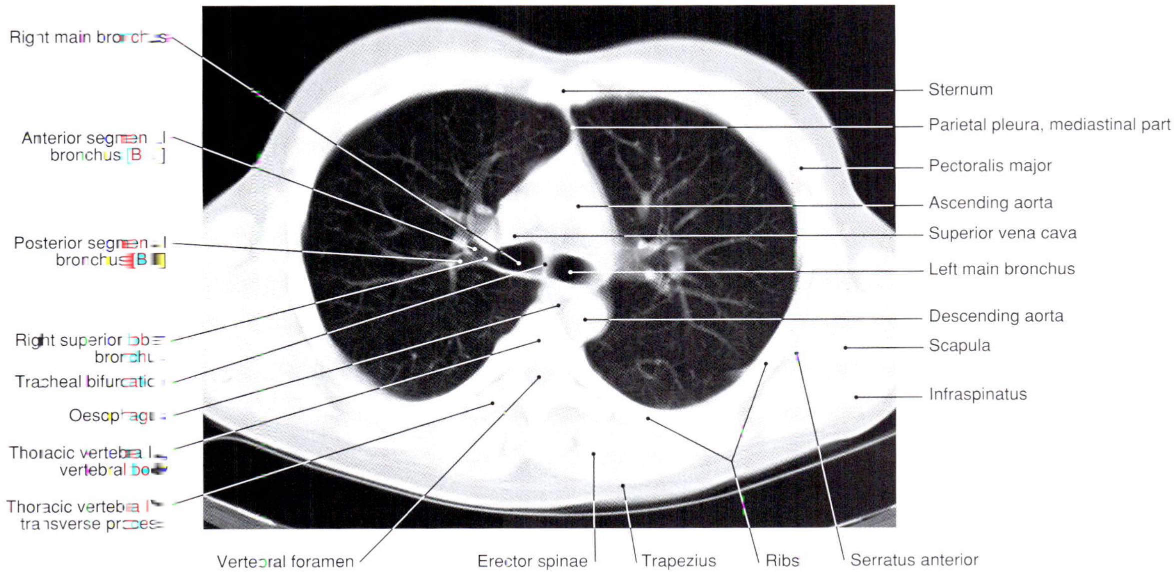

Fig. 703 Thoracic cavity;
computed tomographic cross-section (CT).

Thorax, transverse sections

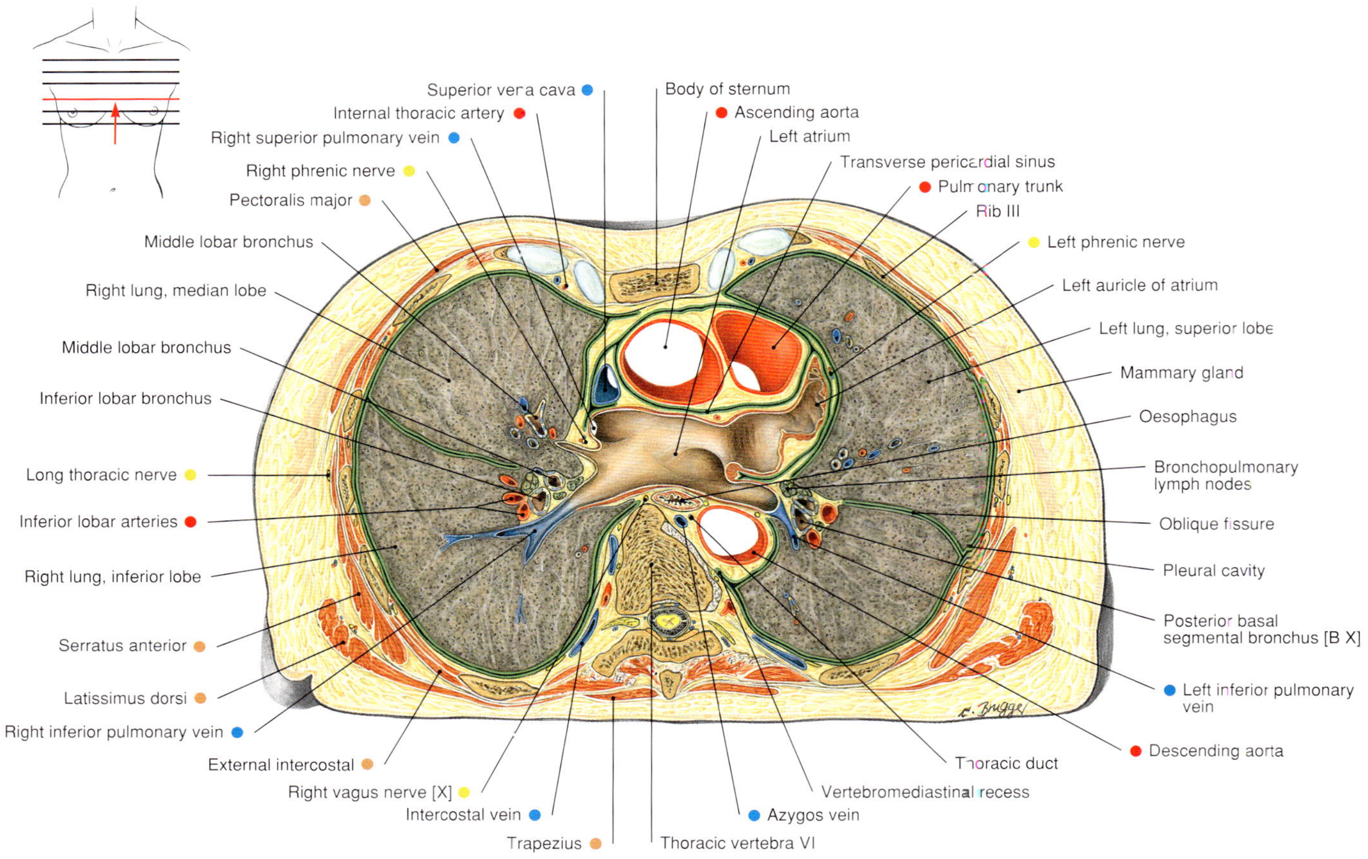

Fig. 704 Thoracic cavity.

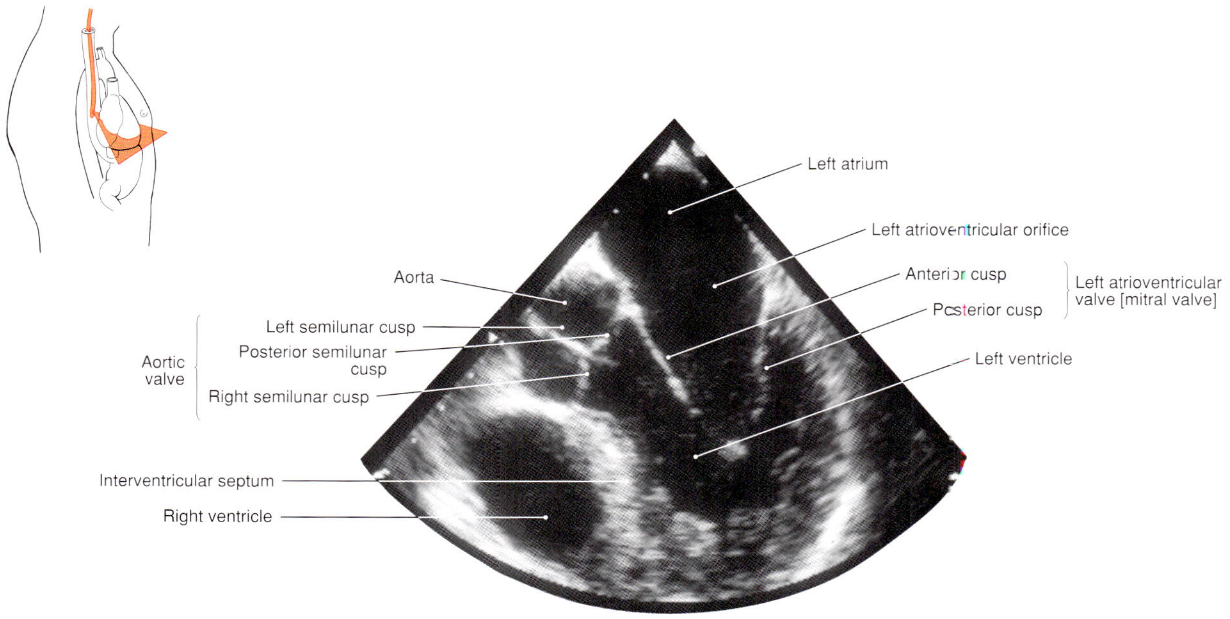

Fig. 705 Heart;
ultrasound image viewed from the oesophagus (transoesophageal echocardiography).

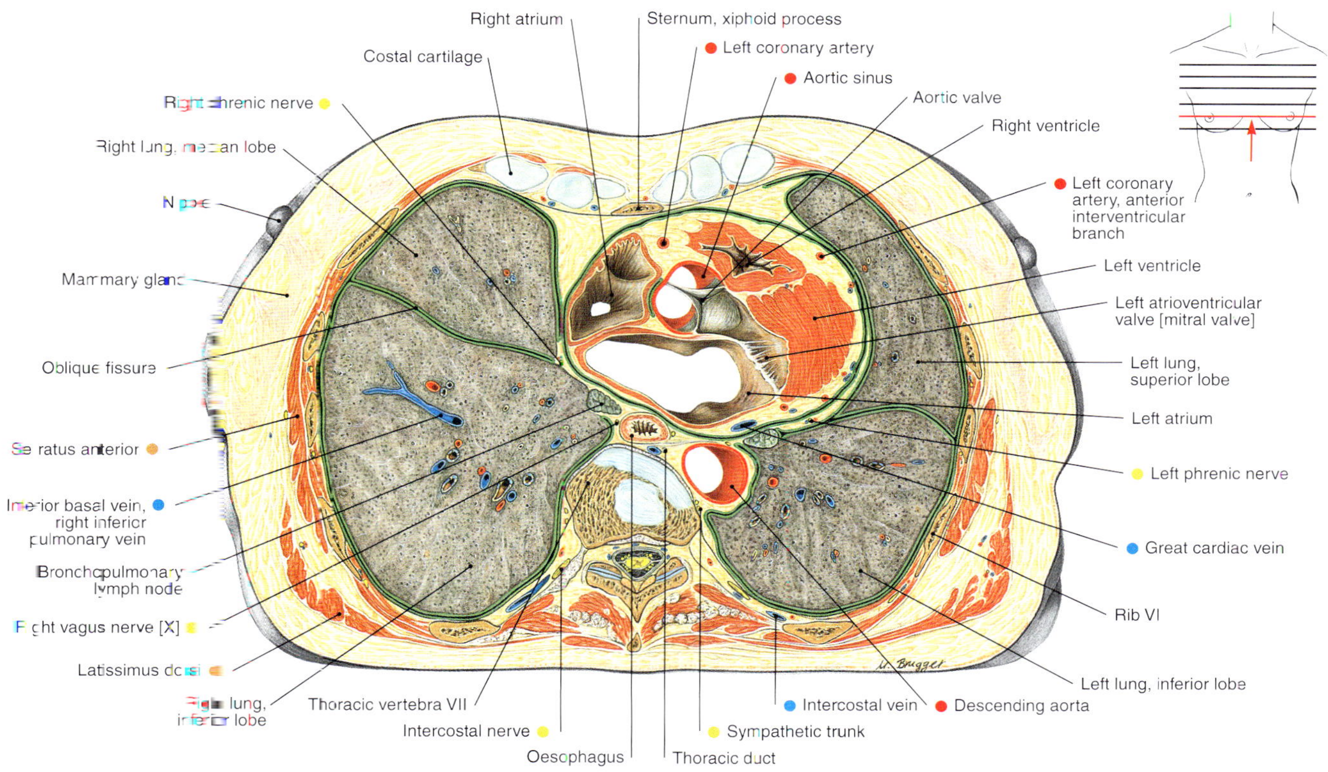

Fig. 706 Thoracic cavity.

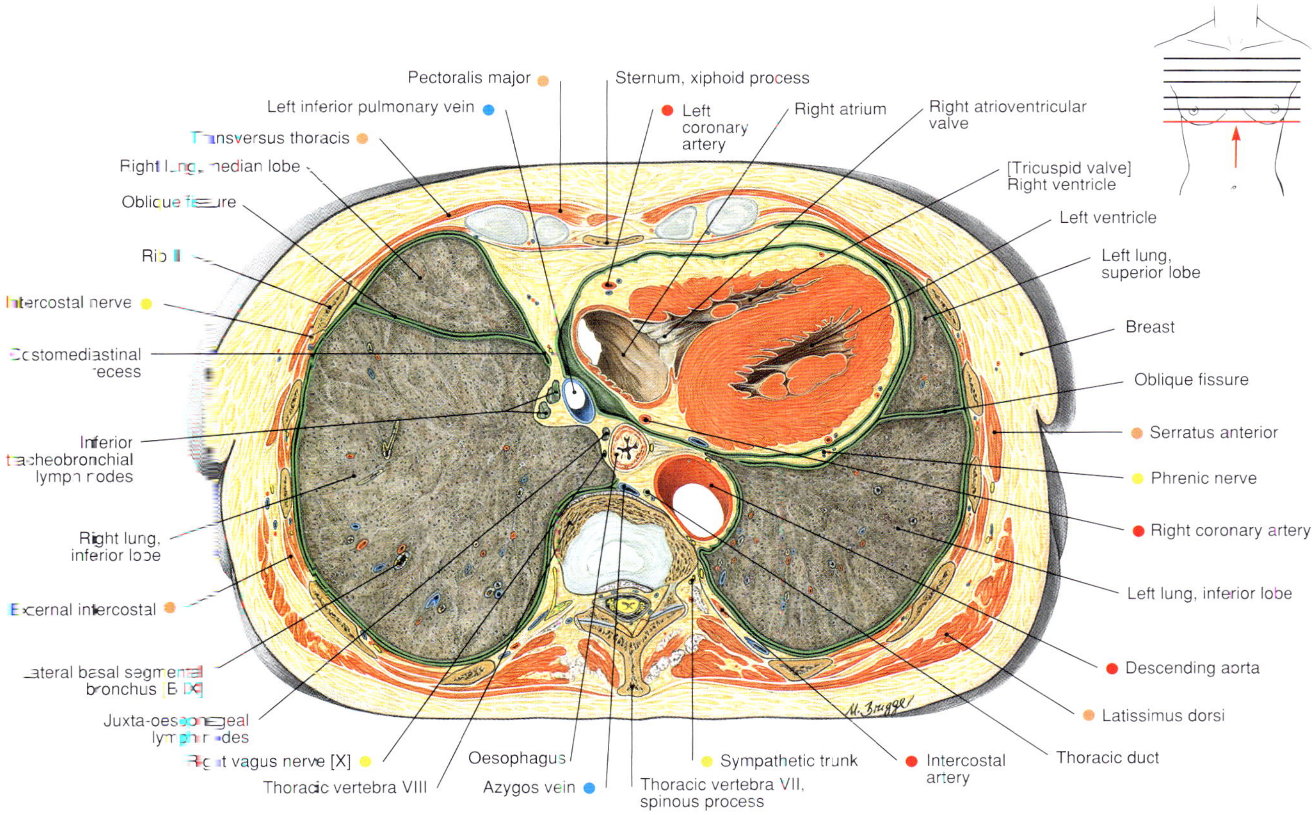

Fig. 707 Thoracic cavity.

Stomach

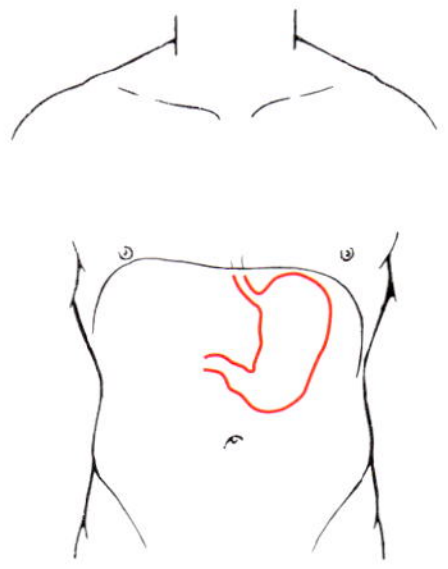

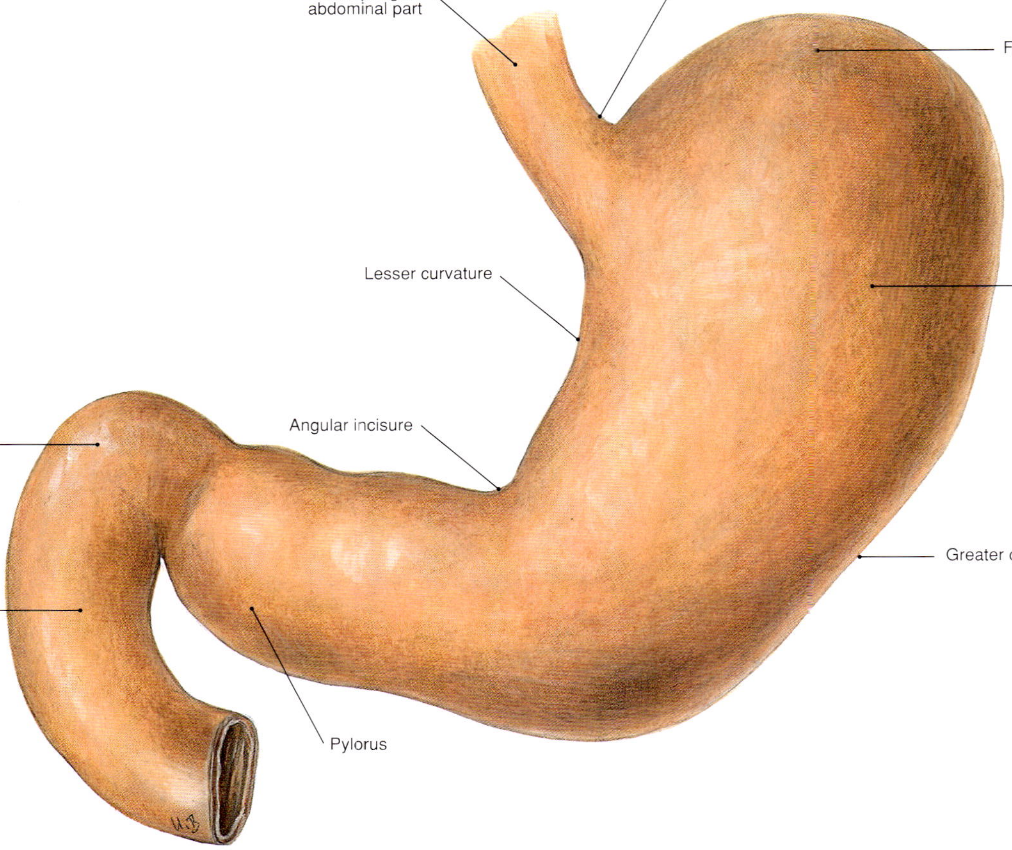

Fig. 708 Stomach;
ventral view.

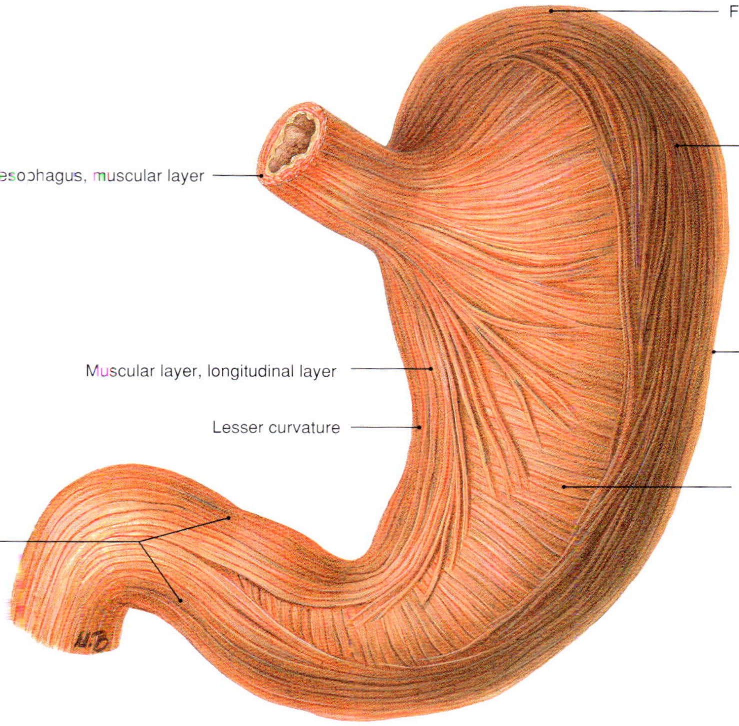

Fig. 709 Stomach; external muscle layers; ventral view.

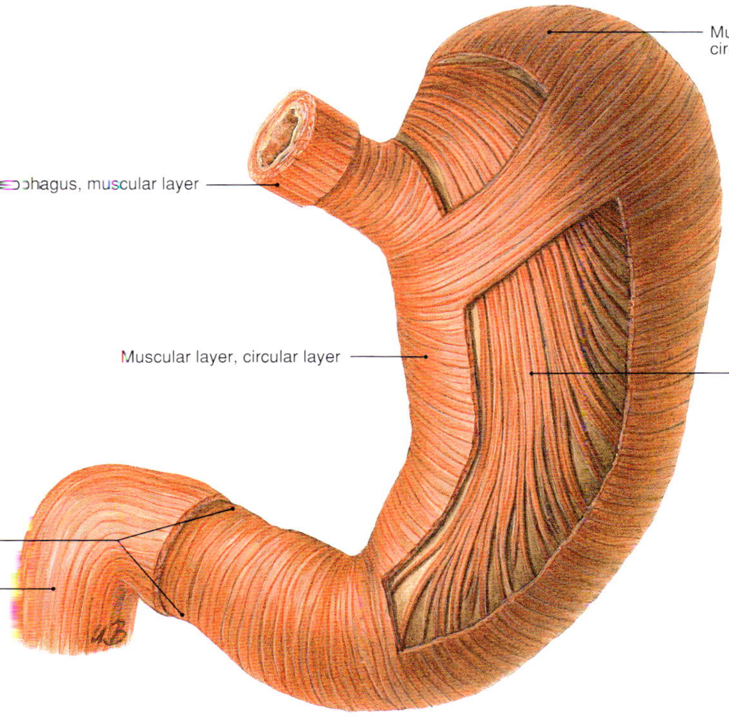

Fig. 710 Stomach; the peritoneum has been removed to demonstrate the internal muscle layers; ventral view.

Stomach, structure

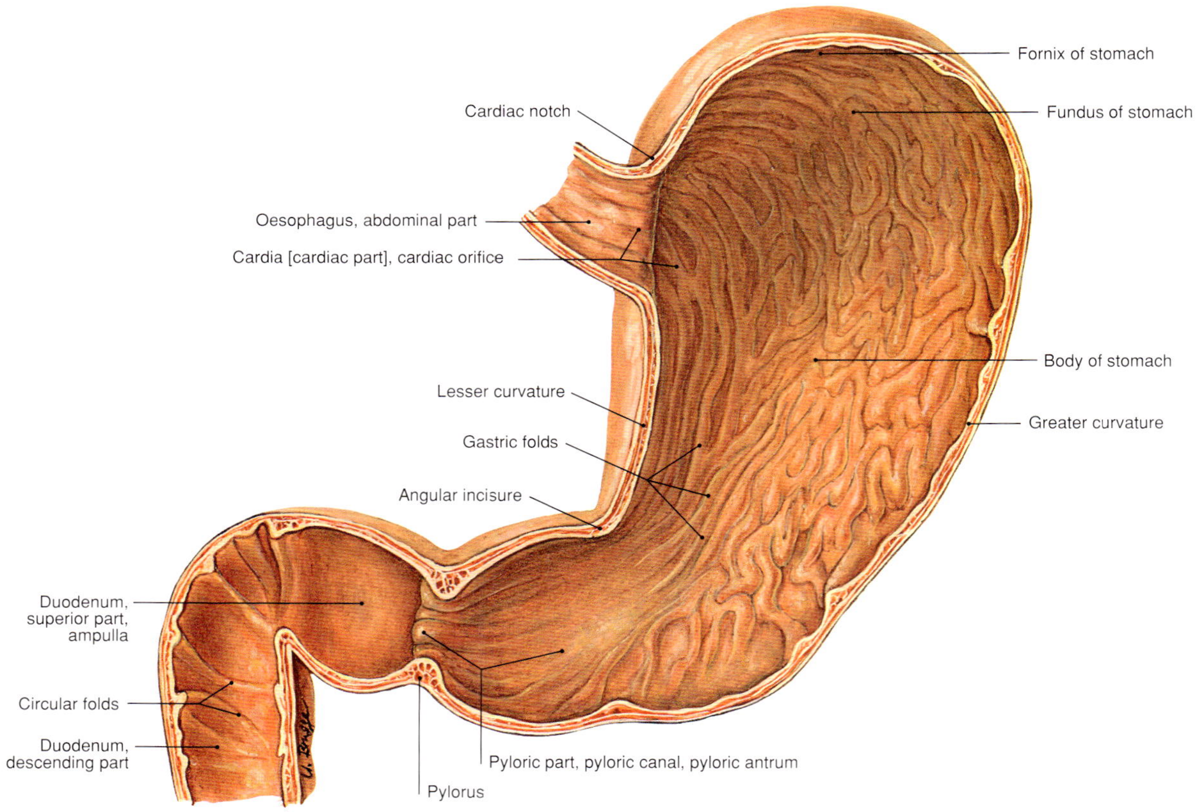

Fig. 711 Stomach and duodenum; ventral view.

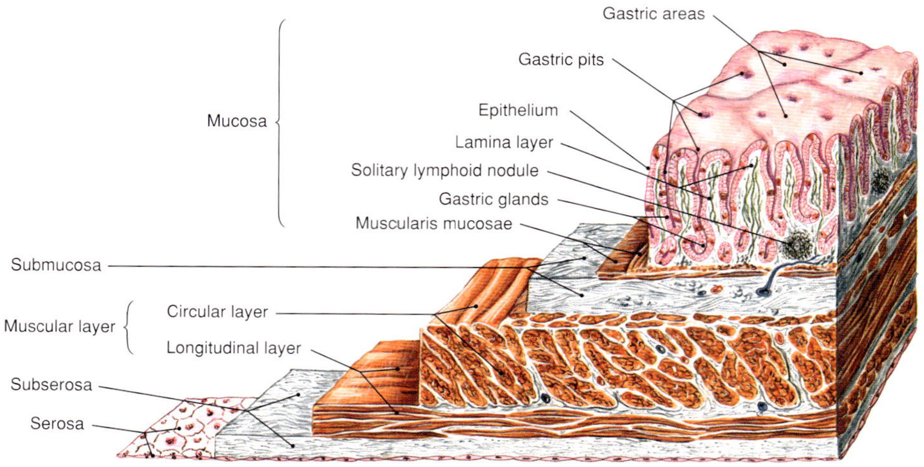

Fig. 712 Diagram of the stomach wall; the layers of the wall have been removed stepwise; microscopic enlargement at low magnification.

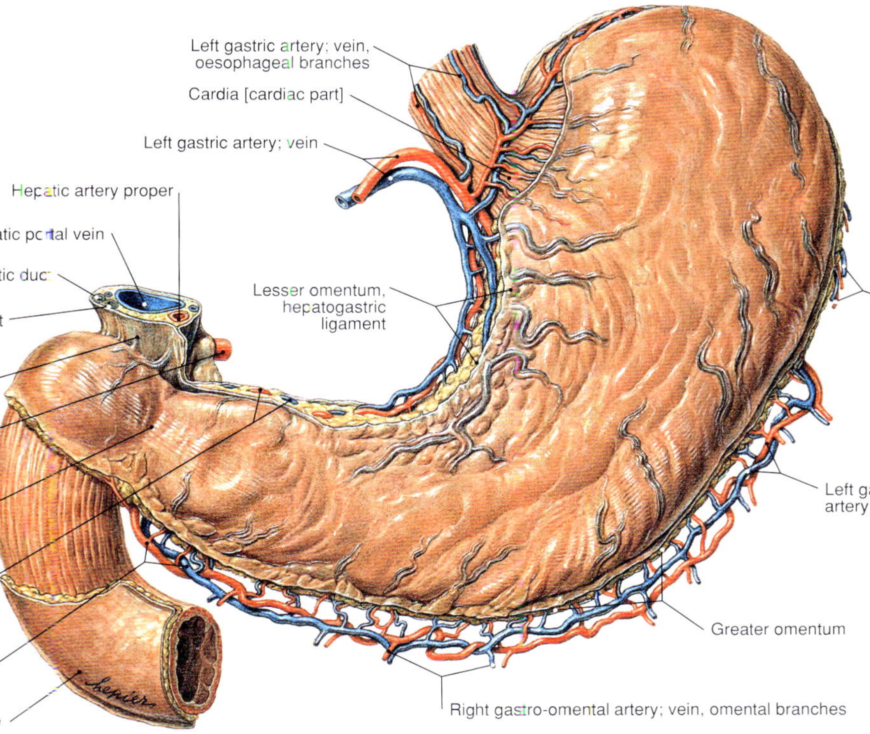

Fig. 713 Blood vessels of the stomach; ventral view.

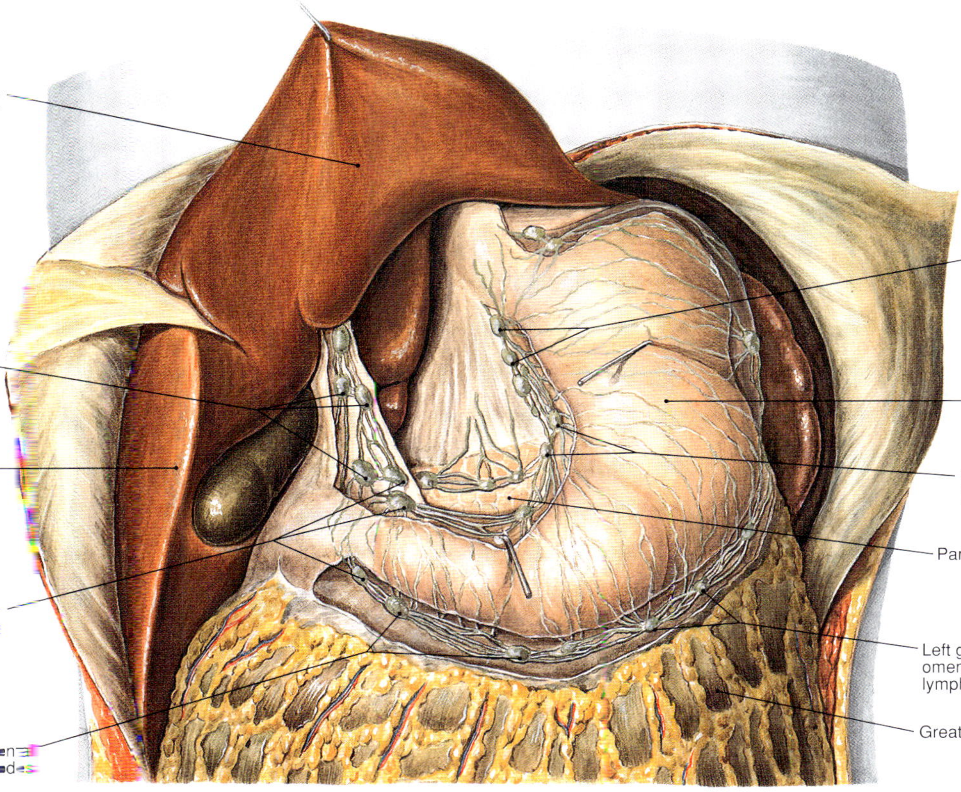

Fig. 714 Stomach and liver with lymph nodes; ventral view.

Stomach, radiography

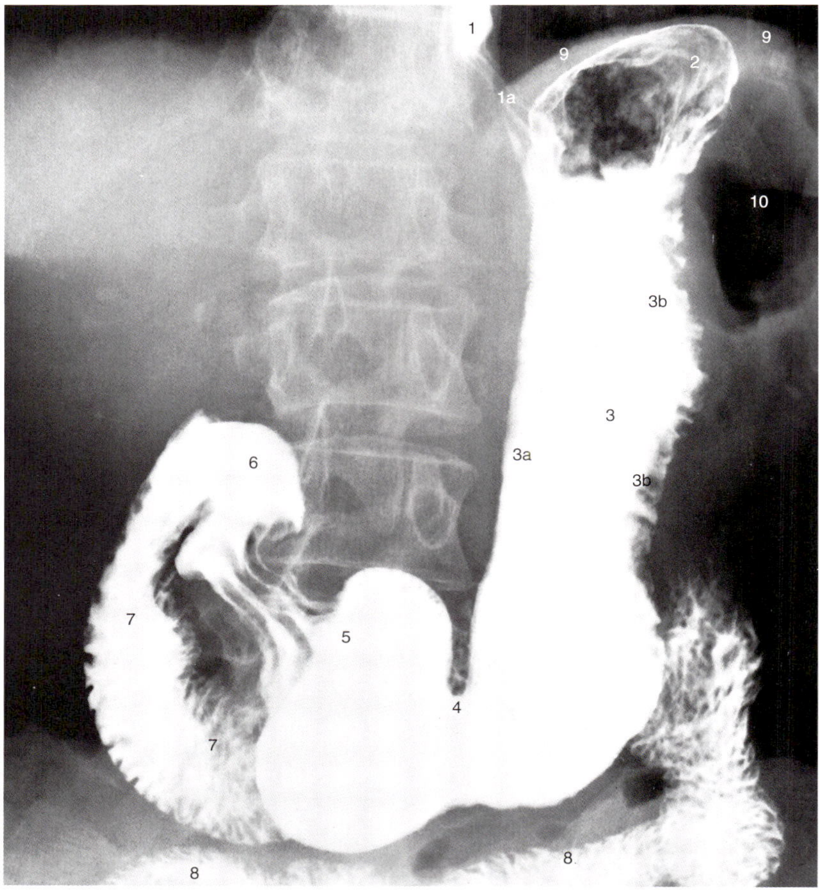

1 = Oesophagus with contrast medium. At the transition (1a) into the fundus of stomach, the grooves between the folds appear as dark striations.
2 = Fundus of stomach with air bubble
3 = Body of stomach
3a = Lesser curvature
3b = Greater curvature. In the linings of the latter, notches corresponding to the contour of the mucous are visible.
4 = Peristaltic constriction at the angular notch
5 = Pyloric part prior to the progression of a portion of the stomach's content
6 = Ampulla of duodenum
7 = Descending part of the duodenum with circular folds
8 = Jejunum
9 = Left „dome" of diaphragm
10 = Left colic flexure (filled with air)

Fig. 715 Stomach and duodenum;
AP-radiograph after oral administration of a contrast medium;
upright position;
ventral view.

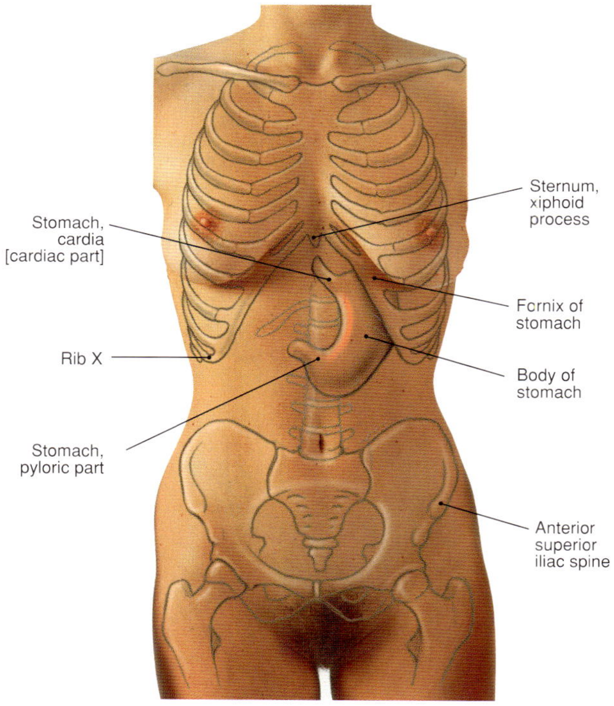

Fig. 716 Stomach;
projection of a „normal" stomach onto the anterior abdominal wall;
upright position.

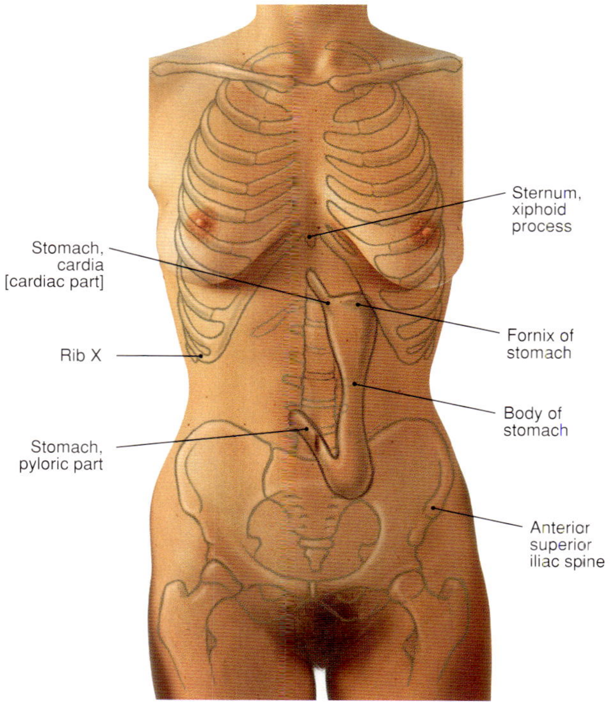

Fig. 717 Stomach;
projection of a „long" stomach onto the anterior abdominal wall;
upright position.

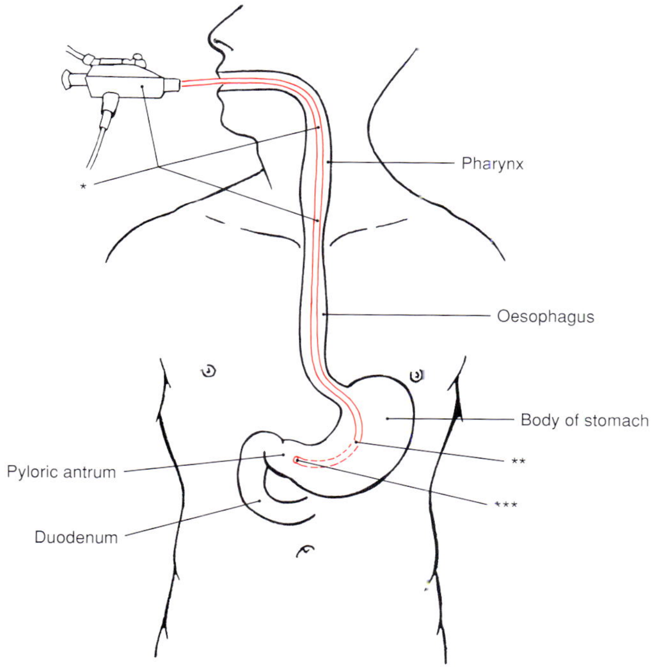

Fig. 718 Technical procedure of oesophagoscopy and gastroscopy.

* Gastroscope
** The gastroscope's tip located in the body of stomach (compare Fig. 719 a)
*** The gastroscope's tip located in the pyloric antrum (compare Fig. 719 b)

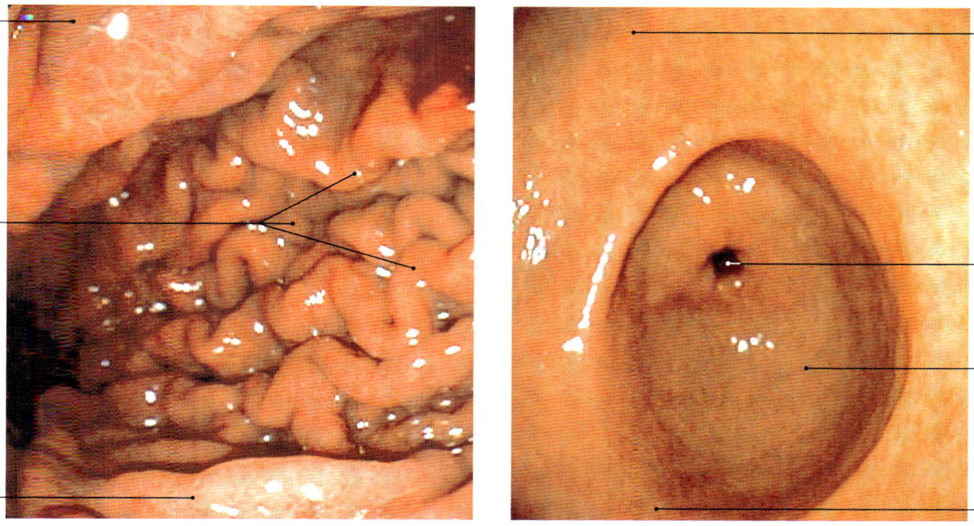

Fig. 719 a, b Stomach endoscopic image of the stomach (gastroscopy); superior view.

a View of the body of stomach with distinct longitudinal folds of the mucosa (Plica gastricae)
b View of the pyloric antrum predominantly covered with smooth mucosa

Duodenum

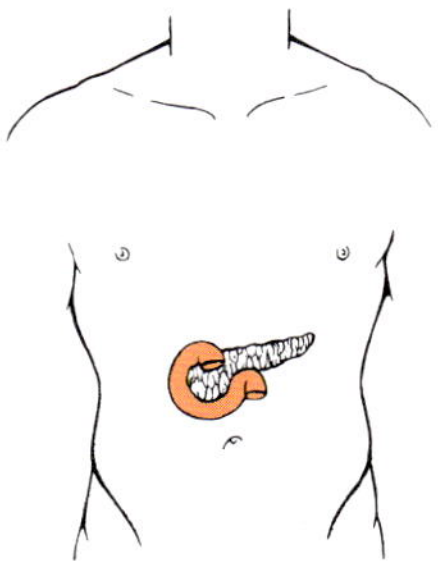

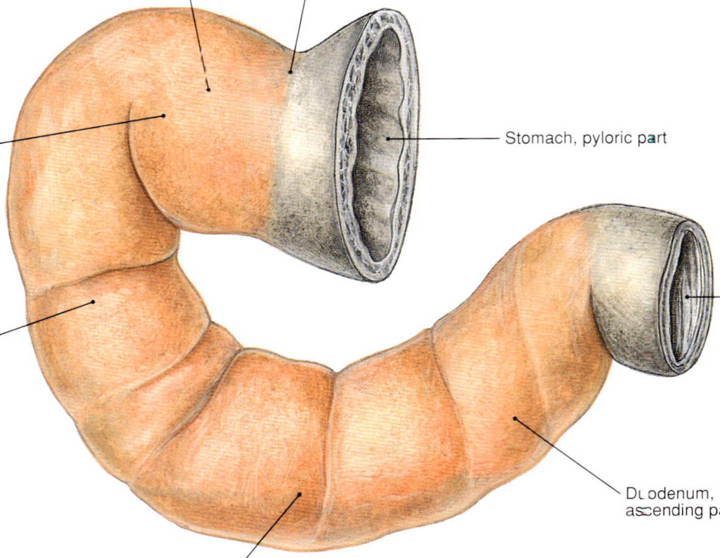

Fig. 720 Duodenum.

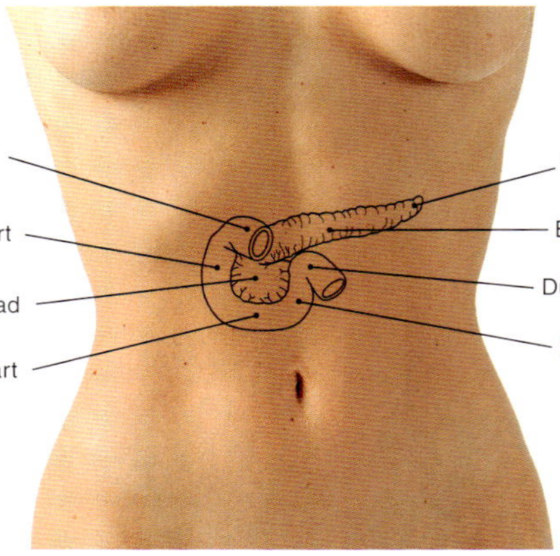

Fig. 721 Duodenum and pancreas; projected onto the anterior abdominal wall.

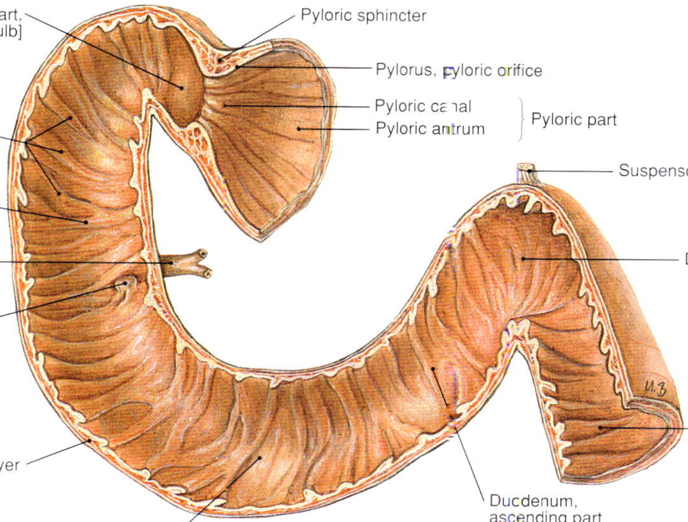

Fig. 722 Duodenum;
ventral view.

* Clinical term: muscle of TREITZ
** Clinical term: papilla of VATER

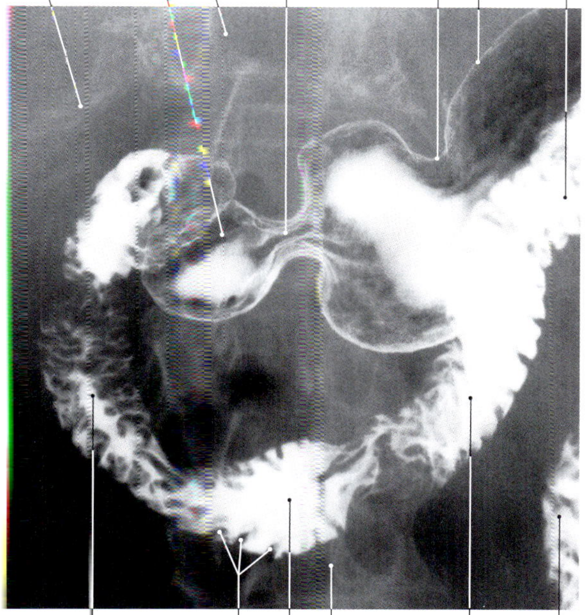

Fig. 723 Duodenum;
AP-radiograph after oral administration of a contrast medium;
upright position;
ventral view.

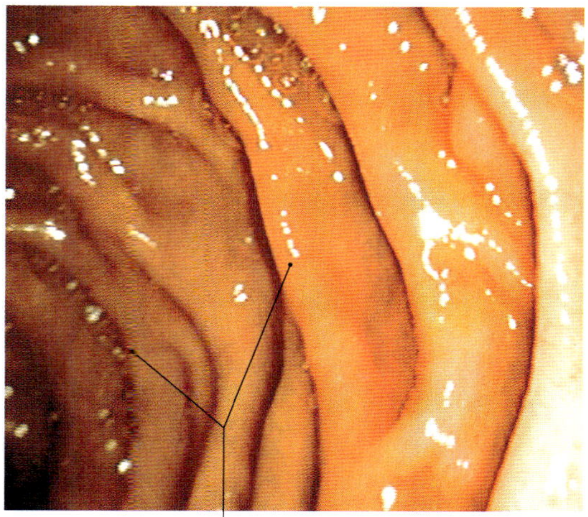

Fig. 724 Duodenum;
endoscopic image.

Small intestine, structure

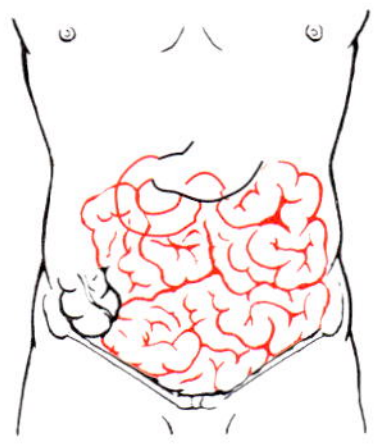

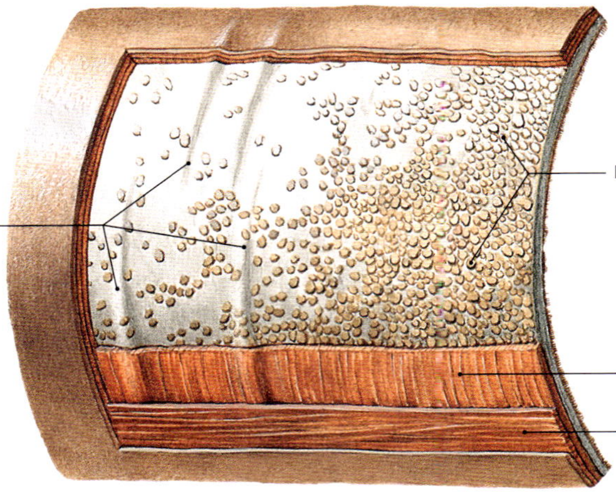

Fig. 725 Superior part of the duodenum; layers of the wall.

* Clinical term: BRUNNER's glands

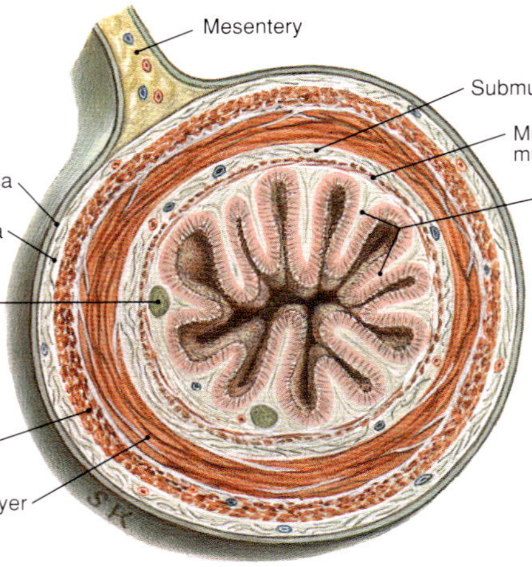

Fig. 726 Small intestine; cross-section through the upper small intestine.

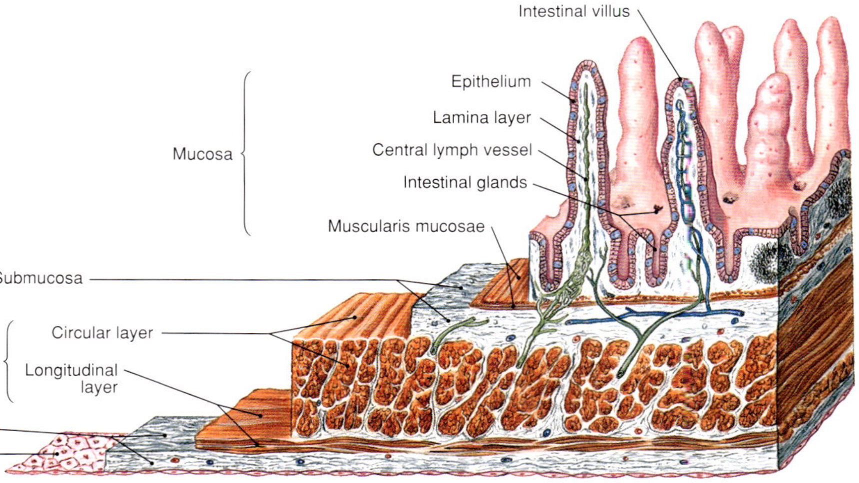

Fig. 727 Small intestine; layers of the wall; microscopic enlargement at low magnification.

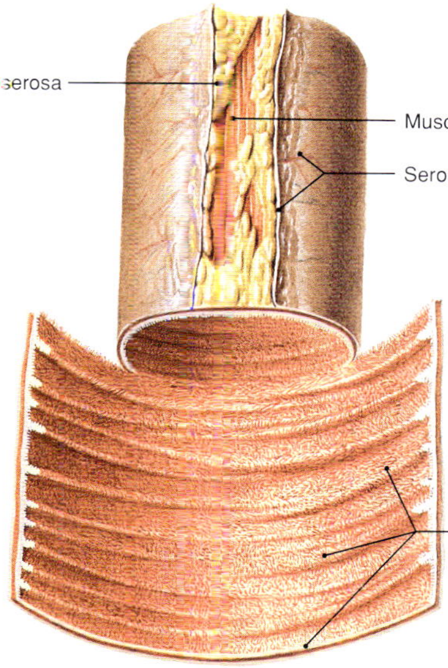

Fig. 728 Jejunum.

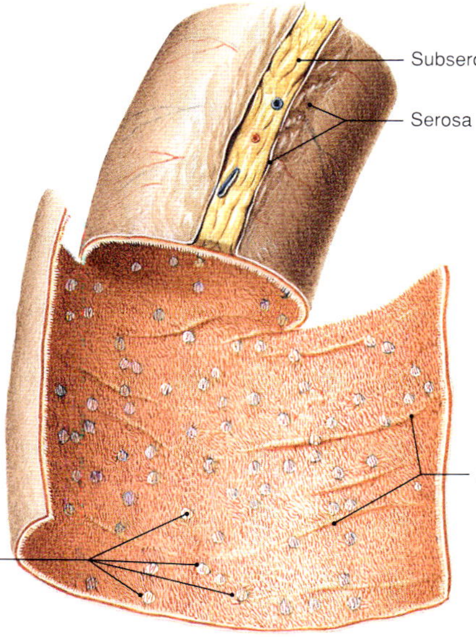

Fig. 729 Ileum.

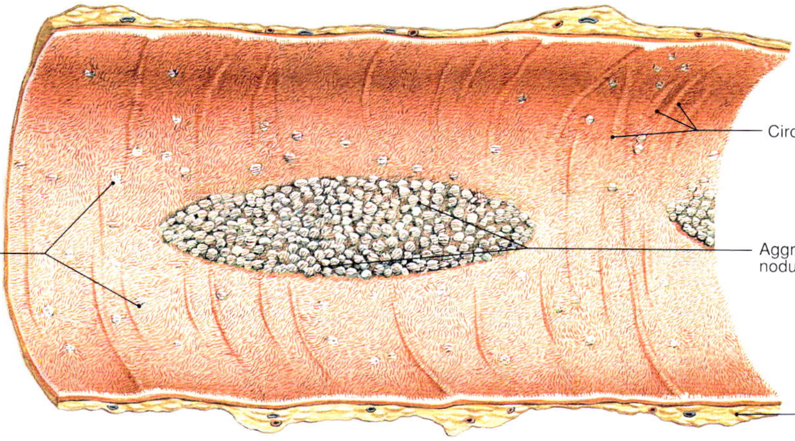

Fig. 730 Terminal ileum.

* Clinical term: PEYER's patches

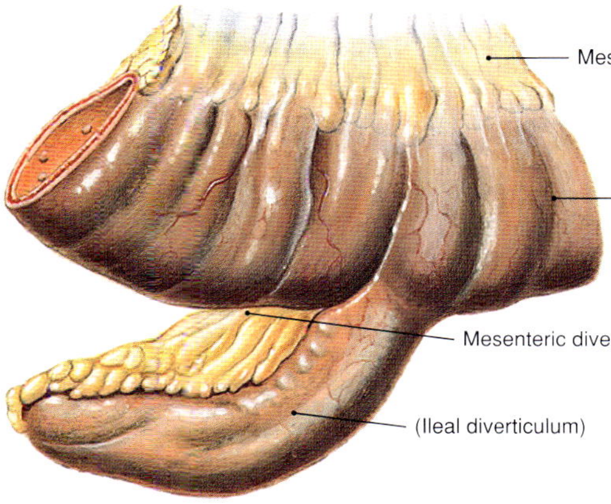

Fig. 731 MECKEL's diverticulum (ileal diverticulum). This vestige of the yolk stalk (omphalomesenteric duct) occurs in 1–3% of cases. It is located 30–70 cm oral to the ileocaecal junction opposite to the attachment of the mesentery.

Large intestine

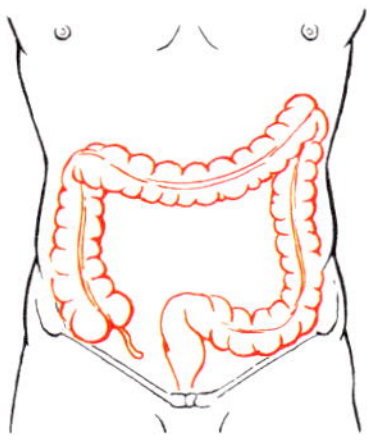

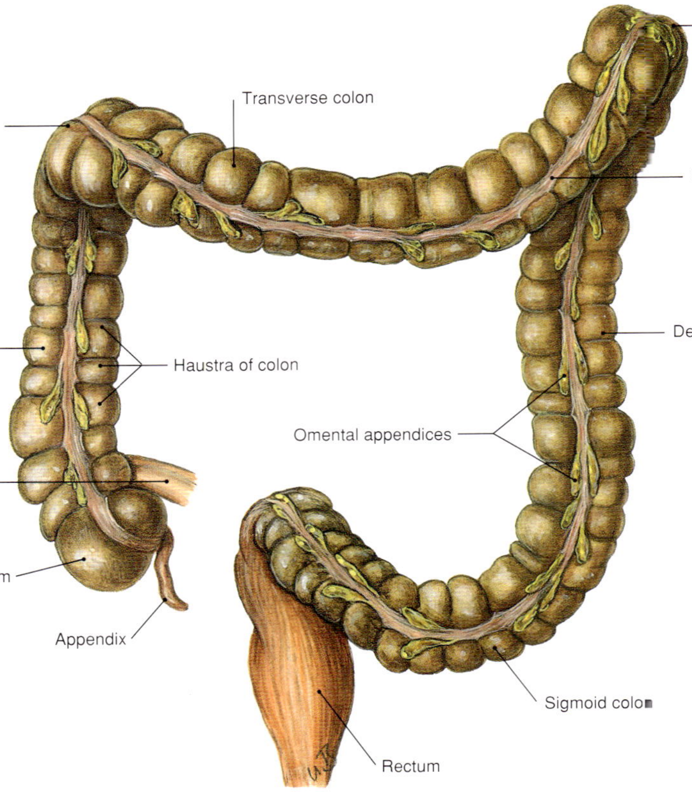

Fig. 732 Large intestine;
ventral view.

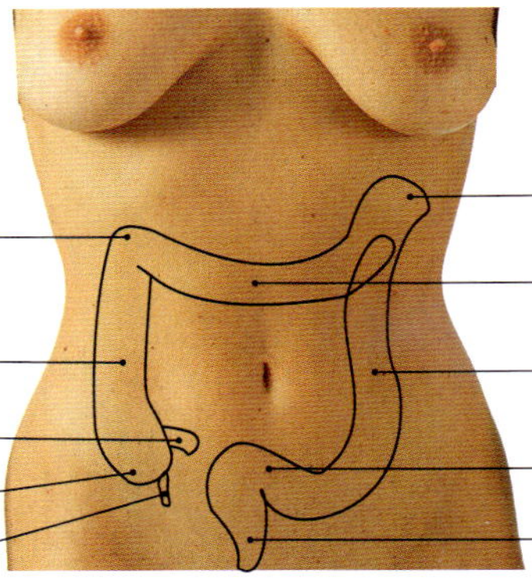

Fig. 733 Large intestine;
projected onto the anterior abdominal wall.
The positions of the transverse colon and of the sigmoid colon are highly variable (compare Fig. 742).

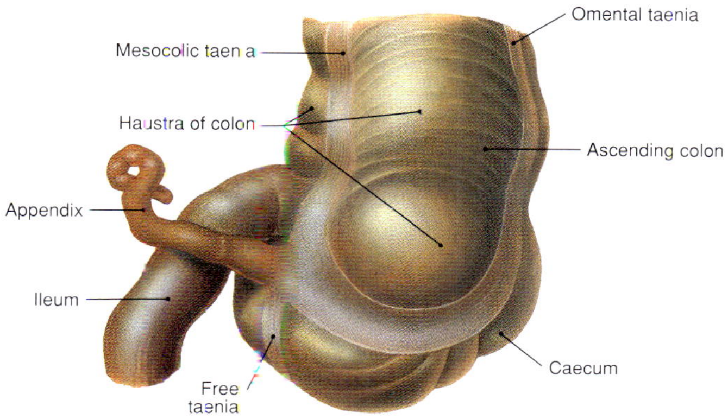

Fig. 734 Caecum; vermiform appendix and terminal ileum; dorsal view.

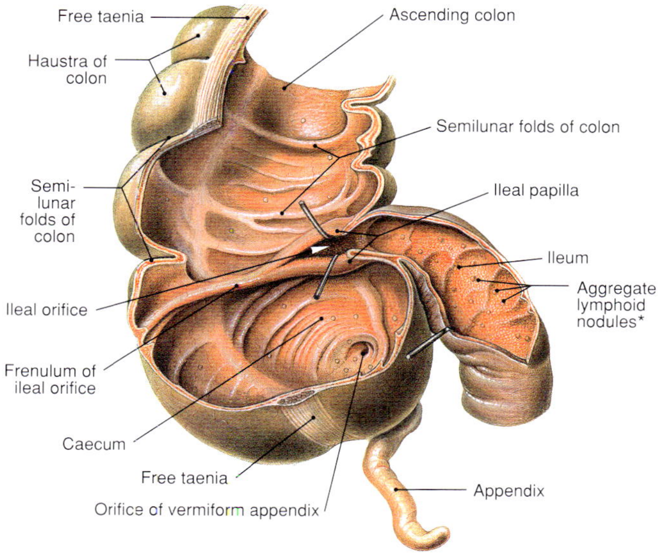

Fig. 735 Ascending colon; caecum, and vermiform appendix; ventral view.

* Clinical term: PEYER's patches

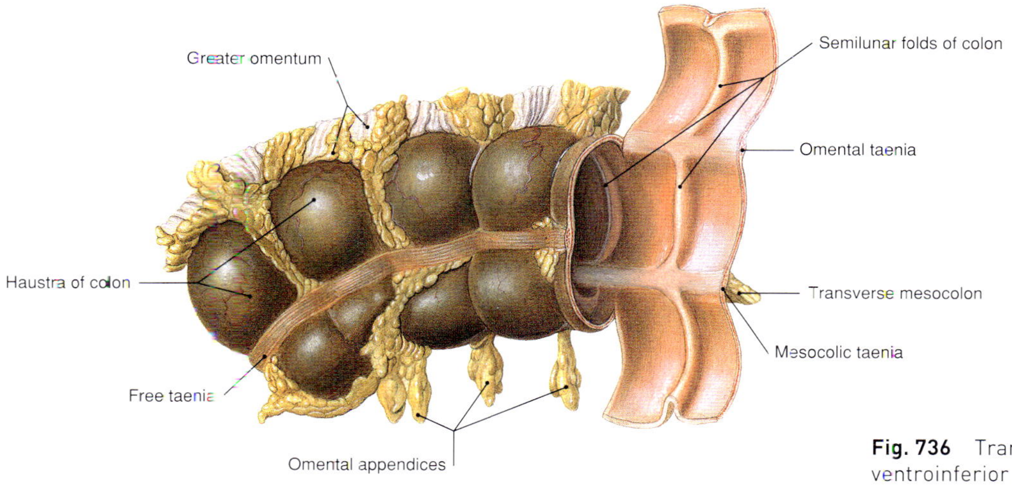

Fig. 736 Transverse colon; ventroinferior view.

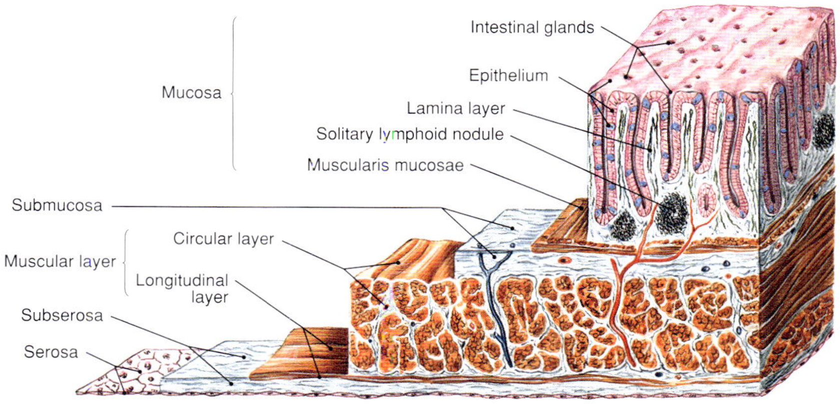

Fig. 737 Colon; layers of the wall; microscopic enlargement at low magnification.

Vermiform appendix

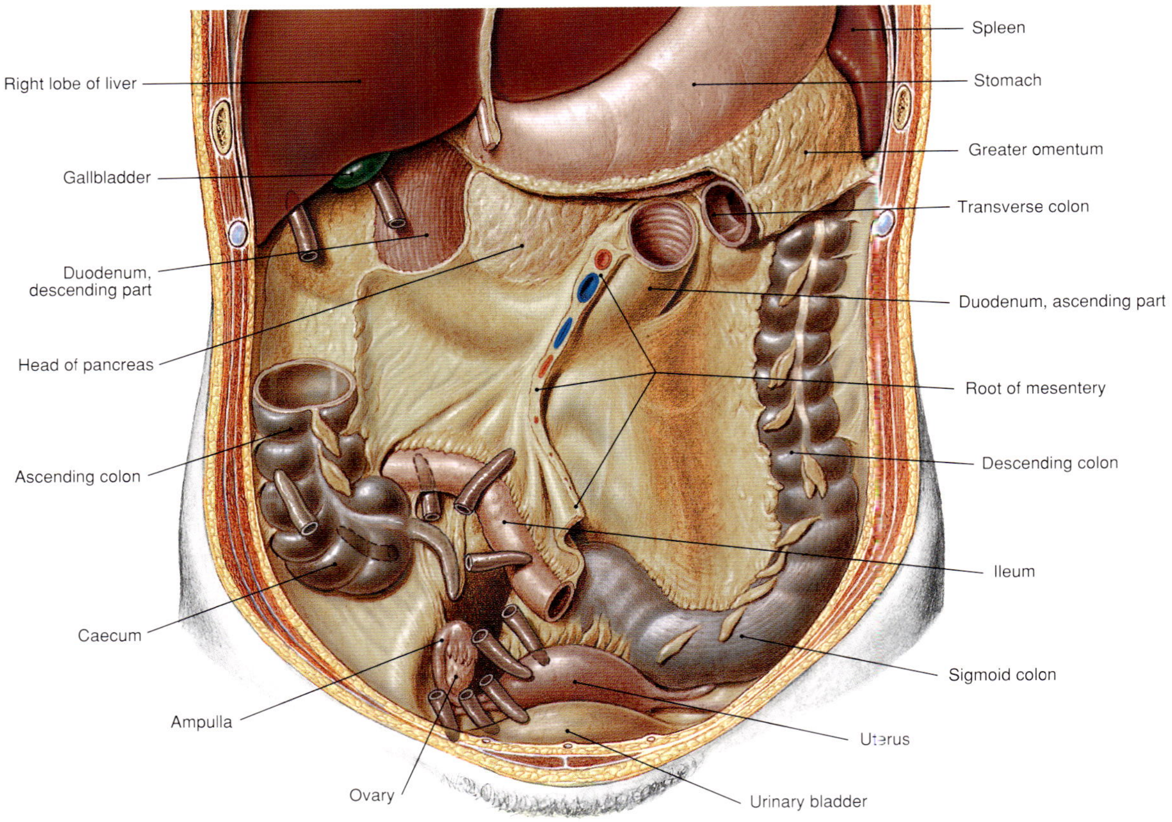

Fig. 738 Vermiform appendix; variations in its position; ventral view.

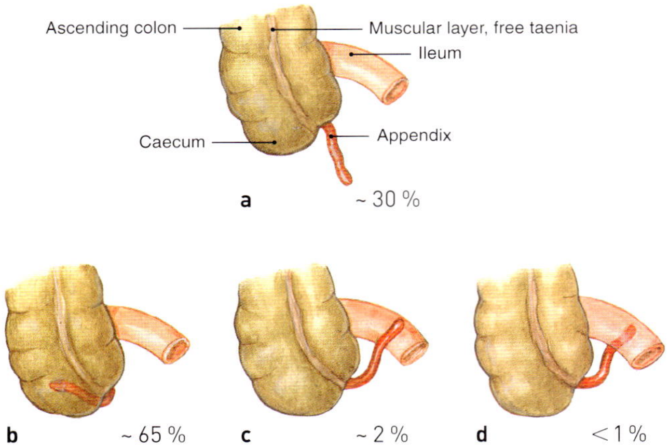

Fig. 739 Vermiform appendix; variations in its position.
a Descending into the lesser pelvis
b Behind the caecum
c In front of the ileum
d Behind the ileum

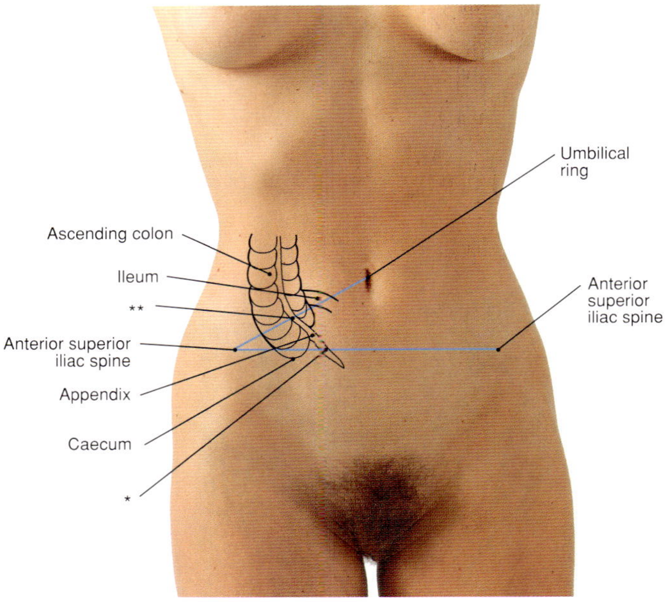

Fig. 740 Caecum and vermiform appendix; projection onto the anterior abdominal wall.

* Clinical term: v. LANZ's point, at the right third of a line connecting the anterior superior iliac spines, locates the tip of the vermiform appendix

** Clinical term: McBURNEY's point, at the outer third of a line connecting the right anterior superior iliac spine and the umbilicus, locates the base of the vermiform appendix

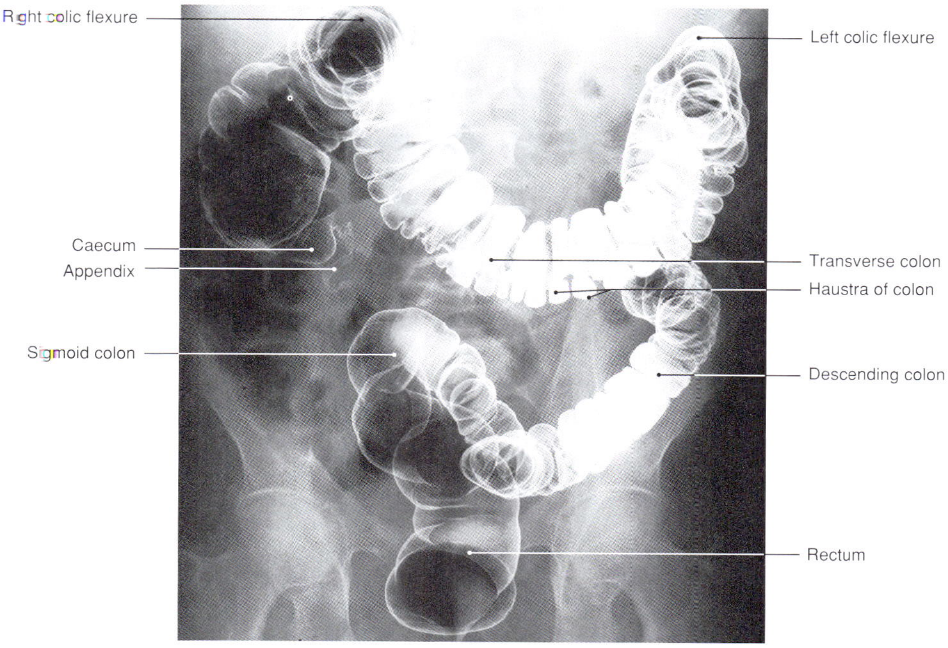

Fig. 741 Colon and rectum;
AP-radiograph after filling with a contrast medium and air (double contrast method).

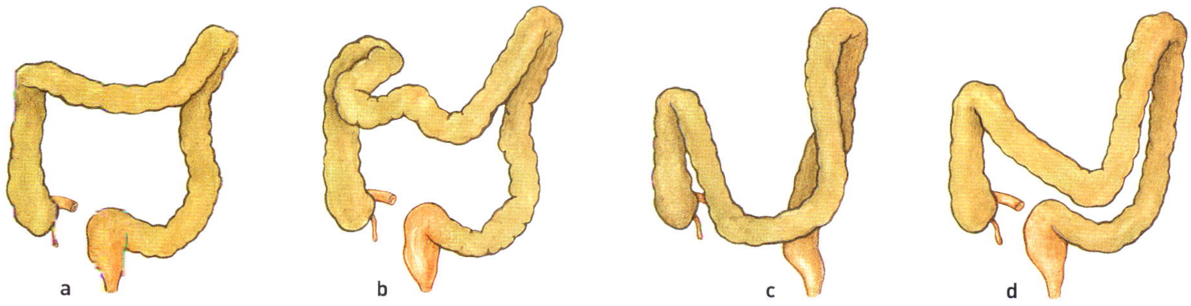

Fig. 742 a–d Transverse colon;
common variations in its position;
ventral view.

a Normal position
b Twisted
c U-shaped
d V-shaped

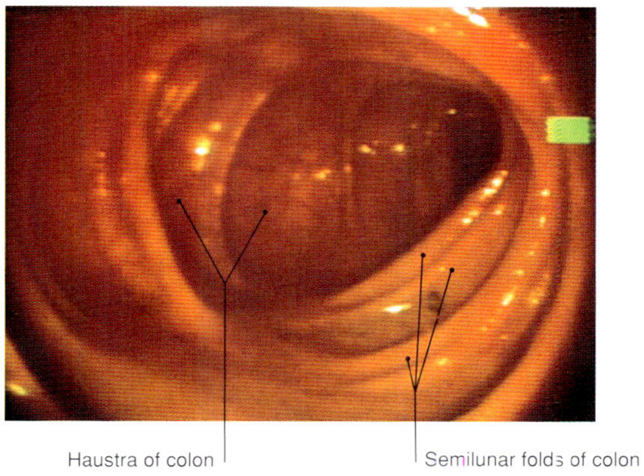

Fig. 743 Ascending colon;
endoscopic image after passage of the rectum, the sigmoid colon, the descending colon and the transverse colon (colonoscopy).

Liver

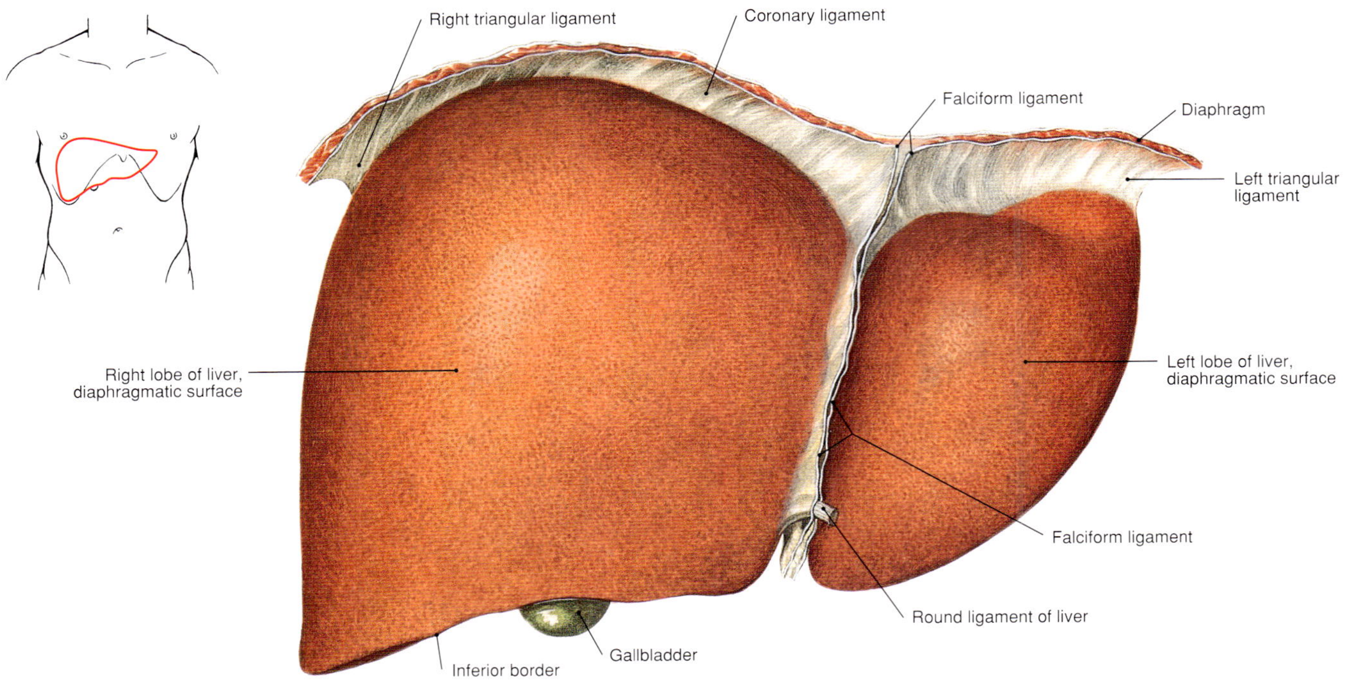

Fig. 744 Liver;
ventral view.

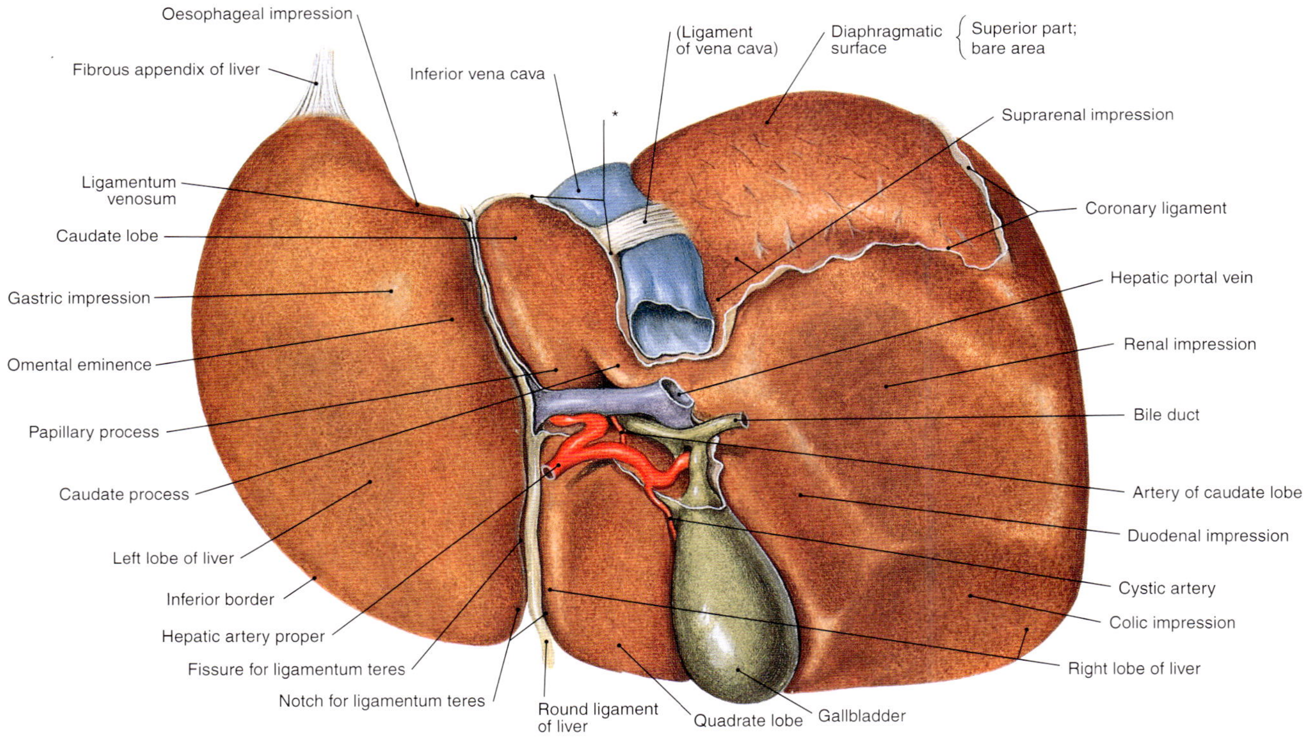

Fig. 745 Liver and porta hepatis;
dorsal view.

* Borders of the superior recess of the omental bursa

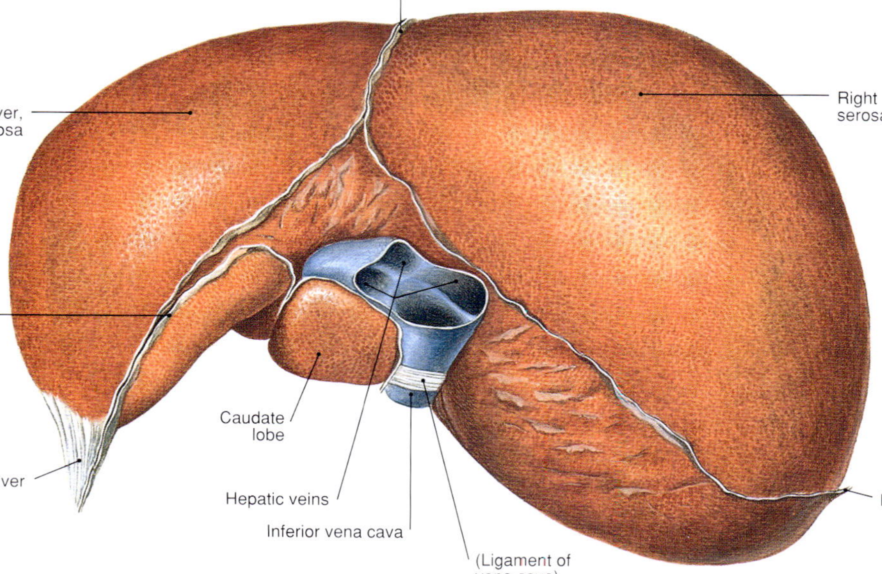

Fig. 746 Liver; superior view.

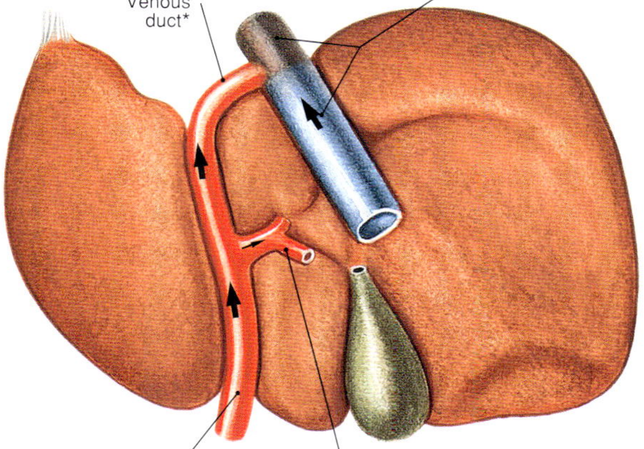

Fig. 747 Liver of a foetus; oxygen content of the blood is shown by different colours and the direction of flow by arrows; dorsal view.

* Also: Ductus ARANTII

Liver puncture

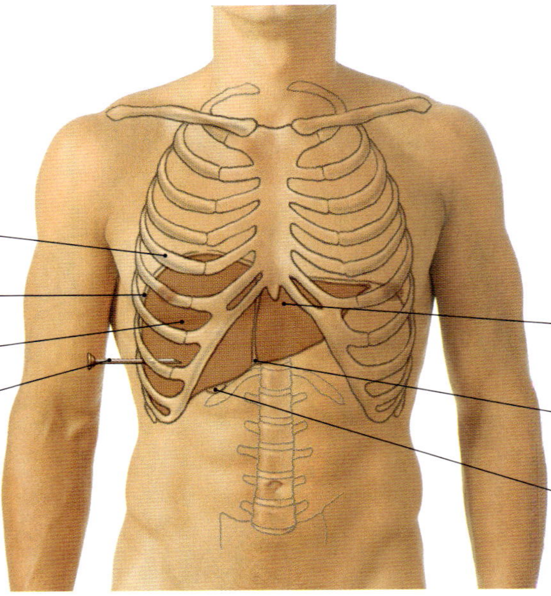

Fig. 748 Liver;
projection onto the anterior abdominal wall;
intermediate position between inspiration and expiration.

* Position of the needle for liver puncture

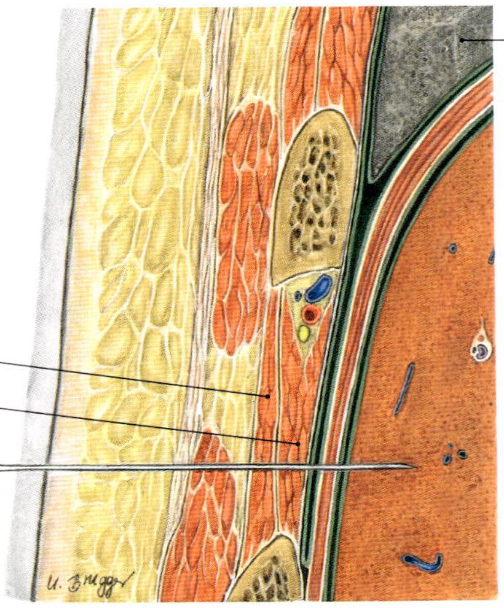

Fig. 749 Layers of the abdominal wall and the liver;
frontal section.

* Position of the needle for liver puncture

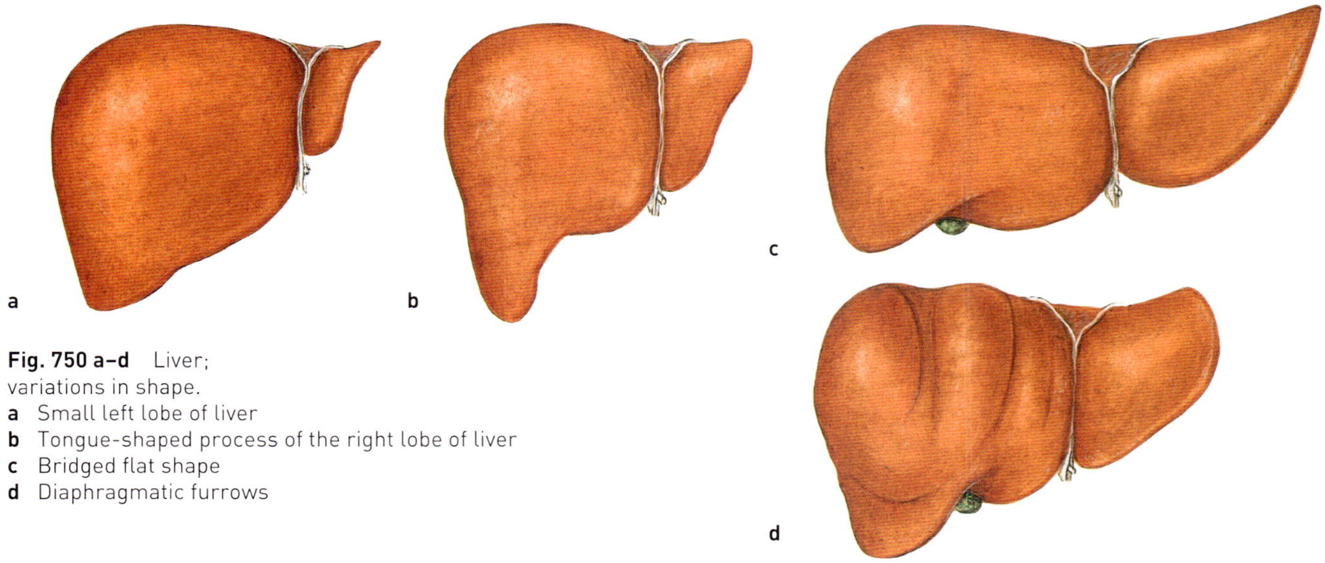

Fig. 750 a–d Liver;
variations in shape.

a Small left lobe of liver
b Tongue-shaped process of the right lobe of liver
c Bridged flat shape
d Diaphragmatic furrows

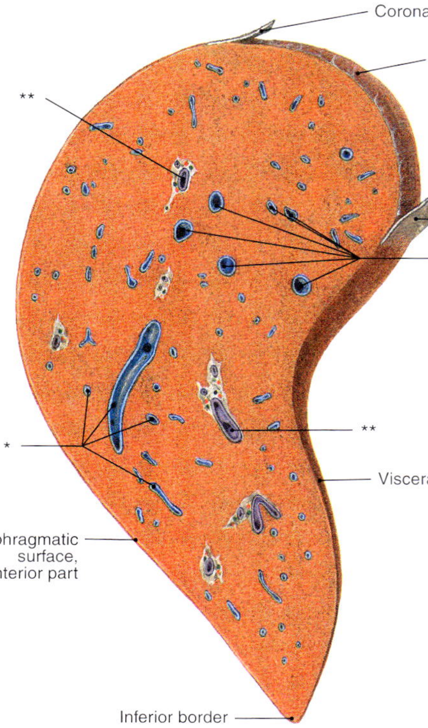

Fig. 751 Liver;
sagittal section through the right lobe of liver to demonstrate the branches of the hepatic veins and the hepatic portal vein.

* Intrahepatic branches of the hepatic veins
** Intrahepatic branches of the hepatic portal vein and the hepatic artery

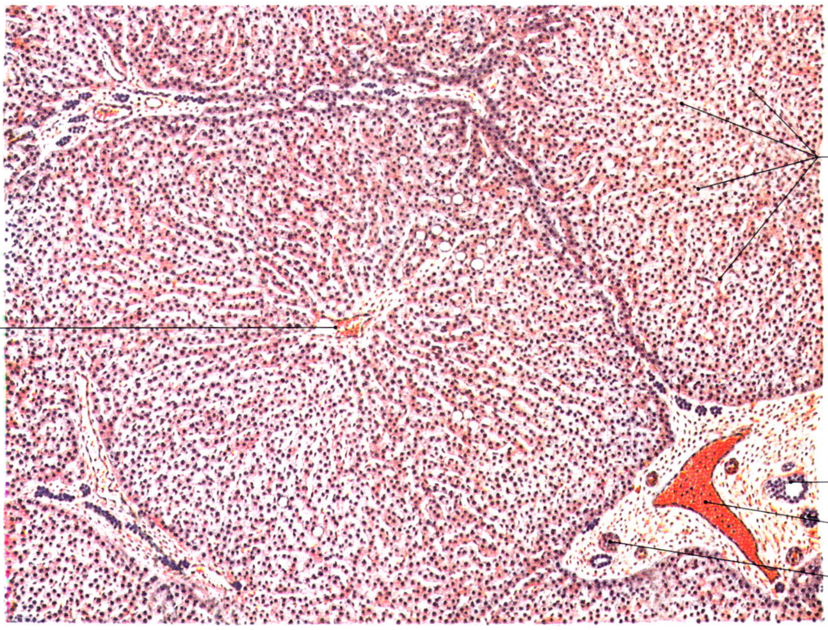

Fig. 752 Liver;
microscopic structure (microscopic enlargement at low magnification); trias of GLISSON (consists of a branch of the hepatic portal vein, a branch of the hepatic artery proper and a small bile duct), and a small liver lobule surrounding a central vein.

Liver puncture

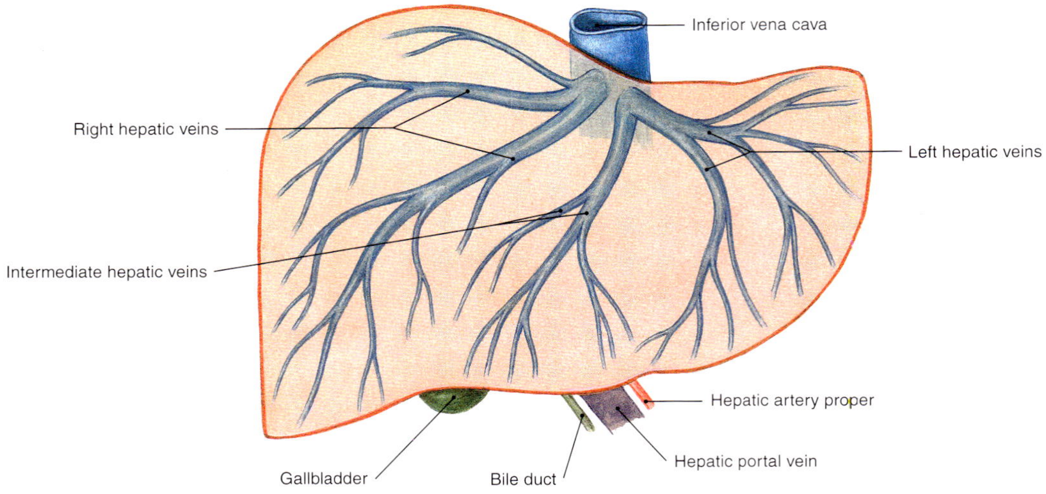

Fig. 753 Liver and hepatic veins; ventral view.

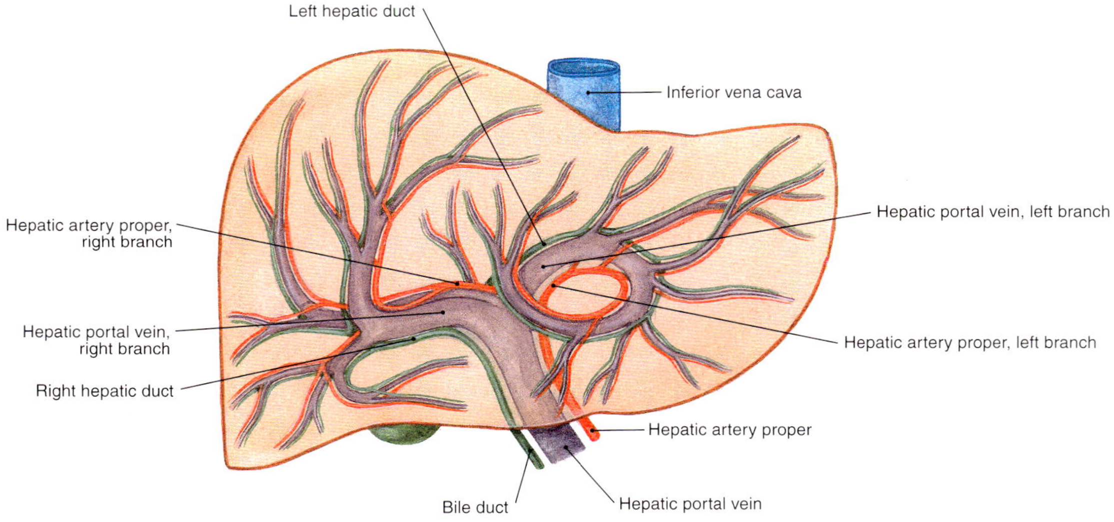

Fig. 754 Liver and the hepatic portal vein; ventral view.

Segments of the liver

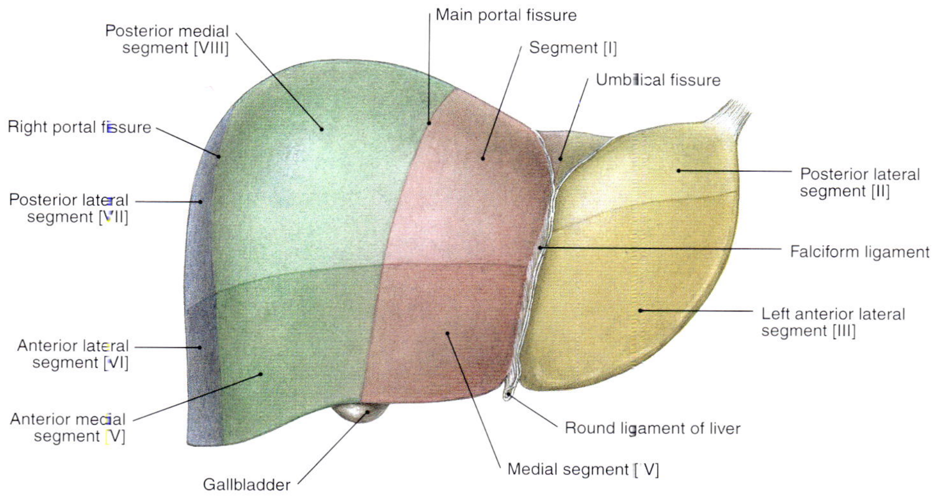

Fig. 755 Liver;
the segments of the lobes are shown in different colours;
ventral view.

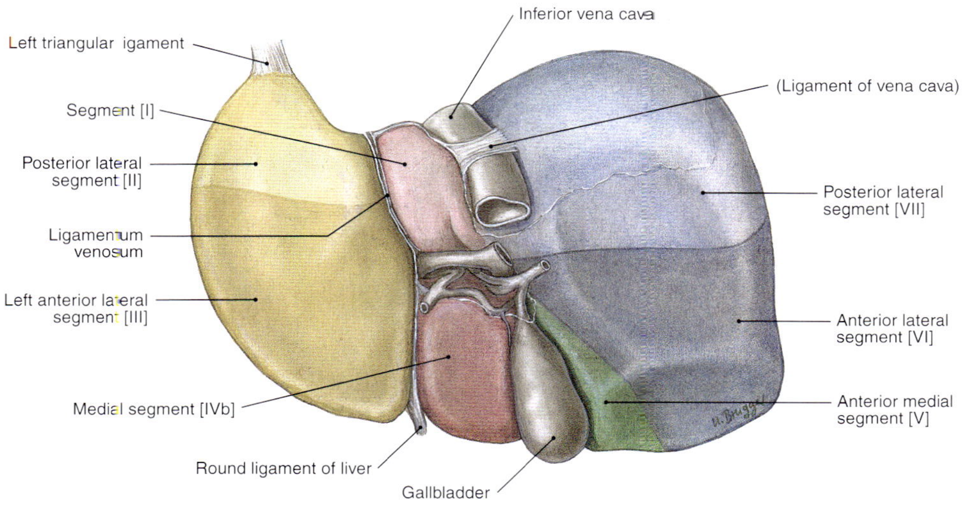

Fig. 756 Liver;
the segments of the lobes are shown in different colours;
dorsal view.

Liver, ultrasound

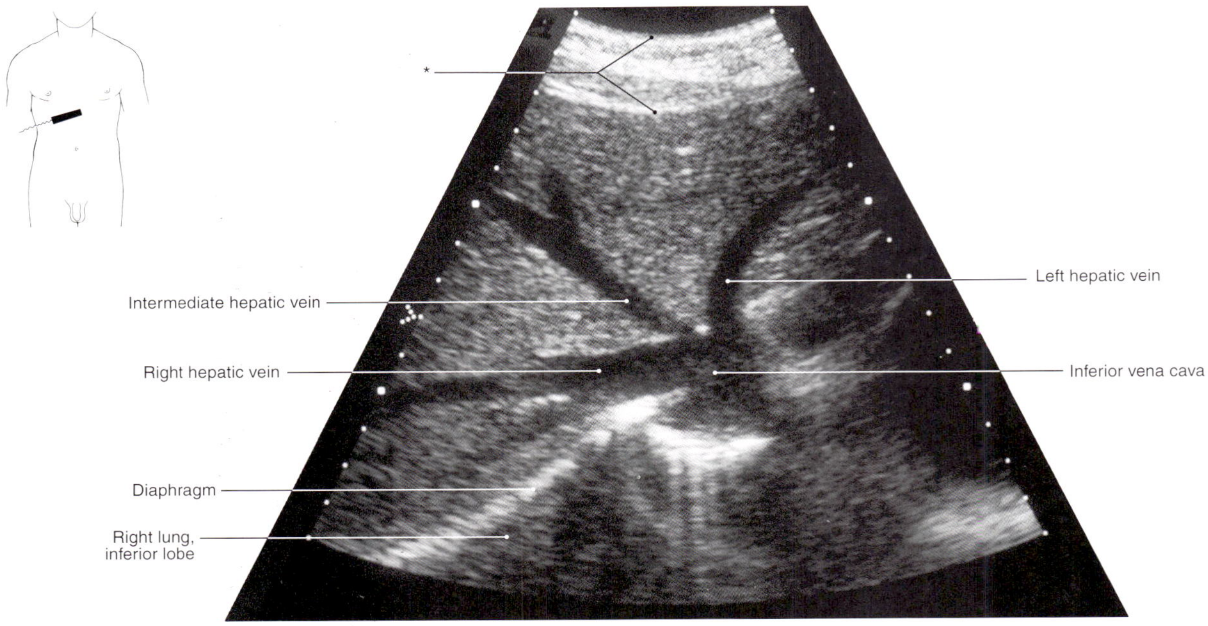

→ 753

Fig. 757 Hepatic veins;
ultrasound image showing the opening of the hepatic veins into the inferior vena cava;
inferior view.

* Abdominal wall

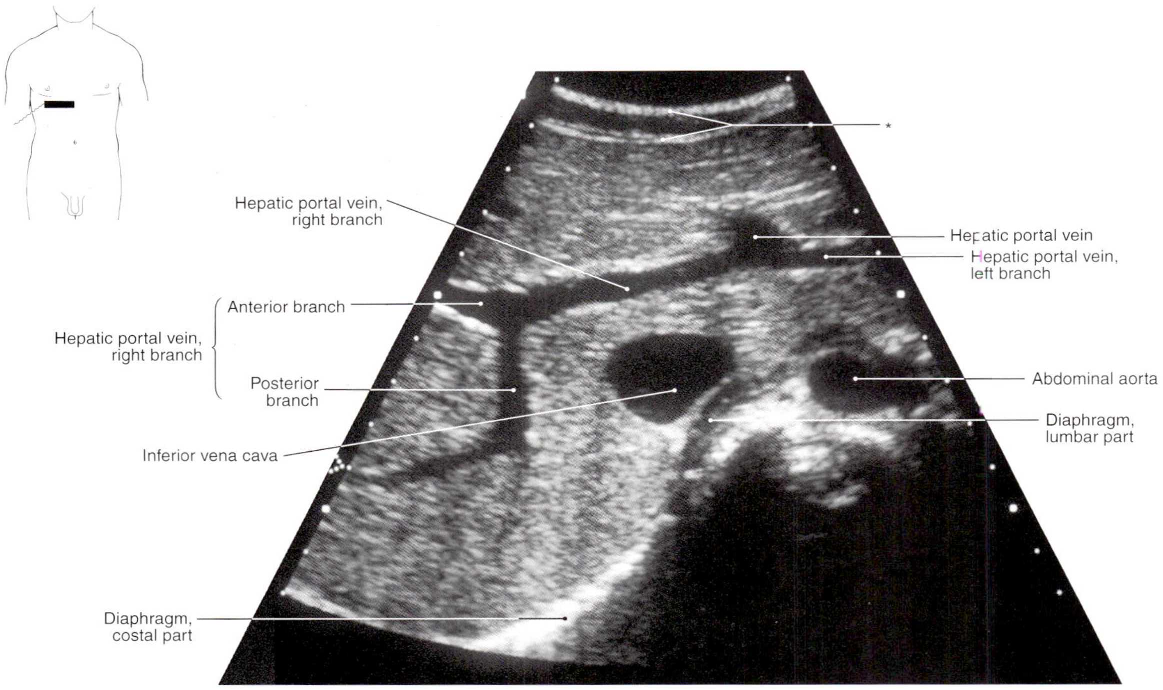

→ 754

Fig. 758 Hepatic portal vein;
ultrasound image showing the division of the hepatic portal vein into the main branches;
inferior view.

* Abdominal wall

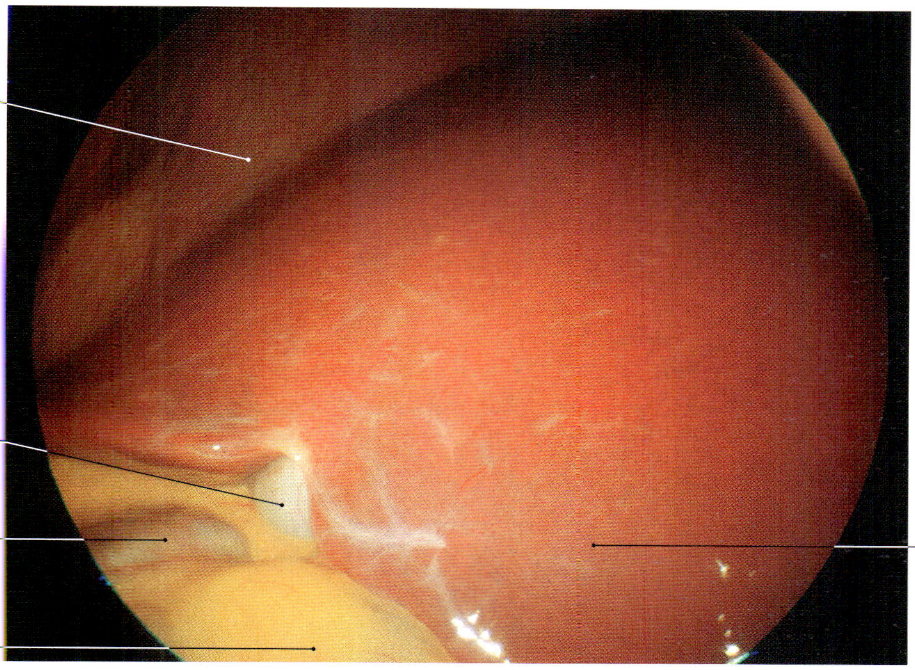

Fig. 759 Liver and gallbladder; laparoscopy; oblique inferior view from the left.

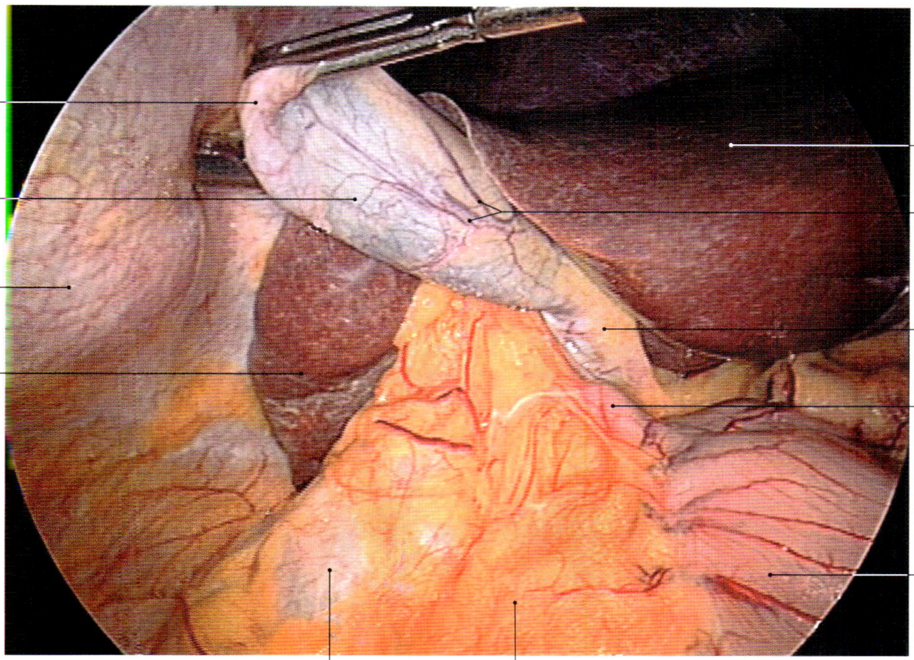

Fig. 760 Gallbladder and liver; laparoscopy; ventral view.

Gallbladder and bile duct system

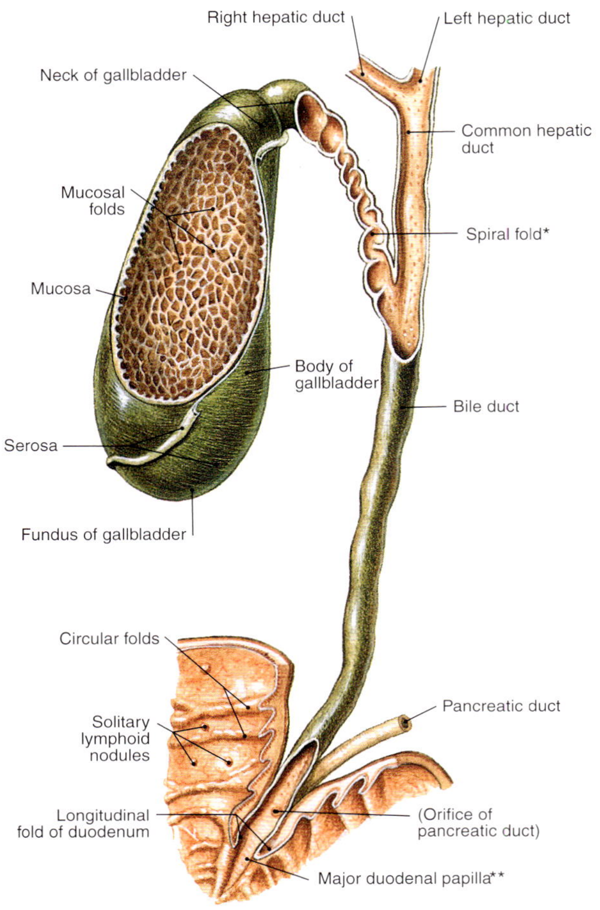

Fig. 761 Gallbladder and bile duct system; ventral view.

* Clinical term: HEISTER's valve
** Clinical term: tubercle of VATER

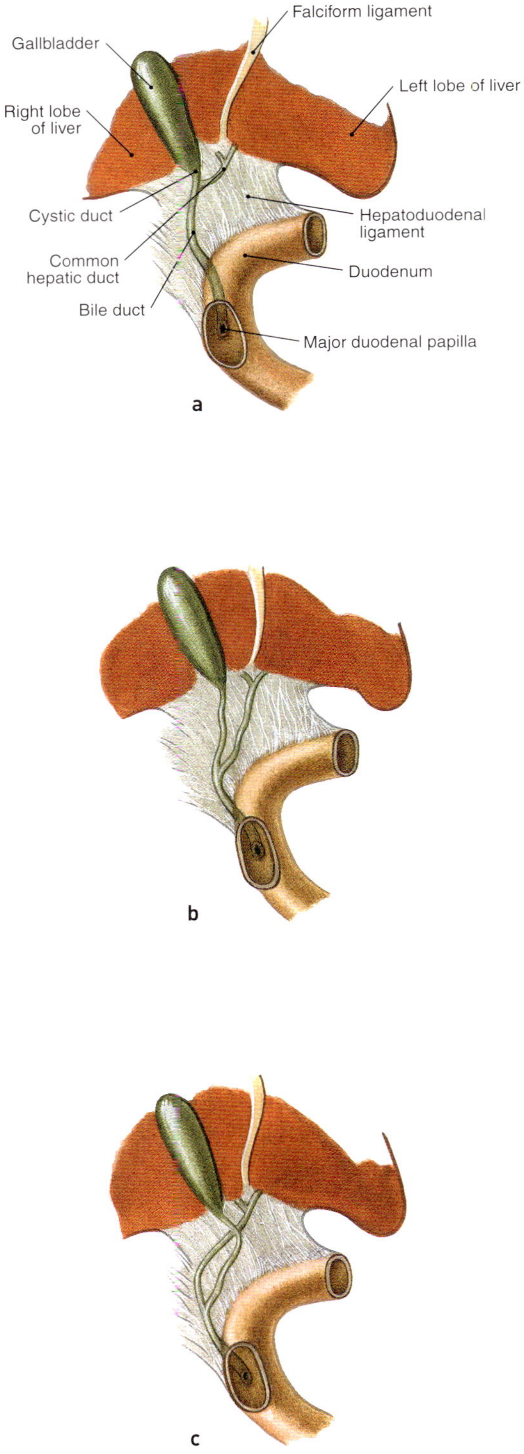

Fig. 762 a–c Variations in the bile duct system: common hepatic duct and bile duct.
a High union of the common hepatic duct and the cystic duct
b Low union of the common hepatic duct and the cystic duct
c Low union after the cystic duct crosses over the common hepatic duct

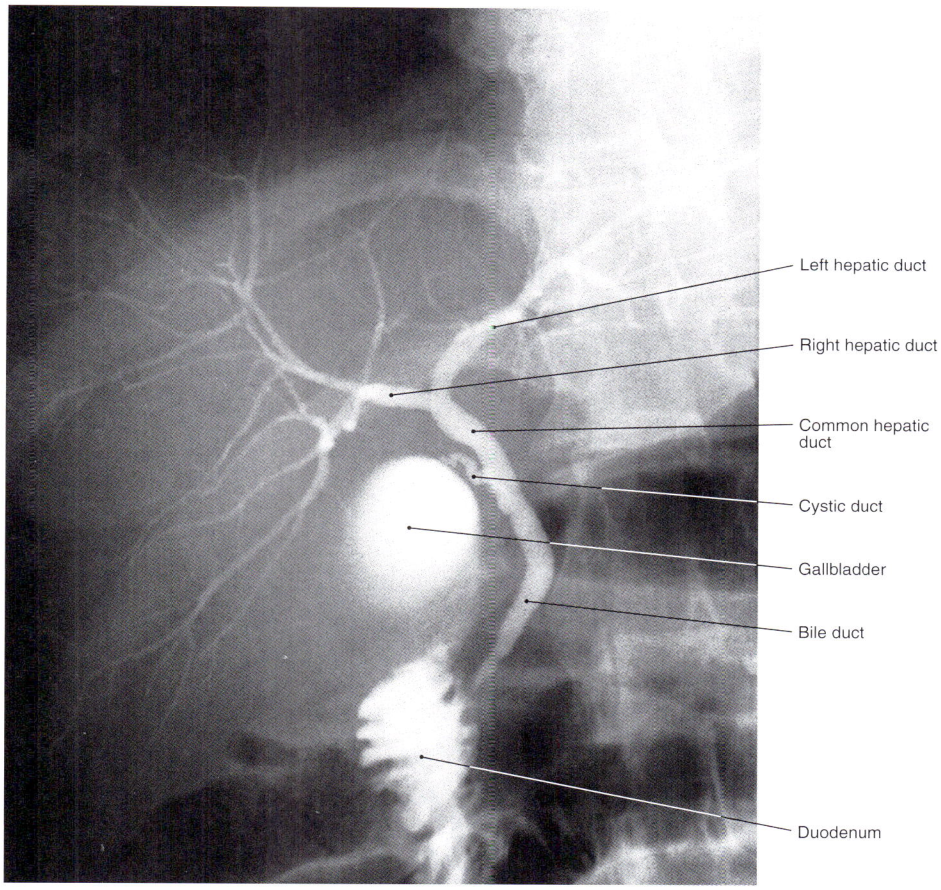

Fig. 763 Bile duct system;
AP-radiograph after administration of a contrast medium;
upright position;
ventral view.

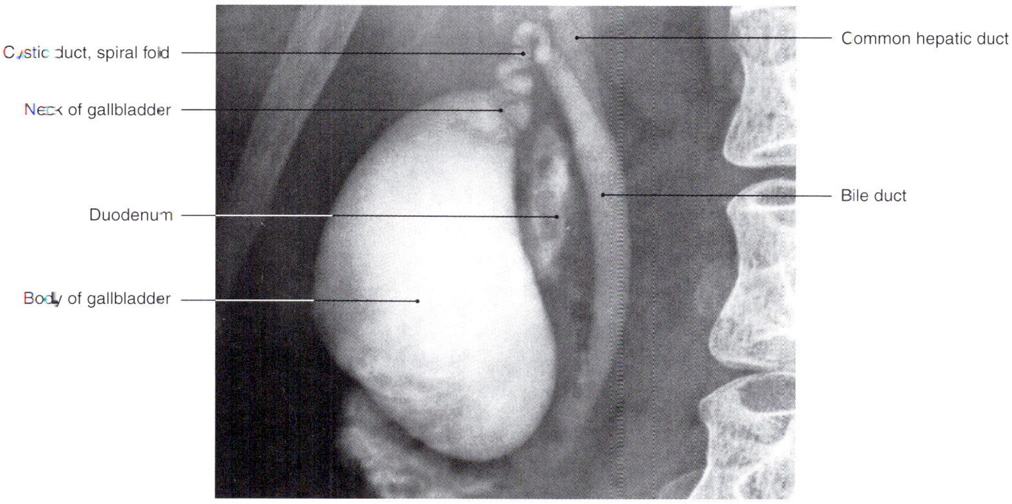

Fig. 764 Gallbladder and bile duct system;
AP-radiograph after administration of a contrast medium;
upright position;
ventral view.

Pancreas

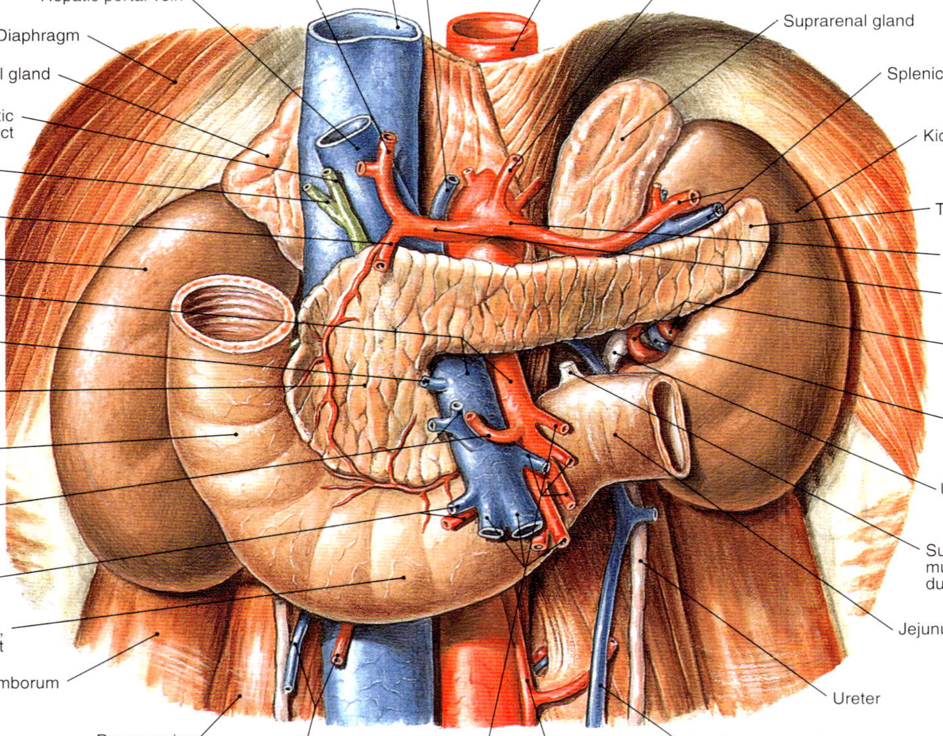

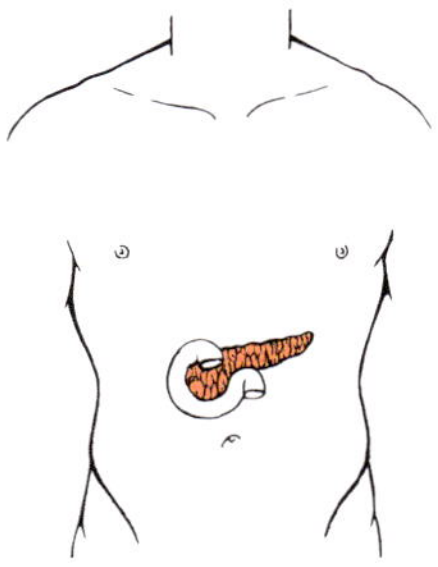

Fig. 765 Retroperitoneal organs and vessels of the upper abdomen; ventral view.

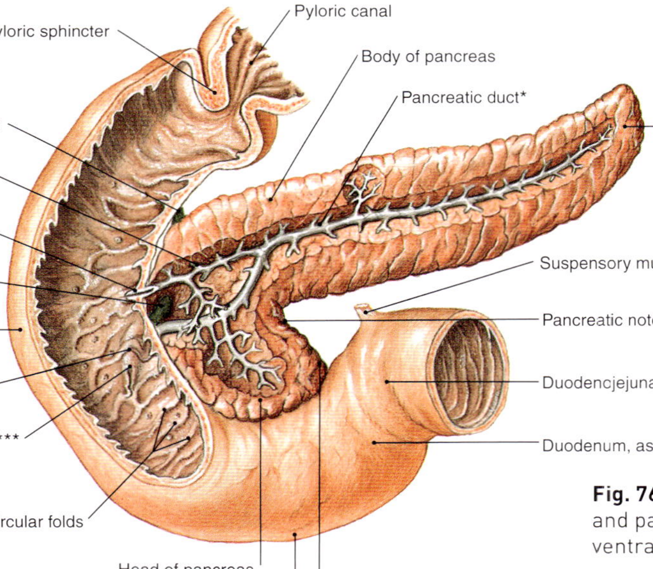

Fig. 766 Duodenum and pancreas; ventral view.

* Clinical term: duct of WIRSUNG
** Clinical term: SANTORINI's duct
*** Clinical term: tubercle of VATER
**** Clinical term: muscle of TREITZ

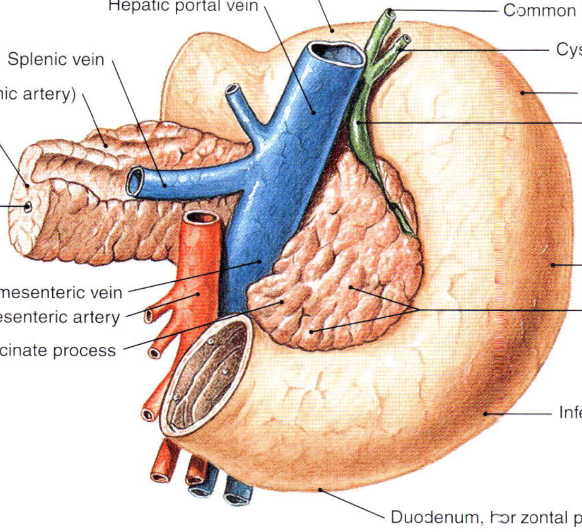

Fig. 767 Duodenum and pancreas; dorsal view.

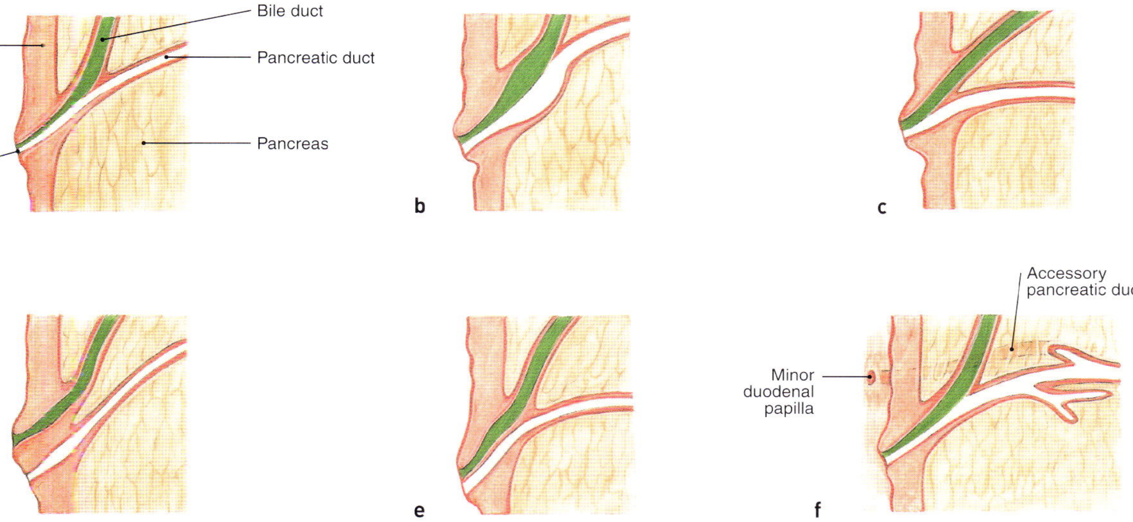

Fig. 768 a–f Variations in the opening of the bile duct and the pancreatic duct.

a Long common part
b Ampullary enlargement at the terminal part
c Short common part
d Separate opening
e Single opening with a septum dividing the common duct
f Accessory pancreatic duct

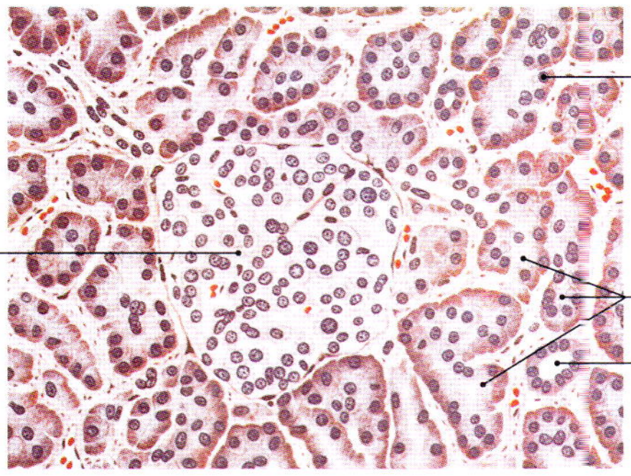

Fig. 769 Pancreas; microscopic enlargement at low magnification.

Pancreas, imaging

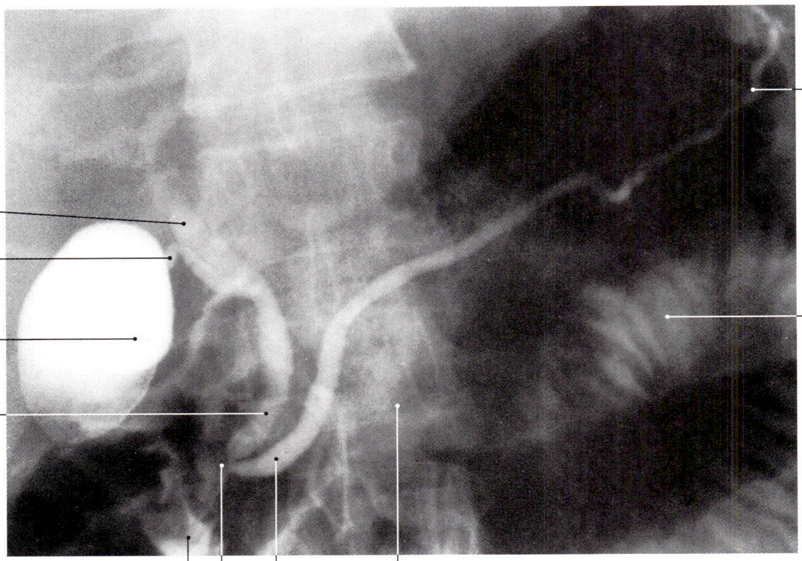

Fig. 770 Pancreatic duct; bile duct and gallbladder; AP-radiograph; supine position; after endoscopic intubation of the common excretory duct of the liver and the pancreas, as well as injection of a contrast medium; ventral view.
Clinical term: ERCP (endoscopic retrograde cholangio-pancreaticography).

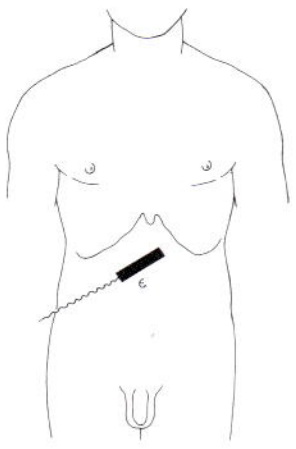

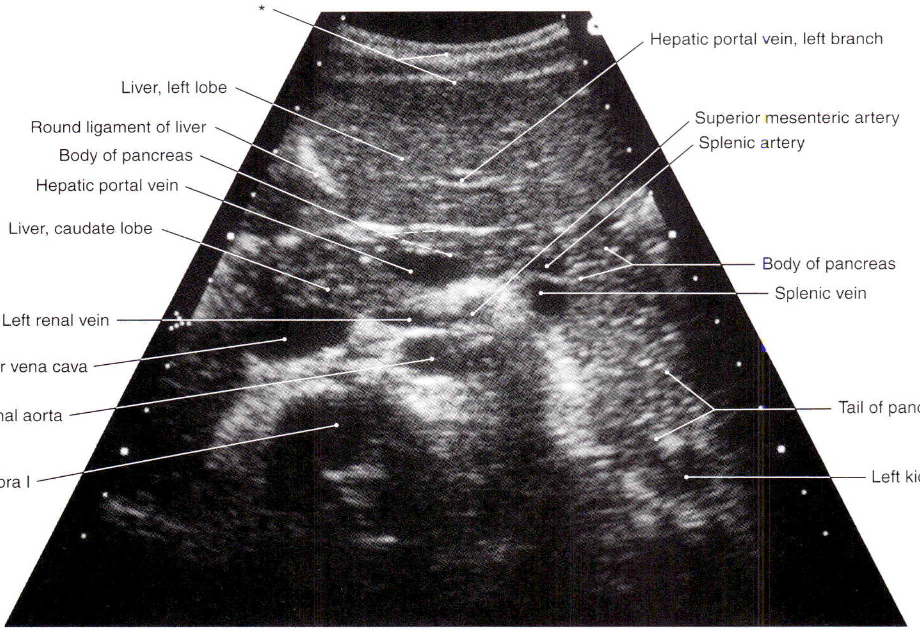

Fig. 771 Pancreas; ultrasound image showing the pancreas and adjacent large vessels in deep inspiration; oblique inferior view.

* Abdominal wall

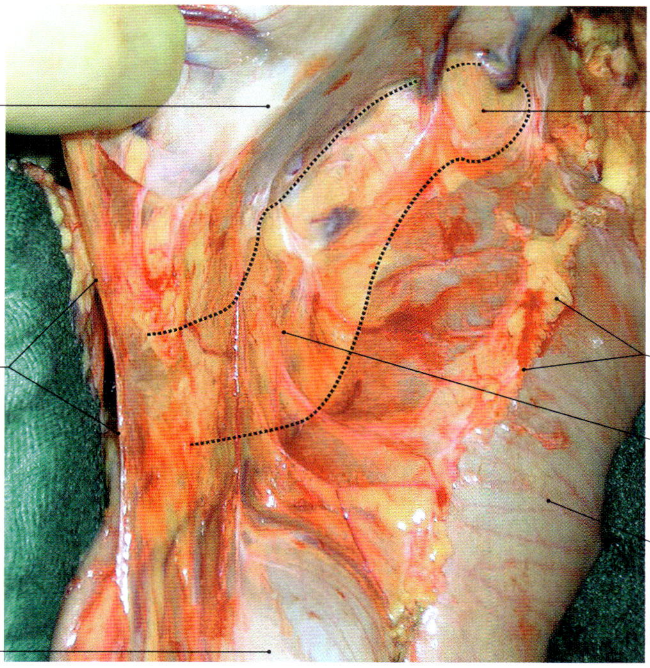

Fig. 772 Pancreas;
the gastrocolic ligament of the greater omentum has been dissected to expose the omental bursa;
photograph taken during surgery.

* Dissection line at the greater omentum

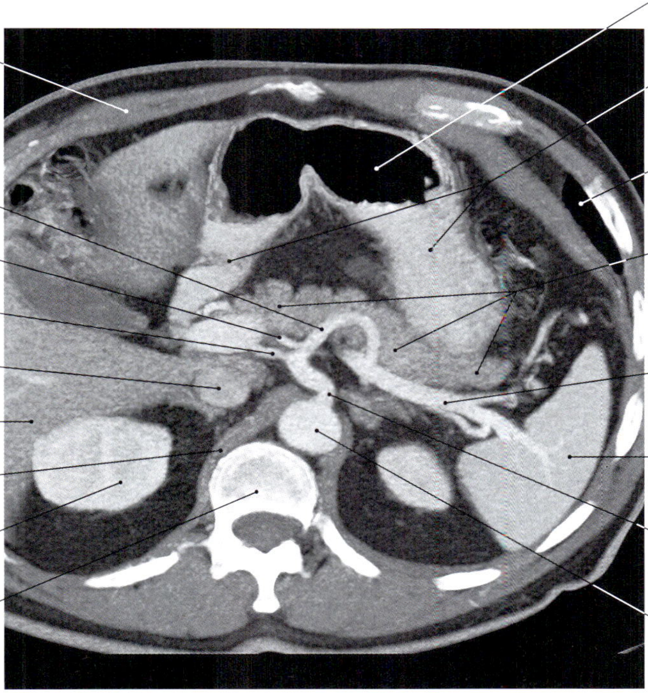

Fig. 773 Pancreas;
computed tomographic horizontal section (CT);
inferior view.
In this subject, the coeliac trunk is located remarkably low.

* Air bubble in the stomach

Spleen

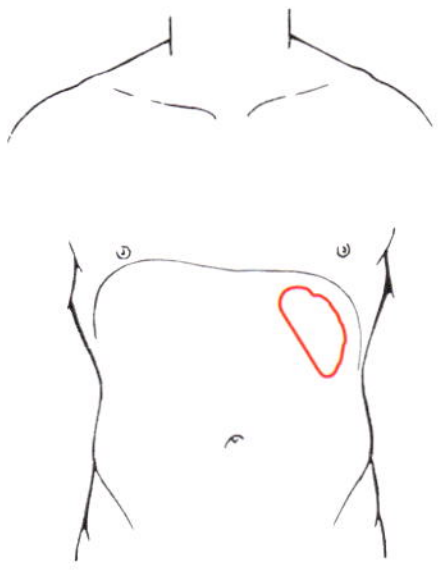

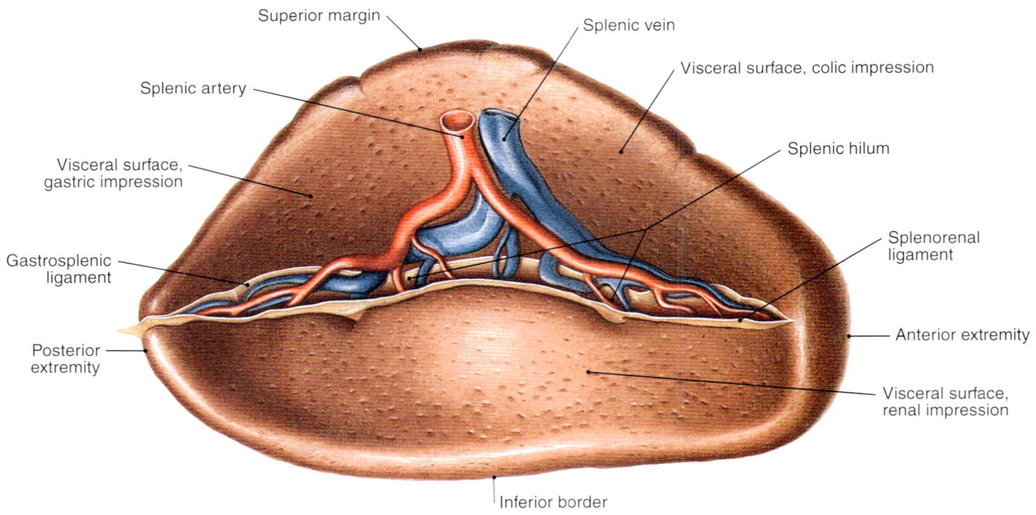

Fig. 774 Spleen; ventromedial view.

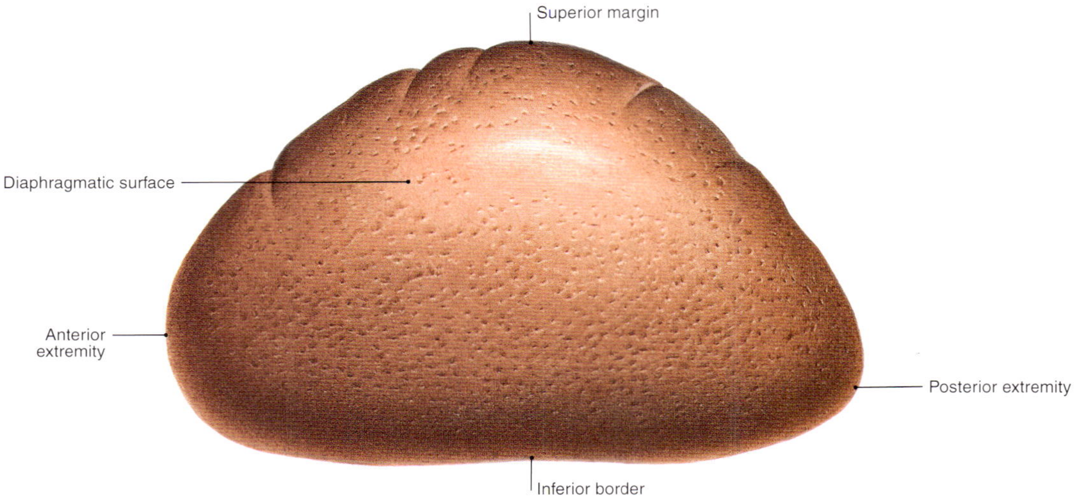

Fig. 775 Spleen; superolateral view.

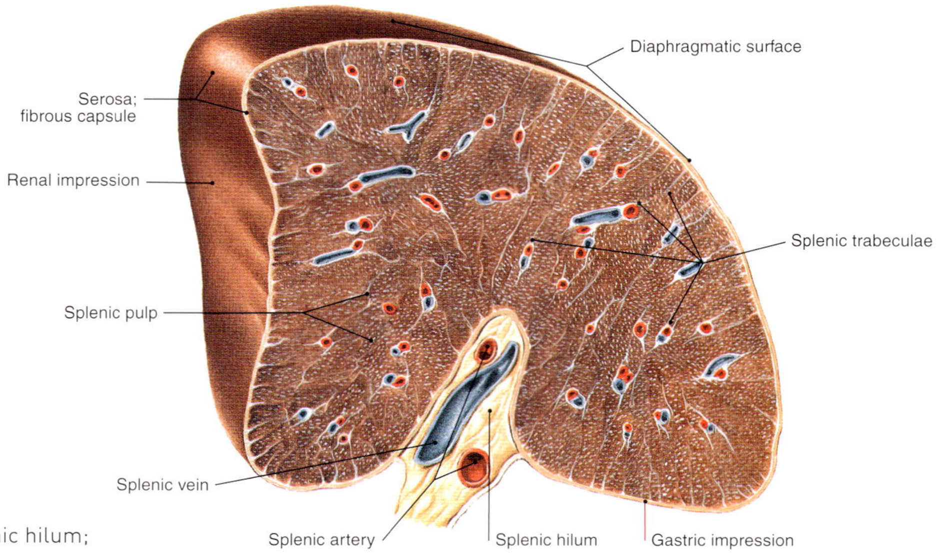

Fig. 776 Spleen; cross-section through the splenic hilum; superomedial view.

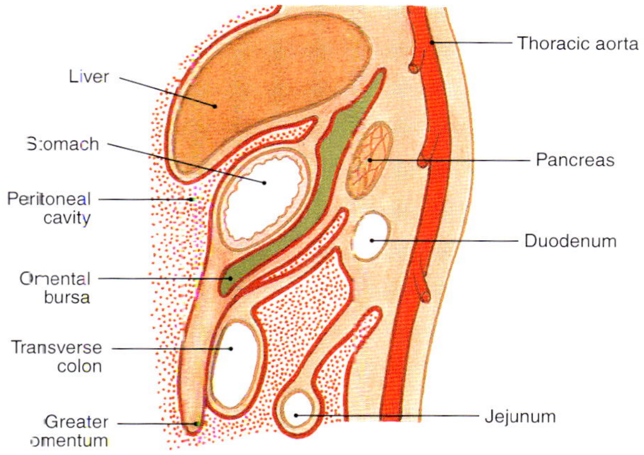

Fig. 777 Development of the peritoneal cavity and the visceral relationships; schematic median section; lateral view.

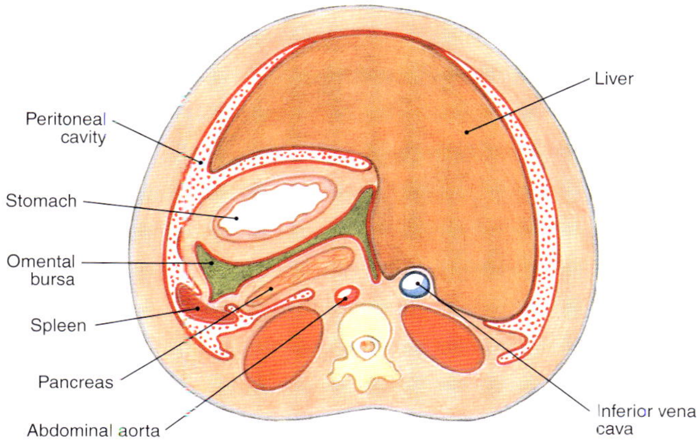

Fig. 778 Development of the peritoneal cavity; schematic horizontal section; superior view.

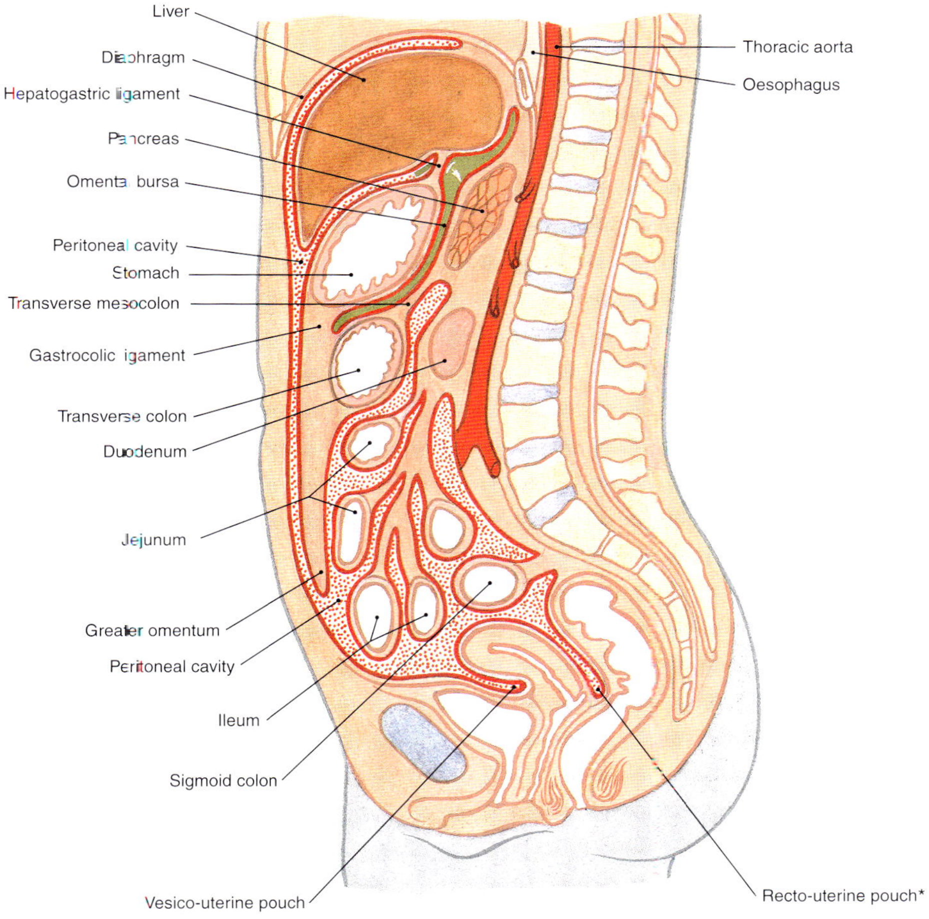

Fig. 779 Development of the peritoneal cavity and the visceral relationships of the female; final state of the peritoneal cavity with adhesion of the greater omentum to the transverse colon; schematic median section; lateral view.
The omental bursa corresponds with the peritoneal cavity via the omental foramen.

* Clinical term: pouch of DOUGLAS

Greater omentum

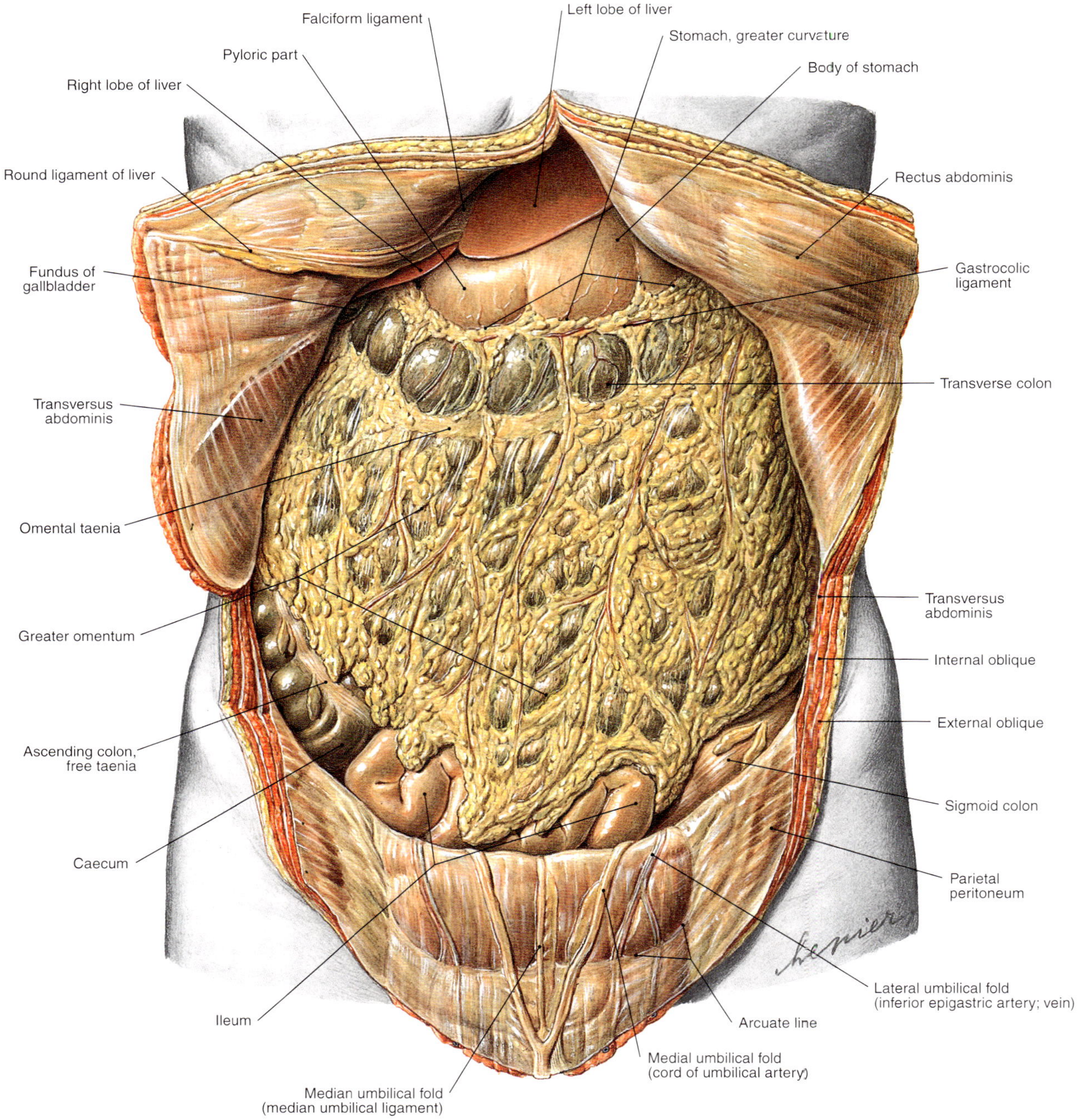

→ 578

Fig. 780 Position of the abdominal viscera and greater omentum.

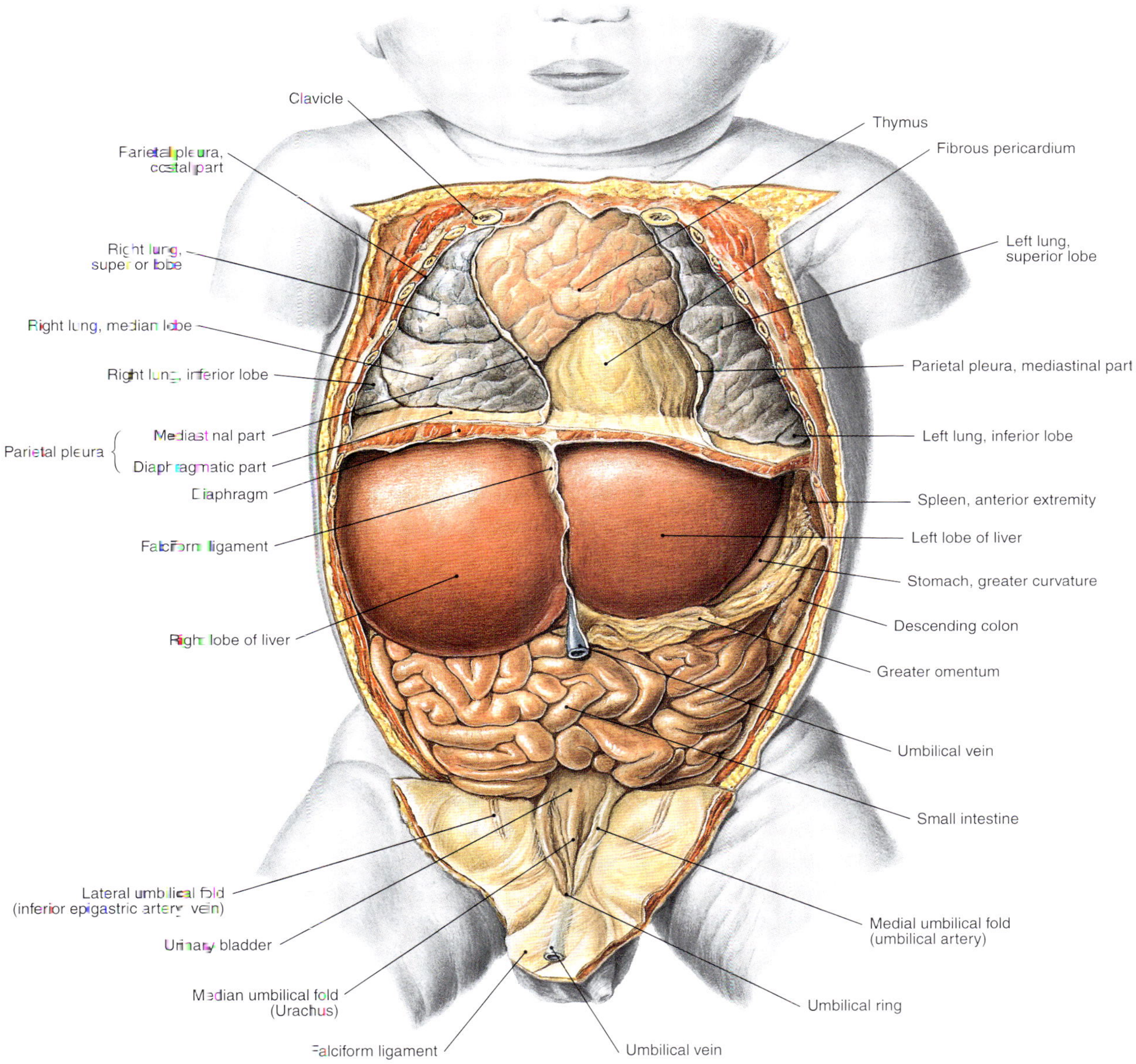

Fig. 781 Position of the abdominal viscera of the neonate

Abdominal viscera in the upper abdomen

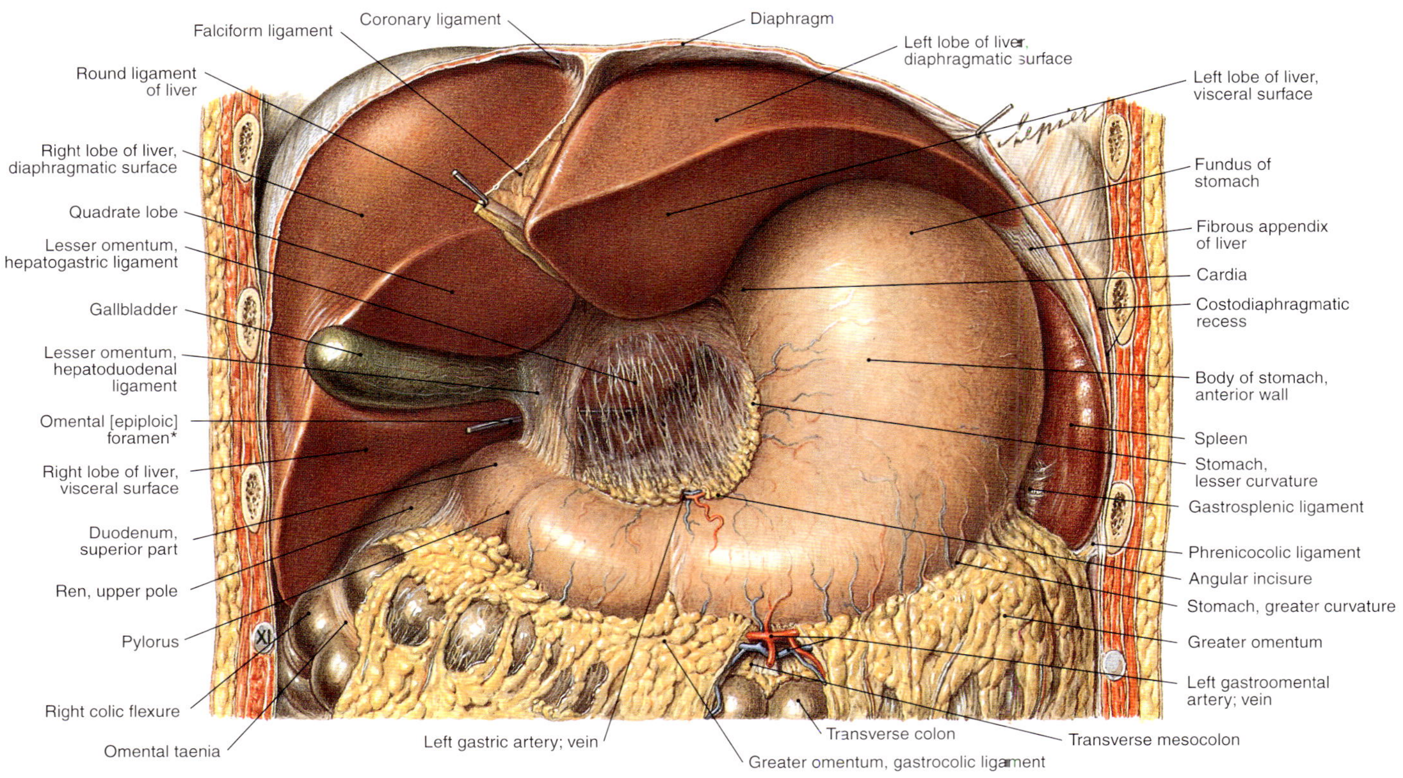

Fig. 782 Position of the abdominal viscera in the upper abdomen; ventral view.

* Also: foramen of WINSLOW

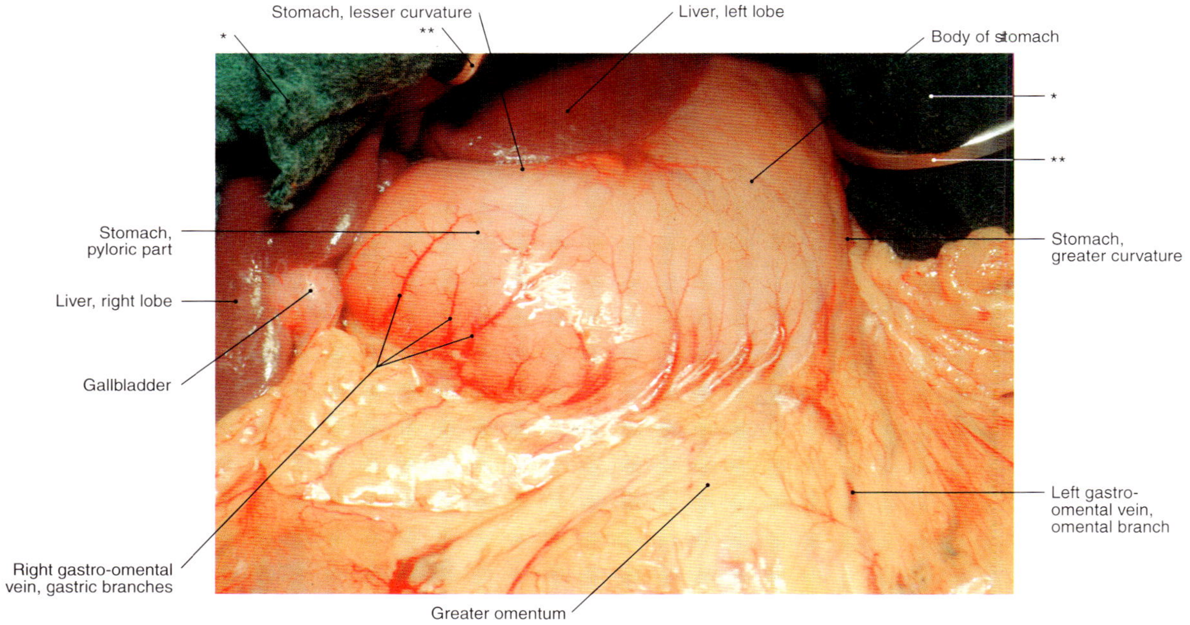

Fig. 783 Stomach and greater omentum; photograph taken during surgery; ventral view.

* Surgical drape

** Surgical retractor

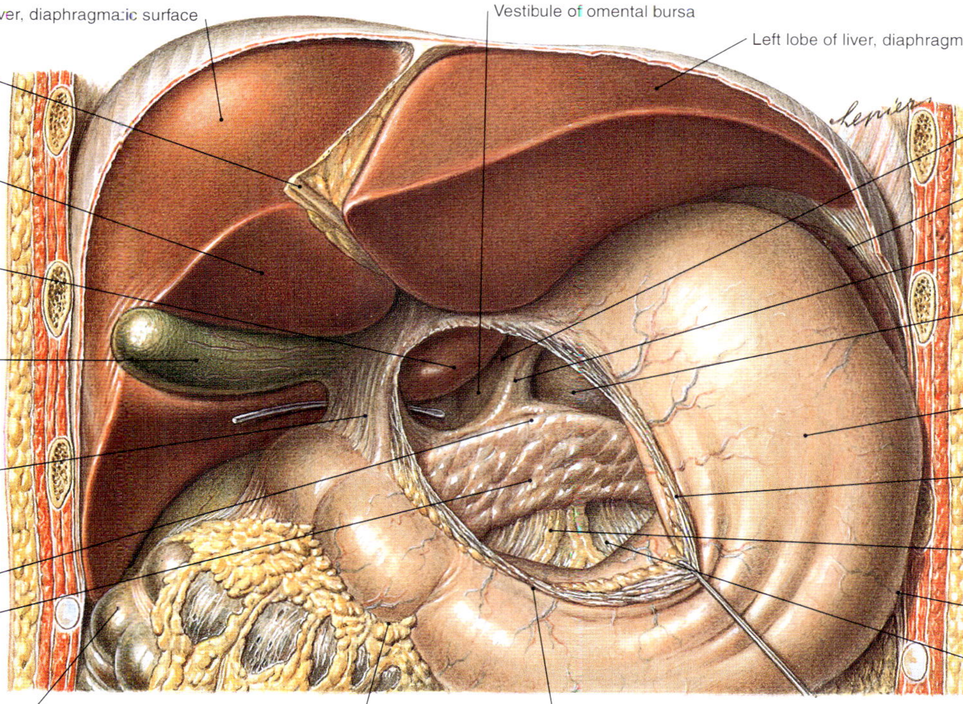

Fig. 784 Abdominal viscera in the upper abdomen;
parts of the lesser omentum have been removed to expose the omental bursa and the pancreas;
oblique view from superior.

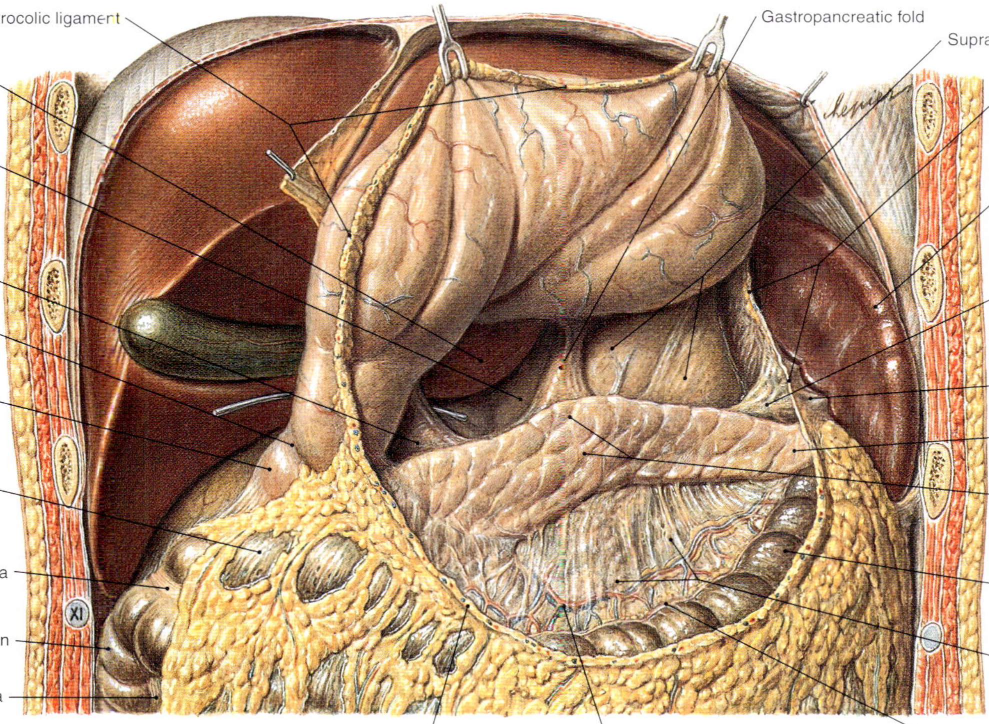

Fig. 785 Omental bursa;
after dissection of the gastrocolic ligament;
oblique view from inferior.

Abdominal viscera in the lower abdomen

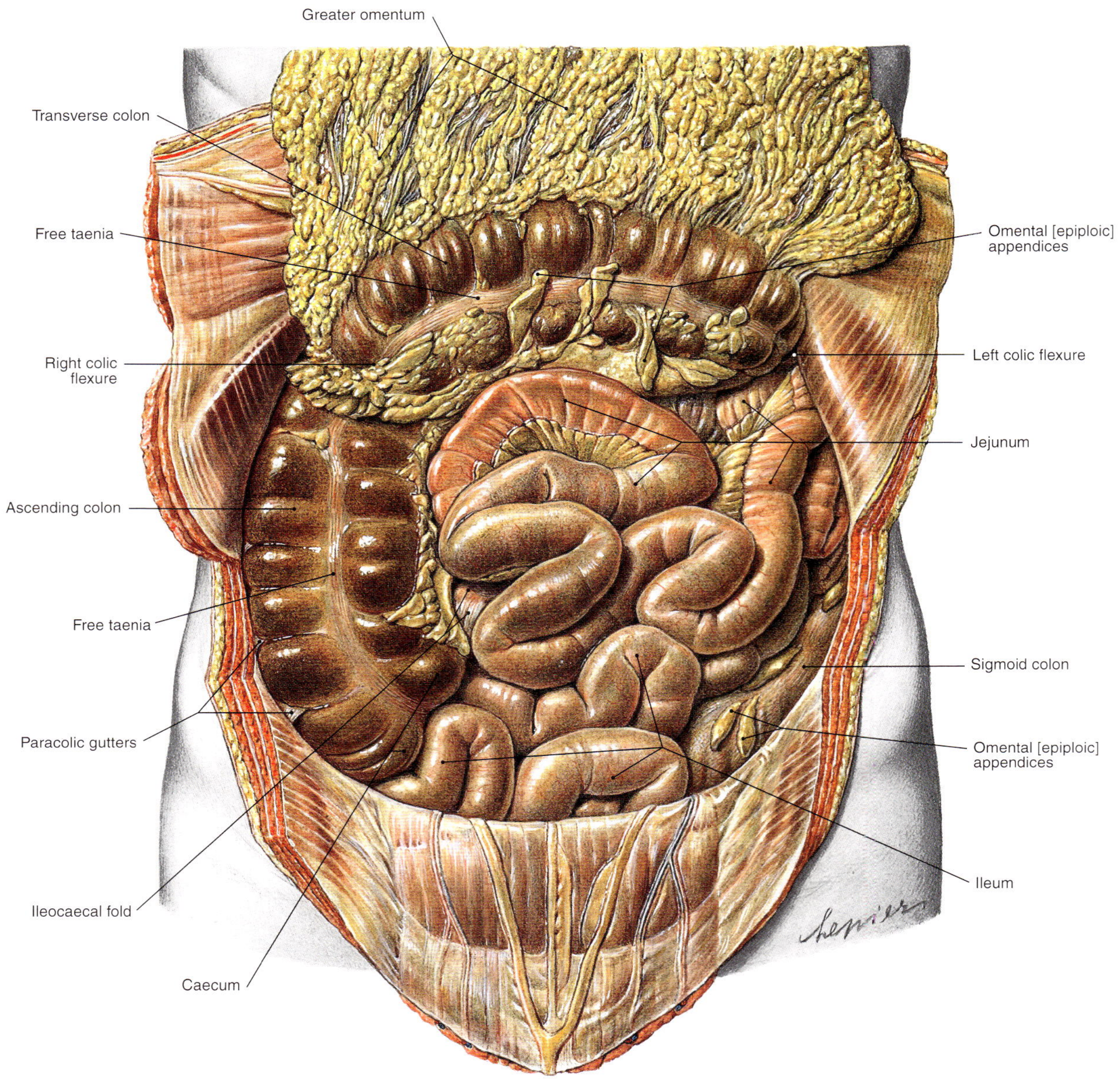

Fig. 786 Position of the abdominal viscera.

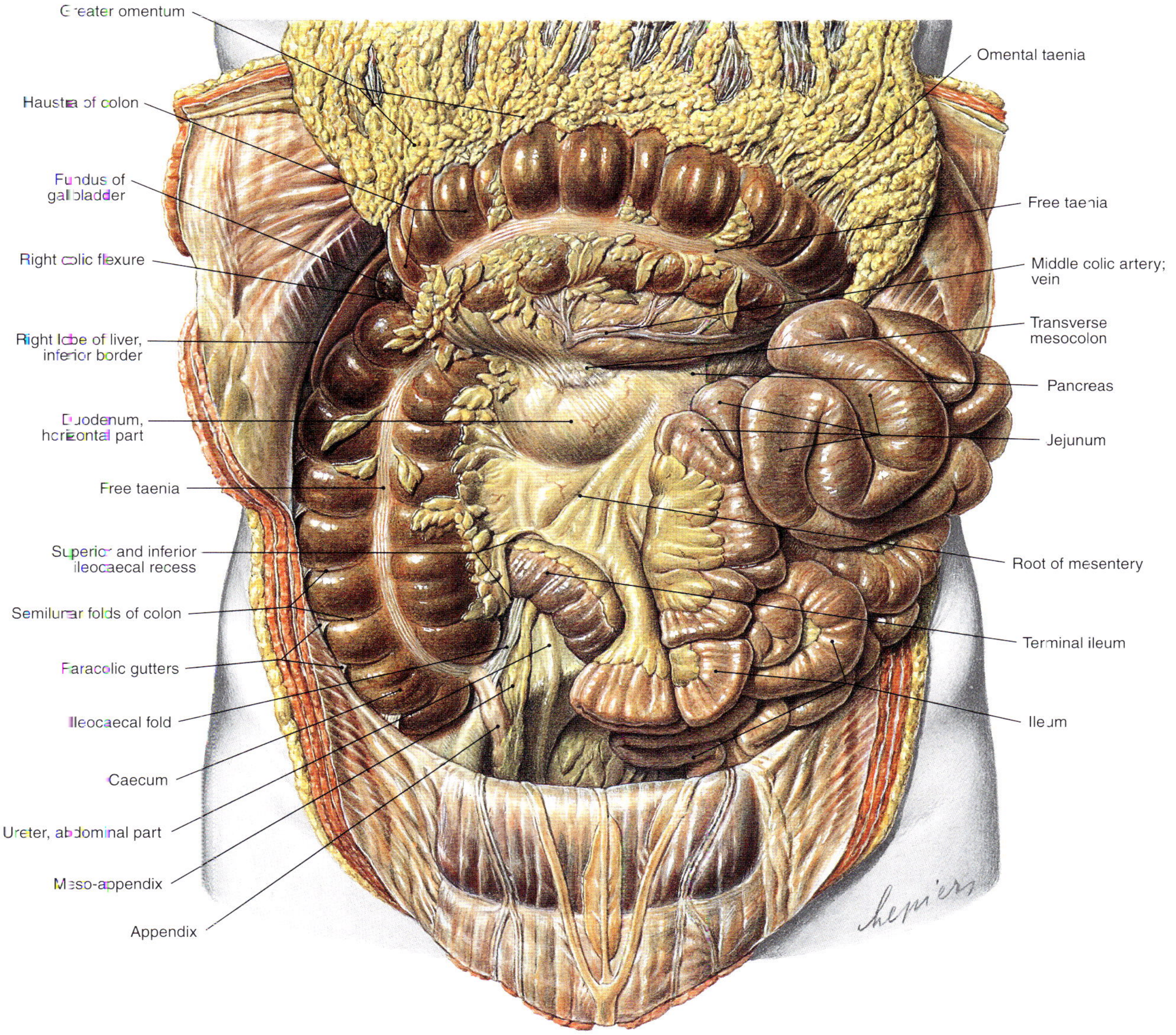

Fig. 787 Small intestine and large intestine.

Abdominal viscera in the lower abdomen

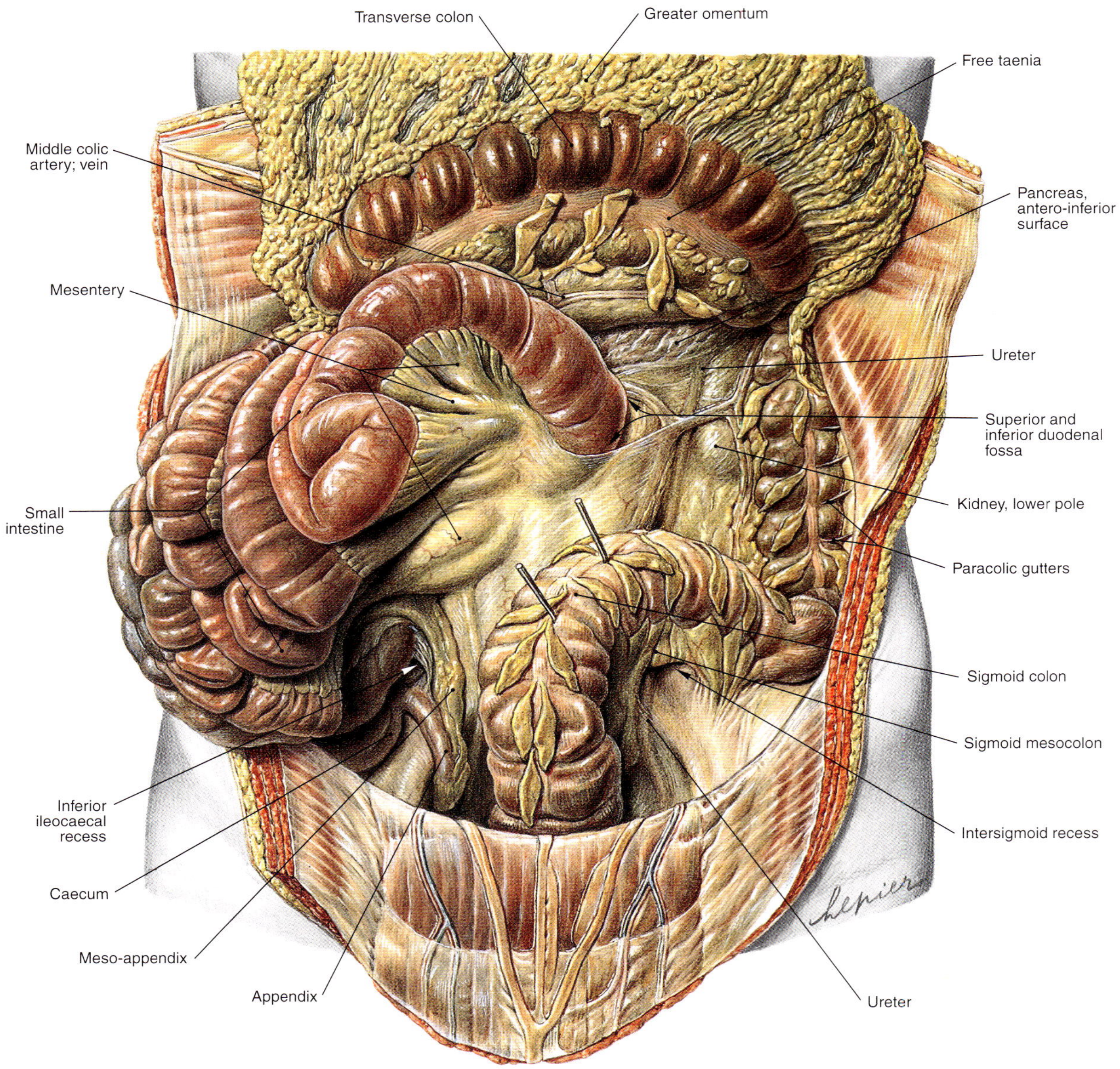

Fig. 788 Small intestine and large intestine.

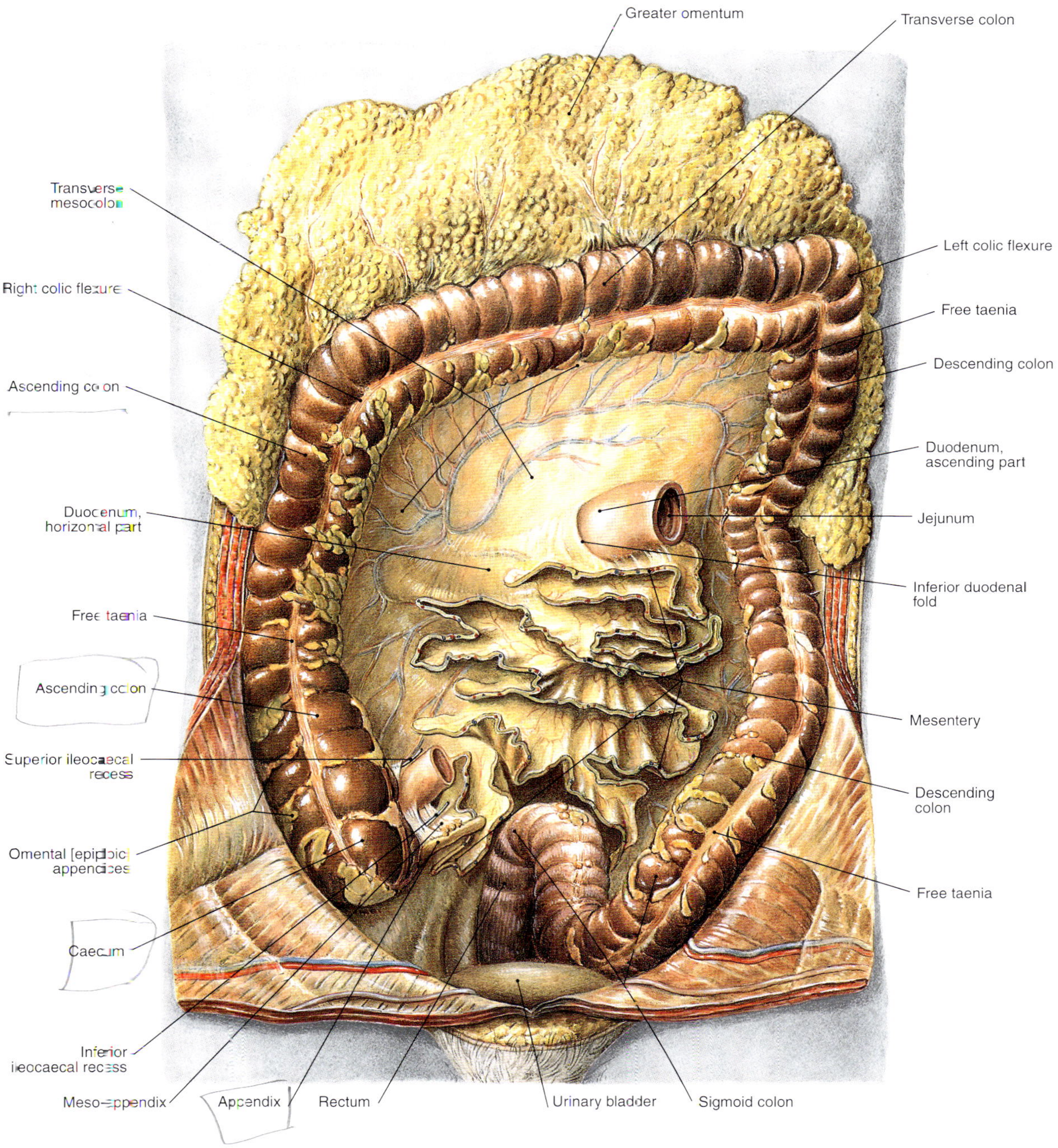

Fig. 789 Mesentery and large intestine.

Mesenteric root and retroperitoneal space

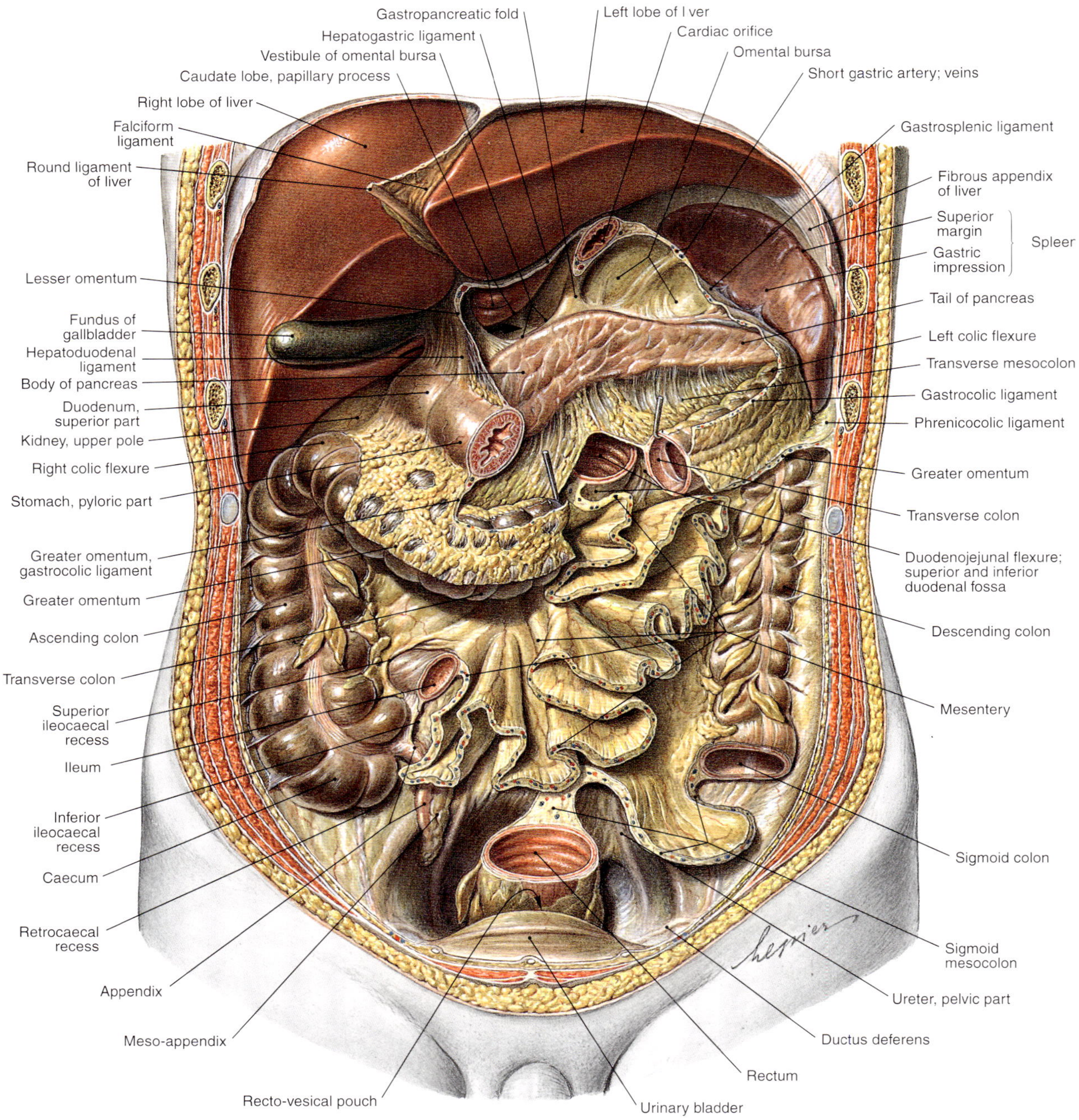

Fig. 790 Position of the abdominal viscera and the omental bursa.
An arrow indicates the omental [epiploic] foramen.

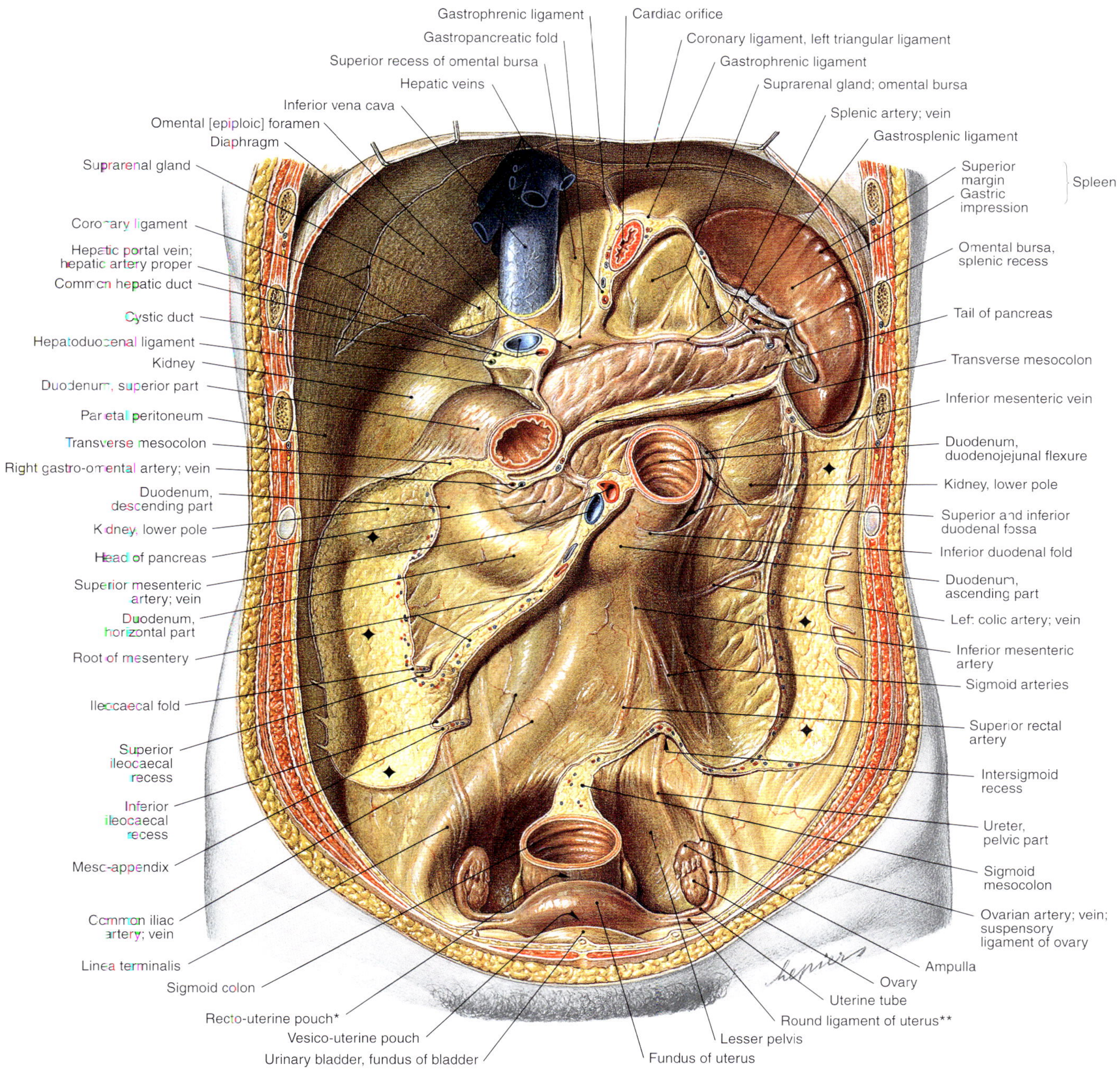

Fig. 791 Posterior wall of the peritoneal cavity and spleen of the female.
Sites of attachment of the ascending and descending colon are indicated (✦).

* Clinical term: pouch of DOUGLAS
** Clinical term: round ligament

Abdominal arteries, overview

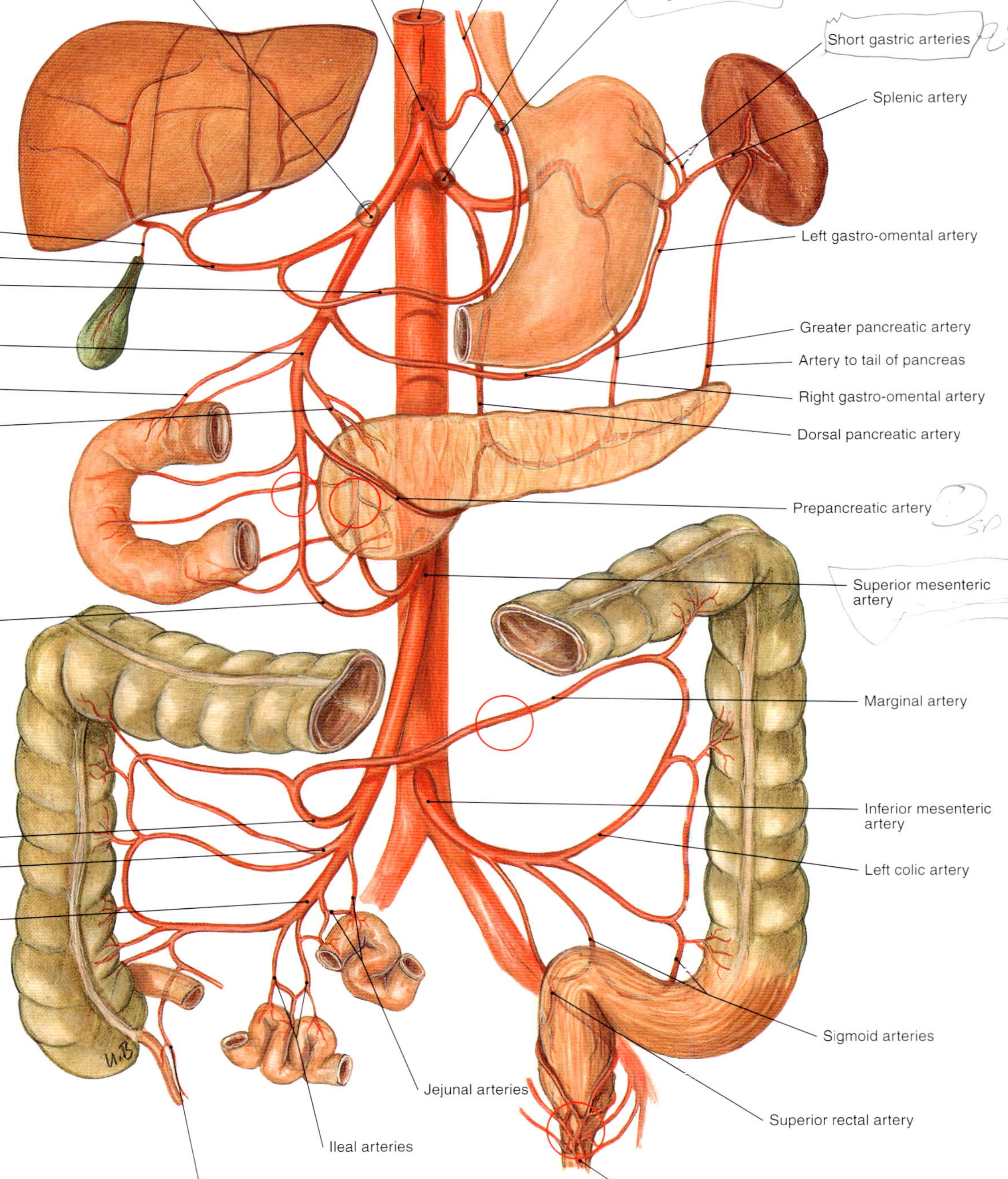

Fig. 792 Arteries of the abdominal viscera;
semi-schematic;
possible anastomoses are indicated (O).

Abdominal veins, overview

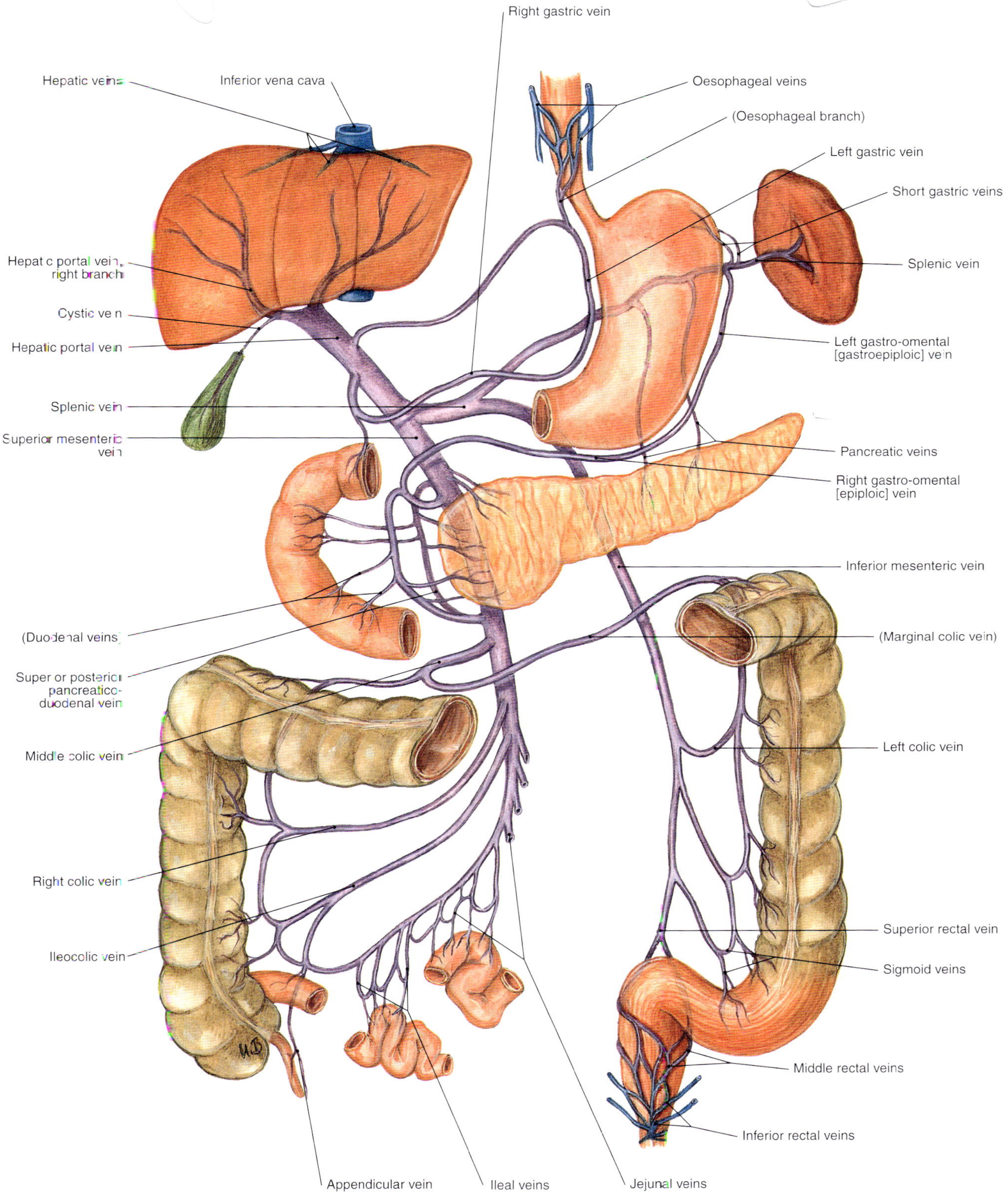

Fig. 793 Hepatic portal vein with tributaries; semi-schematic.

Coeliac trunk

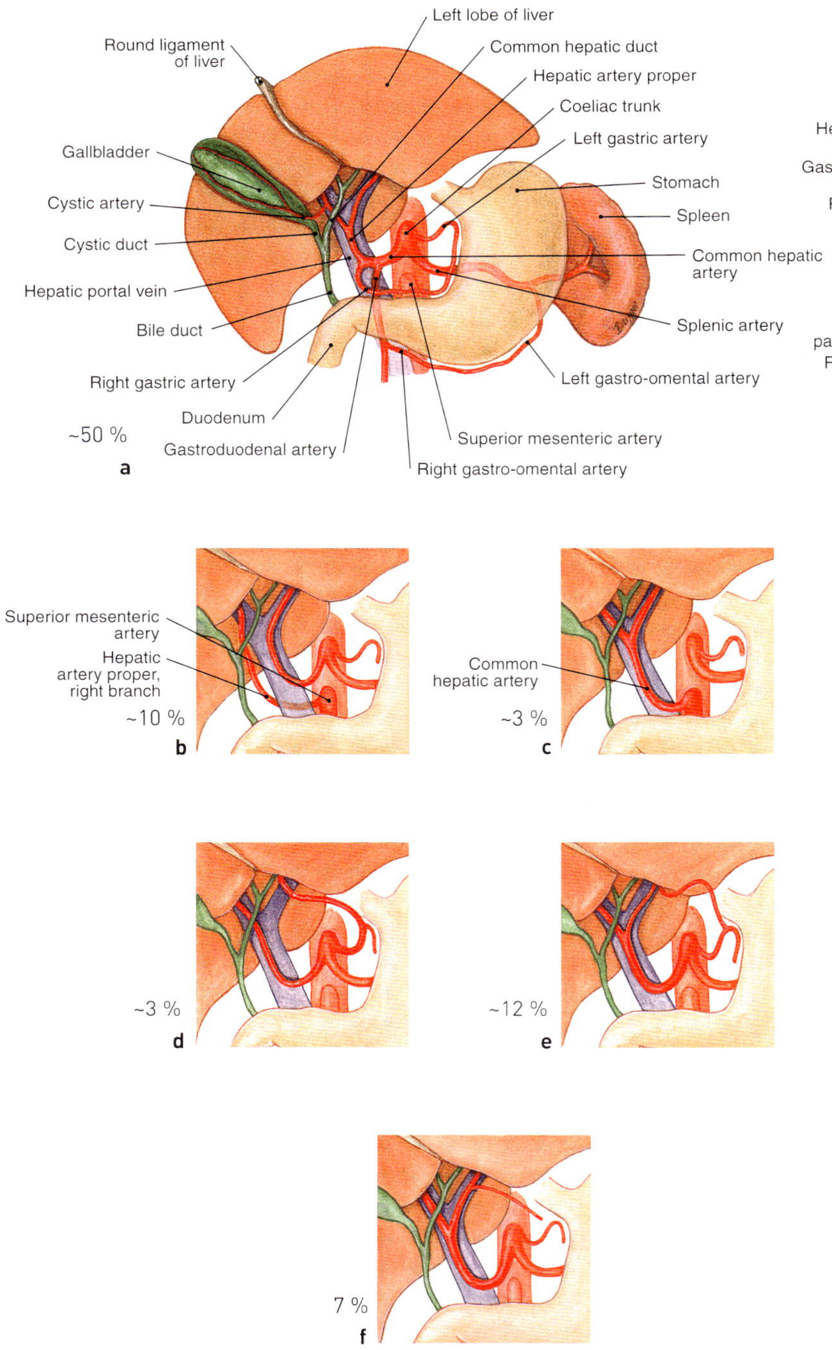

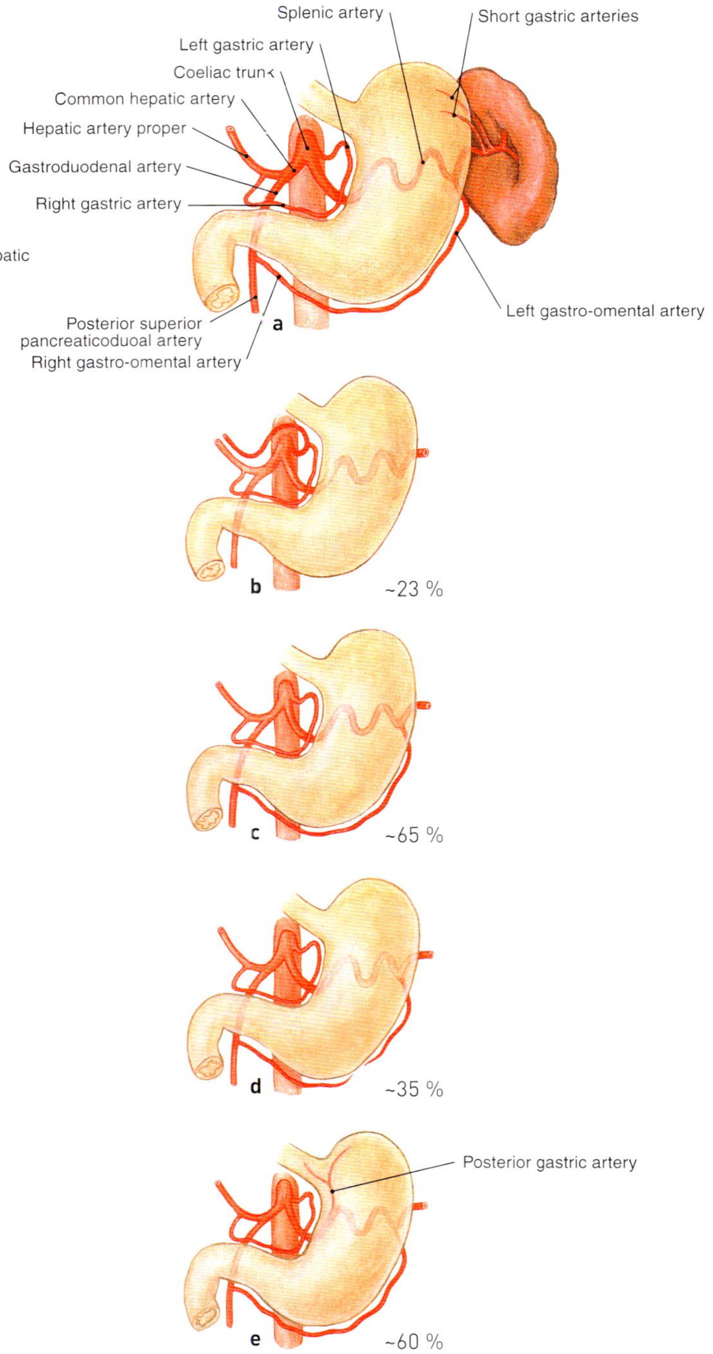

Fig. 794 a–f Variability of the arterial blood supply of the liver.

- **a** "Textbook case"
- **b** The superior mesenteric artery participates in the supply of the right lobe of the liver.
- **c** The common hepatic artery arises from the superior mesenteric artery.
- **d** The left lobe of the liver is supplied by the left gastric artery.
- **e** A branch of the left gastric artery supplies the left lobe of the liver along with the left branch of the hepatic artery proper.
- **f** An accessory branch of the hepatic artery proper supplies the lesser curvature of the stomach.

Fig. 795 a–e Variability of the arterial blood supply of the stomach.

- **a** "Textbook case", closed arterial arcade supplying both the lesser and the greater curvature
- **b** The left gastric artery participates in the supply of the left lobe of the liver.
- **c** Anastomosis between the right and left gastro-omental arteries at the greater curvature
- **d** Absence of an anastomosis between the right and left gastro-omental arteries at the greater curvature
- **e** An accessory posterior gastric artery arising from the splenic artery supplies the posterior wall of the stomach.

Arteries of the upper abdomen, radiography

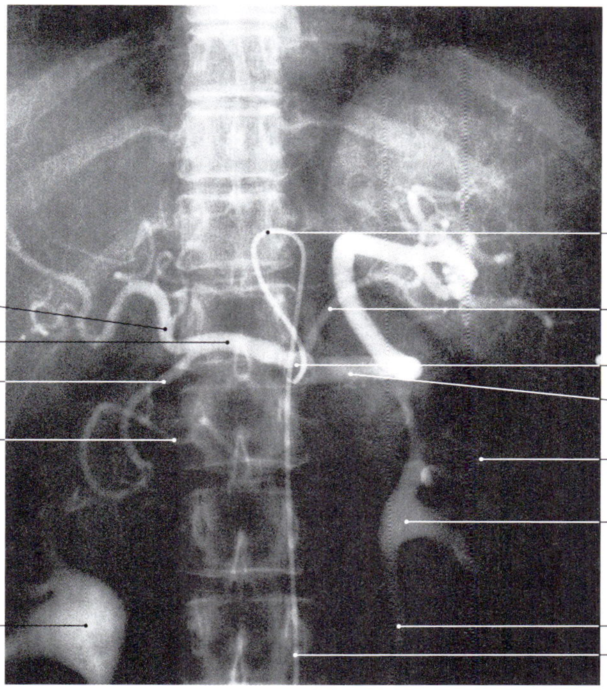

Fig. 796 Arteries of the stomach; the spleen and the liver; AP-radiograph after selective injection of a contrast medium into the coeliac trunk (coeliacography) with concomitant visualization of the renal pelvis due to the renal excretion of the medium; ventral view.

* Catheter loop in the aorta
** Catheter in the aorta

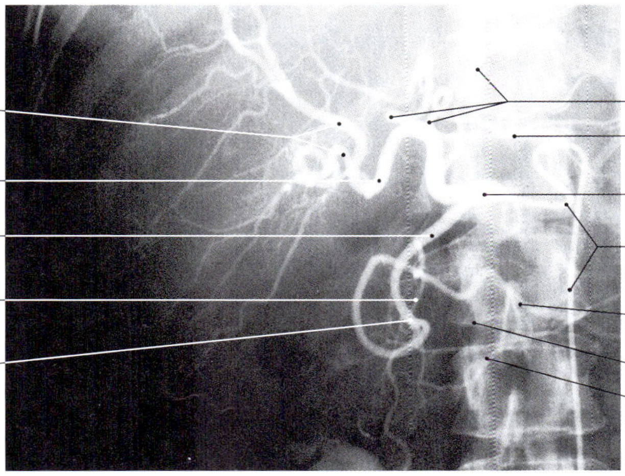

Fig. 797 Common hepatic artery;
AP-radiograph after selective injection of a contrast medium into the common hepatic artery;
ventral view.

* Branches to the left lobe of the liver replacing a single left branch of the hepatic artery proper
** An accessory branch of the hepatic artery to the lesser curvature of the stomach
*** Catheter in the aorta

Vessels of the upper abdomen

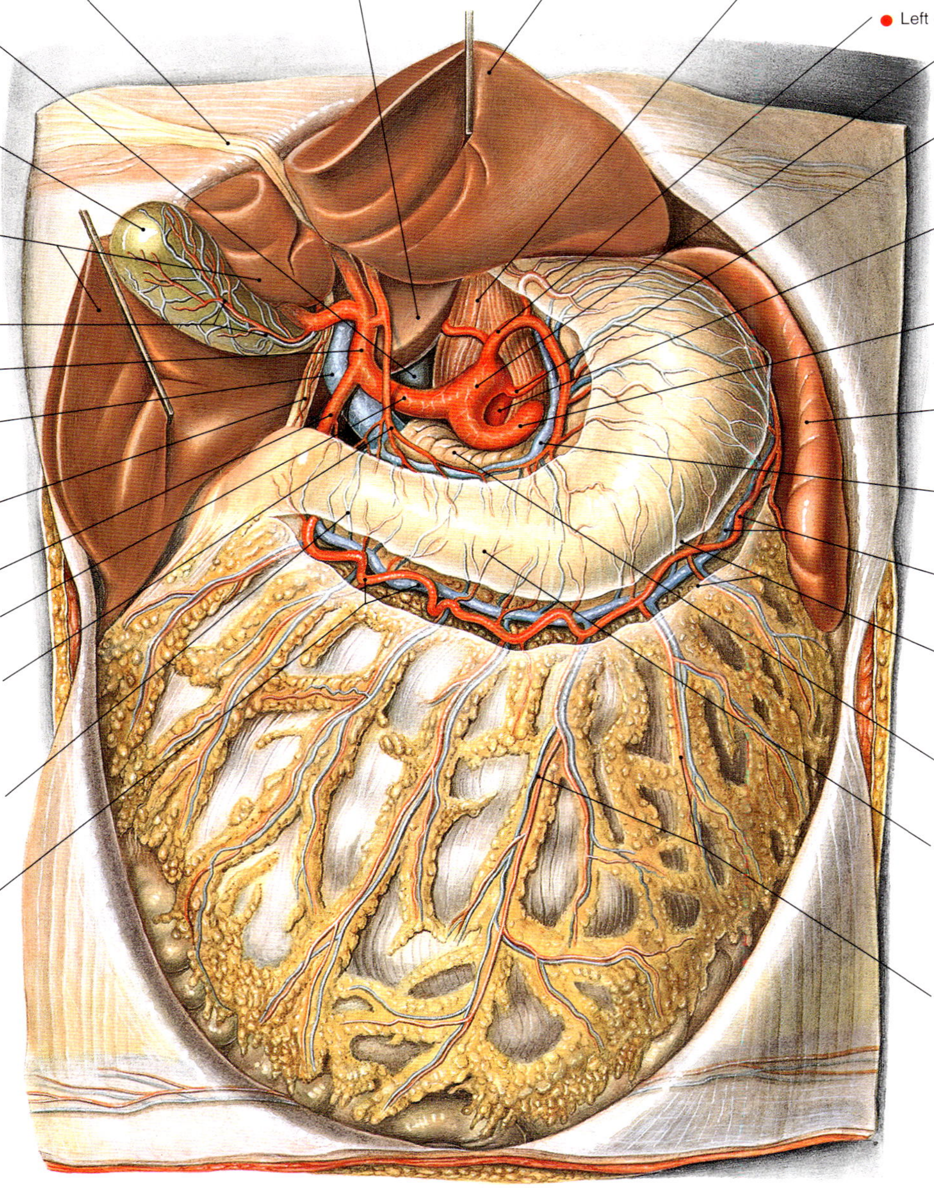

Fig. 798 Vessels of the upper abdomen.

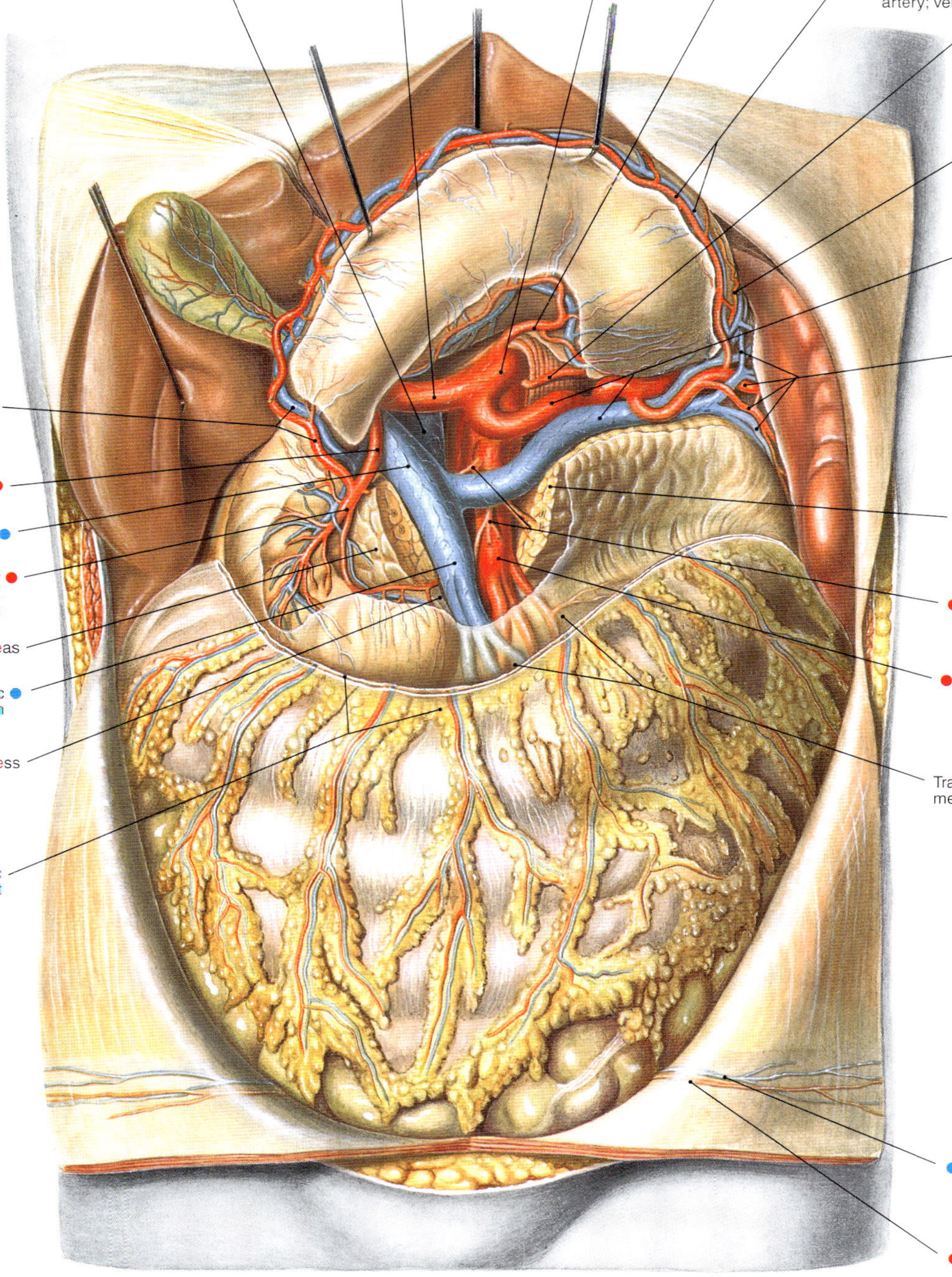

Fig. 799 Vessels of the upper abdomen.

Superior mesenteric artery

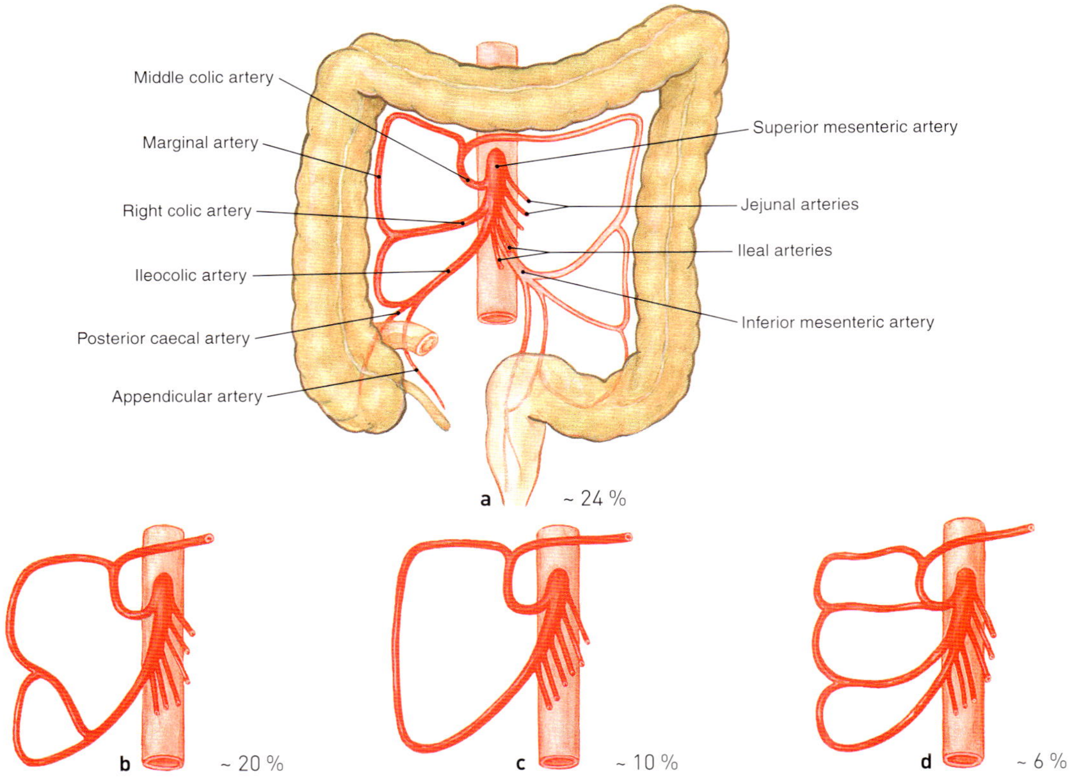

Fig. 800 a–d Variability of the branches of the superior mesenteric artery supplying the large intestine.

a „Textbook case", the ascending and the transverse colon are supplied by three branches.

b The ileocolic artery and the right colic artery form a common trunk.

c Only two branches arise from the mesenteric artery while the right colic artery is absent.

d Duplication of the right colic artery.

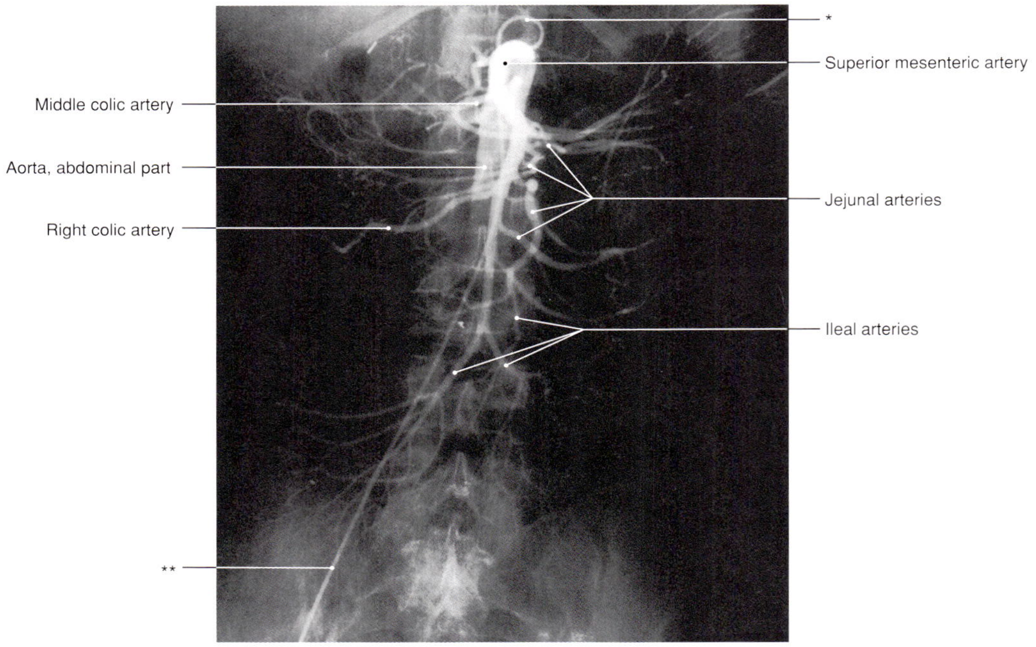

Fig. 801 Superior mesenteric artery; AP-radiograph after injection of a contrast medium into the origin of the superior mesenteric artery; ventral view.

* Catheter in the aorta

** Catheter in the common iliac artery

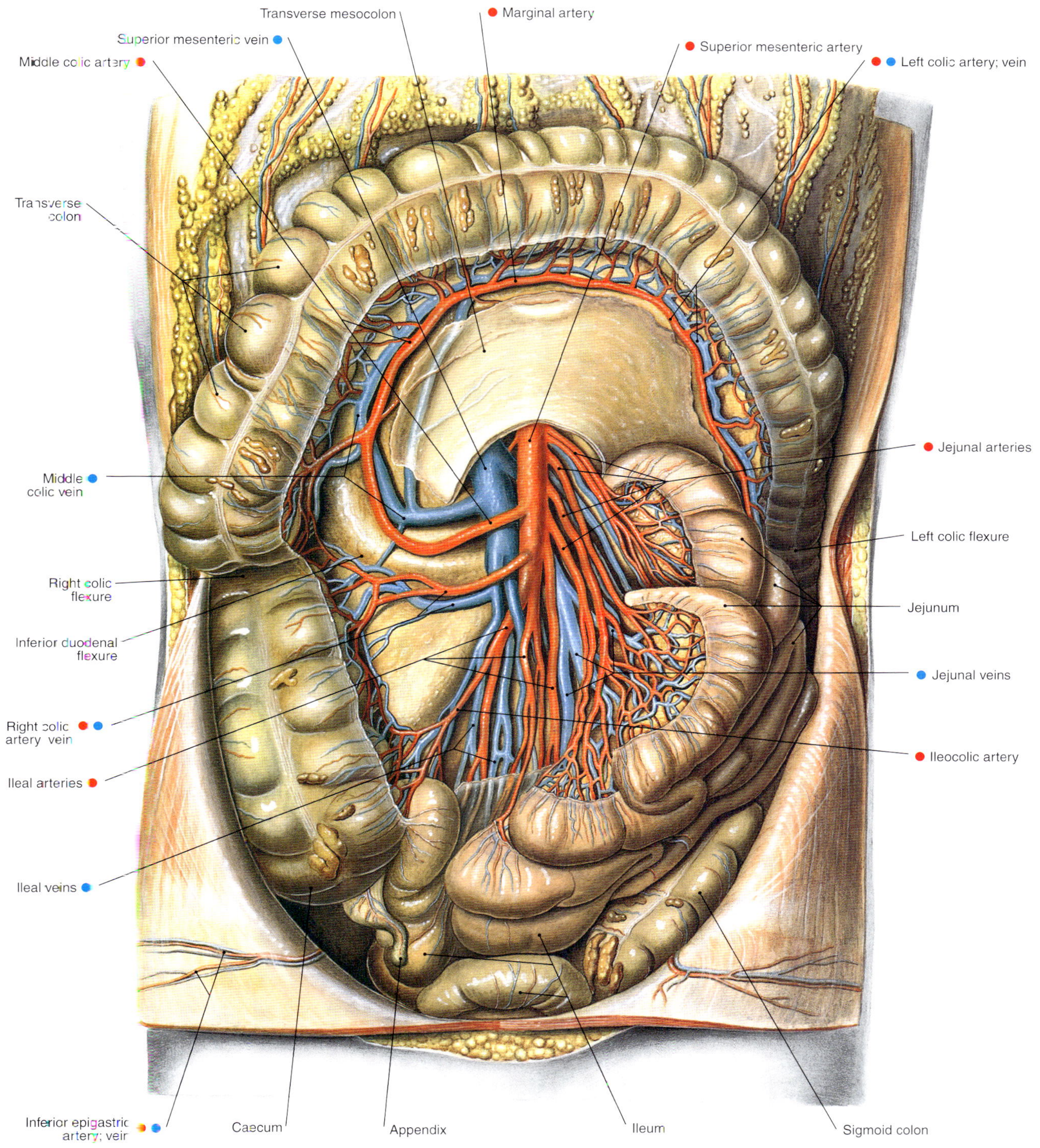

Fig. 802 Superior mesenteric artery and vein.
The arteries supplying the small intestine form a series of arcades.

Inferior mesenteric artery

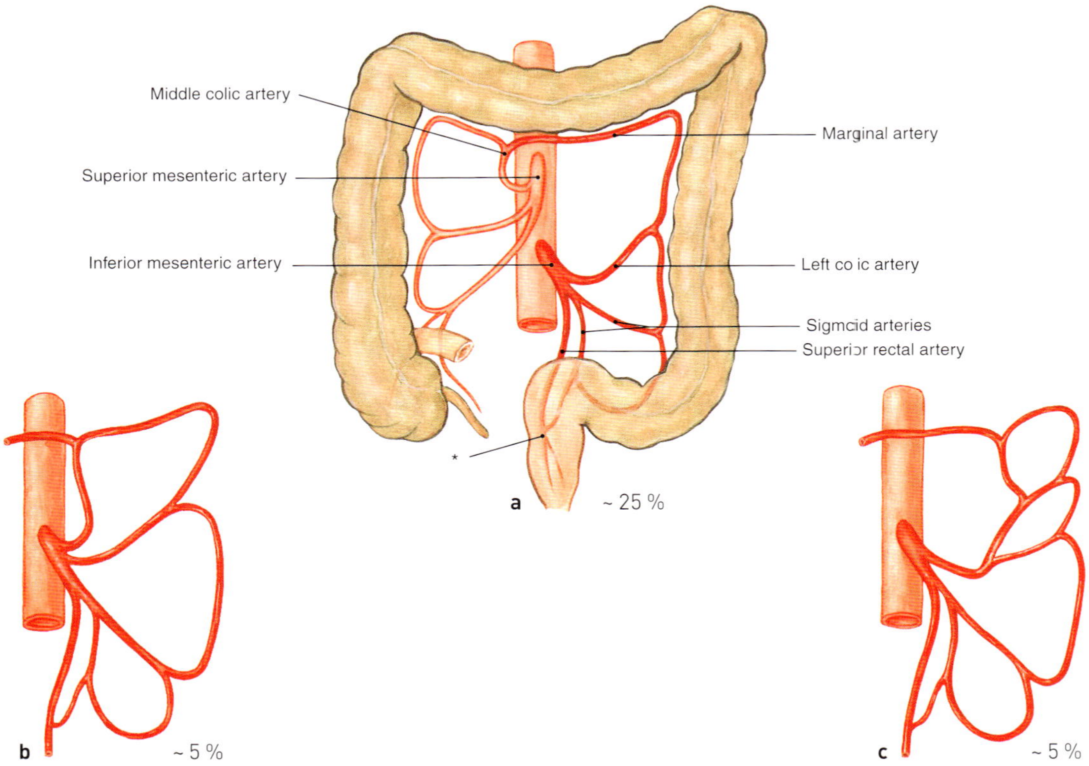

Fig. 803 a–c Variations in the branches of the inferior mesenteric artery.

a The inferior mesenteric artery divides into three parts supplying the descending and sigmoid colon, as well as the rectum.

b An accessory middle colic artery arises from the inferior mesenteric artery.

c An accessory middle colic artery arises from the left colic artery.

* Clinical term: SUDECK's point

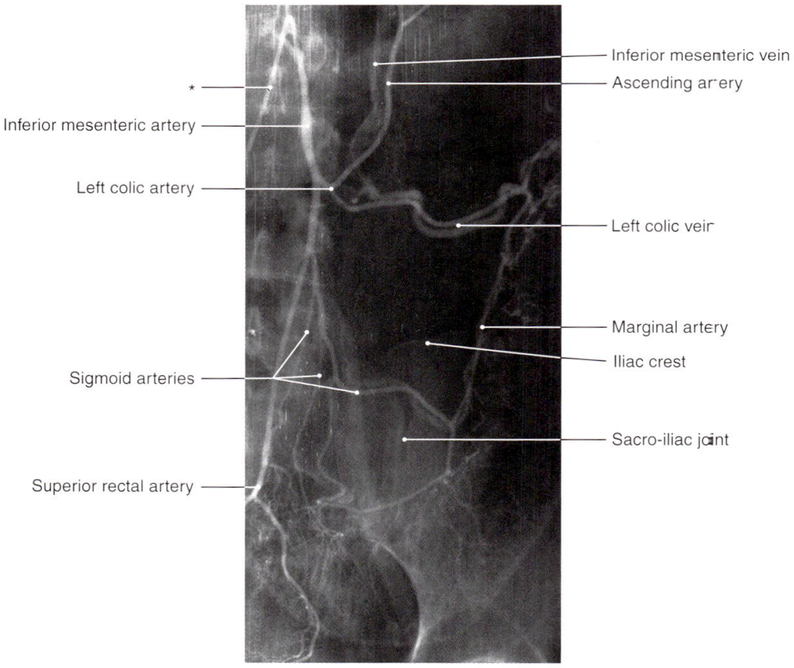

Fig. 804 Inferior mesenteric artery;
AP-radiograph after selective injection of a contrast medium into the origin of the inferior mesenteric artery;
ventral view.

* Catheter in the aorta

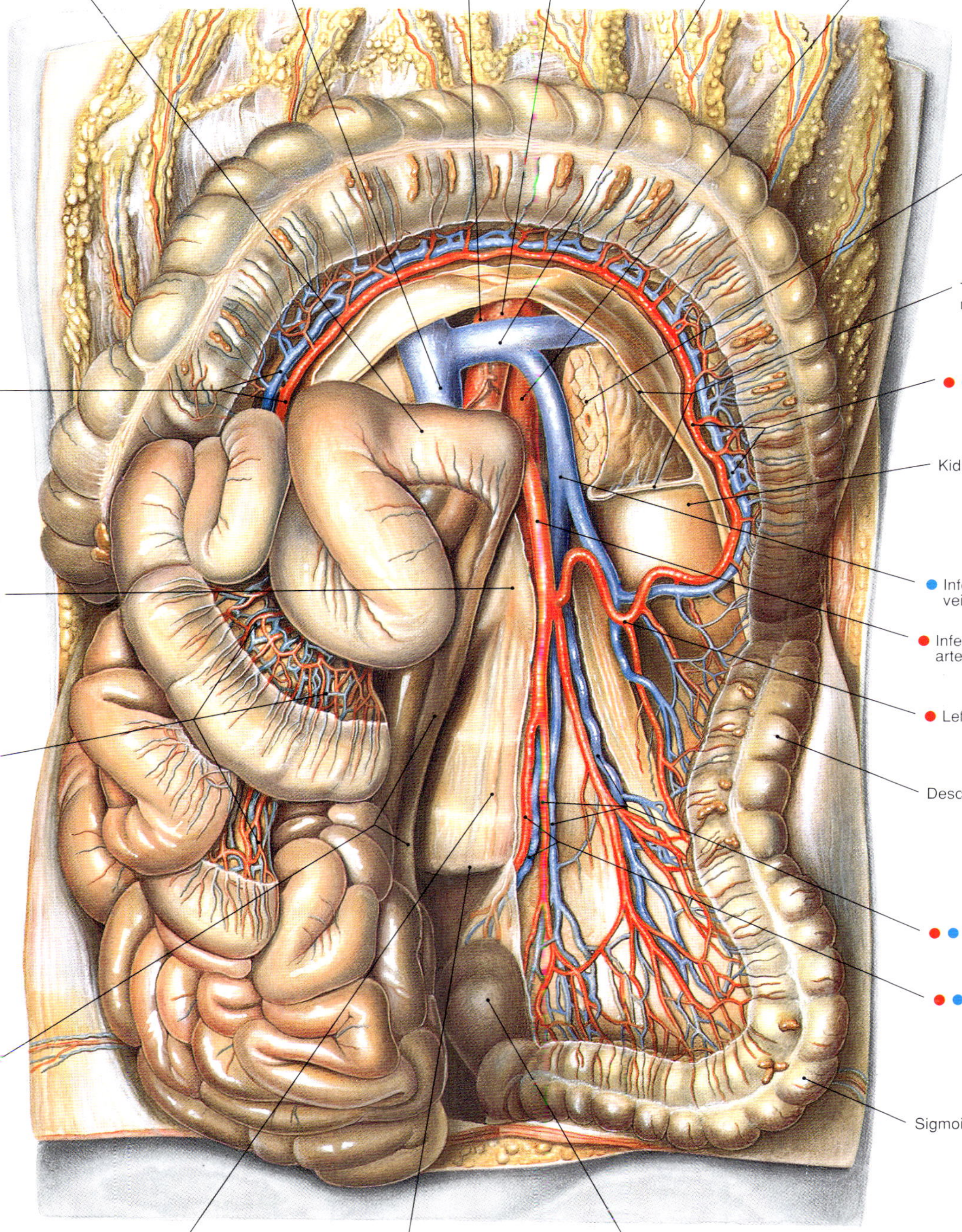

Fig. 805 Inferior mesenteric artery and vein.

Coeliac trunk

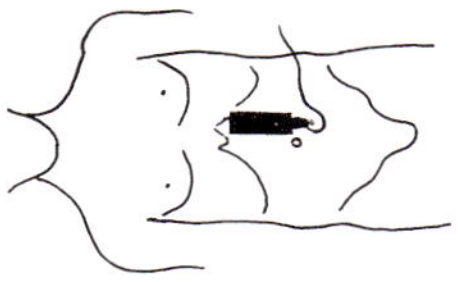

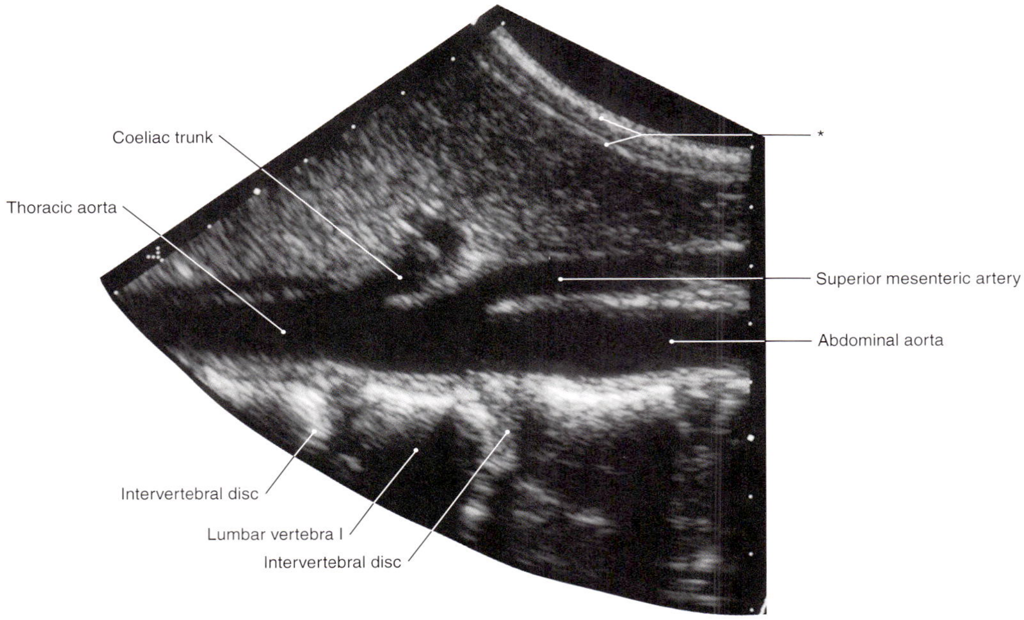

Fig. 806 Abdominal aorta with the coeliac trunk and the superior mesenteric artery; ultrasound image; almost in the sagittal plane.

* Abdominal wall

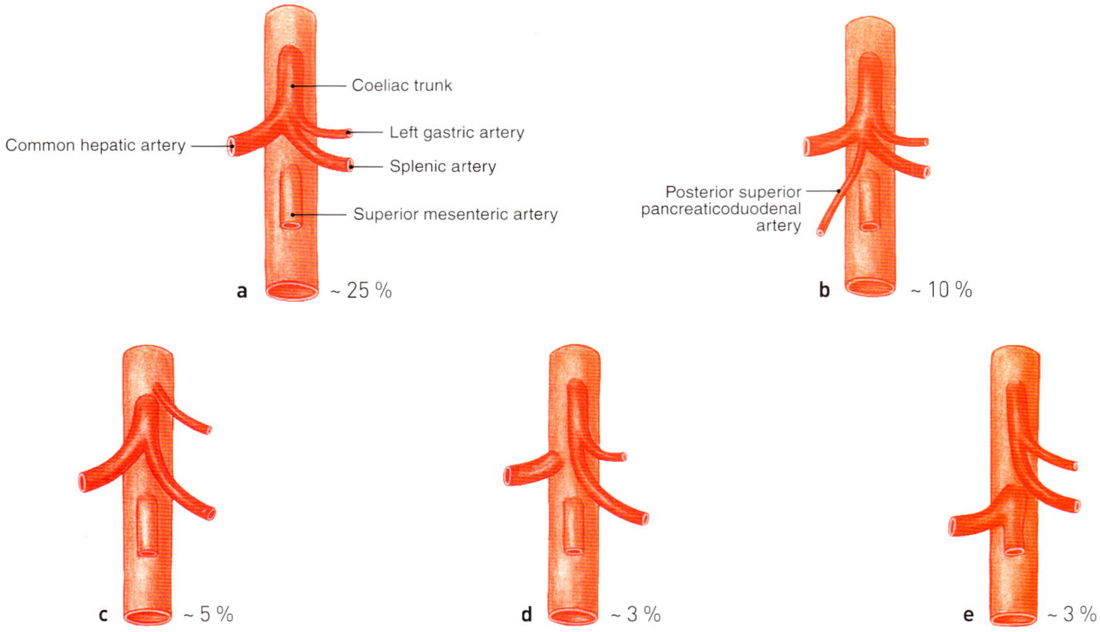

Fig. 807 a–e Variability of the coeliac trunk.

a „Textbook case", division of the trunk into three branches
b Division of the trunk into four branches
c Development of a hepatosplenic trunk
d Development of a gastrosplenic trunk
e Development of a gastrosplenic trunk and a hepatomesenteric trunk

Vessels of the retroperitoneal space

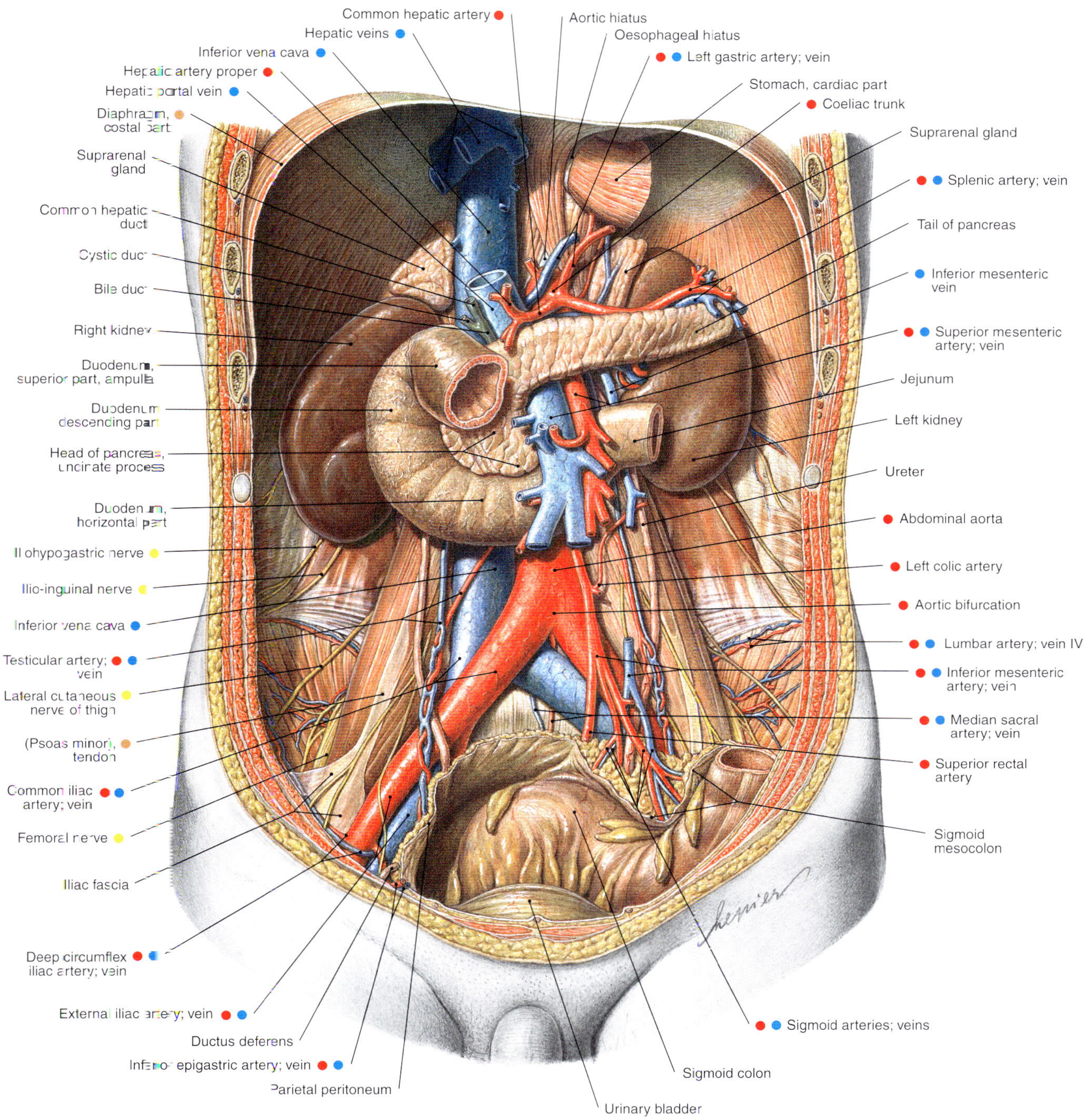

Fig. 808 Vessels of the retroperitoneal space of the male.

Hepatic portal vein, overview

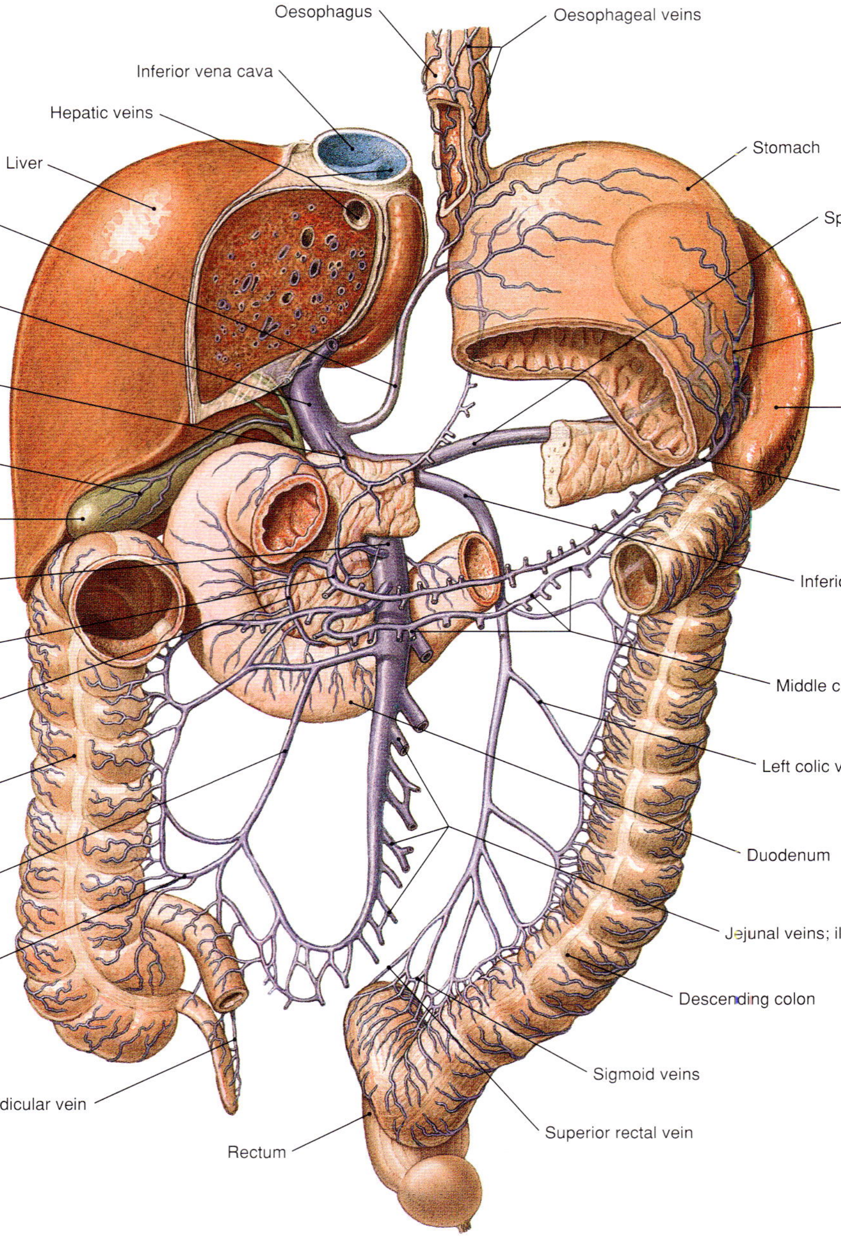

Fig. 809 Hepatic portal vein; ventral view.

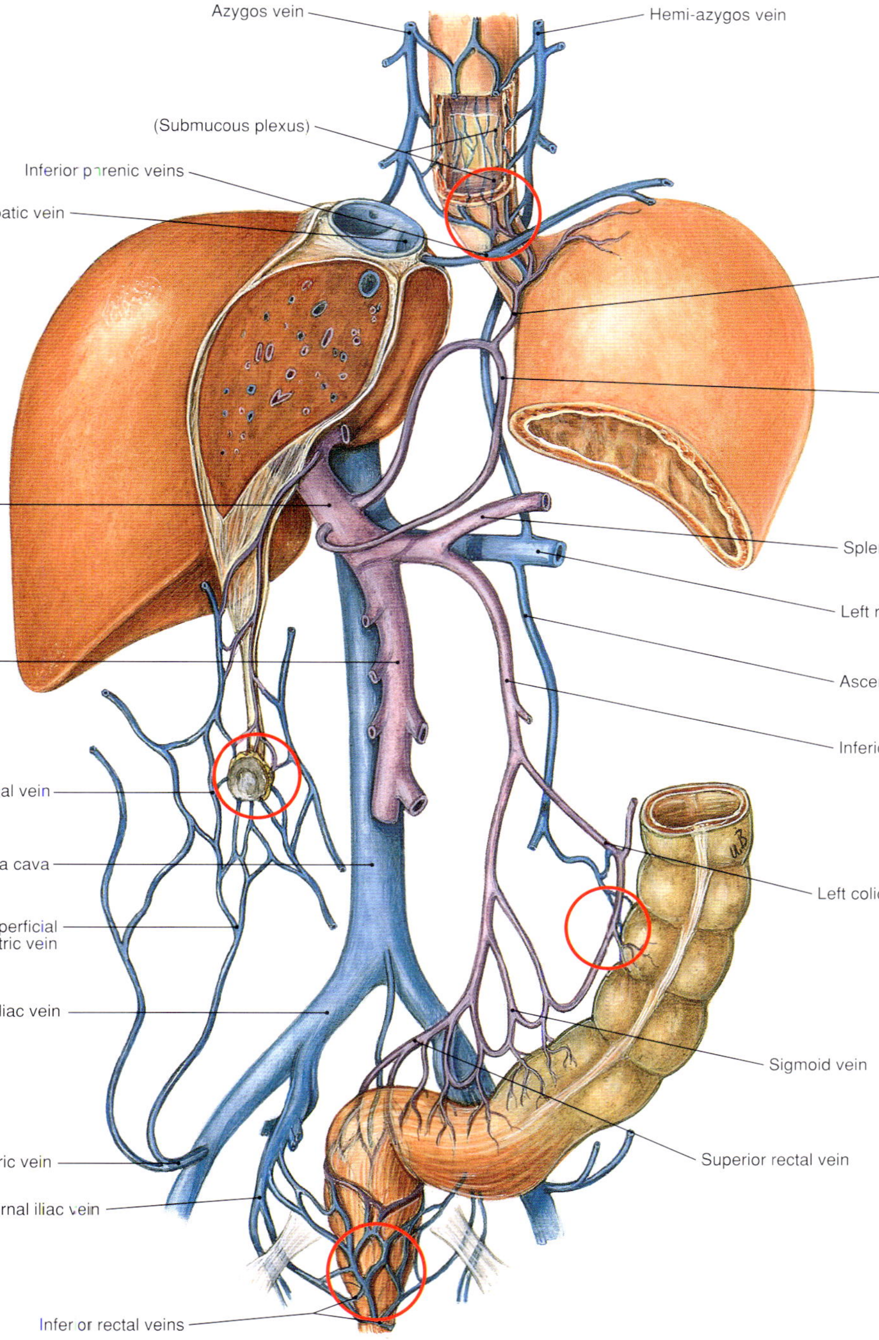

Fig. 810 Hepatic portal vein and inferior vena cava; semi-schematic; tributaries of the inferior vena cava in blue; tributaries of the hepatic portal vein in purple; potential portocaval anastomoses are indicated by circles.

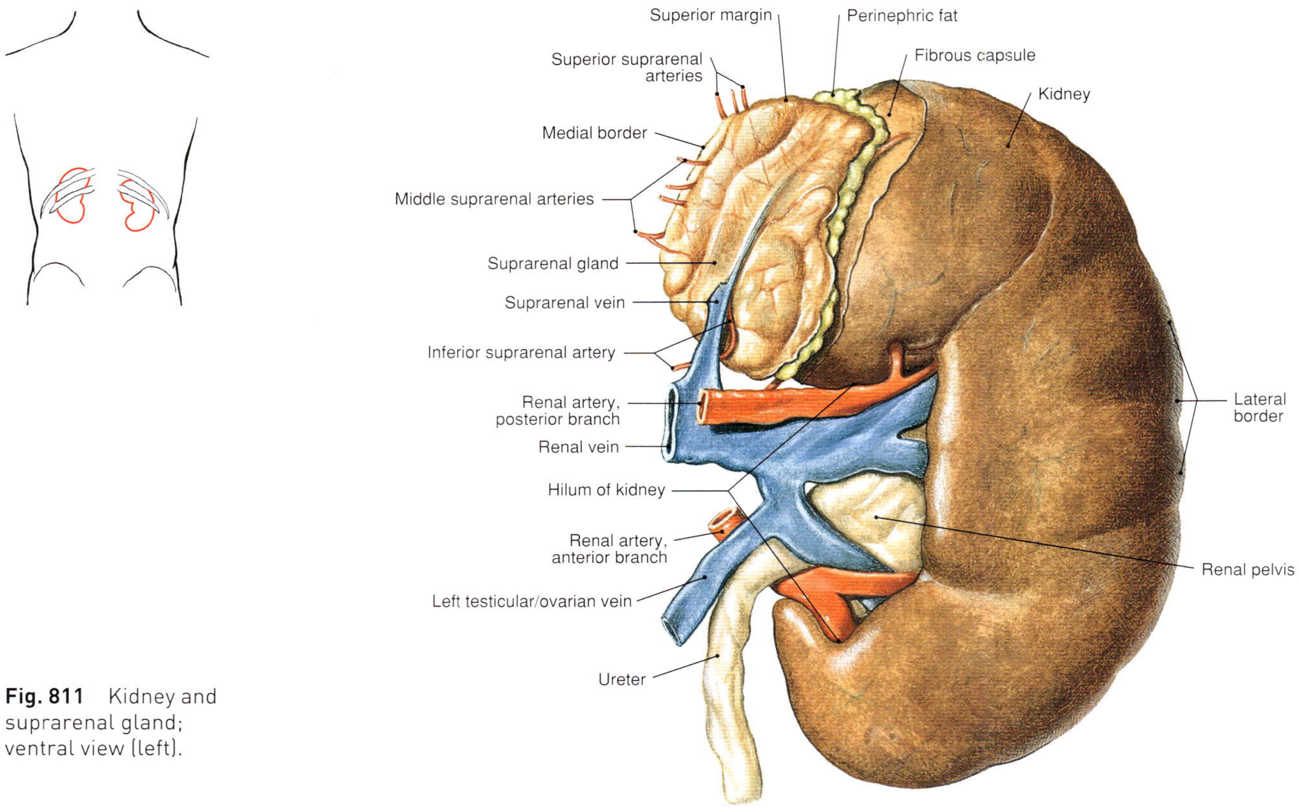

Fig. 811 Kidney and suprarenal gland; ventral view (left).

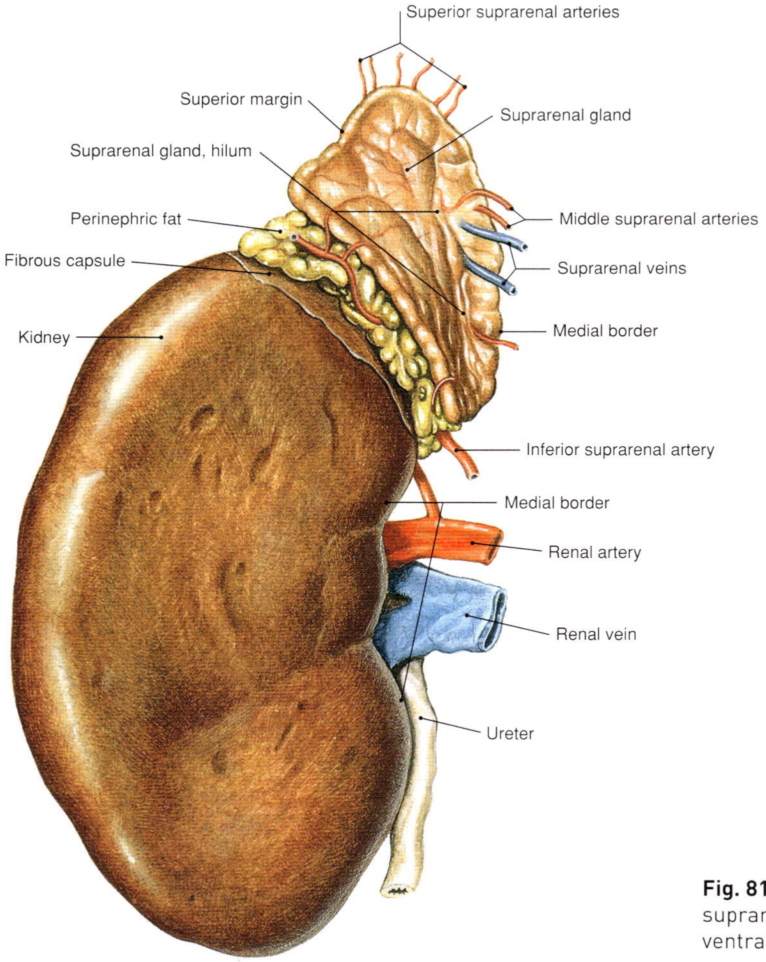

Fig. 812 Kidney and suprarenal gland; ventral view (right).

located at the back of abdomen one on each side of spine at level of lower ribs

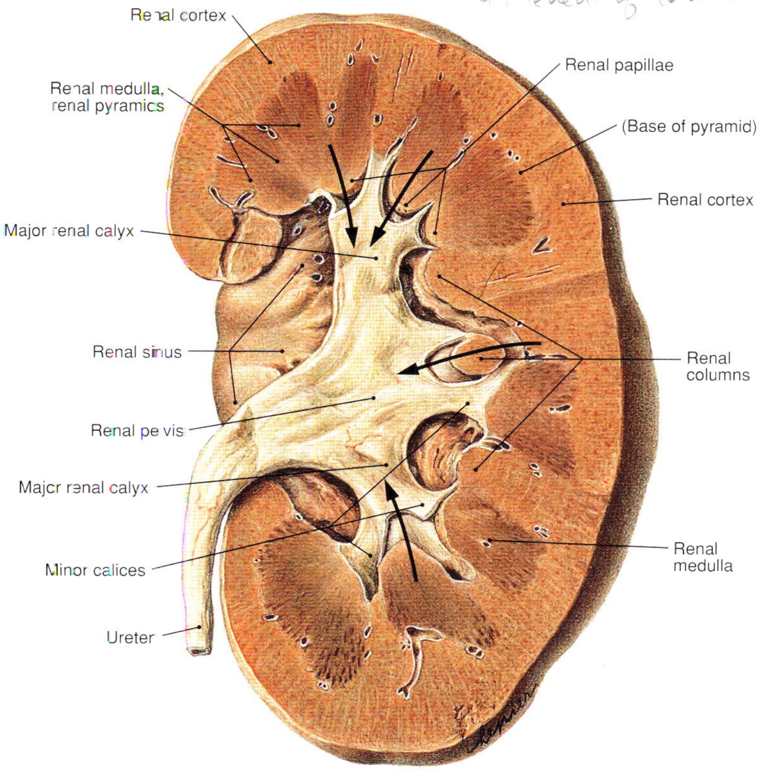

Fig. 813 Kidney;
oblique and vertical hemisection displaying the renal cortex, the medulla and the pelvis;
ventral view (left).
Arrows point from the pyramids to the calyces.

Function of kidneys

1. forming urin
2. maintaining hemostasis
3. hormone secreation (erythropoietin venin)

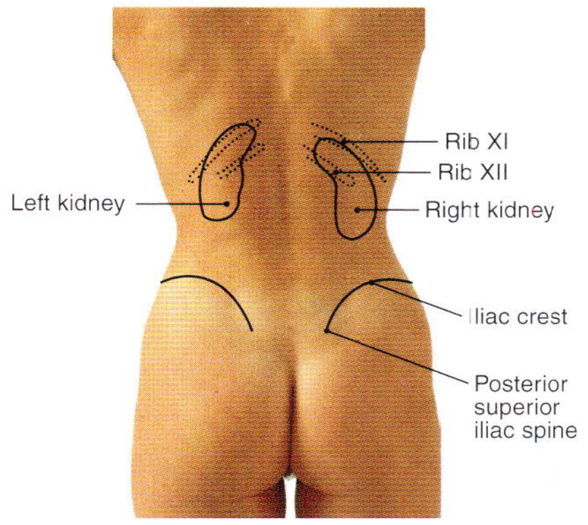

lower ribs

Fig. 814 Projection of the kidneys onto the back.

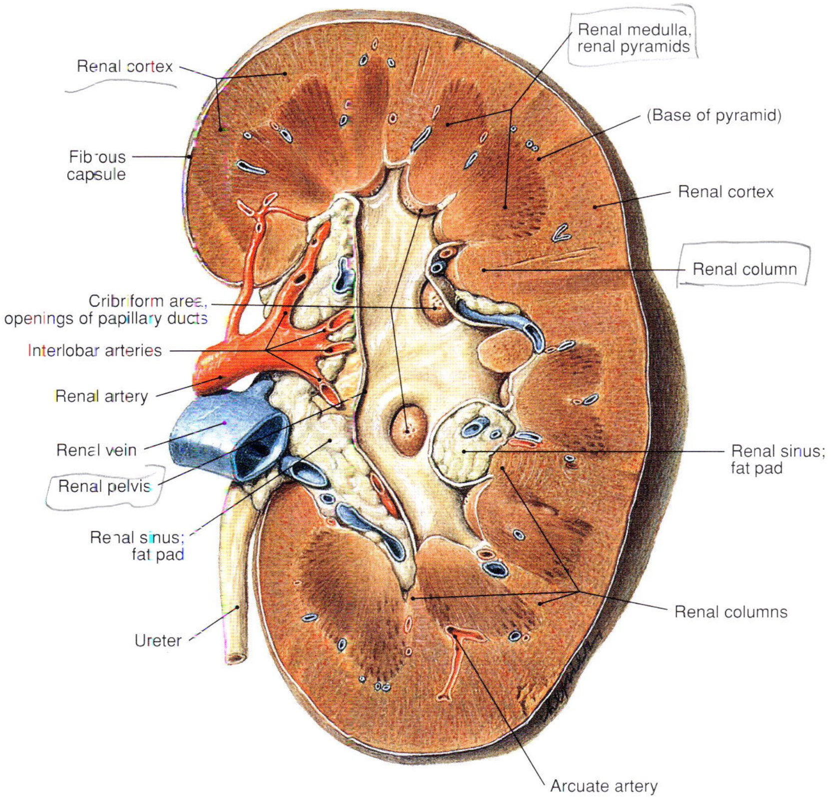

Fig. 815 Kidney;
oblique and vertical hemisection;
ventral view (left).

Kidney, structure

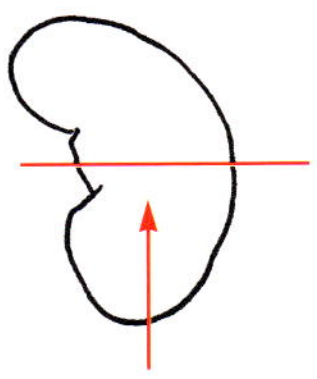

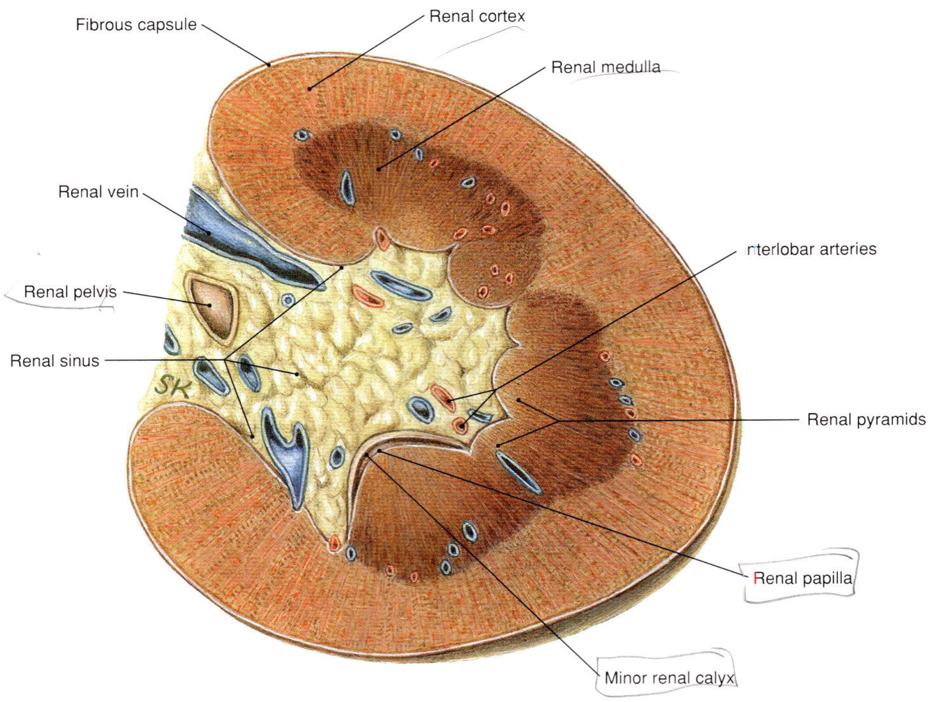

Fig. 816 Kidney;
transverse section through the renal sinus;
inferior view (left).

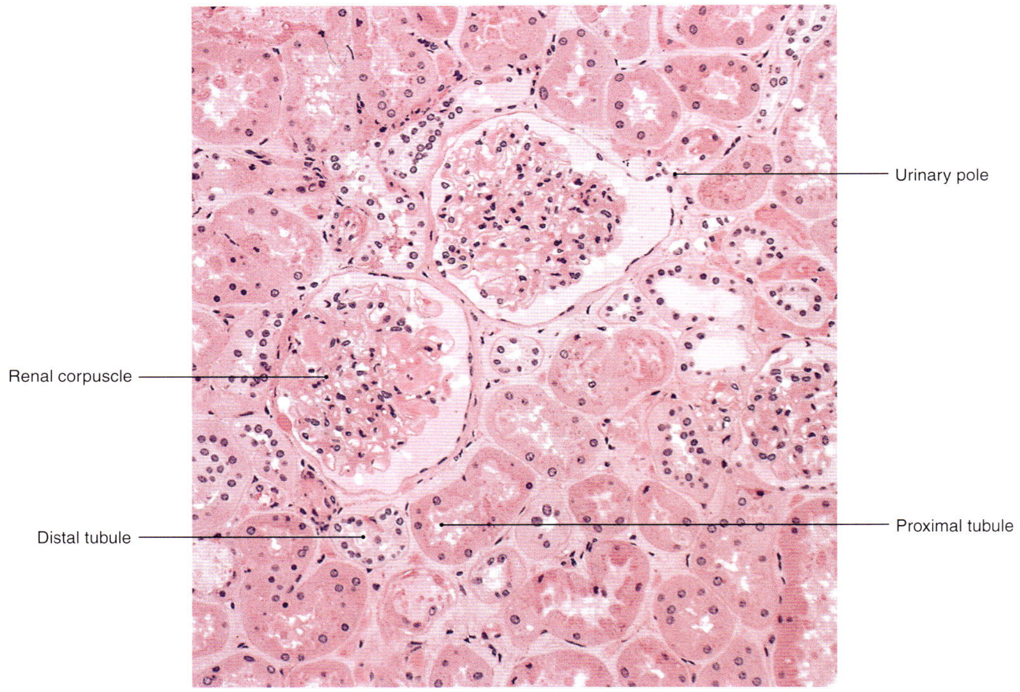

Fig. 817 Kidney;
microscopic section of the cortex (100 x).

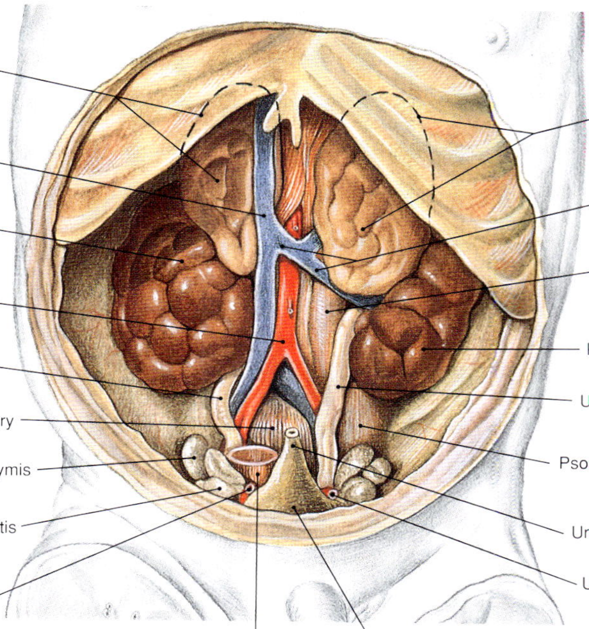

Fig. 818 Kidney and the suprarenal gland of a ~ 5-month-old foetus.

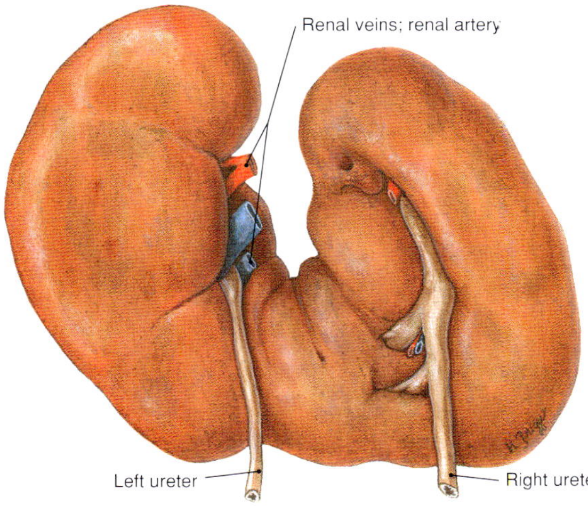

Fig. 819 Kidney;
dorsal view.
The lower poles of both kidneys are fused (= horseshoe kidney).

Renal pelvis and calyces

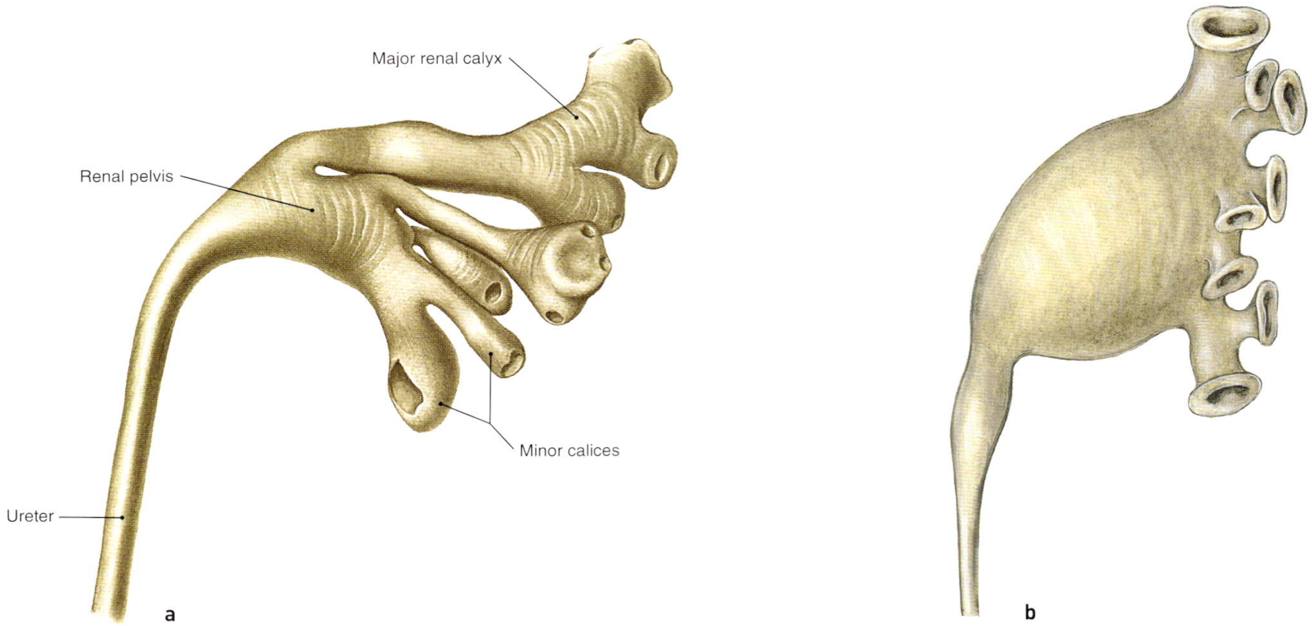

Fig. 820 a, b Renal pelvis;
corrosion casts;
ventral view (left).
a Dendritic type
b Ampullar type

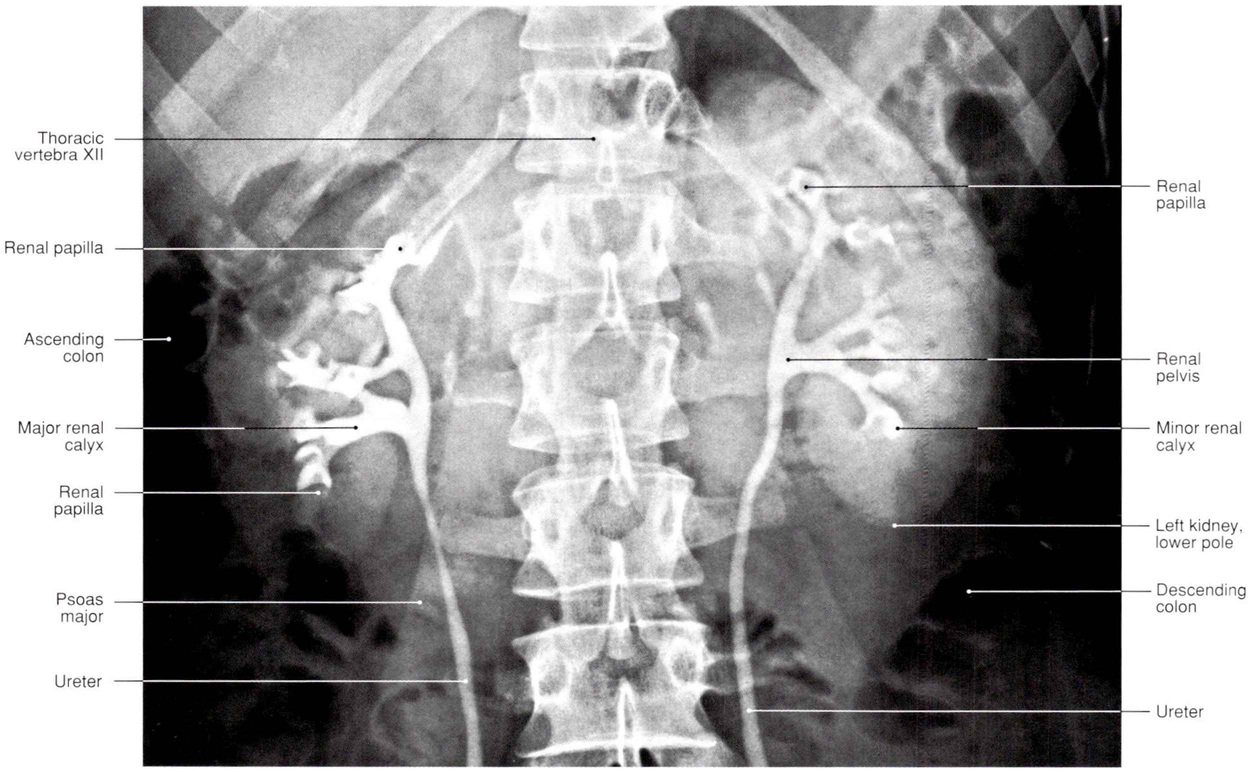

Fig. 821 Kidney;
renal pelvis and ureter;
AP-radiograph after retrograde injection of a contrast medium via both ureters.

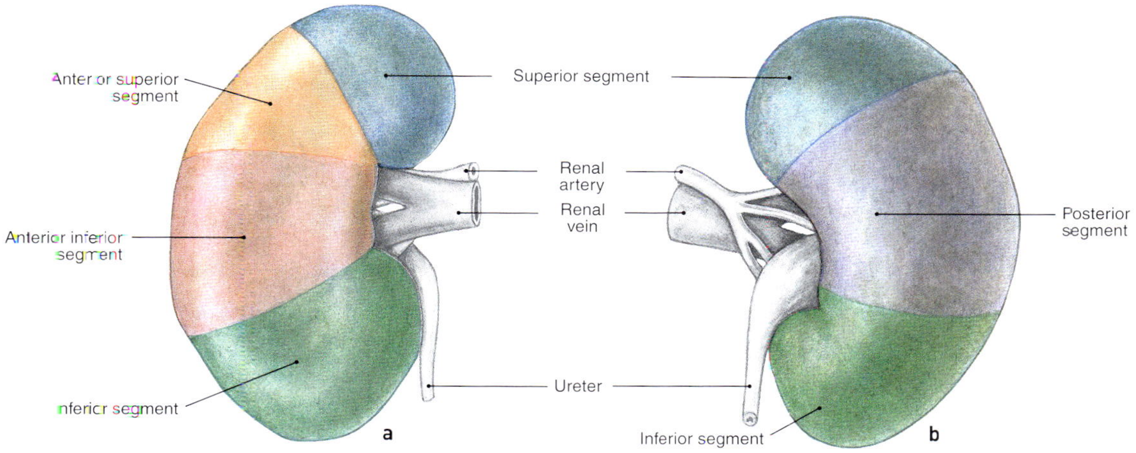

Fig. 822 a, b Renal segments.

a Ventral view (right)
b Dorsal view (right)

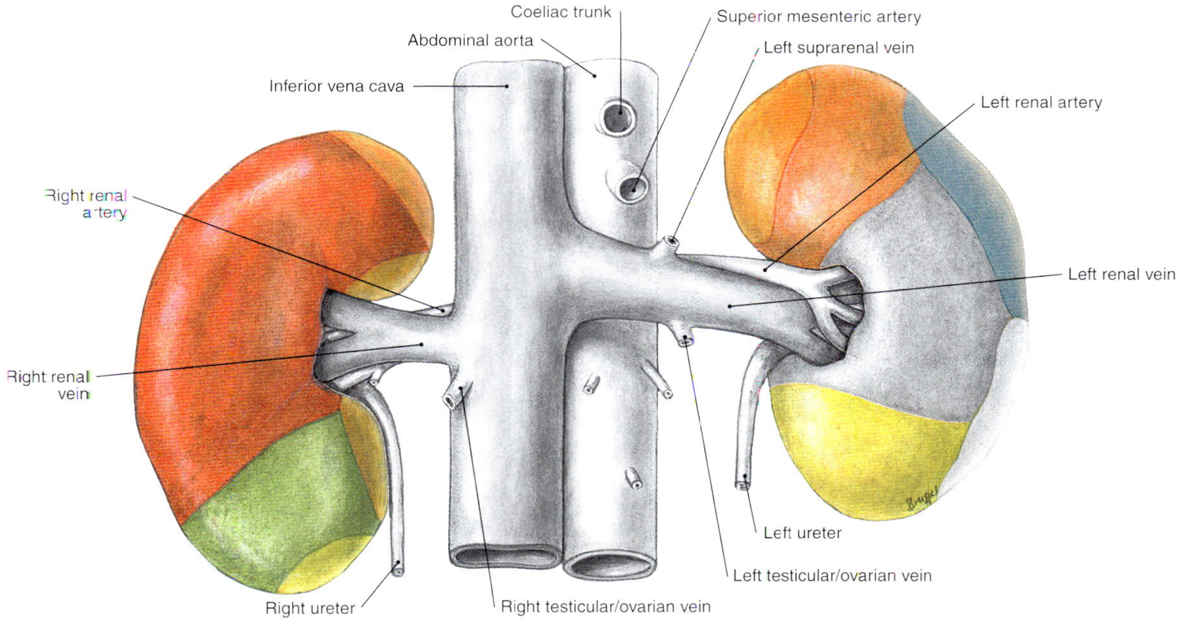

Fig. 823 Kidney;
areas of contact with adjacent organs;
ventral view.

Areas of contact of the Kidneys

Suprarenal glands	Colon, tight flexure	Spleen
liver	Jejunum	Pancreas
Duodenum, descending part	Stomach	Descending colon

Kidney, imaging

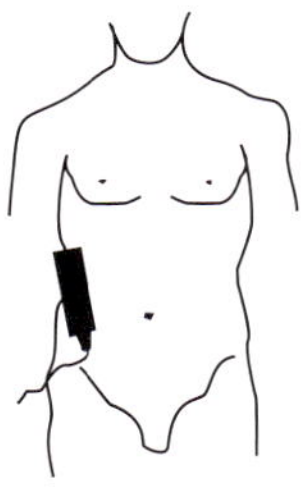

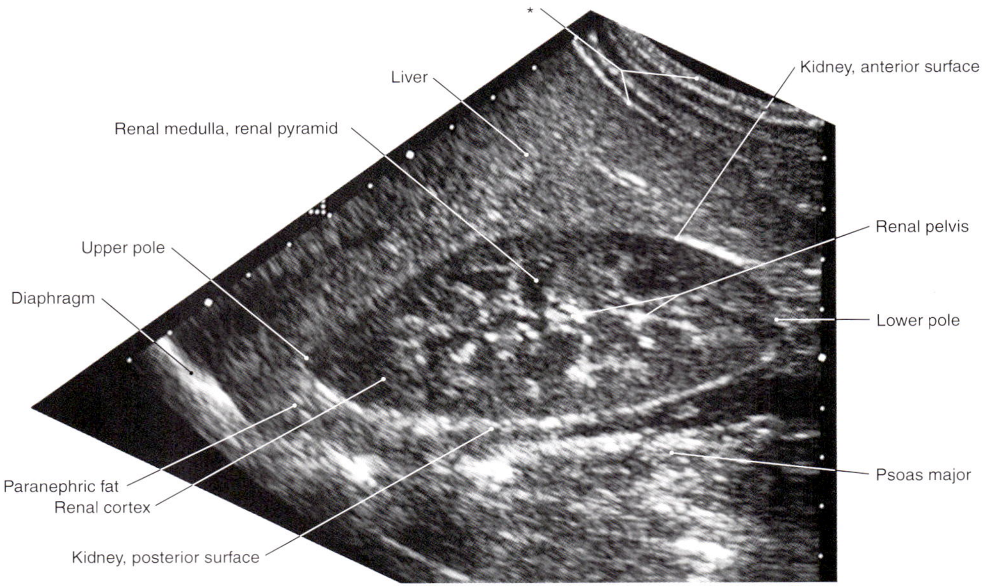

Fig. 824 Kidney;
ultrasound image;
the transducer is directed from ventroinferior to dorsosuperior;
lateral view (right).

* Abdominal wall

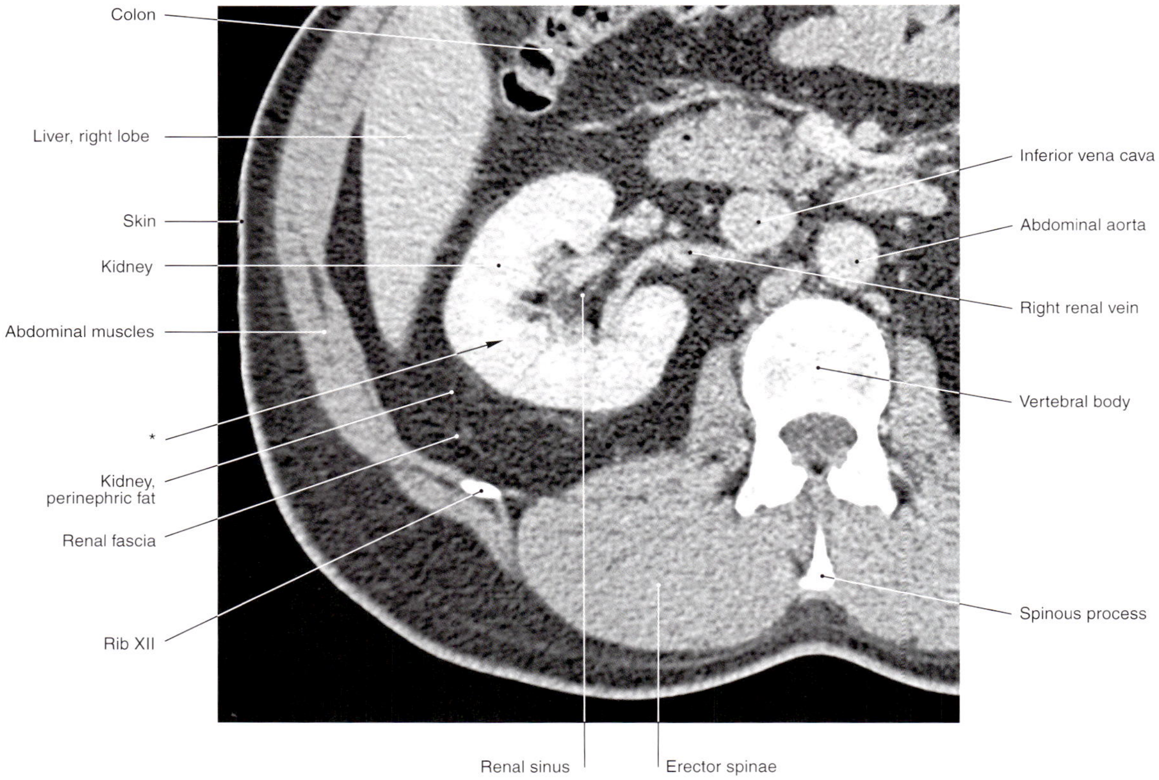

→ 928

Fig. 825 Kidney;
puncture of the right kidney;
computed tomographic cross-section (CT);
inferior view.

* Guidance of a needle for kidney biopsy

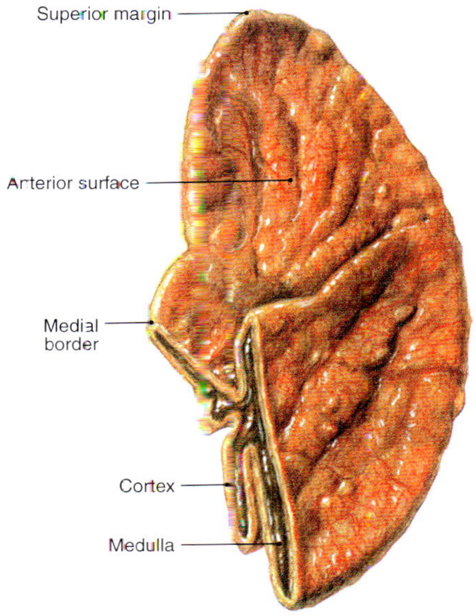

Fig. 826 Suprarenal gland; ventral view (right).

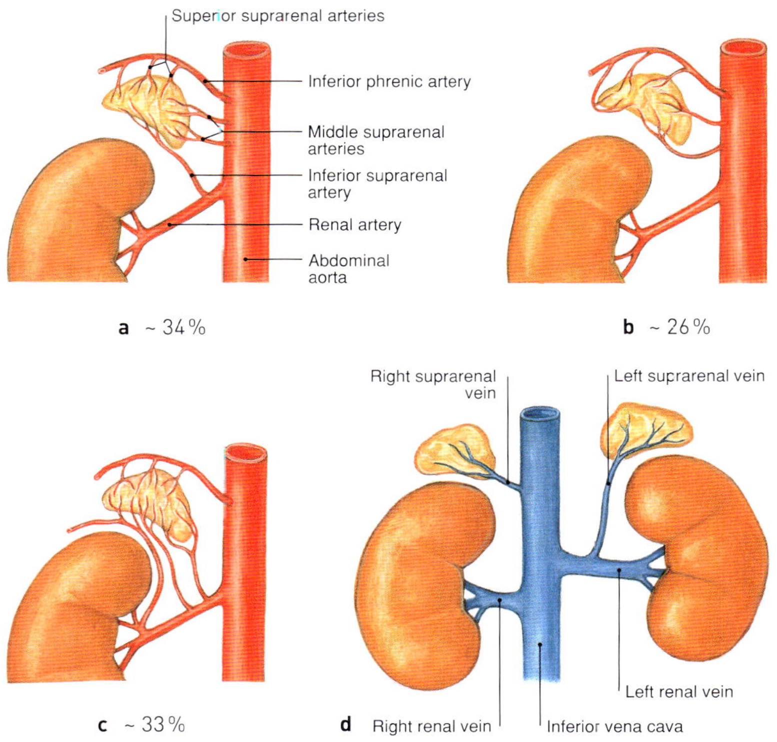

Fig. 827 a–d Variability of the suprarenal arteries and course of the suprarenal veins.

a Arterial supply by three arteries („textbook case")
b Arterial supply without a branch from the renal artery
c Arterial supply without a direct branch from the aorta
d Course of the suprarenal veins

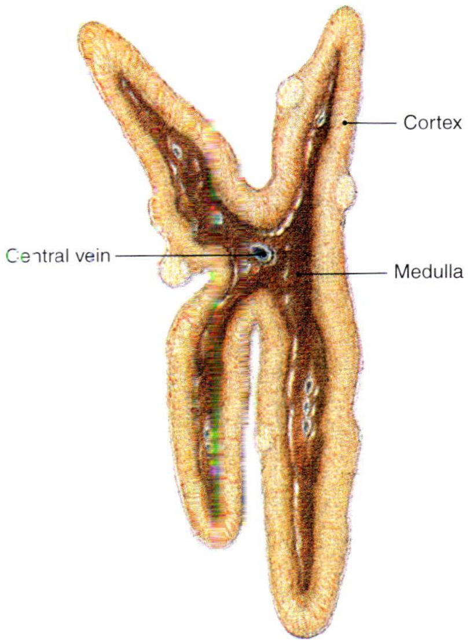

Fig. 828 Suprarenal gland; sagittal section; lateral view (right).

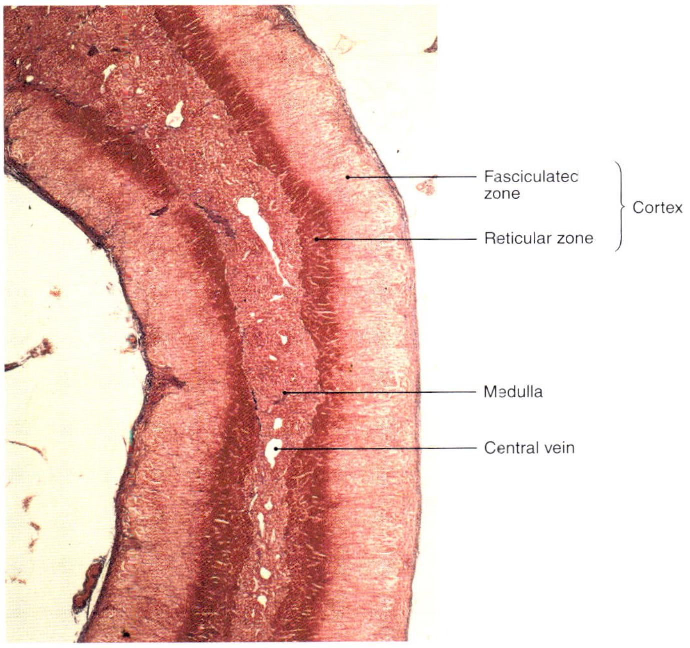

Fig. 829 Suprarenal gland; microscopic enlargement at low magnification.

Urinary bladder

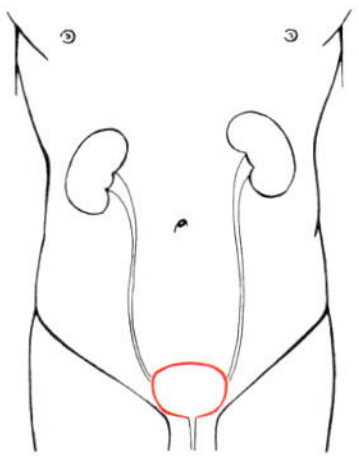

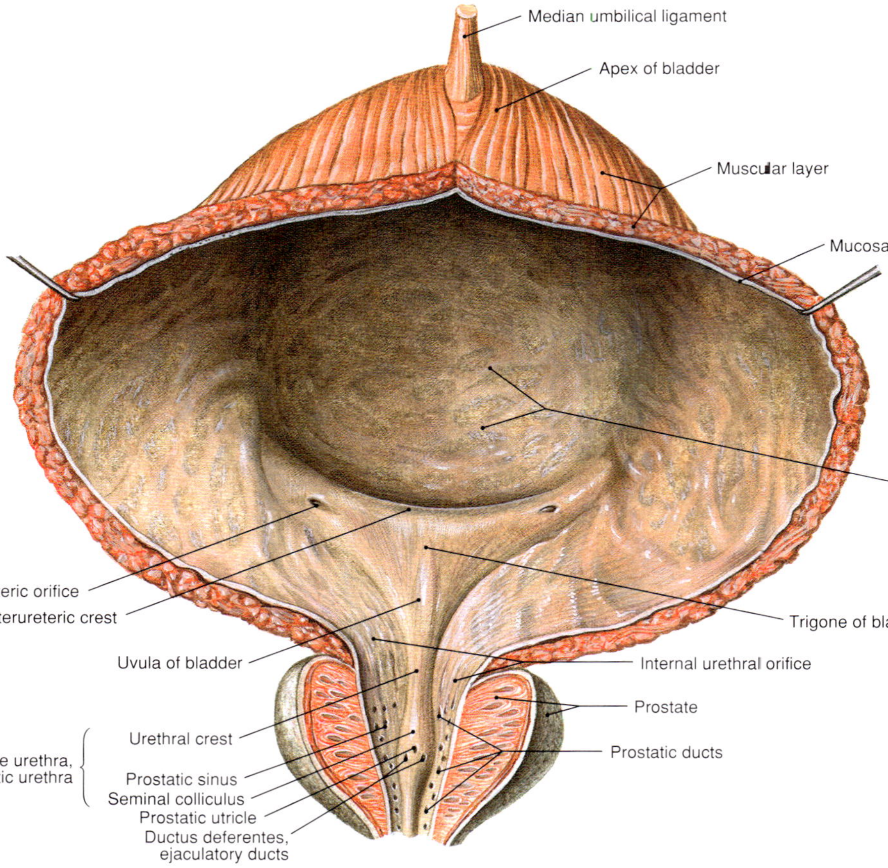

Fig. 830 Urinary bladder; prostate and urethra; ventral view.

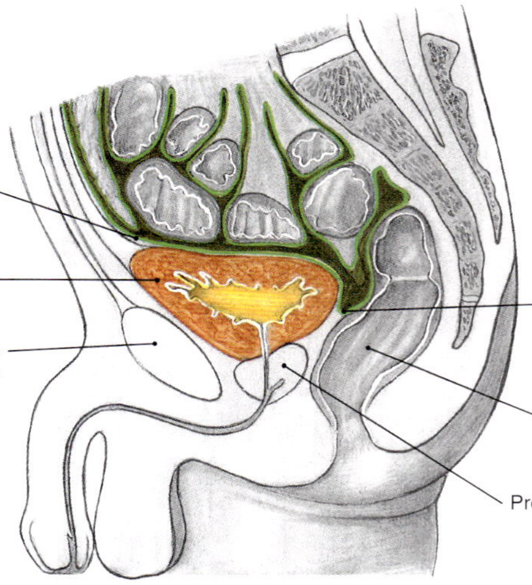

Fig. 831 Urinary bladder almost completely voided.

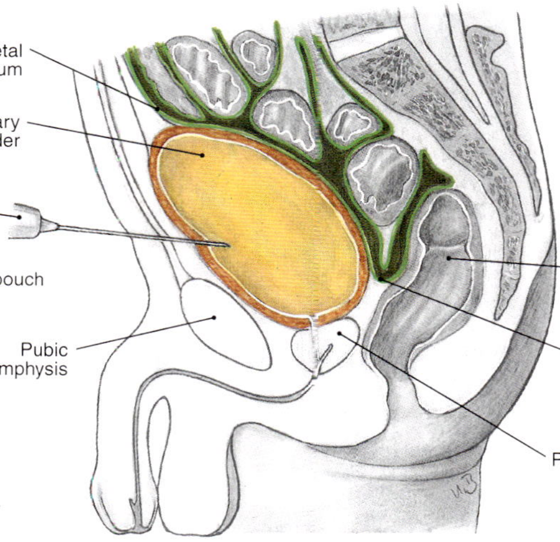

Fig. 832 Urinary bladder filled.
In this situation, the bladder can be punctured from just above the pubic bone without passing through the peritoneal cavity.

* Puncture needle

Urinary bladder, ductus deferens and seminal vesicle

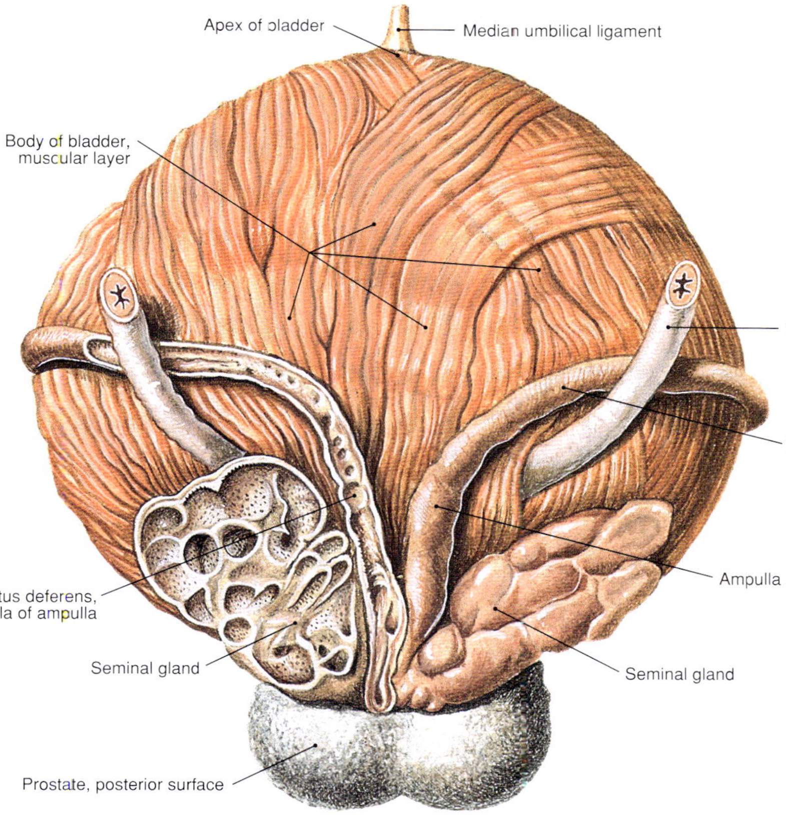

Fig. 833 Urinary bladder, ductus deferentes, seminal vesicles and prostate; dorsal view.

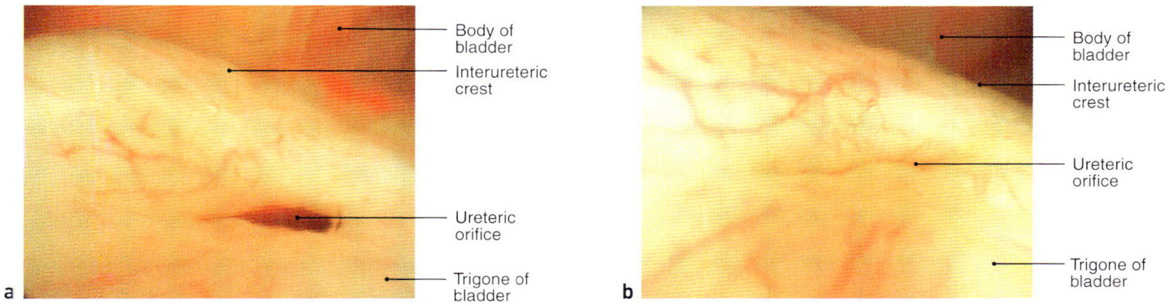

Fig. 834 a, b Urinary bladder; endoscopic view of the opening of the ureter (cystoscopy).

a Open ostium of the ureter with a peristaltic wave transporting urine into the bladder

b Closed ostium of the ureter

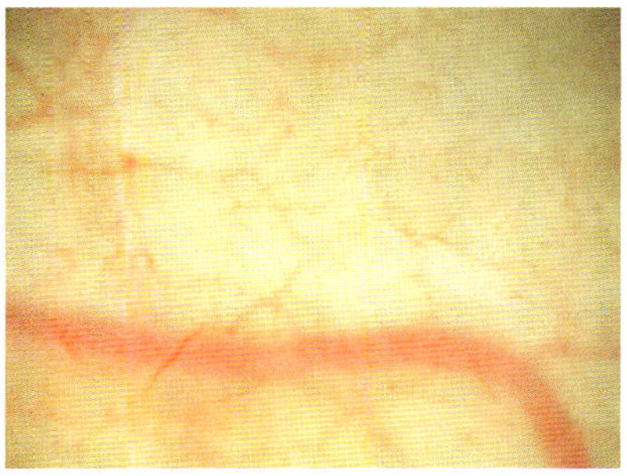

Fig. 835 Urinary bladder; endoscopic view of the mucosa in the body of the bladder (cystoscopy); inferior view.

Male urinary and genital organs, overview

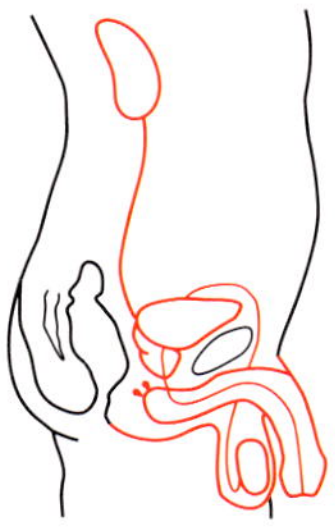

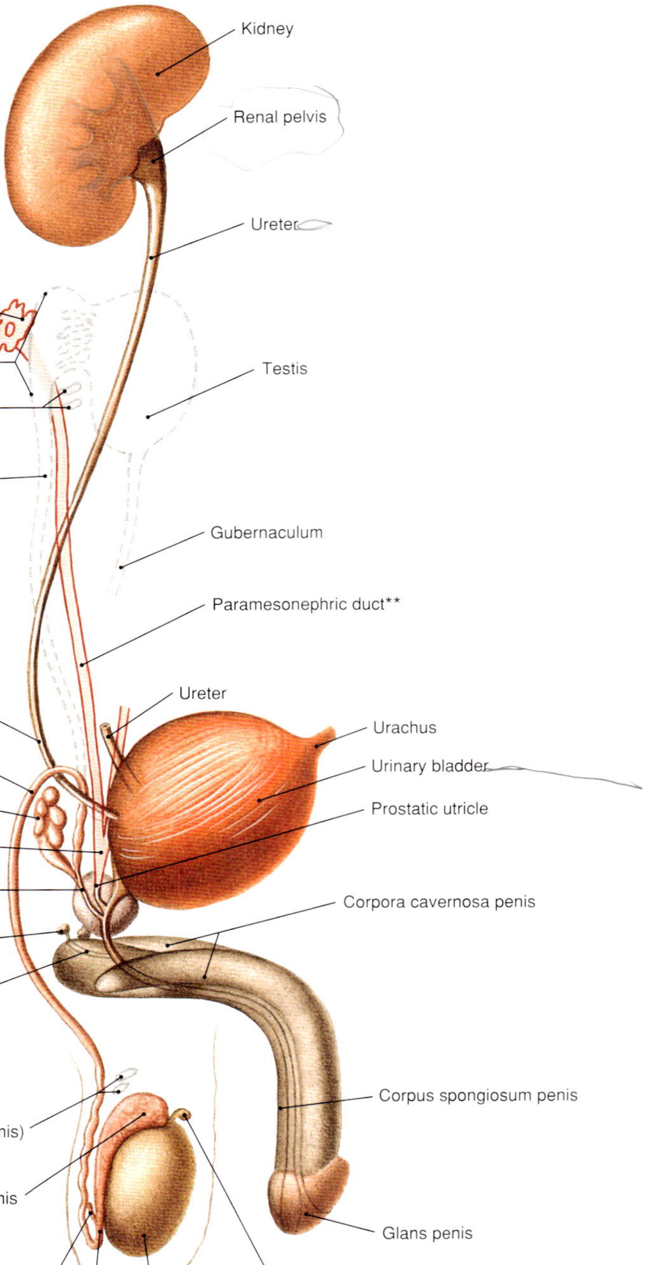

→ 851

Fig. 836 Male urinary and genital organs;
diagram of the development: the parts that degenerate are displayed in pale pink, and the position of the testis prior to its descent is indicated by the dashed line;
viewed from the right.

Epididymis = genital part of the mesonephros;
Paradidymis = remnants of tubules of the mesonephros

* WOLFFian duct
** MÜLLERian duct
*** Junction of the MÜLLERian ducts, paramesonephric duct

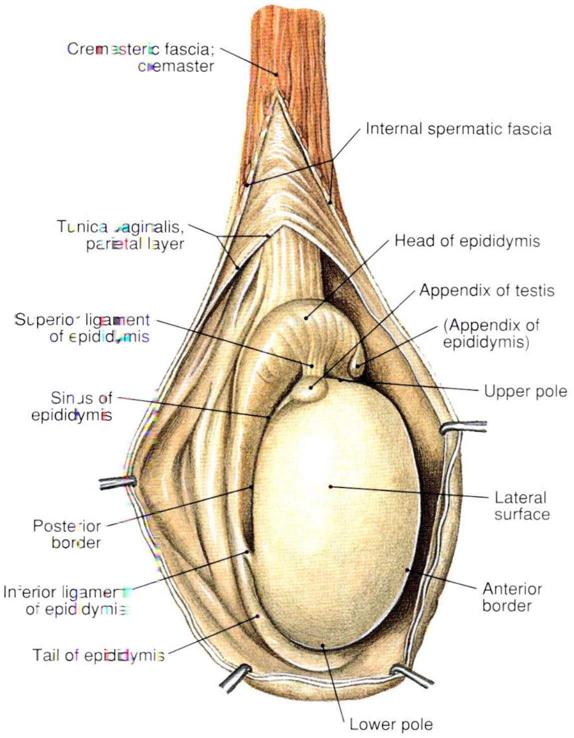

Fig. 837 Testis and epididymis; viewed from the right.

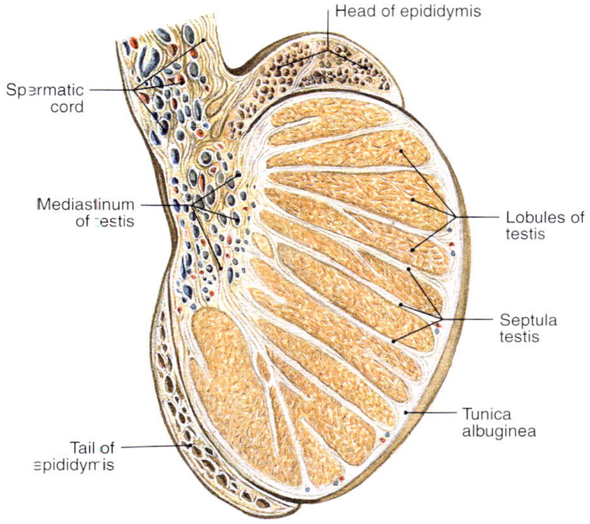

Fig. 838 Testis and epididymis; viewed from the right.

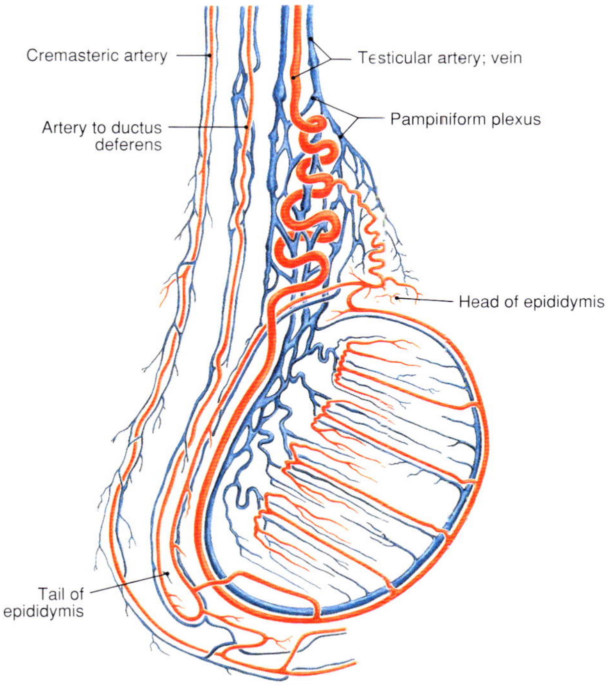

Fig. 839 Blood vessels of the testis, the epididymis and the spermatic cord; viewed from the right.

Testis and epididymis

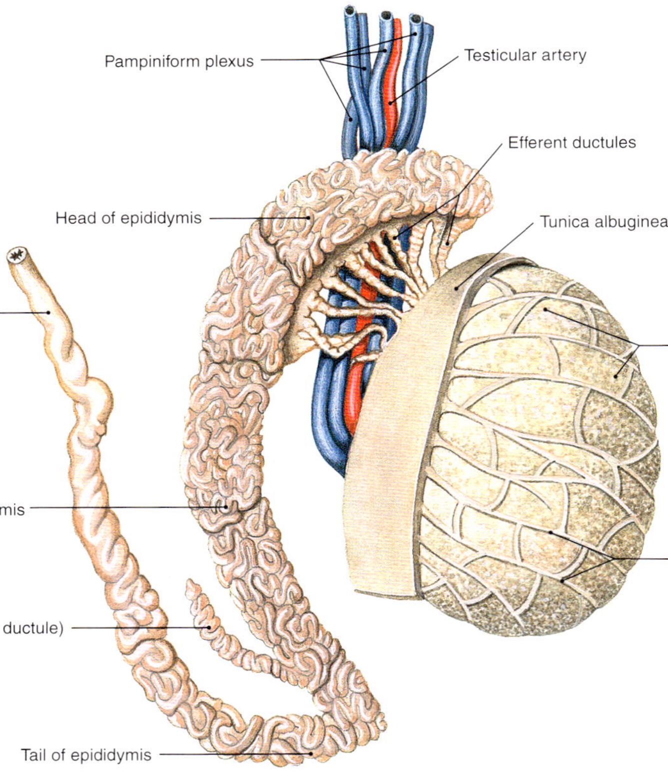

Fig. 840 Testis; epididymis and ductus deferens (vas deferens); lateral view.

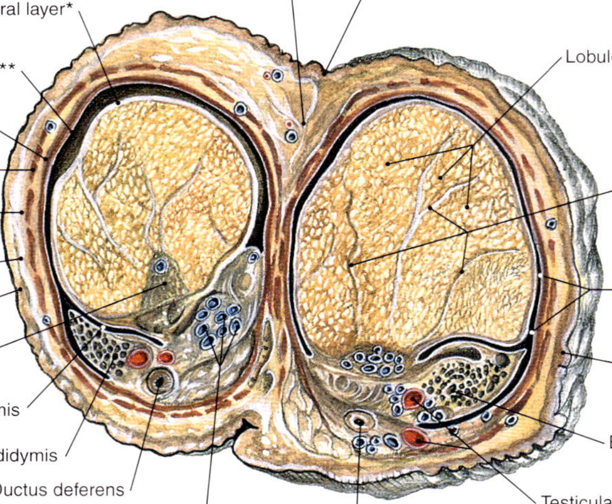

Fig. 841 Testis; epididymis and scrotum; superior view.

* Also: Epiorchium
** Also: Periorchium

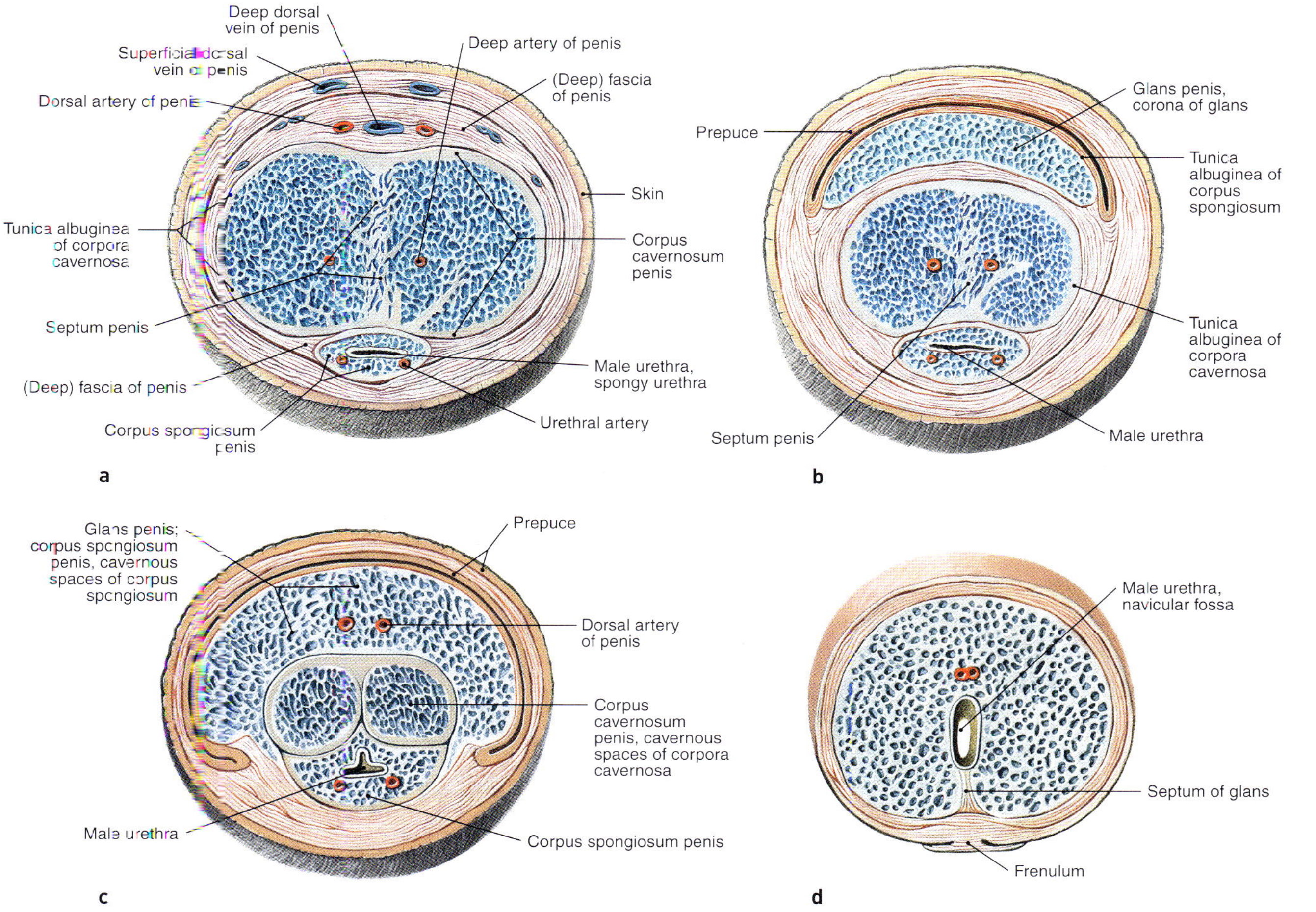

Fig. 849 a–d Penis; cross-sections; planes indicated in Fig. 850; ventral view.

a Cross-section through the middle of the shaft
b Cross-section at the level of the proximal part of the glans penis
c Cross-section through the middle of the glans penis
d Cross-section at the level of the distal part of the glans penis

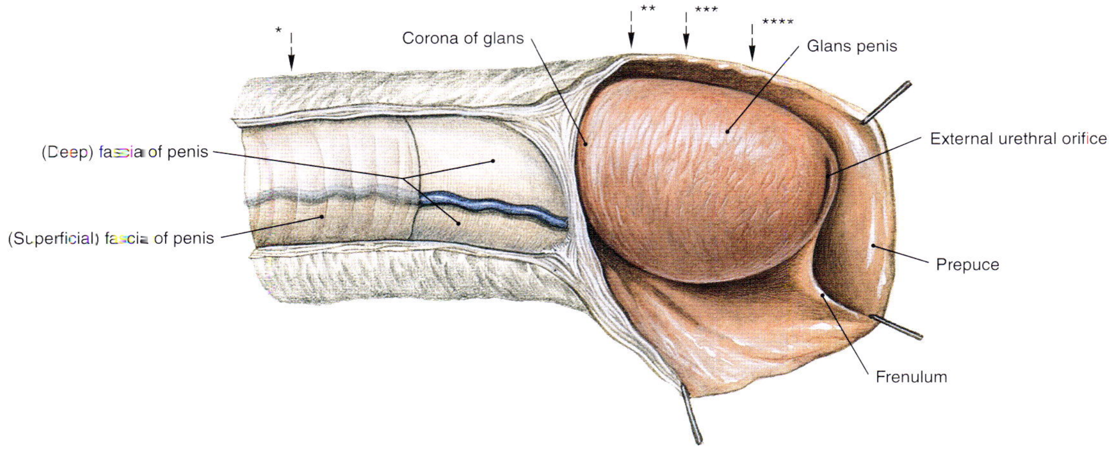

Fig. 850 Penis with glans penis and prepuce.

* Level of section of Fig. 849 a
** Level of section of Fig. 849 b
*** Level of section of Fig. 849 c
**** Level of section of Fig. 849 d

Female urinary and genital organs, overview

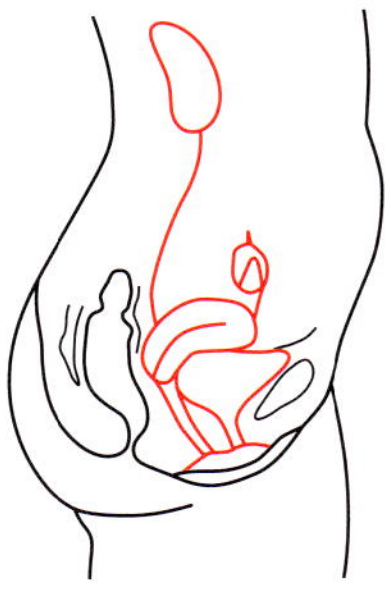

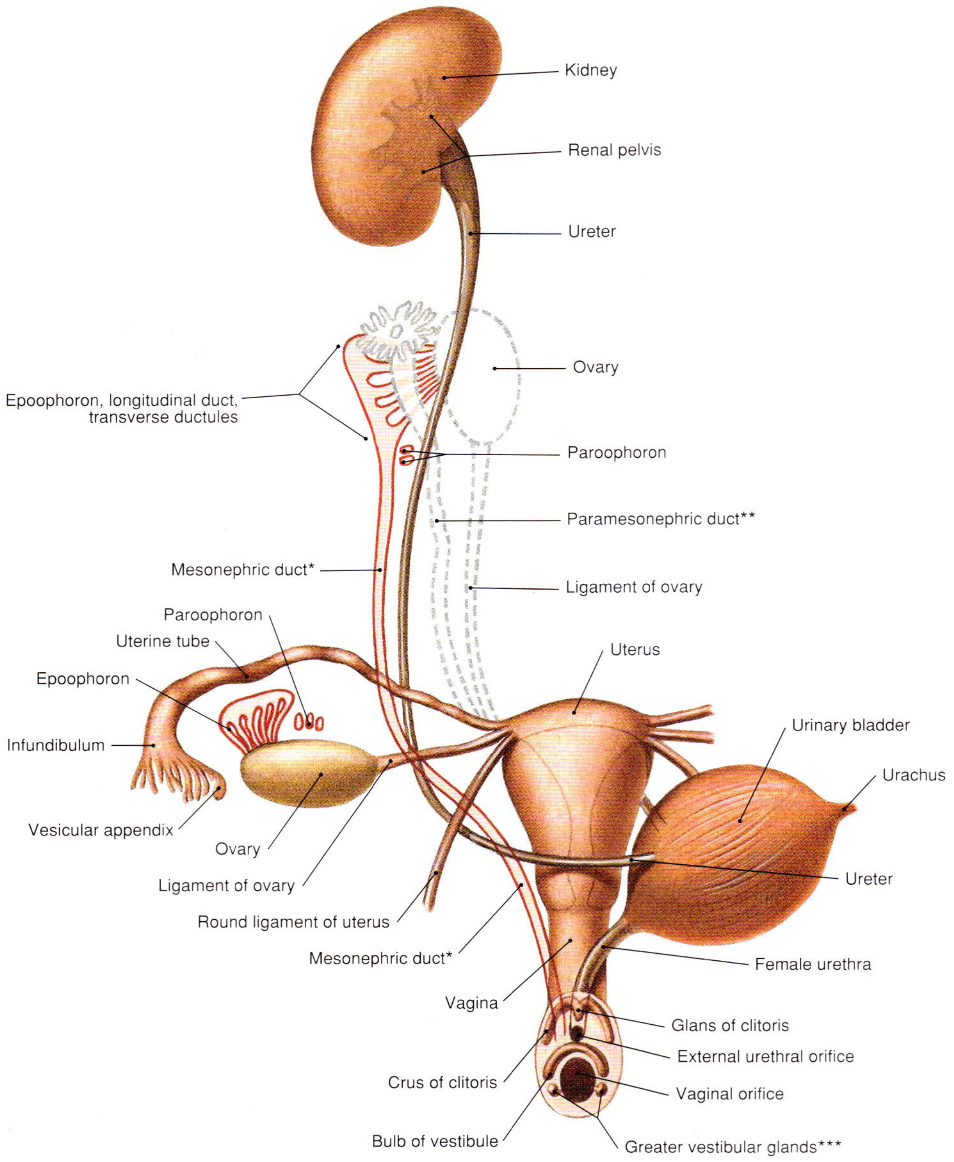

→ 836

Fig. 851 Female urinary and genital organs;
diagram of the development: the parts that degenerate are displayed in pale pink, and the position of the ovary prior to its descent is indicated by the dashed line;
ventral view.

Epoophoron = genital part of the mesonephros;
Paroophoron = remnants of the tubules of the mesonephros

* WOLFFian duct
** MÜLLERian duct
*** BARTHOLIN's glands

Uterus and ovaries

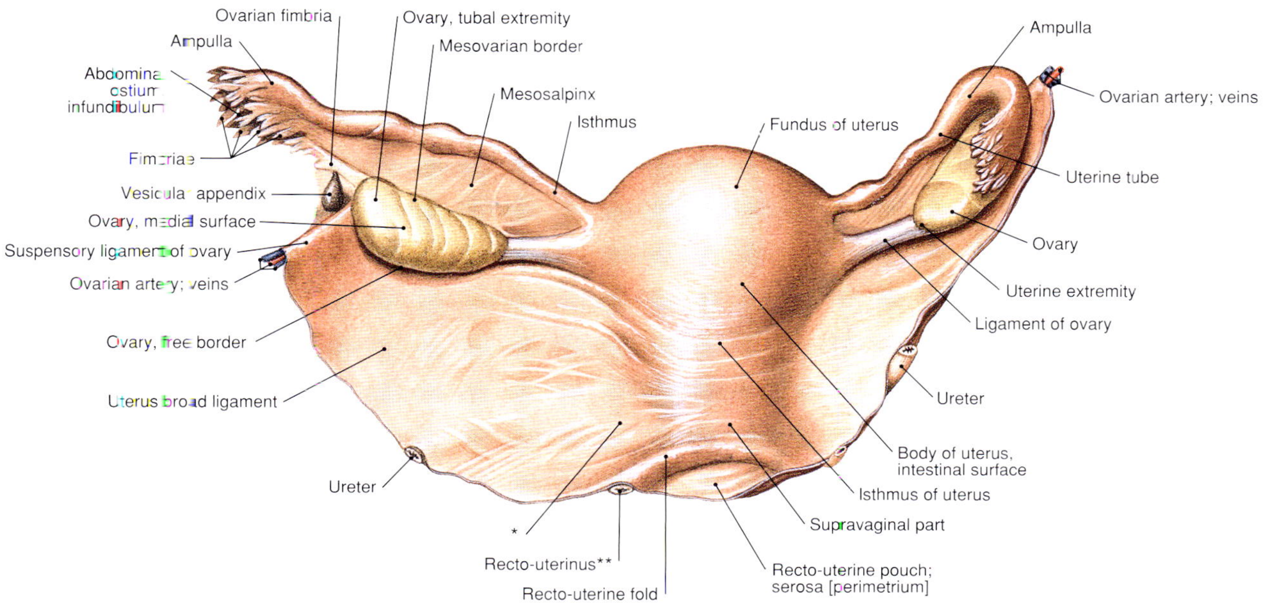

Fig. 852 Uterus; ovary and uterine tube; dorsal view.

* Clinical term: cardinal ligament
** Clinical term: sacrouterine ligament

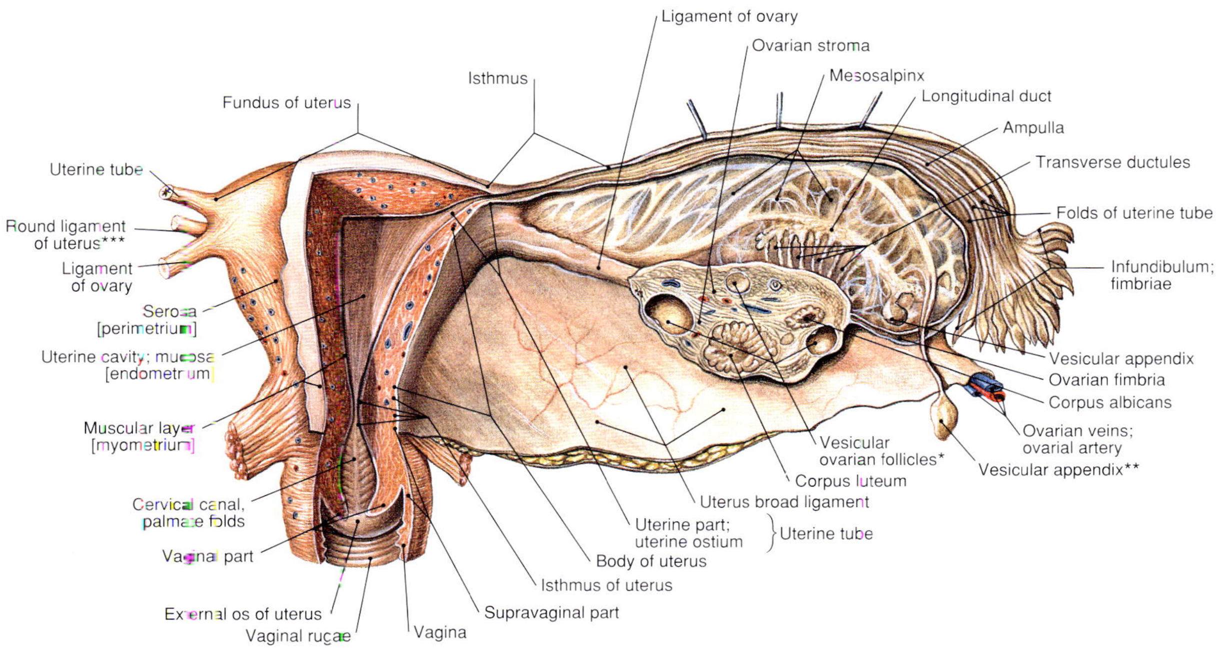

Fig. 853 Uterus; ovary and uterine tube; dorsal view.

* Clinical term: GRAAFian follicle
** Stalked hydatid
*** Clinical term: round ligament

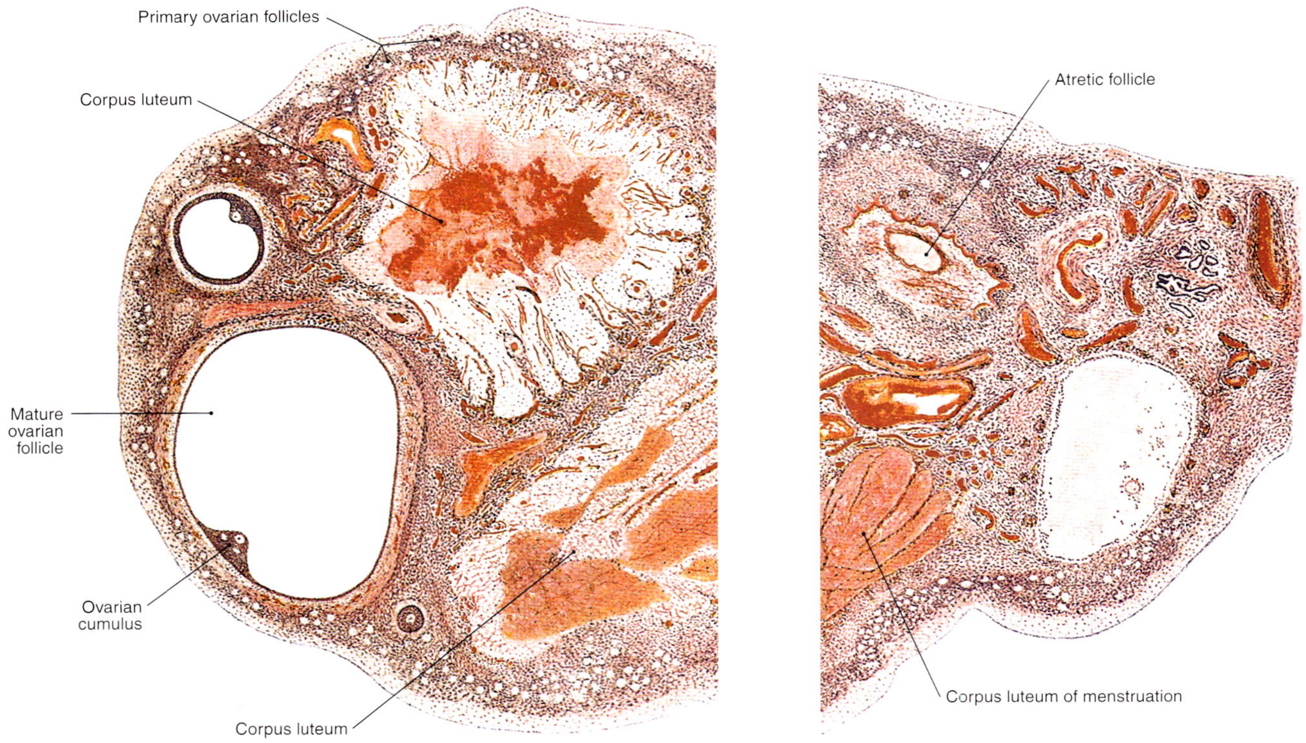

Fig. 854 Ovary;
microscopic enlargement at low magnification.

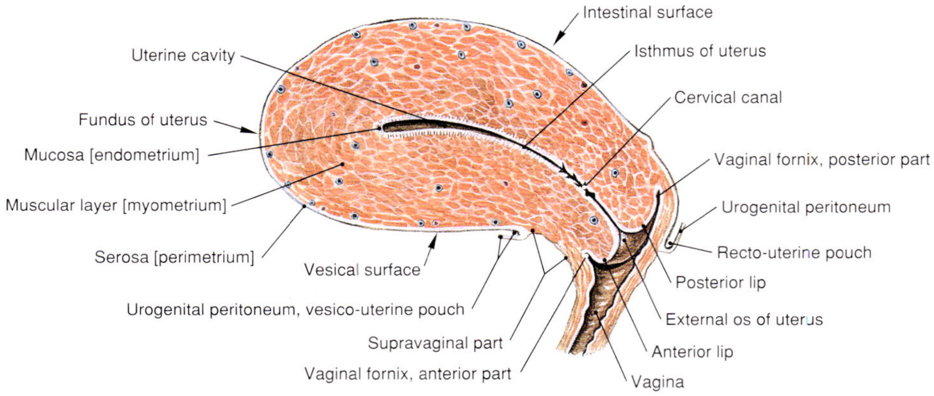

Fig. 855 Uterus and vagina;
viewed from the right.

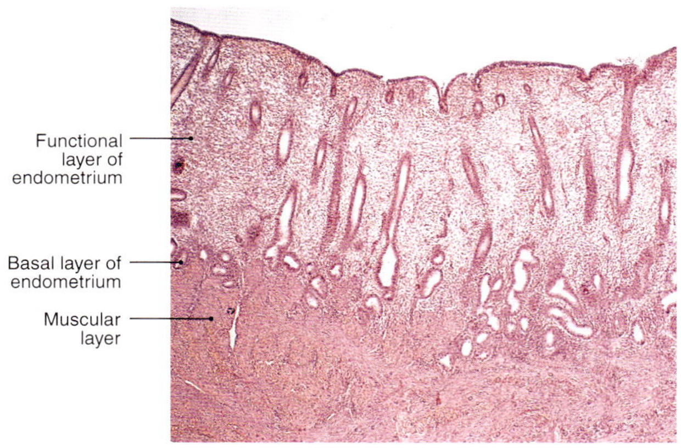

Fig. 856 Mucosa of the uterus;
early phase of proliferation.

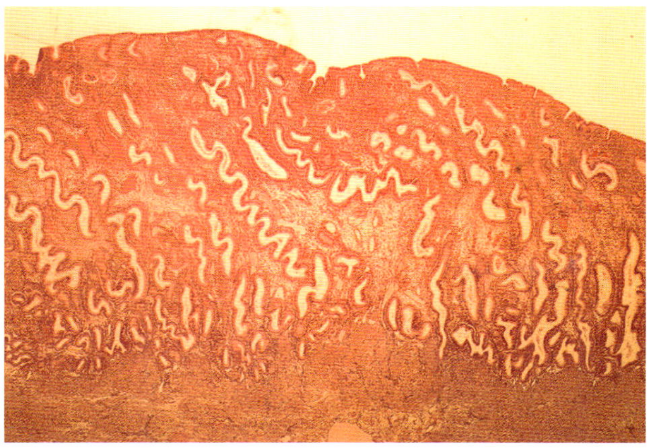

Fig. 857 Mucosa of the uterus;
late phase of proliferation with excretory glands.

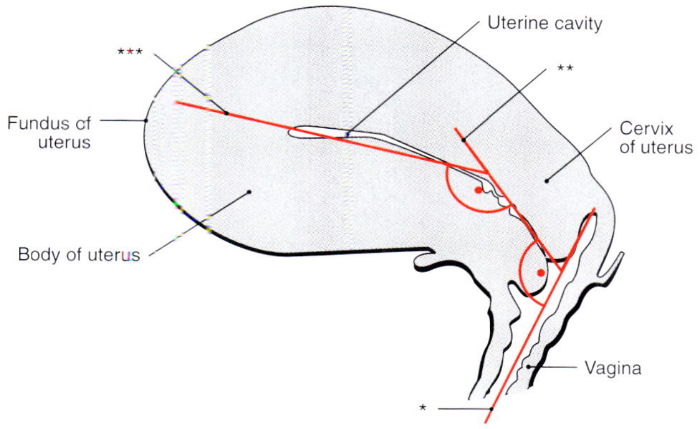

Fig. 858 Uterus and vagina;
normal angles between the vagina, the cervix, and the body of uterus;
viewed from the right.

* Longitudinal axis of the vagina
** Longitudinal axis of the cervix of uterus
*** Longitudinal axis of the body of uterus

Angle between vagina and cervix of uterus = version
Angle between cervix and body of uterus = flexion
Normal topographical situation of the uterus: anteversion, anteflexion
Relation to the median plane = position

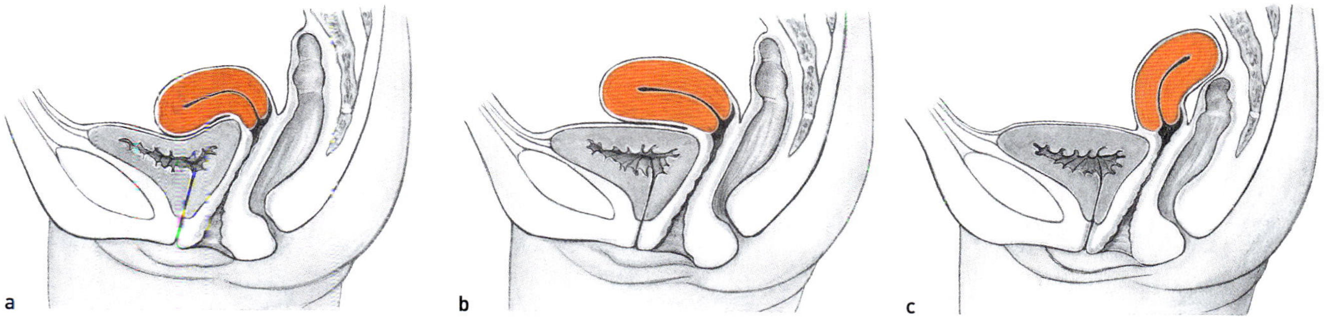

Fig. 859 a–c Uterus and vagina.
a Anteversion, anteflexion = normal position
b Anteversion, but no anteflexion
c Retroversion, retroflexion

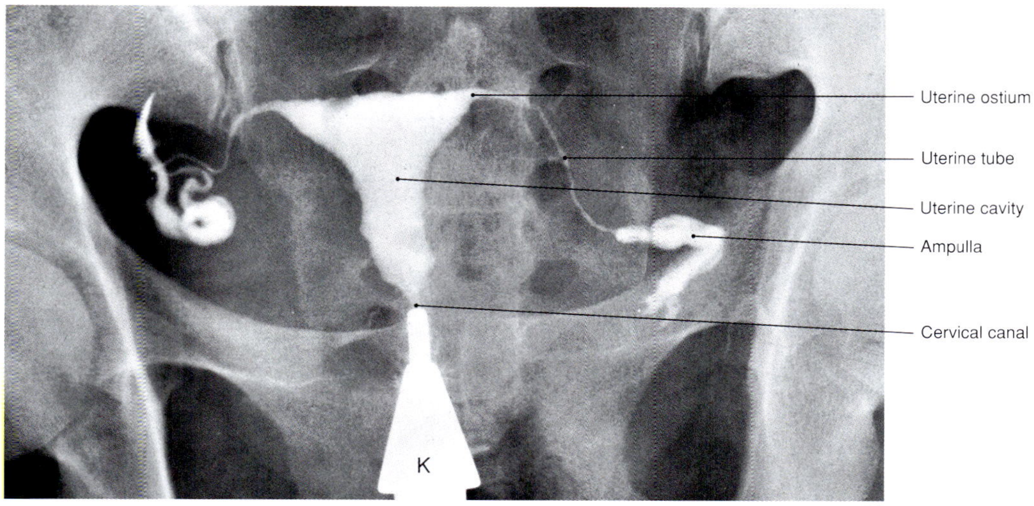

Fig. 860 Uterus and uterine tube;
AP-radiograph after injection of to contrast medium into the cervix of uterus (hysterosalpingography);
uterus in dextroposition;
ventral view.

This formerly clinically applied technique allows to determine the position of the organs and the patency of the tubes.
K = tube adaptor for injection of the contrast medium

Arteries of the femal internal genitalia

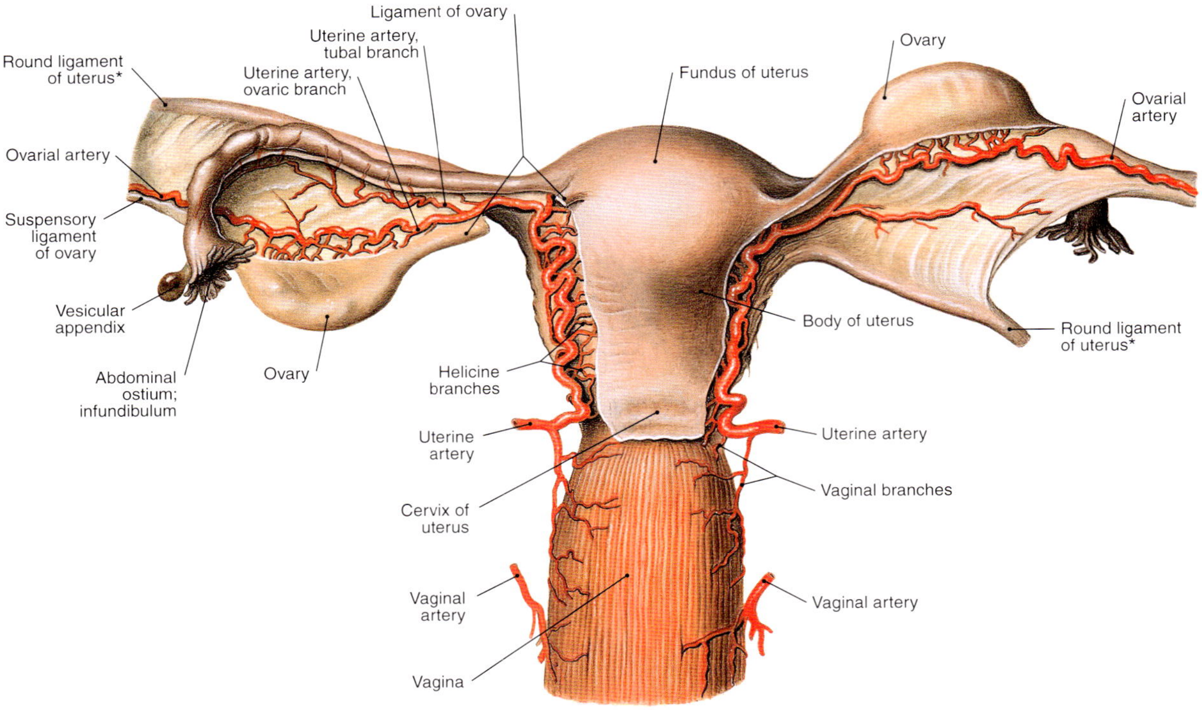

Fig. 861 Arteries of the female internal genitalia; dorsal view.

* Clinical term: round ligament

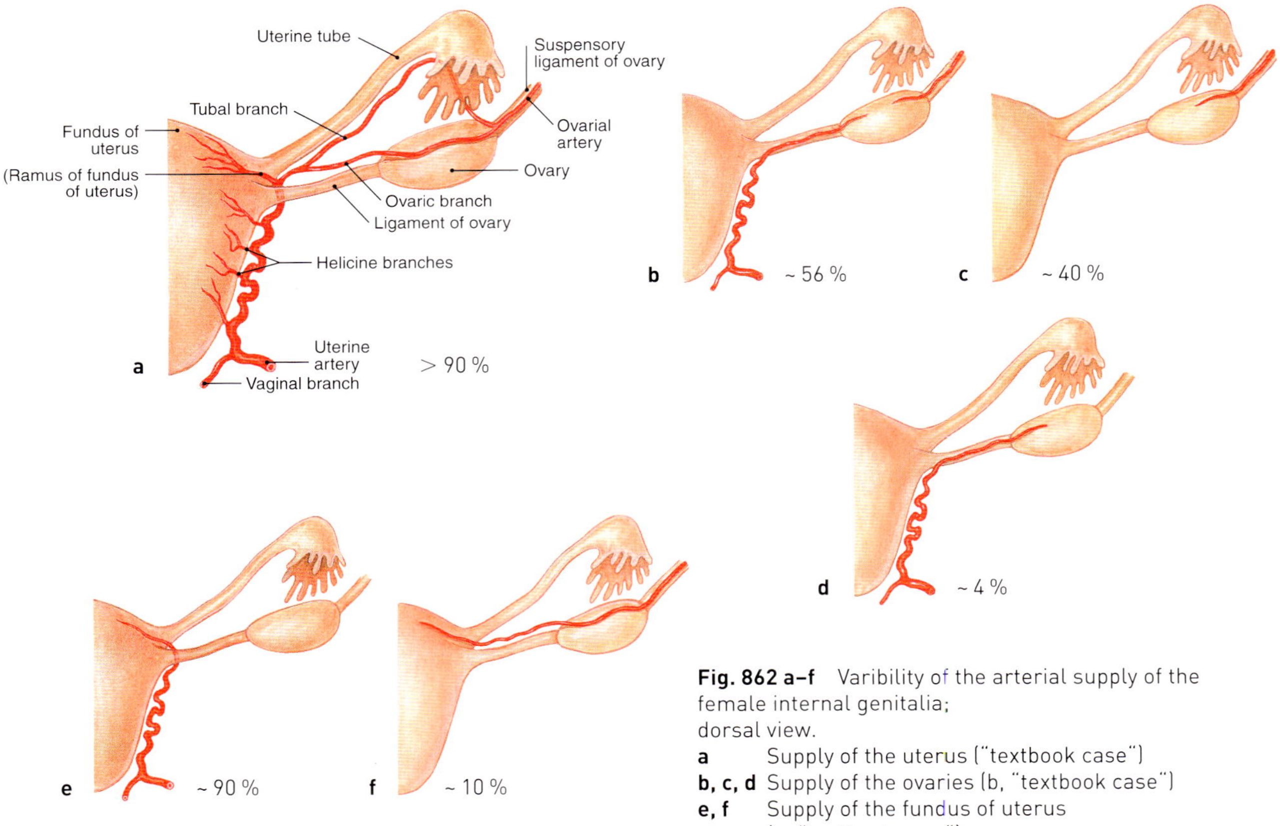

Fig. 862 a–f Varibility of the arterial supply of the female internal genitalia; dorsal view.

a Supply of the uterus ("textbook case")
b, c, d Supply of the ovaries (b, "textbook case")
e, f Supply of the fundus of uterus (e, "textbook case")

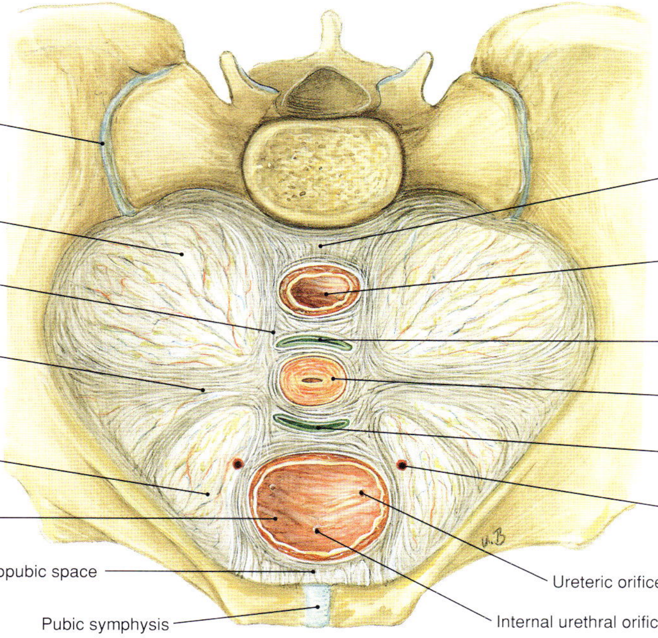

Fig. 863 Uterus;
uterine ligaments and connective tissue spaces;
semi-schematic transverse section at the level of the cervix of uterus;
superior view.

* Clinical term: Paraproctium
** Clinical term: Parametrium
(existence of this structure is controversial)
*** Clinical term: Paracystium

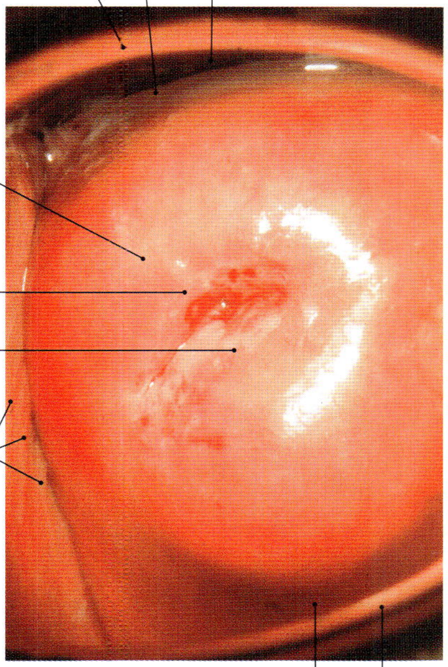

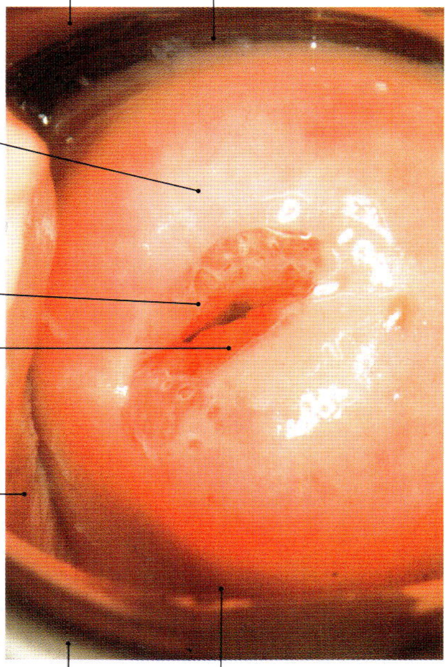

Fig. 864 Vaginal portion of the cervix of uterus.
a Photograph of the cervix of a young nulliparous woman
b Photograph of the cervix of a young woman who has given birth to two children

For the inspection of the vaginal portion of the cervix the normally slit-like vagina is spreaded by means of a bivalve speculum (*);
inferior view.

Pregnancy, ultrasound

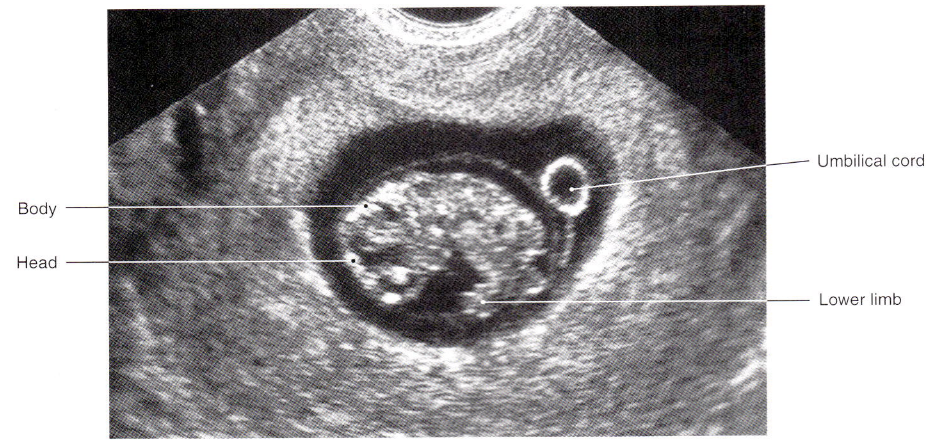

Fig. 865 Uterus with an embryo;
ultrasound image taken in the eighth week of pregnancy;
lateral view (right).

The embryo is immersed in the amniotic fluid of the chorionic cavity.

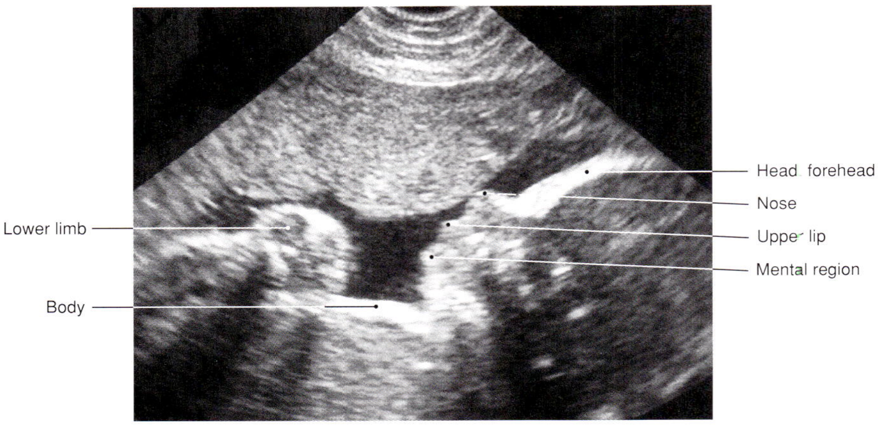

Fig. 866 Uterus with a foetus;
ultrasound image taken in the 28th week of pregnancy;
lateral view (left).

Ultrasound examination allows the visualization of movements of the extremities and the opening of the mouth.

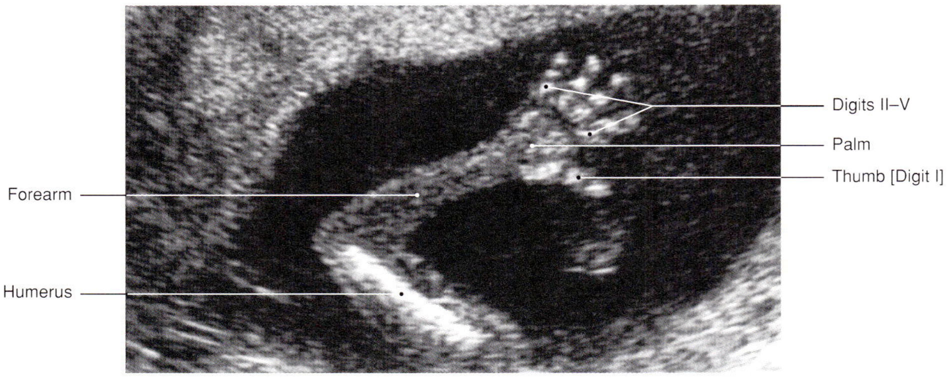

Fig. 867 Hand of a foetus;
ultrasound image taken in the 18th week of pregnancy;
lateral view.

Details such as fingers can be observed.

Pregnancy

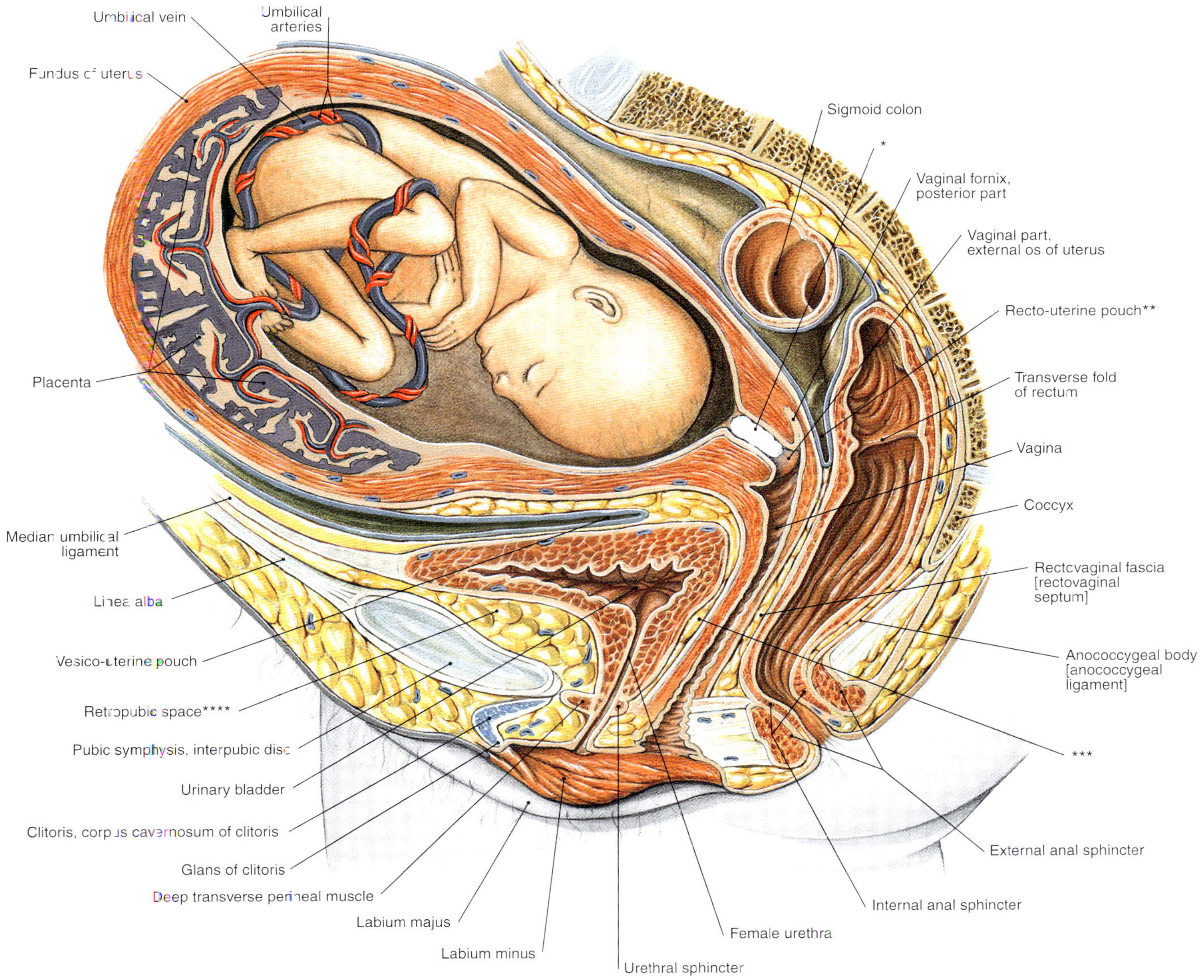

Fig. 868 Uterus with a foetus;
the pelvis has been sectioned in the median plane.

* Mucous plug (of KRISTELLER) in the cervical canal of the uterus
** Clinical term: pouch of DOUGLAS
*** Clinical term: vesicovaginal septum
**** Clinical term: cave of RETZIUS

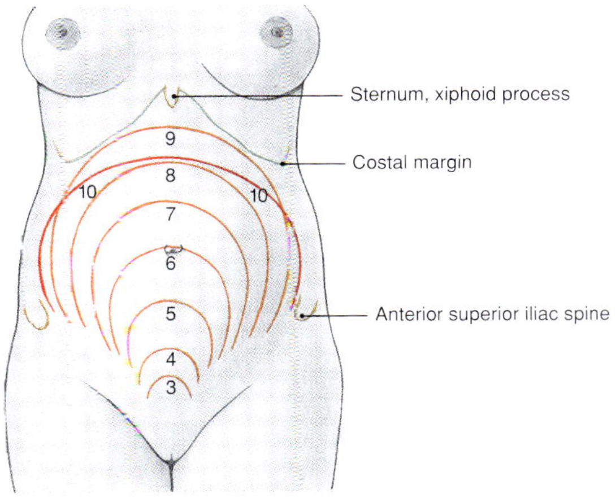

Fig. 869 Uterus;
position of the fundus of uterus during pregnancy.
Numbers refer to the end of the respective month of pregnancy (= 28 days).

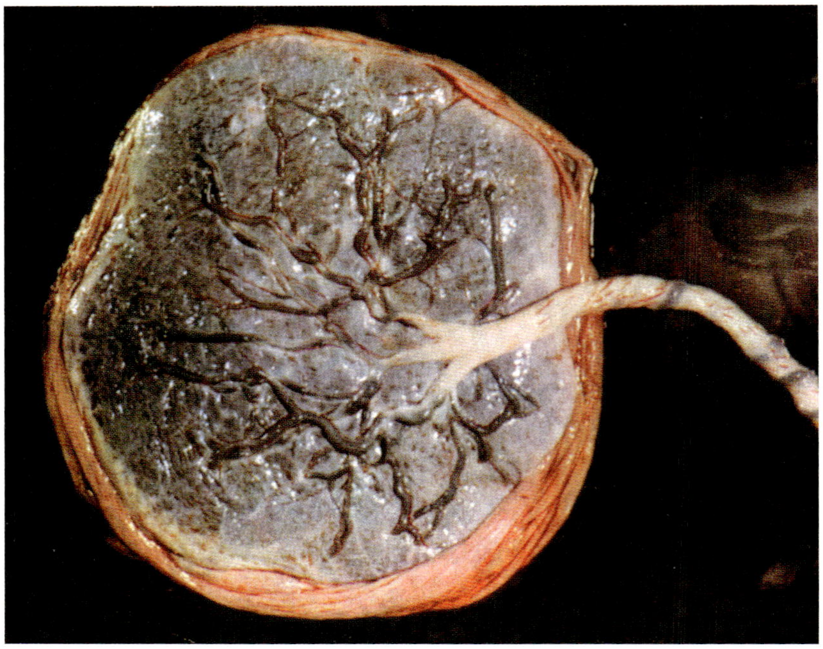

a

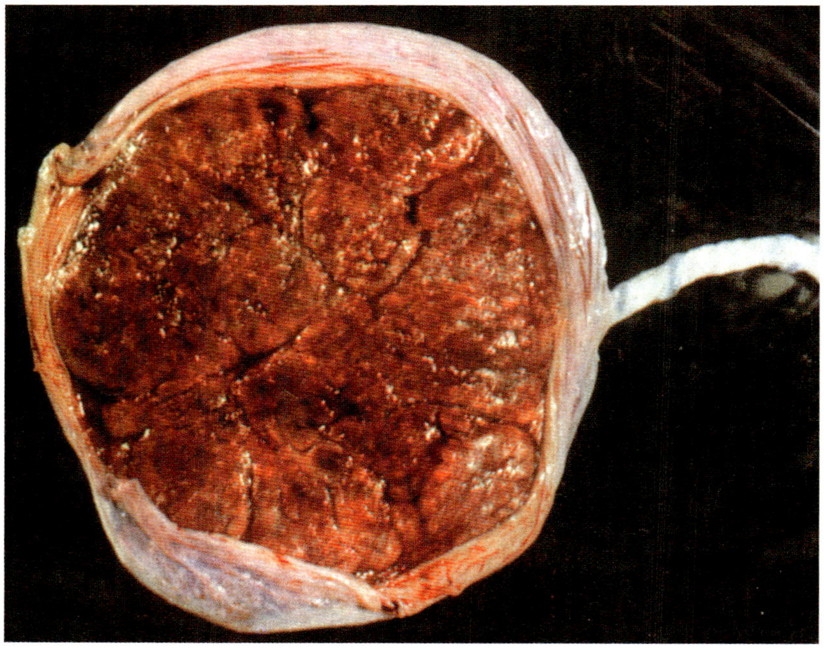

b

Fig. 870 a, b Placenta and umbilical cord.
a View of the foetal surface
b View of the maternal surface of a parturient placenta

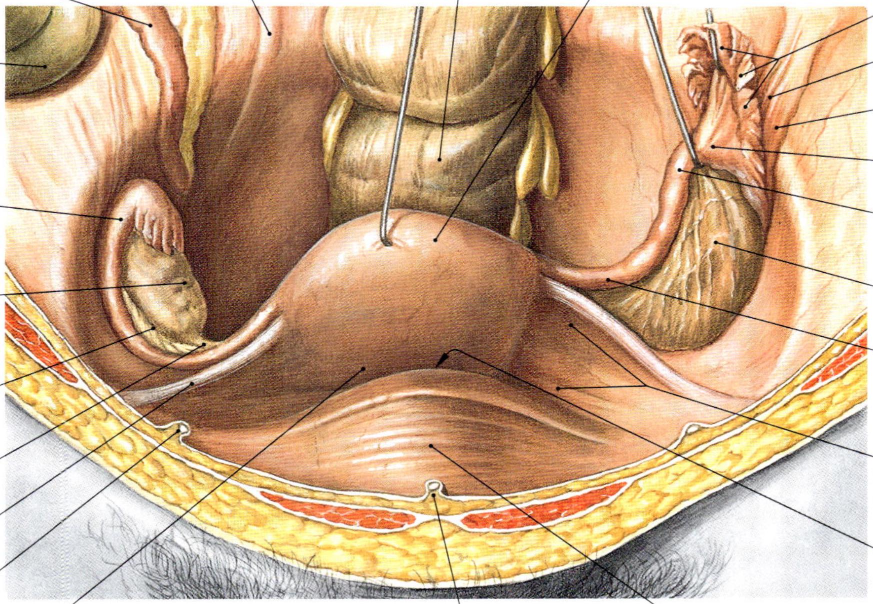

Fig. 871 Female internal genitalia; ventral view.

* Clinical term: infundibulopelvic ligament

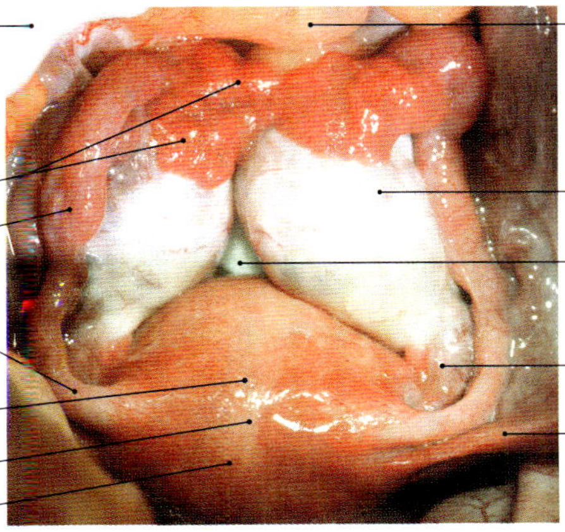

Fig. 872 Female internal genitalia; surgical exposure in a young woman; ovaries displaced both medially and superiorly by compresses (*) in the pouch of DOUGLAS; ventrosuperior view.

** Swab

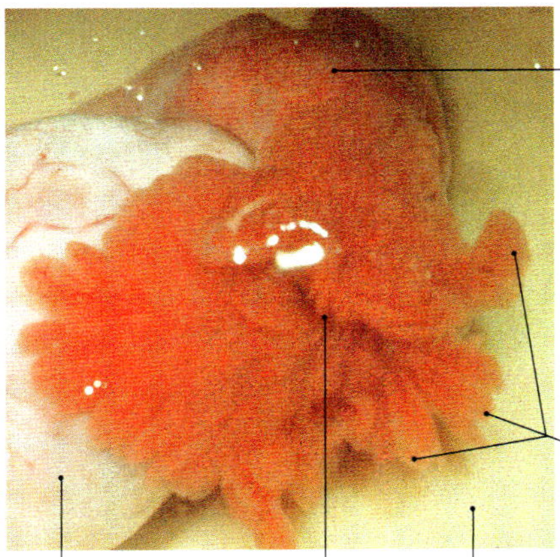

Fig. 873 Abdominal ostium of the uterine tube; surgical exposure in a young woman; the pelvic cavity is filled with saline to demonstrate the fimbria; dorsosuperior view.

* Plastic tray to support the uterine tube

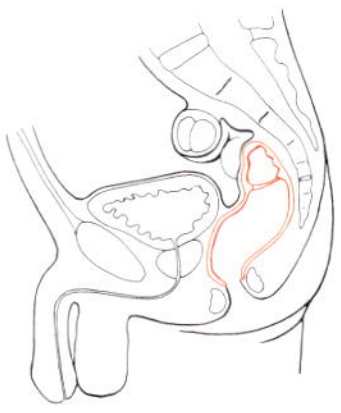

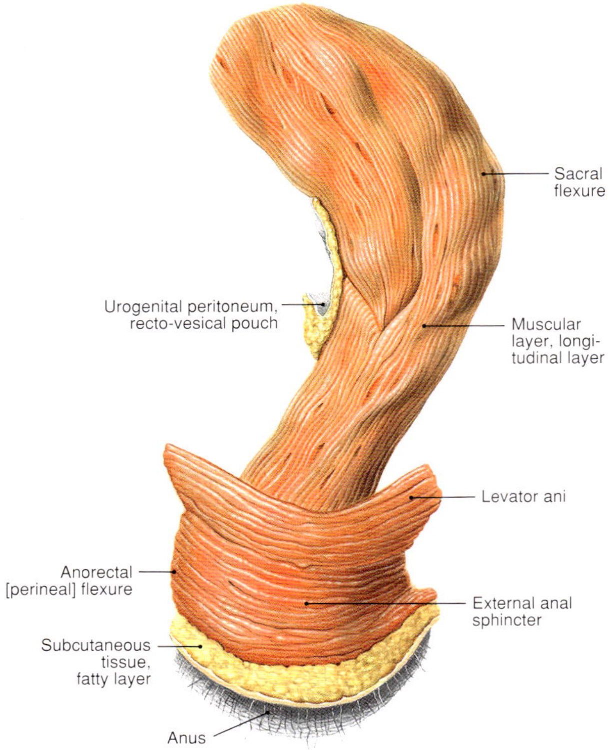

Fig. 874 Rectum;
viewed from the left.

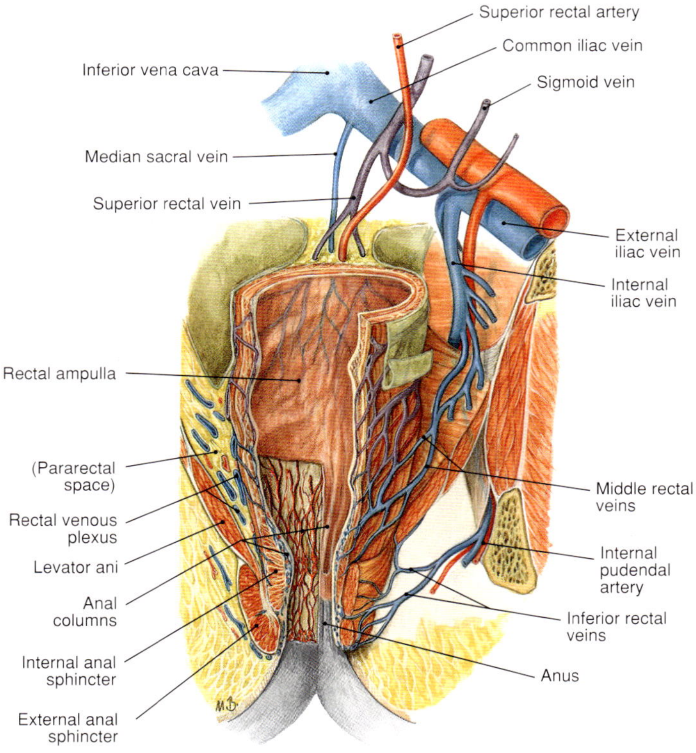

Fig. 875 Rectum;
blood supply; the mucosa and the pararectal adipose tissues have been partly removed; openings into the hepatic portal vein in purple.

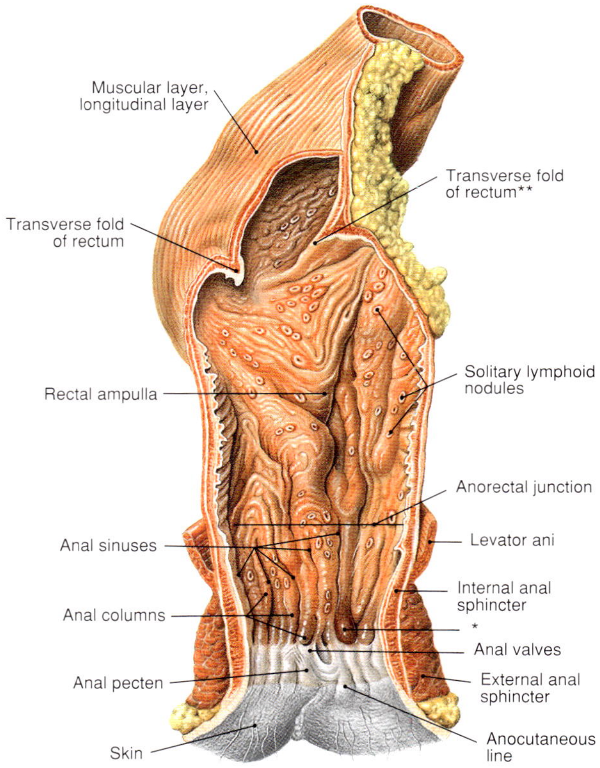

Fig. 876 Rectum and anus;
ventral view.

* Haemorrhoidal node
** KOHLRAUSCH's fold

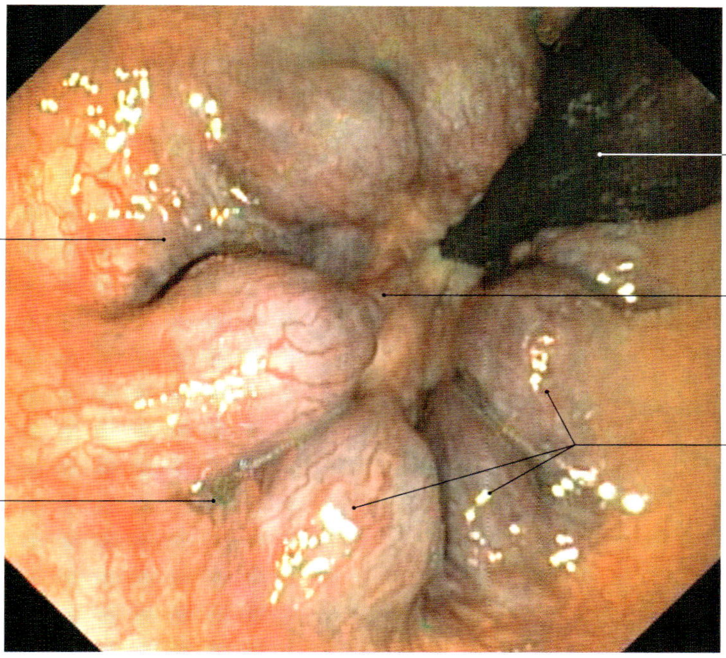

Fig. 877 Rectum;
endoscopic image of the anal canal with six enlarged nodes of the cavernous rectal body, haemorrhoids; superior view.

* Colonoscope
** Three haemorrhoidal nodes

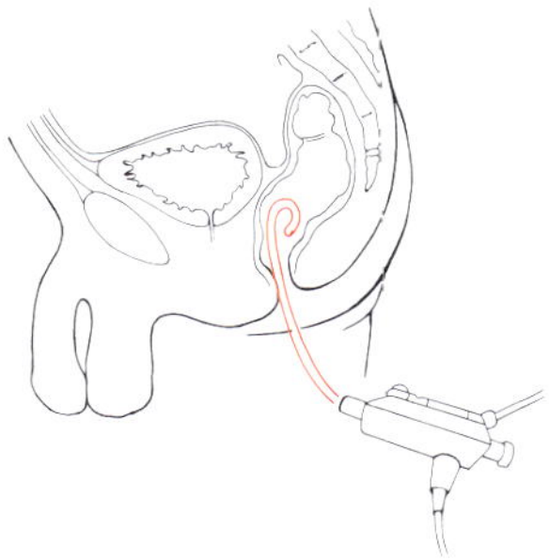

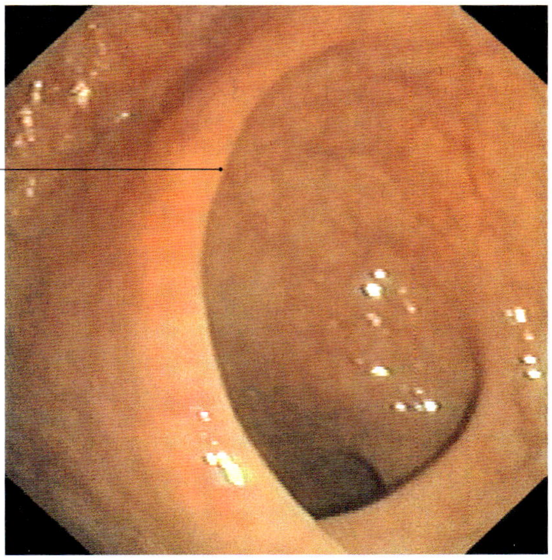

Fig. 878 Rectum;
endoscopic image of the rectal ampulla (rectoscopy); inferior view.

Arteries of the rectum

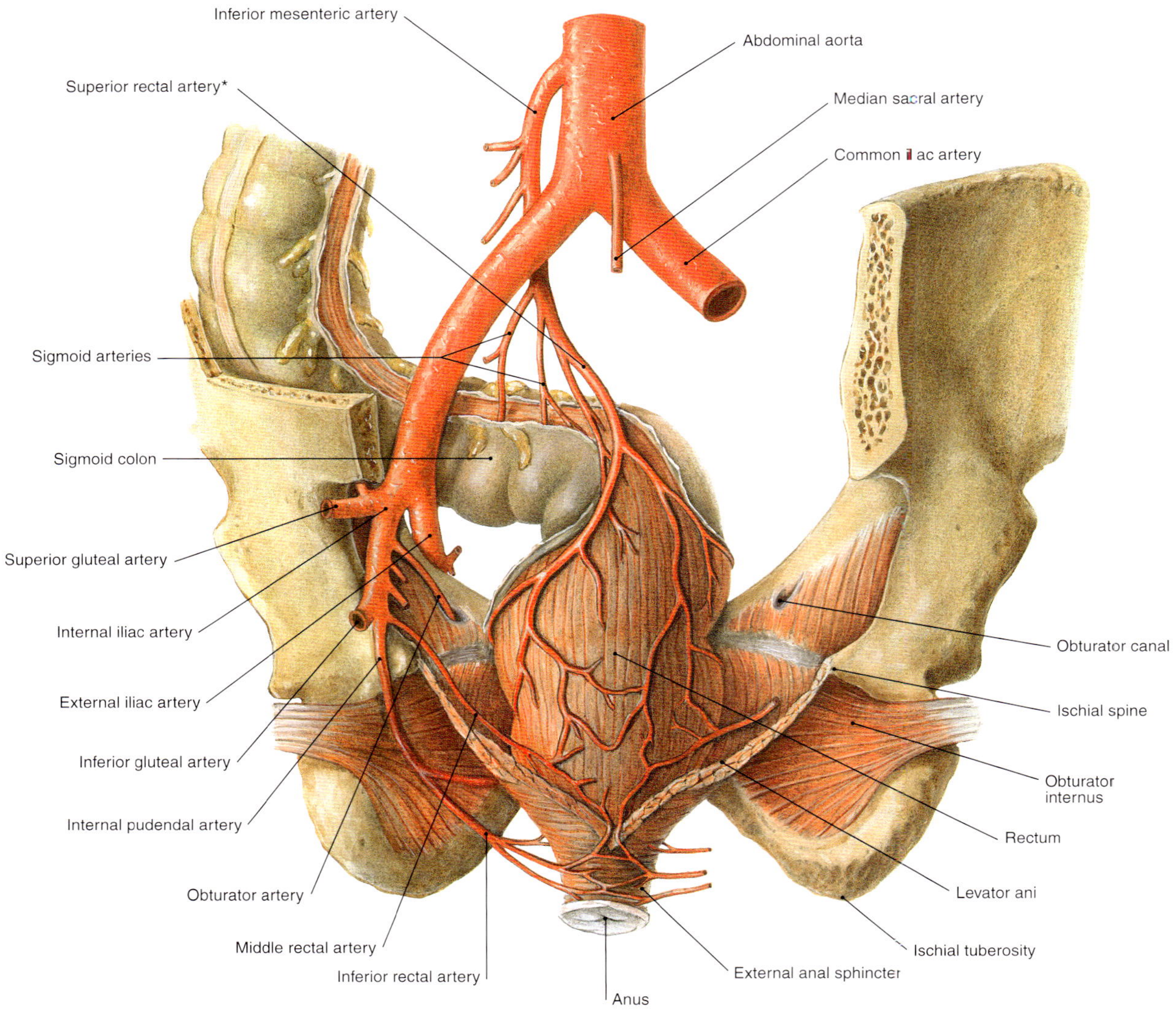

Fig. 879 Rectal arteries;
dorsal view.

* Clinical term: SUDECK's point (from this point on there are no further anastomoses with the sigmoid arteries)

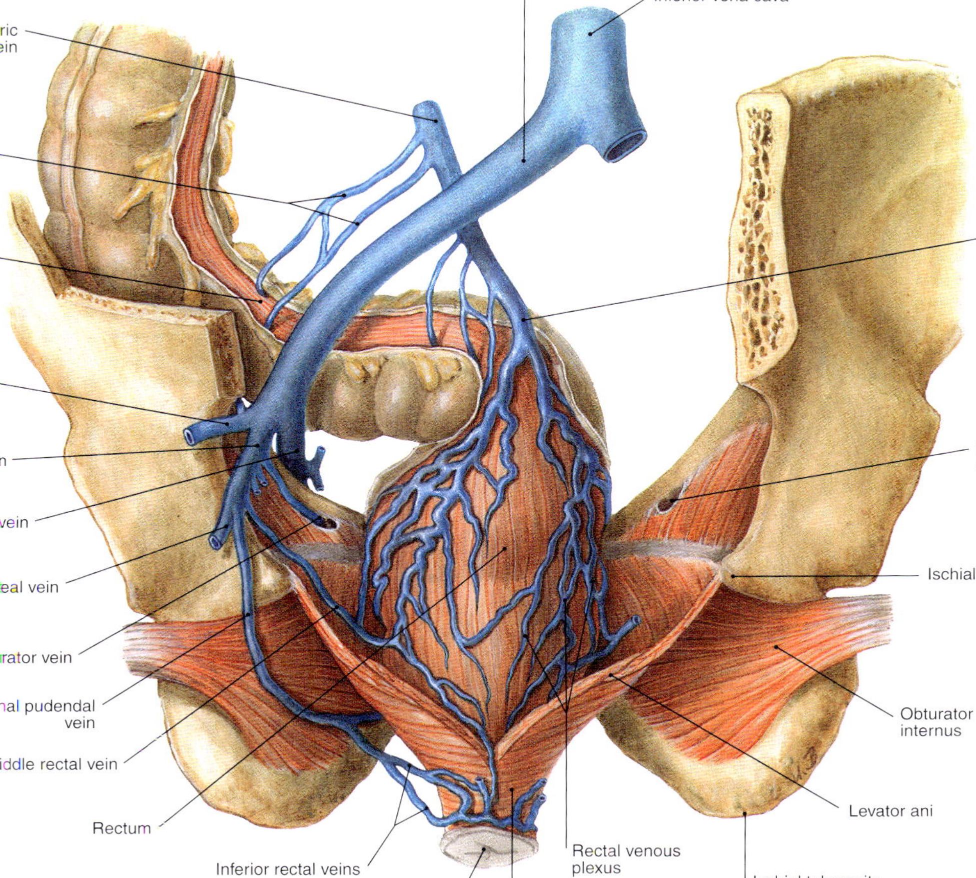

Fig. 880 Rectal veins;
diagram with parts of the pelvis and the pelvic diaphragm;
dorsal view.
There are numerous connections between the veins draining into the hepatic portal vein (superior rectal vein) and those draining into the inferior vena cava (middle and inferior rectal veins). They form the portocaval anastomoses, which are of particular clinical importance.

→ 809, 810

Innervation of the rectum

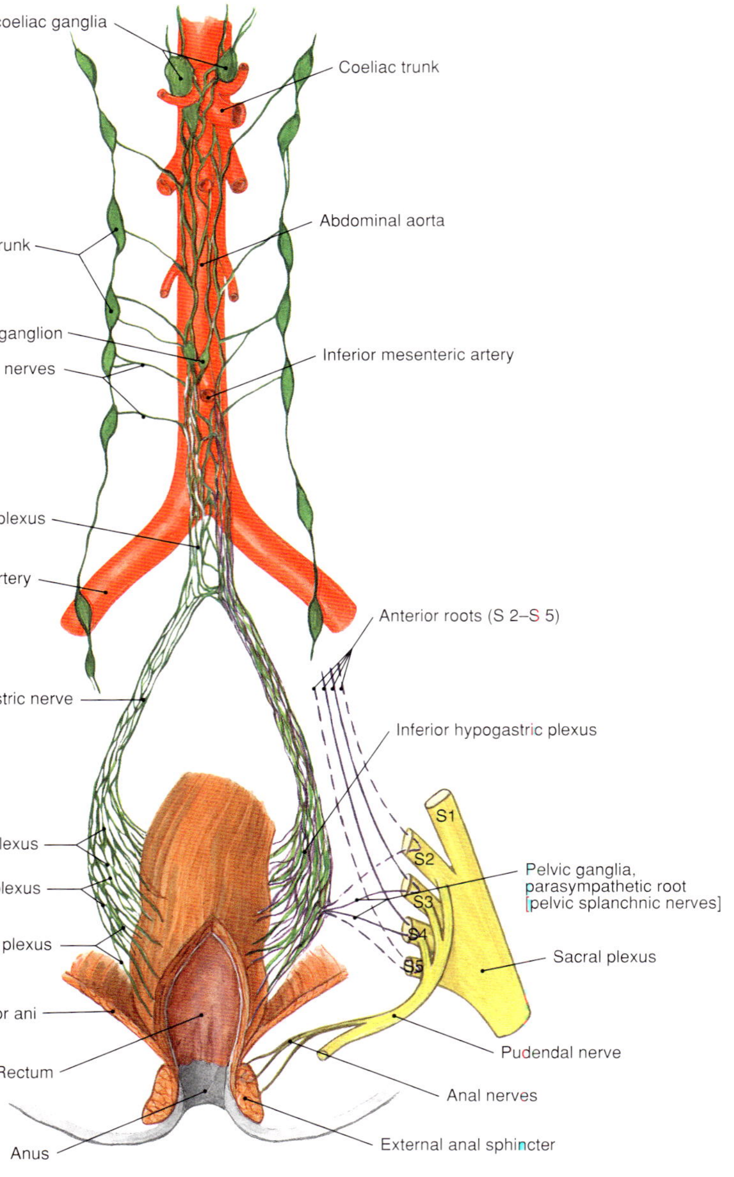

Fig. 881 Rectum;
schematic overview of the innervation;
ventral view.
Green = sympathetic nervous system
Purple = parasympathetic nervous system

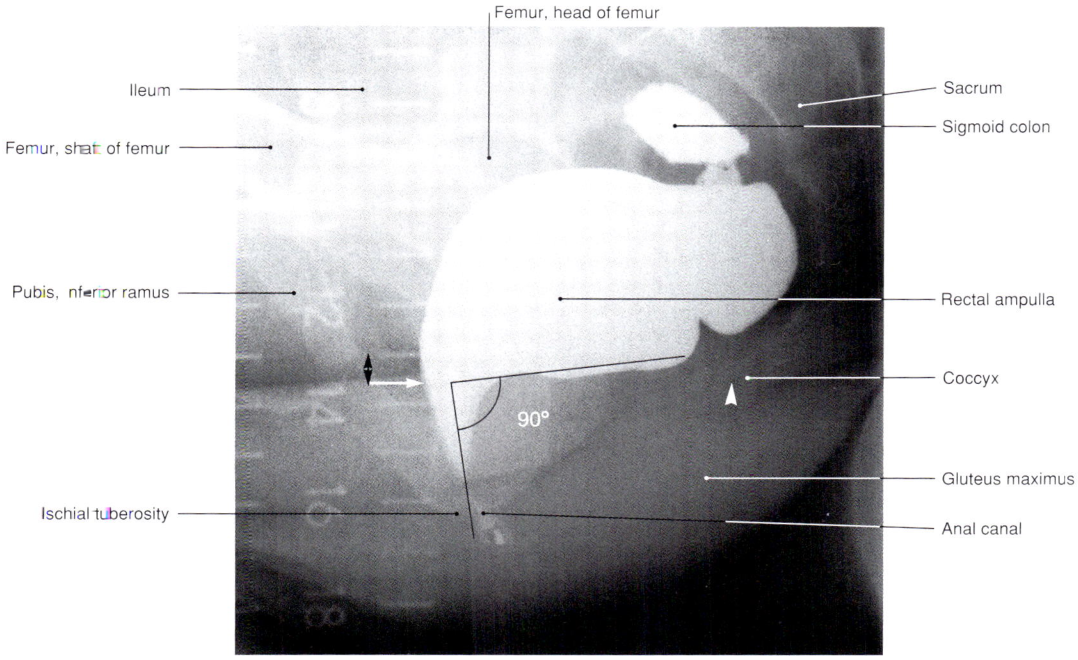

Fig. 882 Rectum;
lateral radiograph in voluntary closure of the anus after filling with a contrast medium (defaecography).

The transitional zone between the anus and the rectum (arrow) is located at the level of the tip of the coccyx (triangle). The angle between the axes of the anus and the rectum (∡) is approximately 90° and depends upon the curvature of the levator ani muscle (puborectal muscle). Scale in cm.

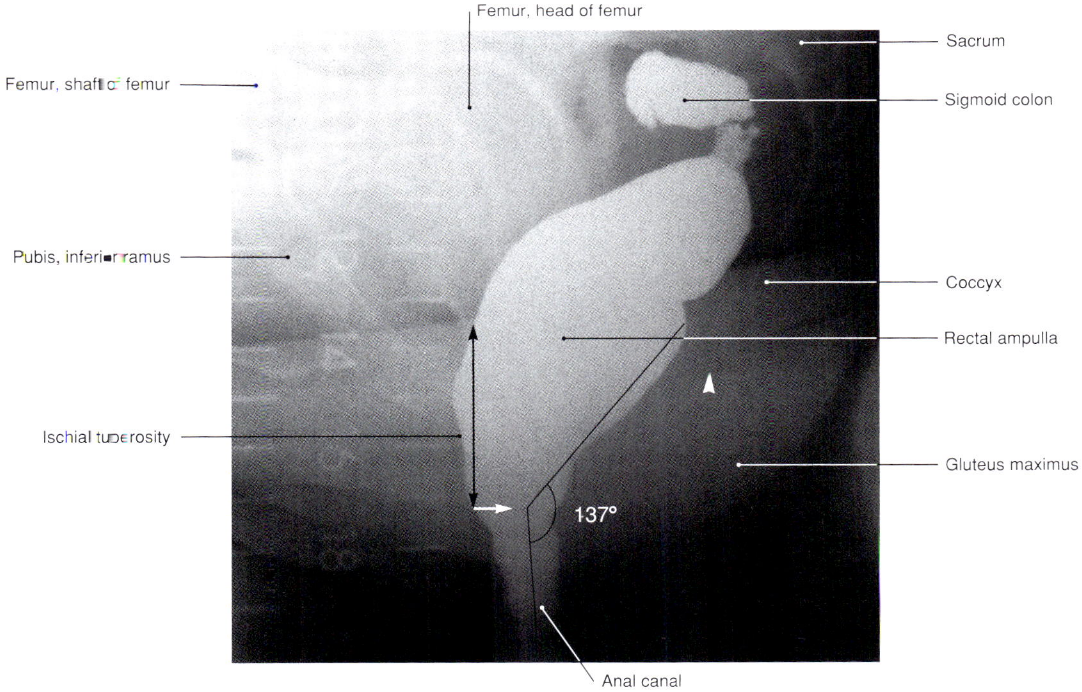

Fig. 883 Rectum;
lateral radiograph of the defaecation after filling with a contrast medium (defaecography).

In comparison to Fig. 882, the anorectal transitional zone has descended and the angle (∡) increased to 137° due to the relaxation of the curvature of the levator ani muscle. As the bending acts like a valve, the elongation results in an unimpeded pressure of the faeces on the anal canal leading to defaecation.

Arterial supply of the kidney

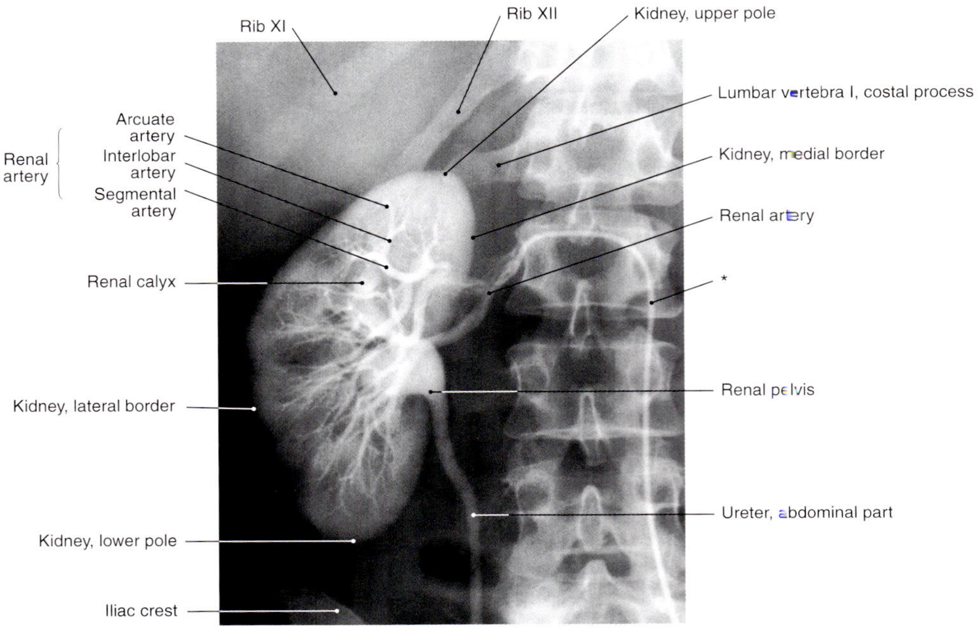

Fig. 884 Kidney;
AP-radiograph after intravenous injection of a contrast medium which is excreted via the kidneys to demonstrate the renal pelvis and the ureters (intravenous pyelography); concomitant visualization of the arteries by injection of a contrast medium into the renal artery through a catheter* introduced into the aorta (arteriography).

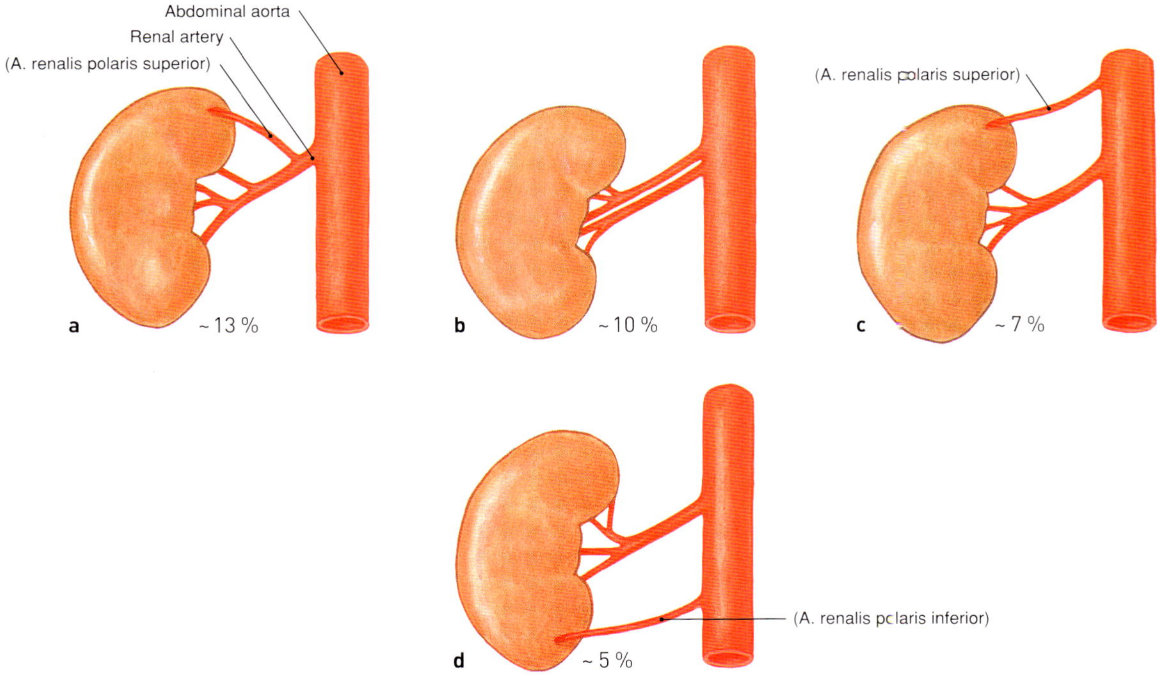

Fig. 885 a–d Variations in the arterial supply of the kidney.
a One renal artery with a branch to the superior pole
b Two renal arteries to the renal hilum
c Two renal arteries, one of which supplies the superior pole
d Two renal arteries, one of which supplies the inferior pole

Retroperitoneal space, overview

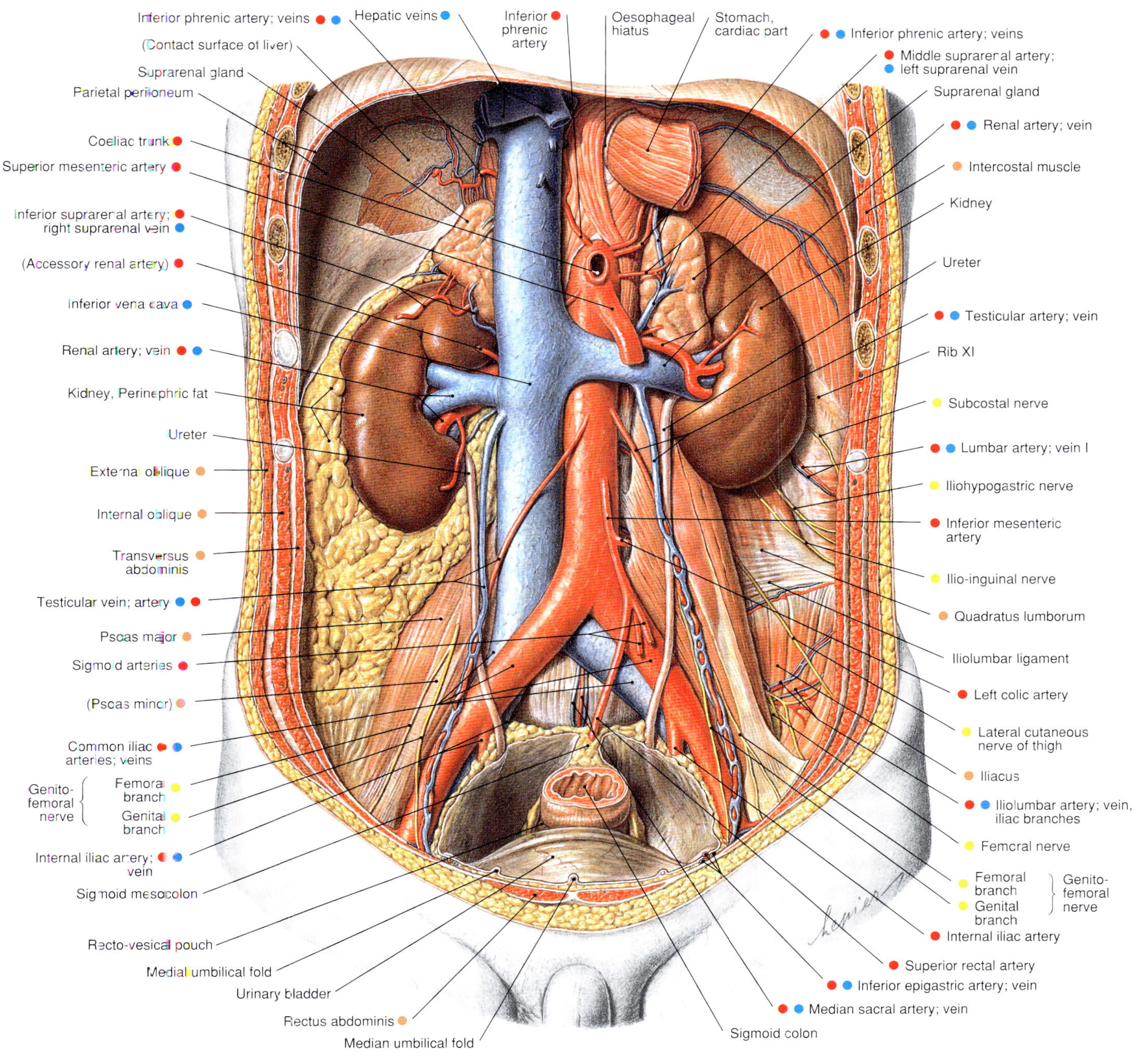

Fig. 886 Position of the retroperitoneal structures of the male.
Whereas the left testicular vein opens into the left renal vein, the right testicular vein drains directly into the inferior vena cava. The same applies to the ovarian veins.

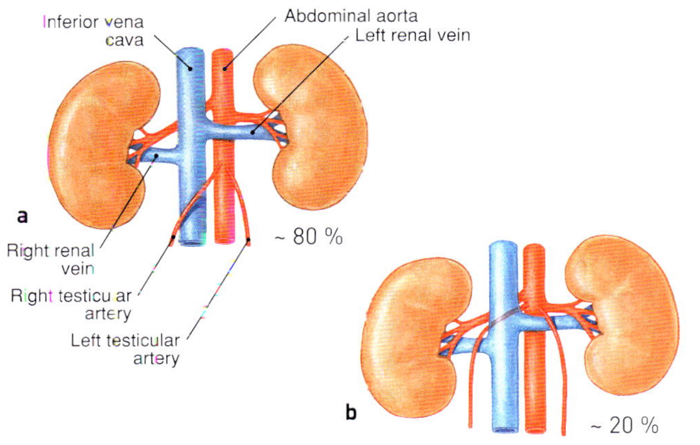

Fig. 887 a, b Variability of the course of the testicular arteries.
a "Textbook case"
b Both testicular arteries branch off cranially to the renal veins; the right artery passes posterior to the inferior vena cava and the left artery passes anterior to the left renal vein.

Lymphatics of the retroperitoneal space

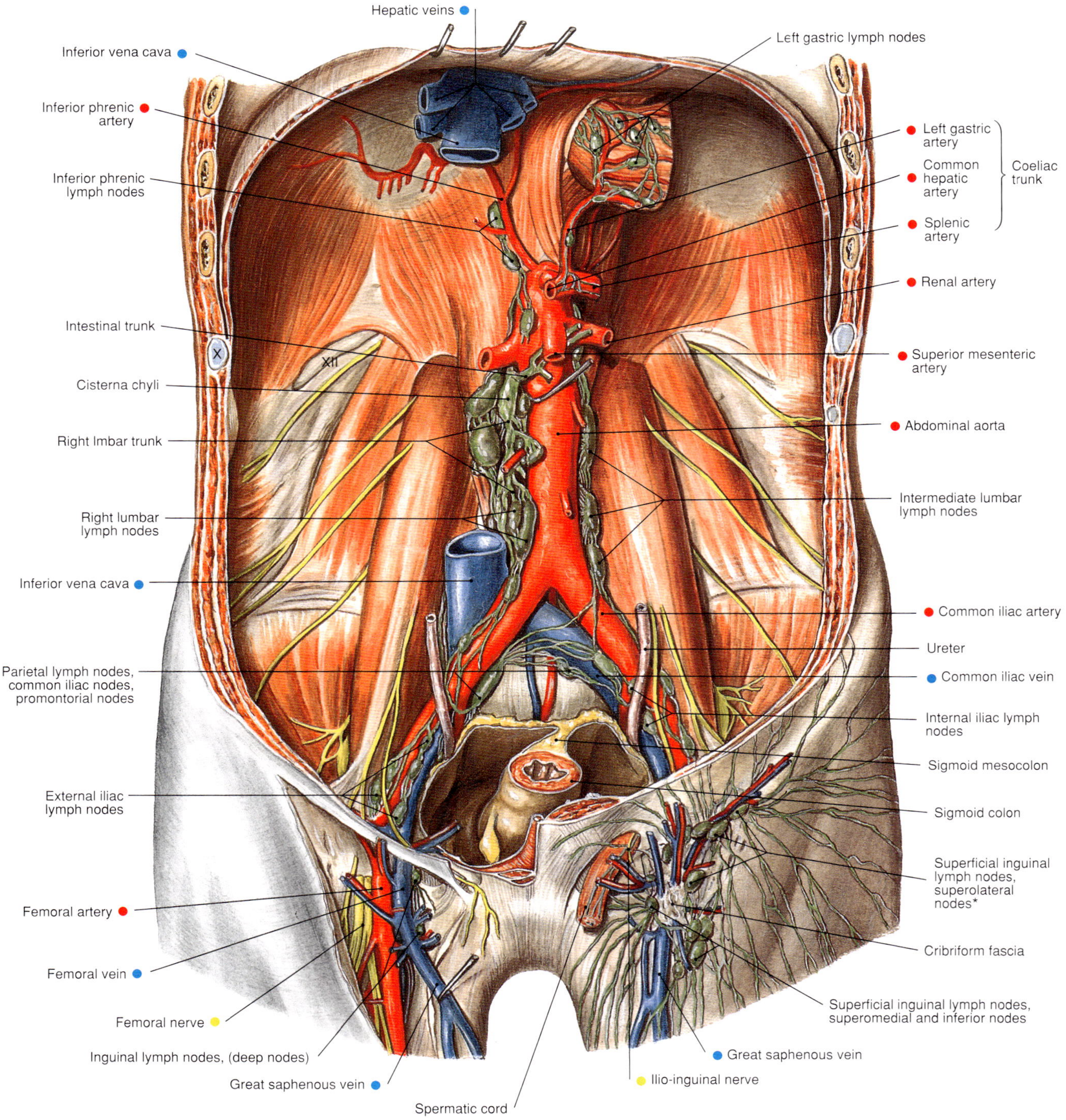

→ 1121

Fig. 888 Lymph nodes and lymphatics of the posterior abdominal wall and the inguinal region; ventral view.

The numbers X and XII indicate the respective ribs.

* Clinical term: „horizontal chain", draining the lower abdominal wall, the gluteal region, the perineum and the external genital

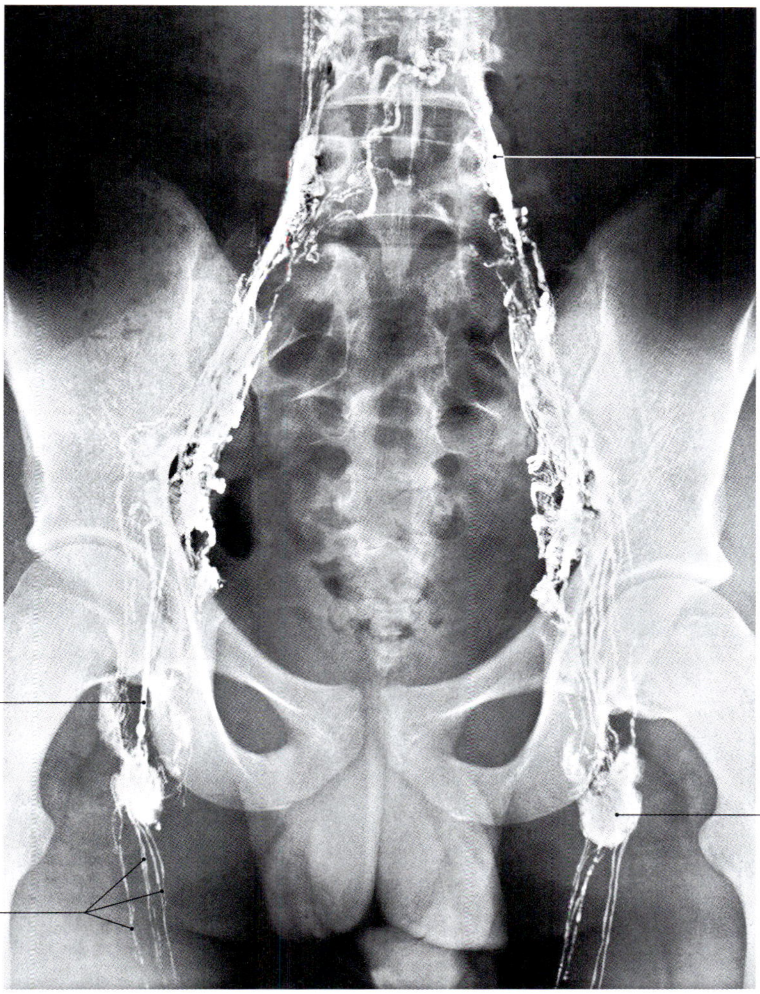

Fig. 889 Lymphatics and lymph nodes of the inguinal, the pelvic and the lumbar region;
AF-radiograph after bilateral injection of a contrast medium into lymphatics of the foot (lymphography).
This formerly applied technique visualizes the position and size of lymphatics and lymph nodes.

Nerves of the retroperitoneal space

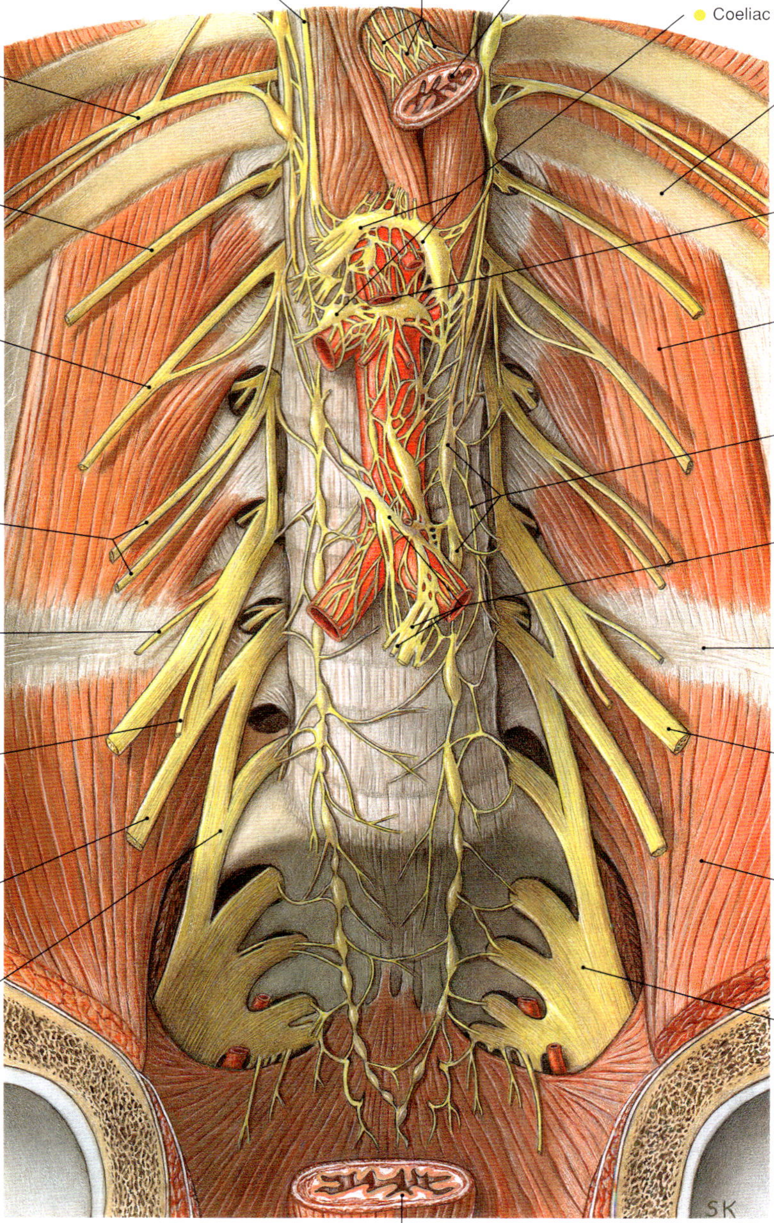

→ 47, 49, 50

Fig. 890 Nerves of the posterior abdominal wall, the lumbosacral plexus and the abdominal part of the autonomous nervous system; ventral view.

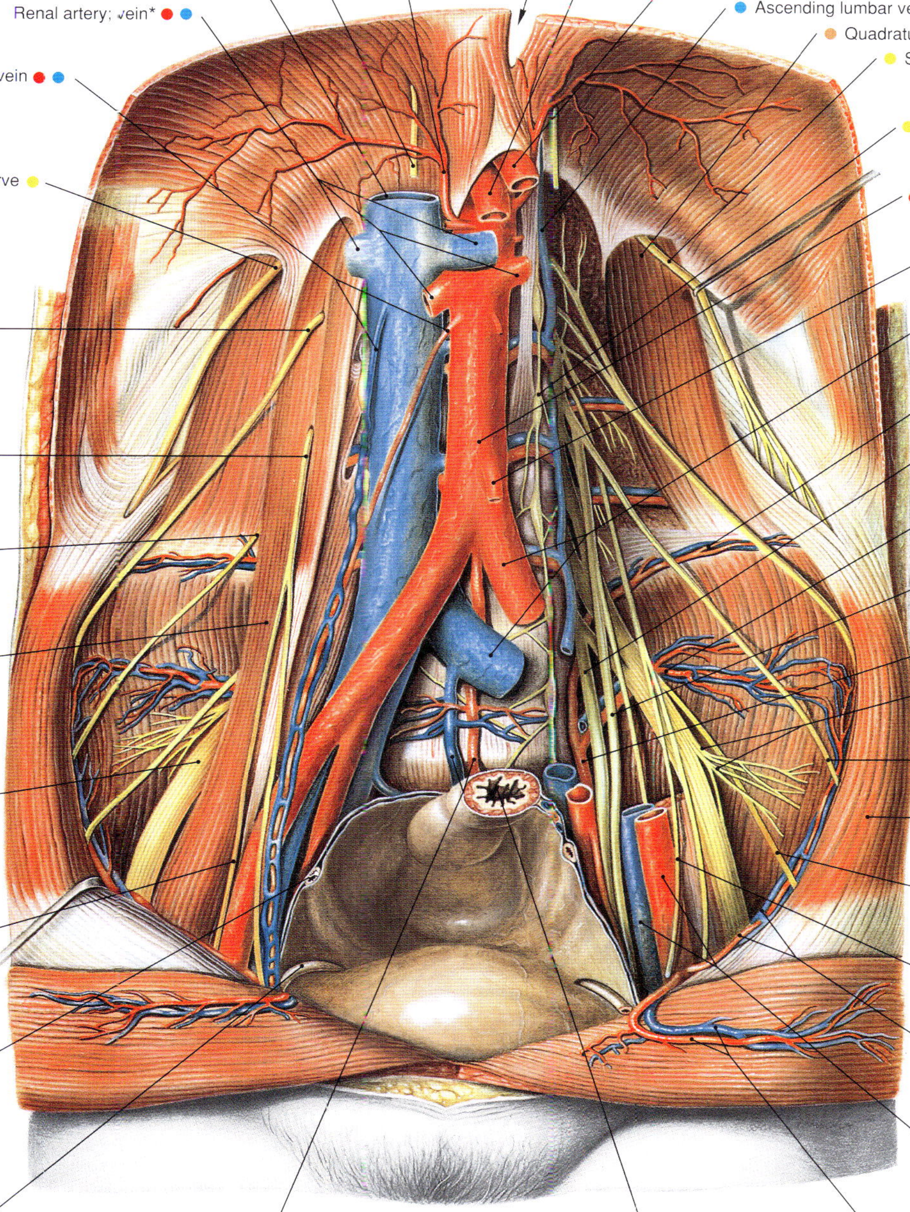

Fig. 891 Vessels and nerves of the posterior abdominal wall of the male.

* In ~10% the left renal vein passes posterior to the aorta.

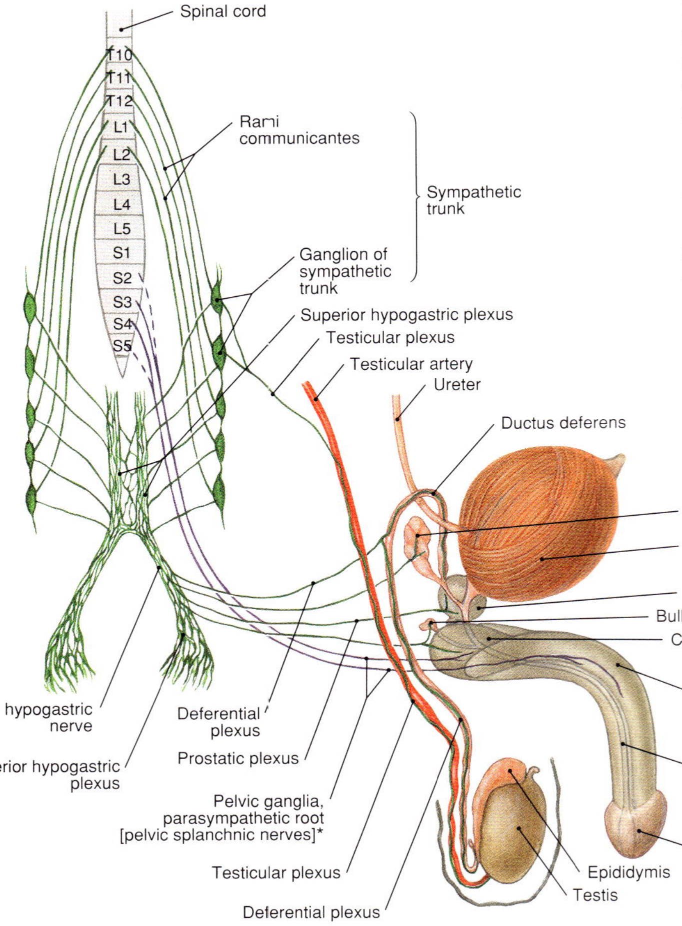

Fig. 892 Male genitalia;
diagram demonstrating the autonomous innervation of the left side;
ventral and lateral view, respectively.
Green = sympathetic nervous system
Purple = parasympathetic nervous system

* Also: erigent nerves

Surgical removal of paraaortic lymph nodes or operations at the abdominal aorta and the large arteries of the pelvis can cause damage to the sympathetic nerves with the consequence of ejaculatory impotency (Impotentia generandi). Prostate operations, in turn, may damage the parasympathetic fibres innervating the penis, thus leading to erectile impotency (Impotentia coeundi).

Innervation of the male genitalia

	Origin	Course	Organ	Function
Parasympathetic	Sacral part of the spinal cord (S2 – S4)	Pelvic ganglia, parasympathetic root (pelvic splanchnic nerves)	Penis Corpus cavernosum	Vasodilatation Erection
Sympathetic	Thoracic part of the spinal cord (T10 – T12)	Superior and inferior mesenteric plexus ↓ Sympathetic trunk ↓ Testicular plexus	Testis	Regulation of blood flow
	Lumbar part of the spinal cord (L1 – L2)	Superior hypogastric plexus ↓ Hypogastric nerve ↓ Inferior hypogastric plexus	Bulbo-urethral glands	Expulsion of its fluid
			Ductus (vas) deferens	Contraction, transport of the sperms into the urethra
			Vesicular gland Prostata	Expulsion of its content into the urethra
Somatomotor, somatosensory	Sacral part of the spinal cord (S2 – S4)	Pudendal nerve	(Sphincter vesicae)	Closure of the urinary bladder to prevent retrograde ejaculation
			Ischiocavernosus Bulbospongiosus	Expulsion of the ejaculate out of the urethra
		Posterior scrotal nerves Dorsal nerve of penis	Scrotal skin Penile skin	

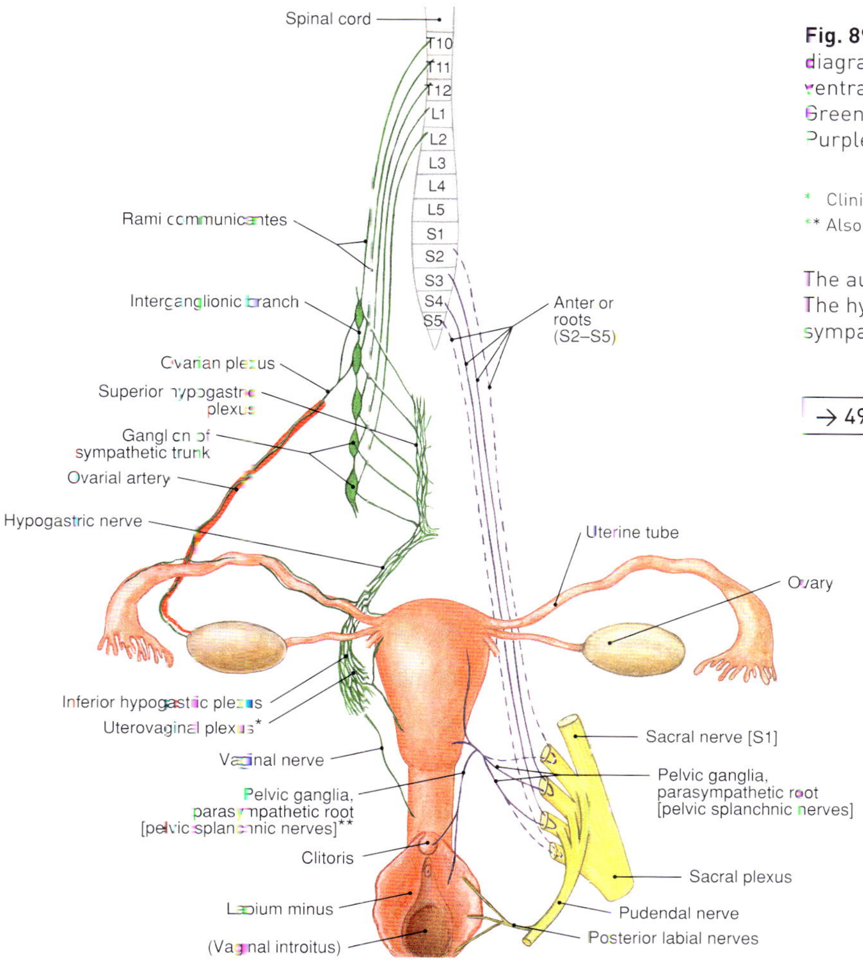

Fig. 893 Female genitalia;
diagram demonstrating the autonomous innervation;
ventral view.
Green = sympathetic nervous system
Purple = parasympathetic nervous system

* Clinical term: FRANKENHÄUSER's ganglion
** Also: erigent nerves

The autonomic plexus are interspersed with ganglia. The hypogastric and uterovaginal plexus contain both sympathetic and parasympathetic fibres.

→ 49, 50

Innervation of the female genitalia

	Origin	Course	Organ	Function
Parasympathetic	Sacral part of the spinal cord (S2 – S4)	Pelvic ganglia, parasympathetic root (pelvic splanchnic nerves)	Uterine tube Uterus	Vasodilatation Vasodilatation
		↓ Cavernous nerves of clitoris	Vagina Clitoris	Transsudation Erection
Sympathetic	Thoracic part of the spinal cord (T10 – T12)	Superior mesenteric plexus ↘ Ovarian plexus ↗ Renal plexus	Ovary	Vasoconstriction
		Sympathetic trunk ↓		
	Lumbar part of the spinal cord (L1 – L2)	Superior hypogastric plexus ↓ Hypogastric nerve Inferior hypogastric plexus	-	
		↓ Uterovaginal plexus (FRANKENHÄUSER's ganglion)	Uteri Uterus Vagina	Contraction
Somatomotor, somatosensory	Sacral part of the spinal cord (S2 – S4)	Pudendal nerve ↗ Dorsal nerve of clitoris	Clitoris	
		Pudendal nerve ↘ Posterior labial nerves	Labia majora Ischiocavernosus Bulbospongiosus	Contraction

Pelvic arteries

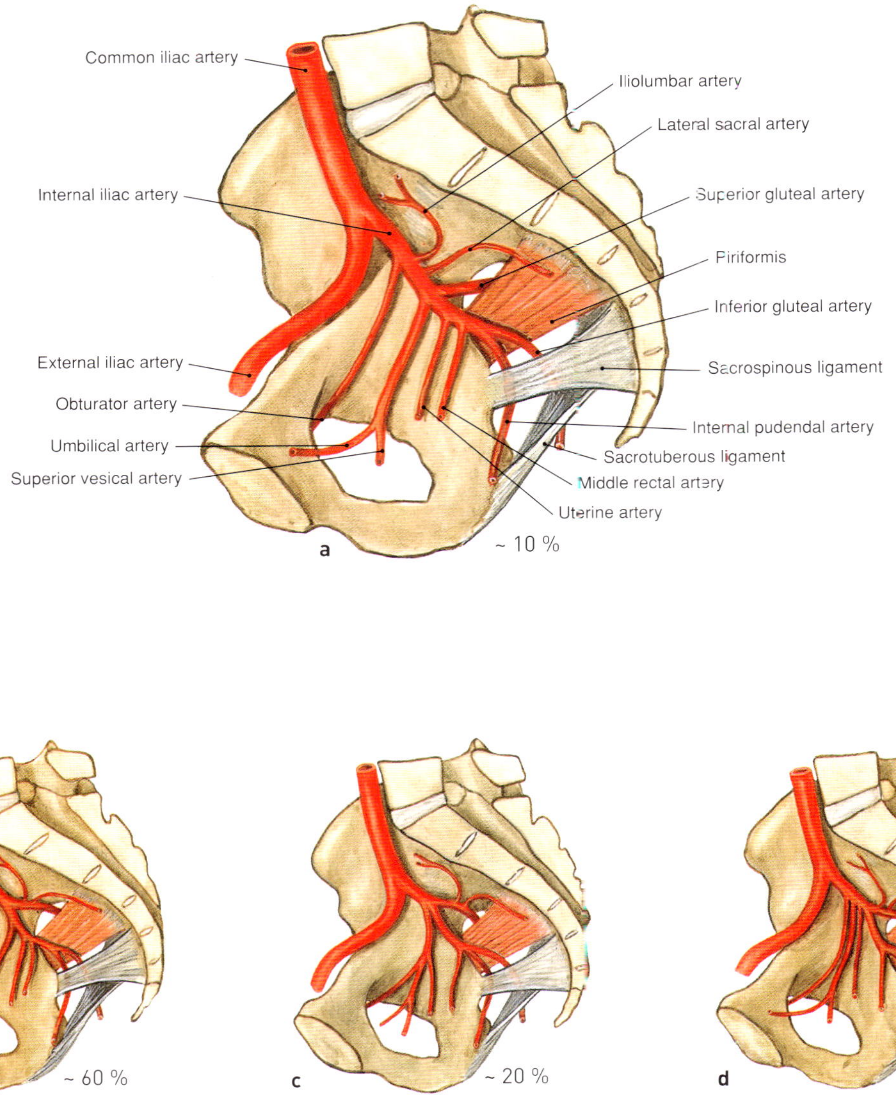

Fig. 894 a–d Variability of the branching pattern of the internal iliac artery; viewed from the left.
a All branches arise from the same stem.
b The internal iliac artery divides into two major branches („textbook case").
c The internal iliac artery divides into three major branches.
d The internal iliac artery divides into more than three major branches.

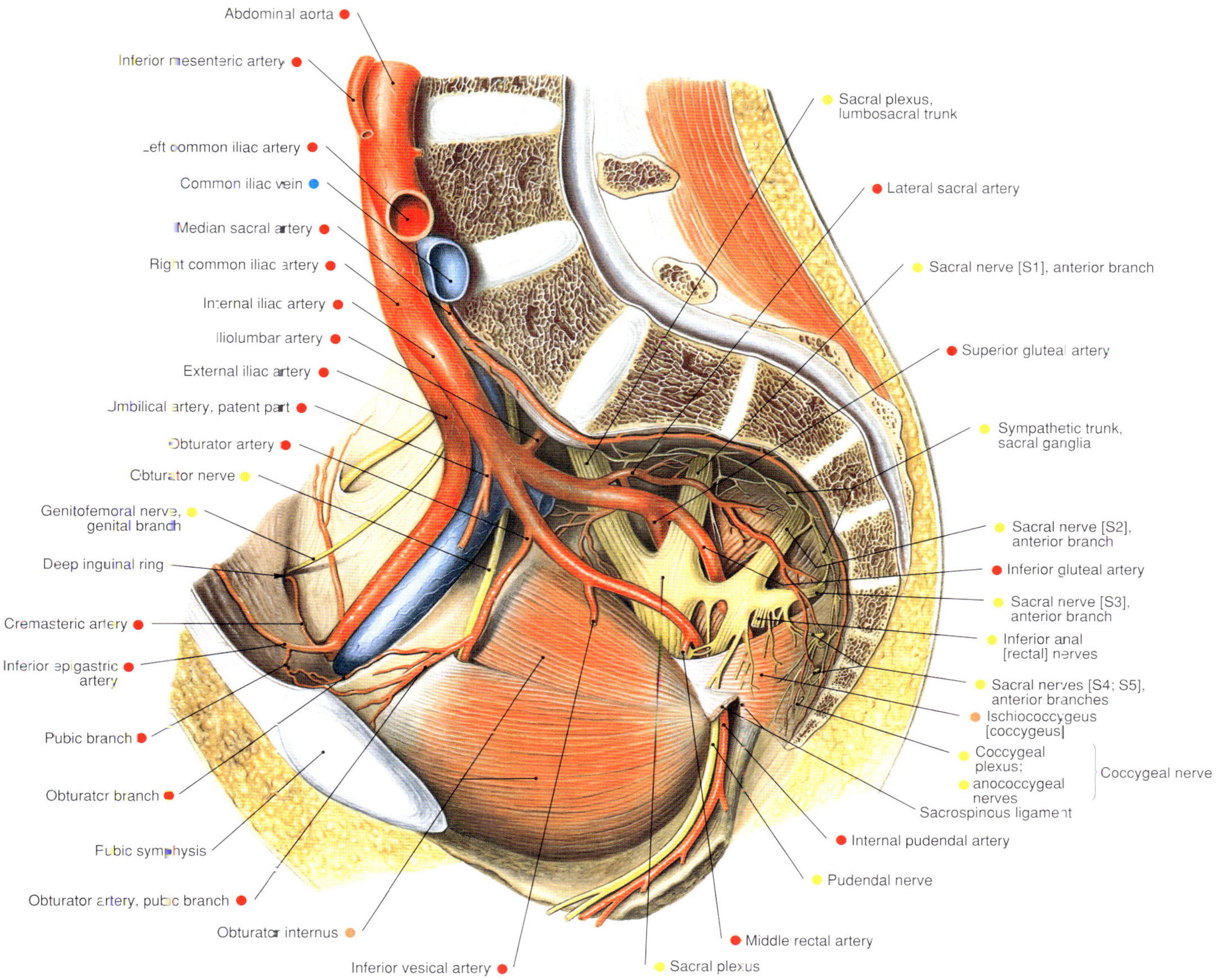

Fig. 895 Internal iliac artery and sacral plexus; viewed from the left.

Organs of the male pelvis

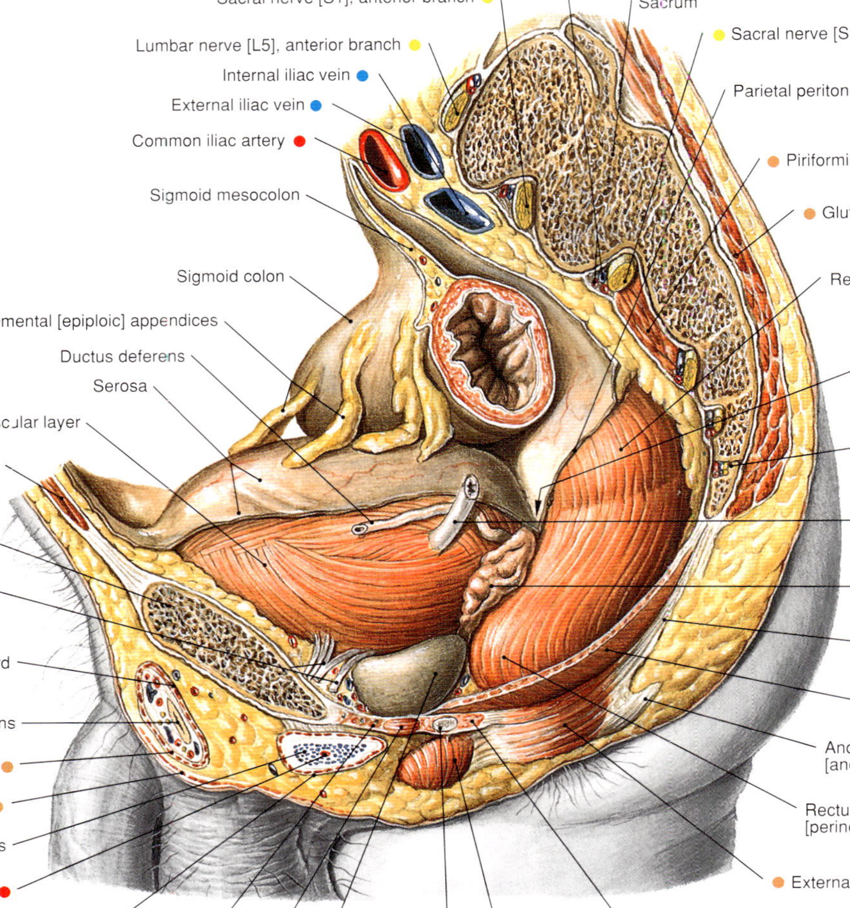

Fig. 896 Organs of the male pelvis.

* Clinical term: COWPER's gland

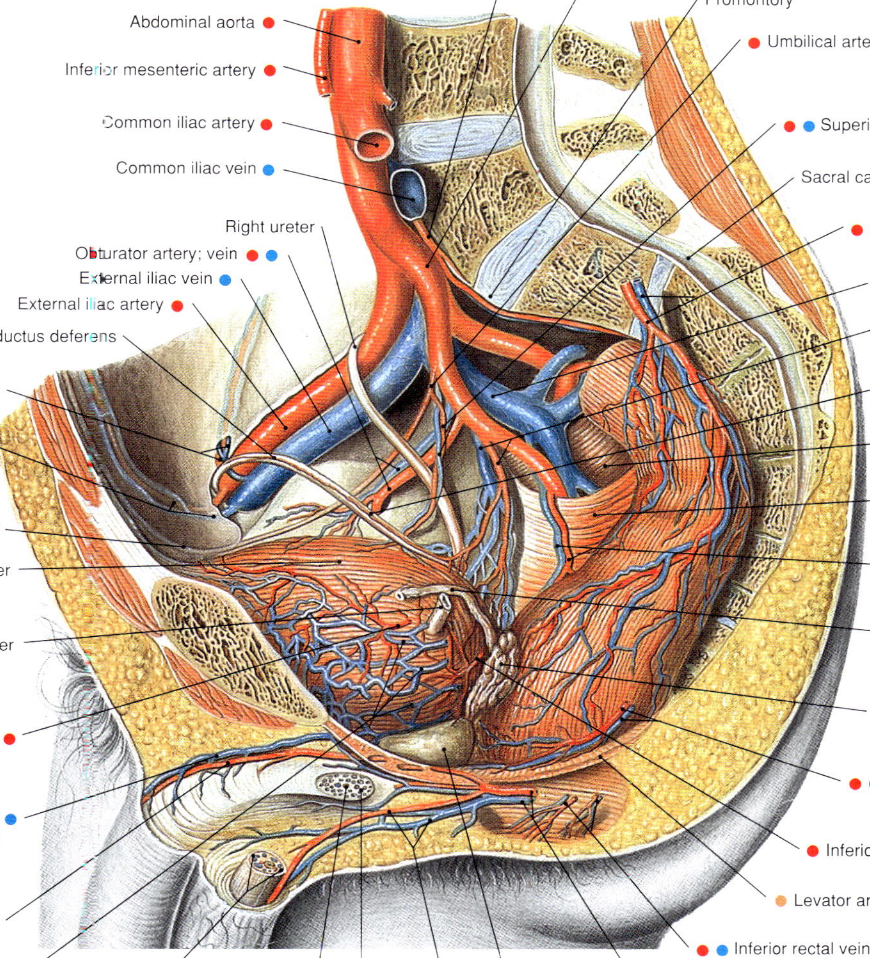

Fig. 897 Blood supply of the male pelvis.

Vessels of the female pelvis

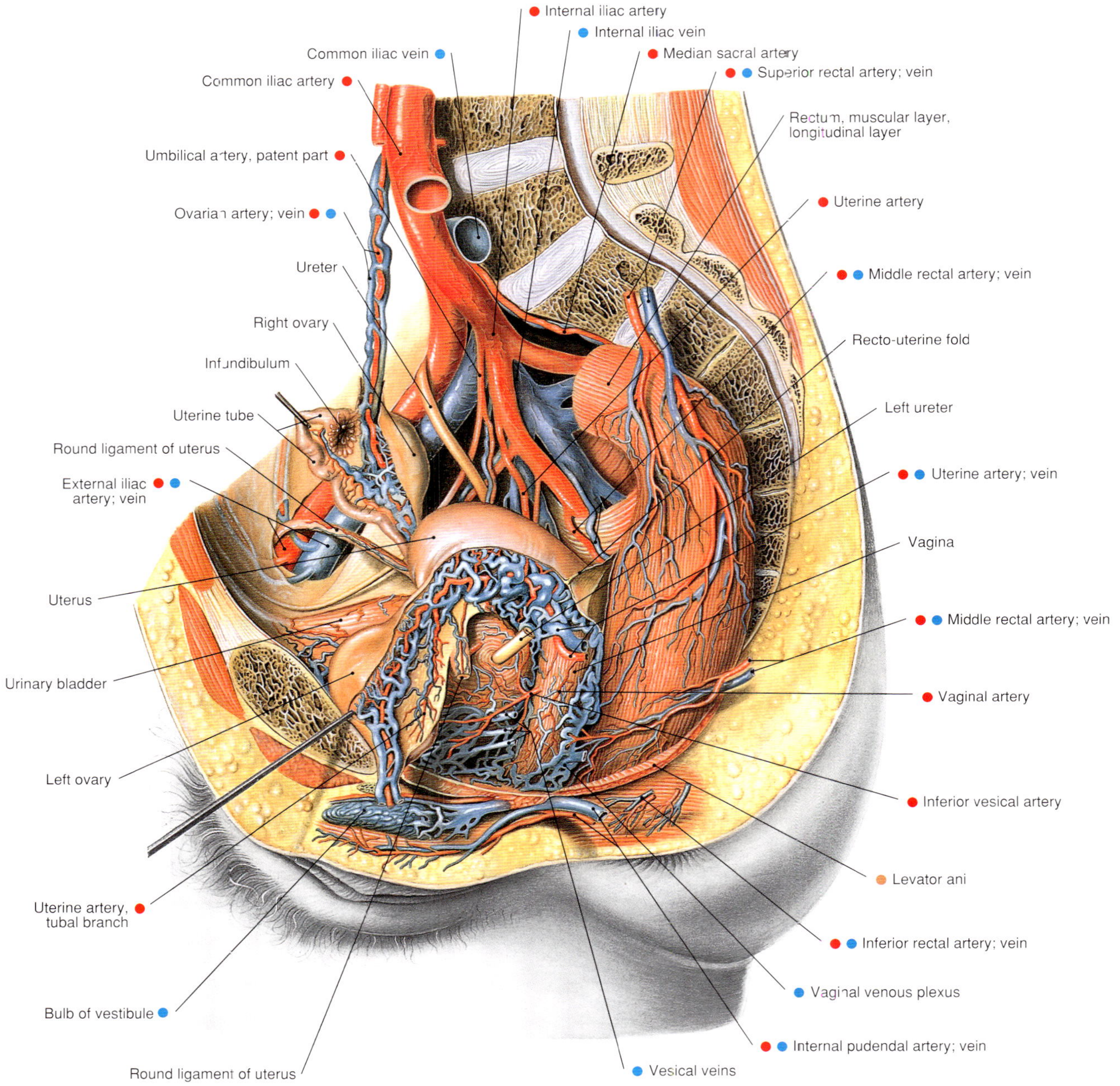

Fig. 898 Blood supply of the female pelvis.

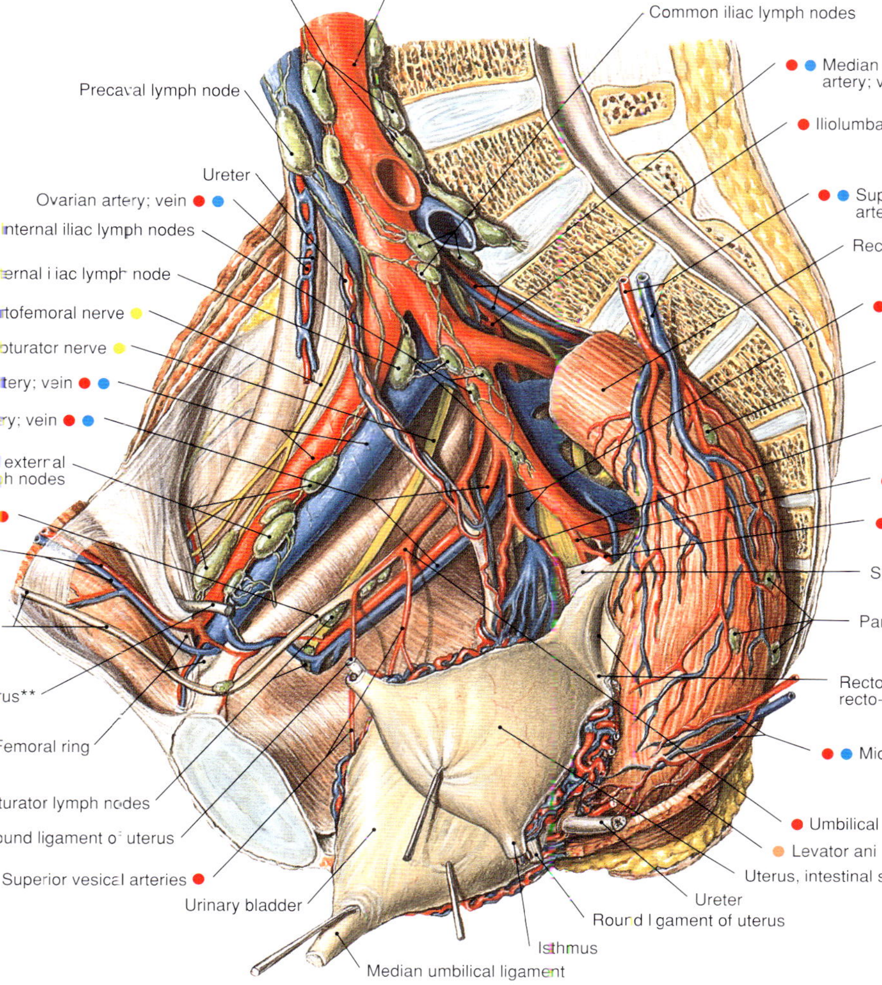

Fig. 899 Lymphatics and lymph nodes of the pelvic wall of the female.

The lymph nodes are frequently much smaller than illustrated but they are always present. Tumour cells from the uterus can reach the superficial inguinal lymph nodes via lymphatics of the round ligament of uterus.

* Clinical term: pouch of DOUGLAS
** Clinical term: round ligament

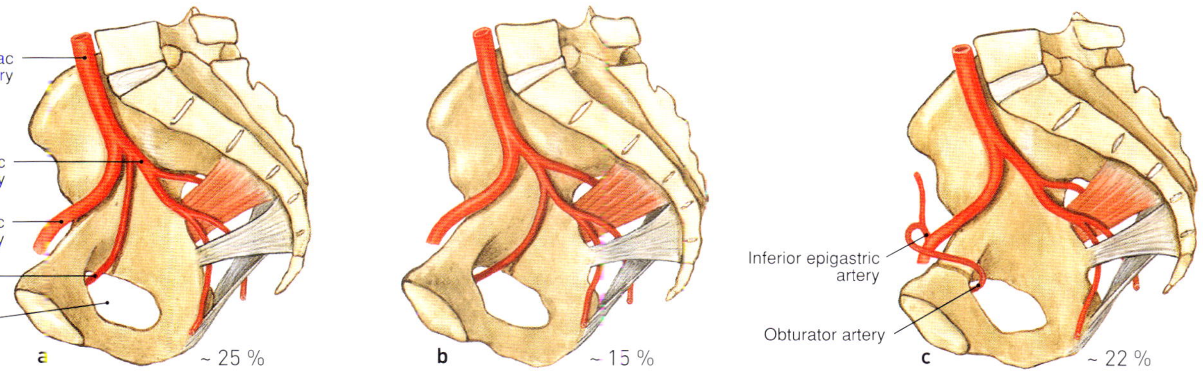

Fig. 900 a–c Variability of the origin of the obturator artery; medial view.

a Origin from the anterior branch of the internal iliac artery („textbook case")

b Origin as an independent branch from the internal iliac artery

c Origin from the external iliac artery

Only in 75% of the cases, the obturator artery originates from the trunk of the internal iliac artery

Female pelvic diaphragm

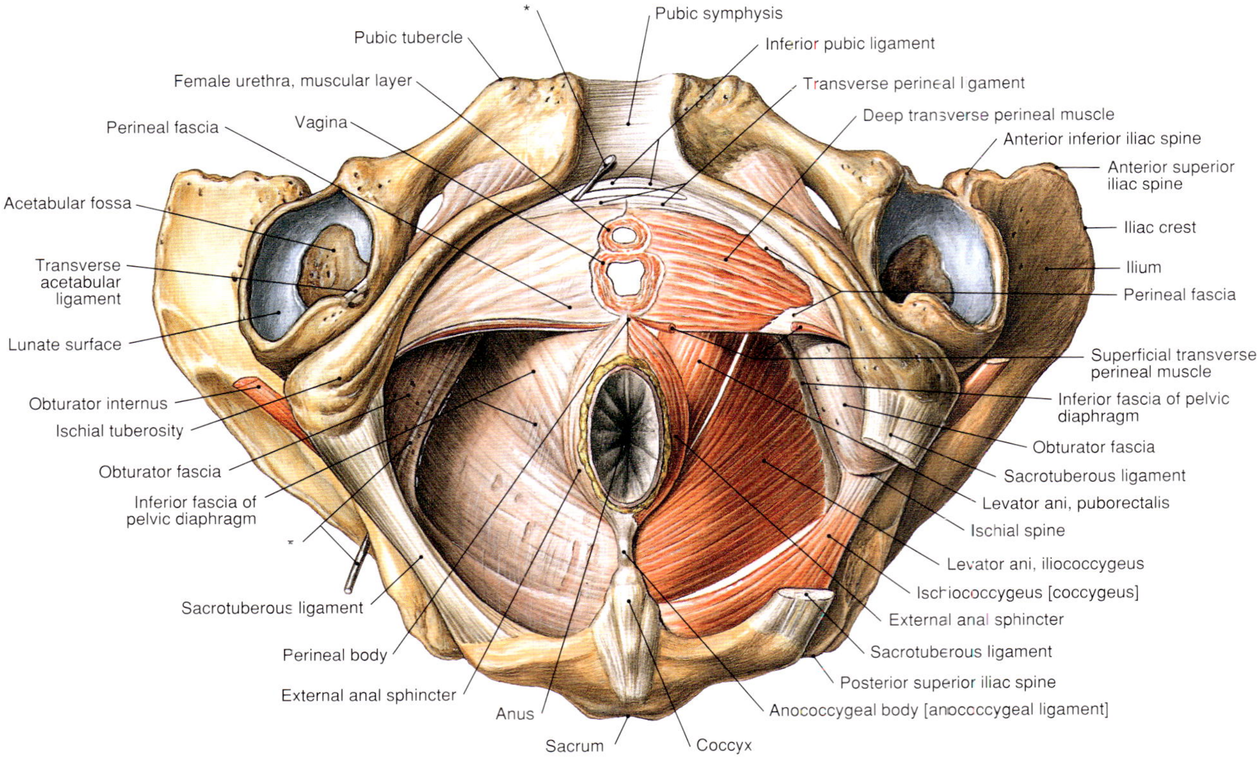

Fig. 901 Perineal muscles and the pelvic diaphragm of the female; inferior view.

* Probe in the pudendal canal (ALCOCK's canal)

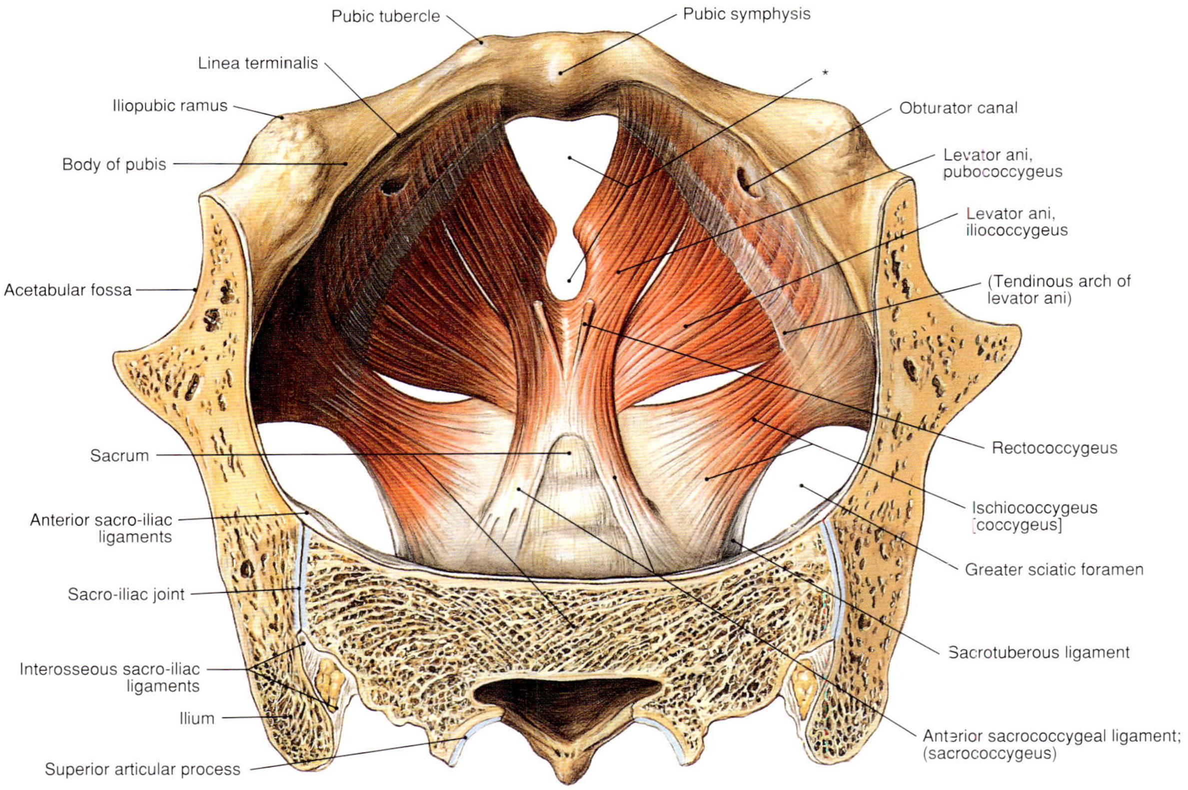

Fig. 902 Pelvic diaphragm of the female; superior view.

* Clinical term: levator hiatus

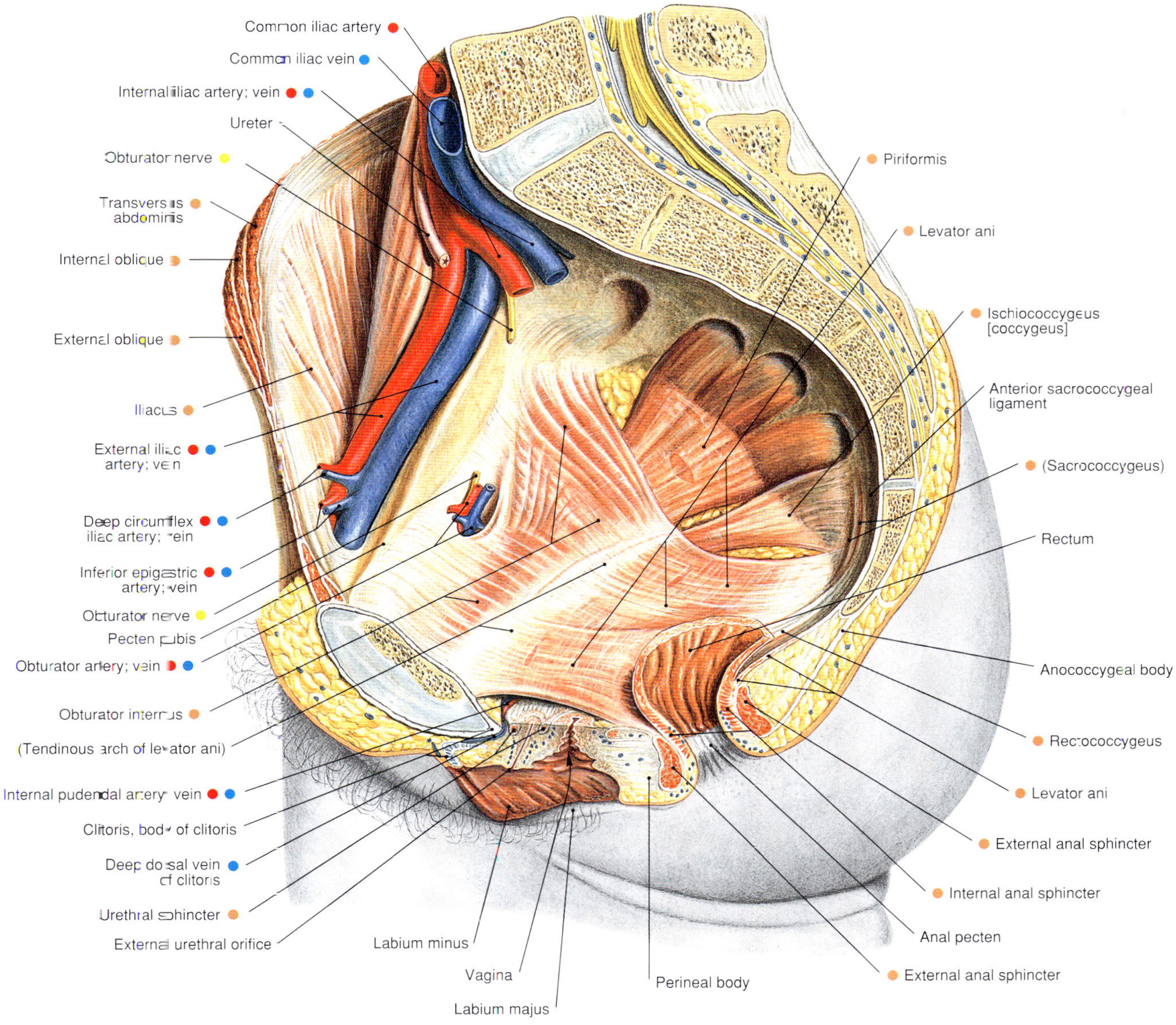

Fig. 903 Muscles of the pelvic diaphragm of the female.

Male pelvic diaphragm

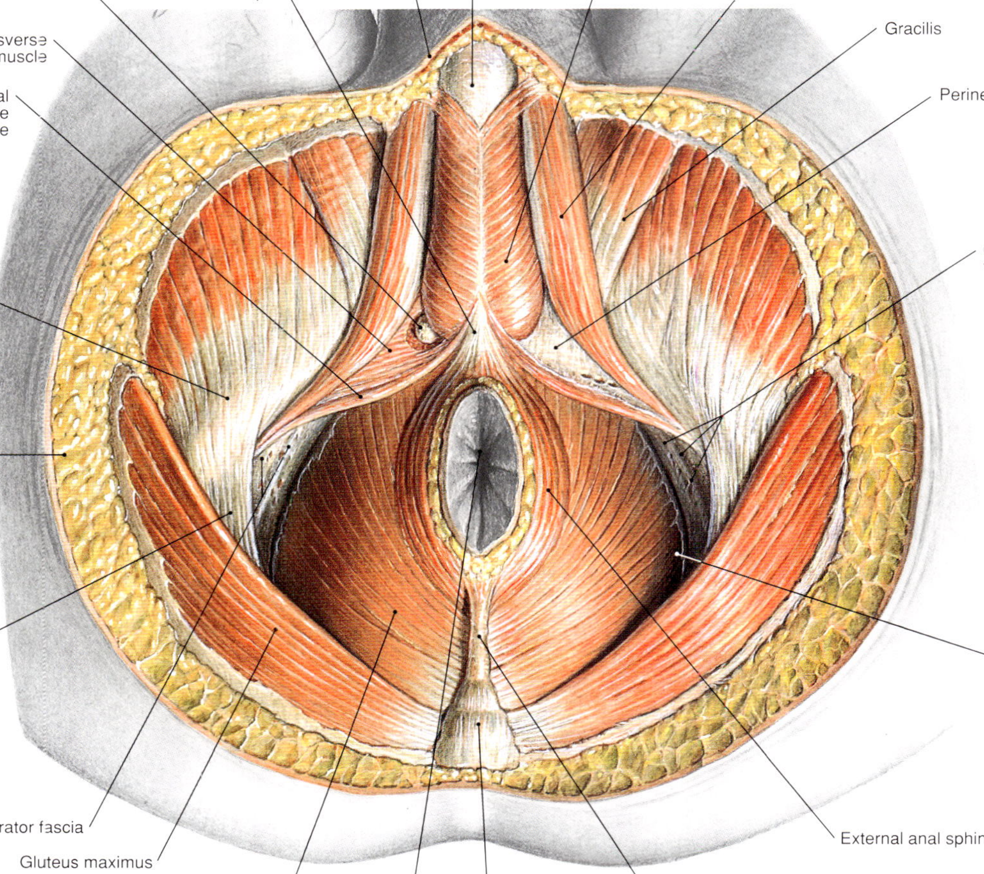

→ T 22

Fig. 904 Perineum and pelvic diaphragm of the male; inferior view.

* Clinical term: COWPER's gland

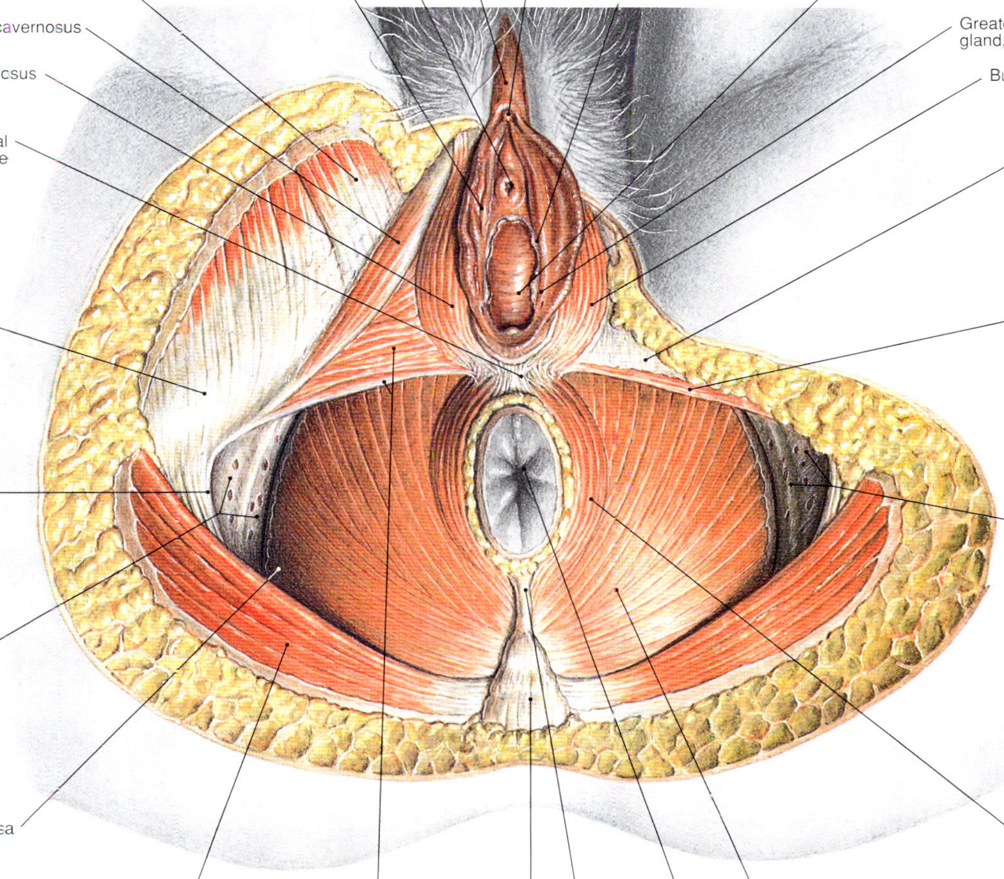

Fig. 905 Perineum; pelvic diaphragm and female external genitalia; inferior view.

* Clinical term: BARTHOLIN's gland

→ T 22

The vaginal and the anal orifices are located in close proximity. During delivery the skin and muscles of the perineum can rupture up to the sphincter muscles of the anus (I. – III. degree perineal lacerations). These can be prevented by surgical incisions directed either laterally or in the median plane (perineal incision = lateral or medial episiotomy).

Urogenital diaphragm

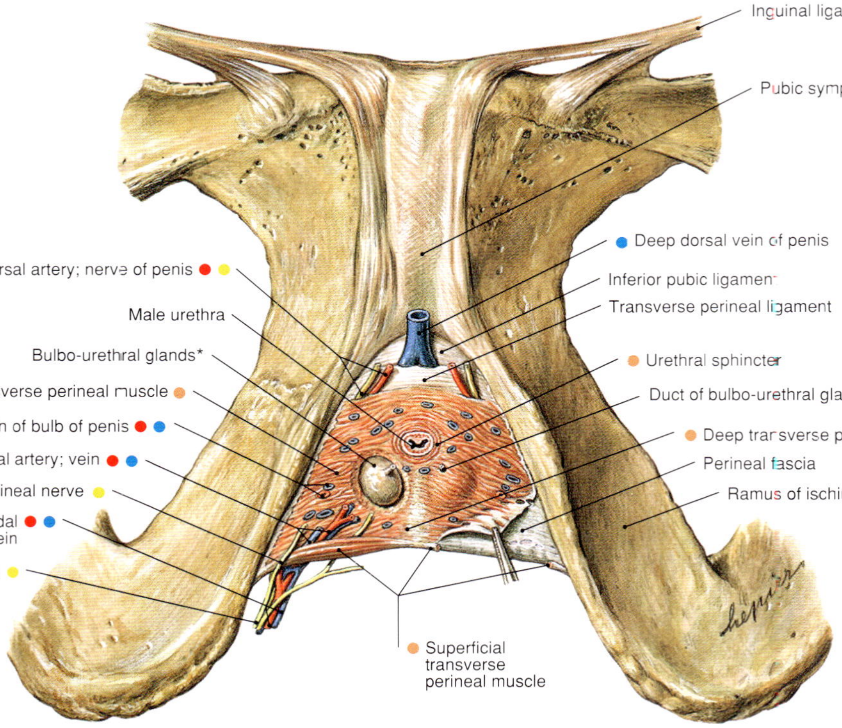

→ T 22

Fig. 906 Urogenital diaphragm of the male; inferior view.

* Clinical term: COWPER's gland

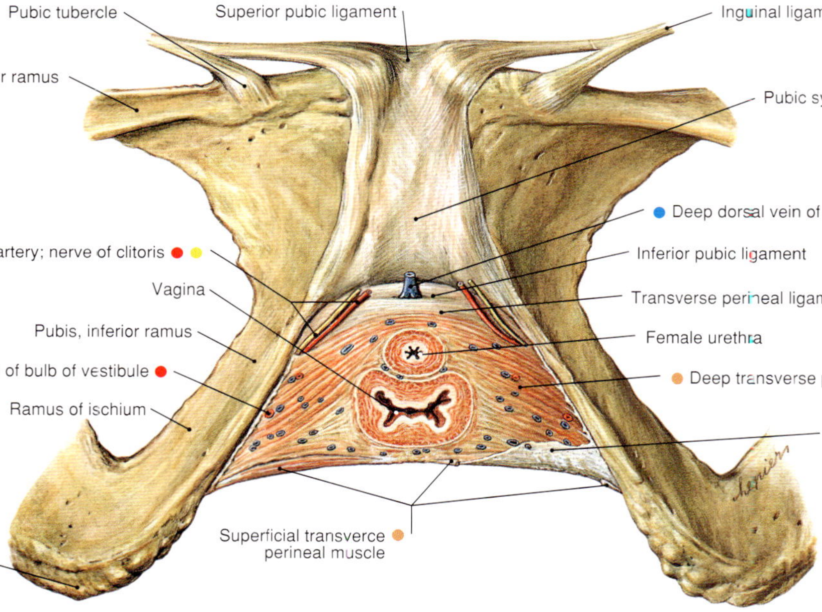

→ T 22

Fig. 907 Urogenital diaphragm of the female; inferior view.

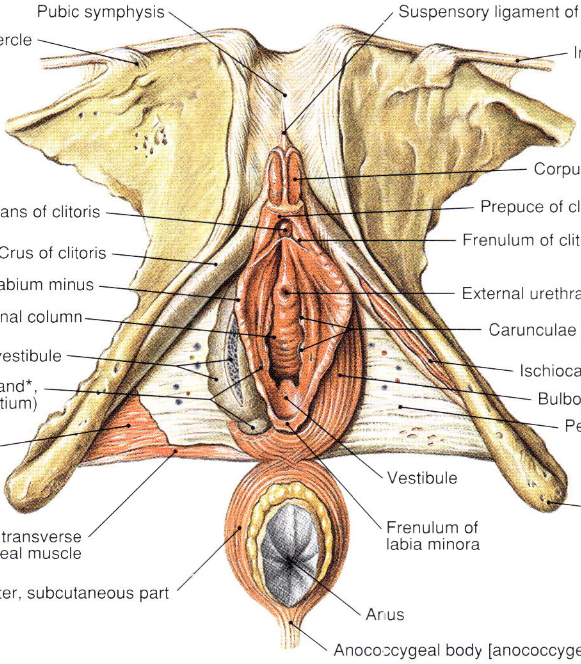

Fig. 908 Female external genitalia; ventroinferior view.

* Clinical term: BARTHOLIN's gland

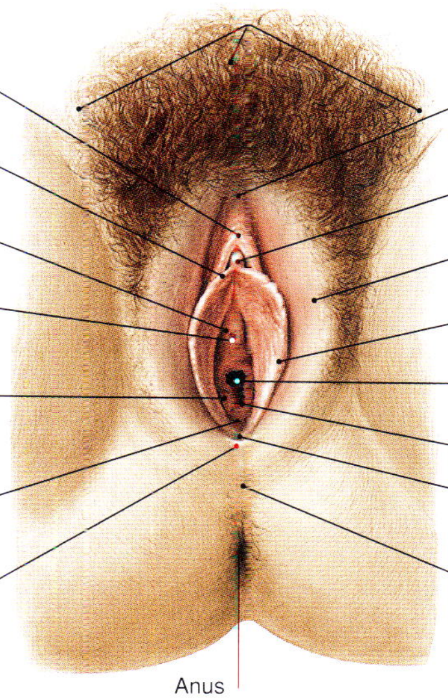

Fig. 909 Female external genitalia; inferior view.

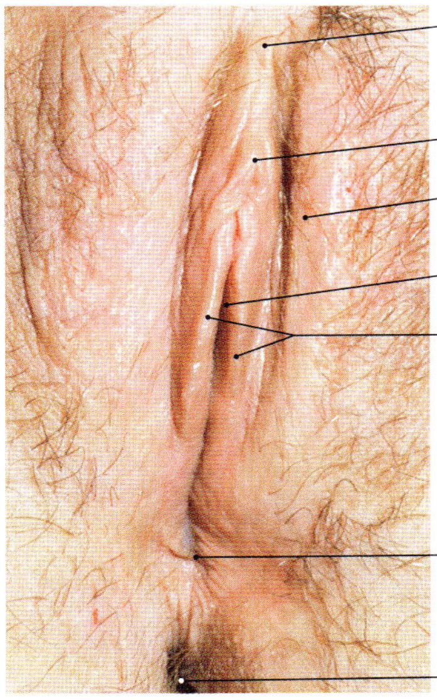

Fig. 910 Female external genitalia; inferior view.

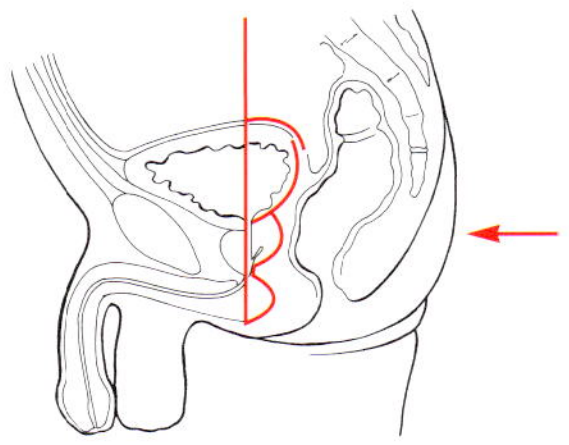

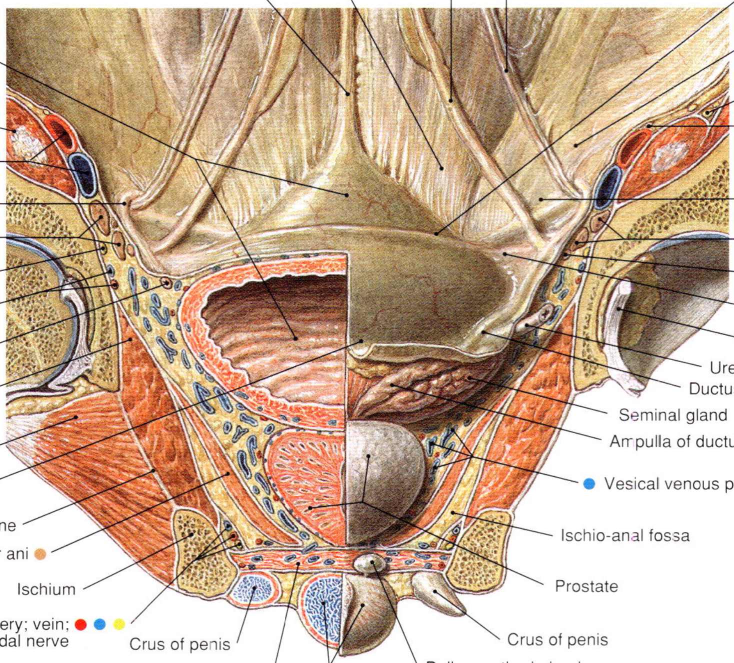

Fig. 911 Pelvic diaphragm;
pelvic organs and anterior abdominal wall of the male;
frontal section through the head of the femur
and the urinary bladder on the left;
dorsal view.

Female pelvic organs and retroperitoneal space

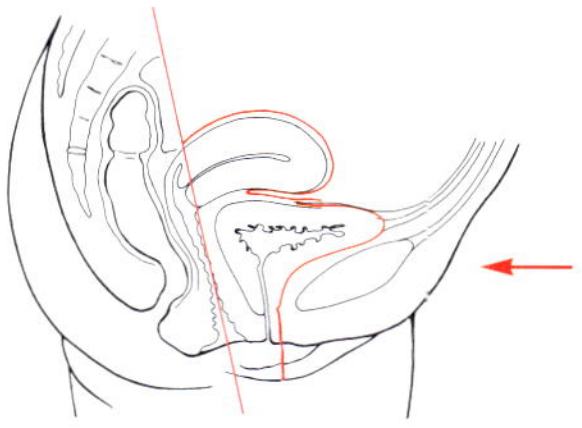

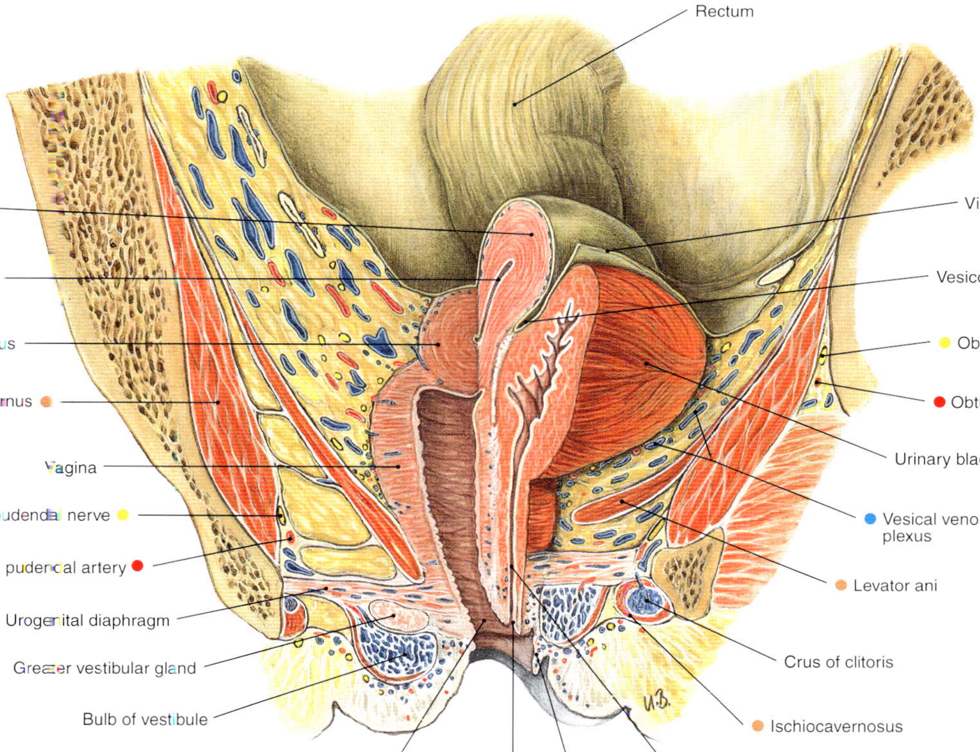

Fig. 912 Pelvic diaphragm and pelvic organs of the female; frontal section (on the right) combined with a median section; ventral view.

Male external genitalia

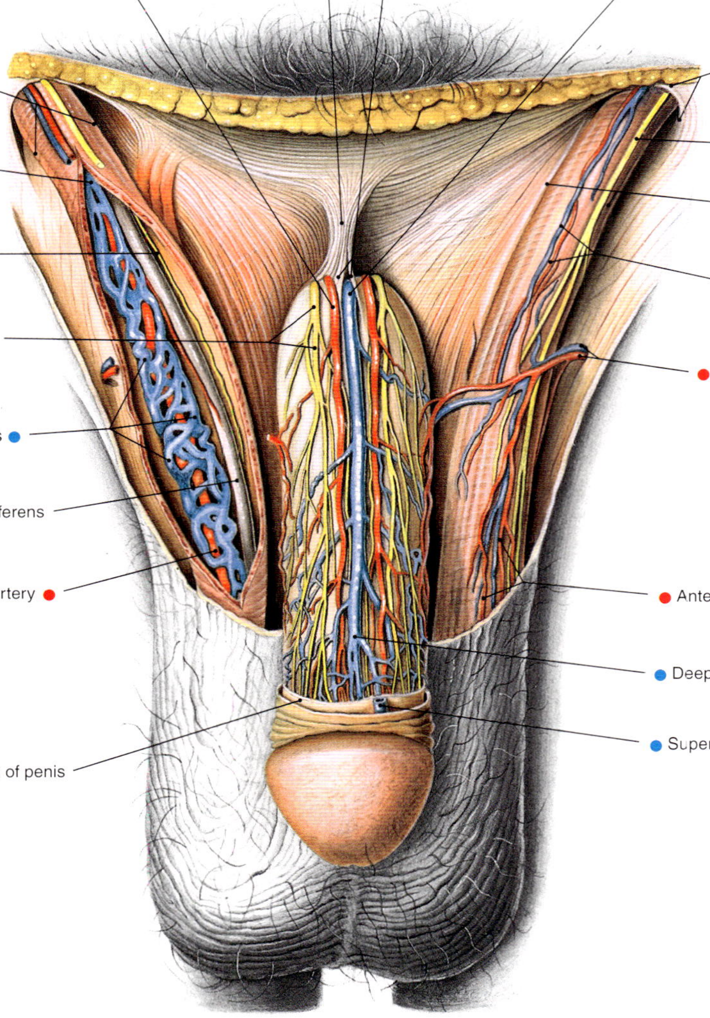

Fig. 913 Male external genitalia.

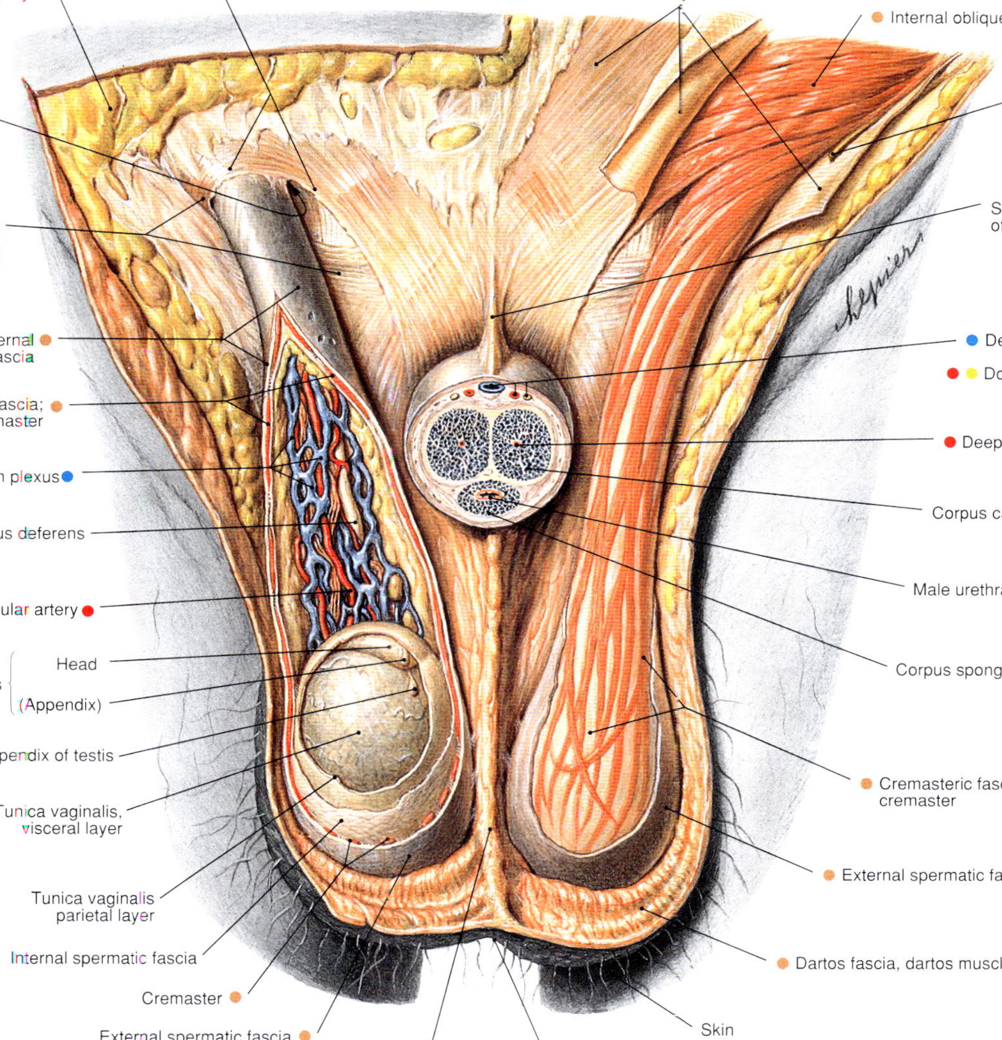

Fig. 914 Male genitalia.

→ 837, 849

Male perineal region

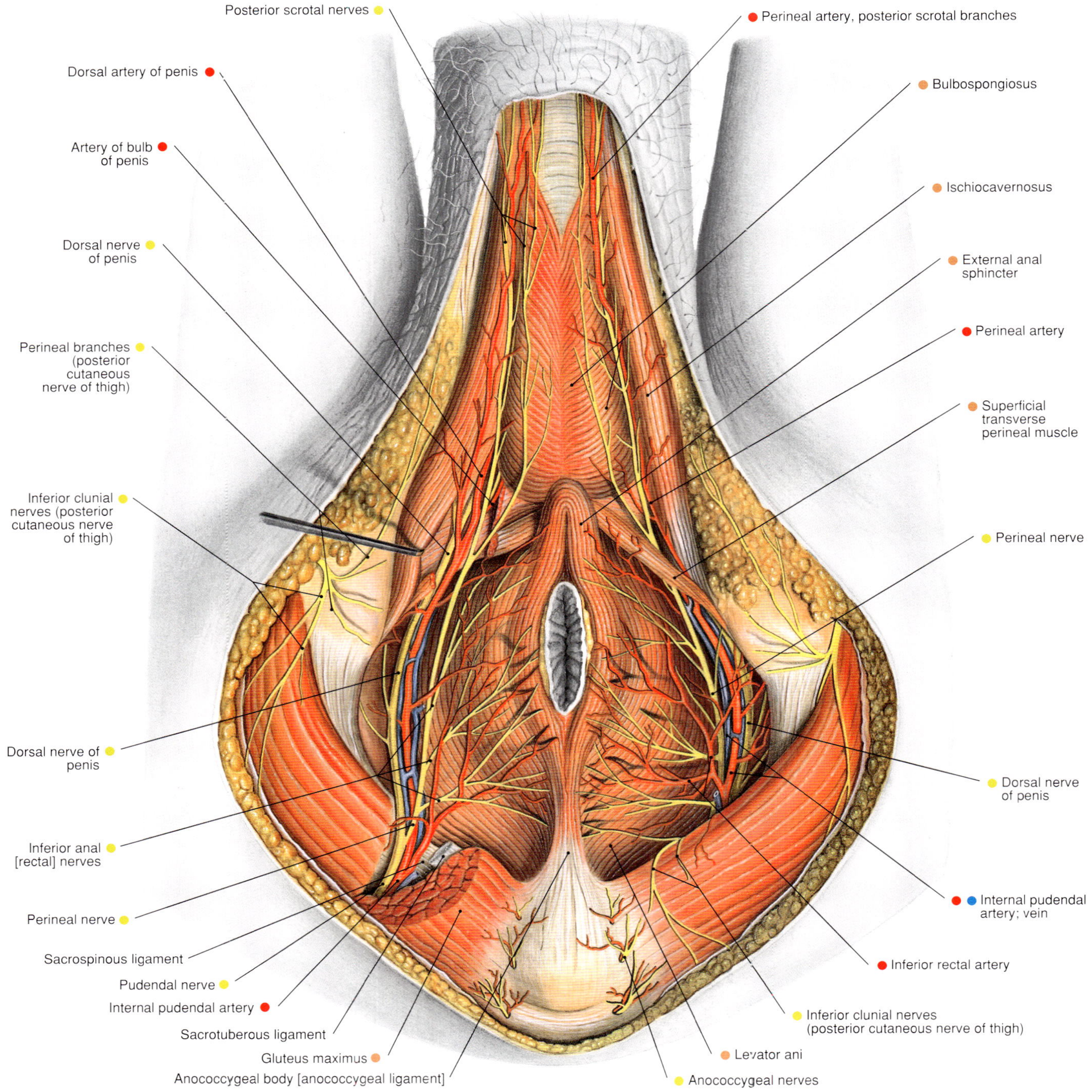

Fig. 915 Vessels and nerves of the perineum and the male external genitalia.

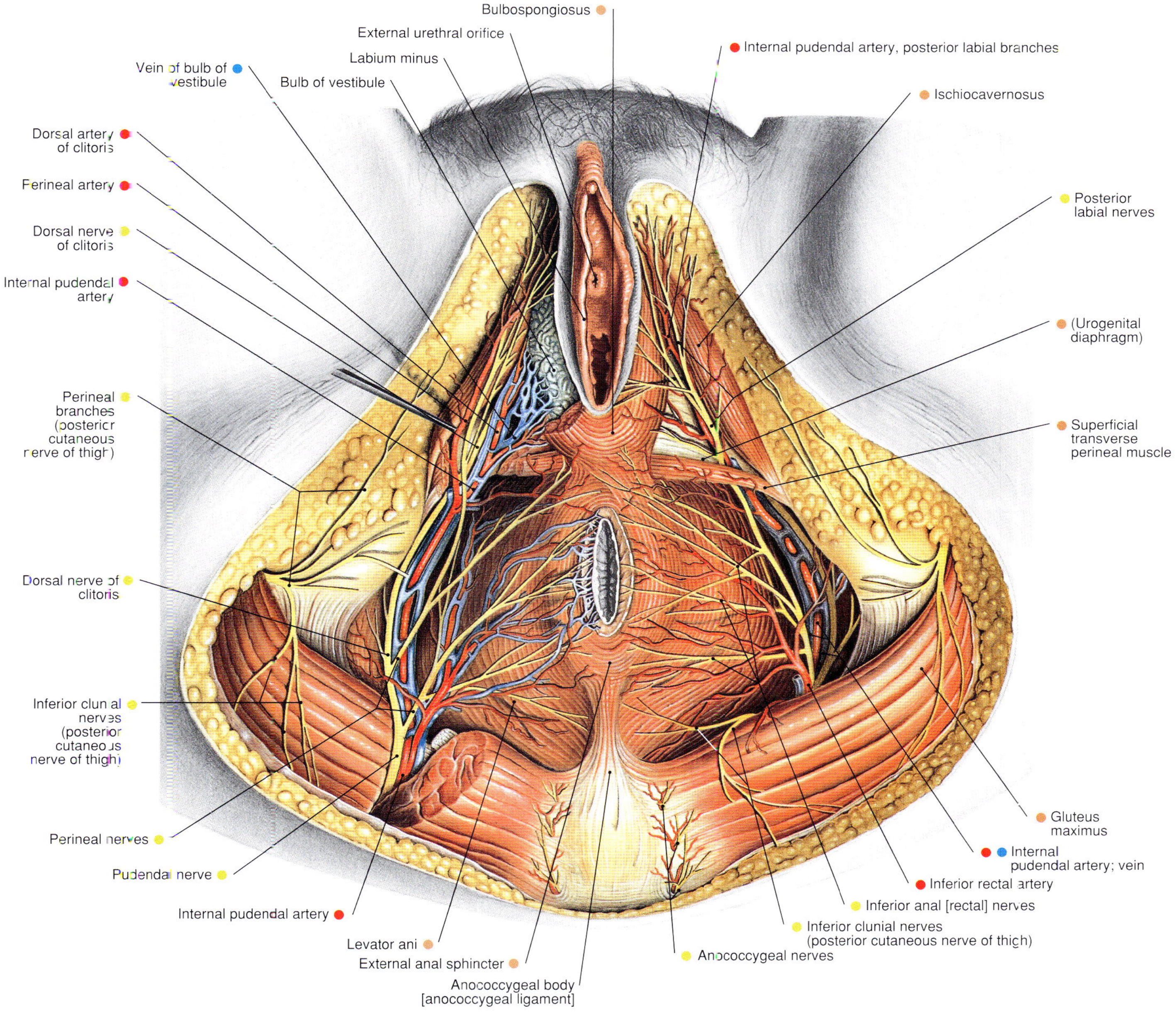

Fig. 916 Vessels and nerves of the perineum and the female external genitalia.

Pelvic viscera and retroperitoneal space

Abdomen, median section

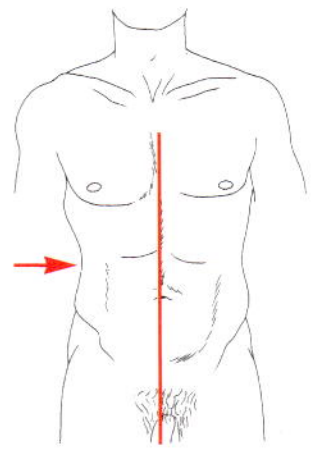

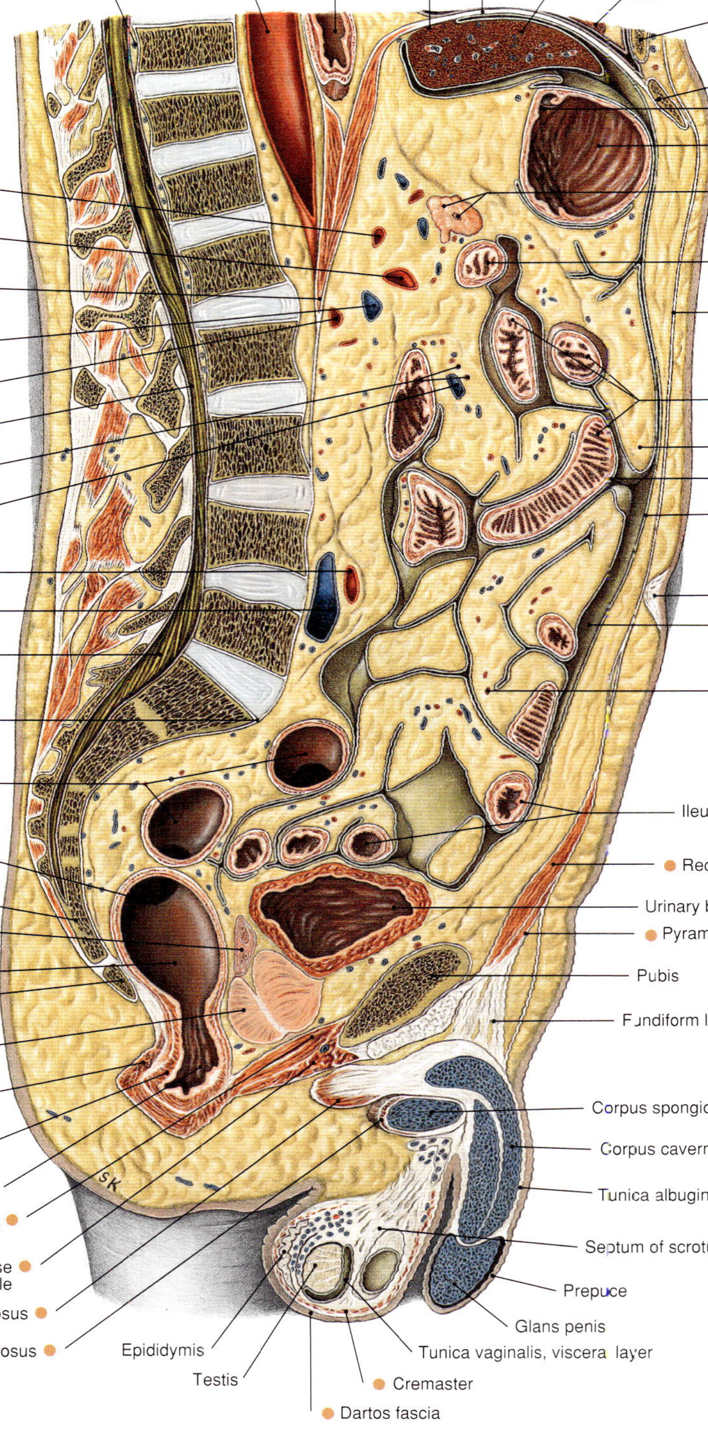

Fig. 917 Abdomen and pelvis of the male; median section.

Abdomen, sagittal section

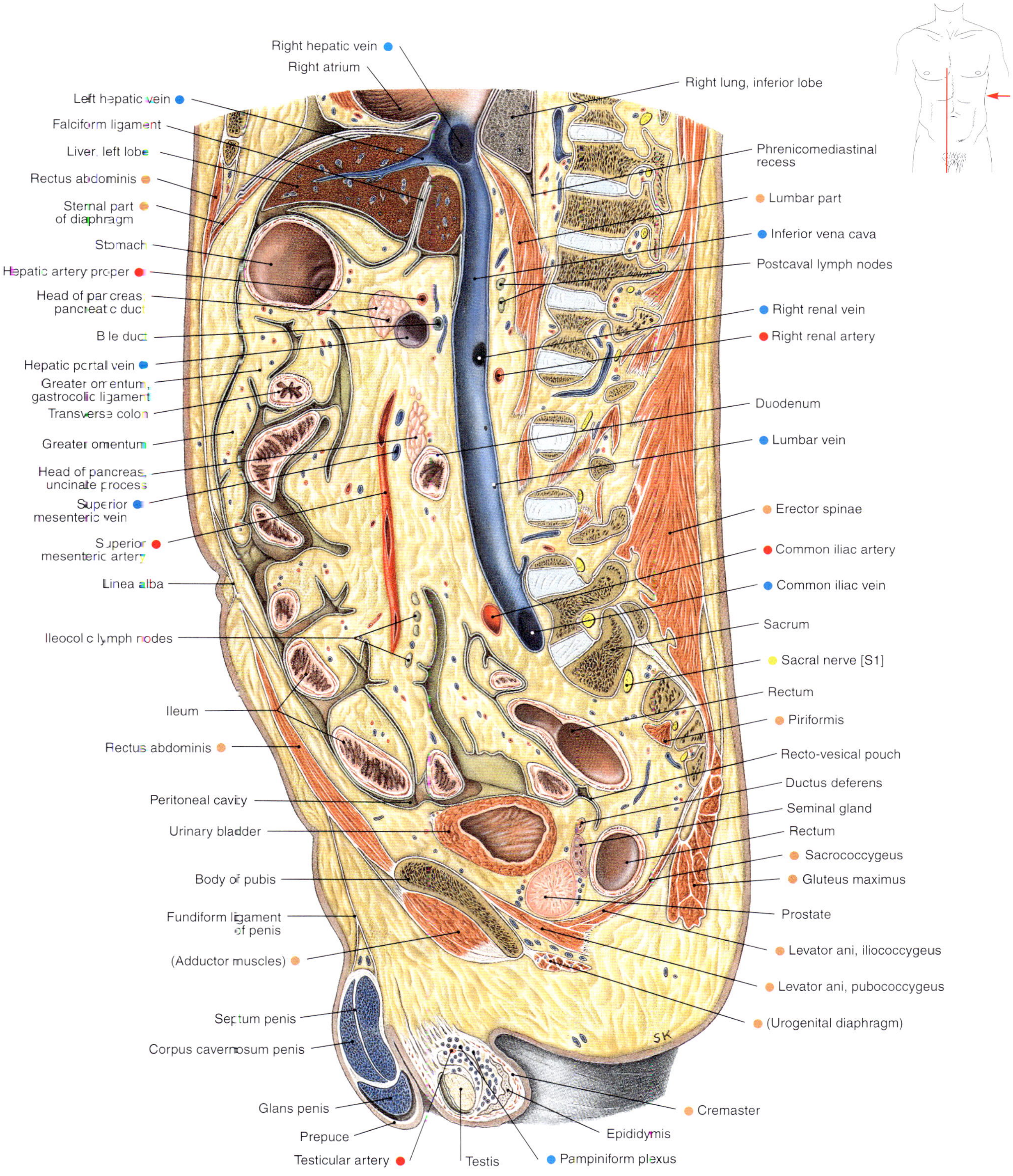

Fig. 918 Abdomen and pelvis of the male; sagittal section to the right of the median plane.

Abdomen, frontal section

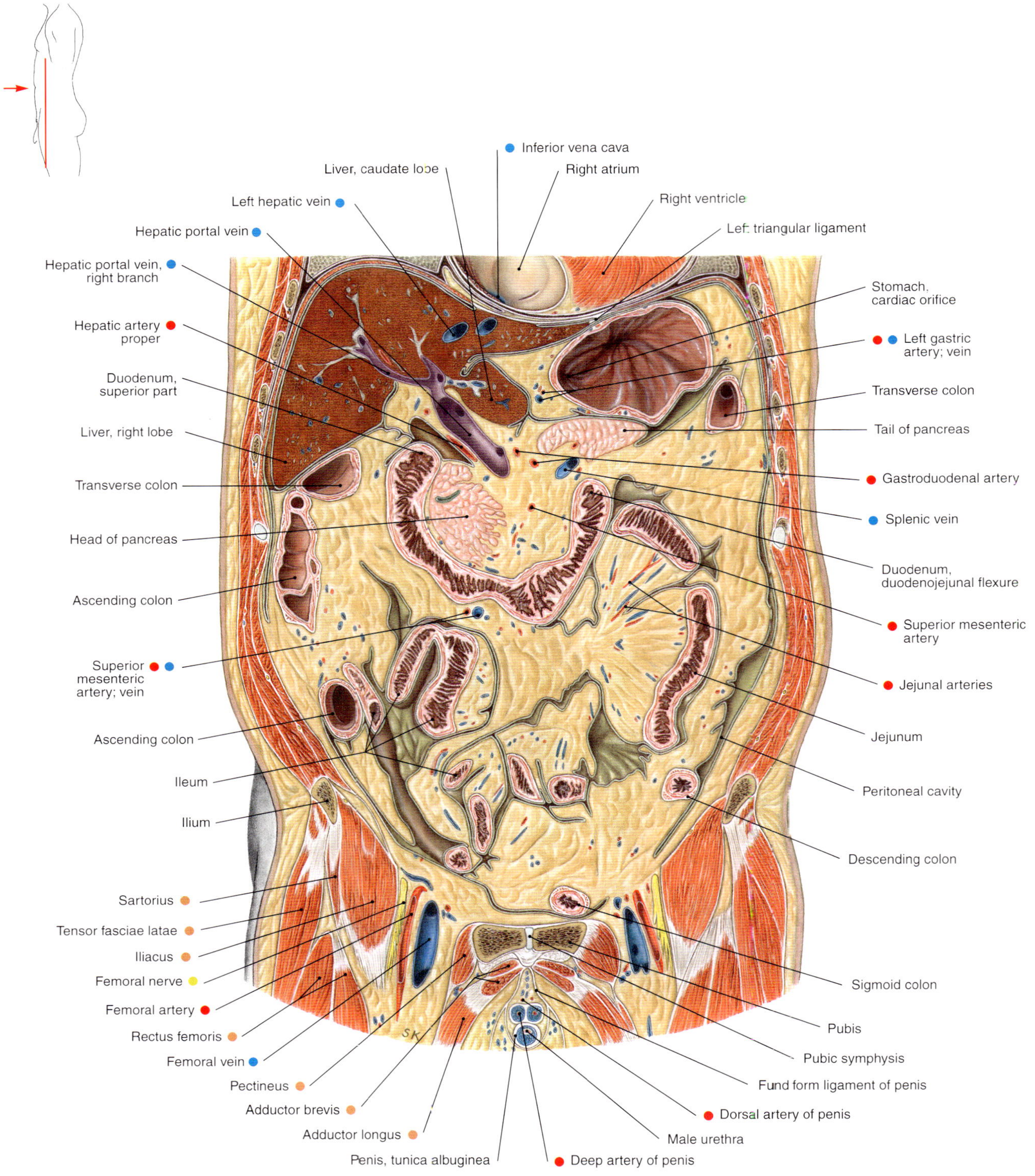

→ 602

Fig. 919 Abdomen;
frontal section through the most anterior part of the abdominal cavity.

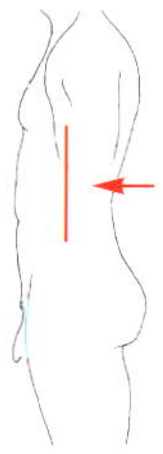

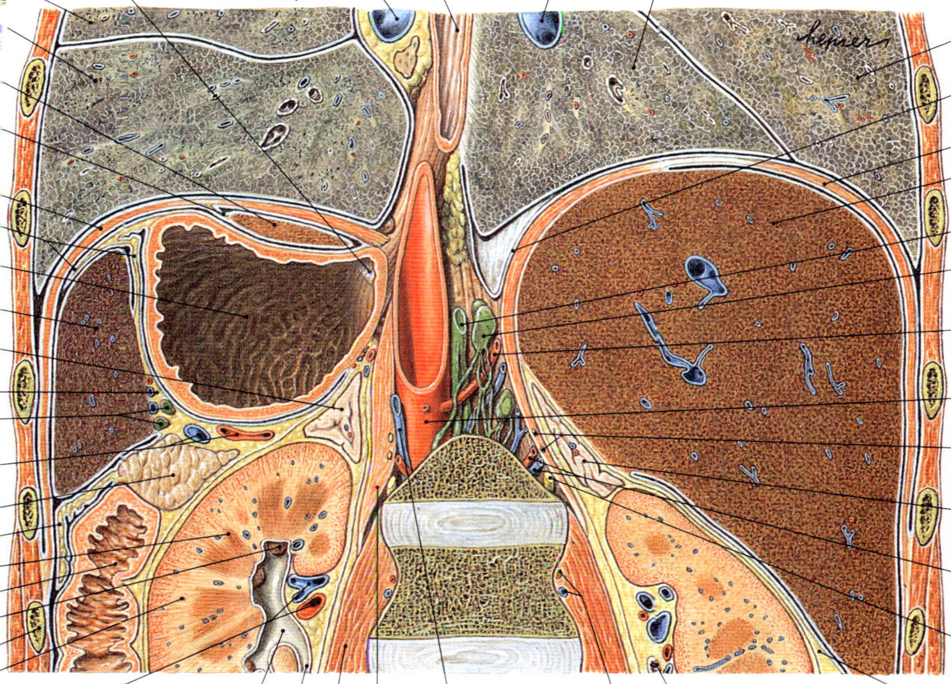

Fig. 920 Abdomen;
frontal section demonstrating the diaphragm,
the organs of the upper abdomen and the kidneys;
dorsal view.

Upper abdomen, sagittal section

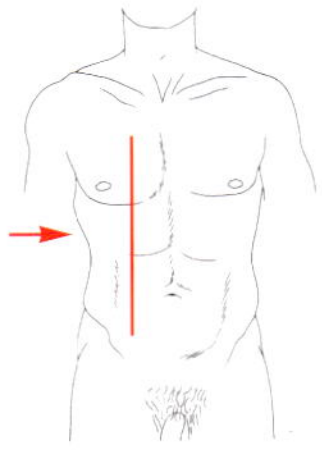

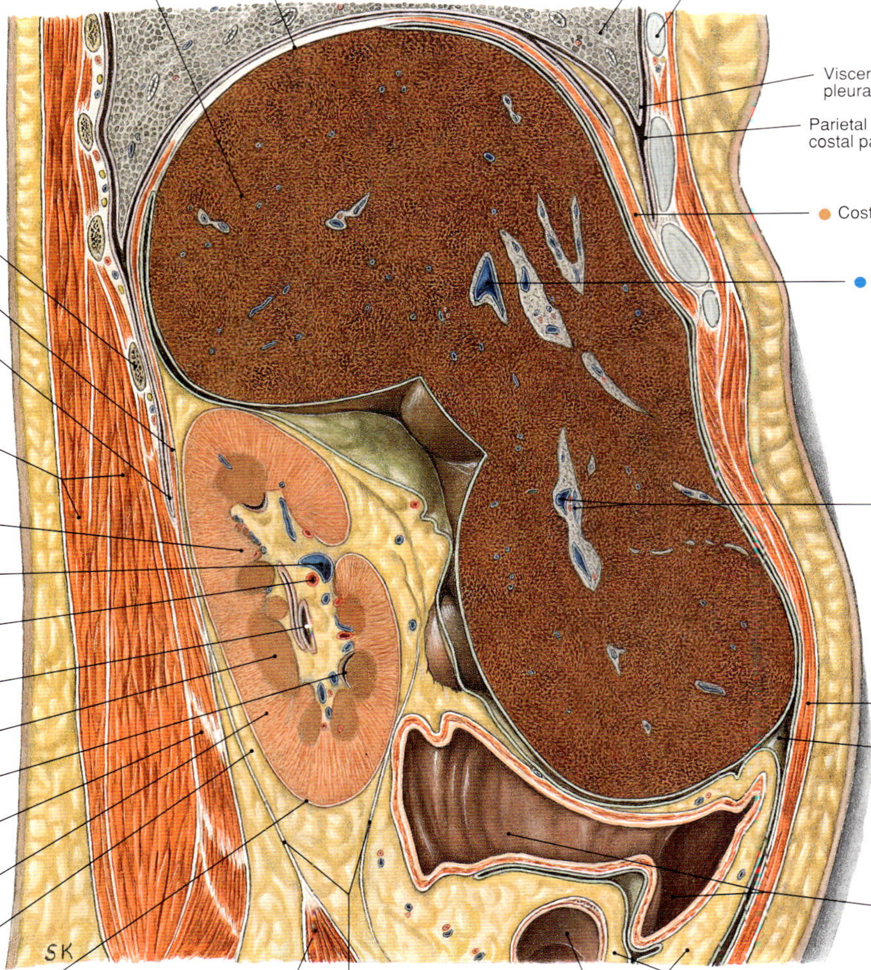

Fig. 921 Abdomen;
sagittal section through the upper abdomen
at the level of the right kidney;
viewed from the right.

Upper abdomen, sagittal section

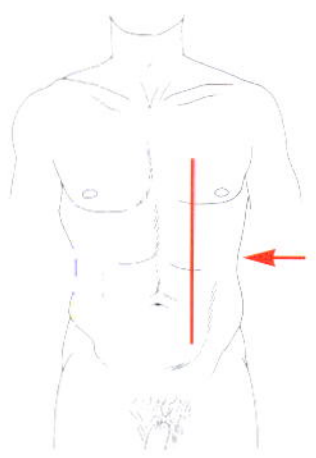

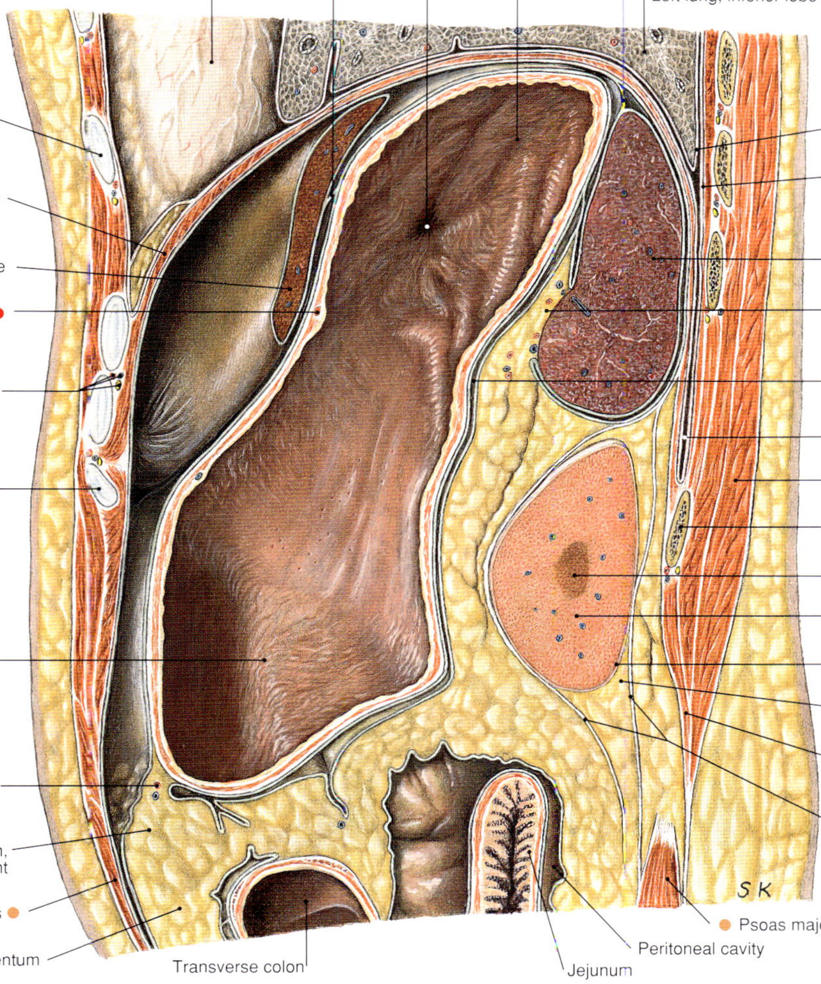

Fig. 922 Abdomen;
sagittal section through the upper abdomen at the level of the spleen; viewed from the left.

Pelvic viscera and retroperitoneal space

Upper abdomen, transverse sections

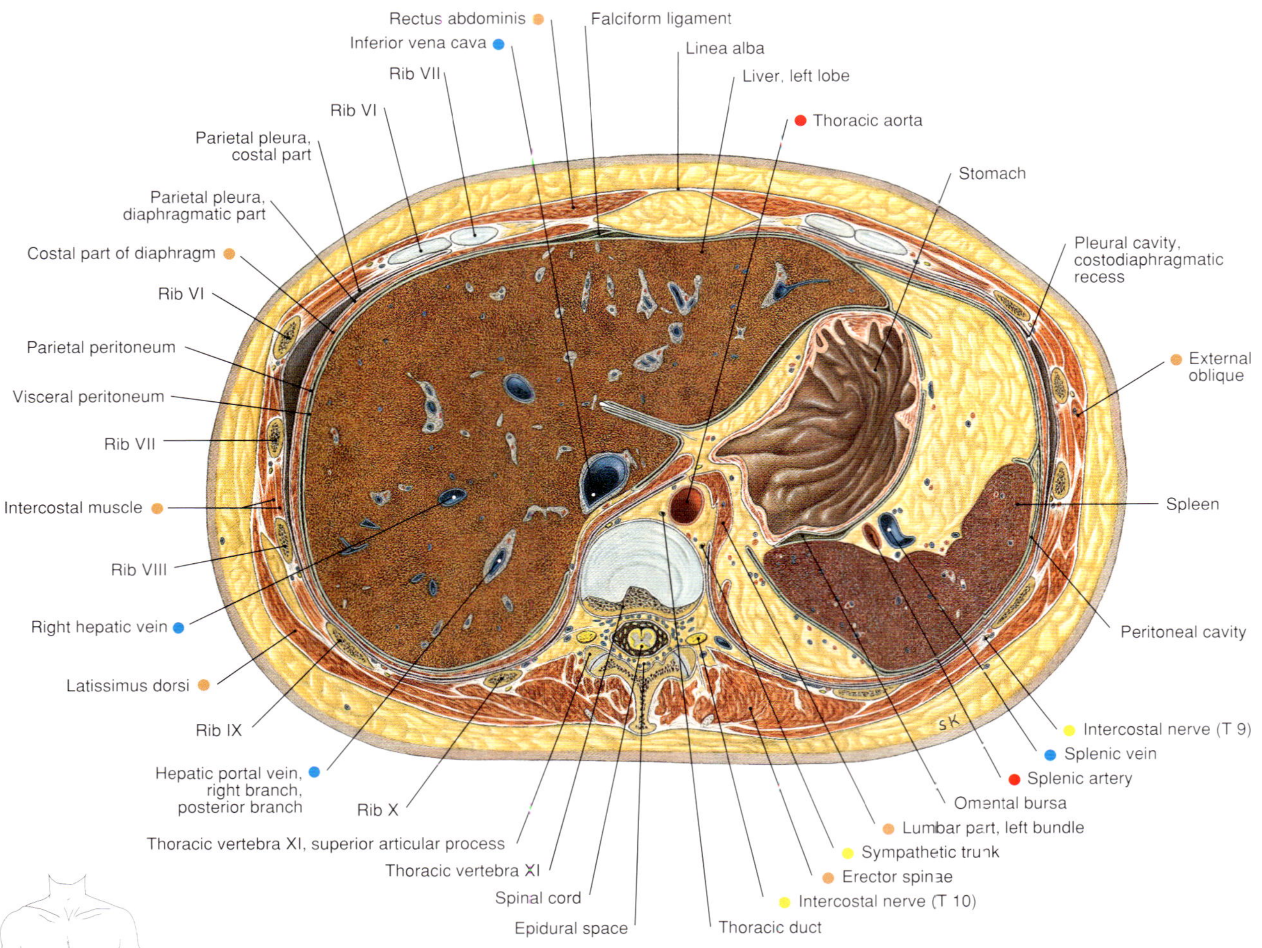

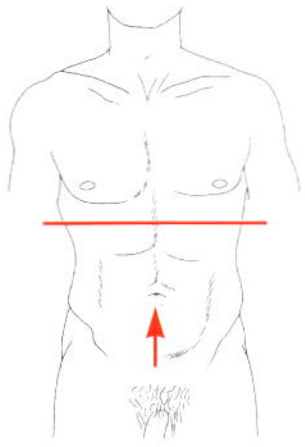

Fig. 923 Abdomen;
transverse section through the upper abdomen at the level of the eleventh thoracic vertebra.

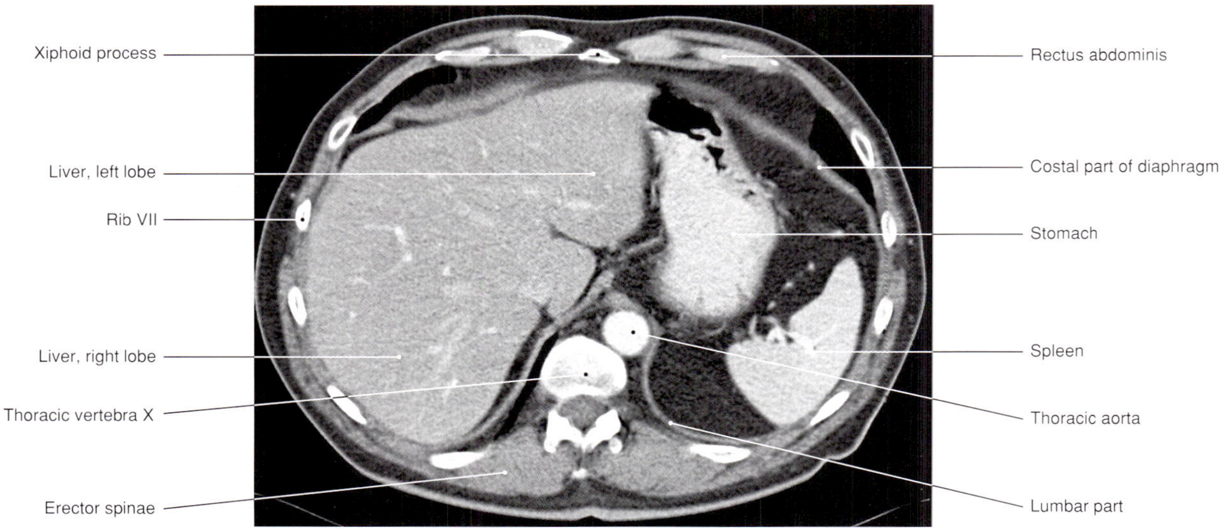

Fig. 924 Abdomen;
computed tomographic cross-section (CT) at the level of the tenth thoracic vertebra; inferior view.

Upper abdomen, transverse sections

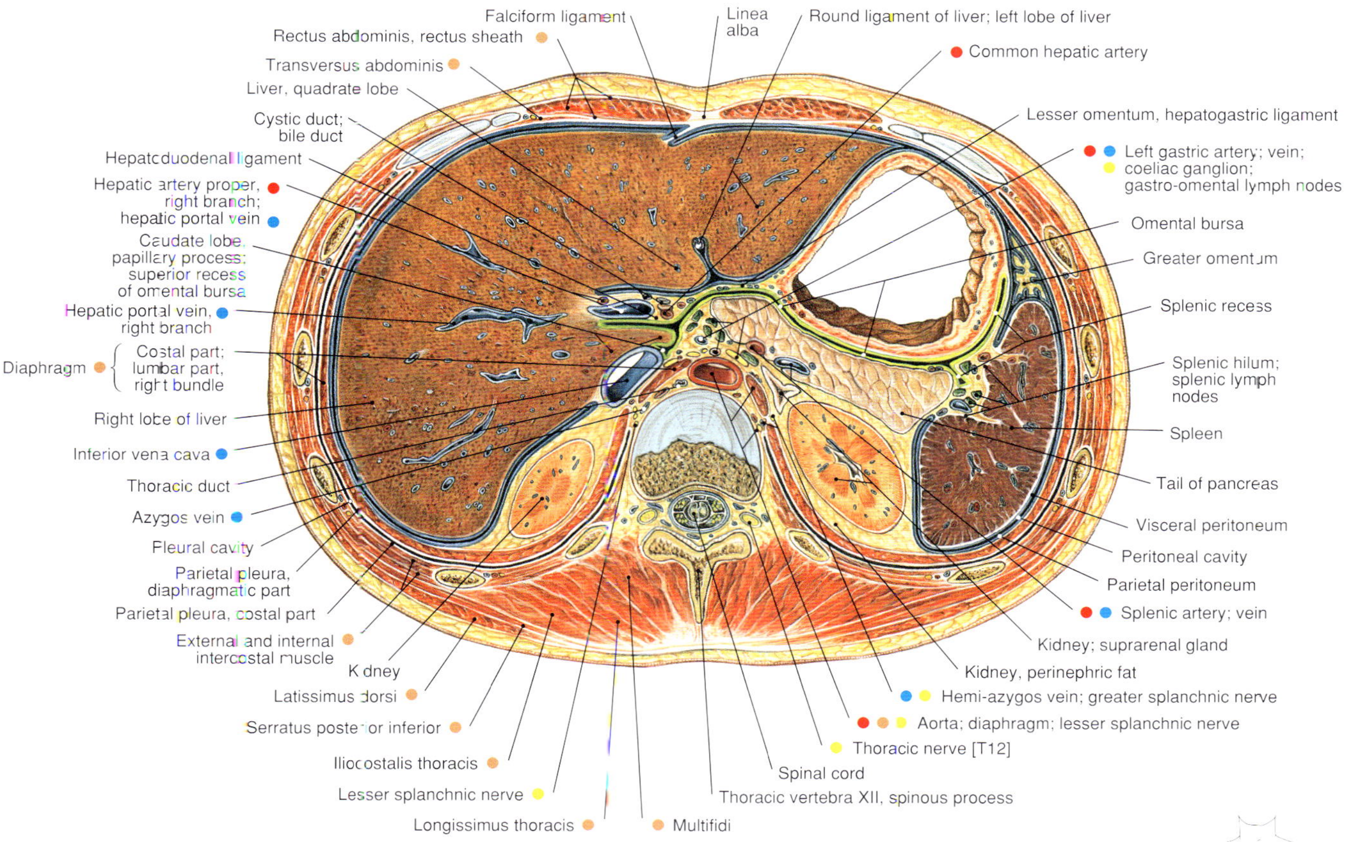

Fig. 925 Abdomen;
transverse section through the upper abdomen at the level of the intervertebral disc between the eleventh thoracic and first lumbar vertebra;
with the exception of the omental bursa highlighted in yellow green the peritoneum is coloured in blue.

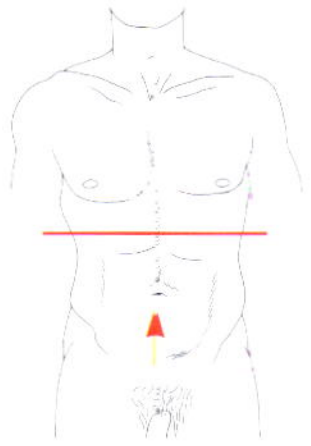

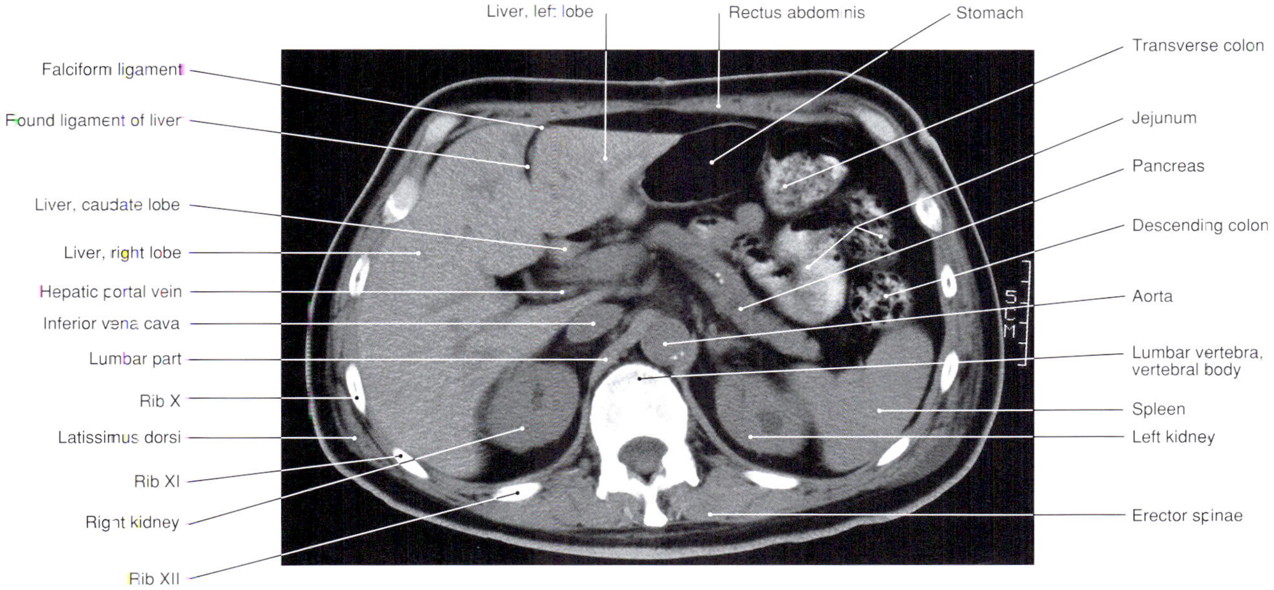

Fig. 926 Abdomen;
computed tomographic section (CT)
at the level of the first lumbar vertebra.
The intestine is partially filled with a contrast medium.

Upper abdomen, transverse sections

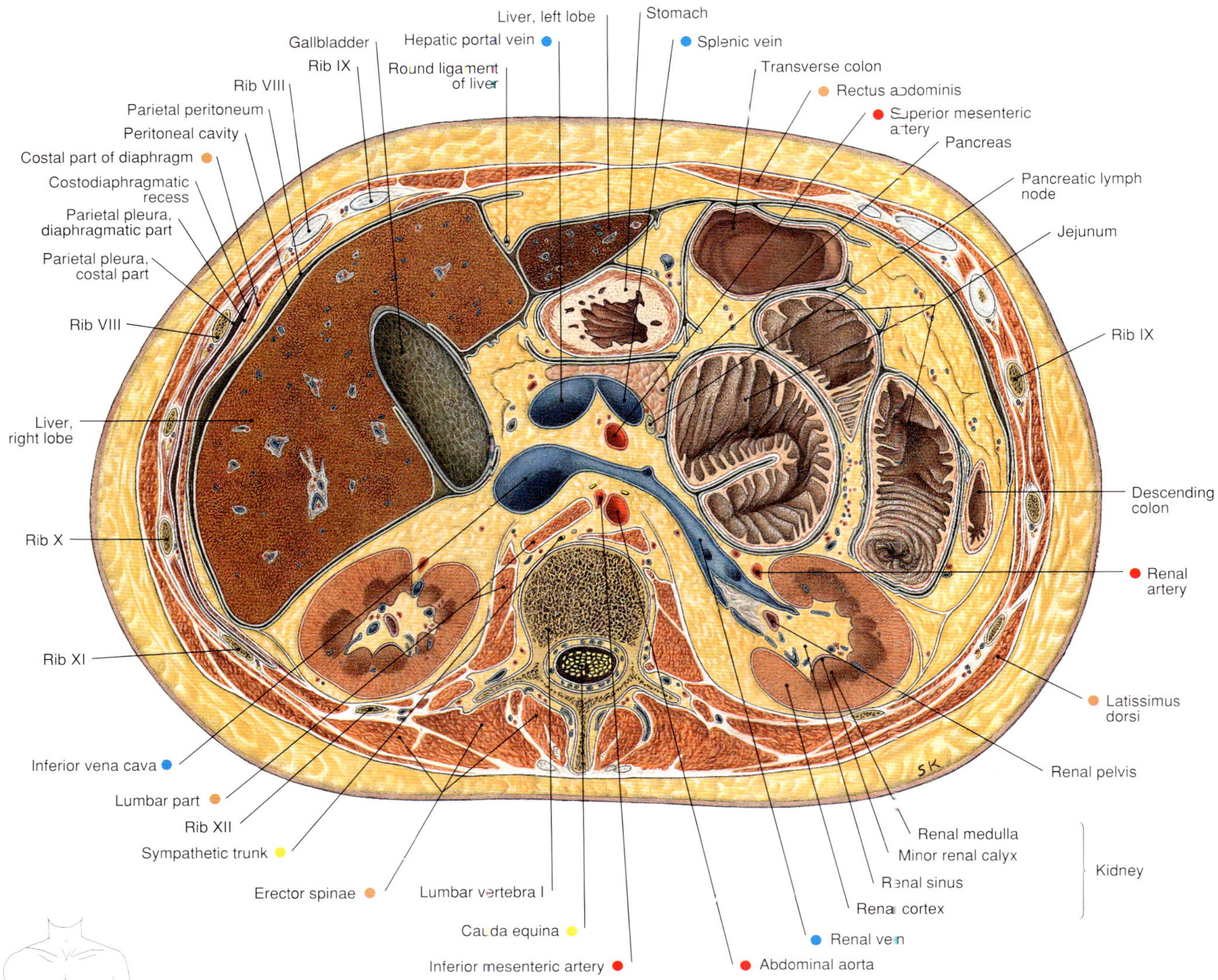

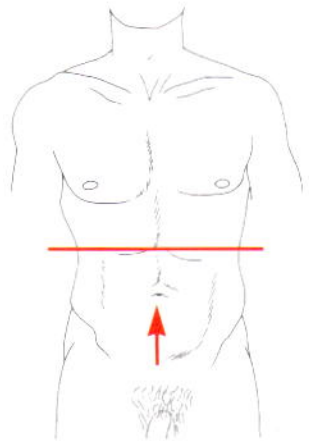

Fig. 927 Abdomen;
transverse section through the upper abdomen
at the level of the first lumbar vertebra.

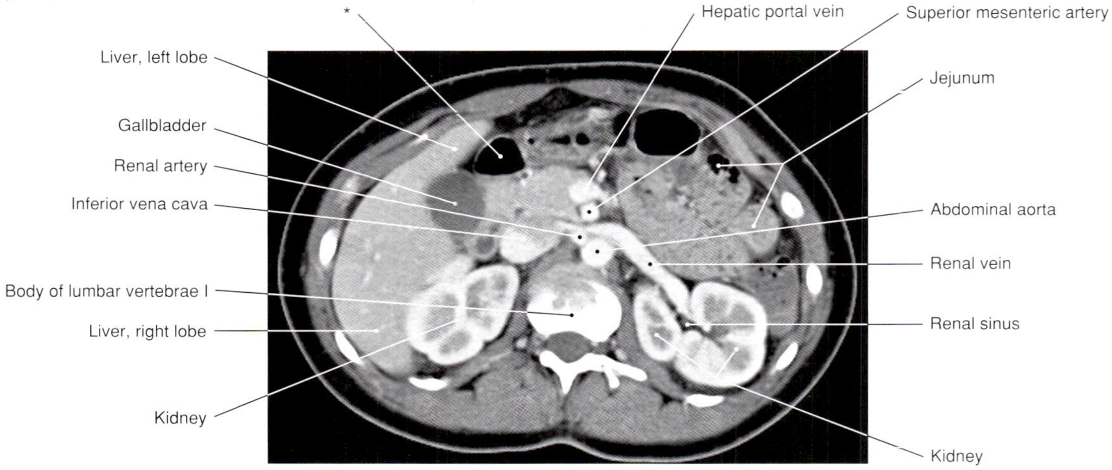

Fig. 928 Abdomen;
computed tomographic section (CT)
at the level of the first lumbar vertebra;
inferior view.

* Intestinal gas

Lower abdomen, transverse sections

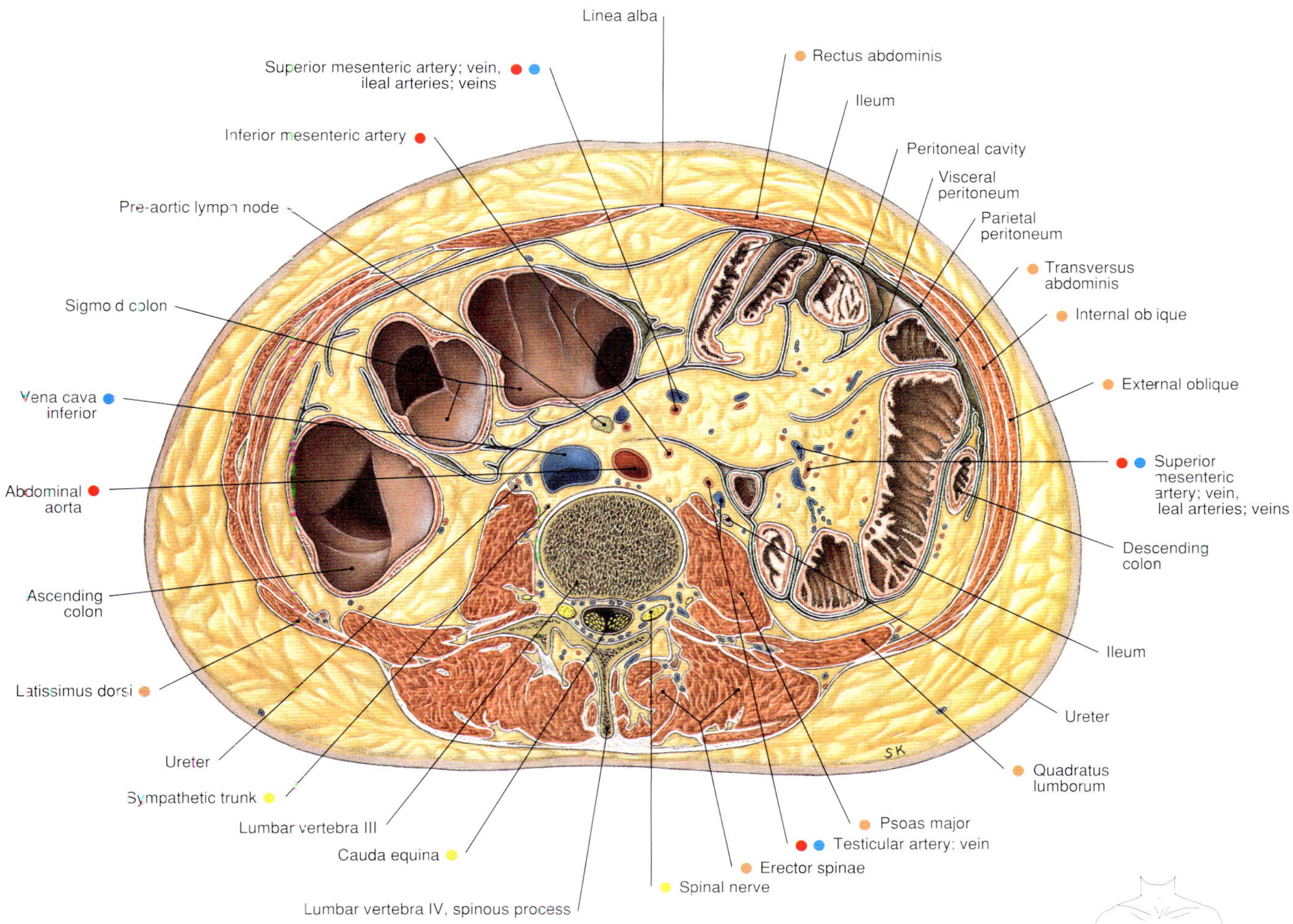

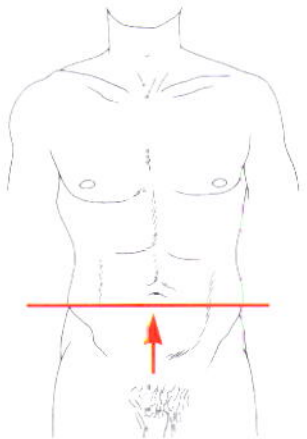

Fig. 929 Abdomen;
transverse section through the lower abdomen
at the level of the third lumbar vertebra.

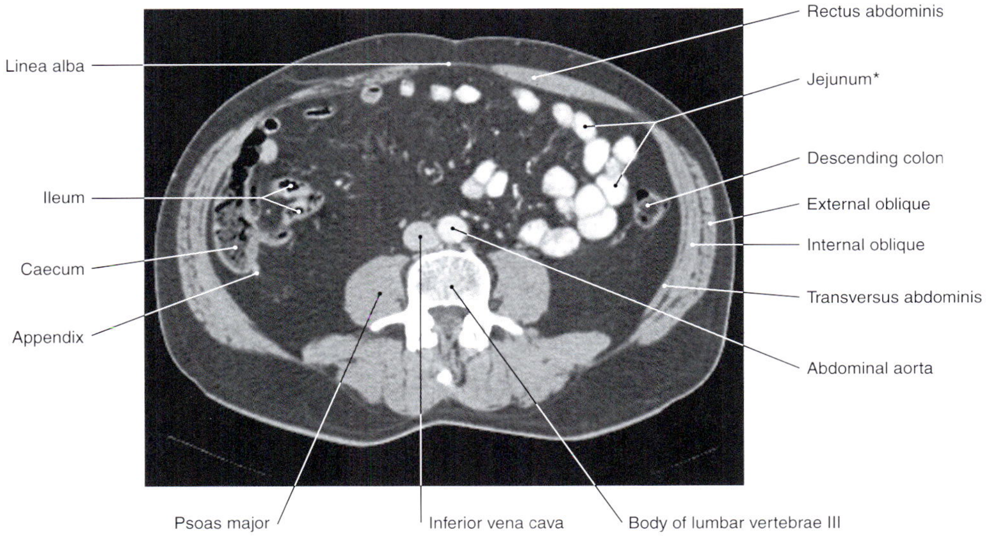

Fig. 930 Abdomen;
computed tomographic section (CT)
at the level of the third lumbar vertebra;
inferior view.

* Jejunum filled with a contrast medium

Male pelvis, median sections

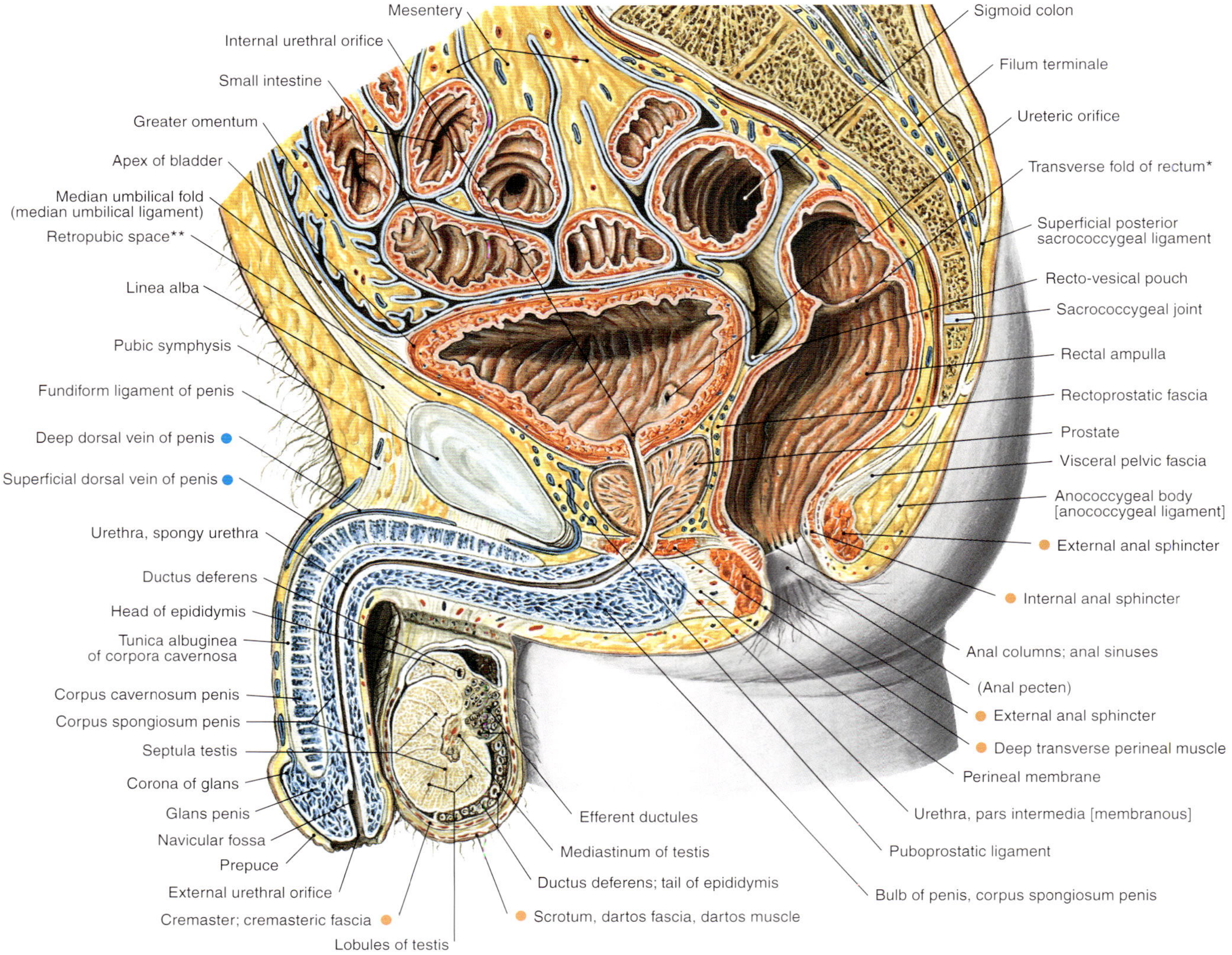

Fig. 931 Pelvis of the male; median section; viewed from the left.

* Clinical term: KOHLRAUSCH's fold
** Clinical term: cave of RETZIUS

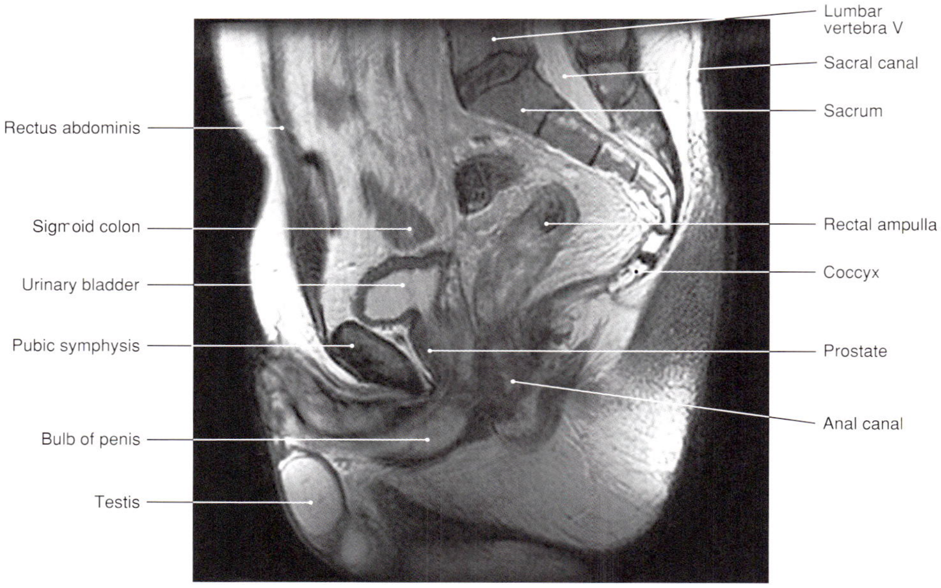

Fig. 932 Pelvis of the male; magnetic resonance tomographic image (MRI); paramedian section; viewed from the left.

Female pelvis, median sections

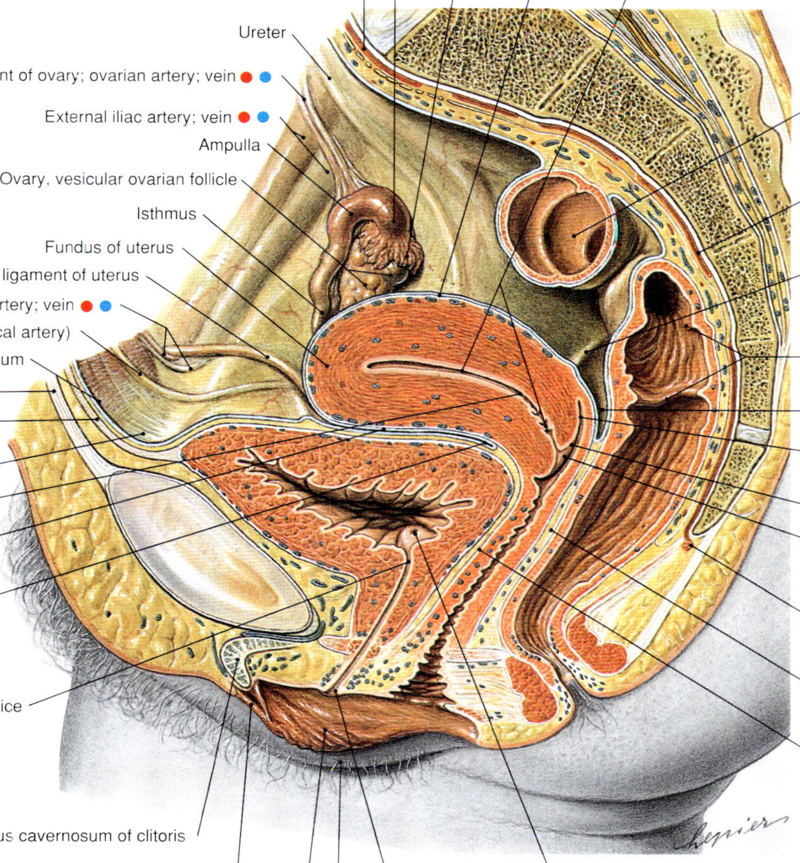

Fig. 933 Pelvis of the female;
median section;
the intestine has been almost completely removed with some remnants of the sigmoid and rectum;
viewed from the left.

* Clinical term: vesicovaginal septum
** Clinical term: sacrouterine ligament
*** Clinical term: pouch of DOUGLAS

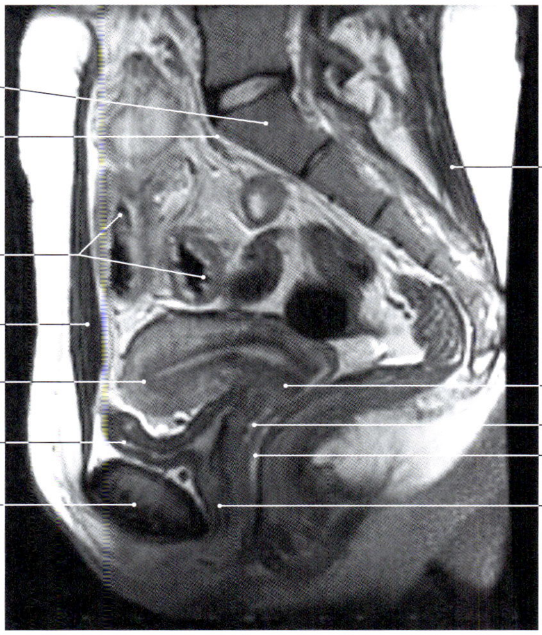

Fig. 934 Pelvis of the female;
magnetic resonance tomographic image (MRI);
paramedian section;
viewed from the left.

Lower abdomen, transverse sections

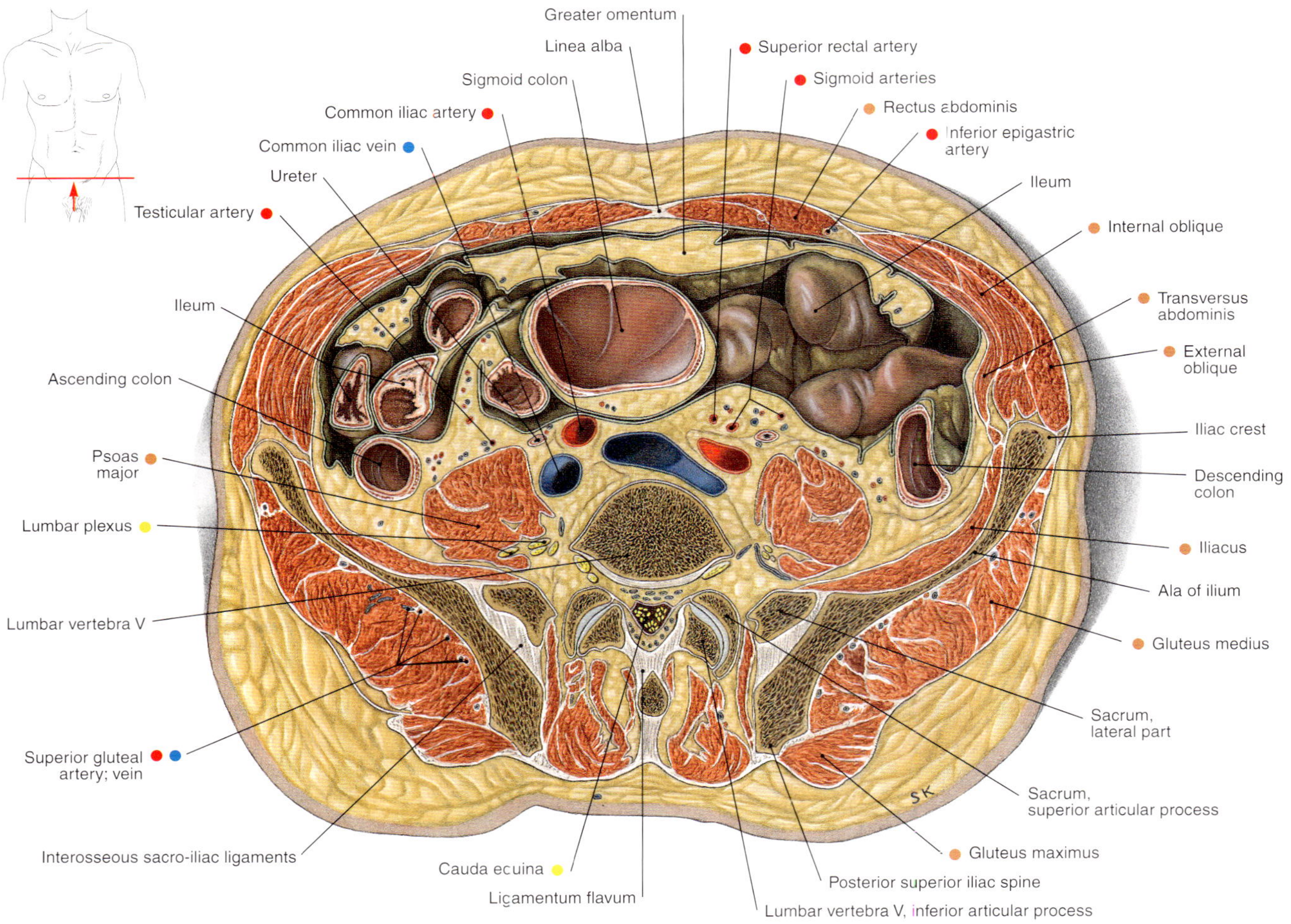

Fig. 935 Pelvis;
transverse section at the level of the fifth lumbar vertebra. This male specimen is different from Fig. 923, 925, 927 and 929.

As the sigmoid reaches far into the upper abdomen the figure also displays the dome of colonic flexure. The thickness of the adipose tissue layer on the gluteus medius muscle must be taken into consideration when injecting intramuscularly.

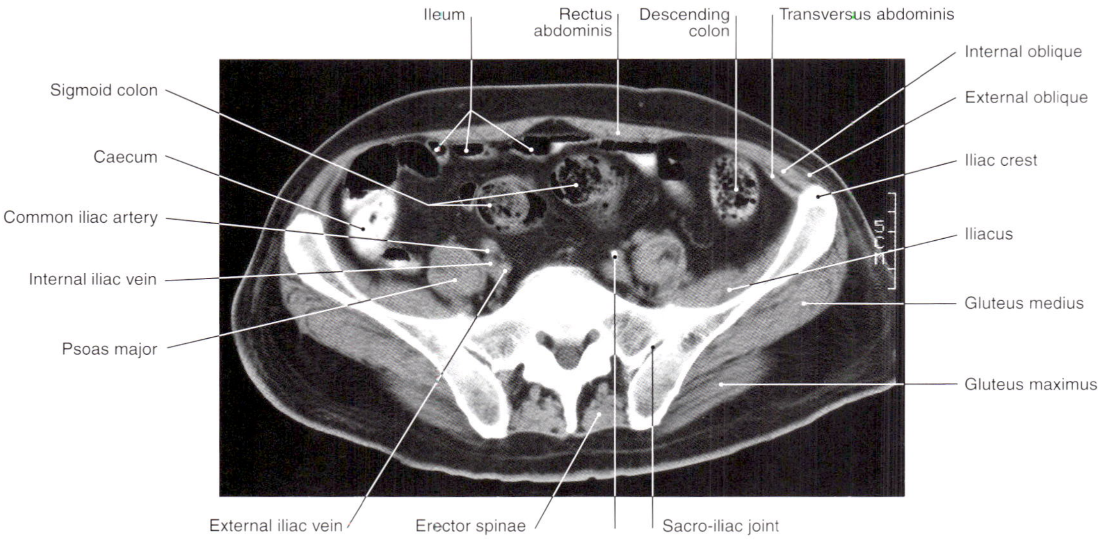

Fig. 936 Pelvis;
computed tomographic cross-section (CT) at the level of the first sacral vertebra after administration of a contrast medium into the colon; supine position; inferior view.

* Calcification in the wall of the iliac artery.

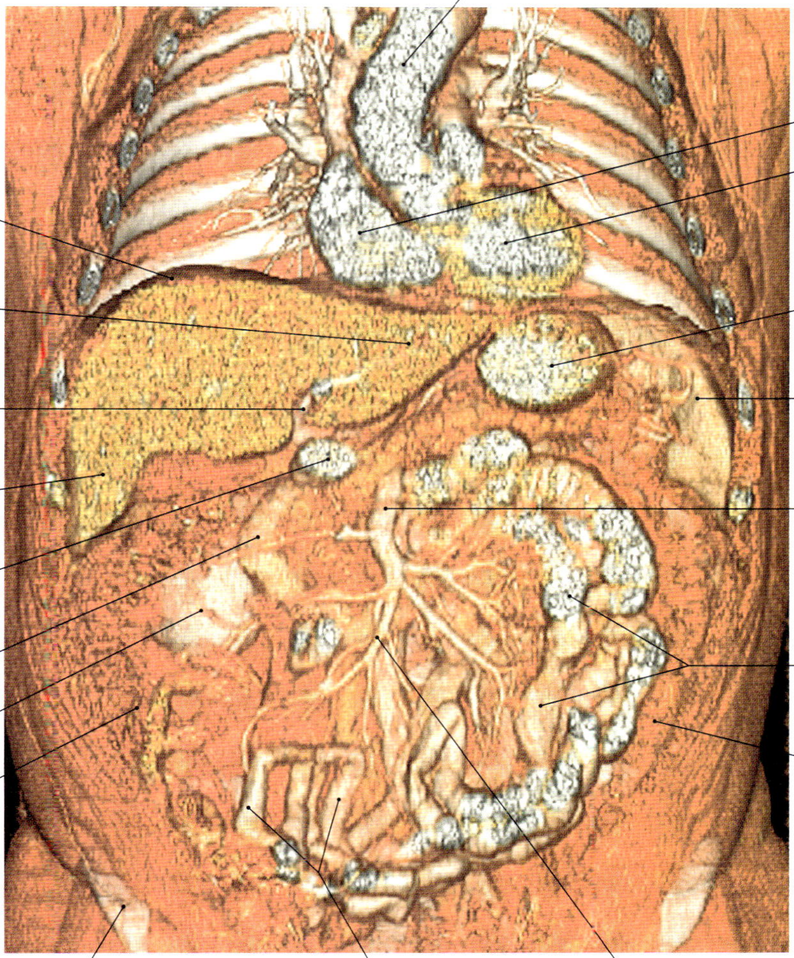

Fig. 937 Abdomen;
volume-guided reconstruction in the frontal plane based on horizontal computed tomographic sections (CT). The section planes of organs such as the heart, the stomach, the liver and parts of the small intestine, appear granulate

→ 802, 919

Male pelvis, transverse sections

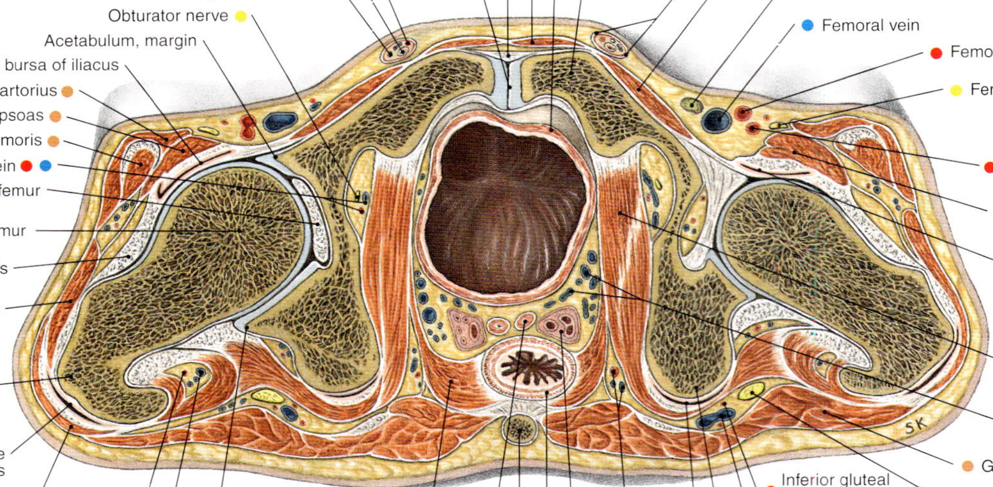

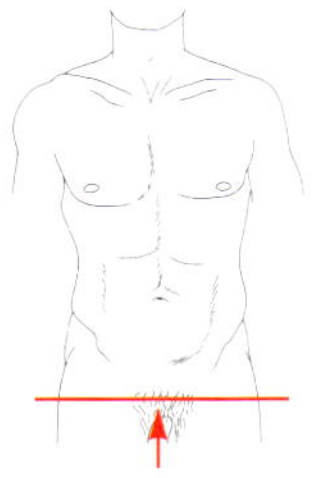

Fig. 938 Pelvis of the male;
transverse section through the lesser pelvis.

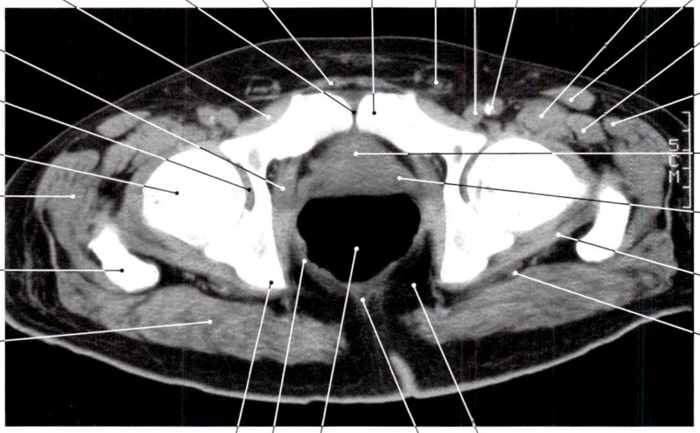

Fig. 939 Pelvis of the male;
computed tomographic cross-section (CT) through the lesser pelvis with the subject in supine position.

* Calcification in the medial part of the femoral artery

Female pelvis, transverse sections

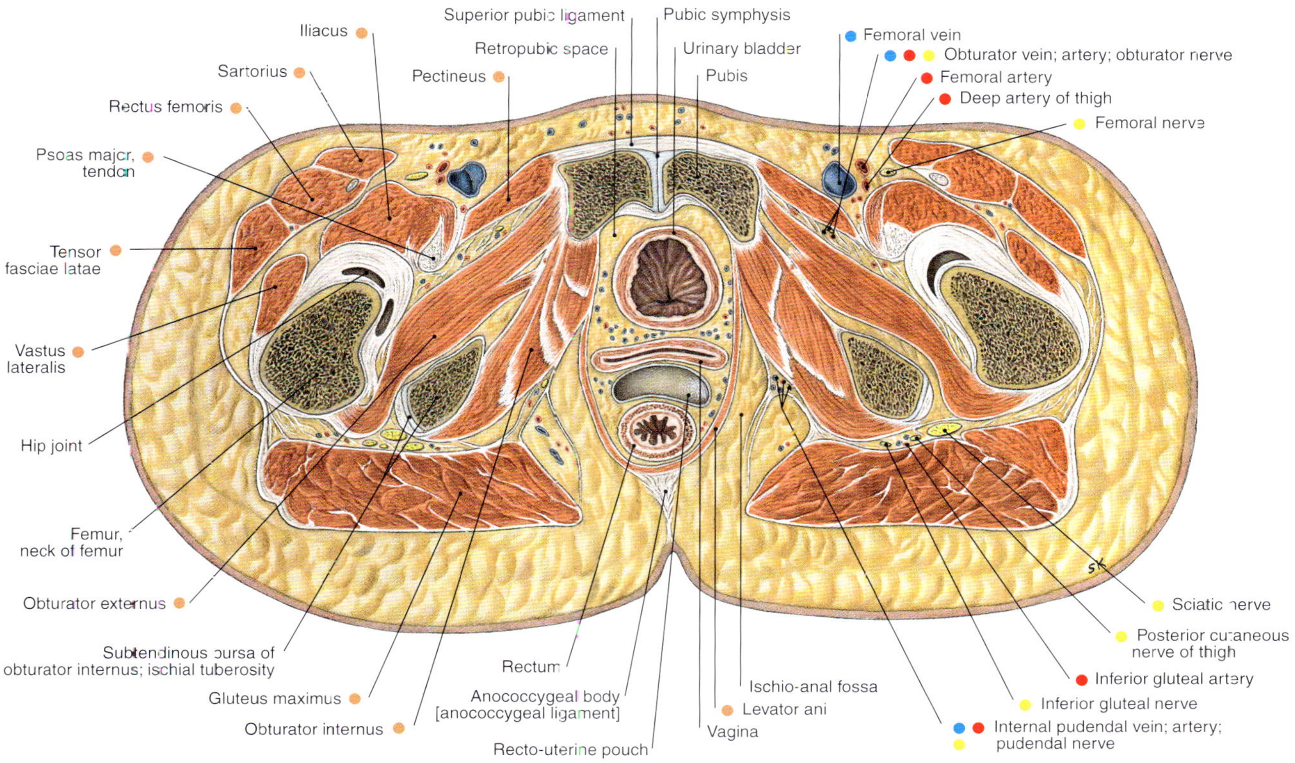

Fig. 940 Pelvis of the female; transverse section through the lesser pelvis at the level of the symphysis.

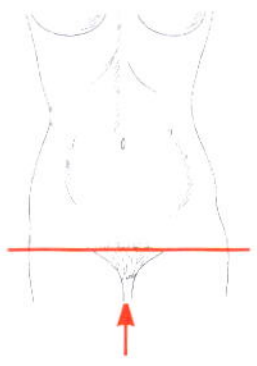

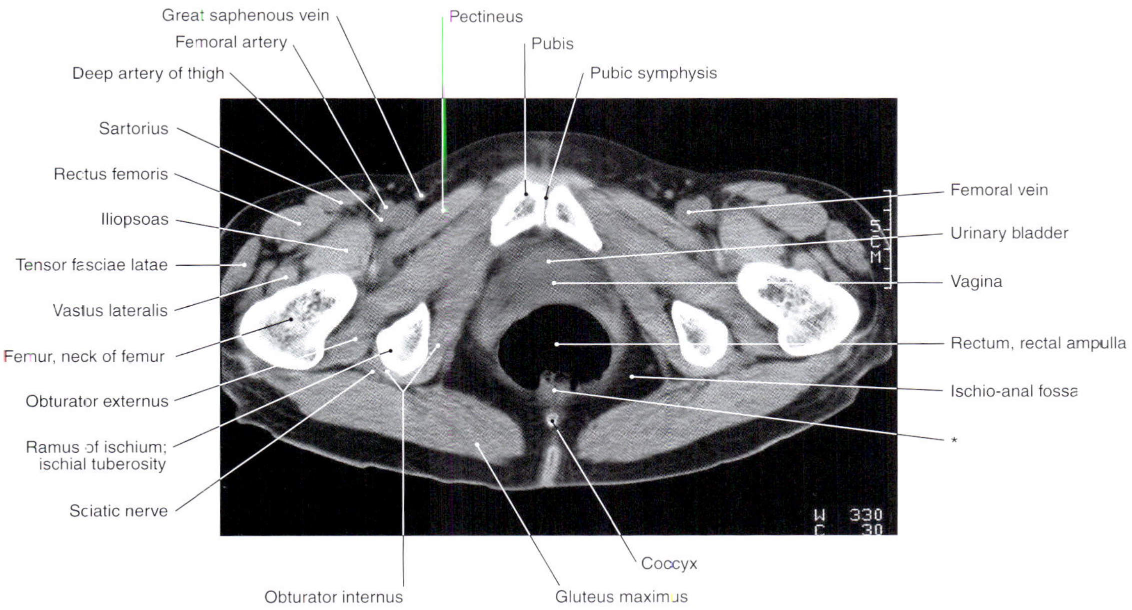

Fig. 941 Pelvis of the female; computed tomographic cross-section (CT) through the lesser pelvis with the subject in supine position.

* Remnants of contrasting intestinal contents

Male pelvis, oblique frontal section

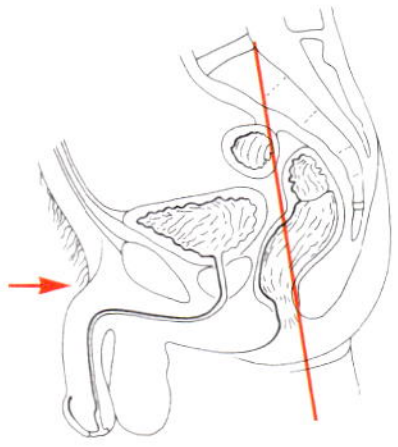

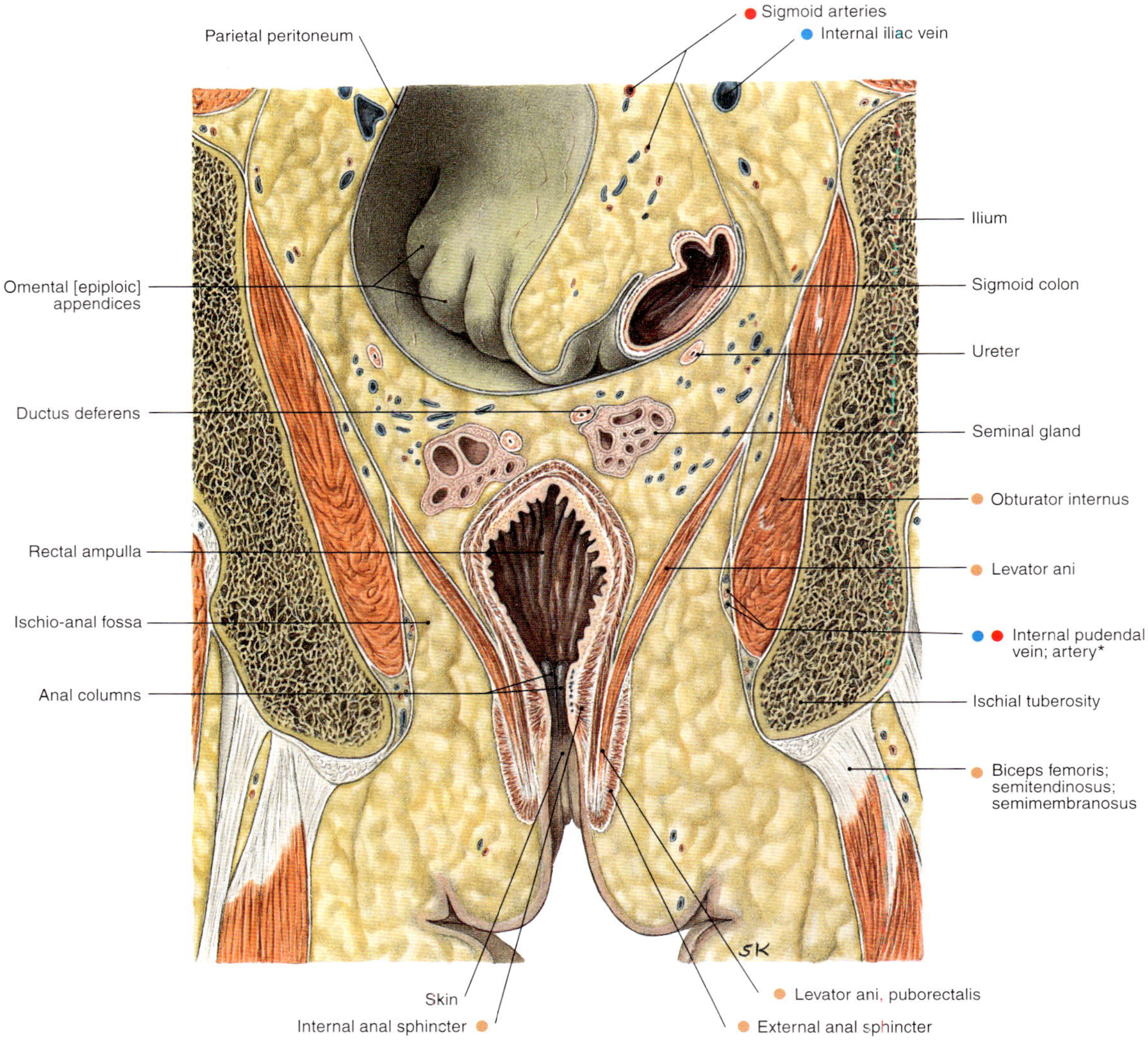

Fig. 942 Pelvis of the male;
oblique frontal section through the lesser pelvis.

* Clinical term: ALCOCK's canal

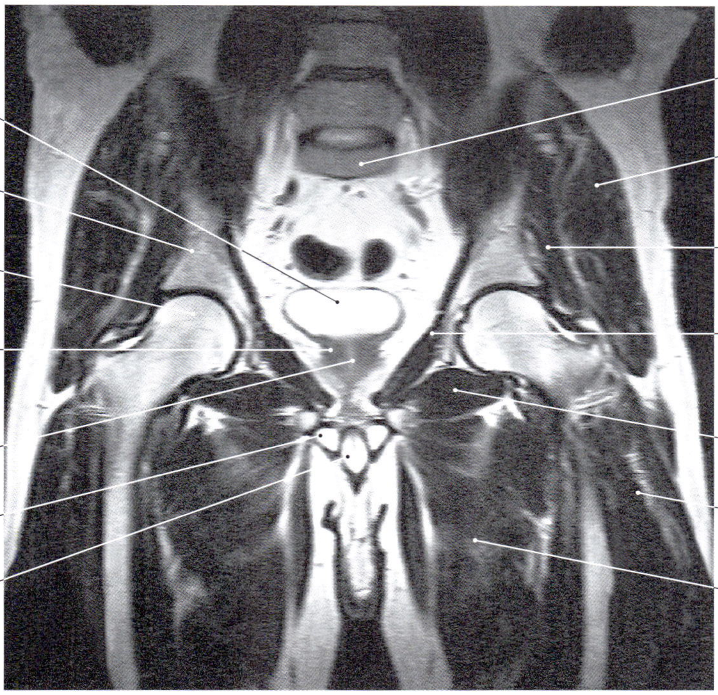

Fig. 943 Pelvis of the male;
magnetic resonance tomographic image (MRI);
frontal section at the level of the hip joints;
ventral view.

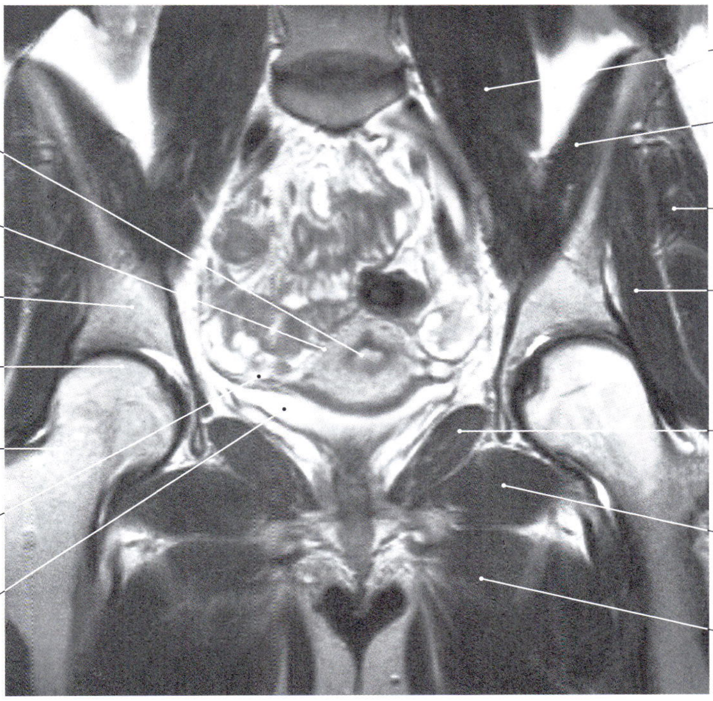

Fig. 944 Pelvis of the female;
magnetic resonance tomographic image (MRI);
frontal section at the level of the hip joints;
ventral view.

When the urinary bladder is empty, the uterus lies on the apex of the bladder due to its anteflexion.

Male pelvis diaphragm, angled-frontal section

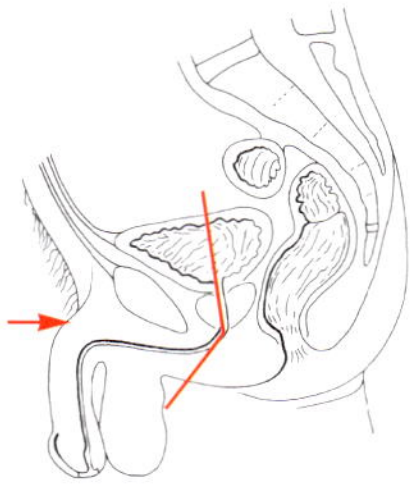

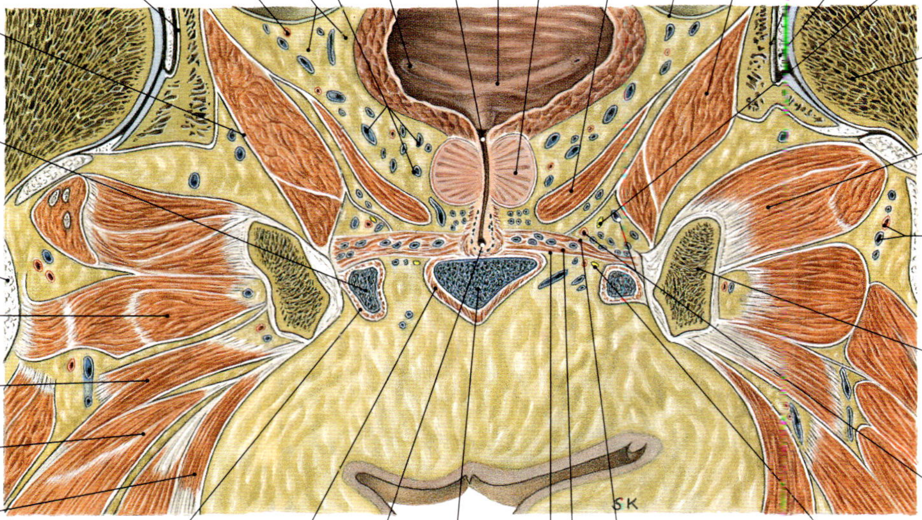

Fig. 945 Pelvis of the male;
angled-frontal section through the urinary bladder.

* Clinical term: paracystium

** Clinical term: prostatic venous plexus

Female pelvic diaphragm, angled-frontal section

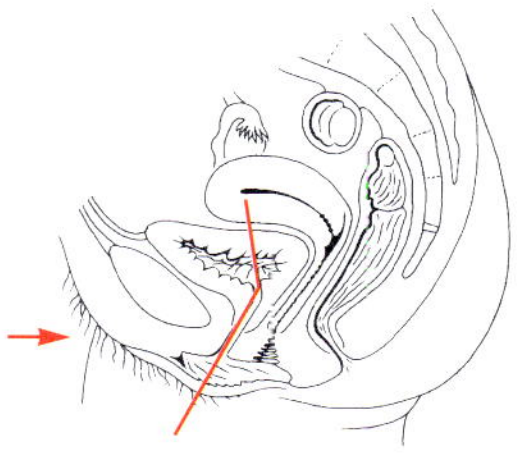

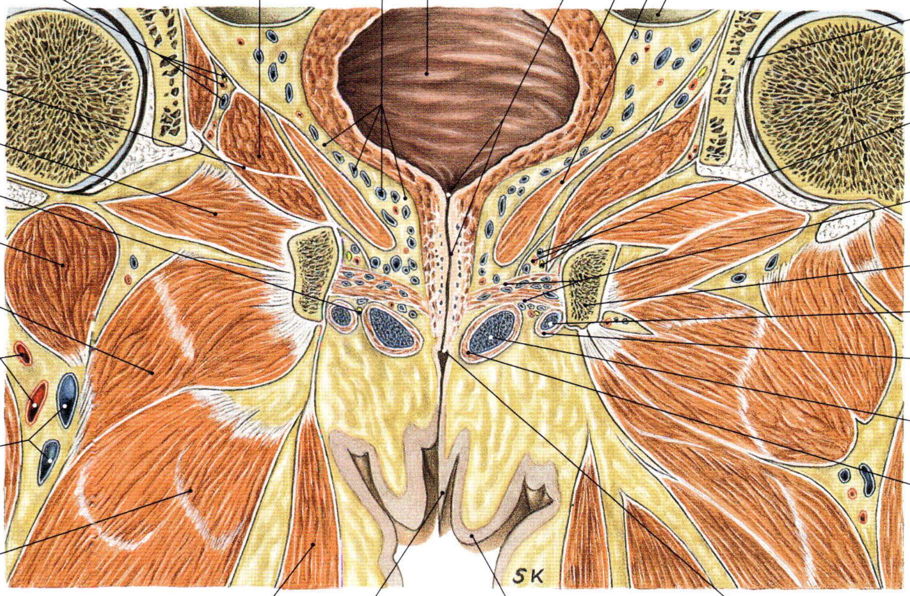

Fig. 946 Pelvis of the female;
angled-frontal section through the urinary bladder.

* Paracystium with venous plexus

Surface anatomy

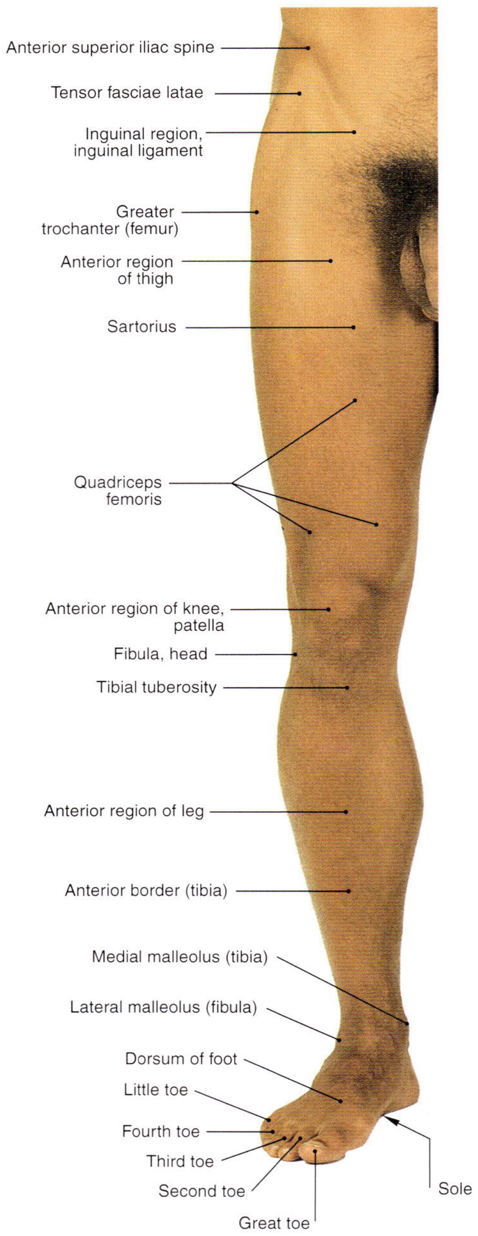

Fig. 947 Lower limb.

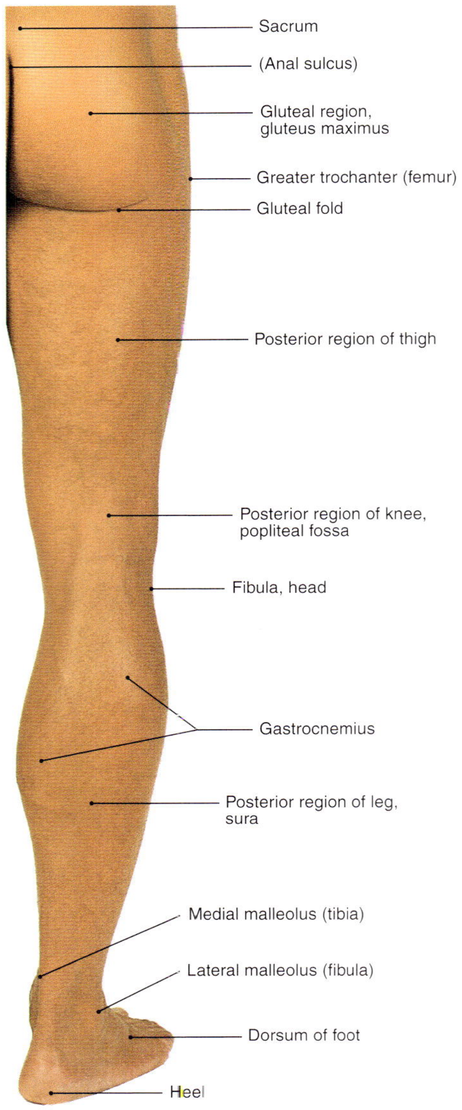

Fig. 948 Lower limb.

Skeleton of the lower limb, overview

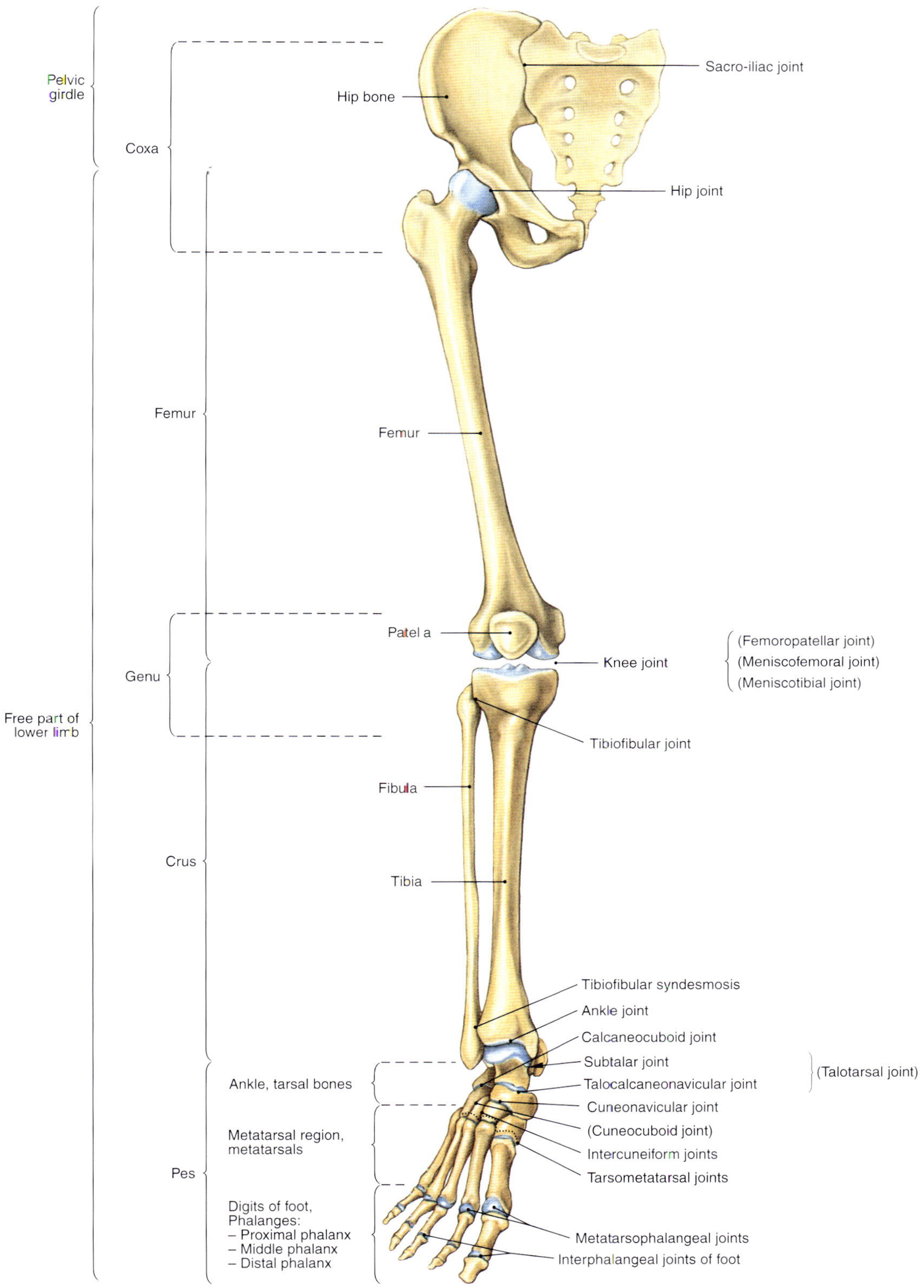

Fig. 949 Lower limb; skeleton and joints.

Pelvis

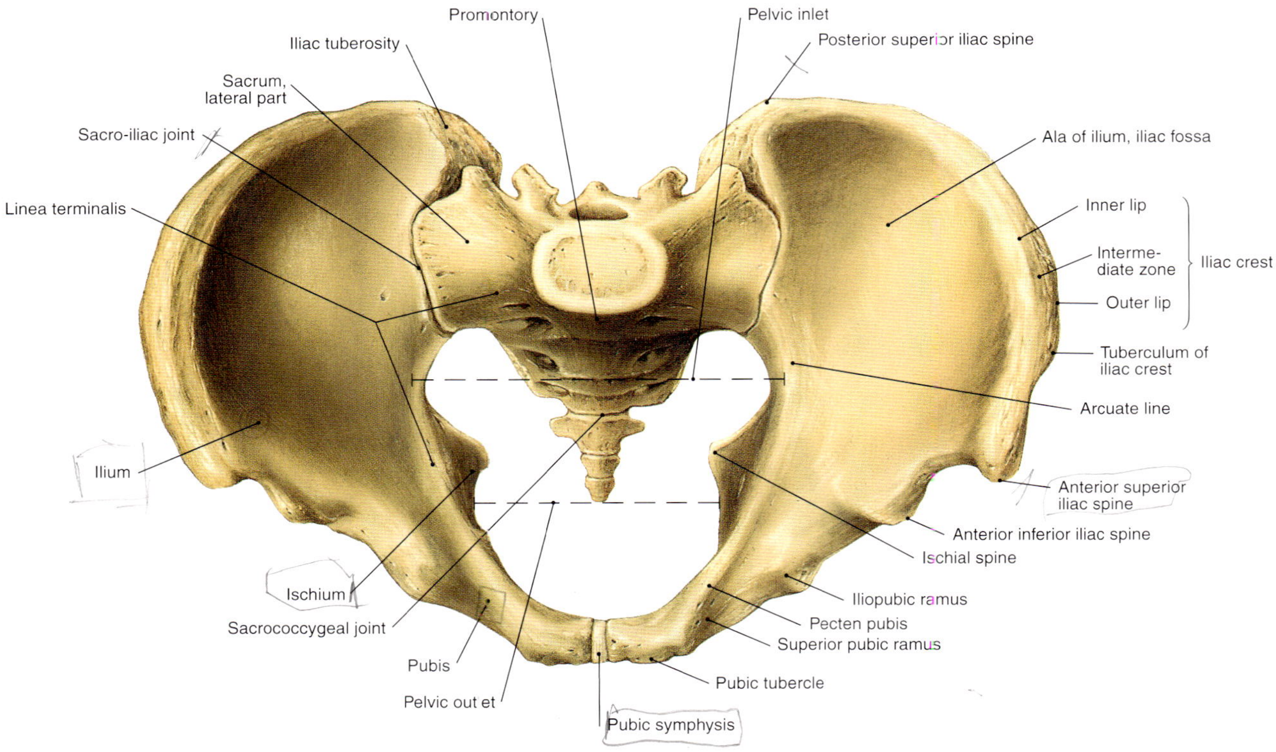

Fig. 950 Sacrum and pelvic girdle.
The region cranial to the linea terminalis is referred to as the greater pelvis and the region caudal to it is known as lesser pelvis.

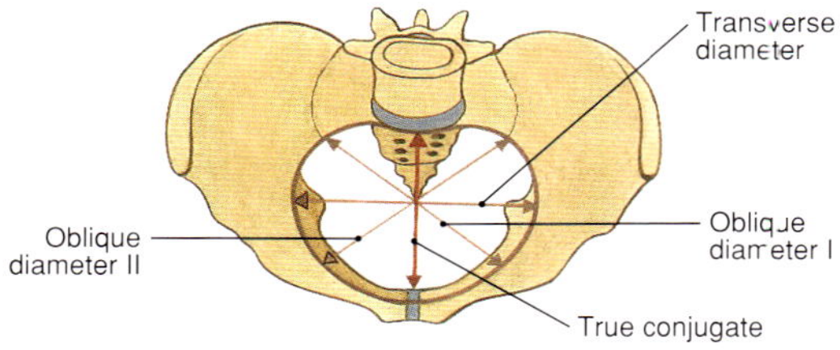

Fig. 951 Pelvis;
shape and dimensions of the pelvic inlet of the female.

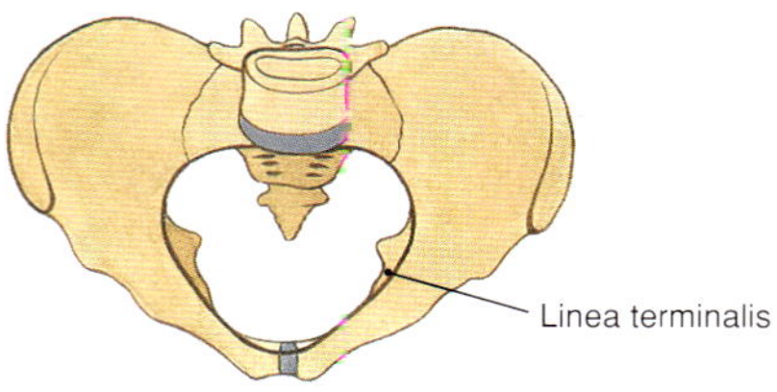

Fig. 952 Pelvis;
shape of the pelvic inlet of the male.

k – k = Pelvic axis
a – b = Anatomical conjugate
a – e = Diagonal conjugate 12.5–13 cm
a – c = True conjugate 10.4–11 cm

h – d = Sagittal diameter of the pelvic brim 12–12.5 cm
e – g = Sagittal diameter of the pelvic constriction 11–11.5 cm
e – f = Sagittal diameter of the pelvic outlet (= pubococcygeal distance) 9–10 cm

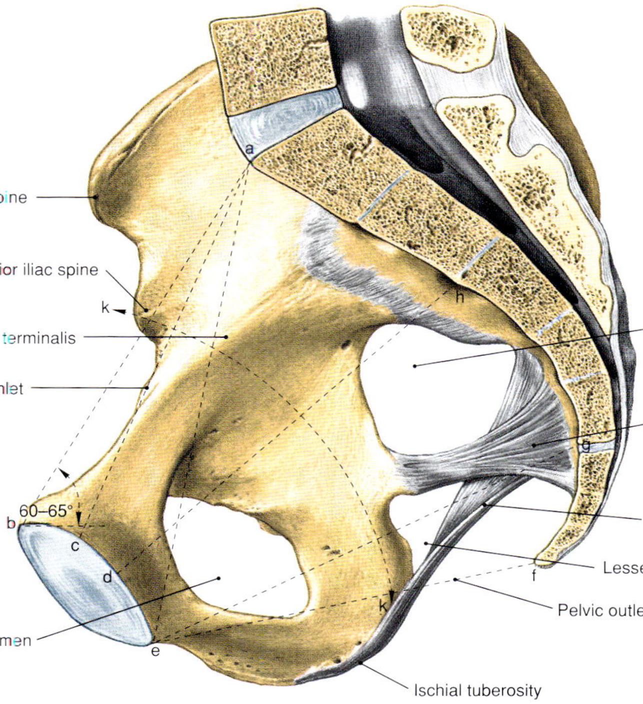

Fig. 953 Pelvis; dimensions in the female; median section.

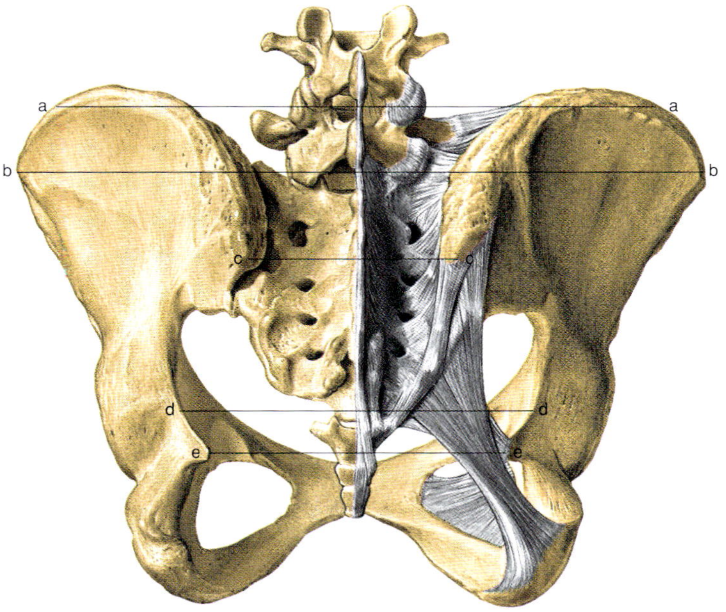

a – a = Crestal distance 28–29 cm*
b – b = Anterior spinal distance 25–26 cm*
c – c = Posterior spinal distance (width of the sacrum) 10 cm
* In this perspective, the crestal distance appears shorter than the anterior spinal distance.

Fig. 954 Pelvis; dimensions in the female.

d – d = Transverse diameter of the pelvic brim (= interacetabular line) 12–12.5 cm
e – e = Transverse diameter of the pelvic constriction (= interspinal line) 10.5 cm
f – f = Transverse diameter of the pelvic outlet (= tuberal diameter) 11–12 cm)

Hip bone

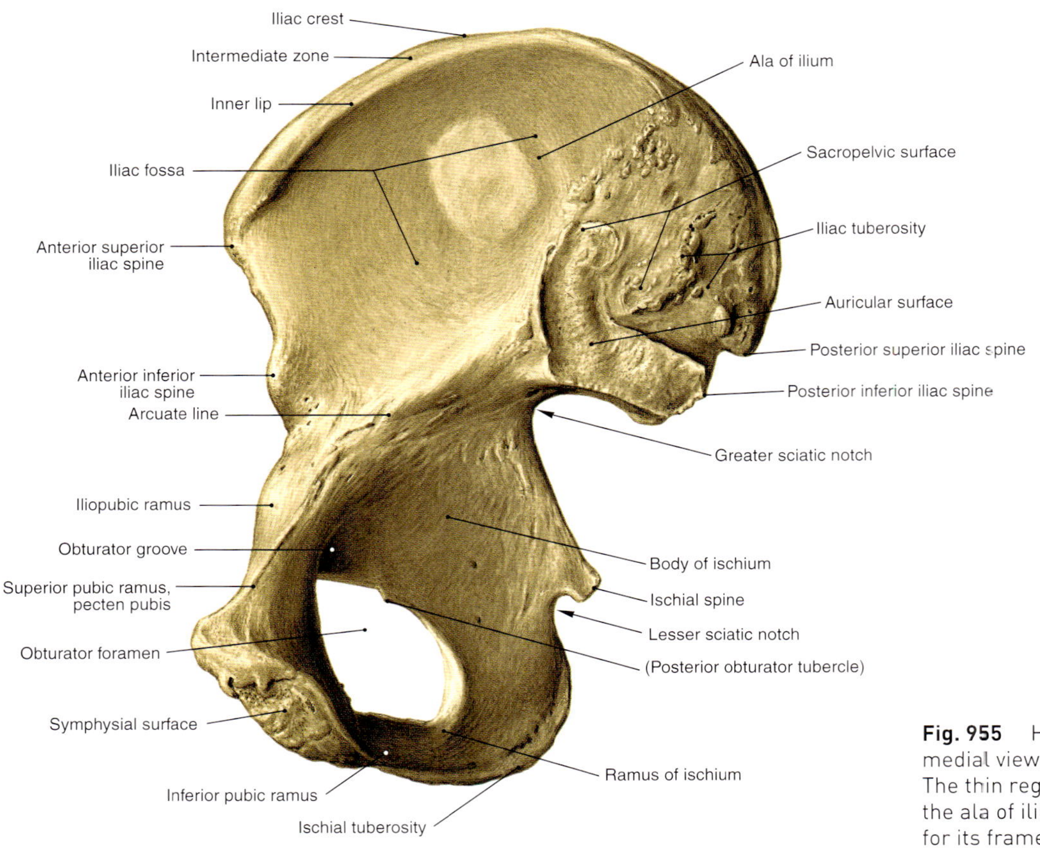

Fig. 955 Hip bone; medial view.
The thin region in the centre of the ala of ilium is characteristic for its frame-like structure.

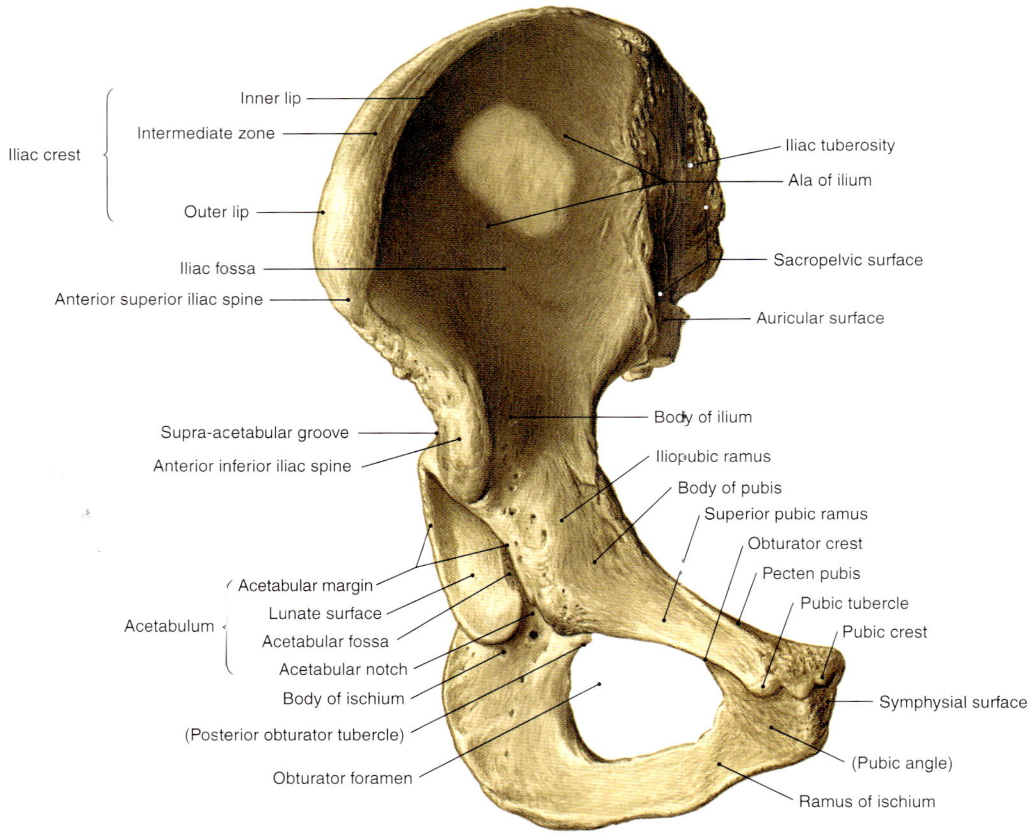

Fig. 956 Hip bone; ventral view.

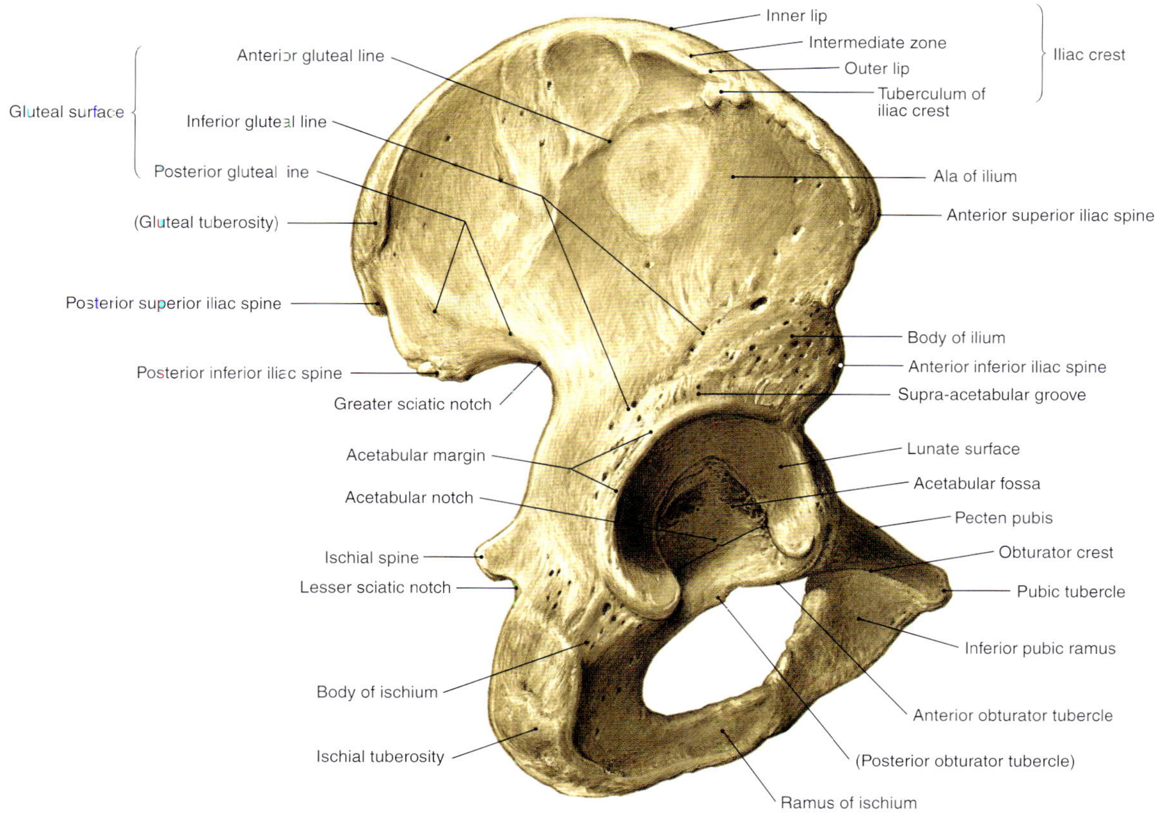

Fig. 957 Hip bone;
dorsolateral view.

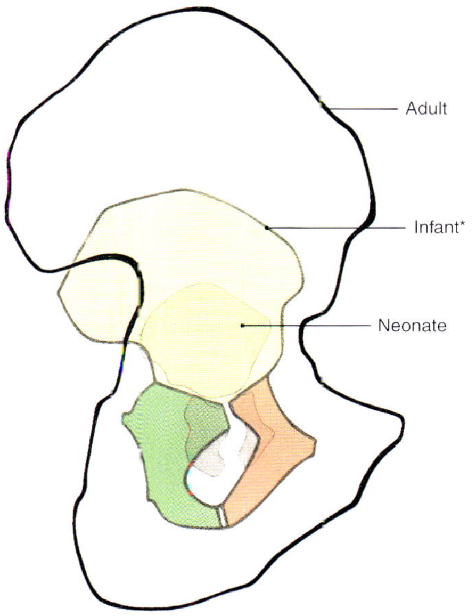

Fig. 958 Hip bone;
development.

* Approximately sixth year of life

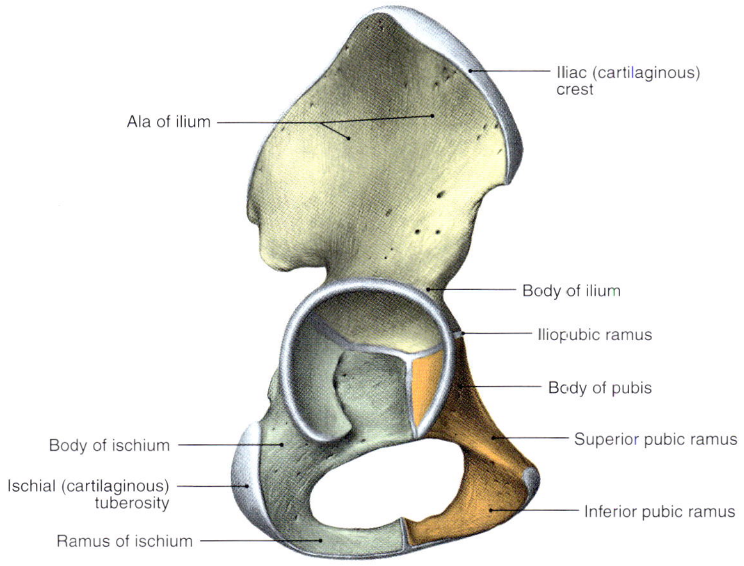

Fig. 959 Hip bone;
stage of development in a 6-year-old child.
In the acetabulum, the three parts of the hip bone are fused to a Y-shaped cartilaginous junction. This junction ossifies at the age of 13–18 years.

Joints of the pelvic girdle

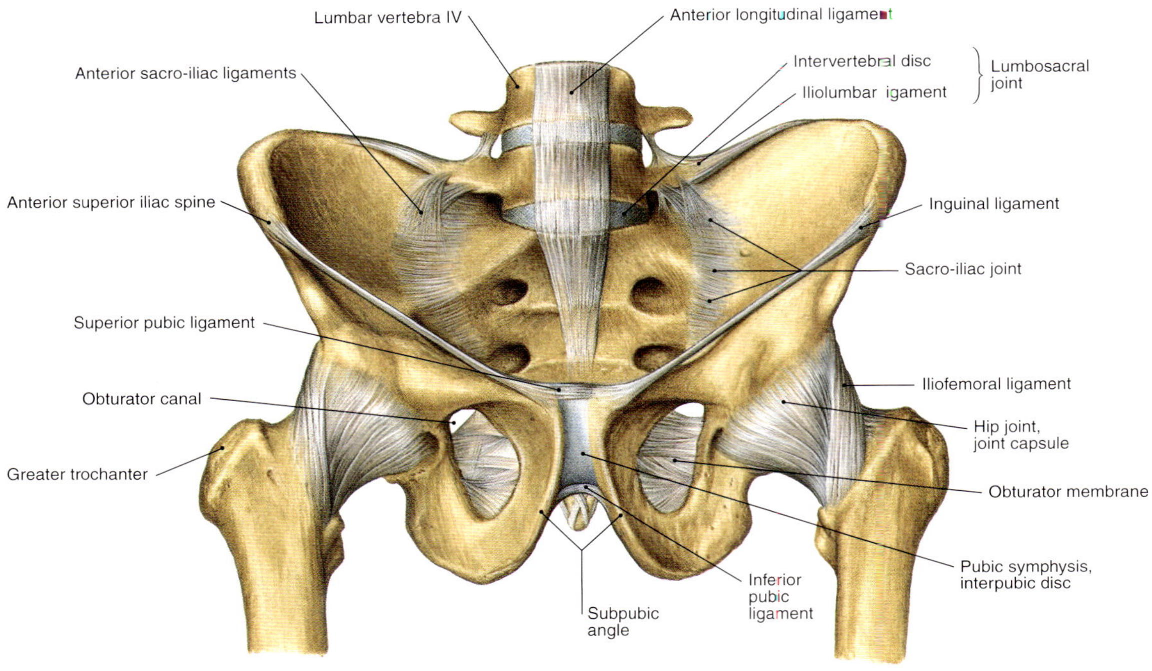

Fig. 960 Joints of the pelvic girdle and the lumbosacral joint of the male.

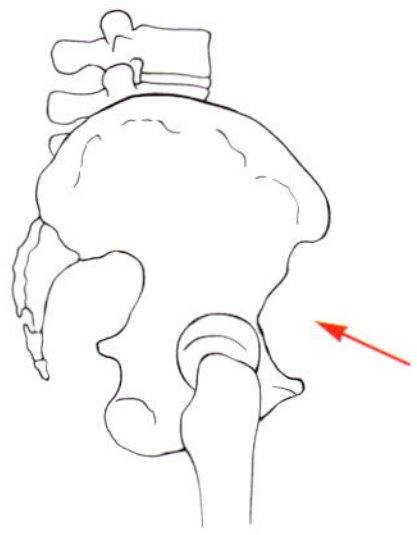

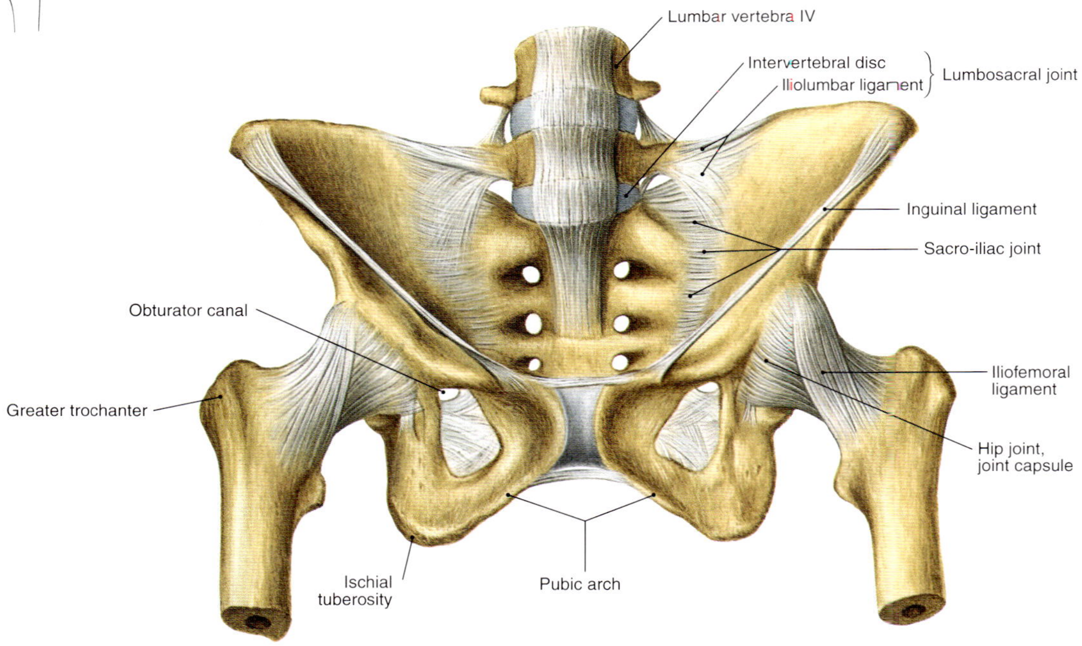

Fig. 961 Joints of the pelvic girdle and the lumbosacral joint of the female.

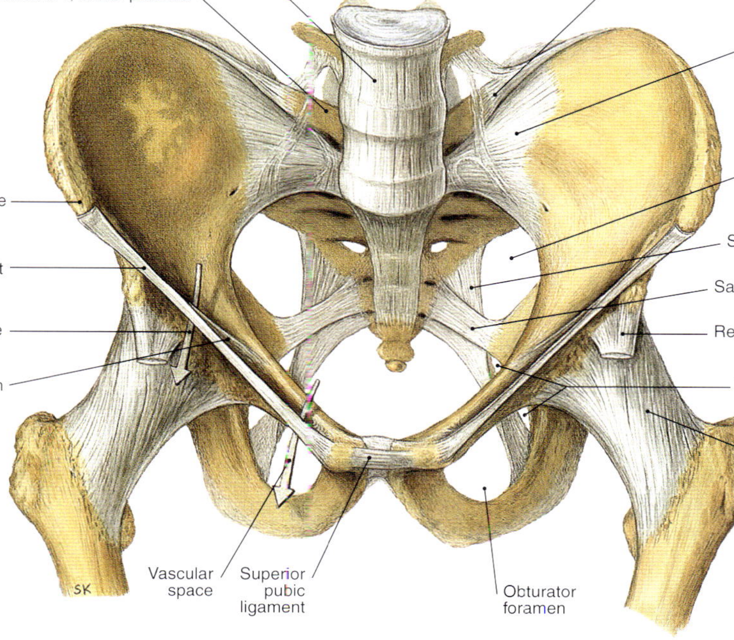

Fig. 962 Joints of the pelvic girdle and the lumbosacral joint of the male.

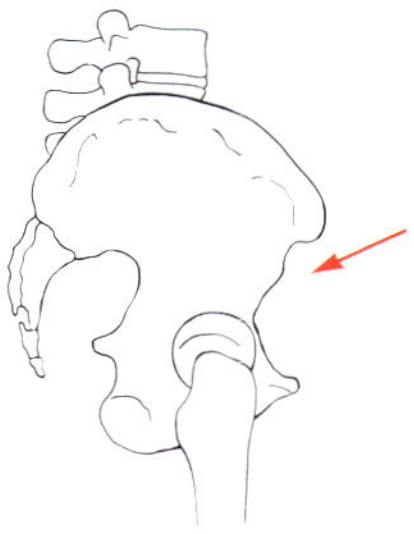

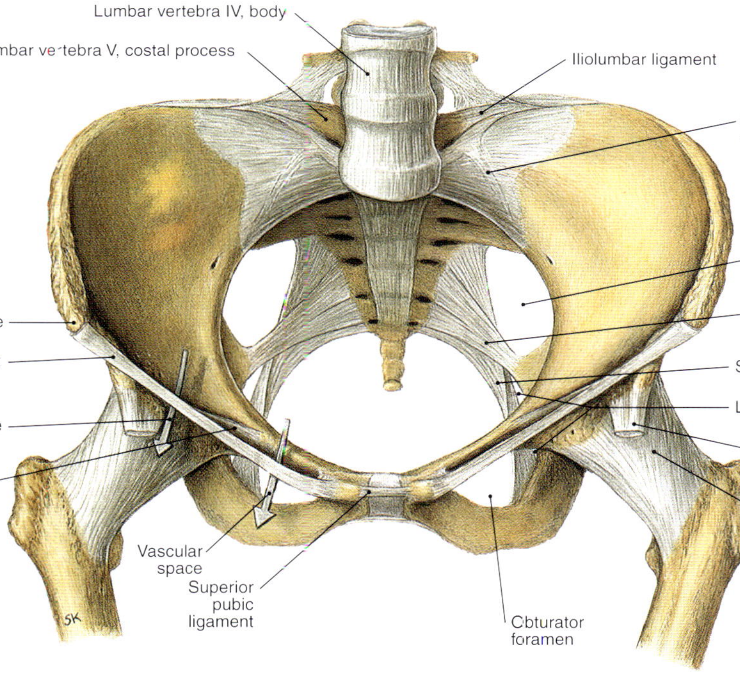

Fig. 963 Joints of the pelvic girdle and the lumbosacral joint of the female.

Joints of the pelvic girdle

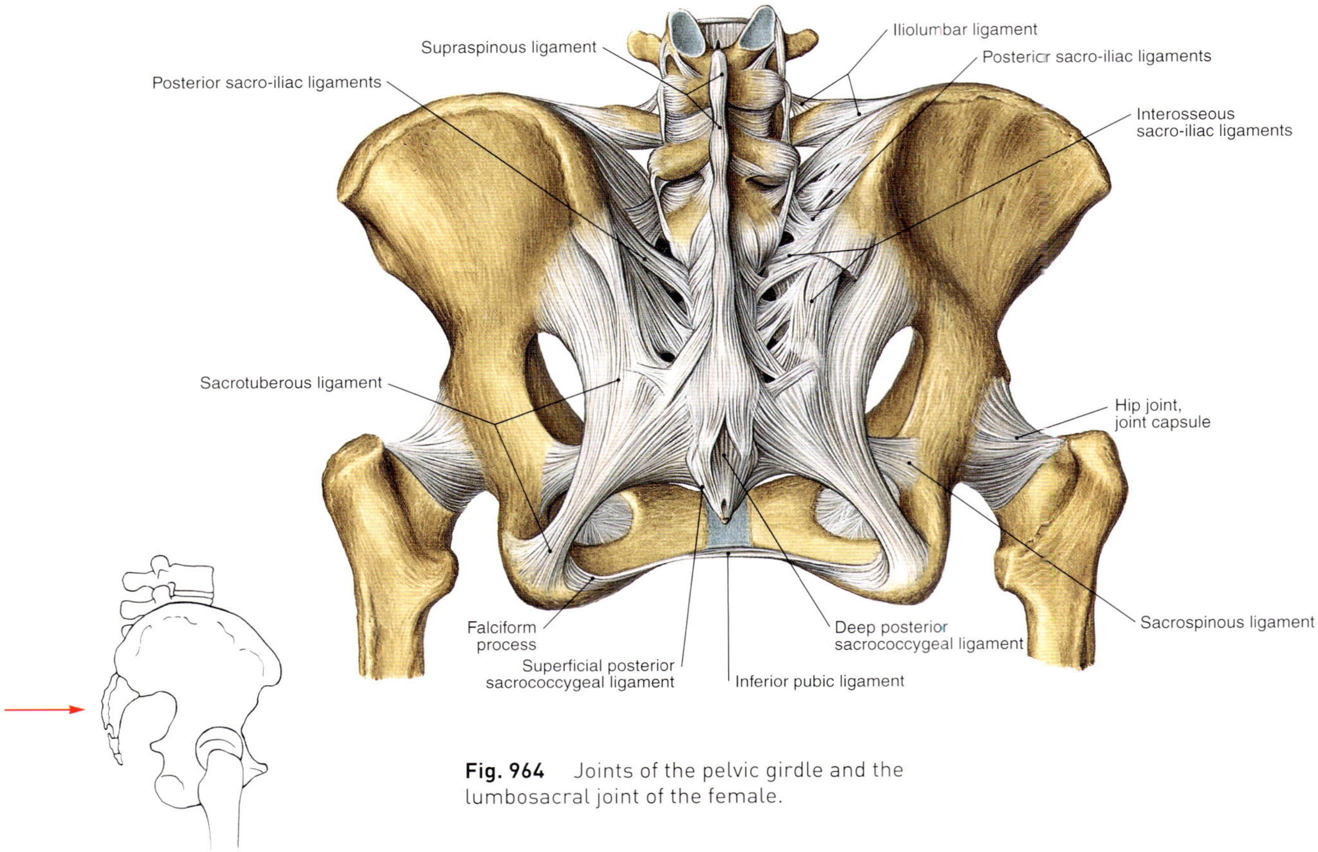

Fig. 964 Joints of the pelvic girdle and the lumbosacral joint of the female.

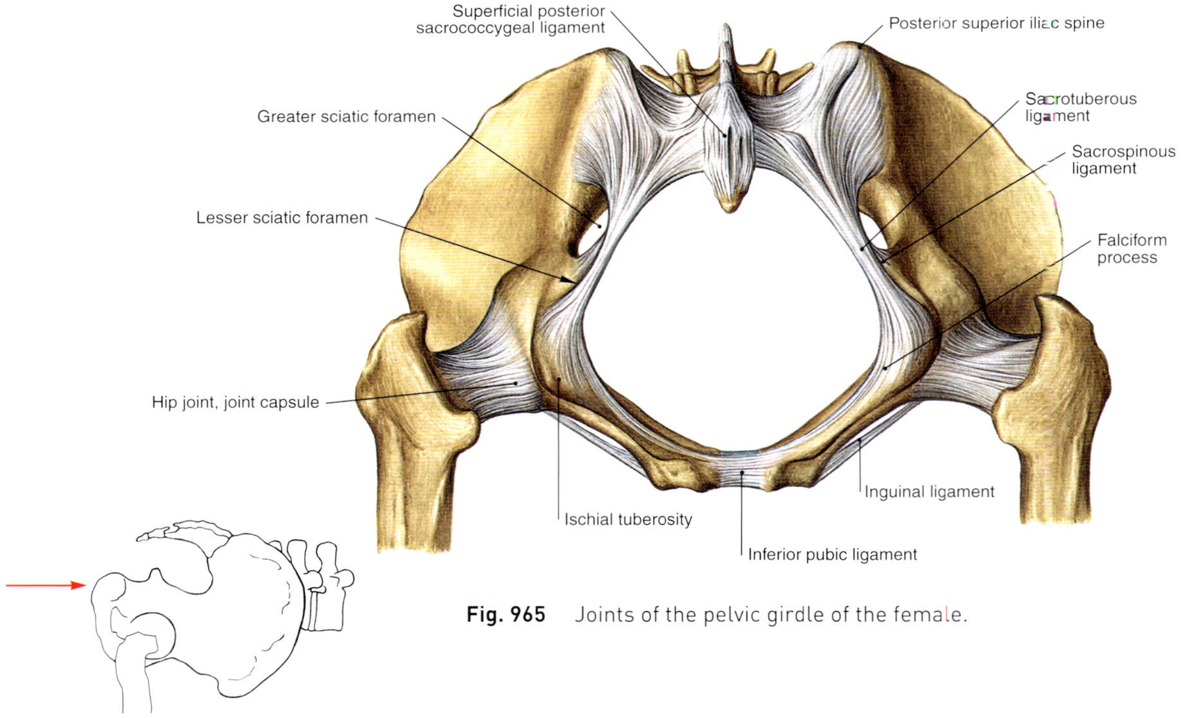

Fig. 965 Joints of the pelvic girdle of the female.

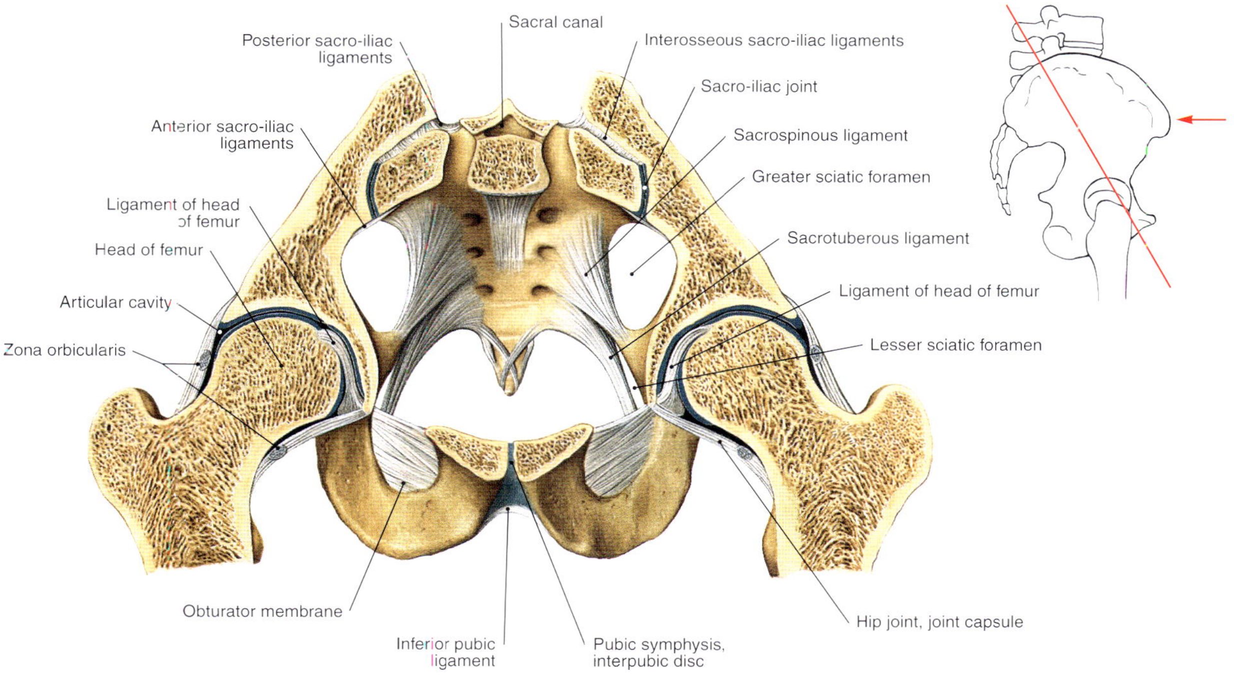

Fig. 966 Joints of the pelvic girdle of the female.

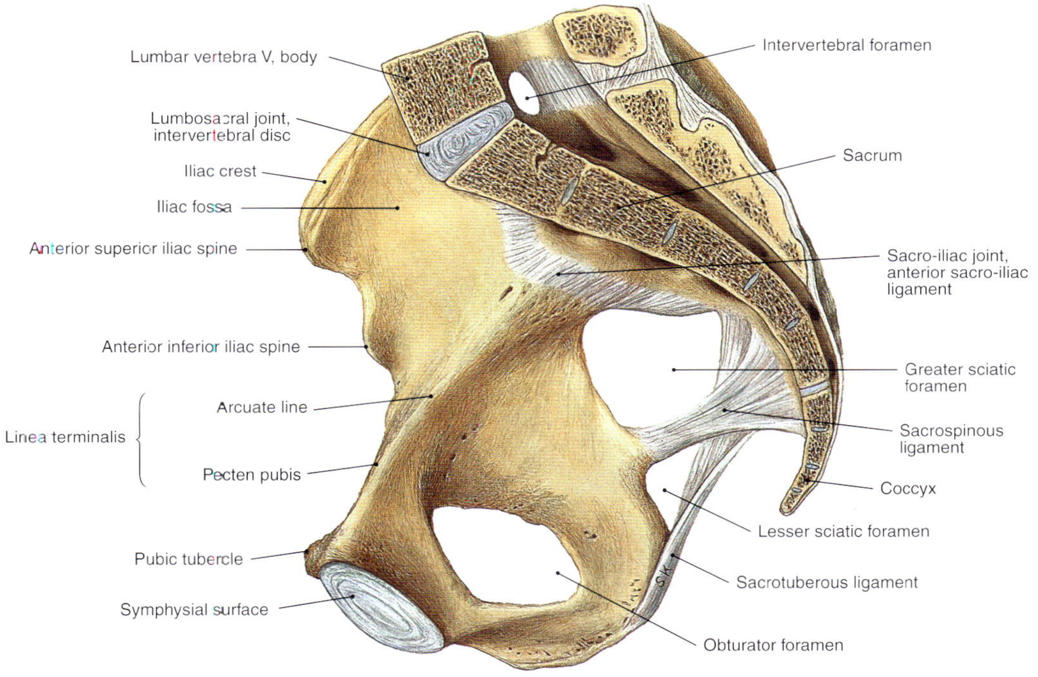

Fig. 967 Joints of the pelvic girdle and the lumbosacral joint of the female; median section.

Normally, the anterior border of the lowest intervertebral disc forms the furthest projecting point of the posterior circumference of the pelvic inlet. Radiographically, the most anterior part of the sacrum is referred to as promontory.

Joints of the pelvic girdle

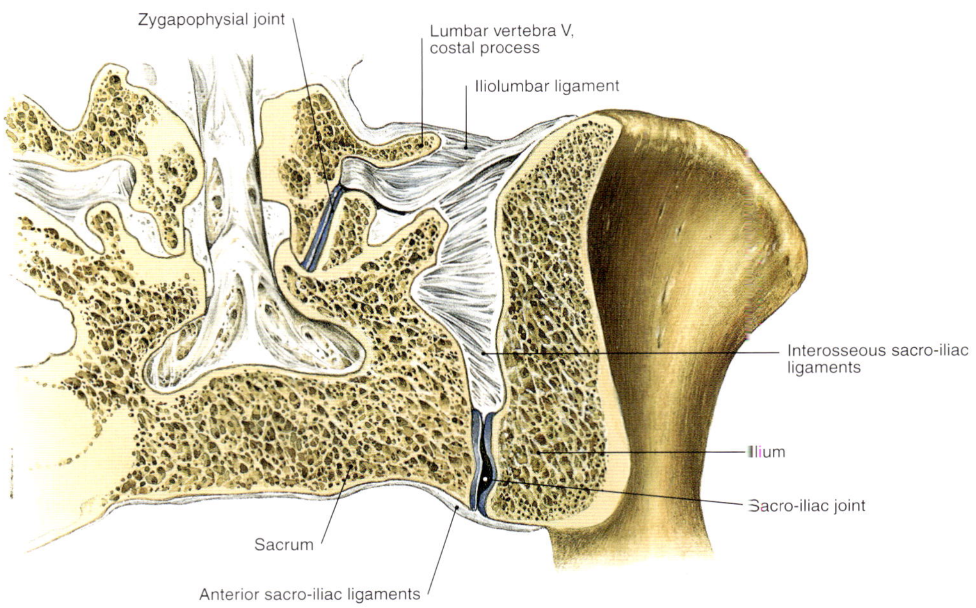

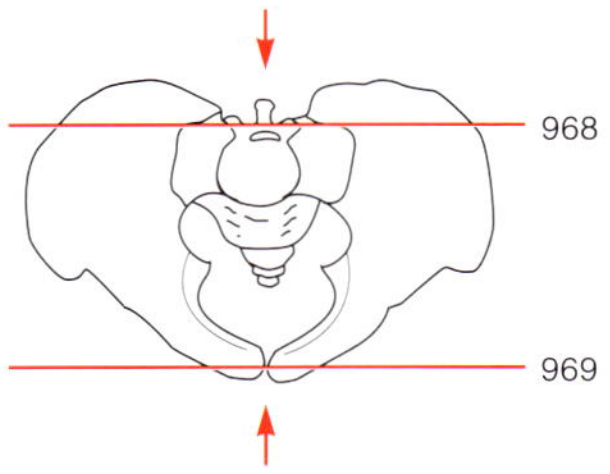

Fig. 968 Sacroiliac joint; frontal section.

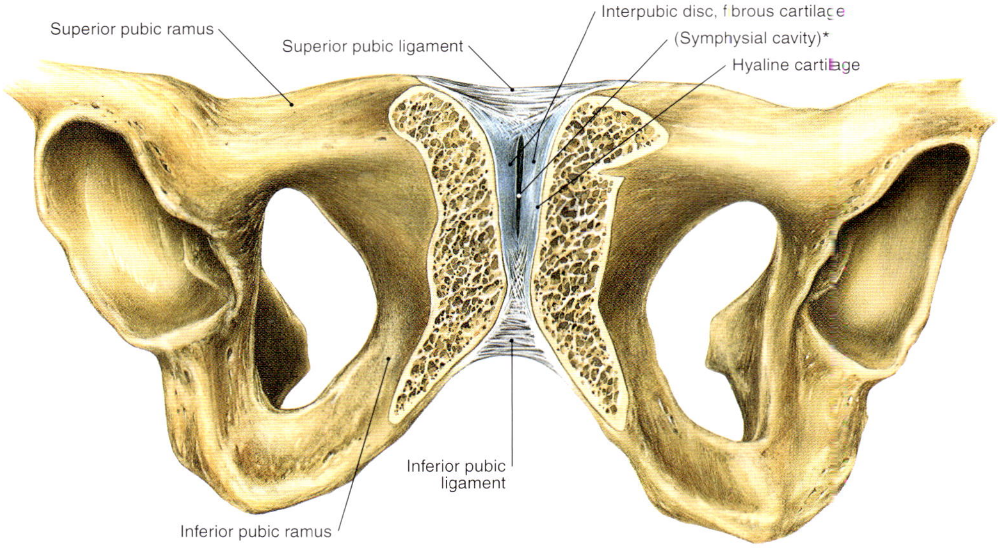

Fig. 969 Pubic symphysis; oblique section in the direction of the longitudinal axis of the symphysis.
The interpubic disc consists of fibrous cartilage, with the exception of the articular symphysial surfaces of both pubic bones that are covered with hyaline cartilage. A longitudinal flat cleft occurs after the first decade of life (*).

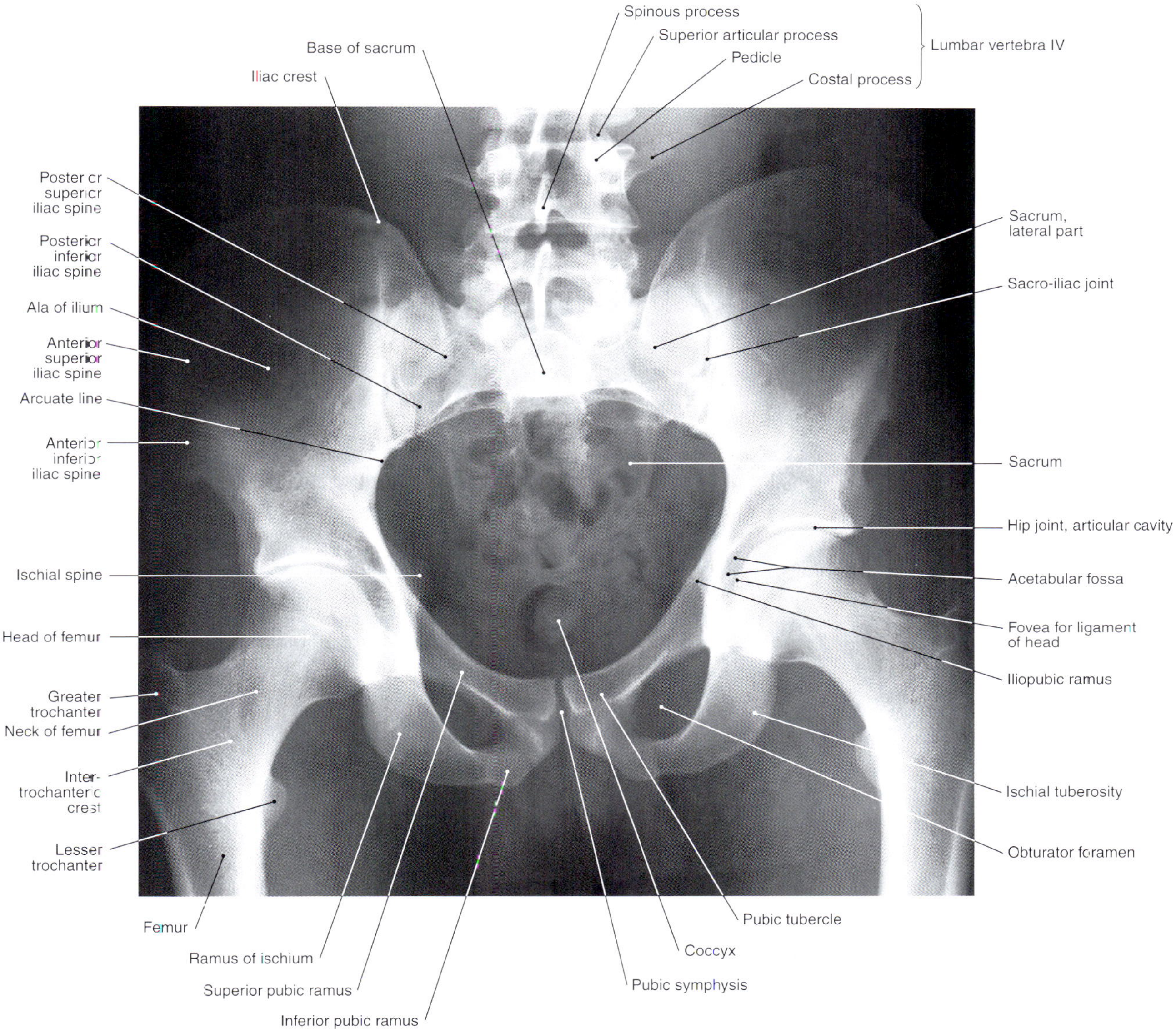

Fig. 970 Pelvis of the male;
AP-radiograph with the central beam directed onto the third sacral segment; upright position.

Pelvis, development

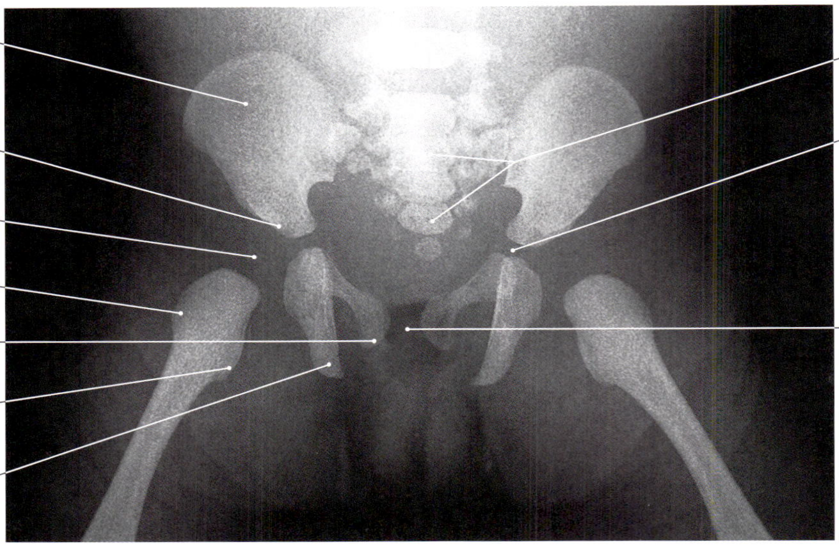

Fig. 971 Pelvis and femur; AP-radiograph of a female, premature baby (eighth month of pregnancy).

- * Osseous roof of the acetabulum
- ** Y-shaped junction in the acetabular fossa
- *** The ossification centre in the head of the femur does not appear before the third to fifth month of life.
- \+ At this age, both greater trochanters only become apparent as small protuberances of the bone of the diaphysis.

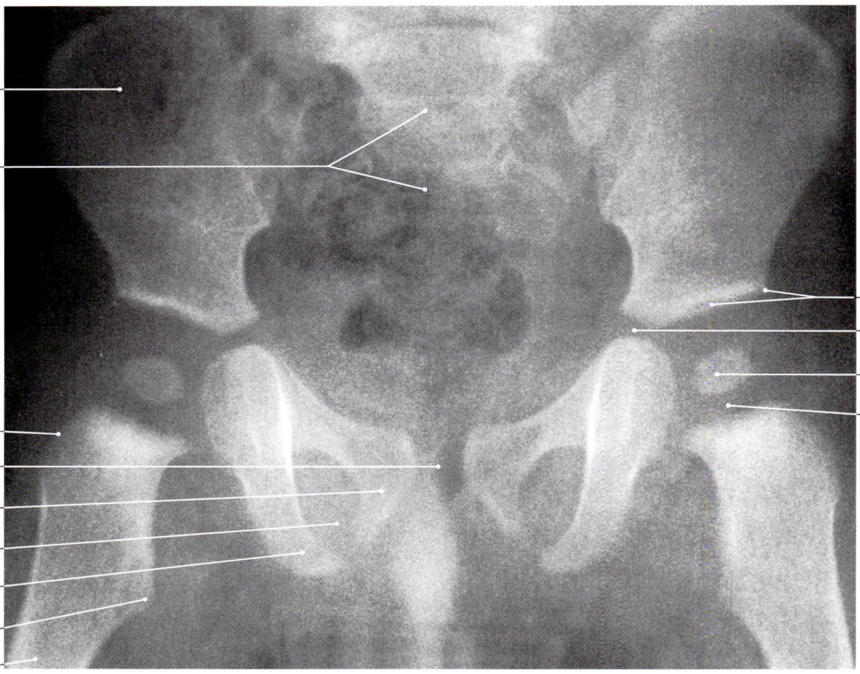

Fig. 972 Pelvis and femur; AP-radiograph of a 12-month-old boy.

- * Osseous roof of the acetabulum
- ** Y-shaped junction in the acetabular fossa
- *** Ossification centre in the epiphysis of the head of the femur
- \+ At this age, both greater trochanters only become apparent as small protuberances of the bone of the diaphysis.

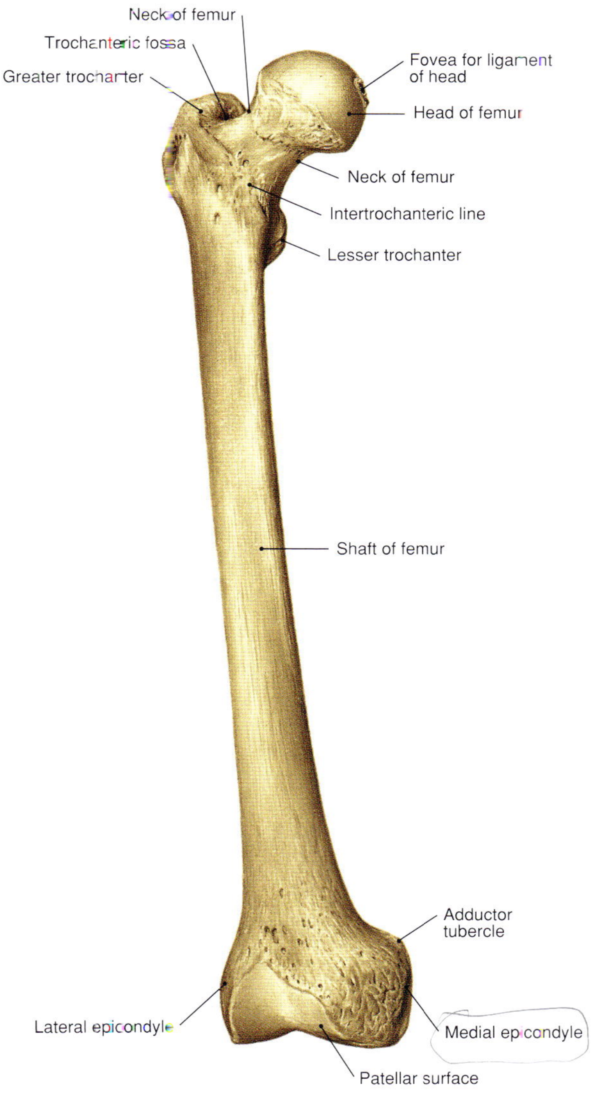

Fig. 973 Femur;
ventral view.

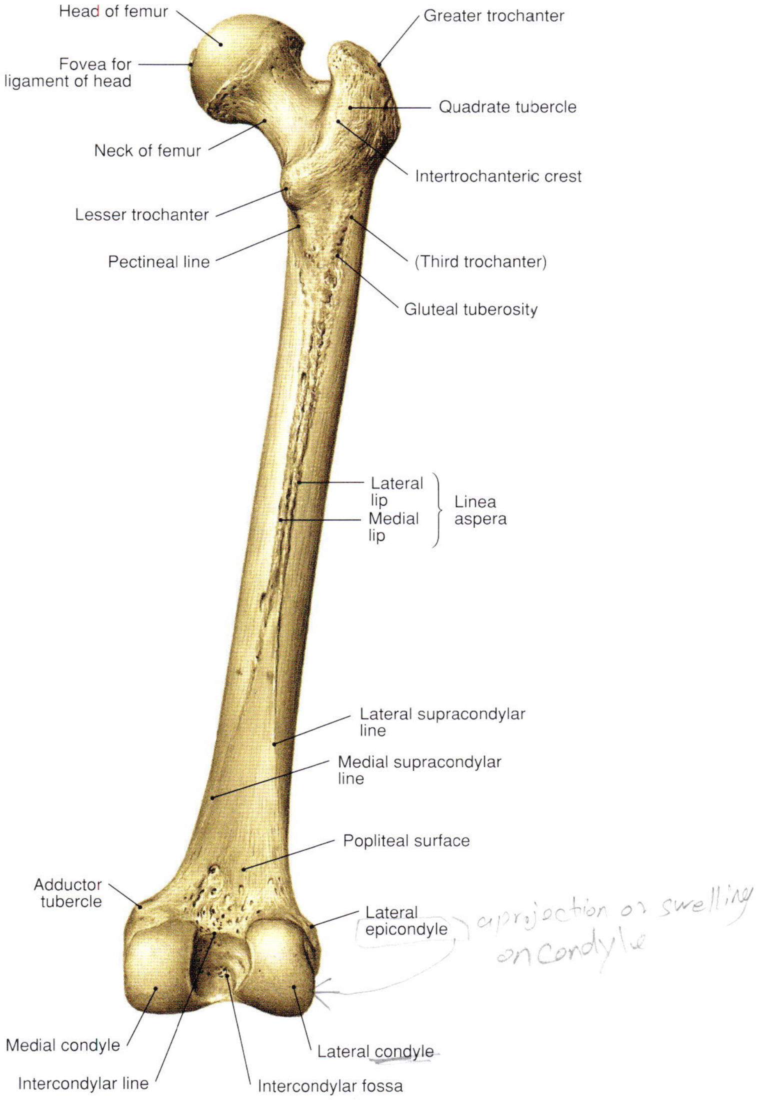

Fig. 974 Femur;
dorsal view.

Femur

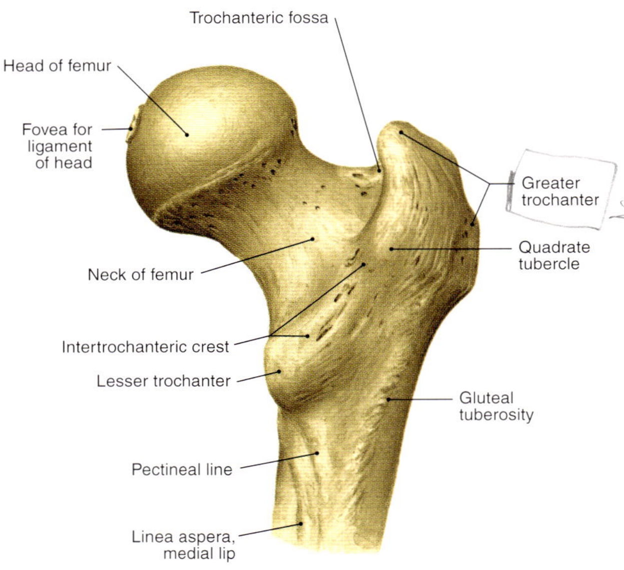

Fig. 975 Femur;
proximal extremity;
dorsal view.

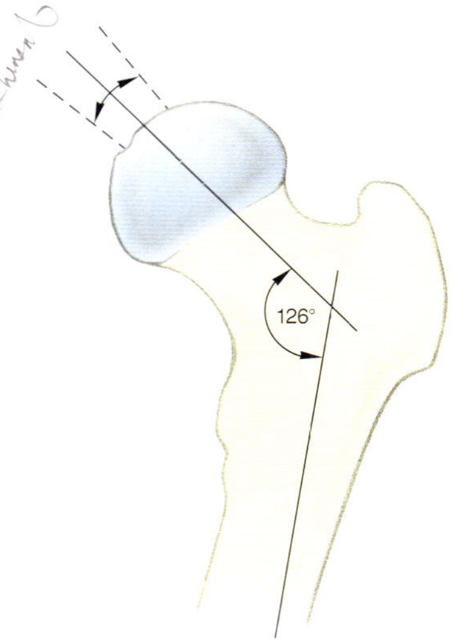

Fig. 976 Femur;
variability of the angle of the neck of the femur;
dorsal view.
The angle between the neck and the shaft of the femur is referred to as neck-shaft angle. It is 150° in infants and about 126° in the adult.

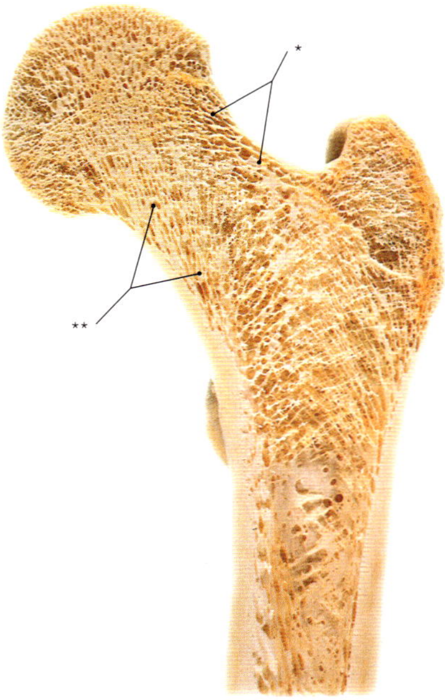

Fig. 977 Femur;
trabecular structure of the femoral bone with a large neck-shaft angle; section in the plane of the angle of anterior torsion (60%).
The lateral plates of the trabecular bone* („tensile system") are only poorly developed, whereas the medial plates** („compressive system") are much stronger.

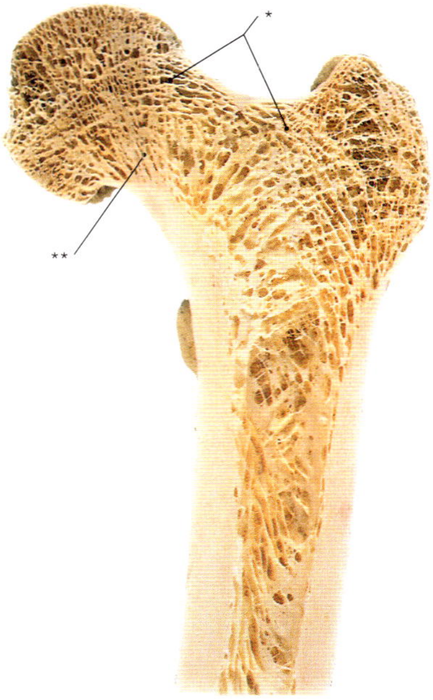

Fig. 978 Femur;
trabecular structure of the femoral bone with a small neck-shaft angle (coxa vara); section in the plane of the angle of anterior torsion (60%).
The lateral plates of the trabecular bone * („tensile system") are well developed, while the medial plates ** („compressive system") are developed less strong. As a result of the high demand of flexion, the cortex on the inner side of the femoral neck is particularly thick.

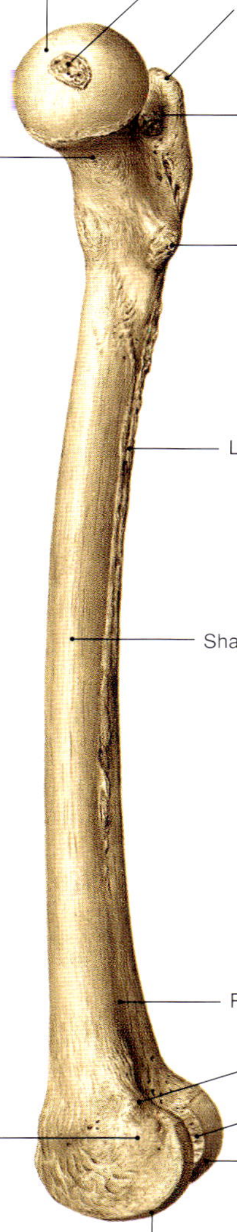

Fig. 979 Femur;
medial view.

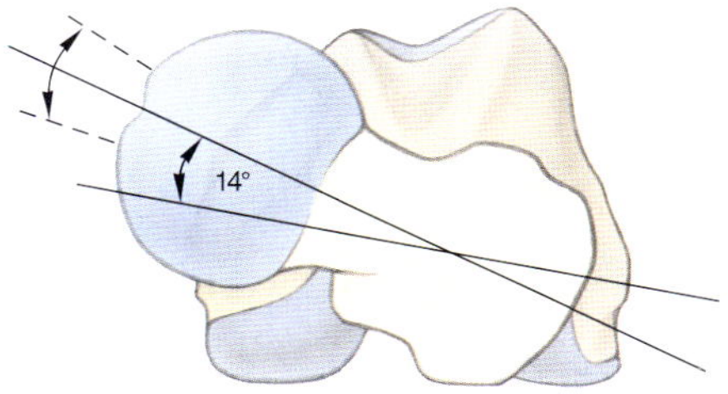

Fig. 980 Femur;
variability of the angle of anterior torsion; the proximal end of the femur has been projected over the distal end; proximal view.
The angle of anterior torsion is about 30° in infants and about 14° in adults.

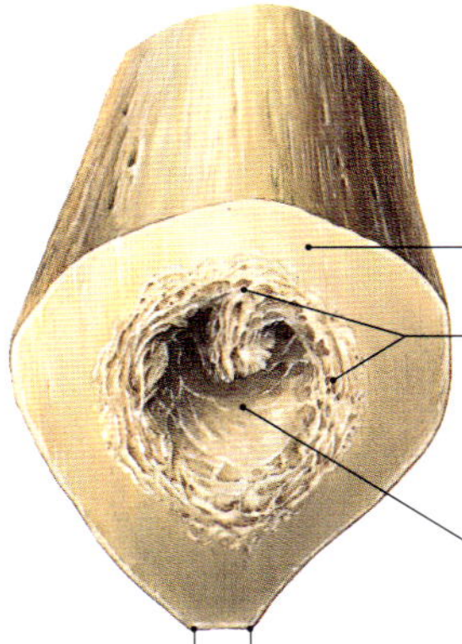

Fig. 981 Femur;
cross-section through the middle of the shaft;
distal view.

Hip joint

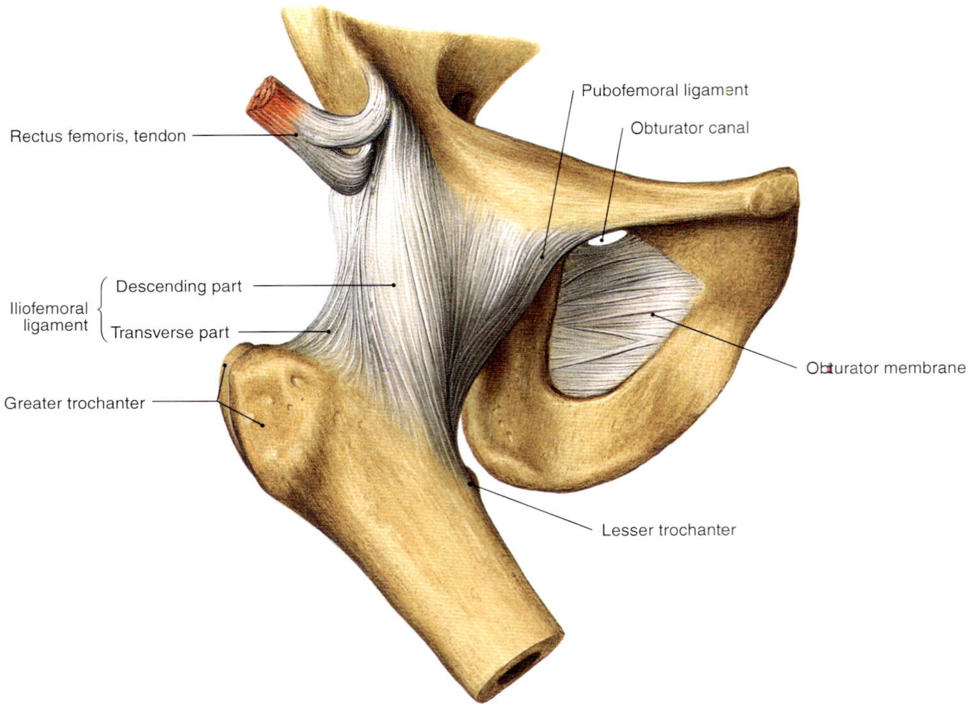

Fig. 982 Hip joint; ventrodistal view.

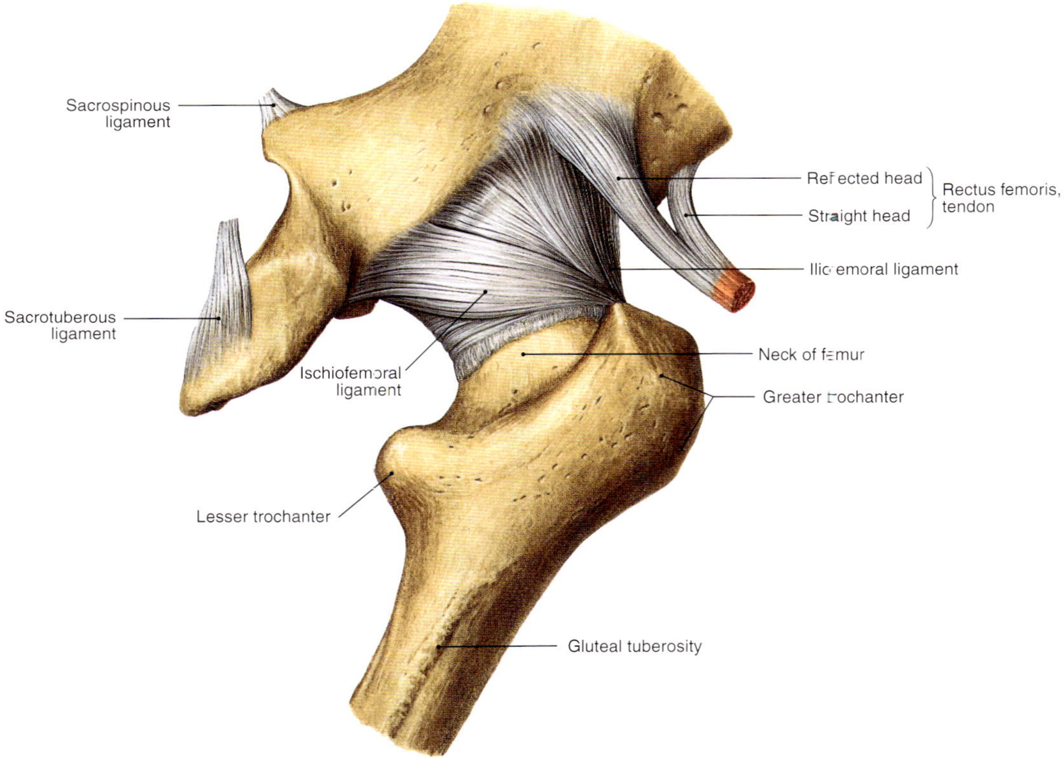

Fig. 983 Hip joint; dorsal view.

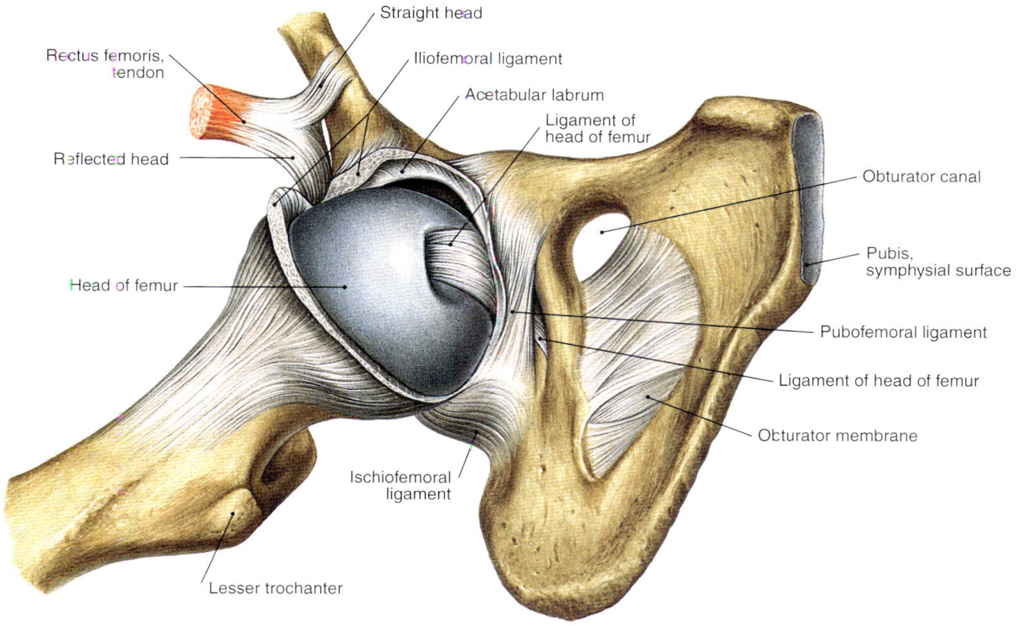

Fig. 984 Hip joint;
the articular capsule has been opened and the head of the femur has been partly exarticulated; laterodistal view.

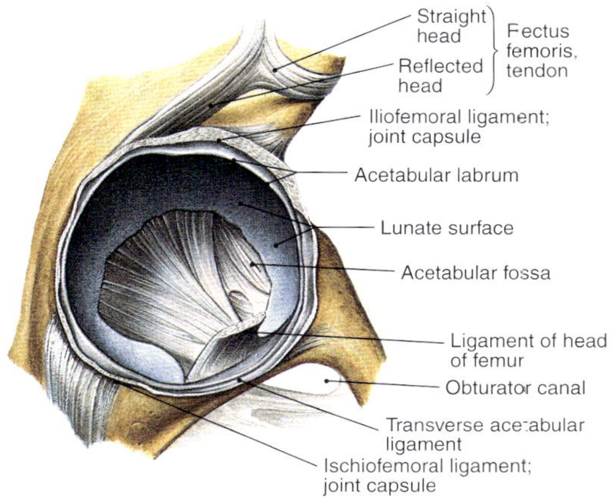

Fig. 985 Hip joint;
aspect of the acetabulum after removal of the articular capsule and exarticulation of the head of the femur; laterodistal view.

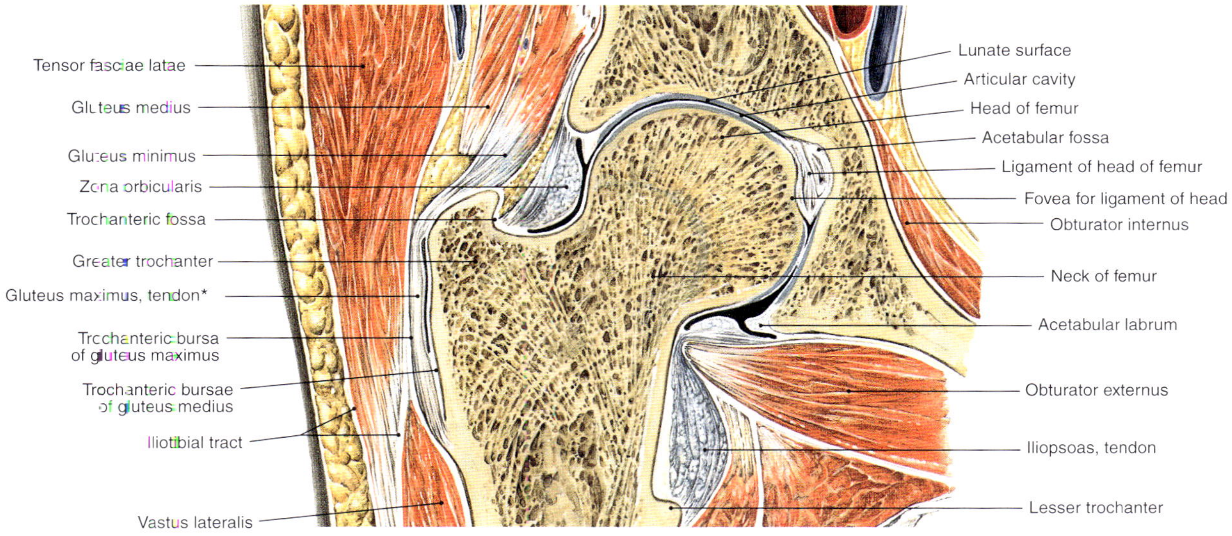

Fig. 986 Hip joint;
vertical section at the plane of the angle of antetorsion.

* Radiations into the iliotibial tract

Hip joint, radiography

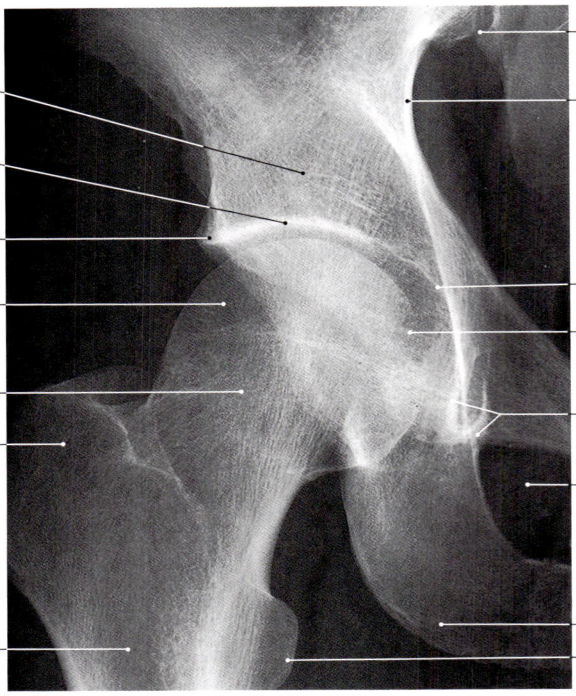

Fig. 987 Hip joint;
AP-radiograph; upright position on both legs.

* Clinical term: acetabular roof = tangential projection of the lunate surface
** Clinical term: edge of the acetabular roof = the most lateral projection of the acetabulum
*** Clinical term: KÖHLER's teardrop = projection of the acetabular fossa

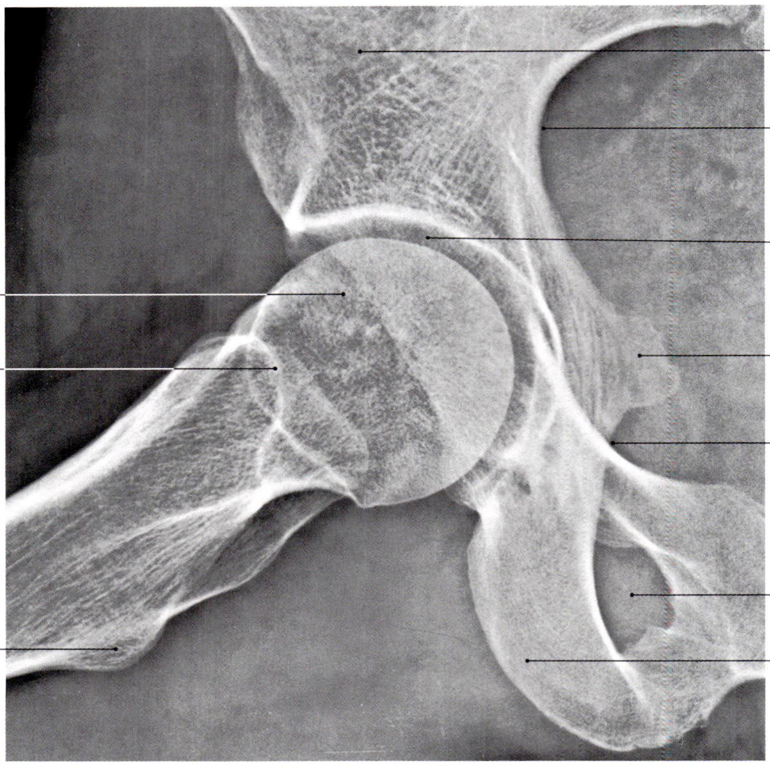

Fig. 988 Hip joint;
AP-radiograph; supine position with the thigh abducted and flexed (so-called LAUENSTEIN projection).

* Due to minimal absorption of X-rays by cartilage, the articular cleft appears abnormally broad.

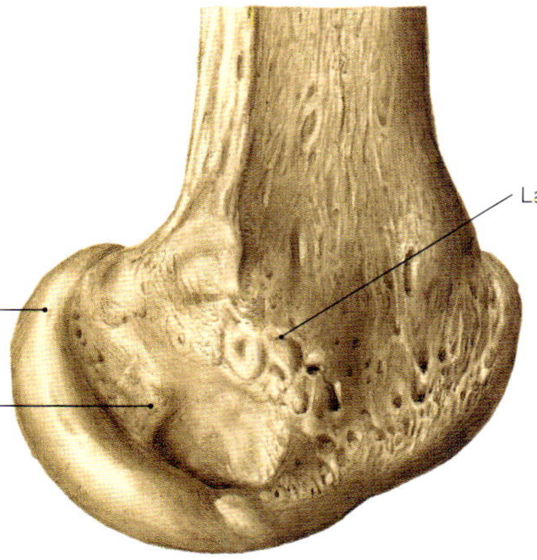

Fig. 989 Femur;
distal extremity;
lateral view.

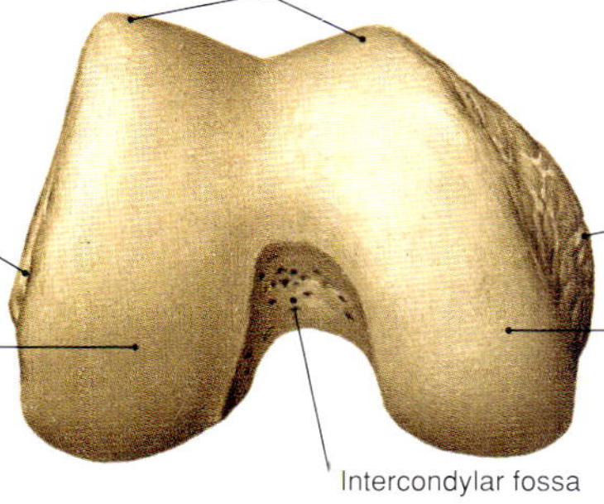

Fig. 990 Femur;
distal extremity;
distal view.

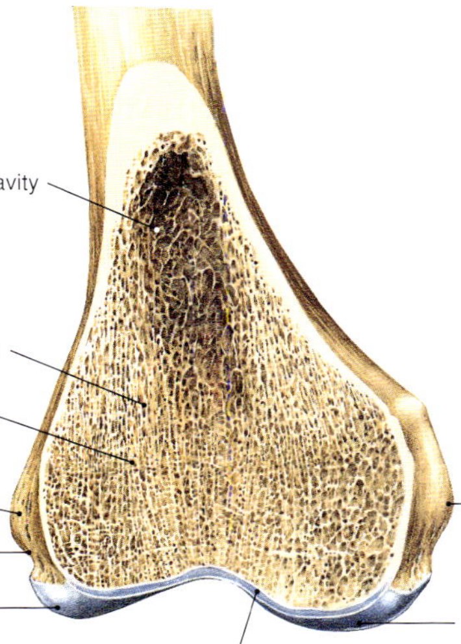

Fig. 991 Femur;
frontal section through the distal part;
ventral view.

Tibia

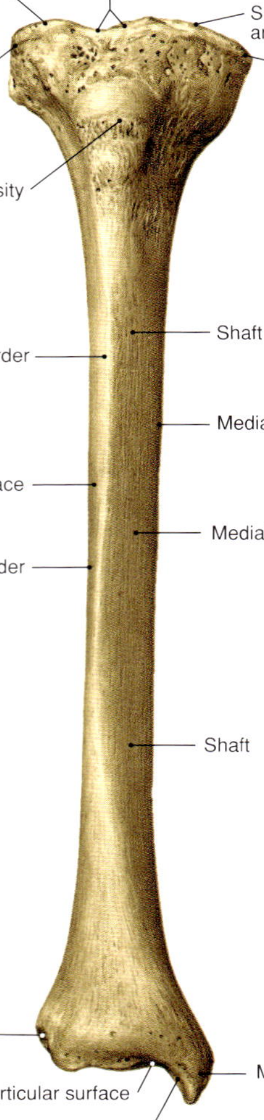

Fig. 992 Tibia; ventral view.

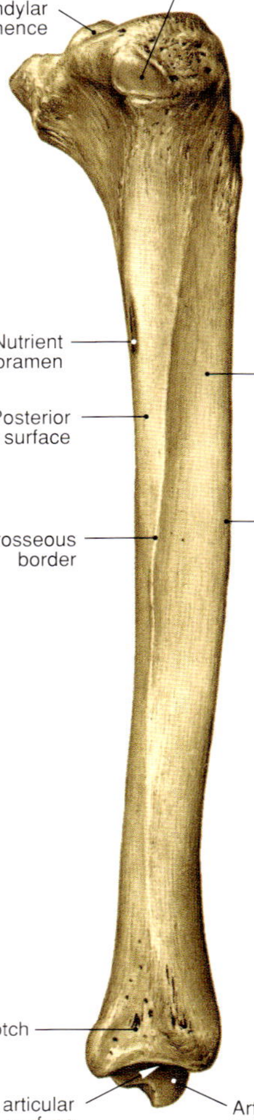

Fig. 993 Tibia; lateral view.

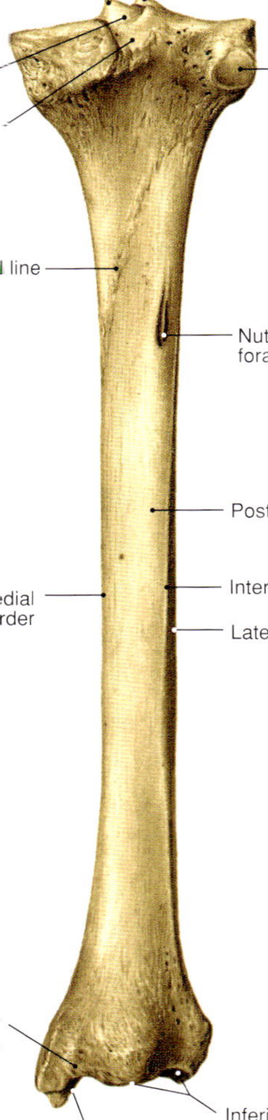

Fig. 994 Tibia; dorsal view.

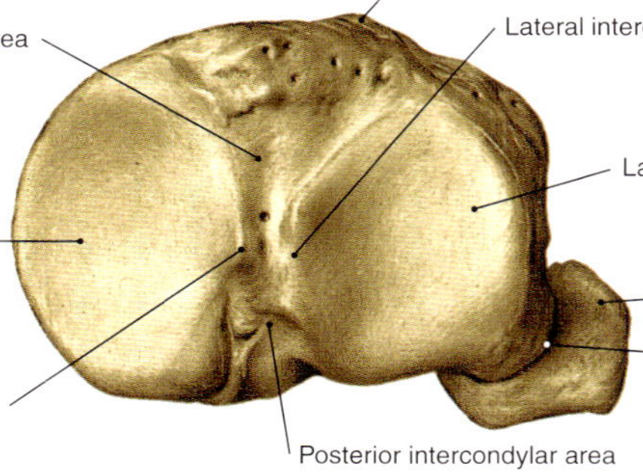

Fig. 995 Tibia and fibula; proximal view.

* The articular surfaces of the condyles together are referred to as superior articular surface.

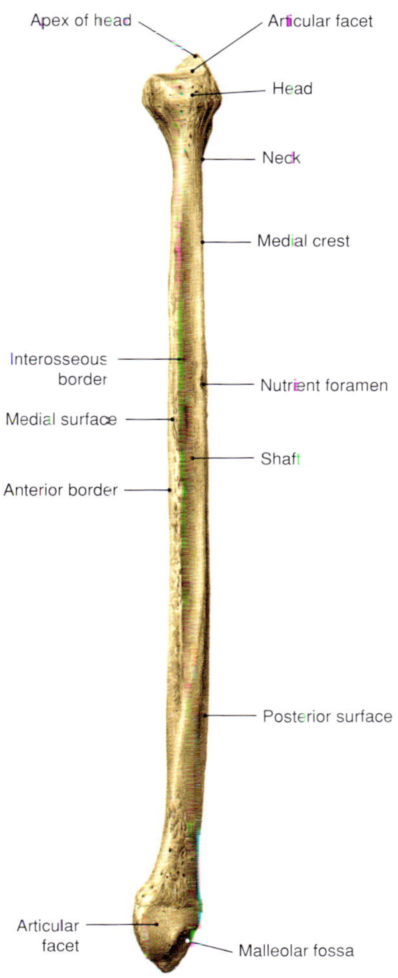

Fig. 996 Fibula; medial view.

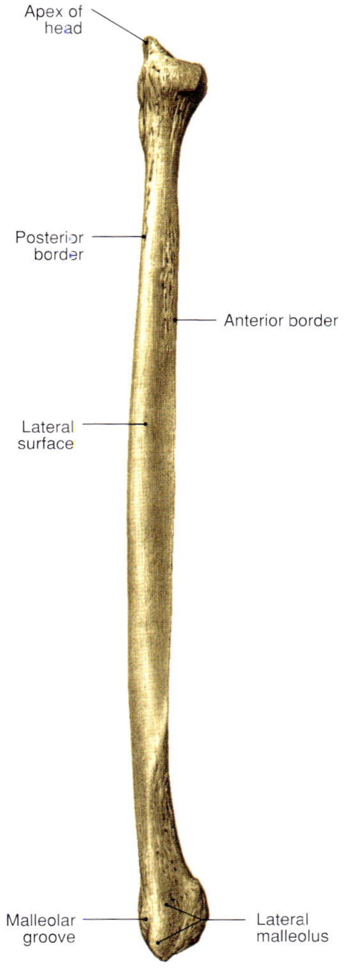

Fig. 997 Fibula; lateral view.

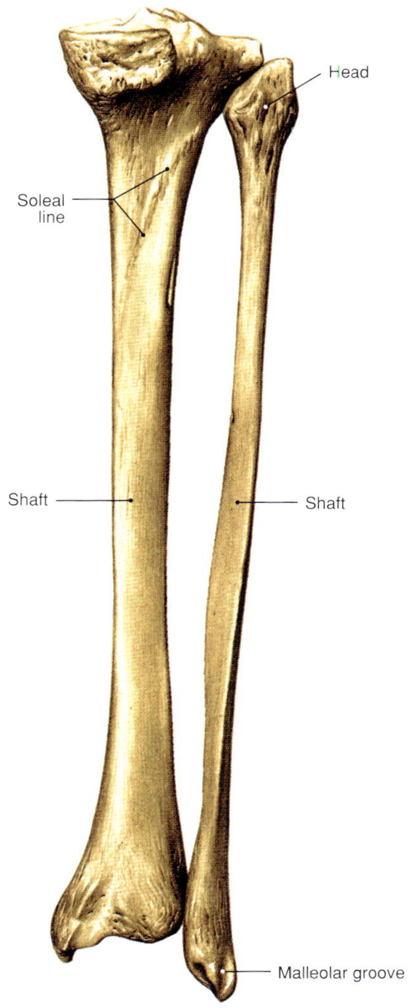

Fig. 998 Tibia, and fibula; dorsal view.

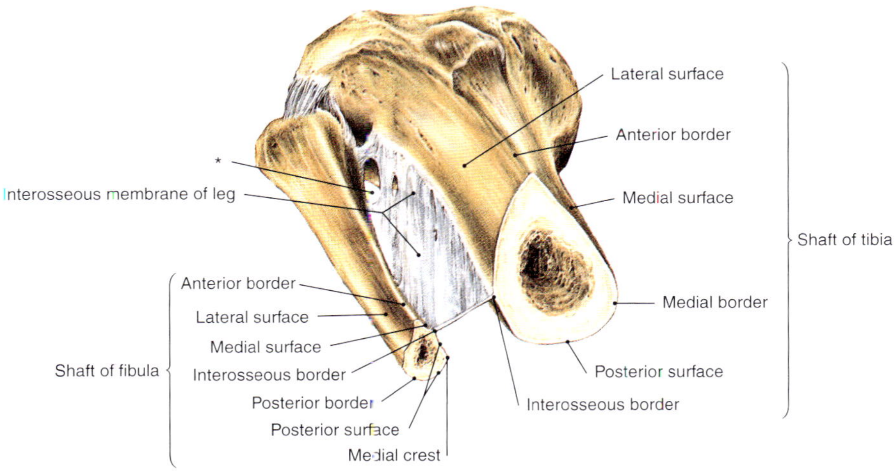

Fig. 999 Tibia and fibula; cross-section with the interosseous membrane of leg; distal view.

* Opening for the anterior tibial artery

Patella and knee joint

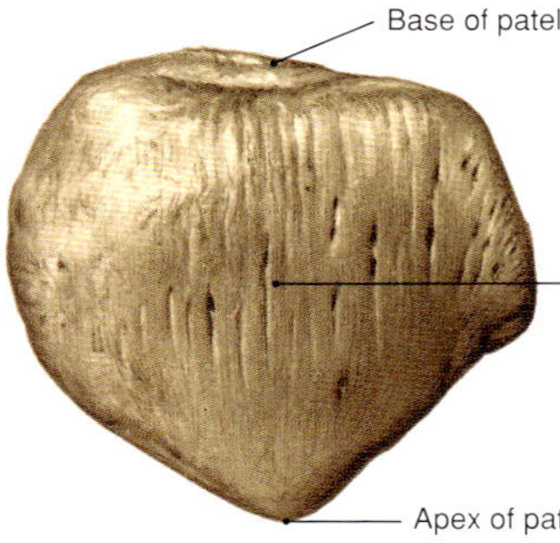

Fig. 1000 Patella;
ventral view.

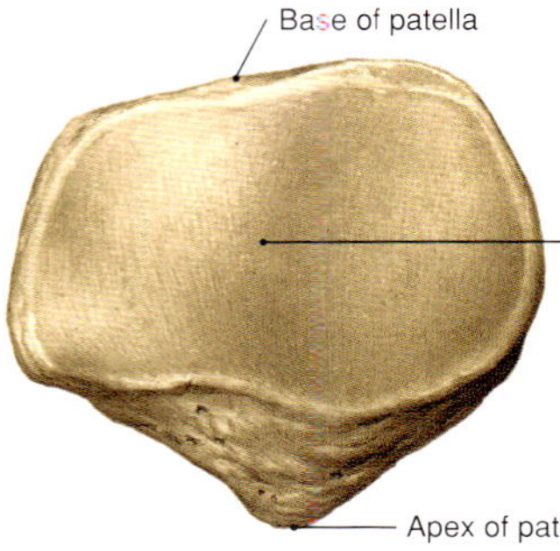

Fig. 1001 Patella;
dorsal view.

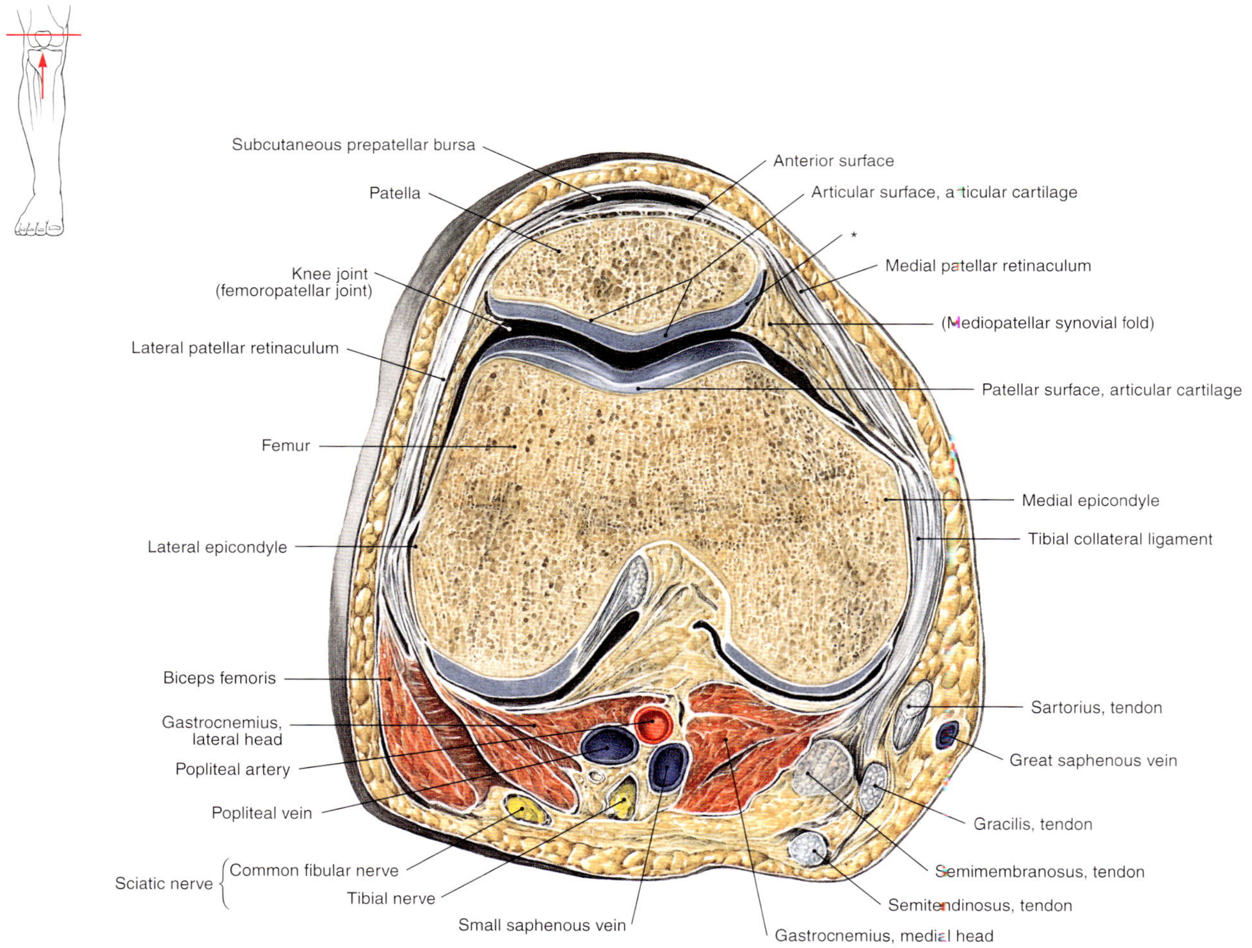

Fig. 1002 Knee joint;
cross-section.

* Medial border facet

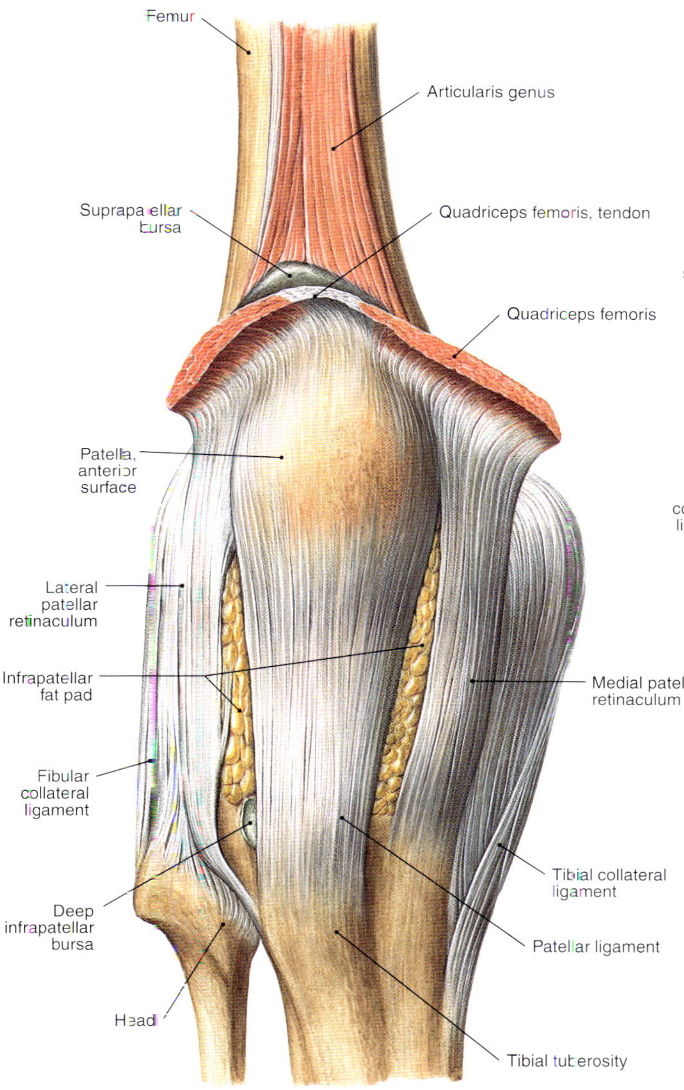

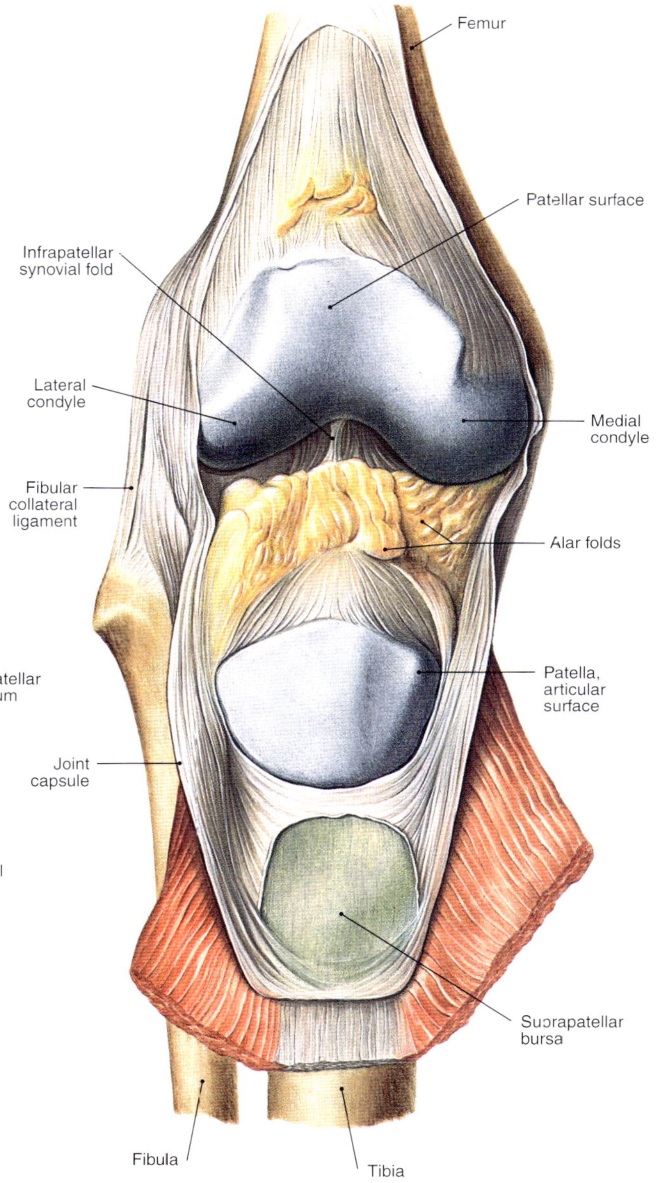

Fig. 1003 Knee joint;
intact articular capsule;
ventral view.

Fig. 1004 Knee joint;
the anterior part of the articular capsule has been reflected downwards after dissection of the quadriceps muscle;
the suprapatellar bursa has been opened;
ventral view.

Knee joint

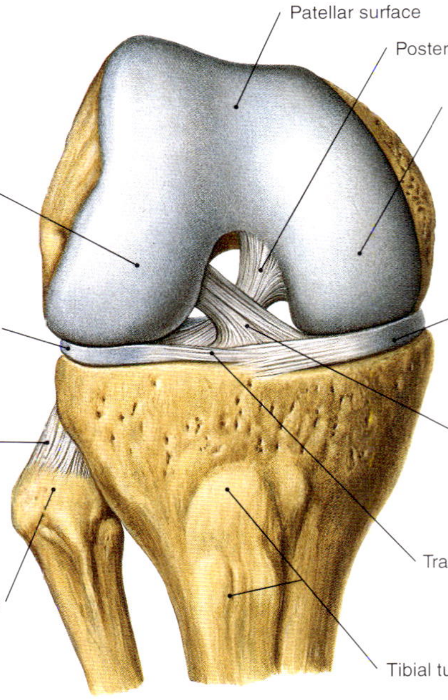

Fig. 1005 Knee joint;
in 90° flexion; the articular capsule and the lateral ligaments have been removed;
ventral view.

* Clinical term: ACL (= anterior cruciate ligament)
** Clinical term: PCL (= posterior cruciate ligament)

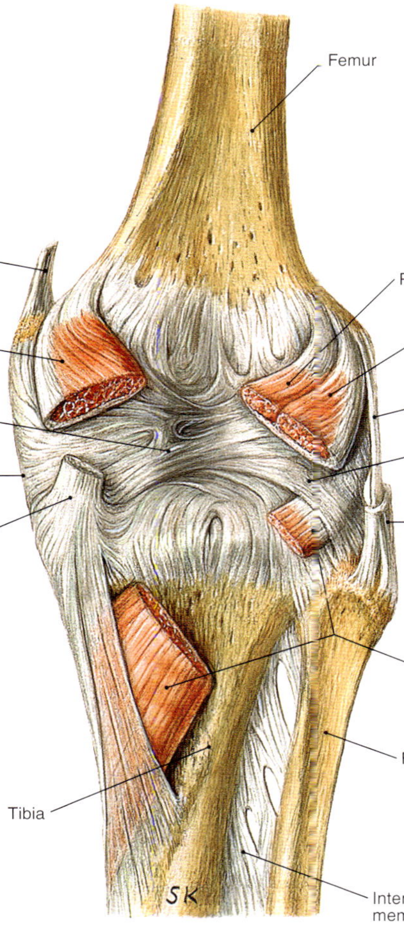

Fig. 1006 Knee joint;
intact articular capsule with muscular origins;
dorsal view.

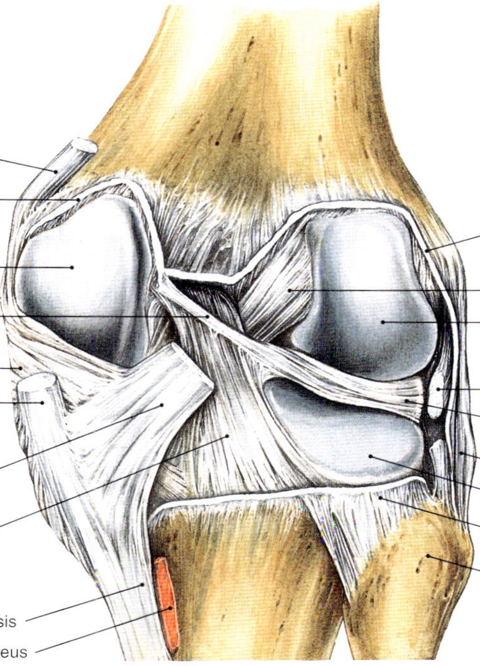

Fig. 1007 Knee joint;
exposure of the cruciate ligaments and the menisci;
dorsal view.

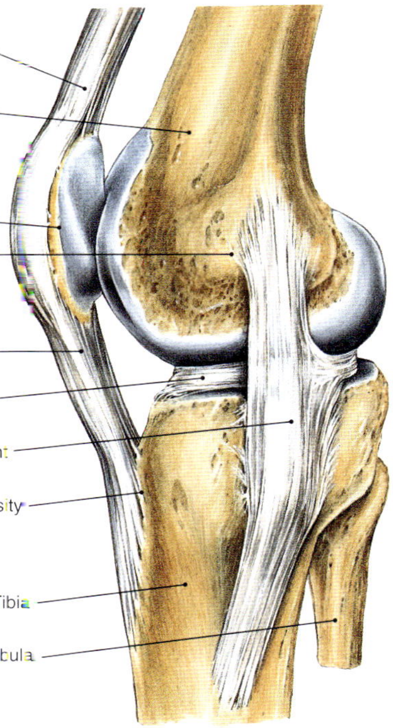

Fig. 1008 Tibial collateral ligament;
knee in extended position;
medial view.
Only the posterior fibres of the tibial collateral ligament are attached to the medial meniscus.

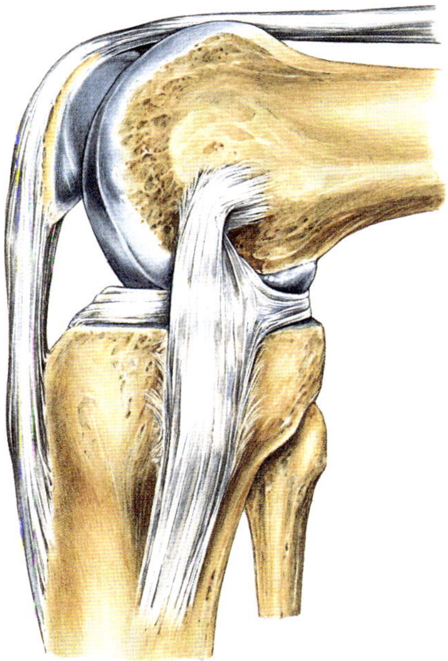

Fig. 1009 Tibial collateral ligament;
knee in flexed position (90°);
medial view.
In the course of flexion, the posterior and proximal fibres of the tibial collateral ligament become twisted, thereby stabilizing the medial meniscus.

Knee joint

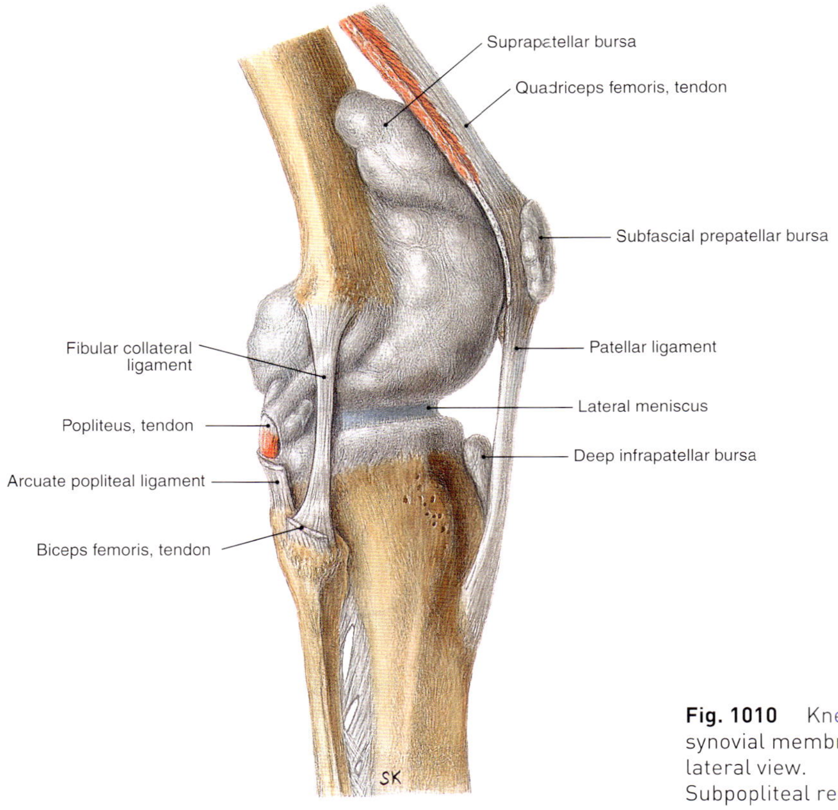

Fig. 1010 Knee joint;
synovial membrane tightly filled after injection of plastic material; lateral view.
Subpopliteal recess not shown (compare Fig. 1011).

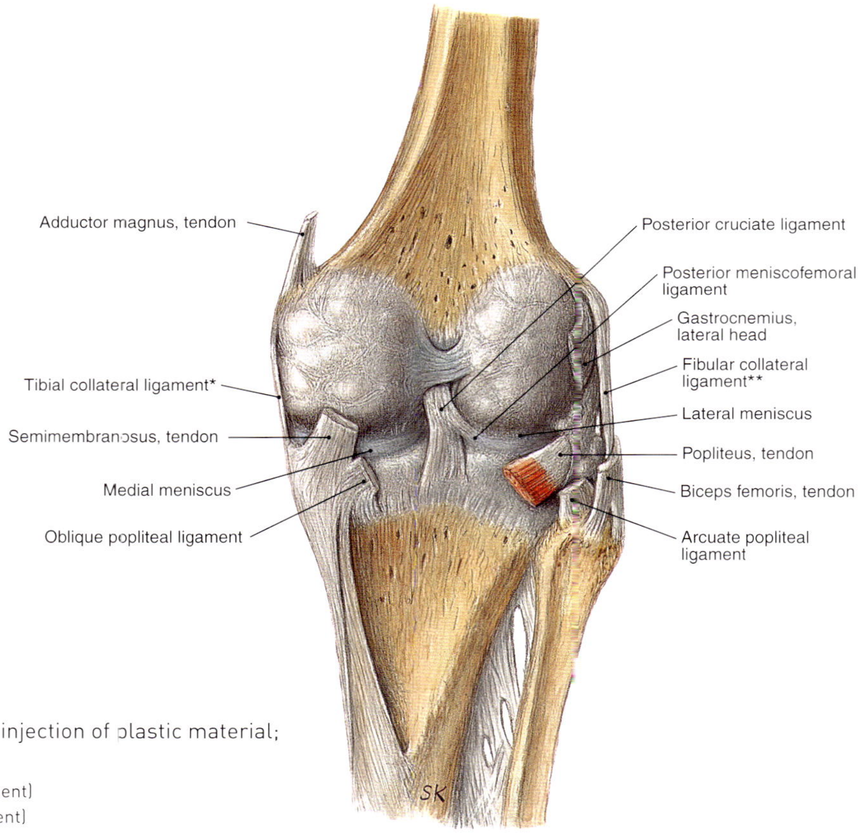

Fig. 1011 Knee joint;
synovial membrane thightly filled after injection of plastic material; dorsal view.

* Clinical term: MCL (= medial collateral ligament)
** Clinical term: LCL (= lateral collateral ligament)

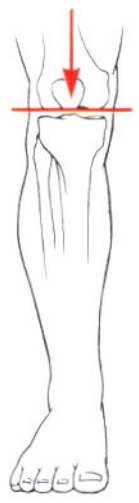

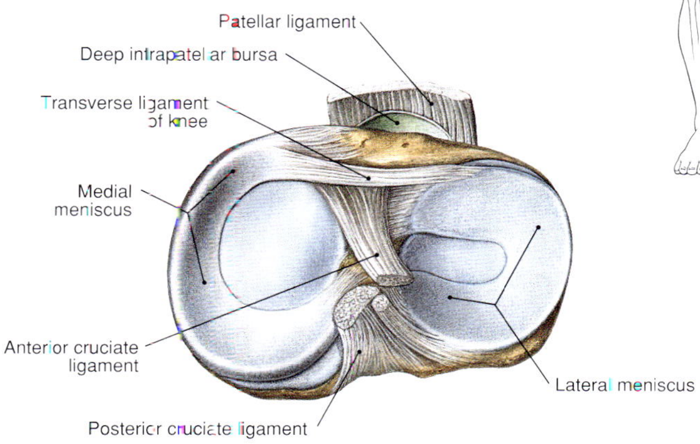

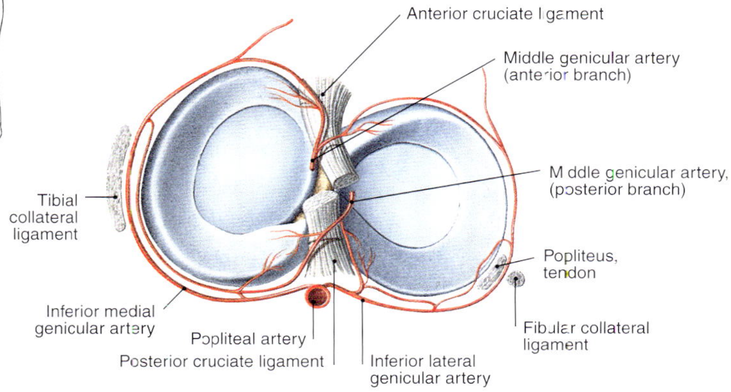

Fig. 1012 Menisci of the knee joint and cruciate ligaments; proximal view.

Fig. 1013 Menisci of the knee joint; arterial supply; proximal view.

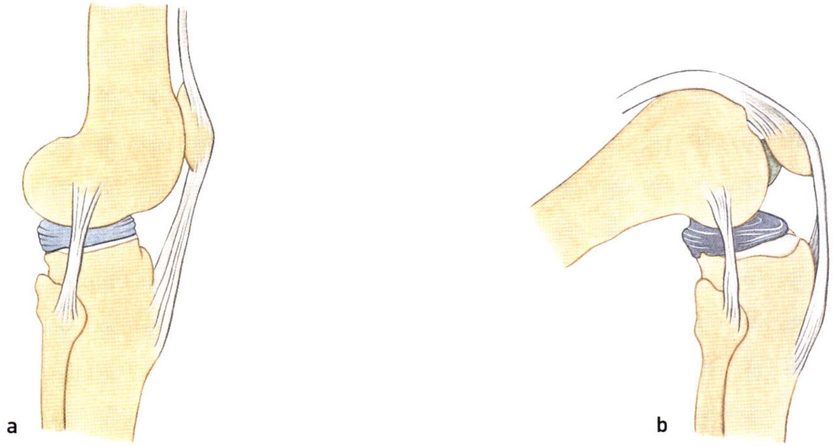

Fig. 1014 a, b Displacement of the menisci during flexion; lateral view.

a Extended position
b Flexed position

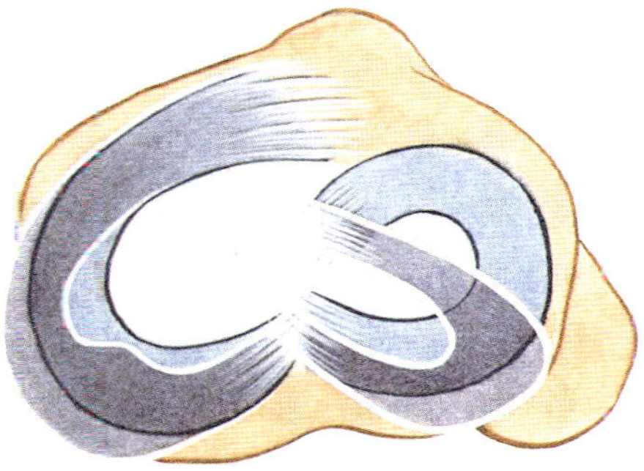

Fig. 1015 Displacement of the menisci during flexion; proximal view.
In flexion, both menisci are displaced posteriorly over the edges of the tibial condyles. The greater mobility of the lateral meniscus accounts for its lesser risk of damage.

Knee joint, sections

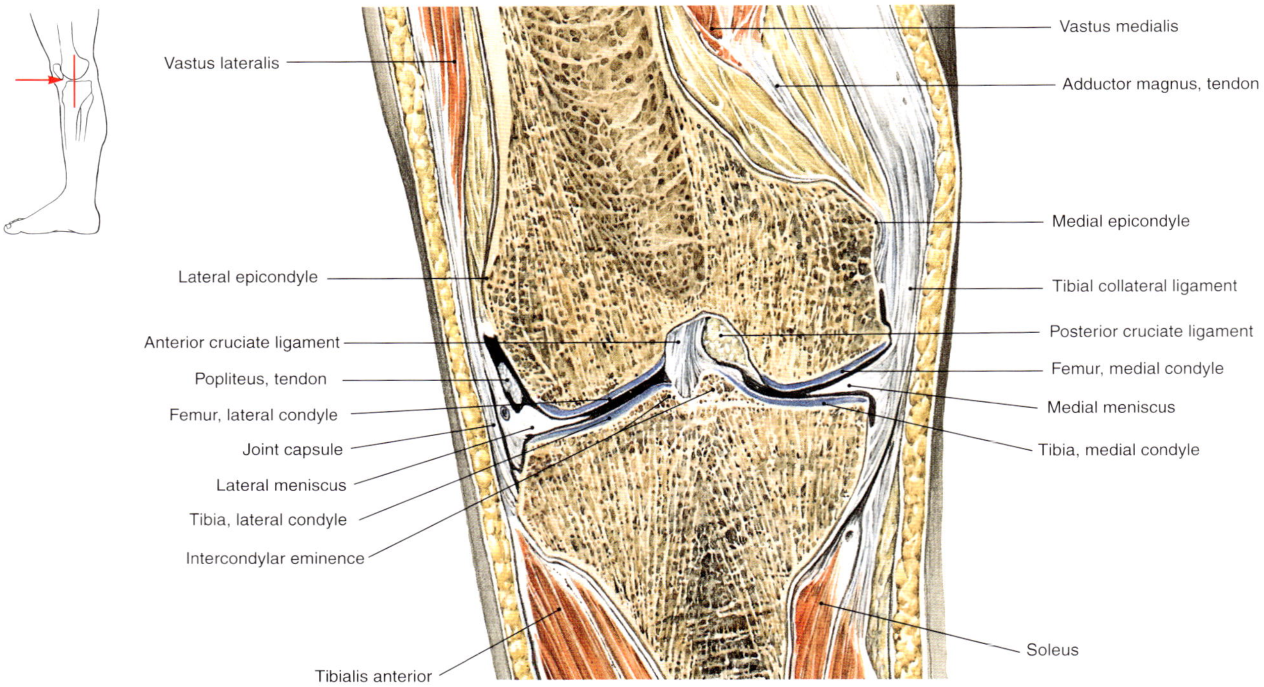

Fig. 1016 Knee joint;
frontal section.

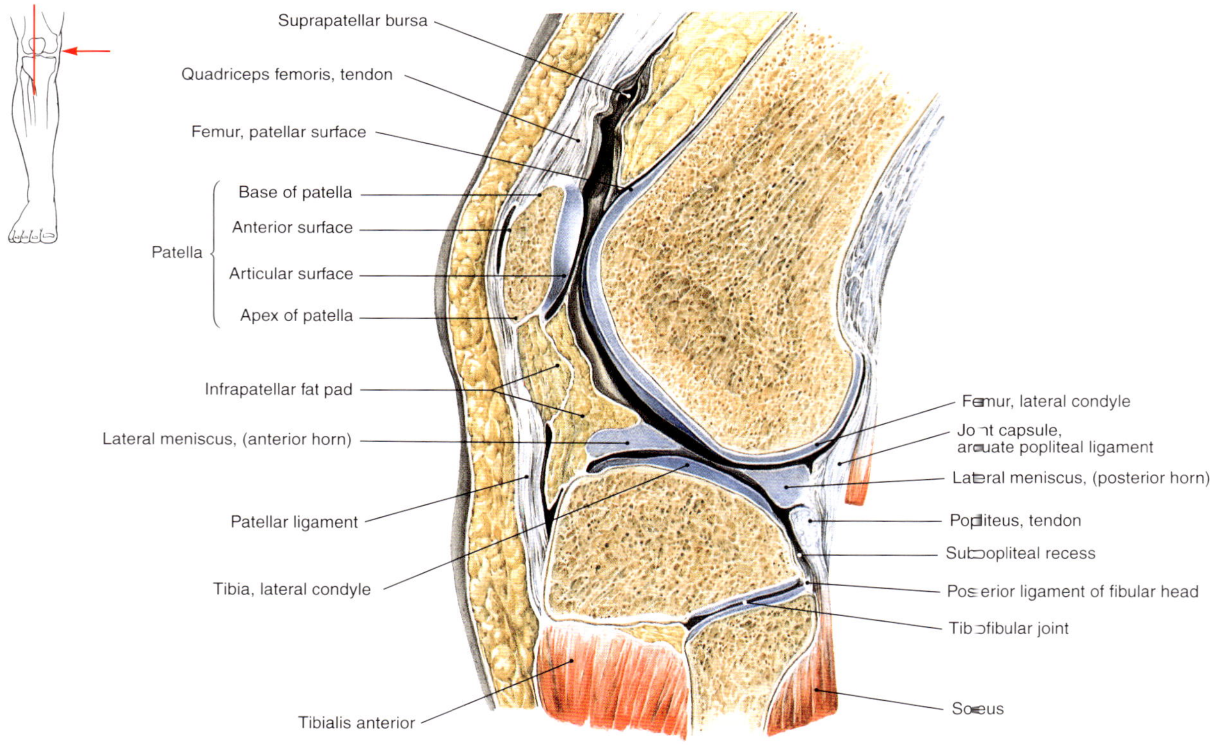

Fig. 1017 Knee joint;
sagittal section through the lateral part of the joint.

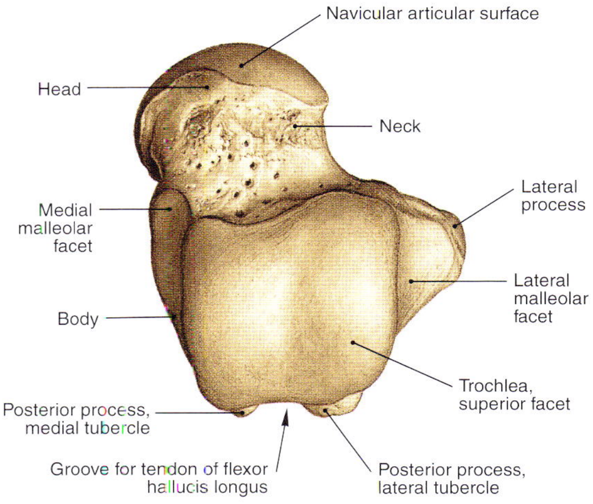

Fig. 1031 Talus; proximal view.

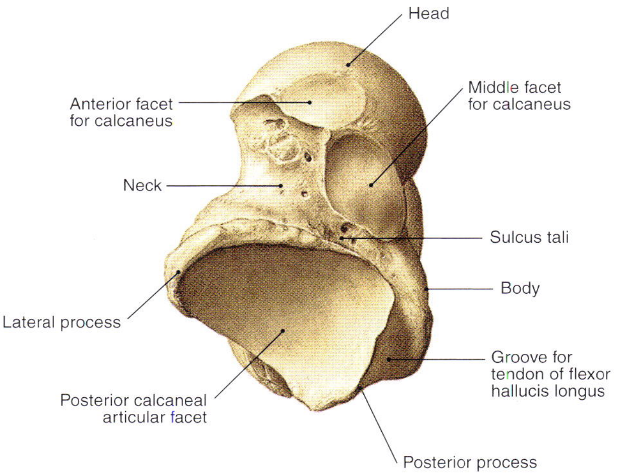

Fig. 1032 Talus; plantar view.

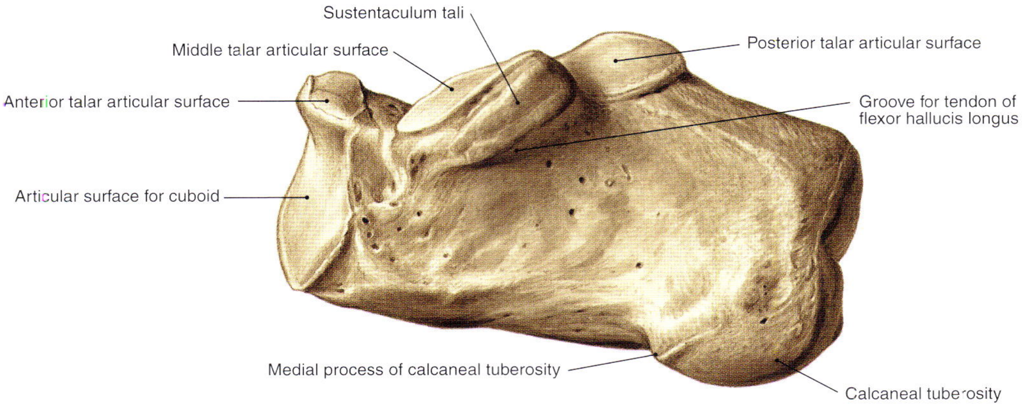

Fig. 1033 Calcaneus; medial view.

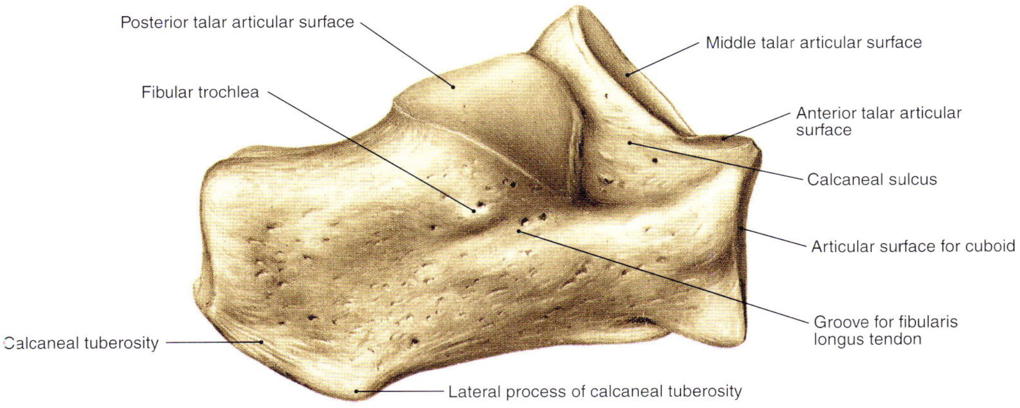

Fig. 1034 Calcaneus; lateral view.

Tarsal bones

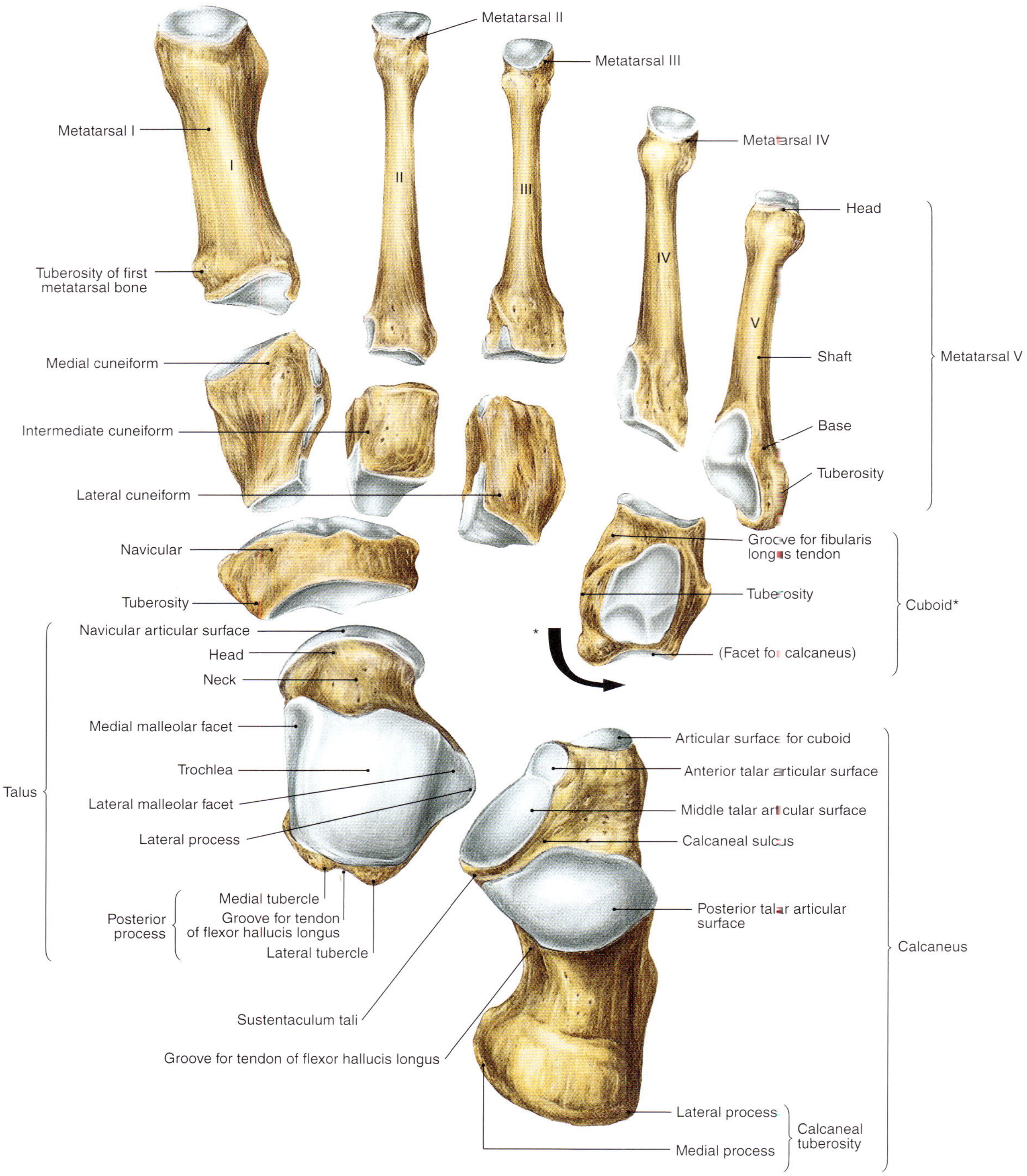

Fig. 1035 Tarsal bones and metatarsal bones; proximal view.

* The cuboid bone is shown in a medial view.

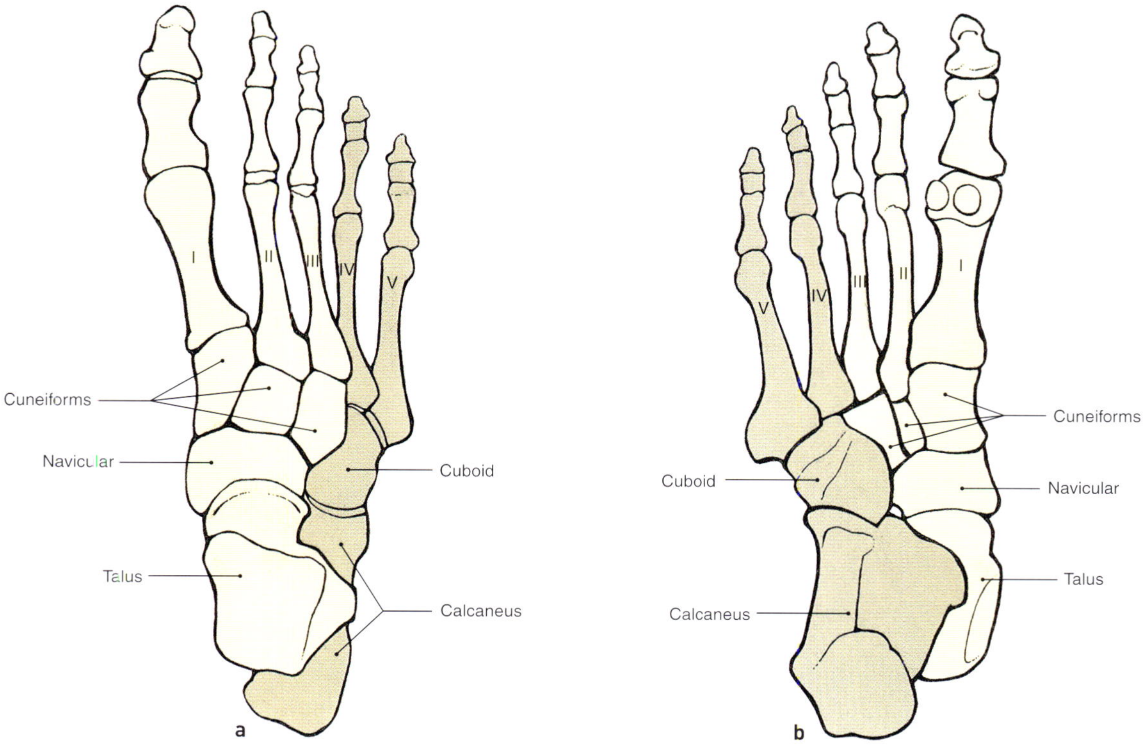

Fig. 1036 a, b Skeleton of the foot; structural organisation.
a Proximal view
b Plantar view

The heads of all metatarsal bones lie in the plantar plane. The cuneiform bones, the navicular bone and the talus rest upon the lateral parts of the skeleton, especially in the posterior part of the foot. The talus is therefore situated above the calcaneus and the longitudinal arch is formed.
The wedge-shaped cross-section of the cuneiform bones and the bases of the metatarsal bones contribute to the formation of the transverse vault.

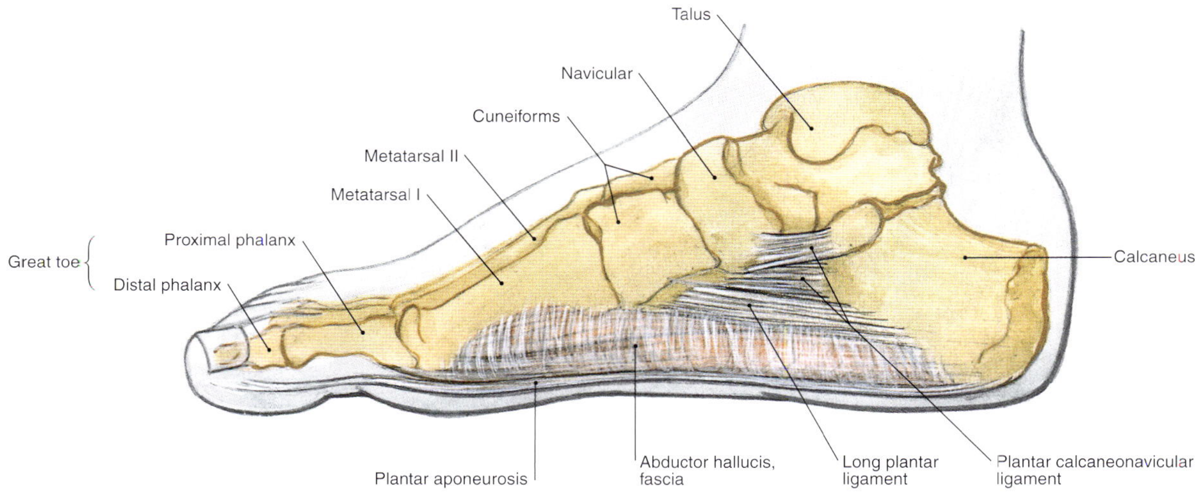

Fig. 1037 Supporting structures of the medial arch of the longitudinal vault of the foot; medial view.

The ligaments shown in this illustration are mostly directed in the longitudinal axis of the foot and support passively the longitudinal vault of the foot. The short muscles of the foot primarily support this construction.

Joints of the foot

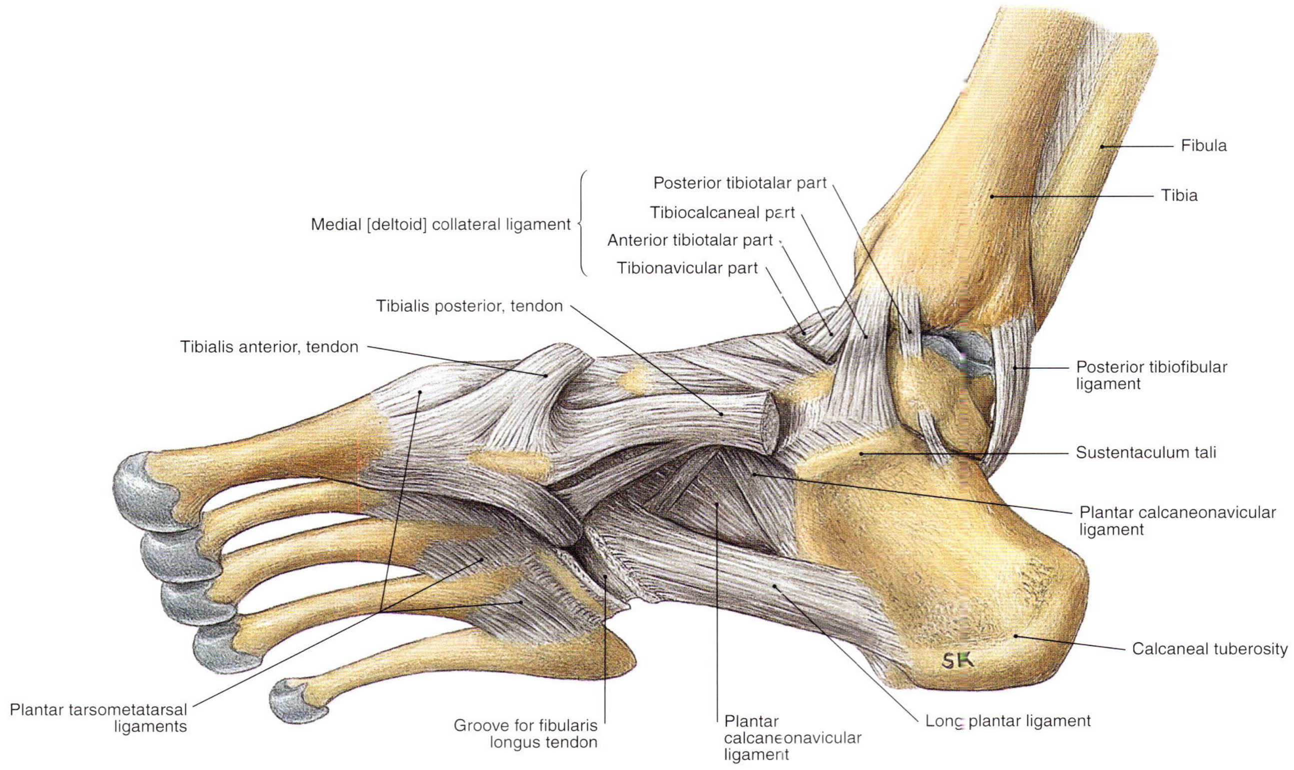

Fig. 1038 Joints of the foot; ligaments and tendons; medial view.

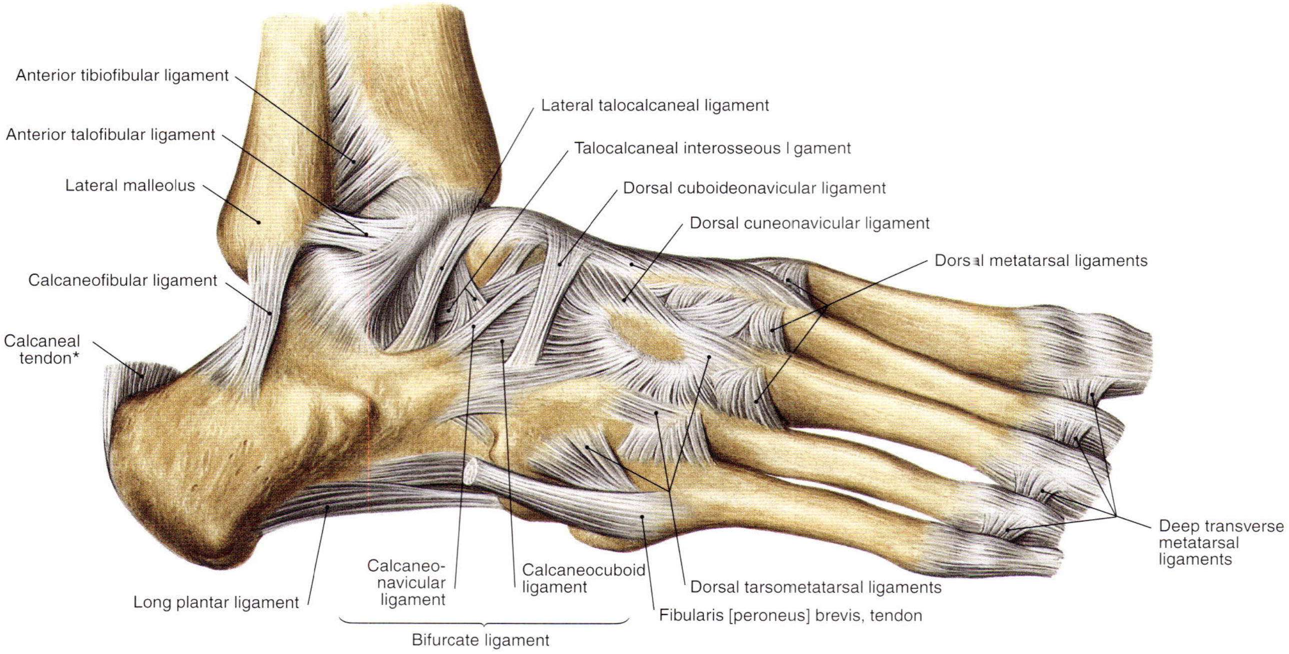

Fig. 1039 Joints of the foot; ligaments and tendons; lateral view.

* Also: Achilles tendon

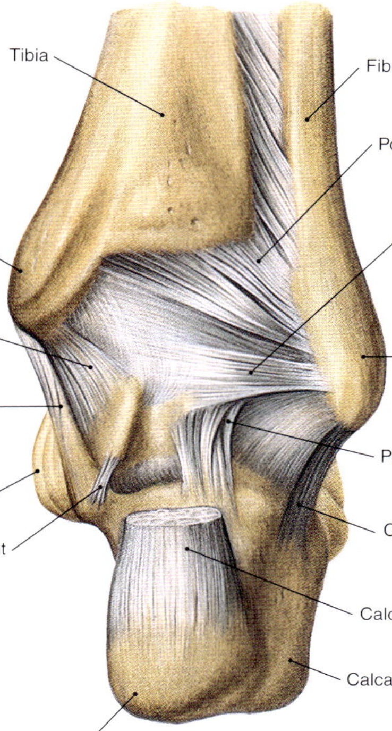

Fig. 1040 Joints of the foot;
ligaments and tendons of the posterior part of the foot.

* Also: Achilles tendon

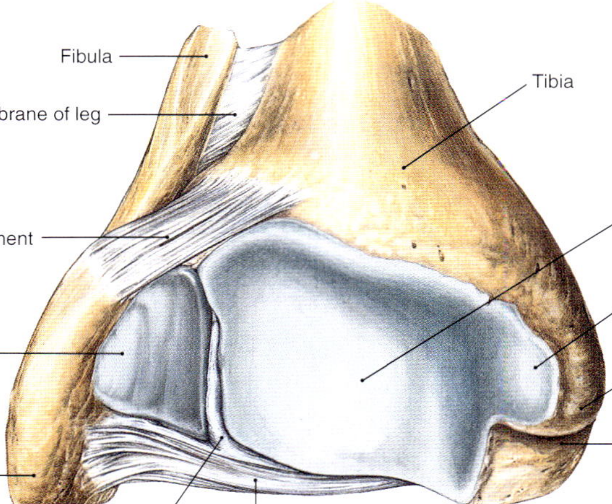

Fig. 1041 Ankle joint;
proximal articular surfaces;
distal view.

Joints of the foot

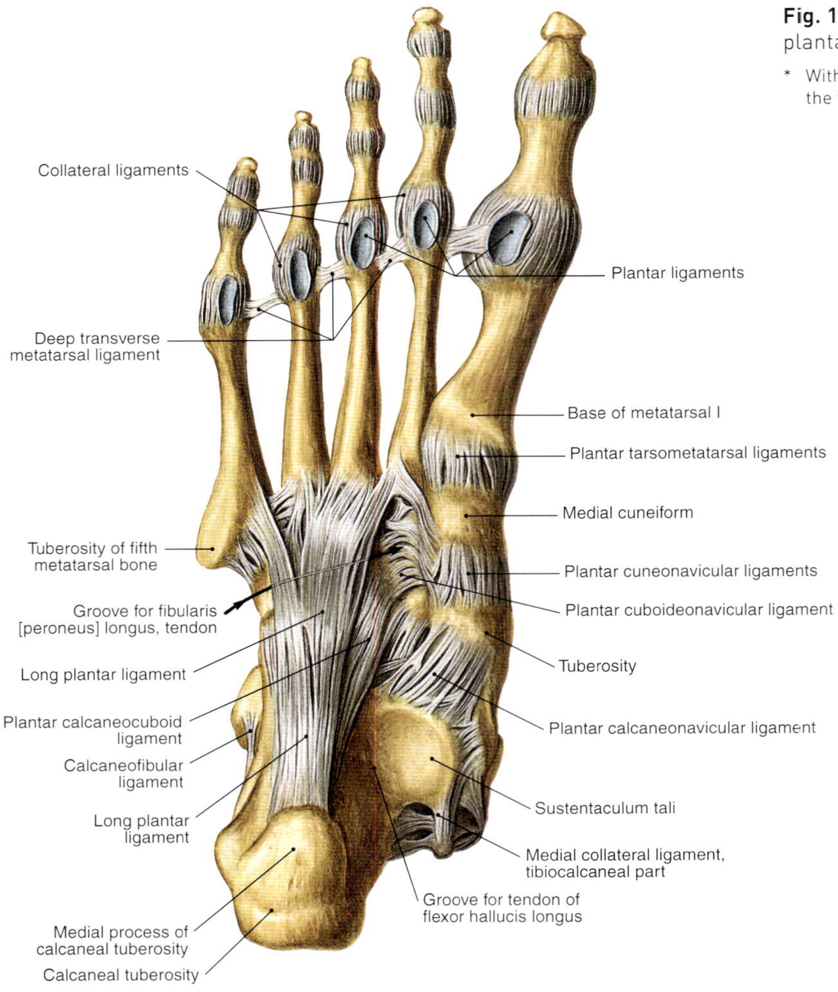

Fig. 1042 Joints of the foot; plantar view.

* With the long plantar ligament the groove for the tendon of the fibularis longus muscle is enclosed in a canal.

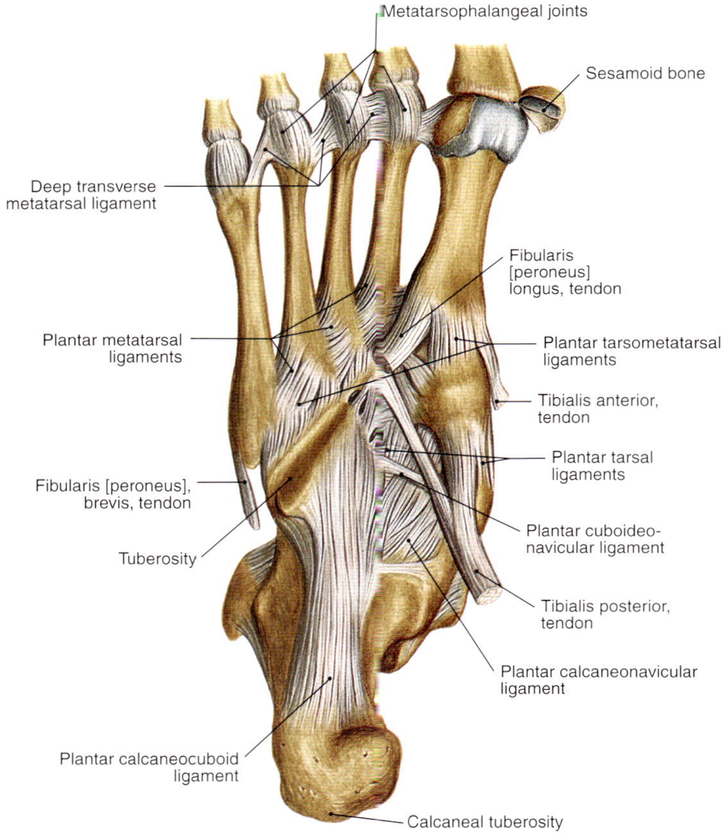

Fig. 1043 Joints of the foot; ligaments and tendons of the tarsus and metatarsus; plantar view.

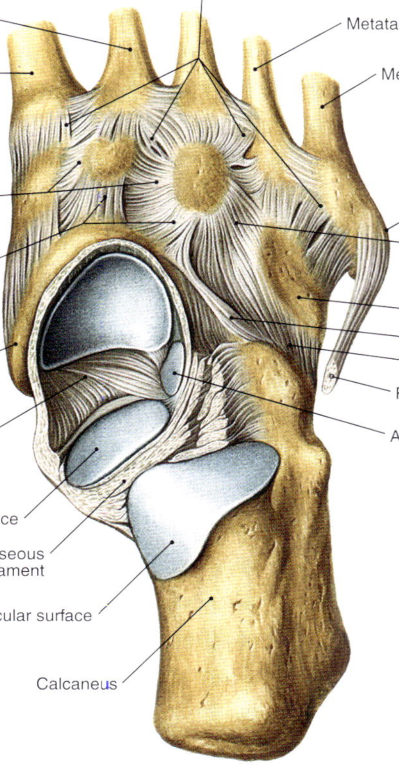

Fig. 1044 Talotarsal joint; distal articular surfaces; proximal view.

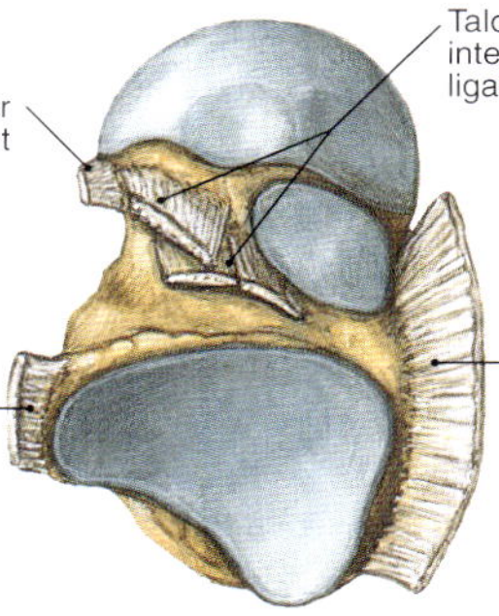

Fig. 1045 Talotarsal joint; proximal articular surfaces; distal view.

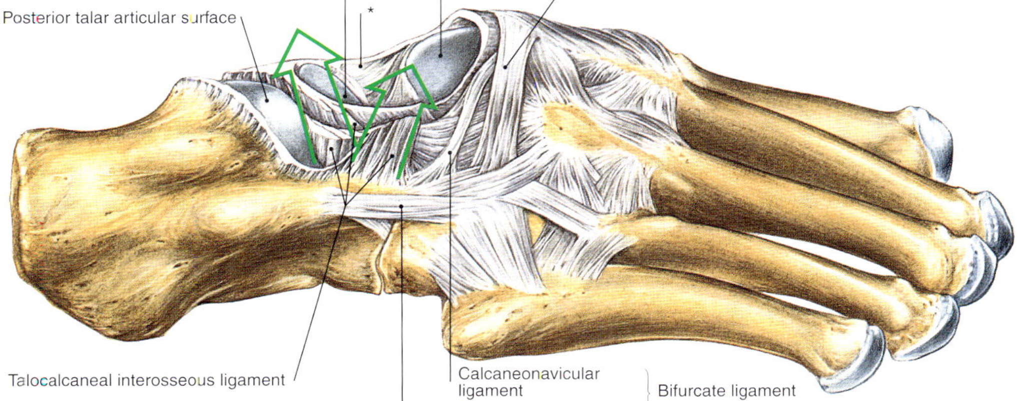

Fig. 1046 Talotarsal joint; the talus and the lateral ligaments have been removed; lateral view.
The two arrows point out the helical distorsion of the talocalcaneal interosseous ligament.

* Tight connective tissue layer between the plantar calcaneonavicular ligament and the tibionavicular part of the deltoid ligament limiting a medially directed gliding of the head of the talus; slackening of this layer results in flattening of the longitudinal vault (flat-foot, pes valgus)

Ankle and talotarsal joint, sections

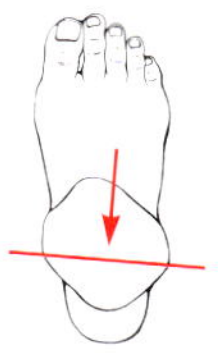

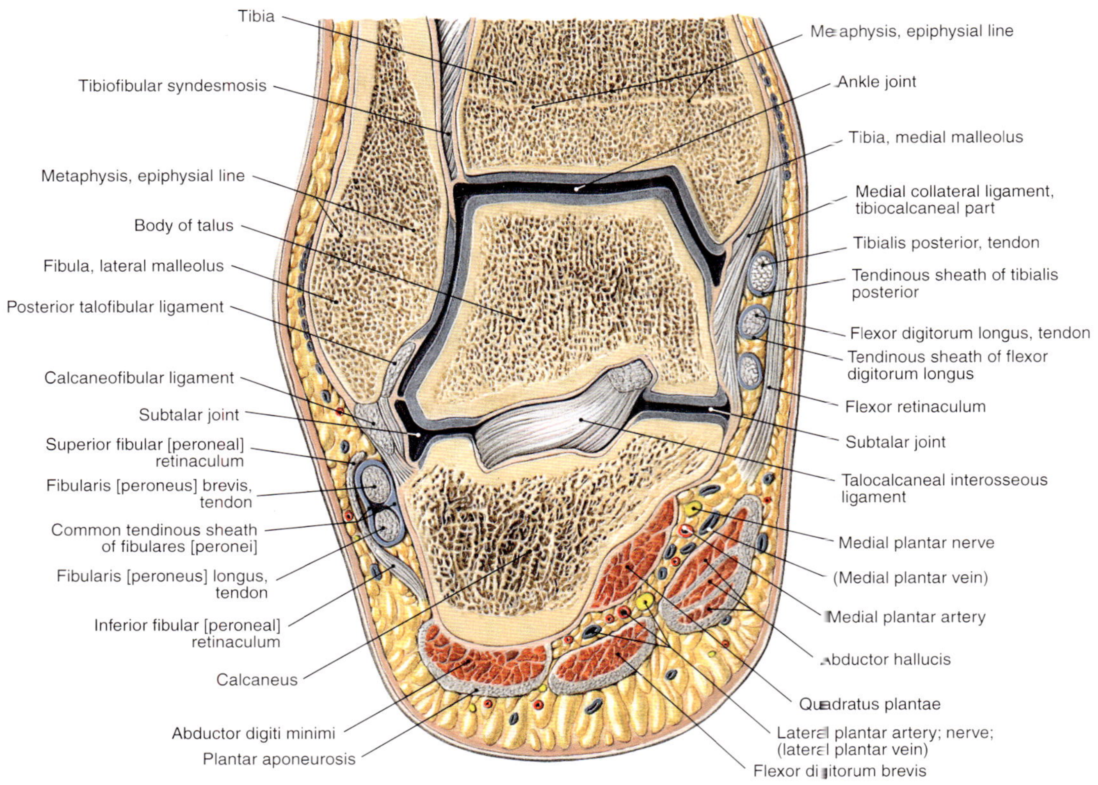

Fig. 1047 Ankle and talotarsal joint; frontal section.

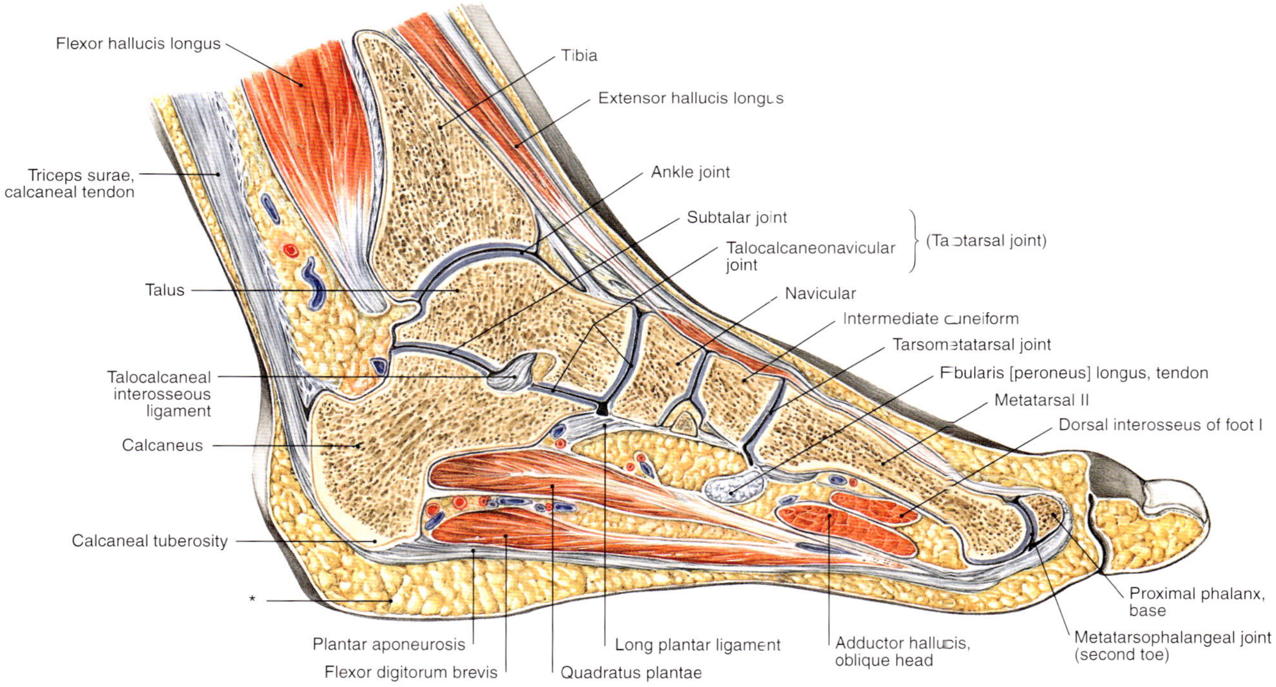

Fig. 1048 Ankle and talotarsal joint; sagittal section.

* Fat pad of the heel

Ankle and talotarsal joint, radiography

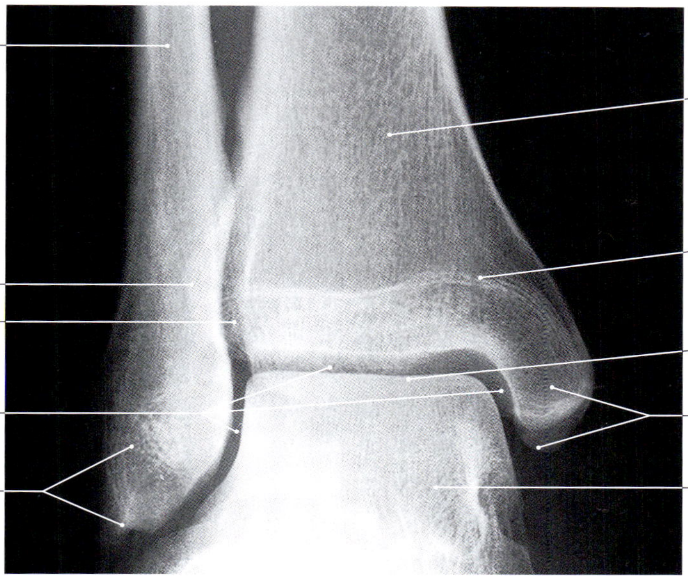

Fig. 1049 Ankle joint;
AP-radiograph with the subject reclined and the central beam directed tangentially onto the trochlea of talus.

* Clinically, the posterior border of the fibular notch is also referred to as the third malleolus.

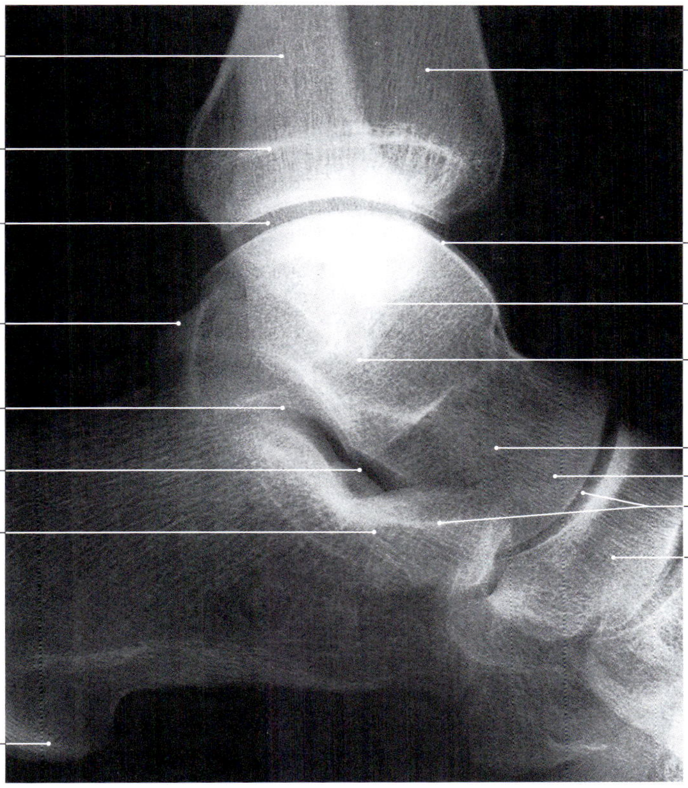

Fig. 1050 Ankle and talotarsal joint;
AP-radiograph with the subject reclined and the central beam directed tangentially onto the apex of the trochlea of talus.

* Due to their helical distorsion, the joint clefts are not displayed orthogonally.
** Overlapping epiphyseal lines of the tibia and fibula

→ 1160, 1162

Fasciae of the lower limb

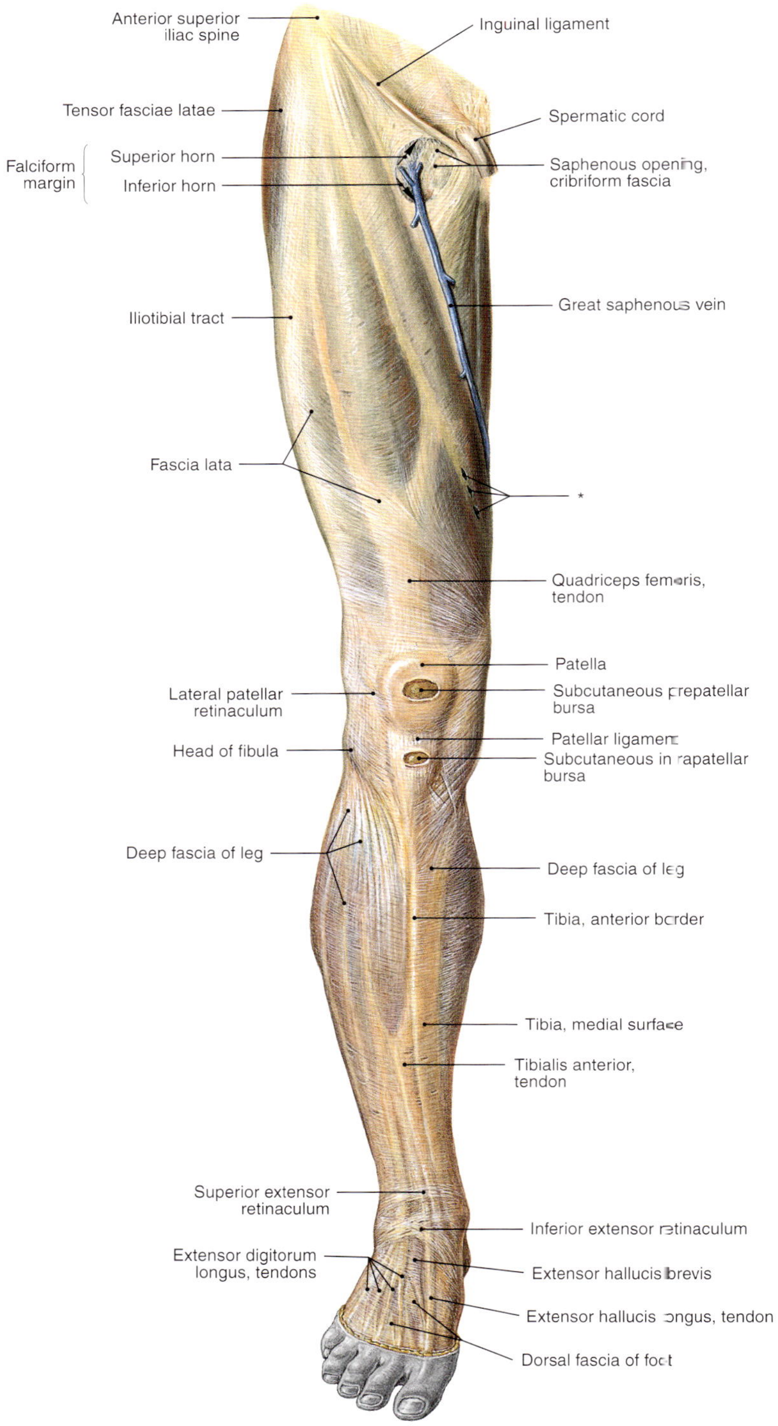

Fig. 1051 Fascia lata and deep fascia of leg.
The transition zone between the aponeurosis of the external oblique abdominal muscle and the fascia lata is known as inguinal ligament. This ligament extends laterally from the anterior superior iliac spine to its attachment on the pubic tubercle medially.

* Openings in the fascia for the perforator veins (DODD's veins)

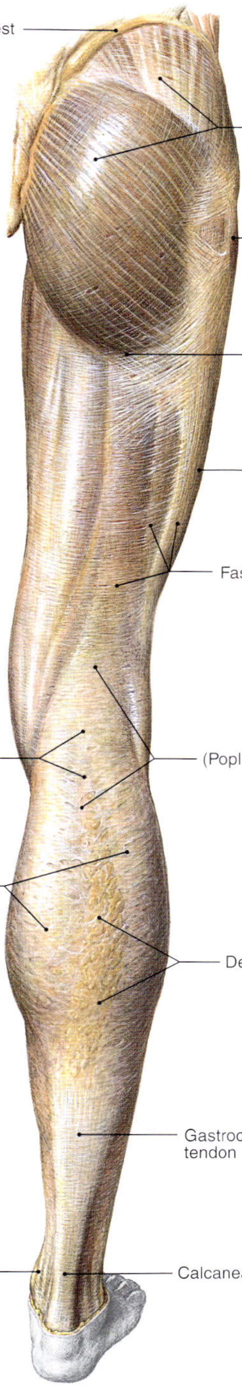

Fig. 1052 Fascia lata and deep fascia of leg.

Muscles of the lower limb, overview

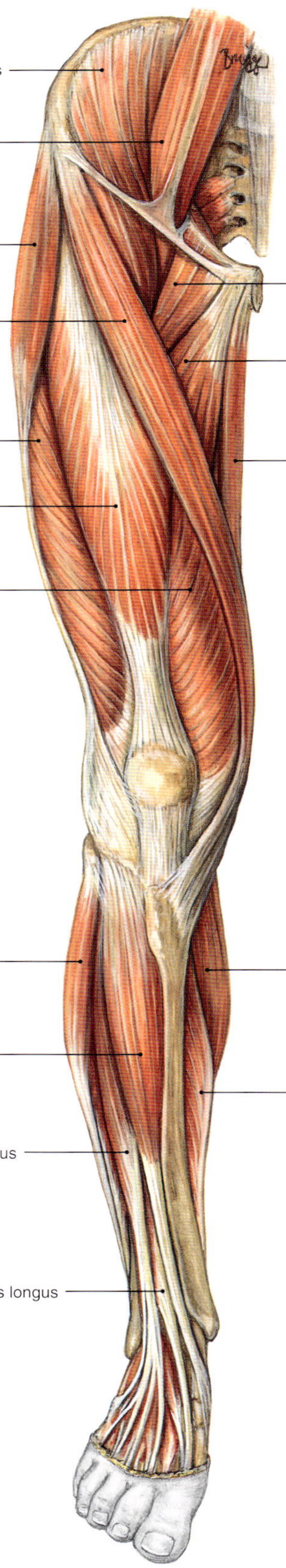

→ T 42, T 44, T 45, T 47, T 48

Fig. 1053 Muscles of the lower limb; overview.

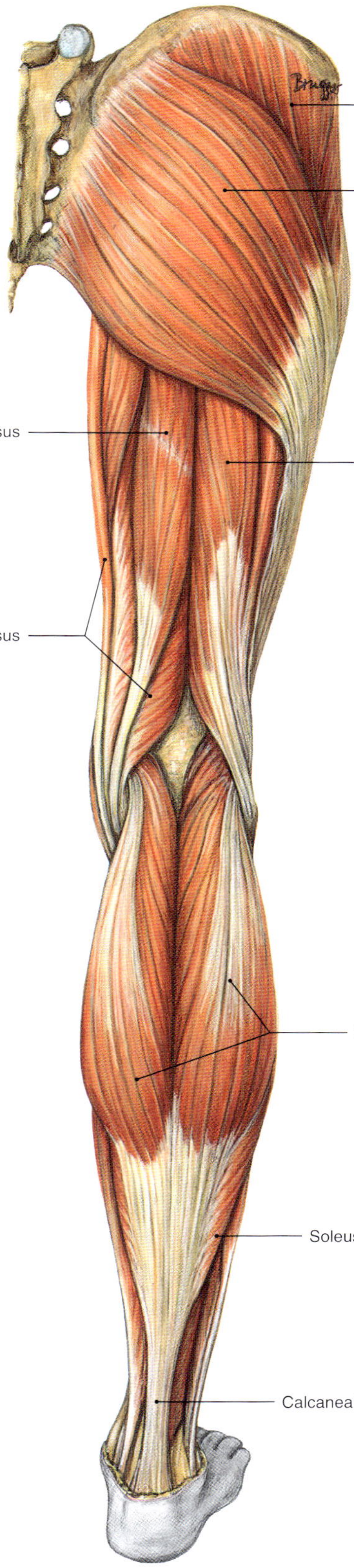

Fig. 1054 Muscles of the lower limb; overview.

→ T 43, T 46, T 49

Origins and insertions of the muscles of the hip, the thigh and the leg

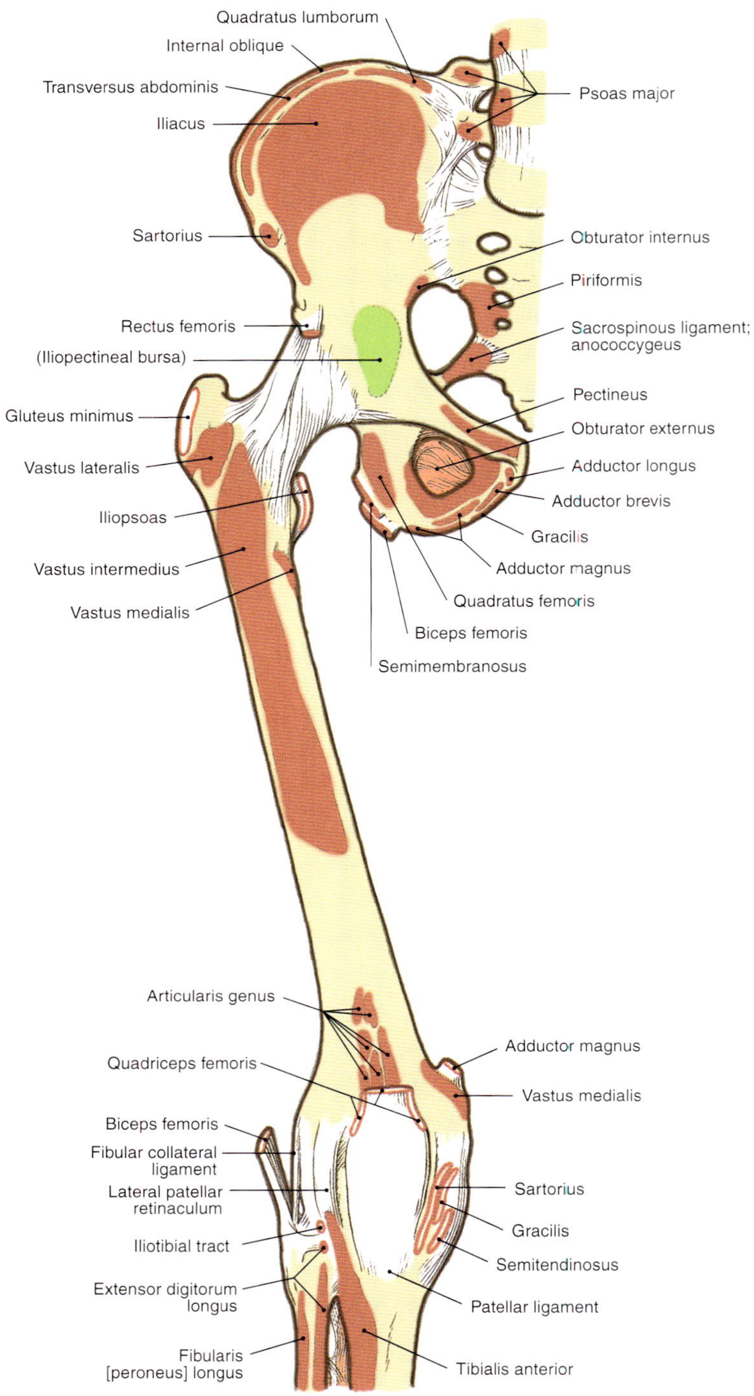

→ T 42–T 48

Fig. 1055 Origins and insertions of the muscles at the lower lumbar vertebrae, the pelvic bones, the femur and the proximal extremities of the bones of the leg; ventral view.

Origins and insertions of the muscles of the hip, the thigh and the leg

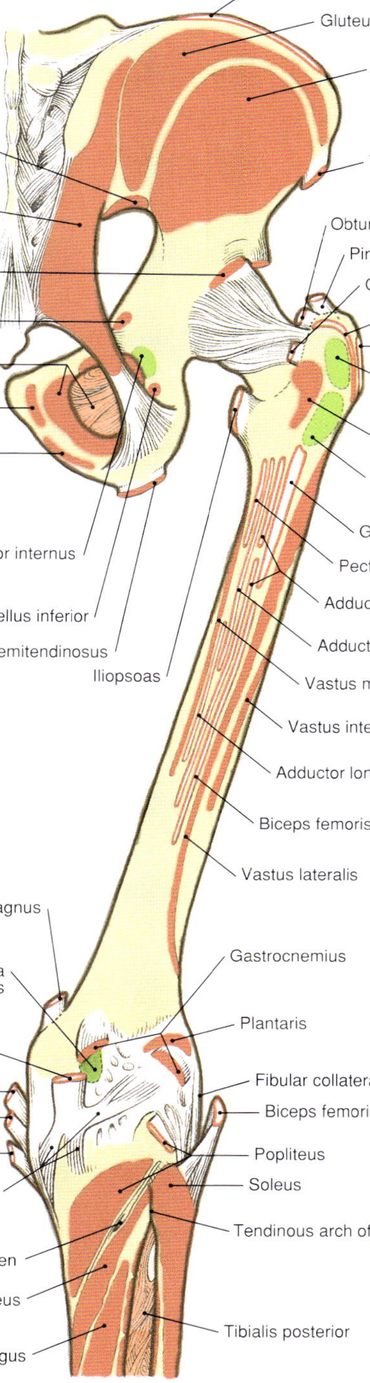

Fig. 1056 Origins and insertions of the muscles at the pelvic bones, the femur and the proximal extremities of the bones of the leg; dorsal view.

→ T 43–T 46, T 49, T 50

Muscles of the thigh

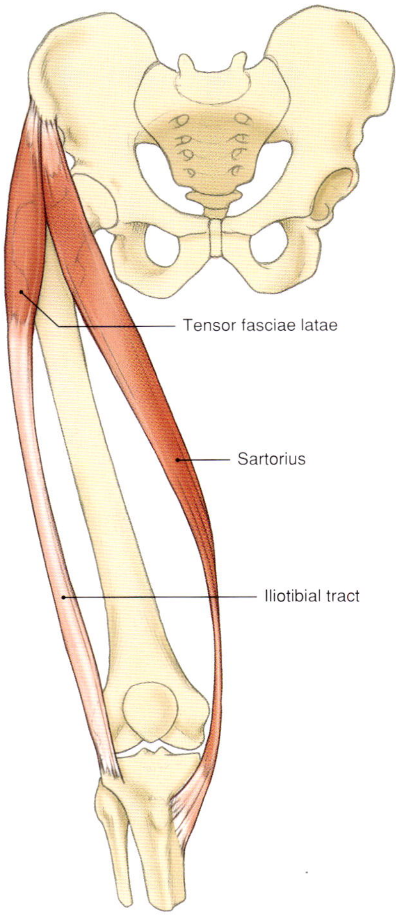

Fig. 1057 Tensor fasciae latae muscle and sartorius muscle.

→ T 44

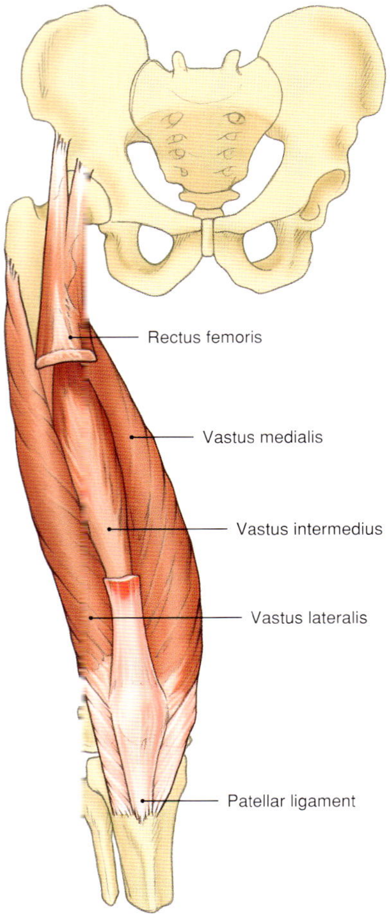

Fig. 1058 Quadriceps femoris muscle.

→ T 44

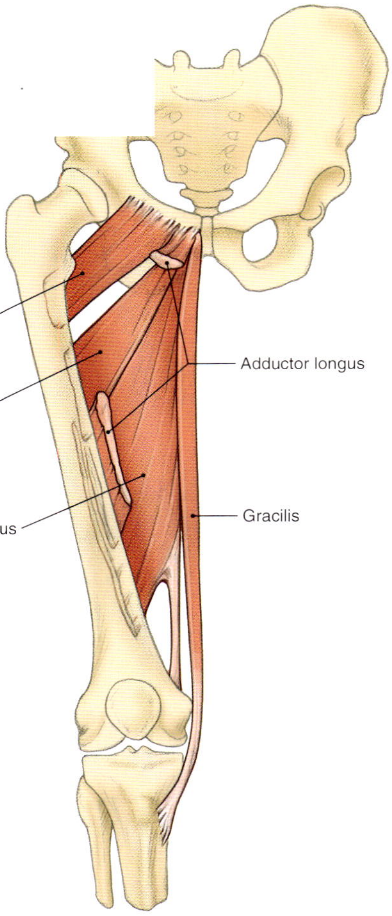

Fig. 1059 Adductor muscles.

→ T 45

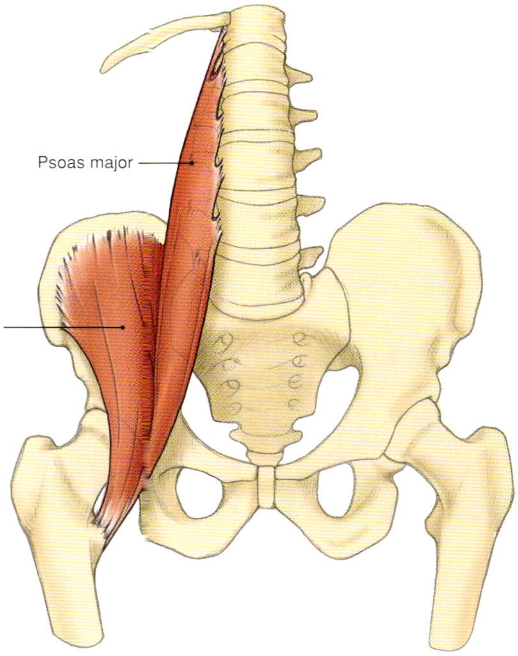

Fig. 1060 Iliopsoas muscle.

→ T 42

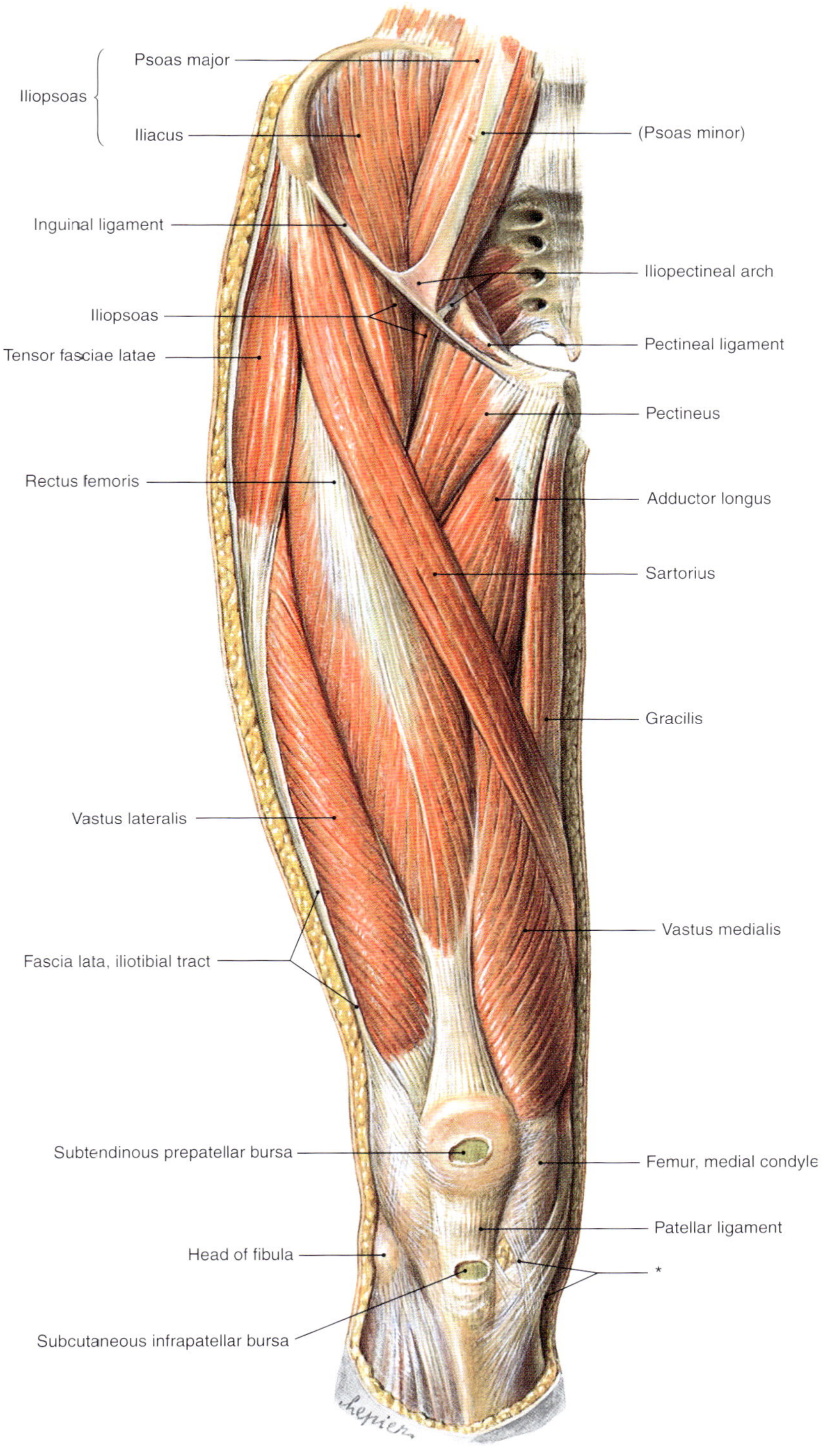

Fig. 1061 Muscles of the thigh and the hip;
after removal of the fascia lata except for the iliotibial tract.

→ T 42, T 44, T 45

* Common insertion of the sartorius, gracilis and semitendinosus muscles just below the medial condyle of the tibia (formerly known as the superficial pes anserinus)

Muscles of the thigh

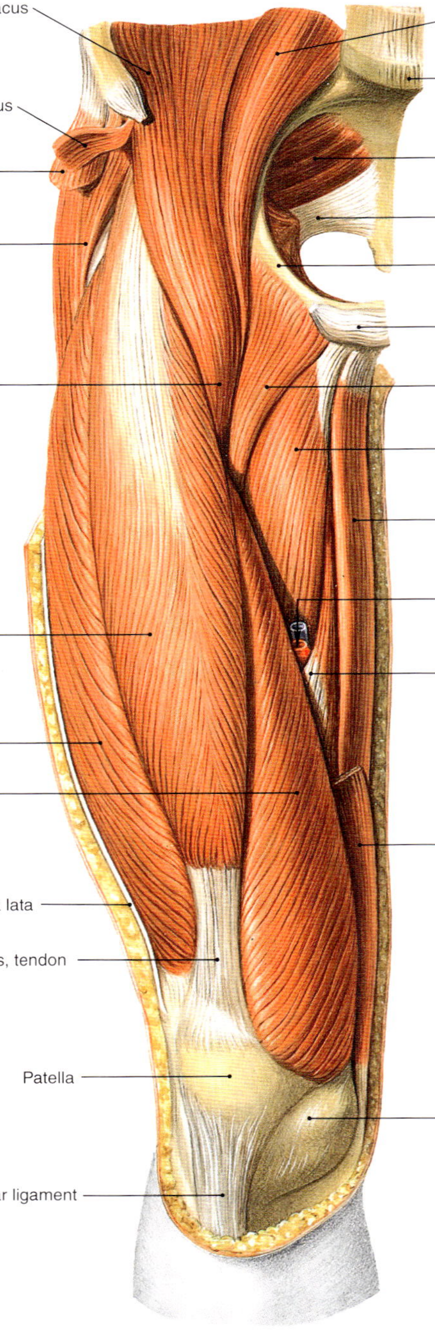

→ T 42, T 44, T 45

Fig. 1062 Muscles of the thigh and the hip; after removal of the fascia lata, the tensor fasciae latae muscle and the sartorius muscle.

* The fourth head of the quadriceps muscle, the vastus intermedius muscle, is covered by the rectus femoris muscle.

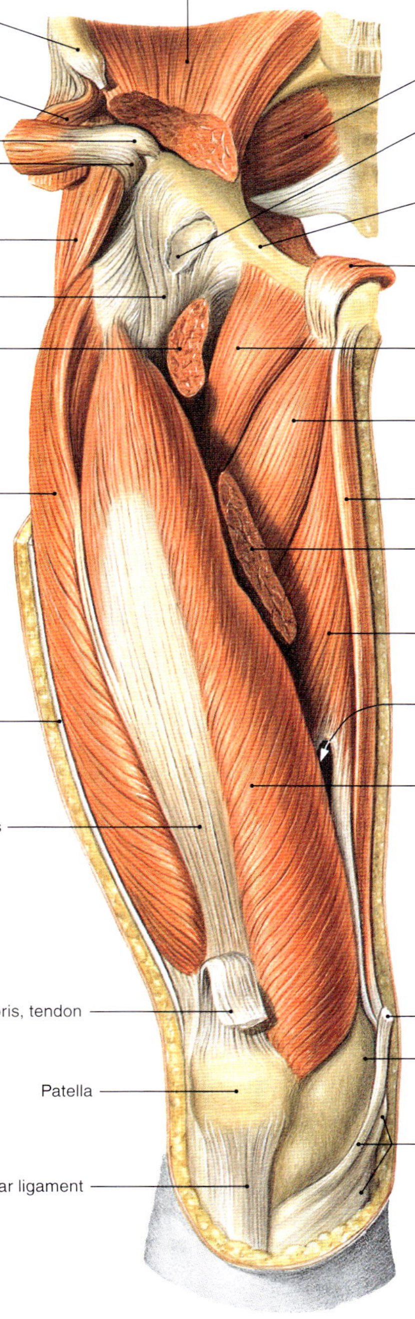

Fig. 1063 Muscles of the thigh and the hip; deep layer after removal of the sartorius, the rectus femoris and the adductor longus muscles as well as parts of the iliopsoas muscle in the joint region.

* Common insertion of the sartorius, gracilis and semitendinosus muscles just below the medial condyle of the tibia

** The origin of the rectus femoris muscle has been flapped laterally upwards.

*** A part of the adductor longus muscle has been flapped upwards.

→ T 42, T 44, T 45

Muscles of the thigh

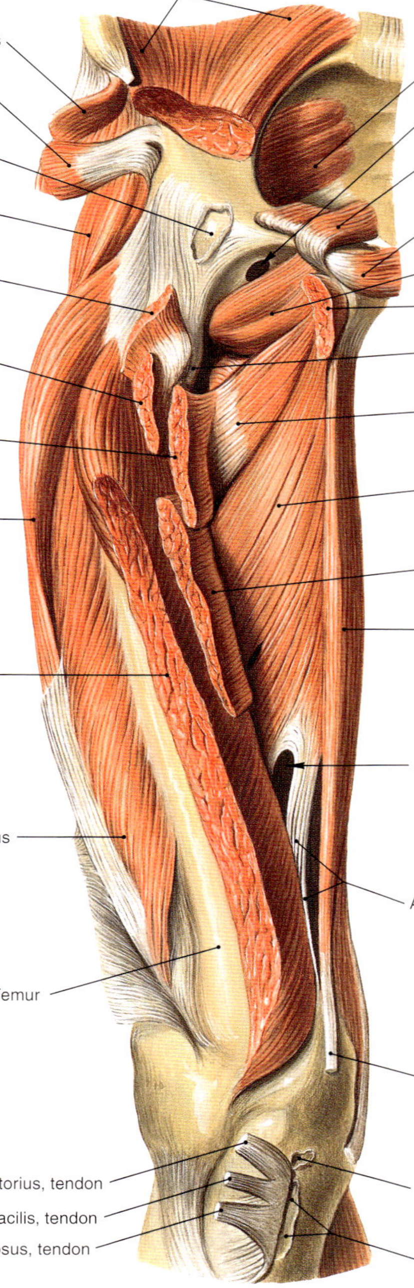

→ T 42, T 44, T 45

Fig. 1064 Muscles of the thigh and the hip; after almost complete removal of superficial and several deeper muscles; ventral view.

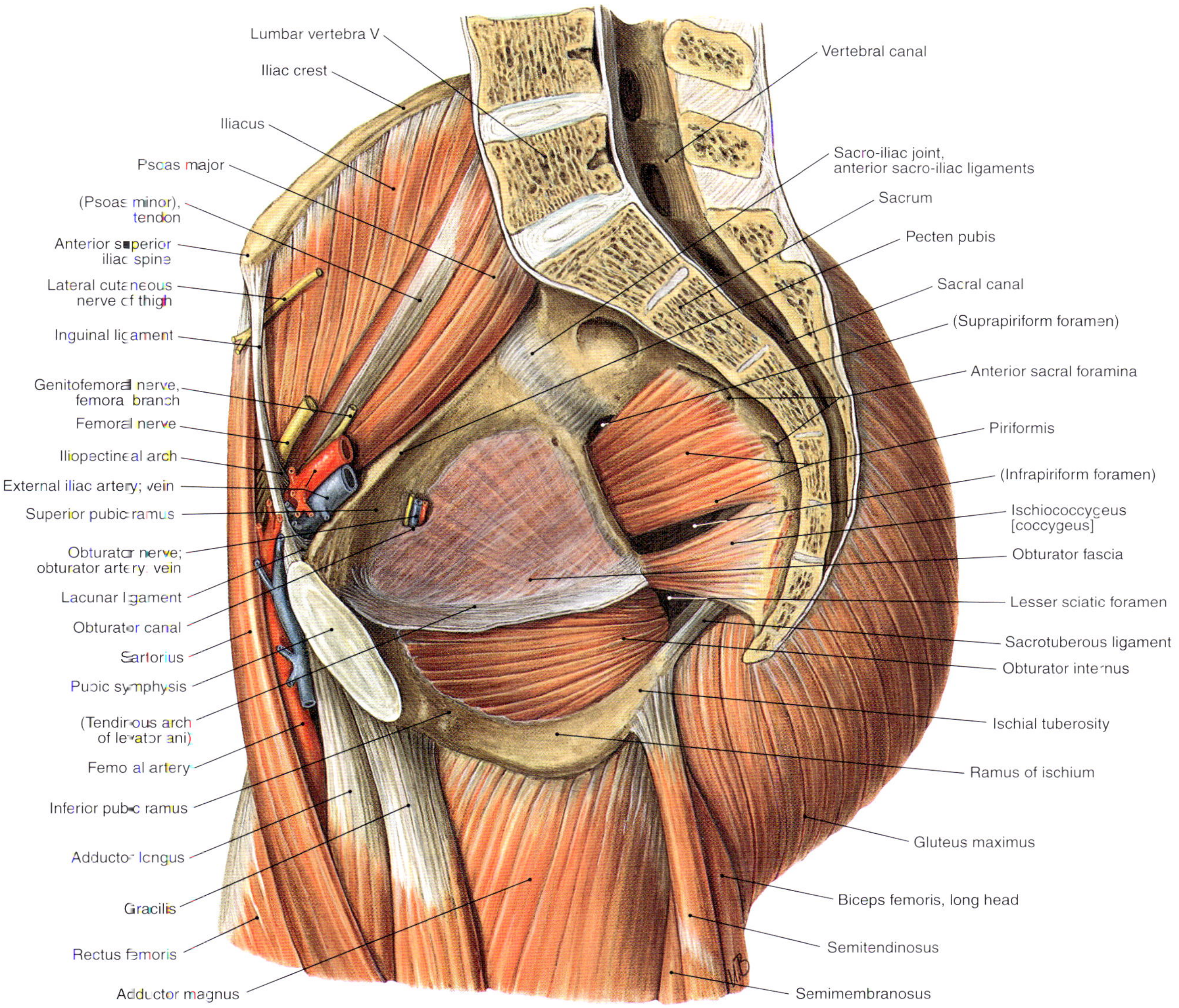

Fig. 1065 Muscles of the thigh and the hip; medial view.

→ T 22 a, T 42–T 46

Muscles of the thigh and the hip

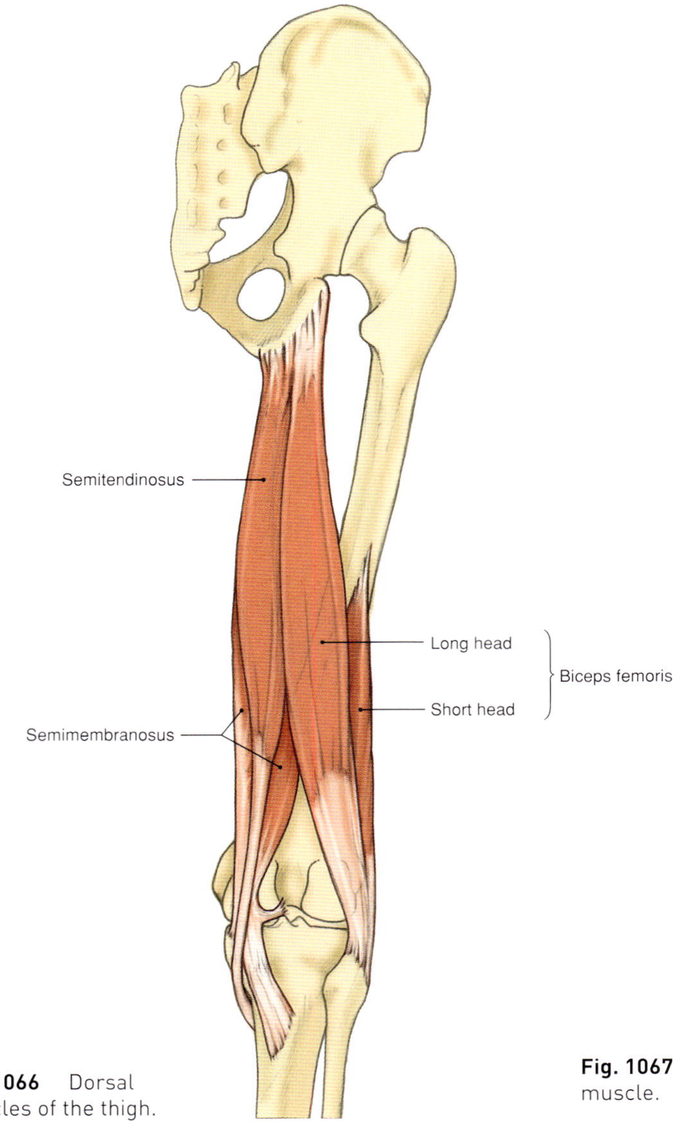

Fig. 1066 Dorsal muscles of the thigh.

→ T 46

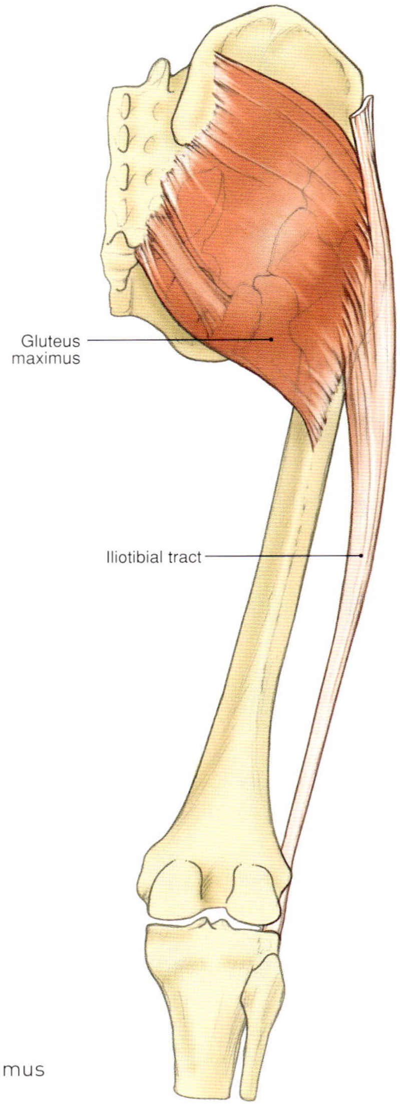

Fig. 1067 Gluteus maximus muscle.

→ T 43

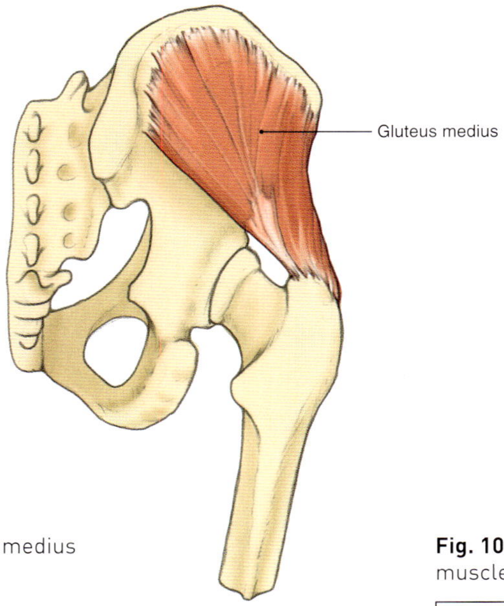

Fig. 1068 Gluteus medius muscle.

→ T 43

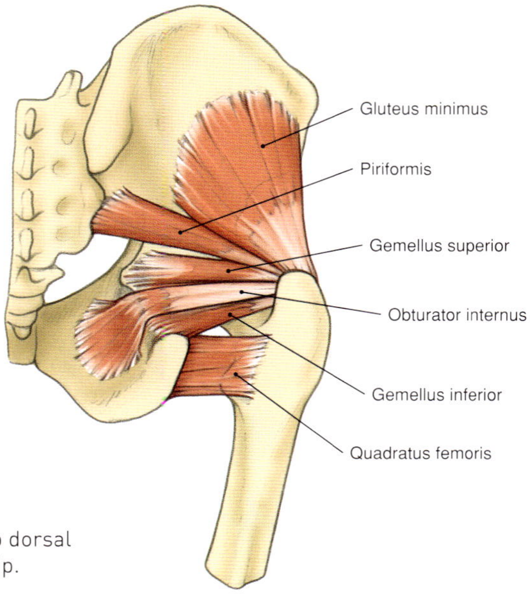

Fig. 1069 Deep dorsal muscles of the hip.

→ T 43

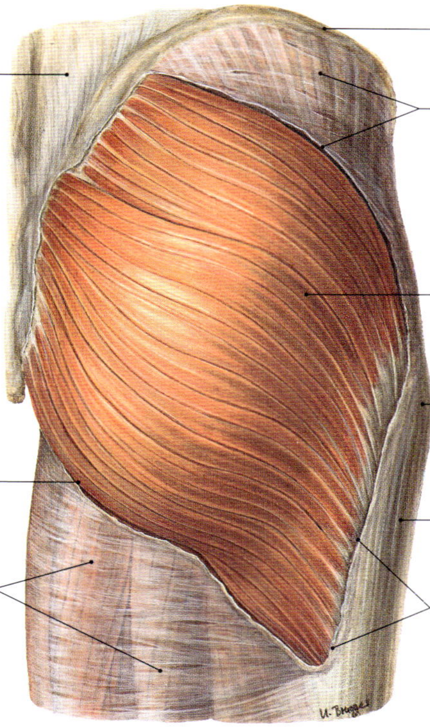

Fig. 1070 Muscles of the thigh and the hip.

→ T 43

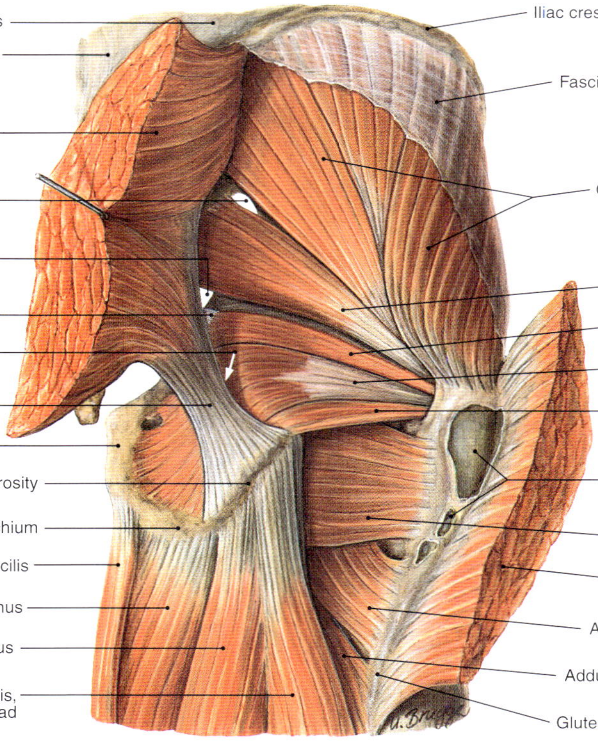

Fig. 1071 Muscles of the thigh and the hip; the gluteus maximus muscle has been sectioned; dorsal view.

* The part of the obturator internus muscle between the curved edge of the lesser sciatic notch and the insertion in the trochanteric fossa frequently consists of tendinous bands.

→ T 43, T 45, T 46

Muscles of the thigh and the hip

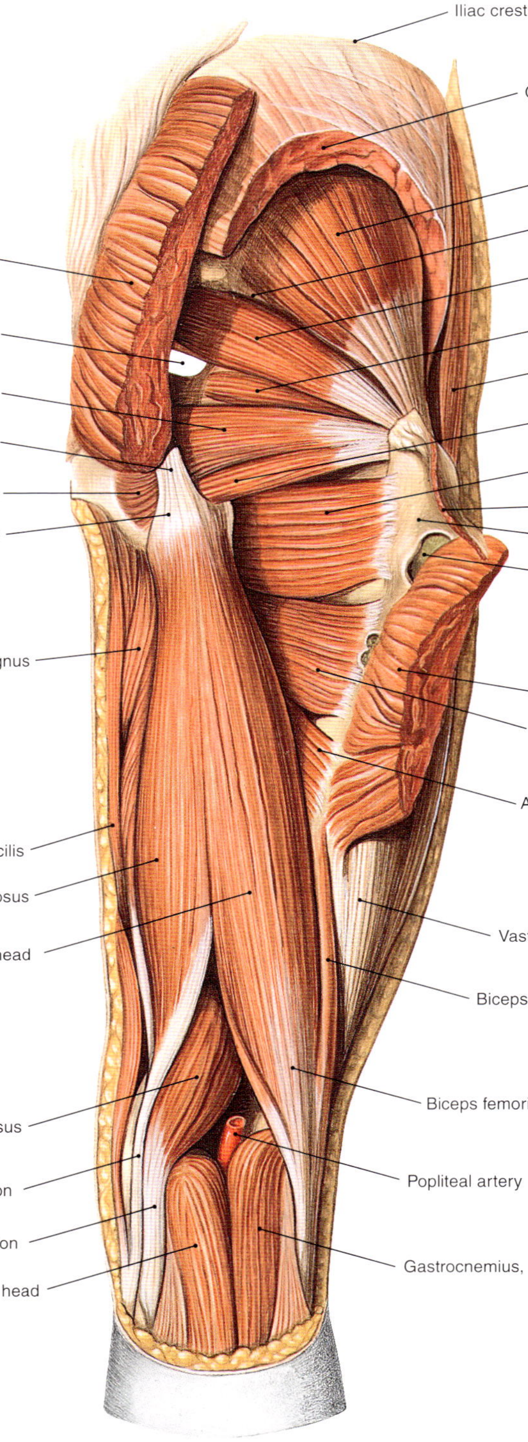

→ T 43, T 45, T 46

Fig. 1072 Muscles of the thigh and the hip; the gluteus maximus and medius muscles have been partially removed; dorsal view.

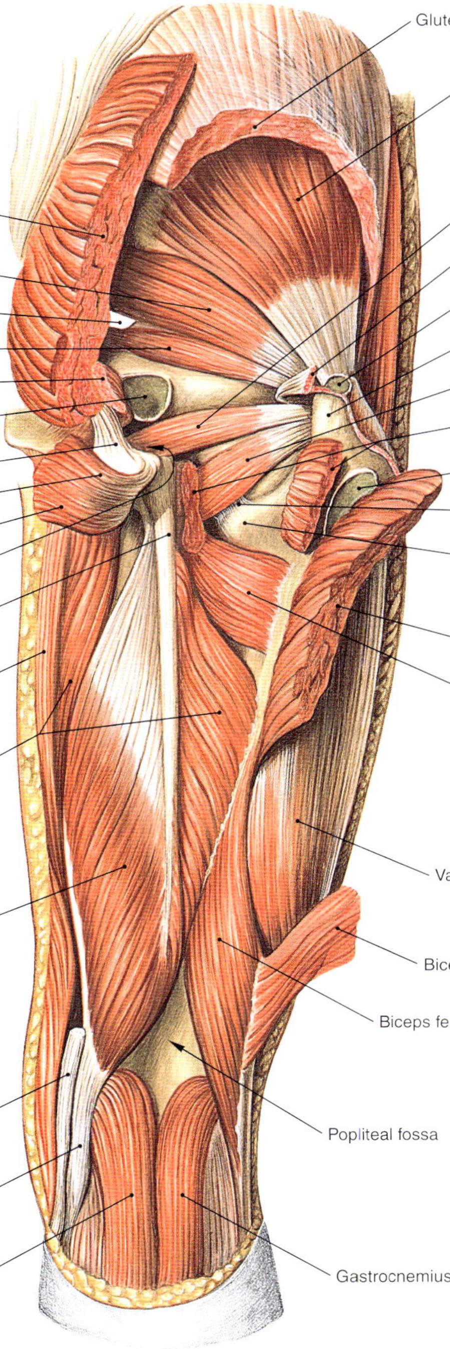

Fig. 1073 Muscles of the thigh and the hip; deep layer after almost complete removal of the superficial gluteal and the ischiocrural muscles; dorsal view.

→ T 43, T 45, T 46

Muscles of the thigh and the hip

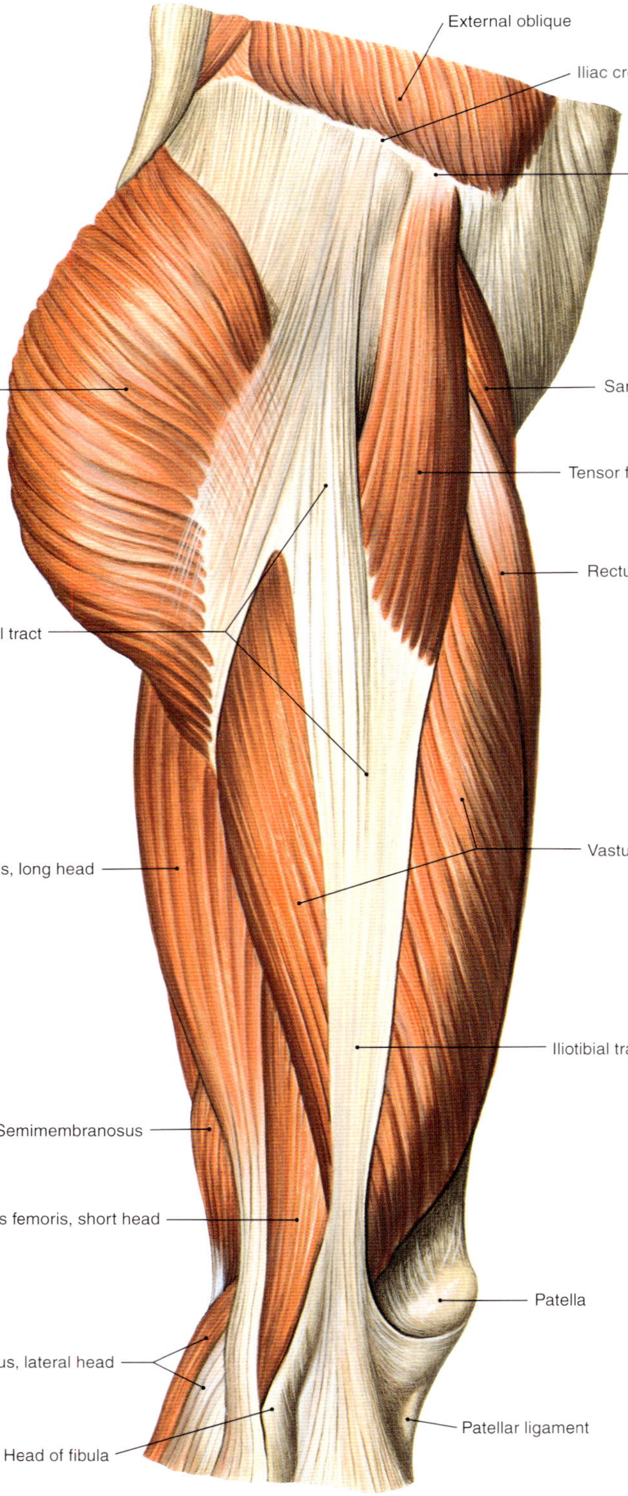

→ T 43, T 44, T 46

Fig. 1074 Muscles of the thigh and the hip; after removal of the fascia lata except for the iliotibial tract.

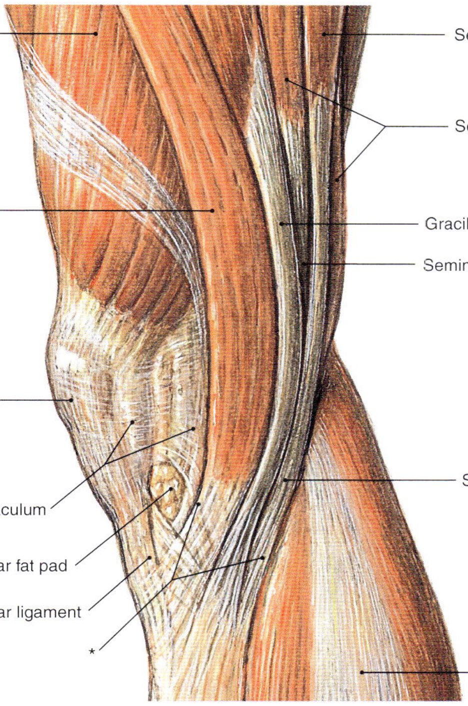

Fig. 1075 Muscles in the region of the knee joint; medial view.

→ T 44–T 46, T 49

* Common insertion just below the medial condyle of the tibia (formerly known as superficial pes anserinus)

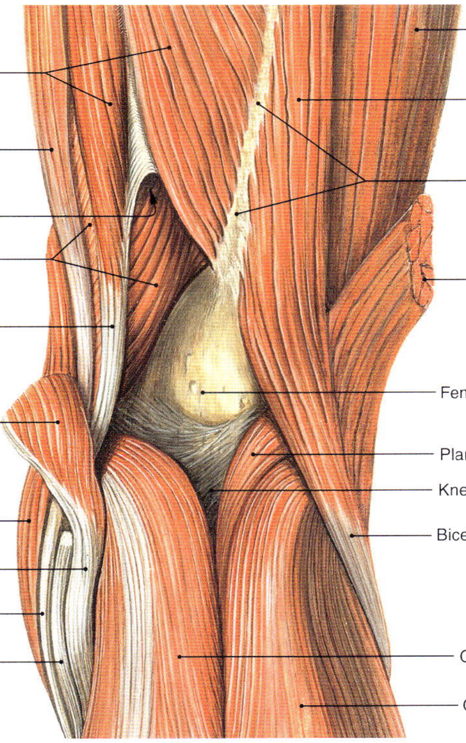

Fig. 1076 Muscles in the region of the knee joint; after almost complete removal of the ischiocrural muscles; dorsal view.

→ T 44–T 46, T 49

Origins and insertions of the muscles of the thigh and the ventral part of the leg

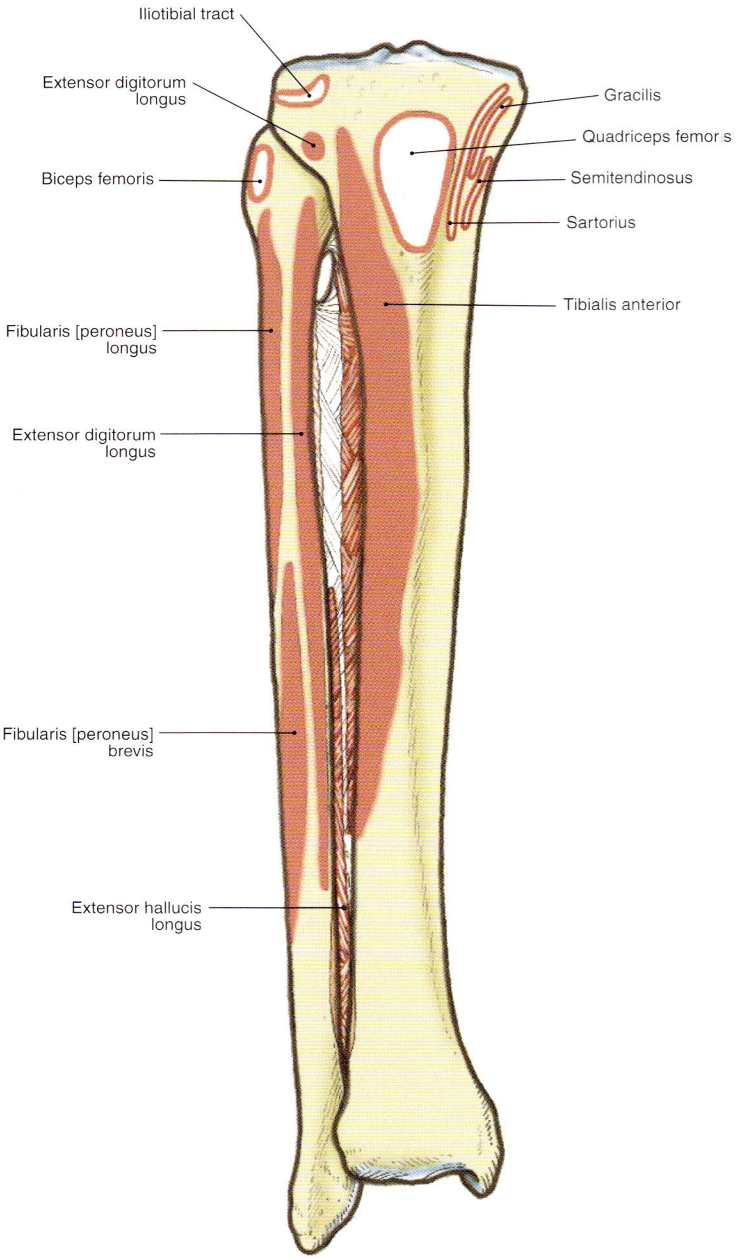

→ T 44–T 47

Fig. 1077 Origins and insertions of the muscles at the bones of the leg; ventral view.

Origins and insertions of the muscles of the thigh and the dorsal part of the leg

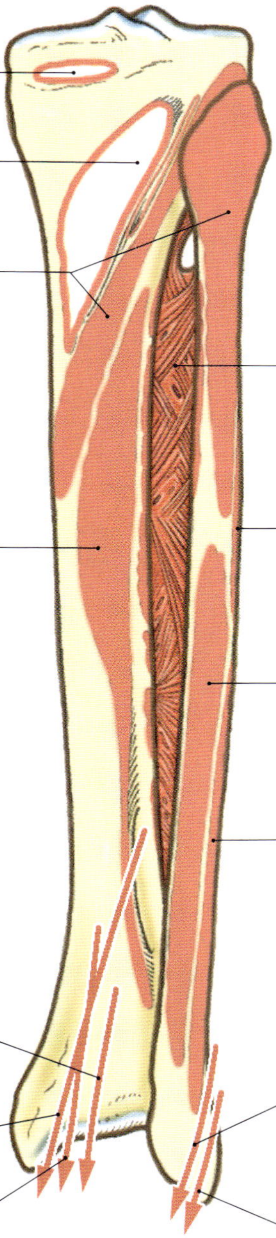

Fig. 1078 Origins and insertions of the muscles at the bones of the leg; dorsal view.

→ T 46, T 48–T 50

Muscles of the leg

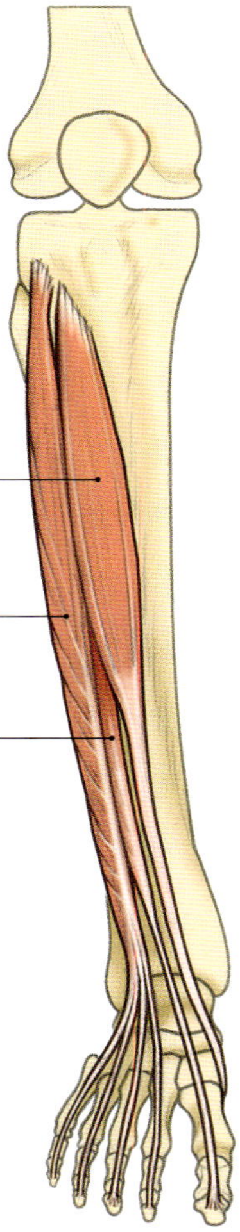

Fig. 1079 Extensor muscles of the leg.

→ T 47

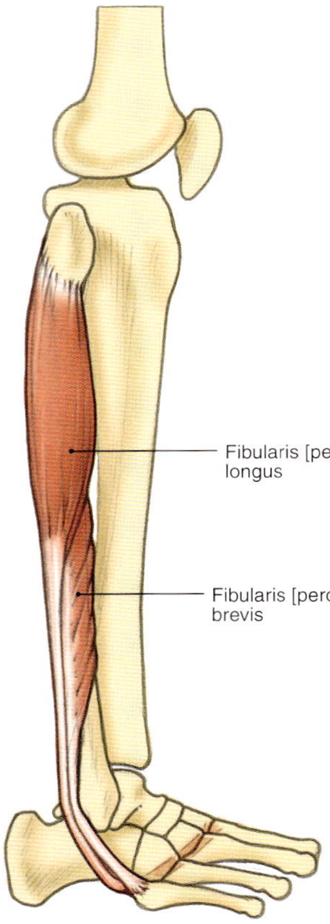

Fig. 1080 Lateral (fibular) muscles.

→ T 48

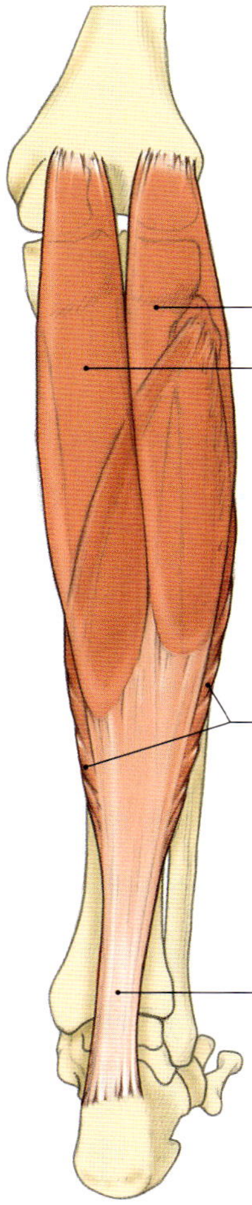

Fig. 1081 Triceps surae muscle.

→ T 49

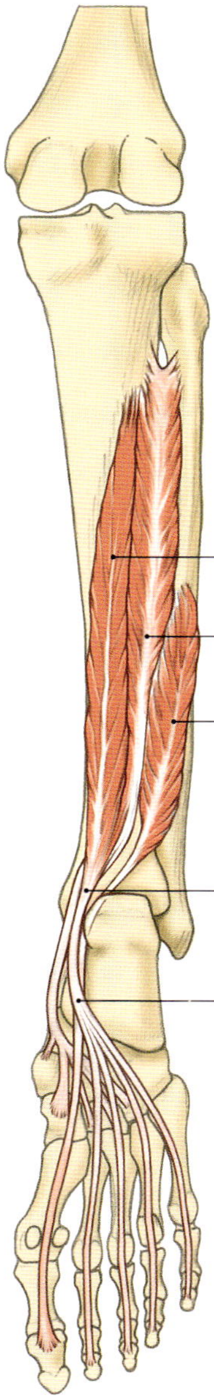

Fig. 1082 Deep flexor muscles of the leg.

→ T 50

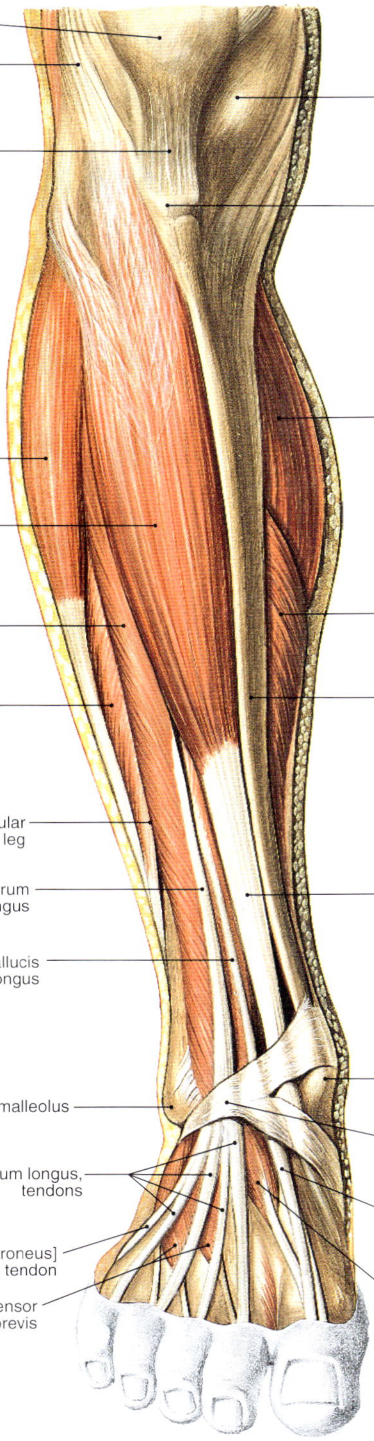

Fig. 1083 Muscles of the leg and the foot.

→ T 47, T 48

Muscles of the leg

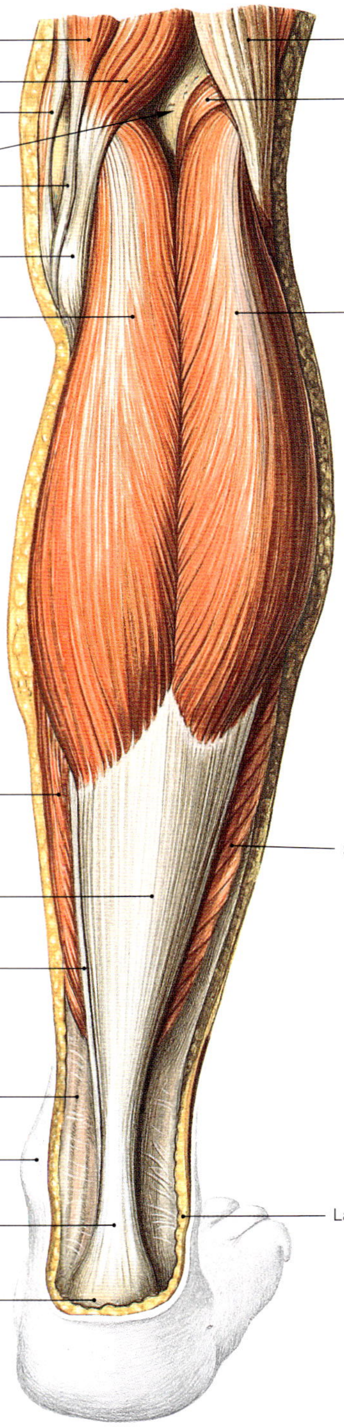

→ T 49

Fig. 1084 Muscles of the leg; superficial layer.

* Also: Achilles tendon

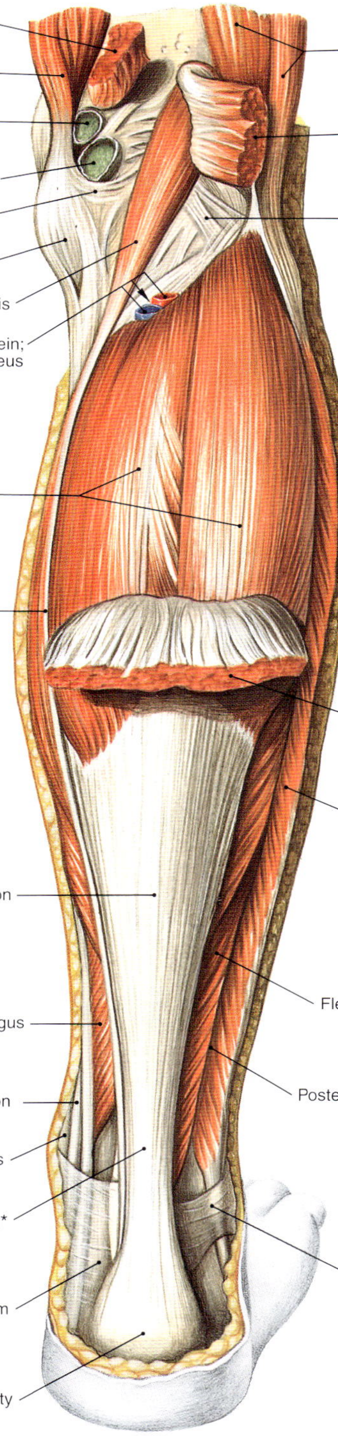

Fig. 1085 Muscles of the leg; superficial layer after partial removal of the gastrocnemius muscle.

* Also: Achilles tendon

→ T 49

Muscles of the leg

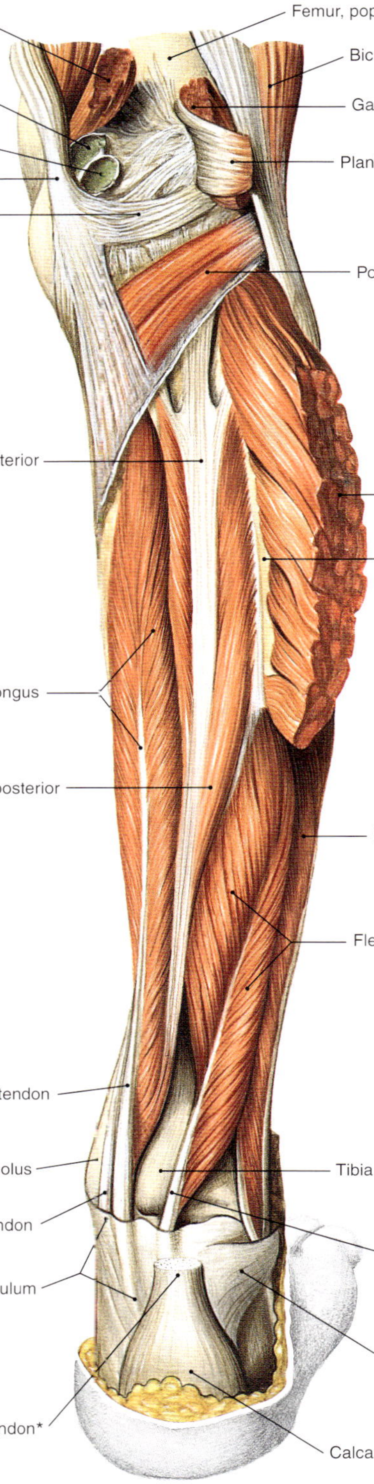

→ T 50

Fig. 1086 Muscles of the leg; deep layer.

* Also: Achilles tendon

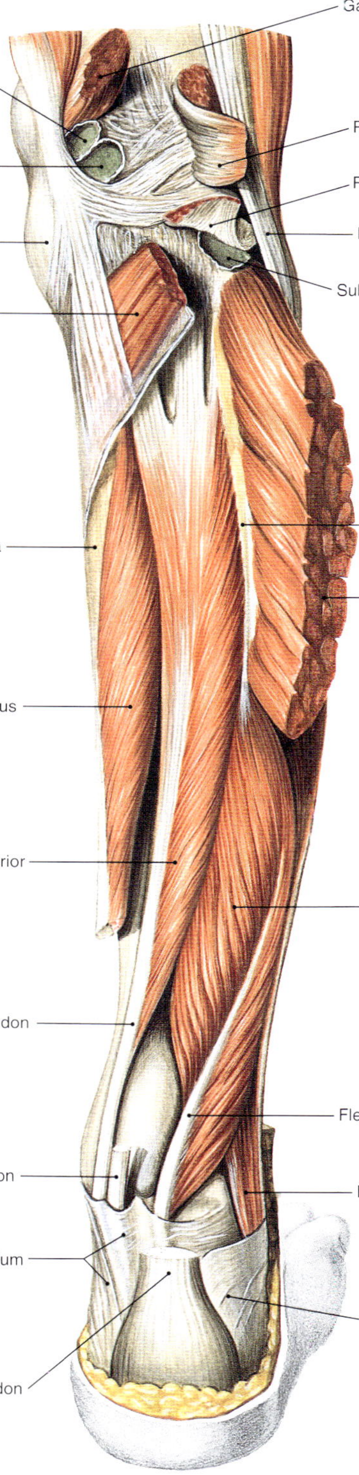

Fig. 1087 Muscles of the leg; deepest layer.

→ T 50

Muscles of the leg

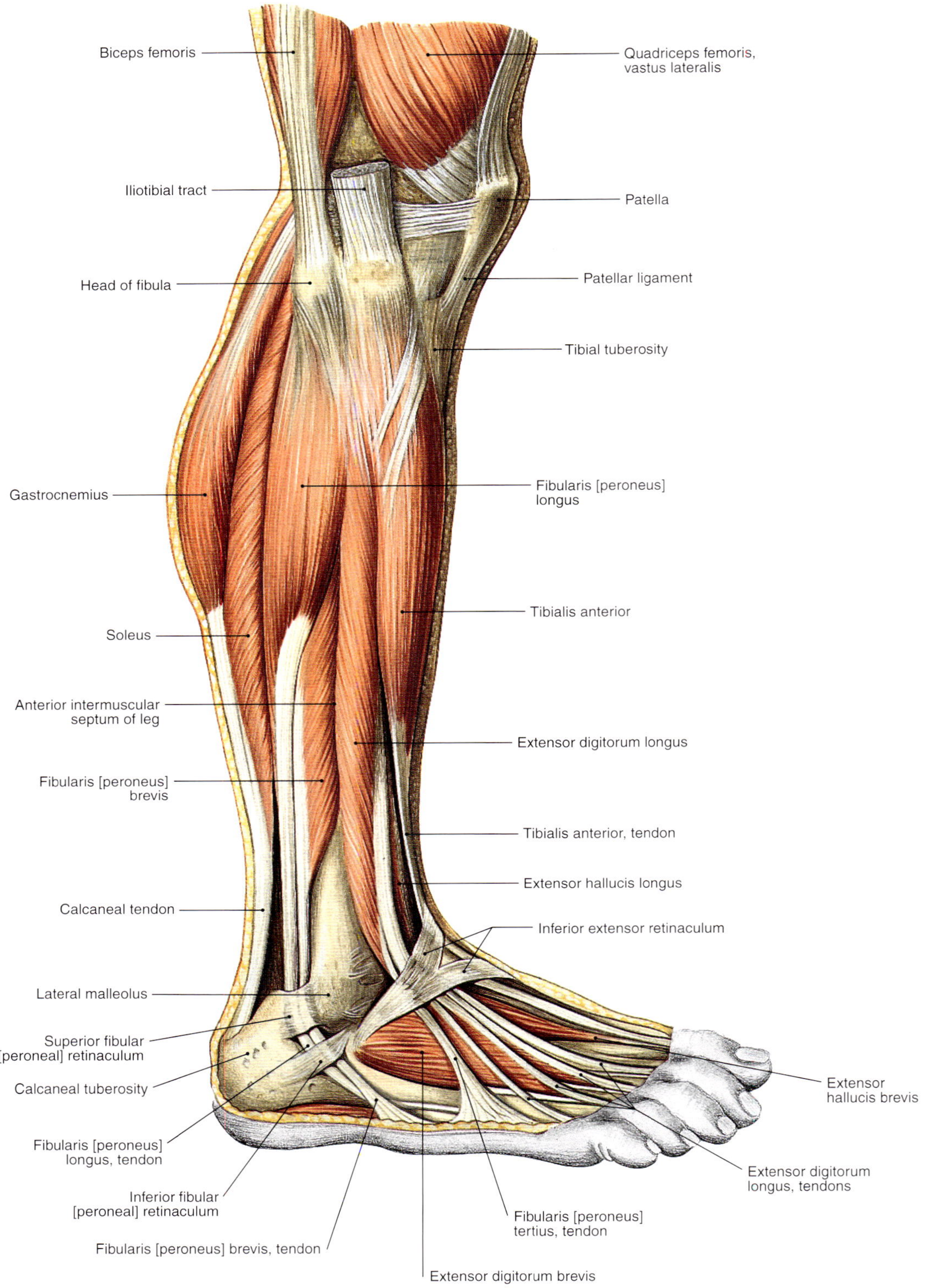

→ T 47–T49, T 51

Fig. 1088 Muscles of the leg and the foot.

Origins and insertions of the muscles of the foot and the leg

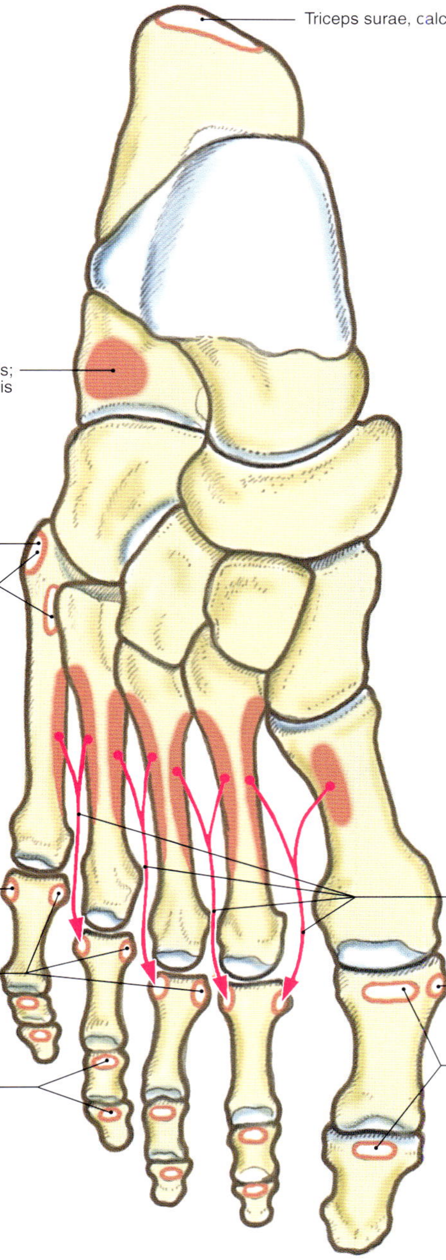

Fig. 1089 Origins and insertions of the muscles at the bones of the foot; dorsal view.

→ T 47, T 48, T 51, T 53, T 54

Tendon sheaths of the foot

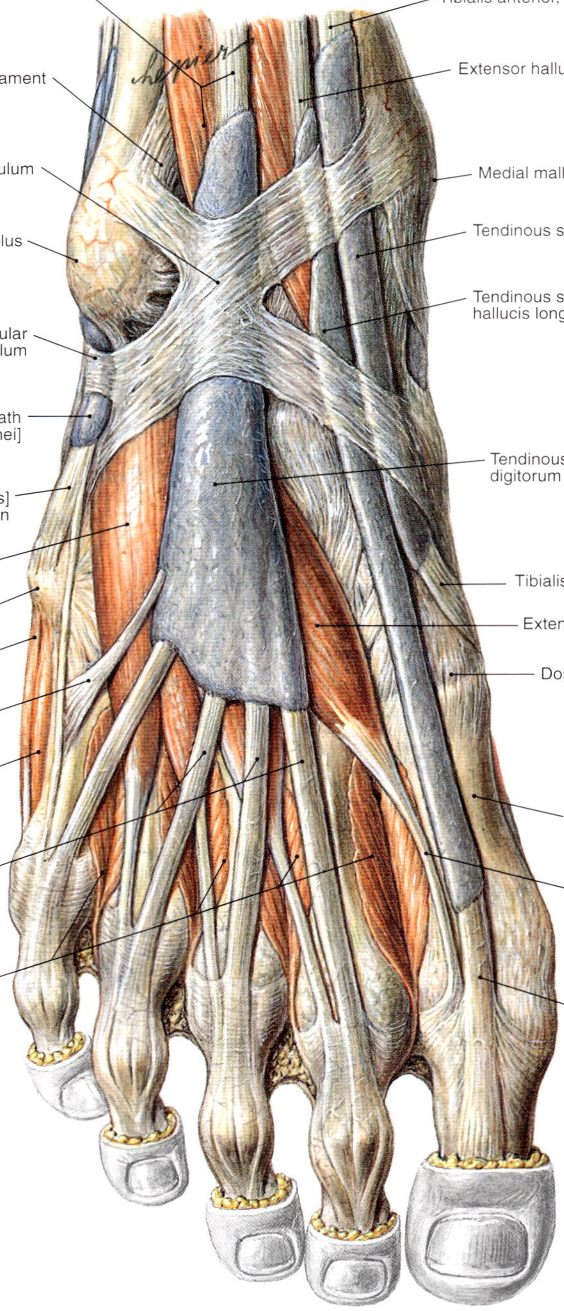

Fig. 1090 Tendon sheaths of the foot.

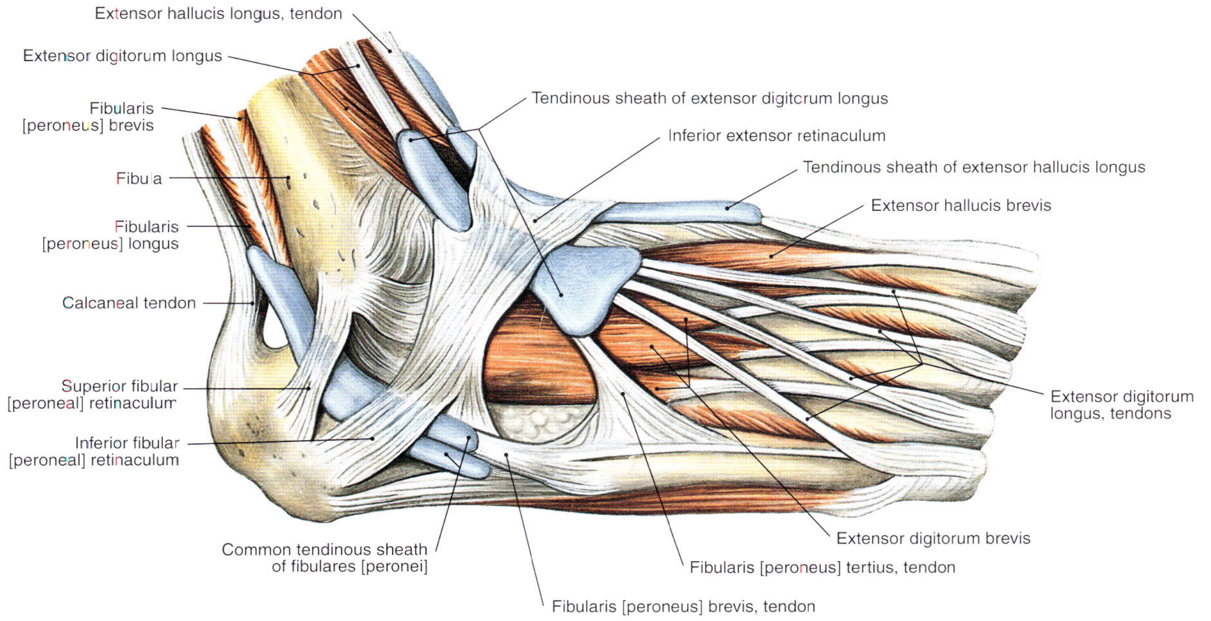

Fig. 1091 Tendon sheaths of the foot.

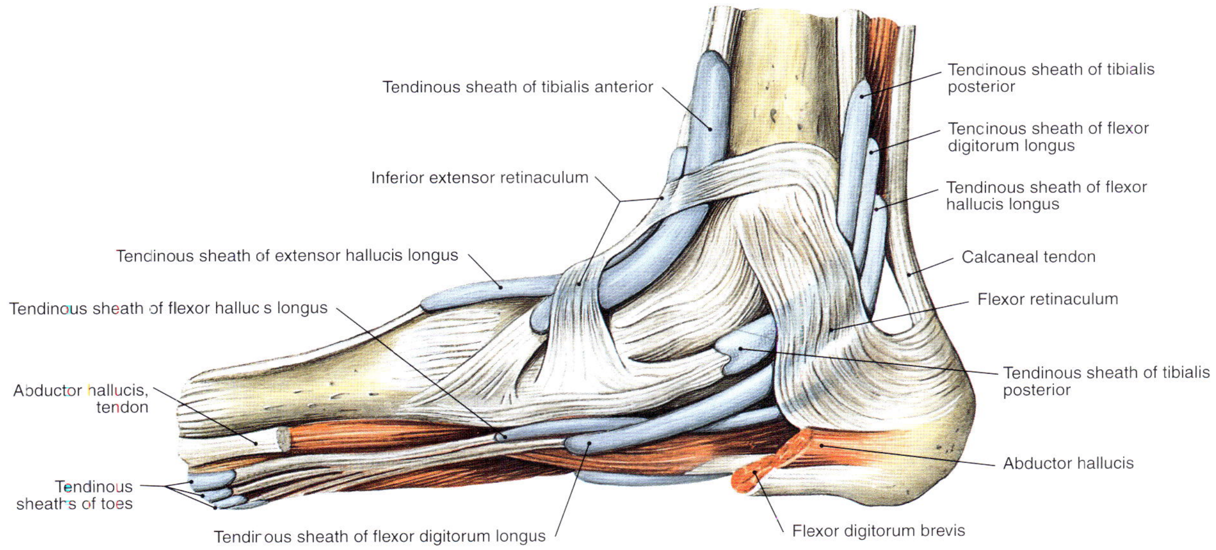

Fig. 1092 Tendon sheaths of the foot.

Muscles of the foot

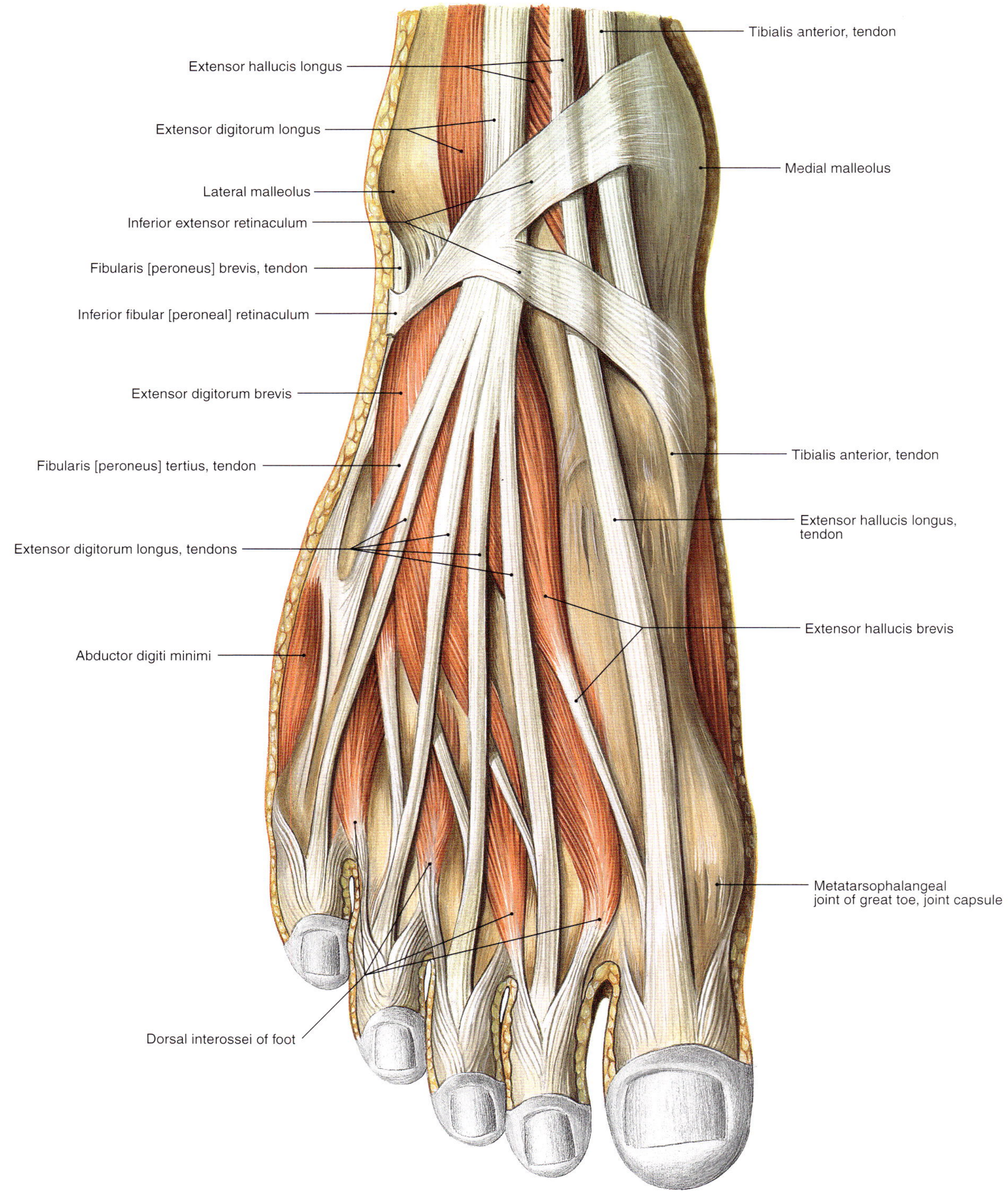

→ T 47, T 51, T 53

Fig. 1093 Muscles of the foot; after removal of the tendon sheaths.

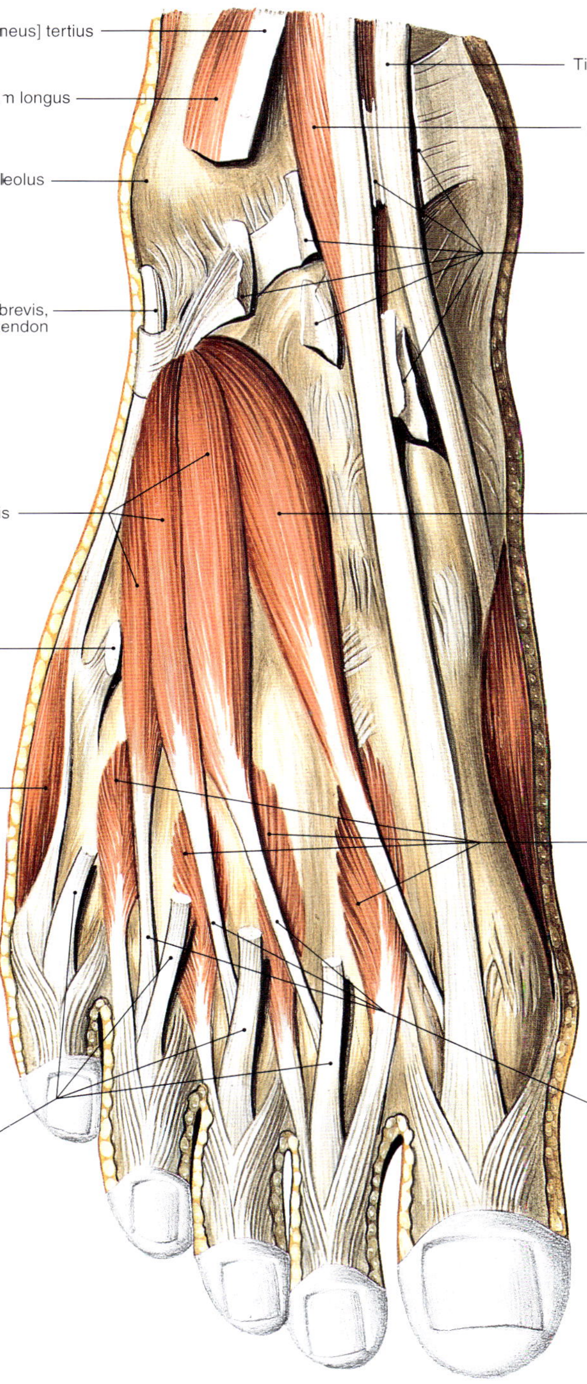

Fig. 1094 Muscles of the foot; after section of the inferior extensor retinaculum.

→ T 47, T 51, T 53

Muscles of the foot

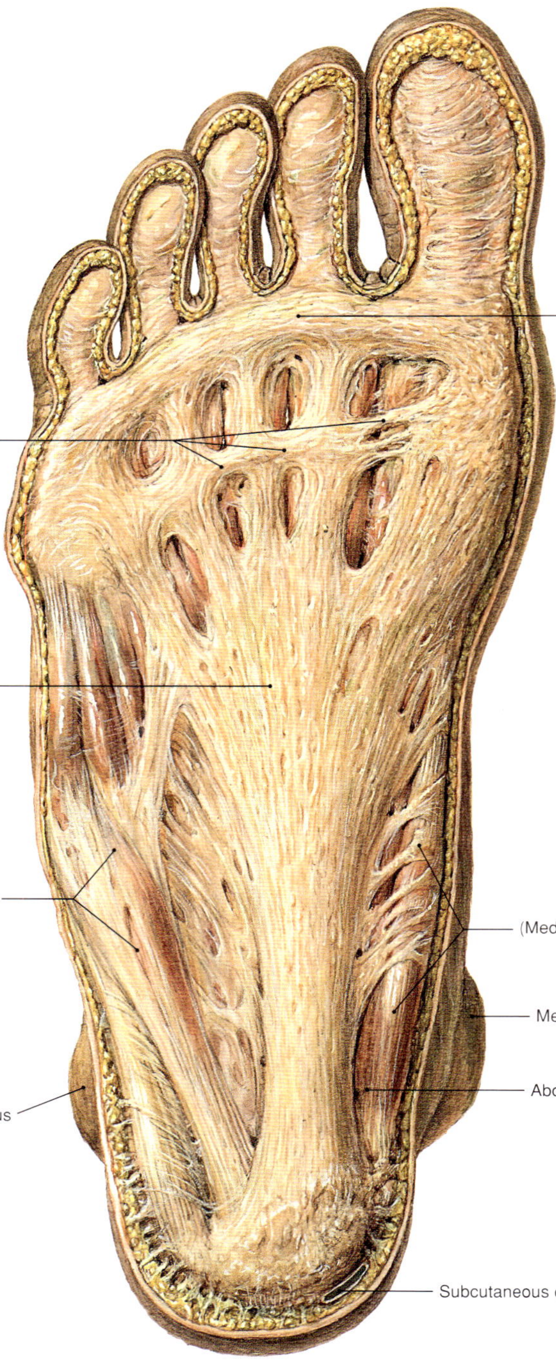

Fig. 1095 Muscles of the foot; plantar aponeurosis.

Origins and insertions of the muscles of the foot and the leg

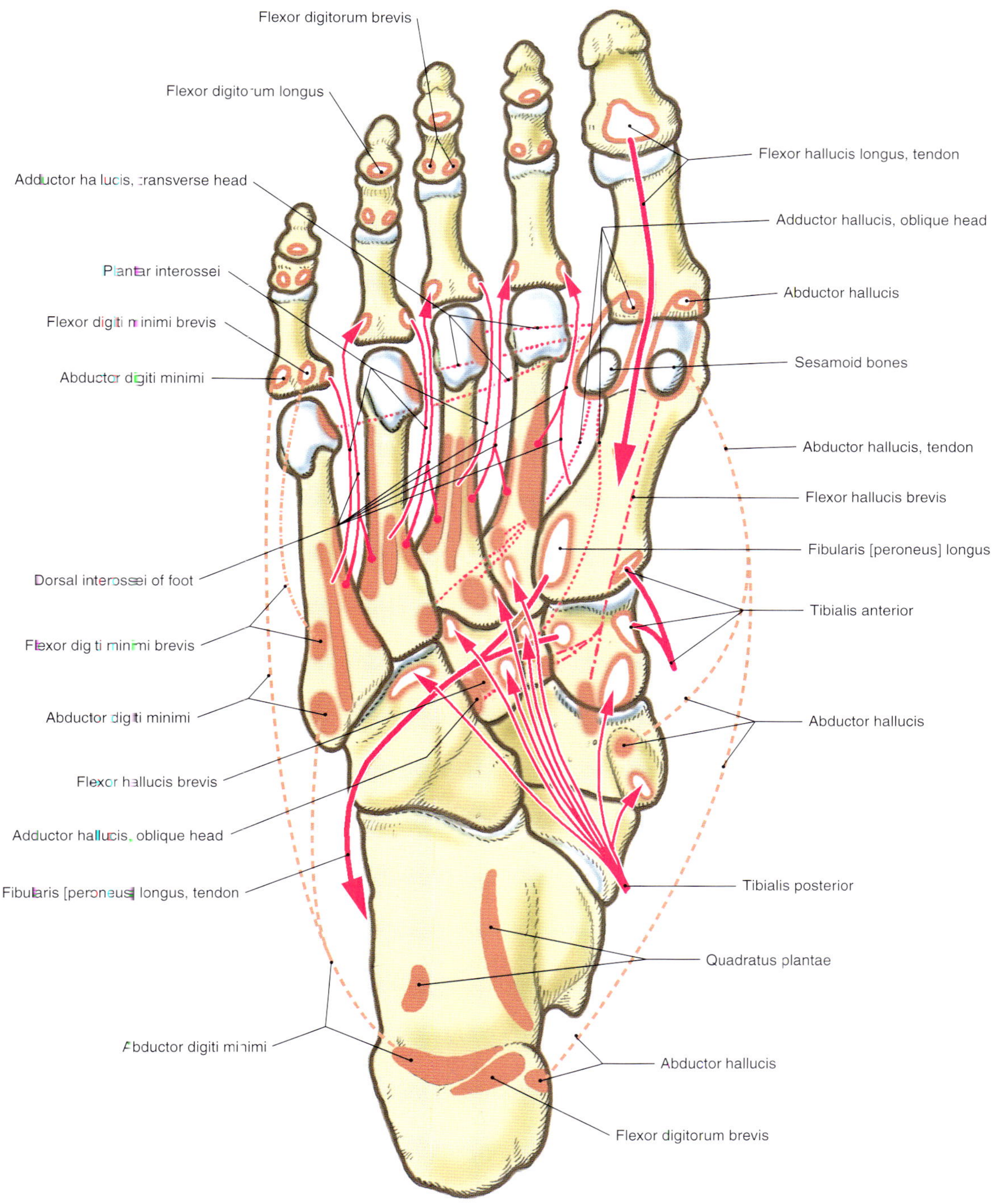

Fig. 1096 Origins and insertions of the muscles at the bones of the foot; plantar view.

→ T 42, T 48, T 50, T 52–T 54

Muscles of the foot

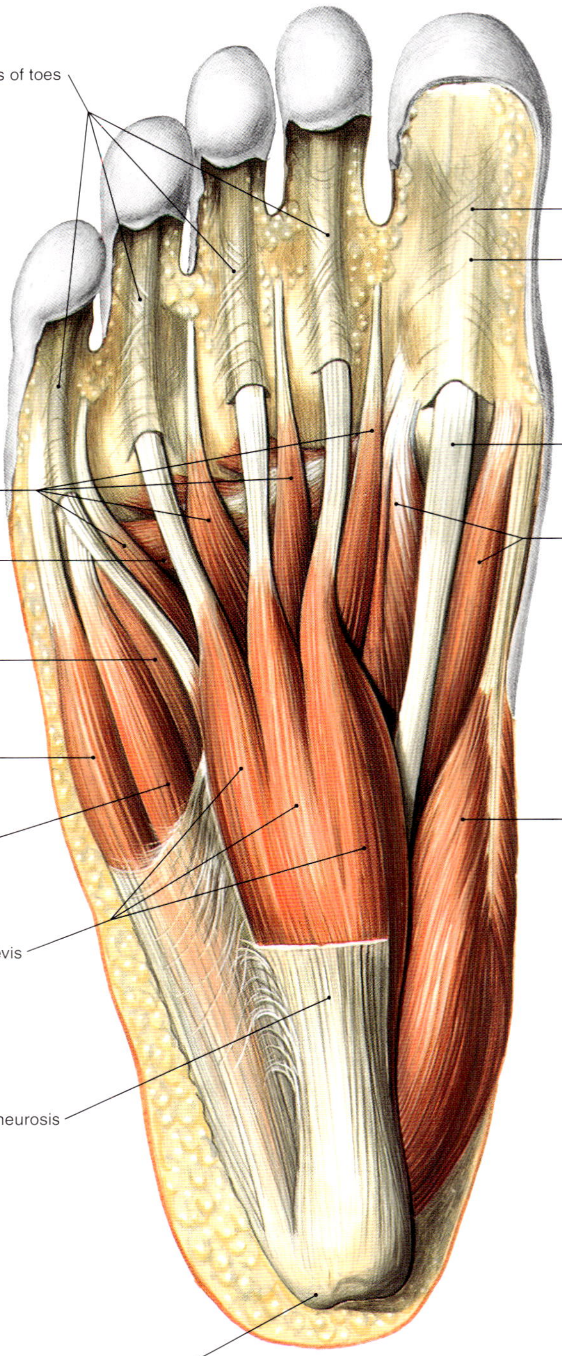

→ T 52–T 54

Fig. 1097 Muscles of the foot;
the plantar aponeurosis has been removed.

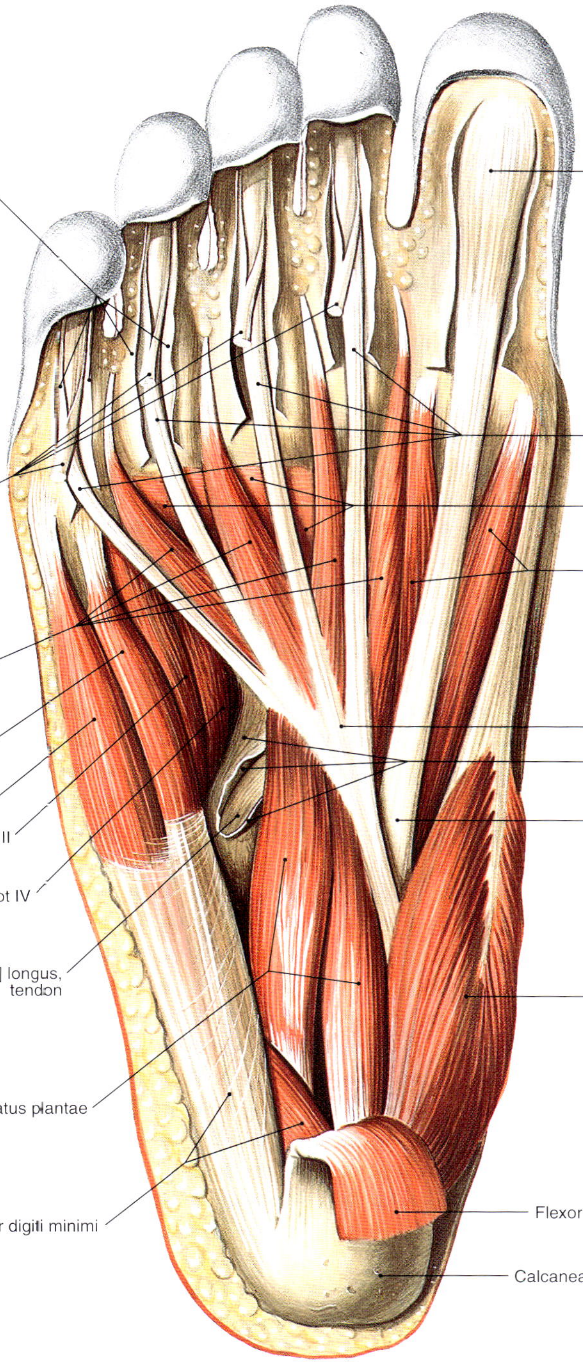

Fig. 1098 Muscles of the foot; middle layer after almost complete removal of the flexor digitorum brevis muscle.

→ T 50, T 52–T 54

Muscles of the foot

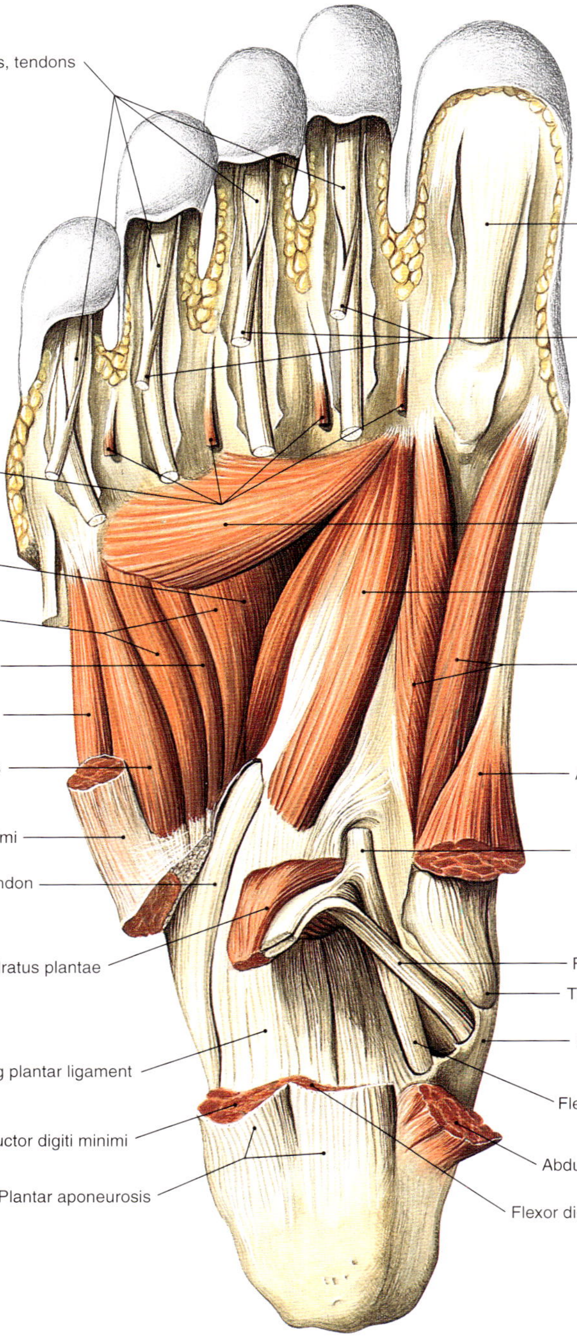

→ T 50, 52–T 54

Fig. 1099 Muscles of the foot; deep layer.

* The site where the tendon of the flexor digitorum longus muscle crosses the tendon of the flexor hallucis longus muscle is commonly referred to as plantar chiasm.

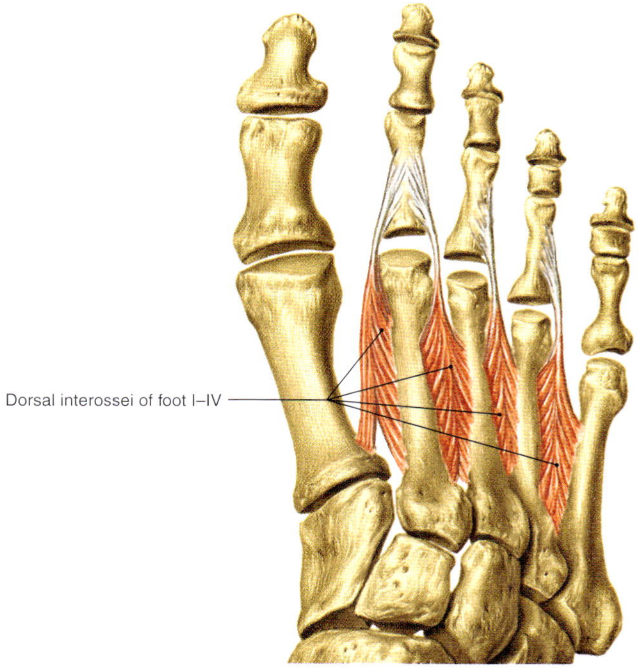

Fig. 1100 Dorsal interossei muscles; dorsal view.

→ T 53

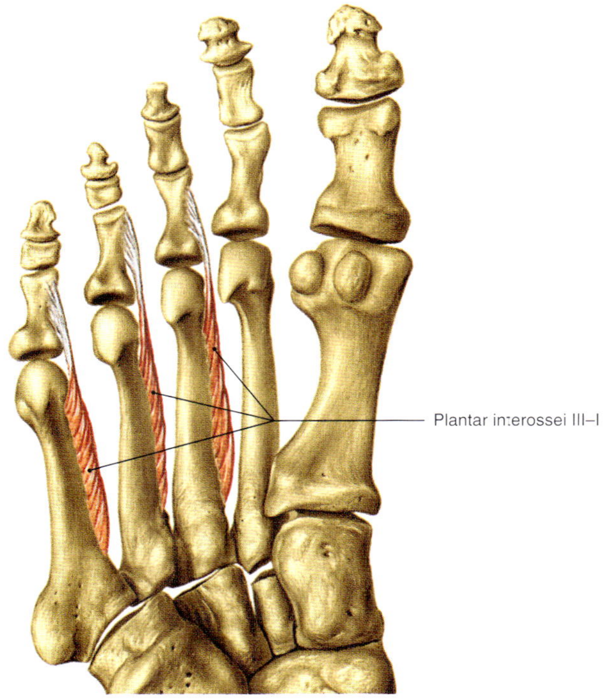

Fig. 1101 Plantar interossei muscles; plantar view.

→ T 53

Lumbosacral plexus

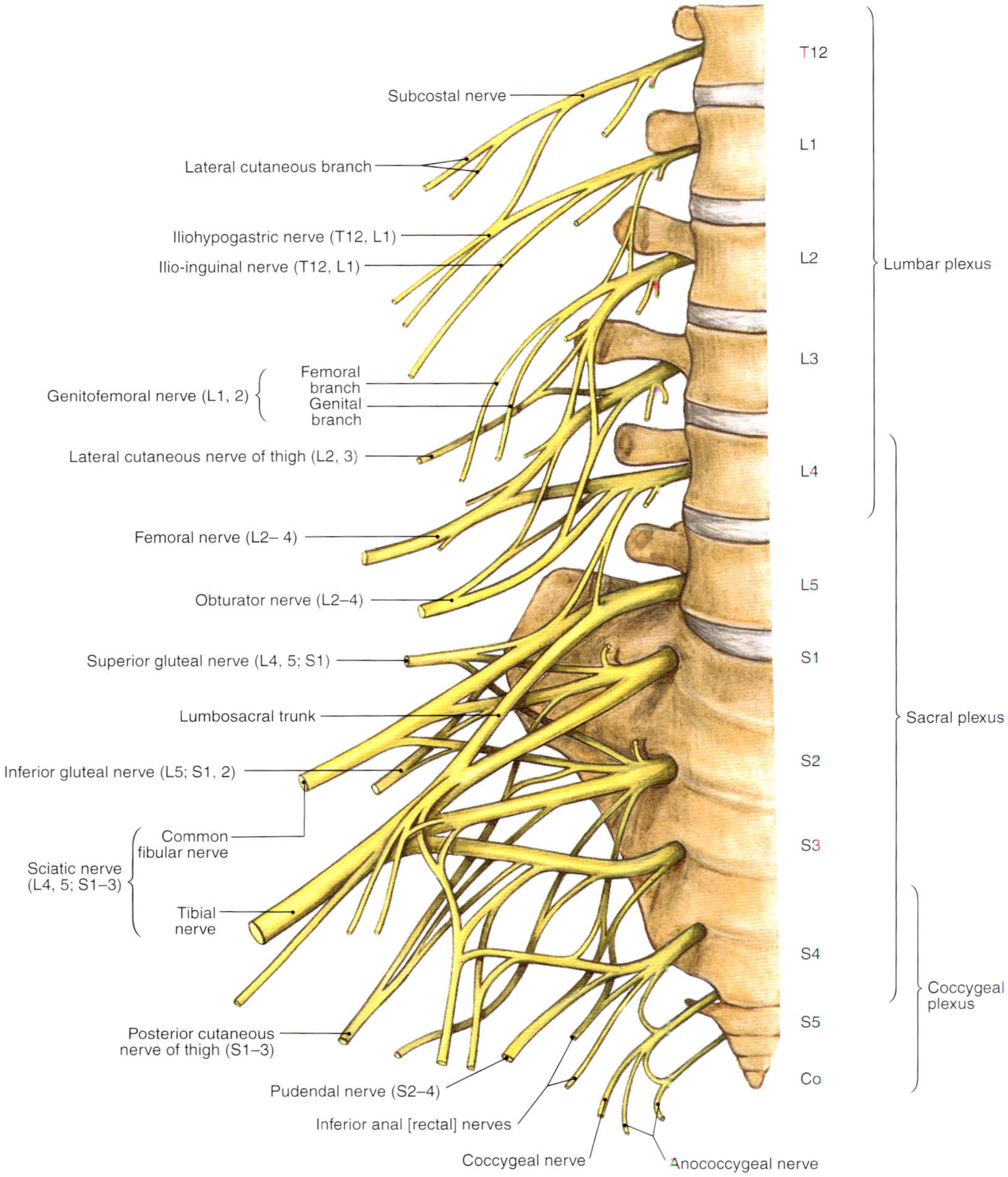

→ 595

Fig. 1102 Lumbosacral and coccygeal plexus; segmental organisation of nerves.

Nerves of the lower limb

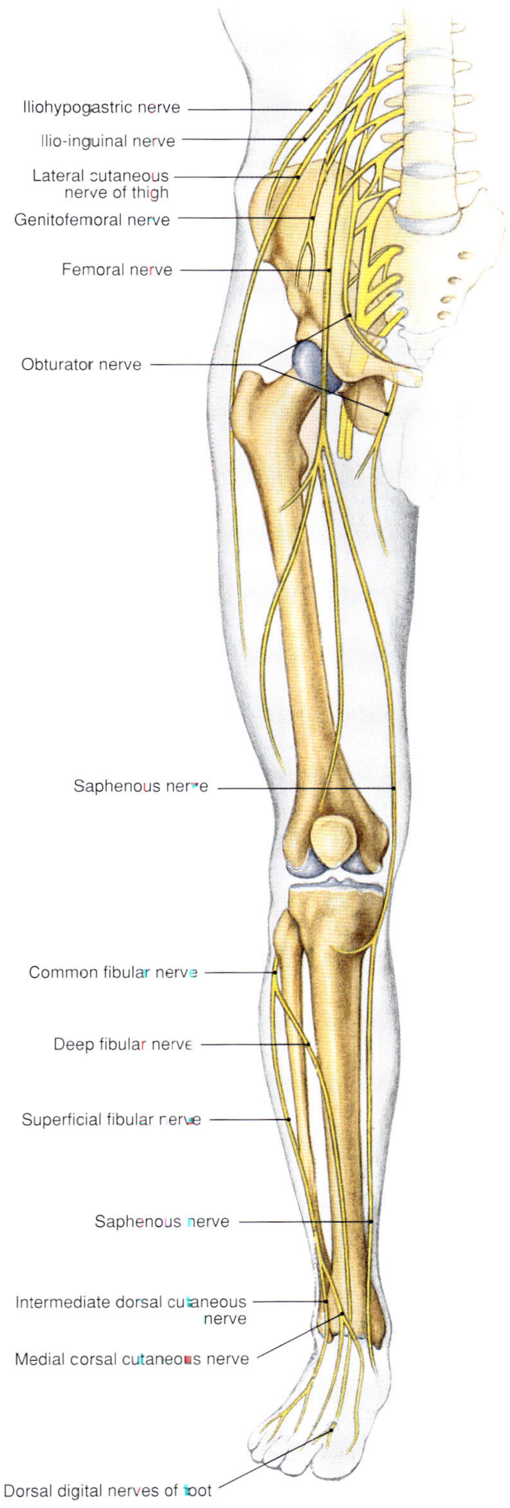

Fig. 1103 Nerves of the lower limb; overview.

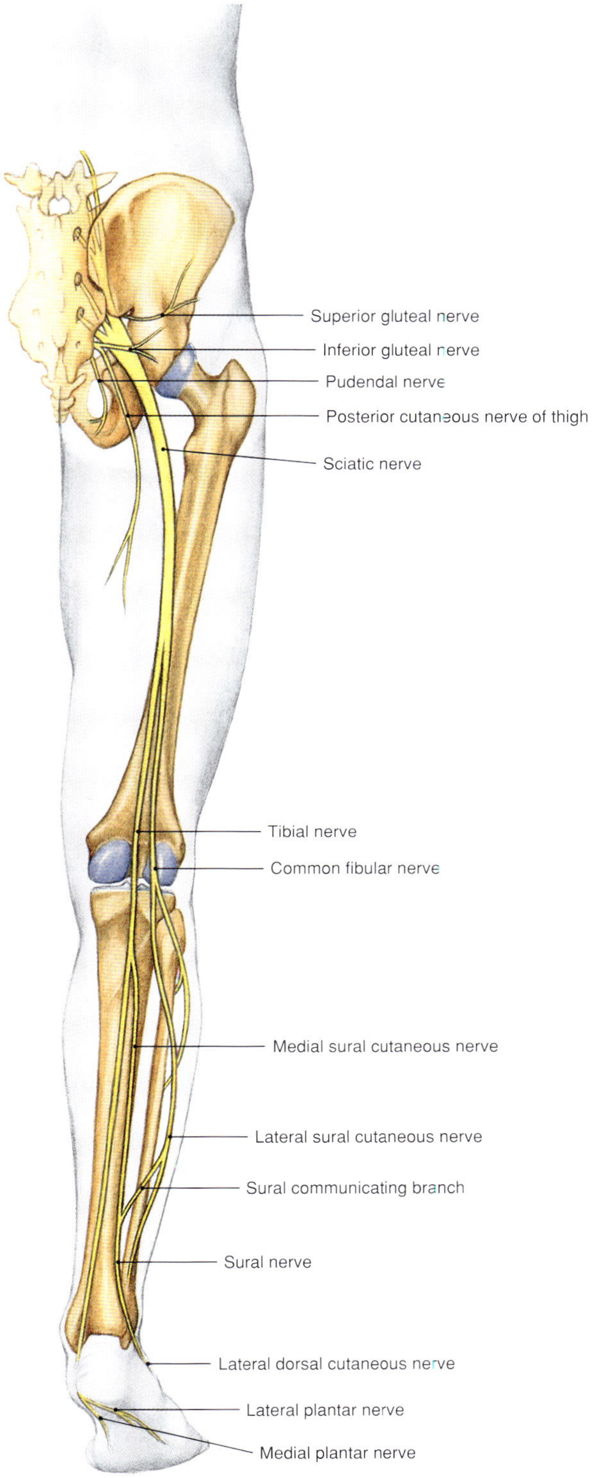

Fig. 1104 Nerves of the lower limb; overview.

Cutaneous innervation

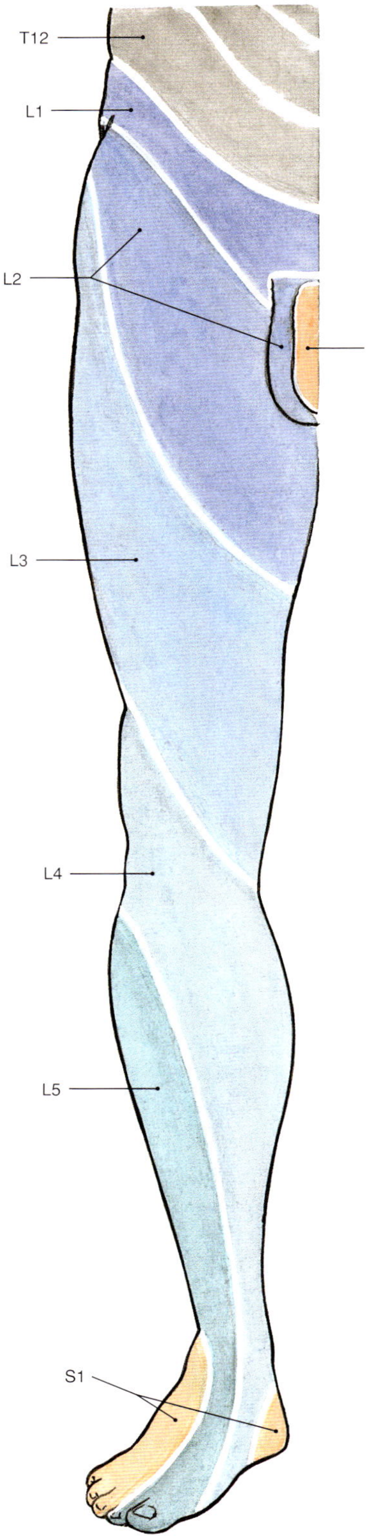

Fig. 1105 Segmental cutaneous innervation (dermatomes) of the lower limb.

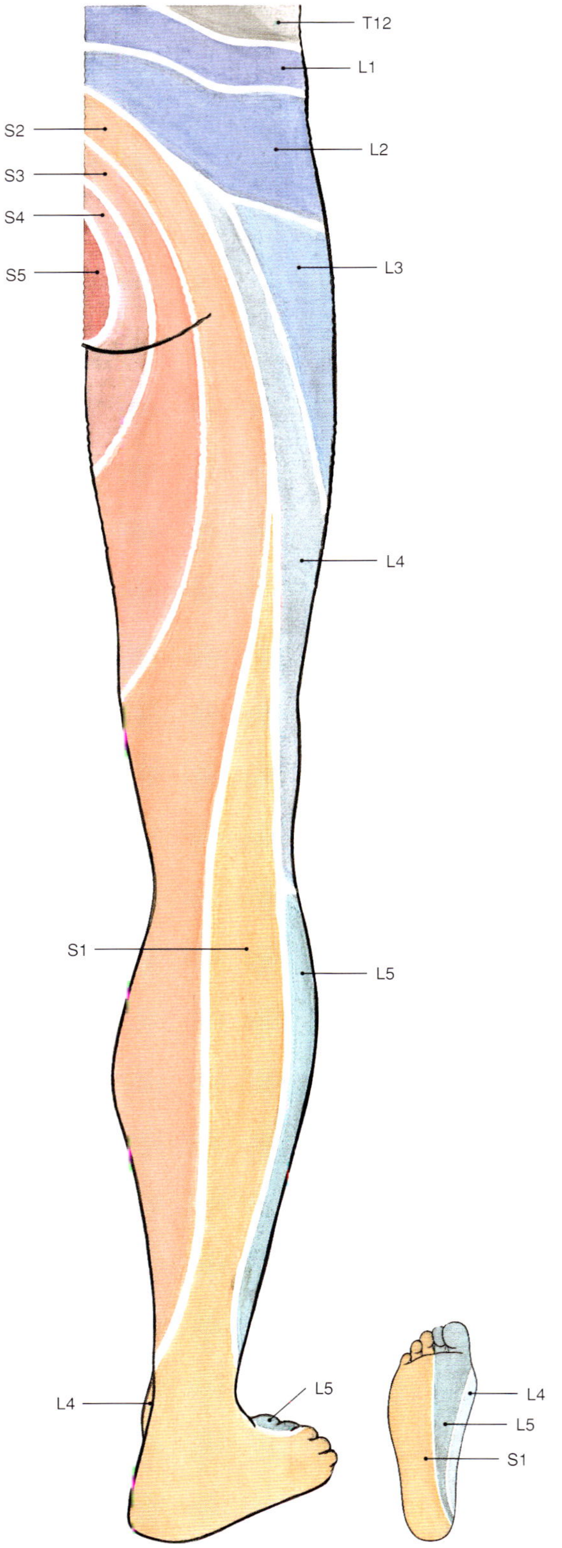

Fig. 1106 Segmental cutaneous innervation (dermatomes) of the lower limb.

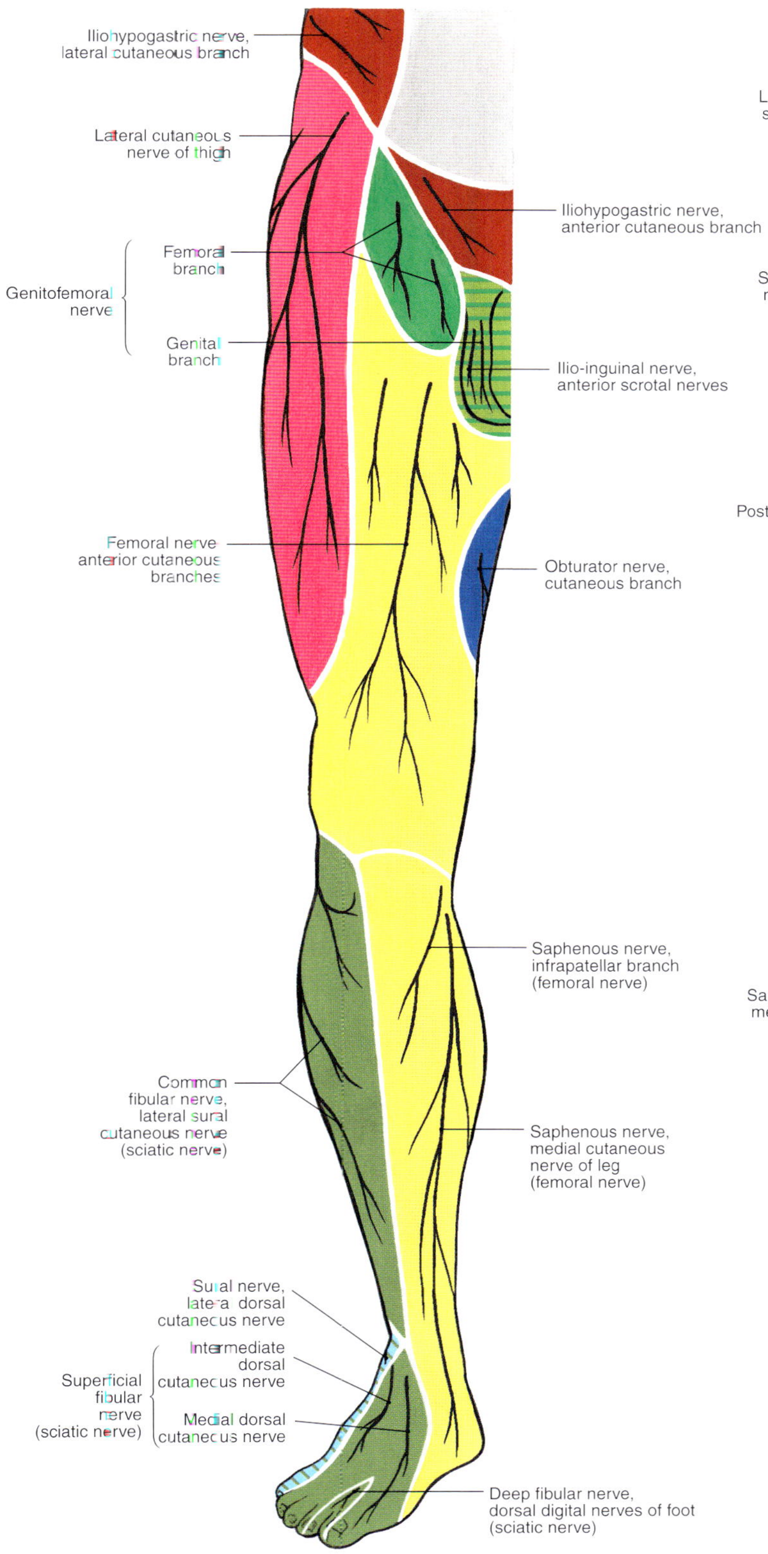

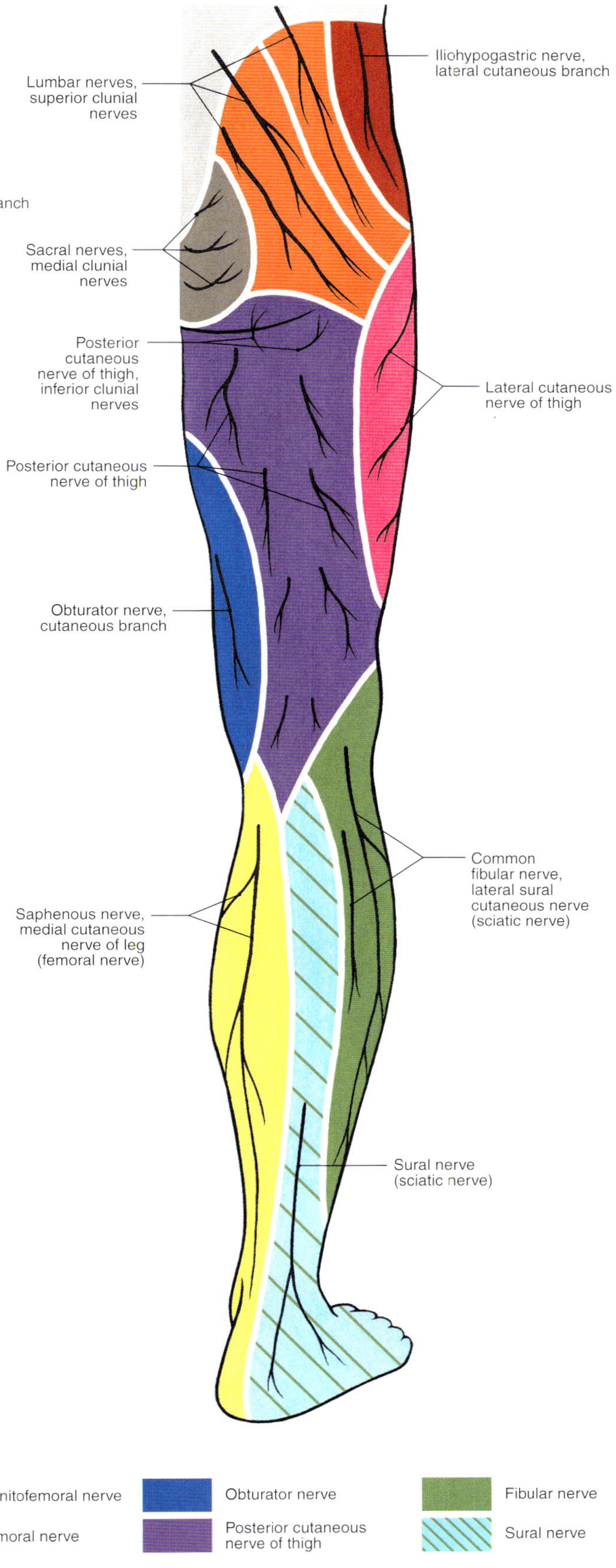

Fig. 1107 Cutaneous nerves of the lower limb.

Fig. 1108 Cutaneous nerves of the lower limb.

Fermoral and obturator nerve

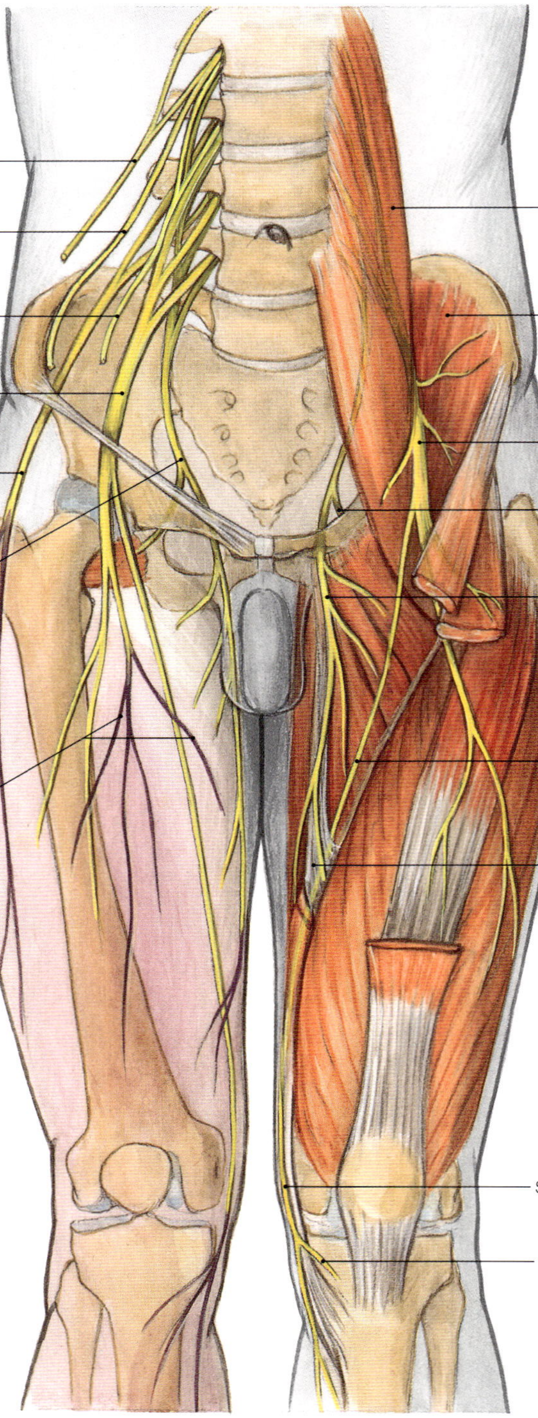

Fig. 1109 Femoral and obturator nerve;
overview;
cutaneous innervation illustrated with purple.

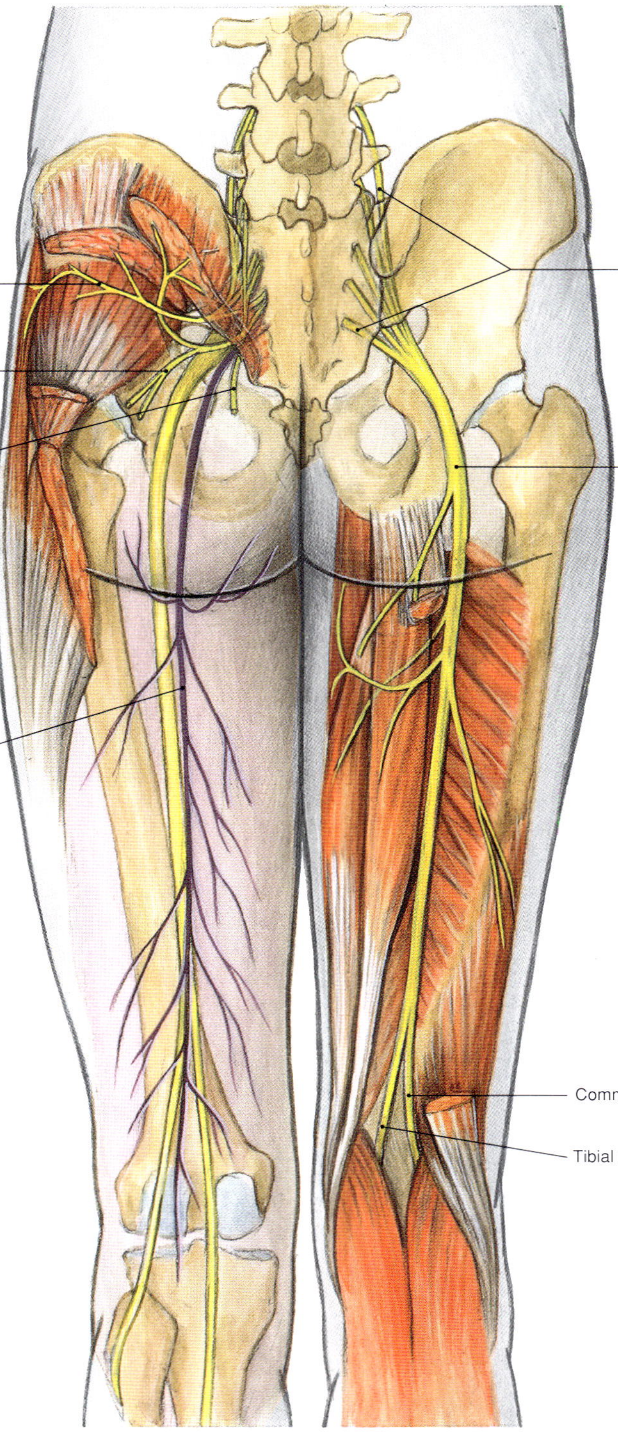

Fig. 1110 Gluteal nerves and sciatic nerve; overview;
cutaneous innervation illustrated with purple.

Tibial and fibular nerve

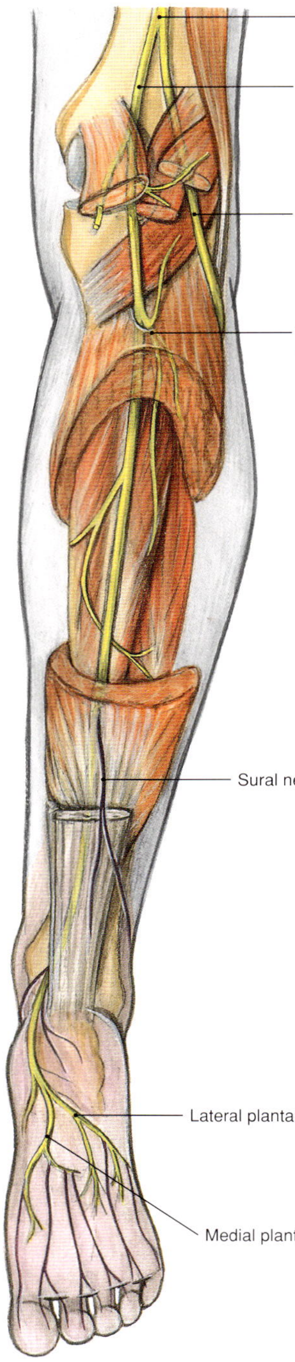

Fig. 1111 Tibial nerve;
overview;
cutaneous innervation illustrated with purple.

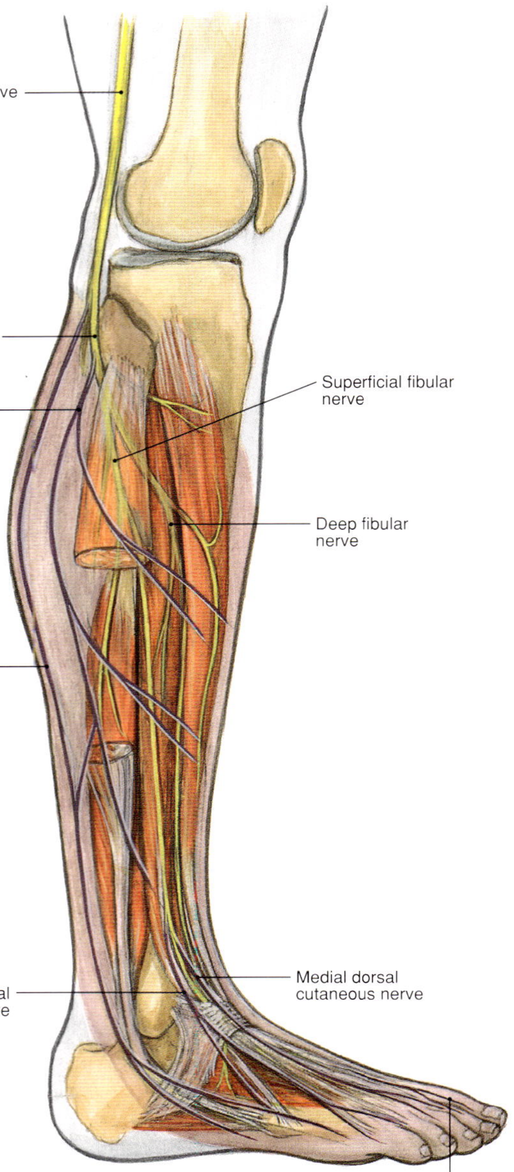

Fig. 1112 Fibular nerve;
overview;
cutaneous innervation illustrated with purple.

Arteries of the lower limb

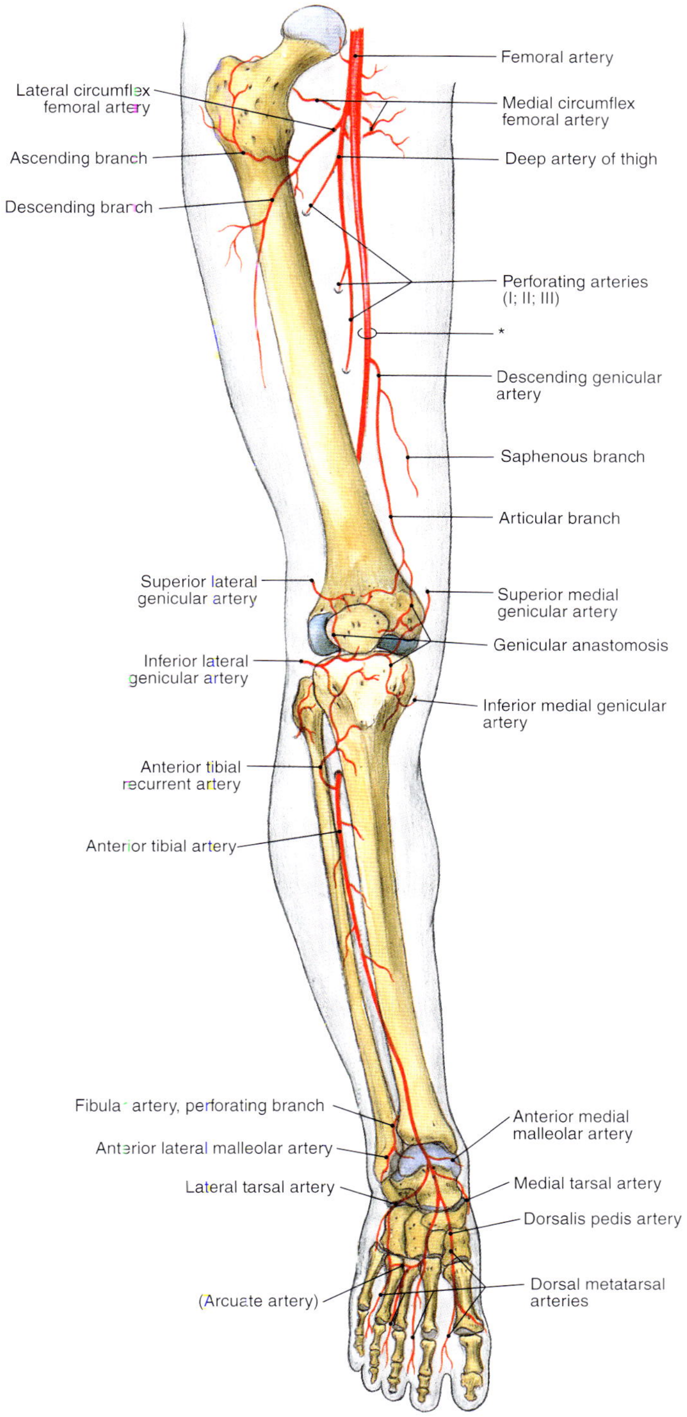

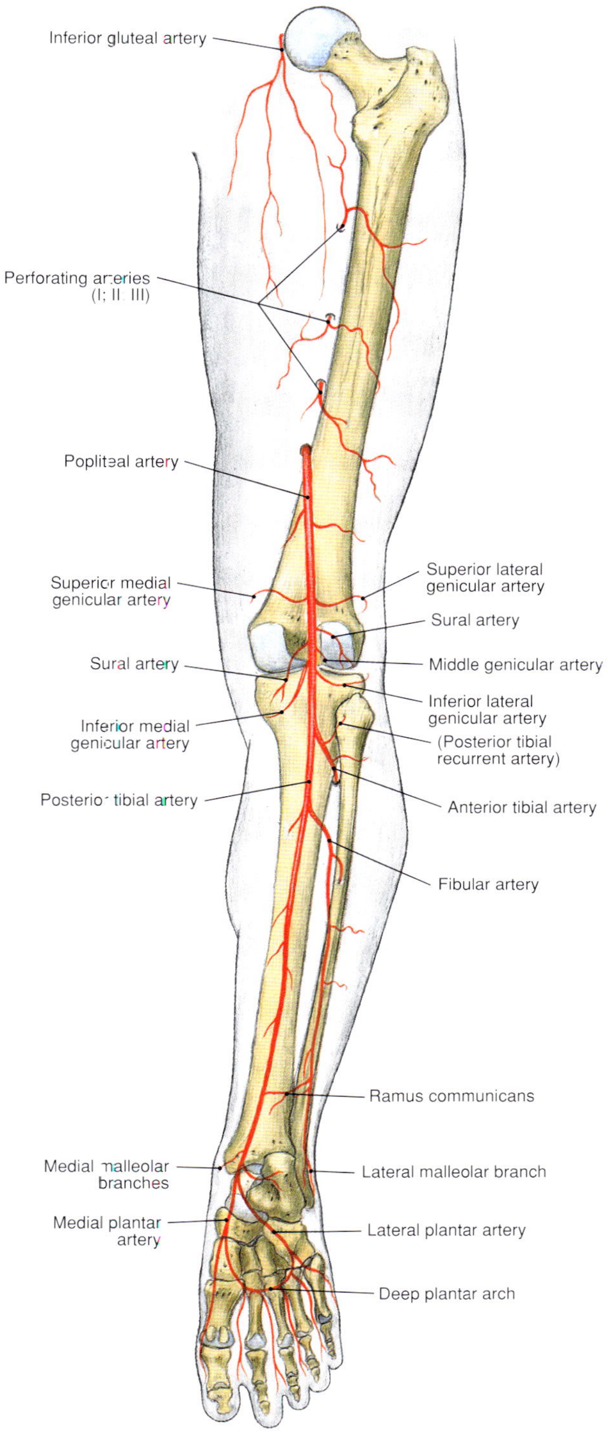

Fig. 1113 Arteries of the lower limb; overview; ventral view.
The segment of the femoral artery between the point where the deep artery of thigh branches off and the point of entry into the adductor canal (*) is known clinically as superficial femoral artery.

Fig. 1114 Arteries of the lower limb; overview; dorsal view.

Veins and lymphatics of the lower limb

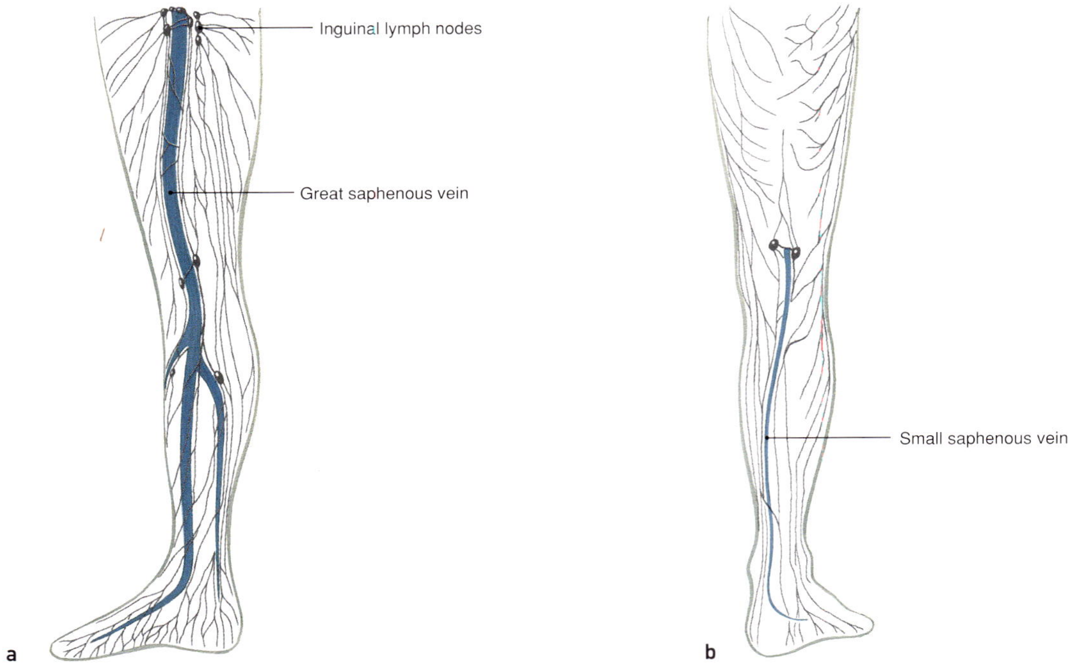

Fig. 1115 a, b Veins and lymphatics of the lower limb; overview.
a Medial view
b Dorsal view

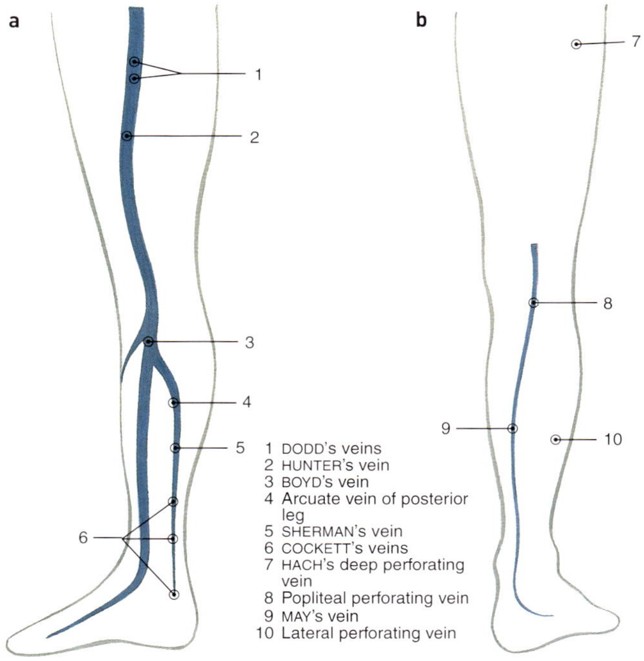

Fig. 1116 a, b Perforating veins; overview (according to HACH, 1986).
a Medial view
b Dorsal view

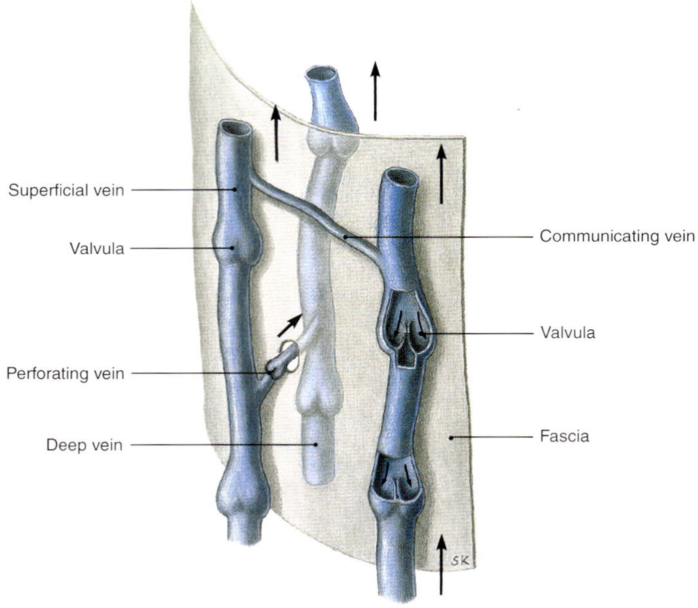

Fig. 1117 Veins of the lower limb; principle of organisation.
Disturbances of the venous flow of the lower limb, especially varicosis, are a common cause of vascular disorders.
If one of the venous systems is entirely occluded, the perforating veins may be of crucial importance to maintain the venous drainage.

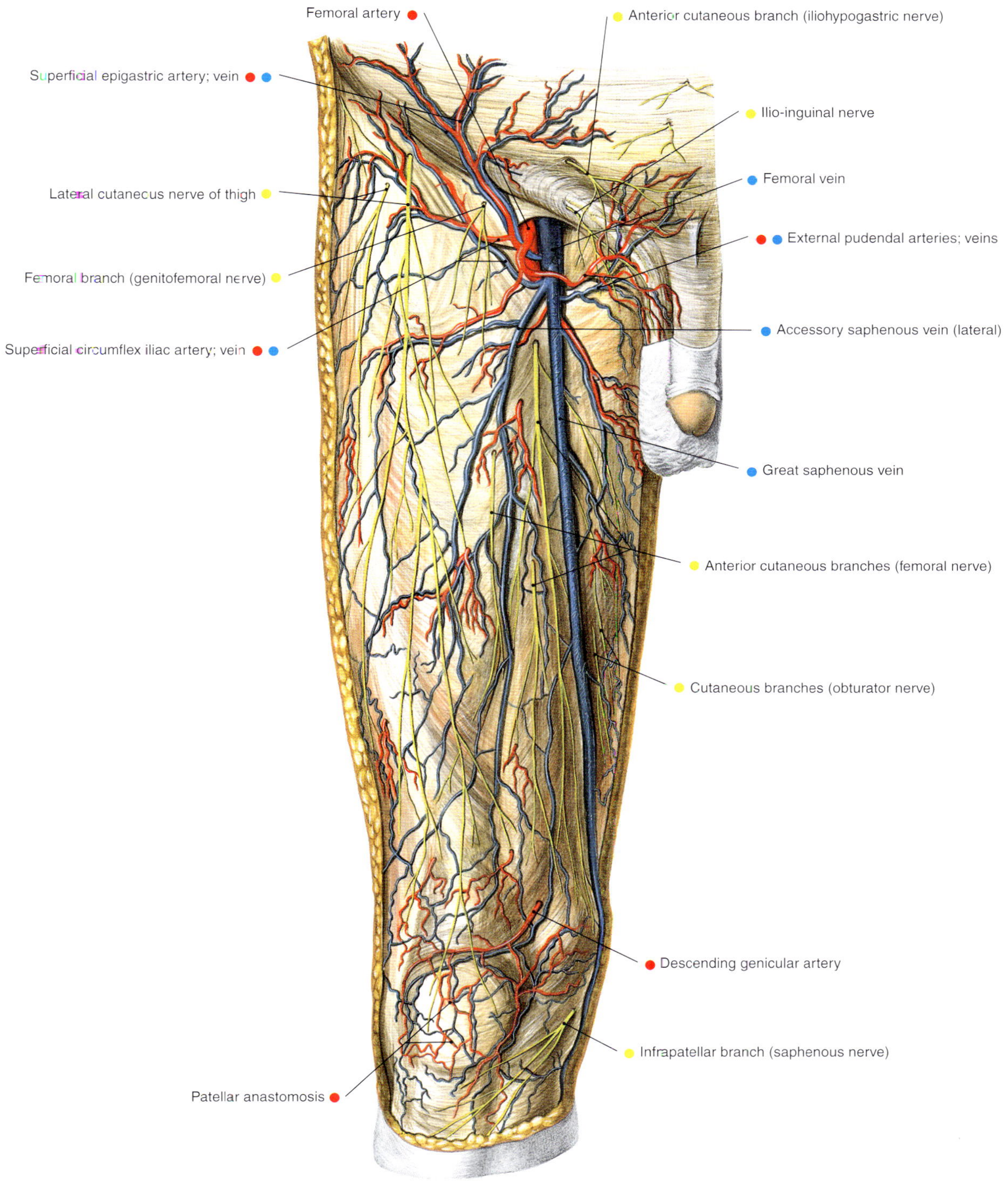

Fig. 1118 Epifascial vessels and nerves of the inguinal region, the anterior region of thigh and the anterior region of knee.

592
1123
1135

Lymphatics of the inguinal region

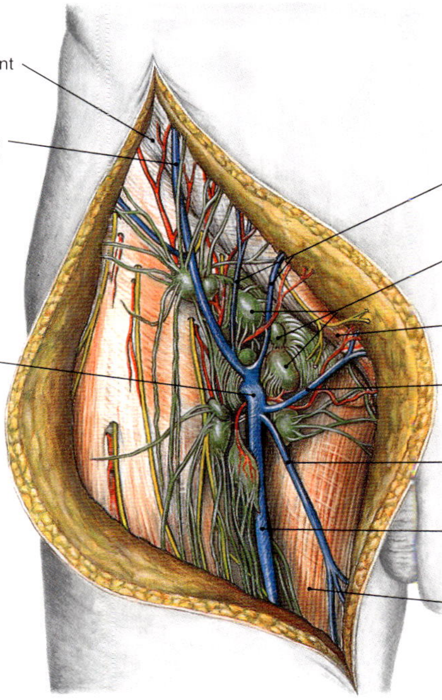

Fig. 1119 Superficial lymphatics, lymph nodes and major veins of the inguinal region.

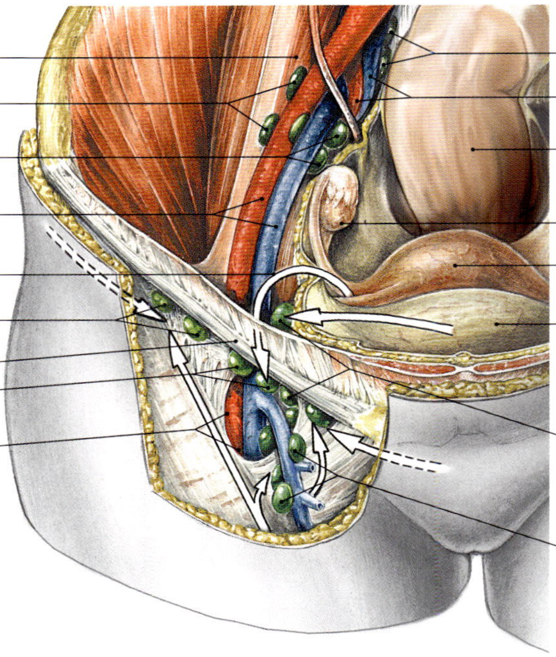

Fig. 1120 Draining areas of the lymph nodes in the inguinal region of the female;
overview.
The arrows indicate possible directions of the flow of lymph.

* In some rare cases, the medial parts of the uterine tube and the fundus of the uterus may be drained by superficial lymph nodes in the inguinal region via the round ligament of uterus.

Vessels and nerves of the inguinal region

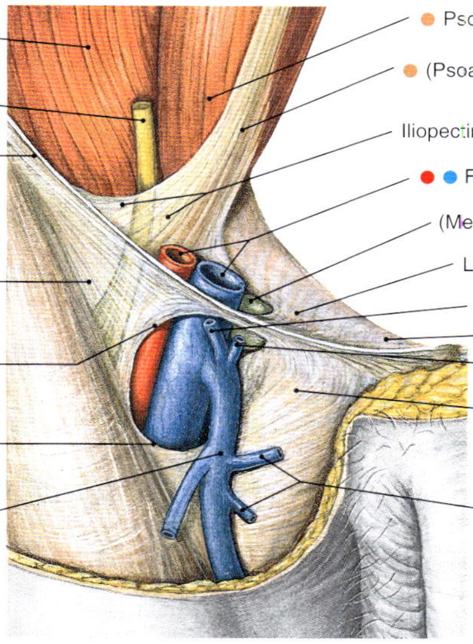

Fig. 1121 Saphenous opening and vascular space; after removal of the anterior abdominal wall and the contents of the abdomen, as well as dissection of the iliac fascia and the femoral septum [CLOQUET].

* Also: ROSENMÜLLER's node
** Also: GIMBERNAT's ligament

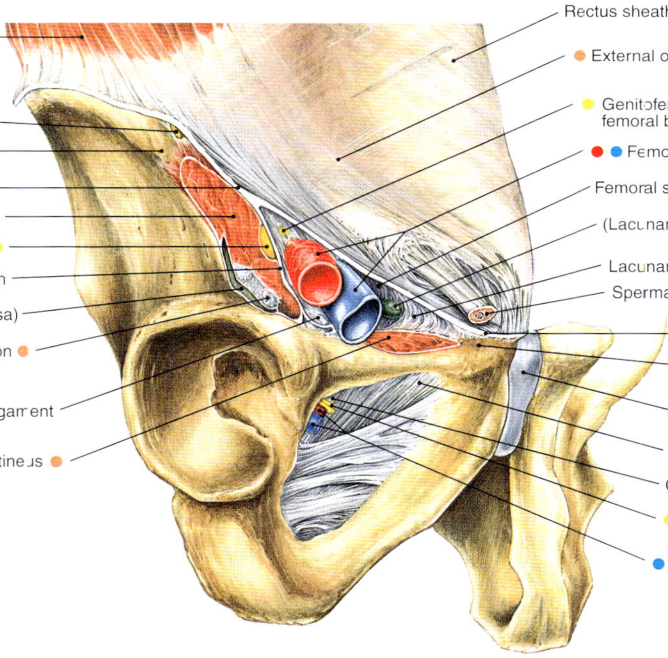

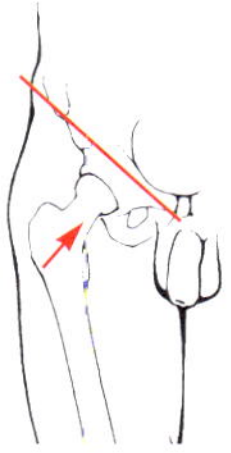

Fig. 1122 Muscular and vascular space; oblique section at the level of the inguinal ligament.

Vessels and nerves of the thigh

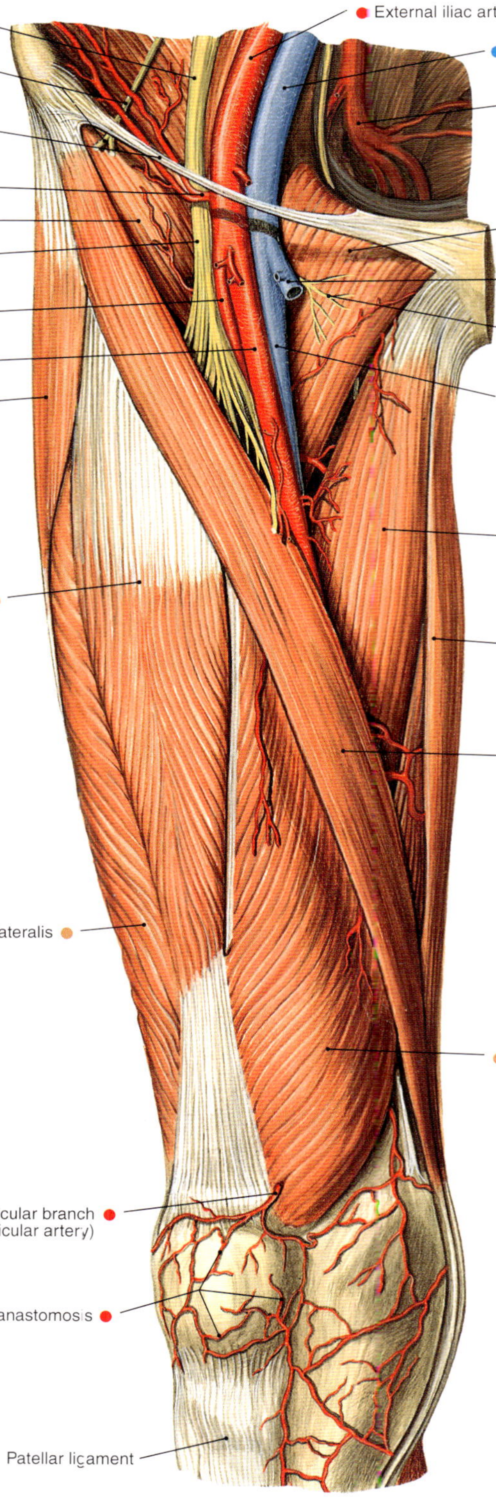

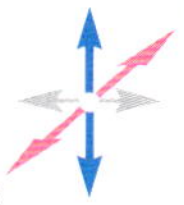

Fig. 1123 Vessels and nerves of the anterior region of thigh; after removal of the fascia lata except for the iliotibial tract.

* Clinically the femoral artery is commonly referred to as superficial femoral artery to distinguish it from the deep artery of thigh.

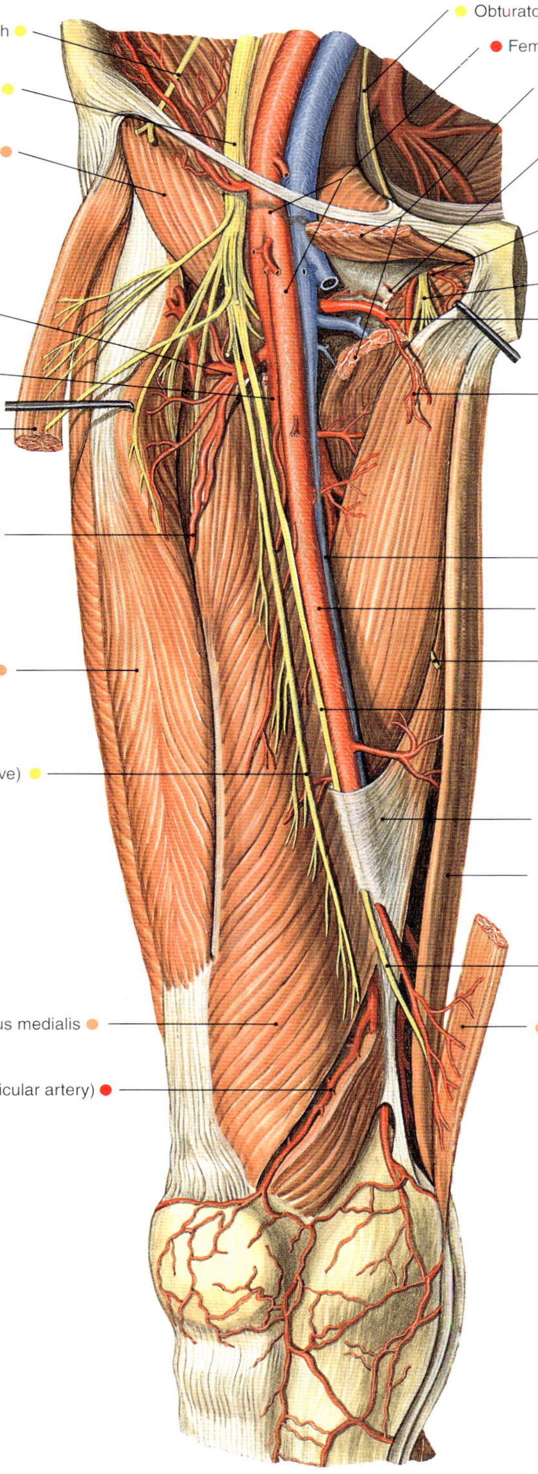

886
888
891
1125
1123
1140

Fig. 1124 Vessels and nerves of the anterior region of thigh; after partial removal of the sartorius muscle and dissection of the pectineus muscle.

* The entrance into the adductor canal is formed by the vastus medialis and adductor longus muscles as well as by the anteromedial intermuscular septum spanning between them.

Vessels and nerves of the thigh

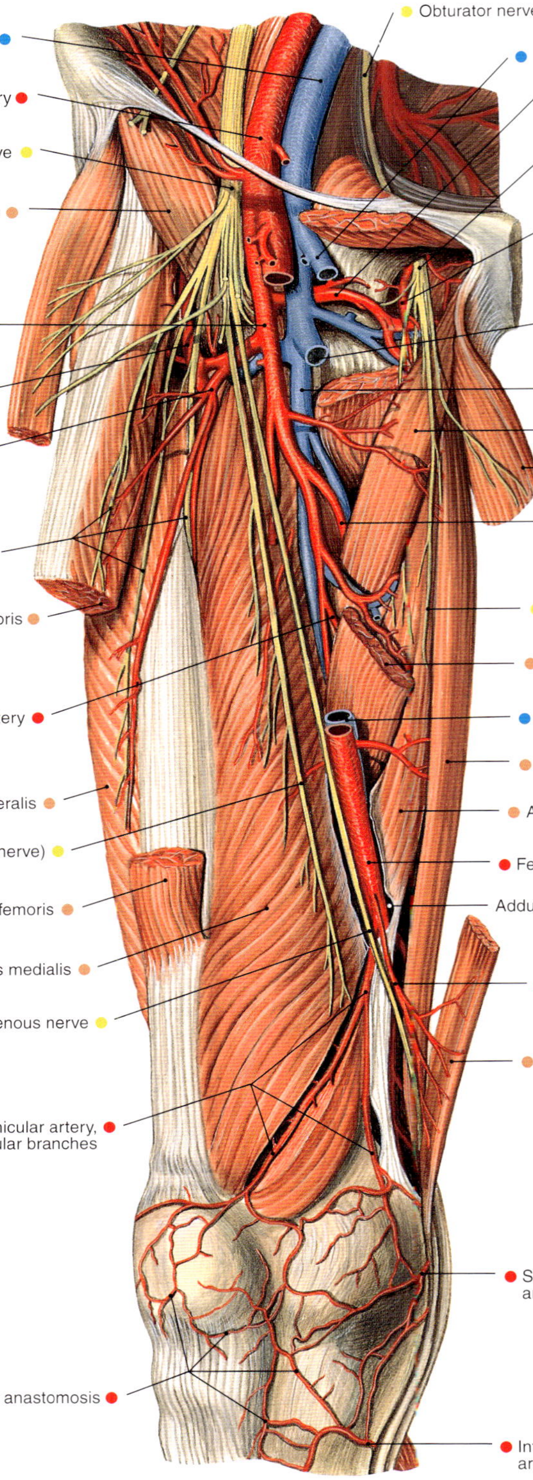

886
888
891
1124
1140

Fig. 1125 Vessels and nerves of the anterior region of thigh; deep layer after partial removal of the sartorius and rectus femoris muscles, the pectineus and adductor longus muscles have been dissected; the adductor canal is almost entirely opened.

Arteries of the pelvis and the hip

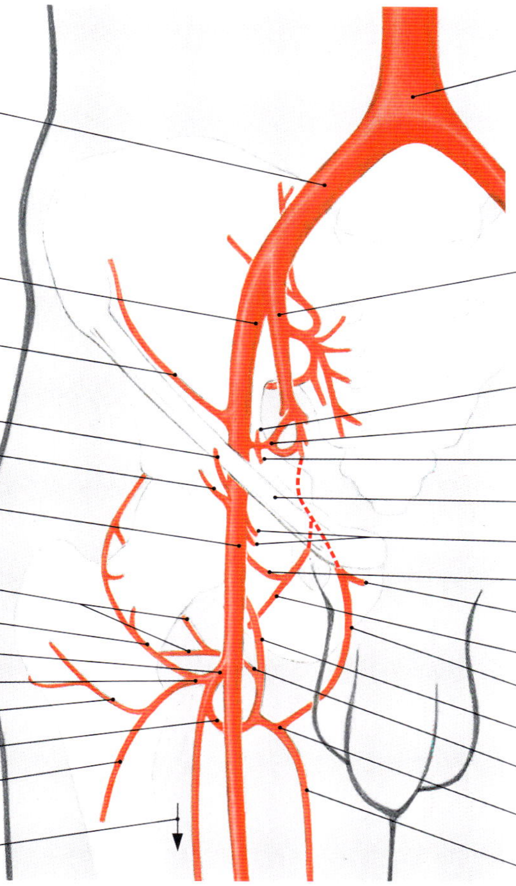

Fig. 1126 Arteries of the hip and the thigh; overview.

The branching pattern of these arteries varies considerably. This type of origin and arborisation of the deep artery of thigh occurs in approximately 58 % of cases.

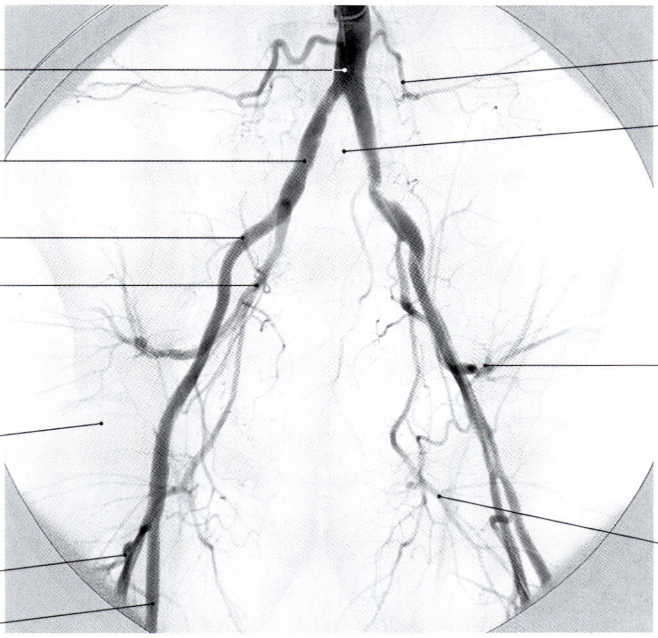

Fig. 1127 Arteries of the pelvis and the thigh; digital subtraction angiography (DSA).

Veins and nerves of the thigh

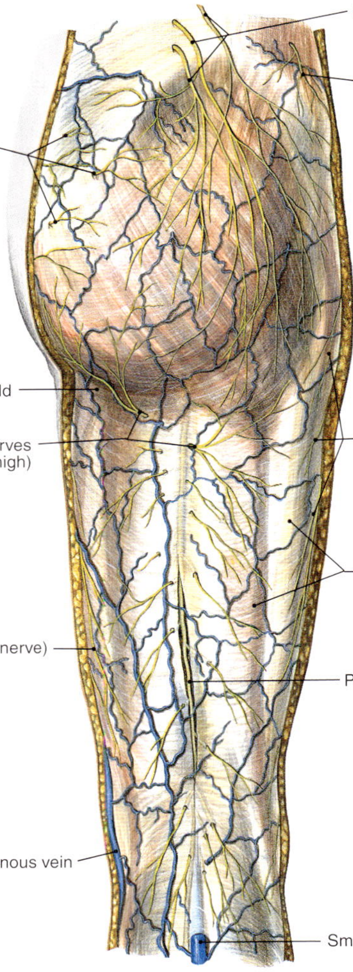

544
1130
1136

Fig. 1128 Epifascial veins and nerves of the posterior region of thigh, the gluteal region and the popliteal fossa.

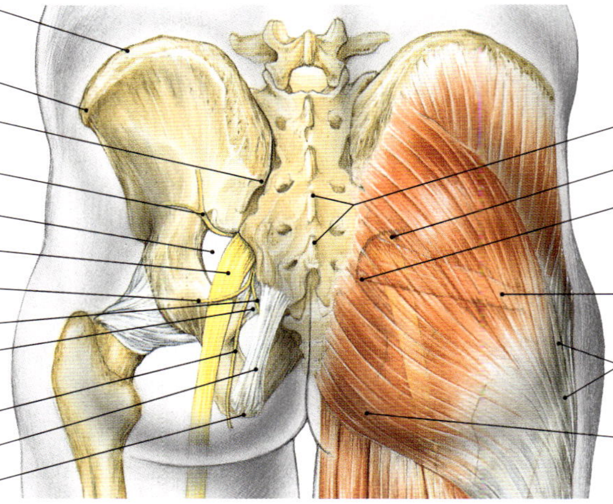

Fig. 1129 Skeleton contour and sciatic nerve projected onto the surface of the gluteal region.

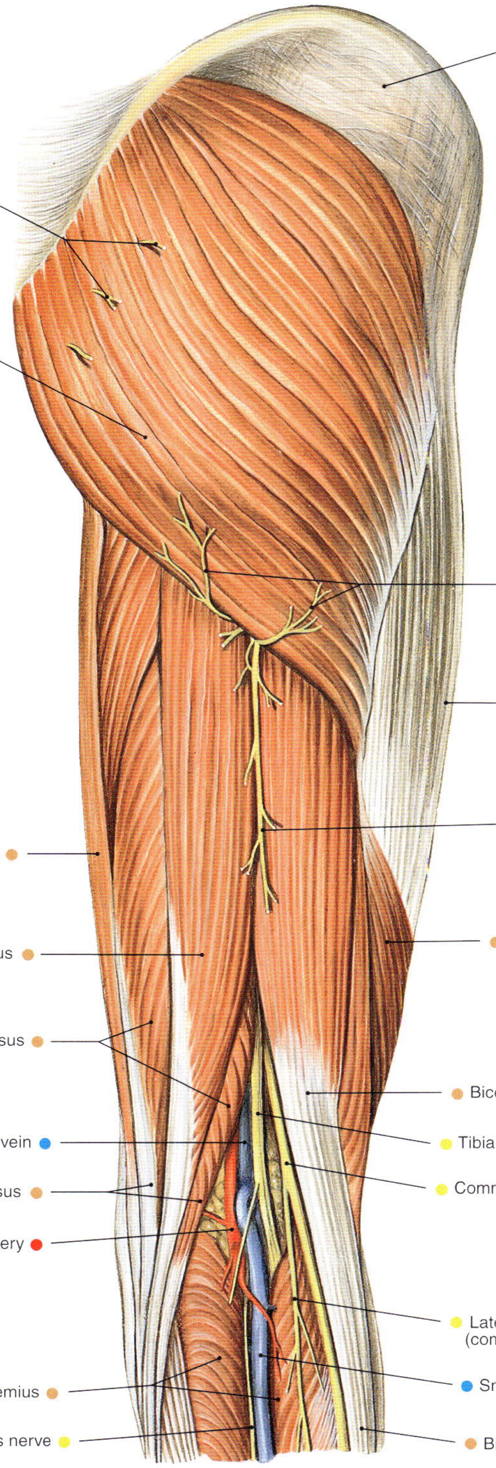

Fig. 1130 Vessels and nerves of the gluteal region, the posterior region of thigh and the popliteal fossa.

1131
1128
1143

Vessels and nerves of the thigh

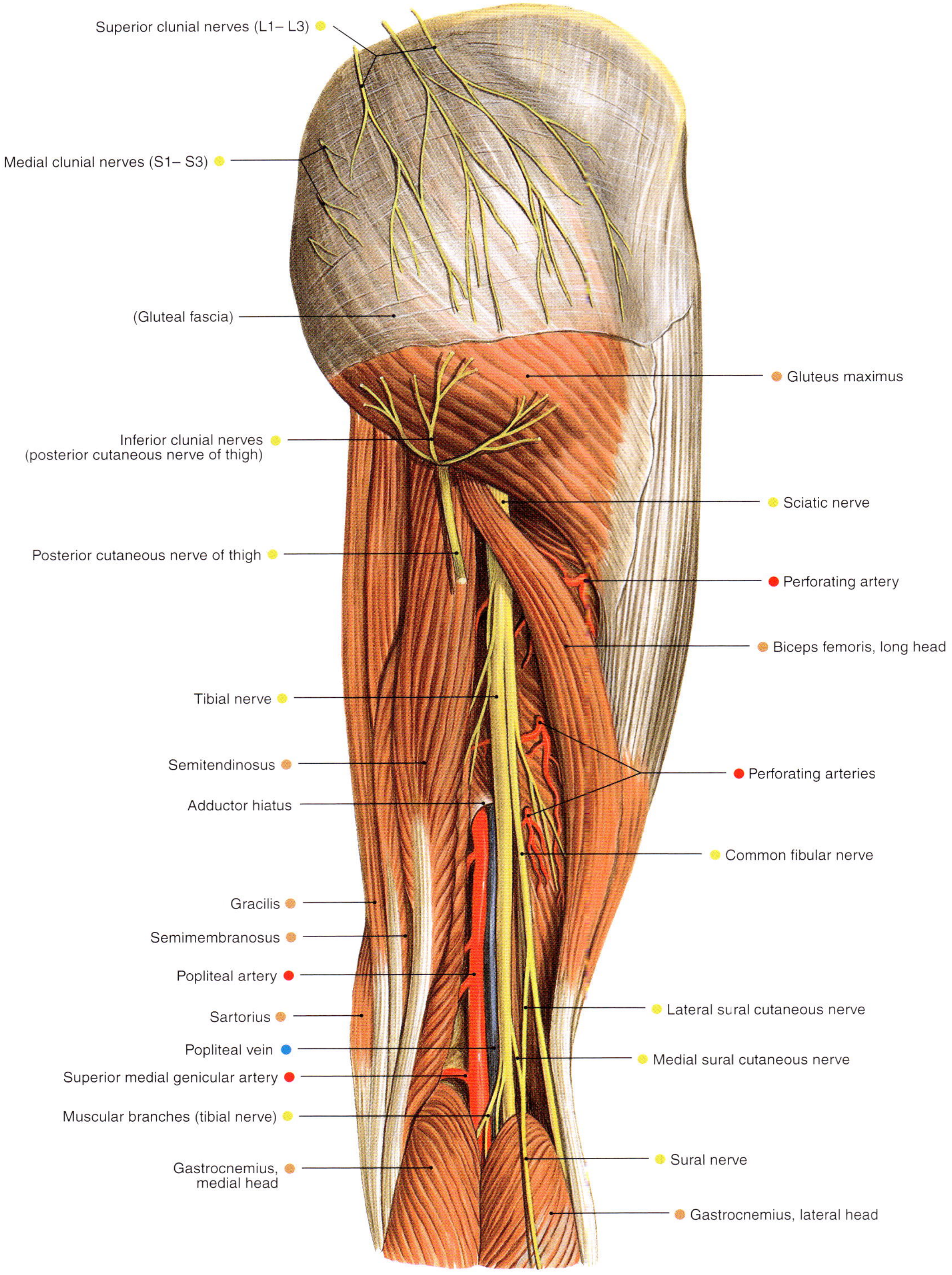

1132
1130

Fig. 1131 Vessels and nerves of the gluteal region, the posterior region of thigh and the popliteal fossa; the long head of the biceps femoris muscle has been retracted laterally. In this specimen, the medial and lateral sural cutaneous nerves branch off quite far proximally.

Vessels and nerves of the thigh

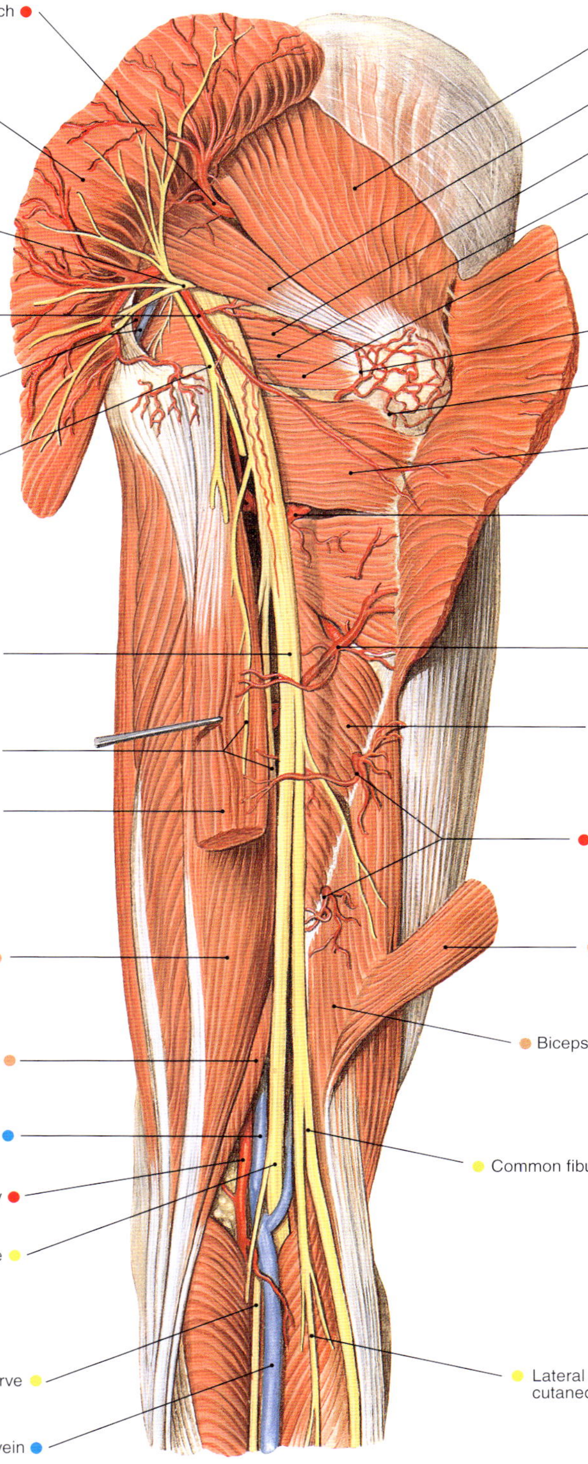

Fig. 1132 Vessels and nerves of the gluteal region, the posterior region of thigh and the popliteal fossa; after dissection of the gluteus maximus muscle and the long head of the biceps femoris muscle.

1131
1143
1145
1146

Vessels and nerves of the gluteal region

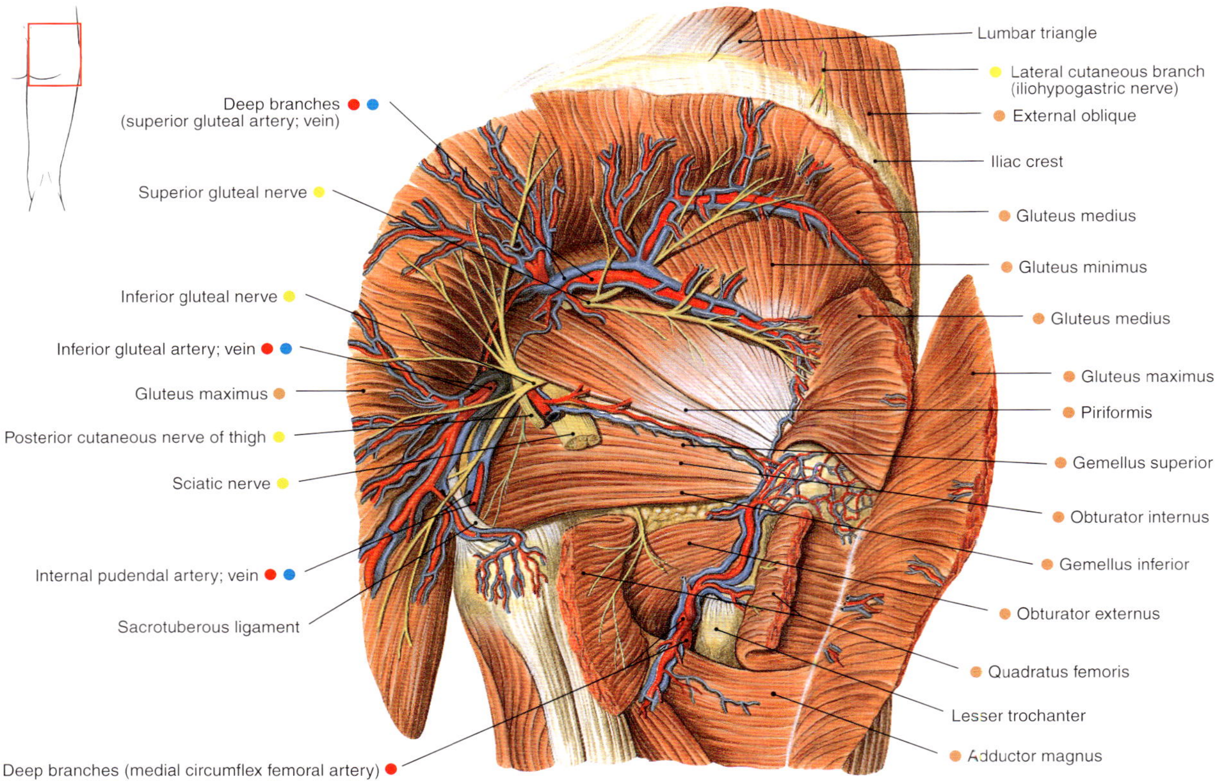

Fig. 1133 Vessels and nerves of the gluteal region;
after dissection and partial removal of the gluteus maximus and medius muscles;
the sciatic nerve has been removed after its passage through the infrapiriform foramen.

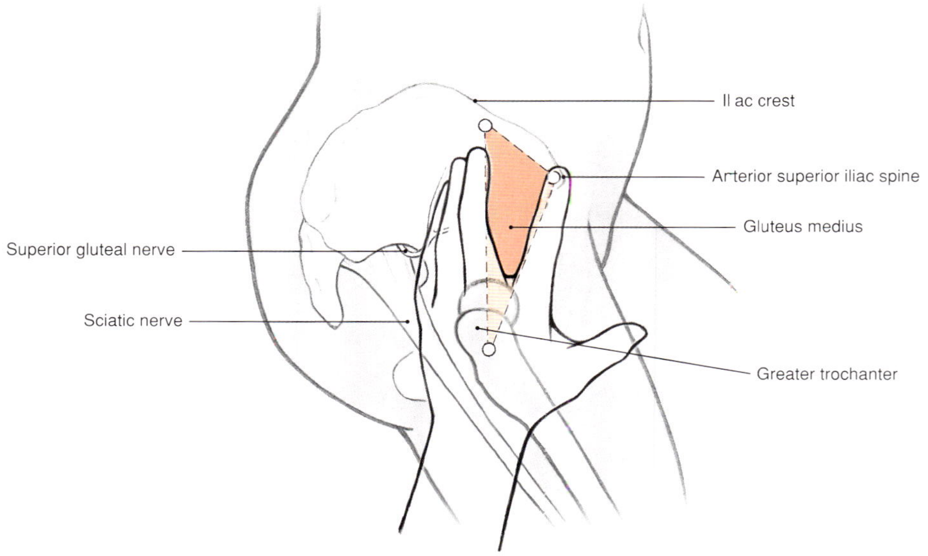

Fig. 1134 Ventrogluteal injection (according to v. HOCHSTETTER). In order to avoid the superior gluteal nerve and, in particular, the superior gluteal artery the injection is made into the triangular field formed by the two spread fingers and the iliac crest. The index finger – or when using the right hand, the middle finger – is placed on the anterior superior iliac spine and the palm of the hand on the greater trochanter. Since the injected material should be deposited within the belly of the gluteus medius muscle as far away as possible from any vessel, the needle should not cross the lines of the triangle. However, some risk remains for the nerve branch that runs from the superior gluteal nerve to the tensor fasciae latae muscle.

Veins and nerves of the leg

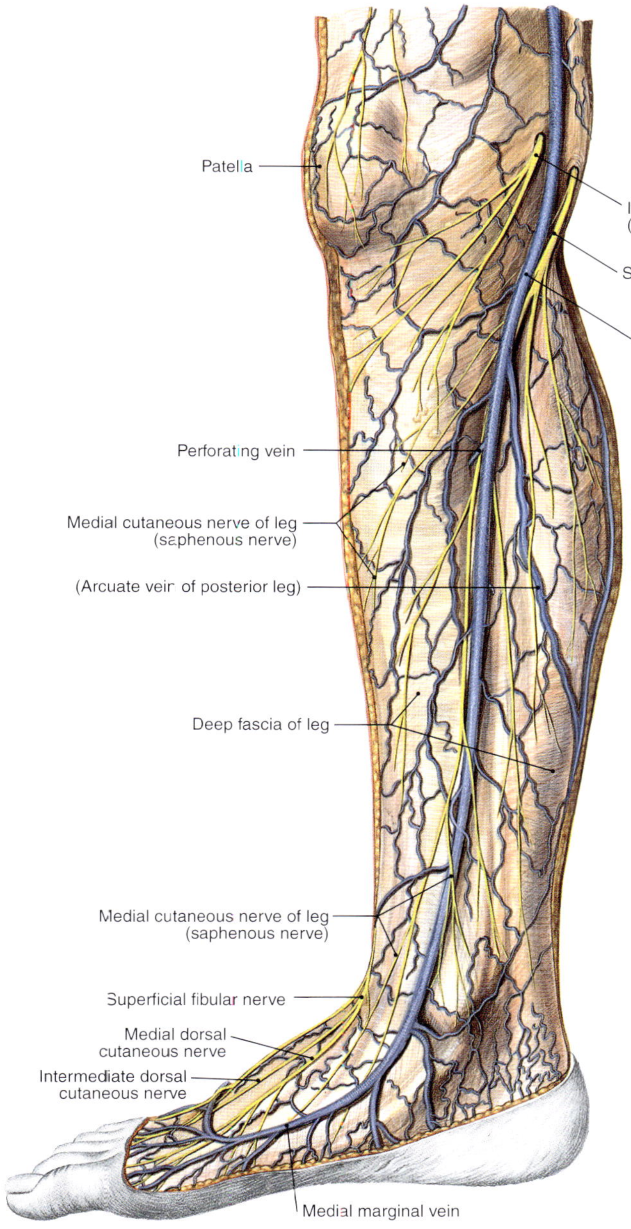

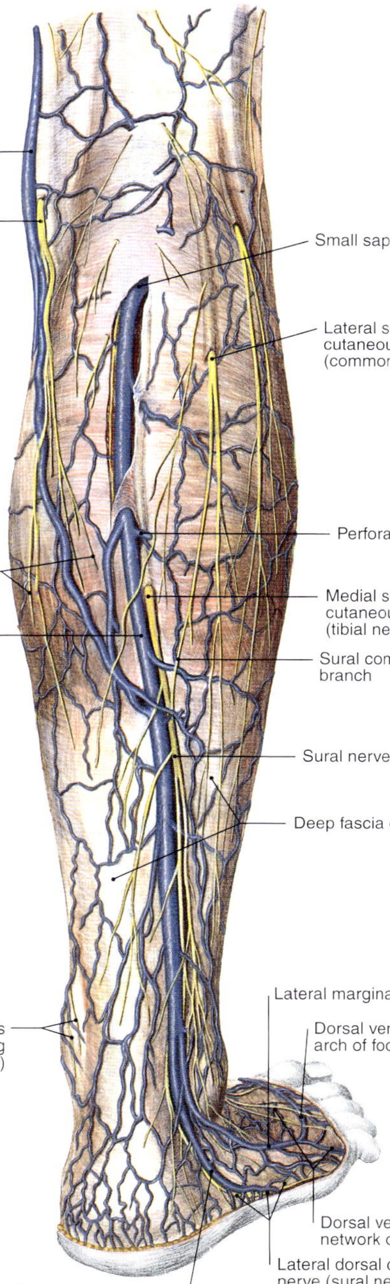

Fig. 1135 Epifascial veins and nerves of the leg and the foot.

Fig. 1136 Epifascial veins and nerves of the leg and the foot;
the deep fascia of leg has been dissected proximally.

* Clinical term: MAY's vein

Vessels and nerves of the leg

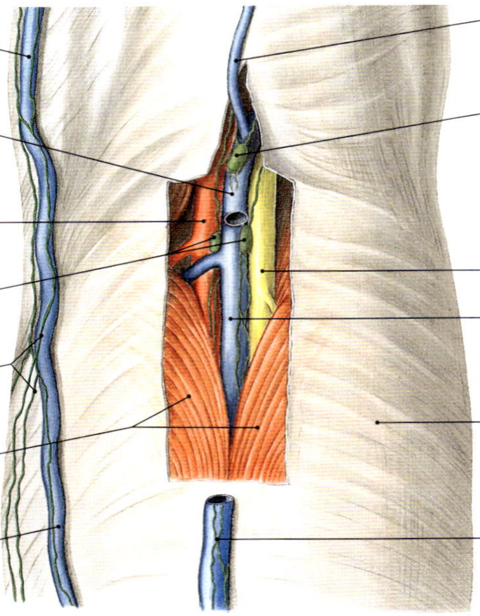

Fig. 1137 Vessels and nerves of the popliteal fossa; after dissection of the deep fascia of leg and partial removal of the small saphenous vein.

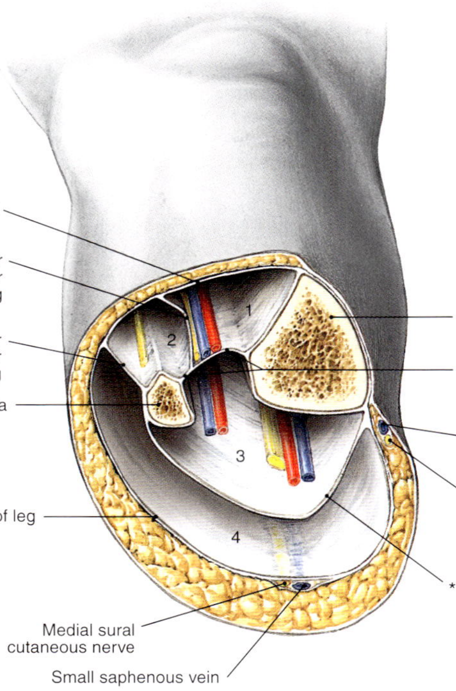

1 Anterior compartment of leg:
Anterior tibial artery; vein
Deep fibular nerve
Tibialis anterior
Extensor digitorum longus
Extensor hallucis longus
Fibularis [peroneus] tertius

2 Lateral compartment of leg:
Superficial fibular nerve
Fibularis [peroneus] longus
Fibularis [peroneus] brevis

3 Posterior compartment of leg, deep part:
Posterior tibial artery; vein
Fibular artery; vein
Tibial nerve
Flexor digitorum longus
Tibialis posterior
Flexor hallucis longus

4 Posterior compartment of leg, superficial part:
Triceps surae
Plantaris

Fig. 1138 Osteofibrous tubes of the leg; cross-section superior to the middle of the leg. These osteofibrous tubes together with their contents are clinically known as compartments.

* Deep part of the deep fascia of leg

→ 1157

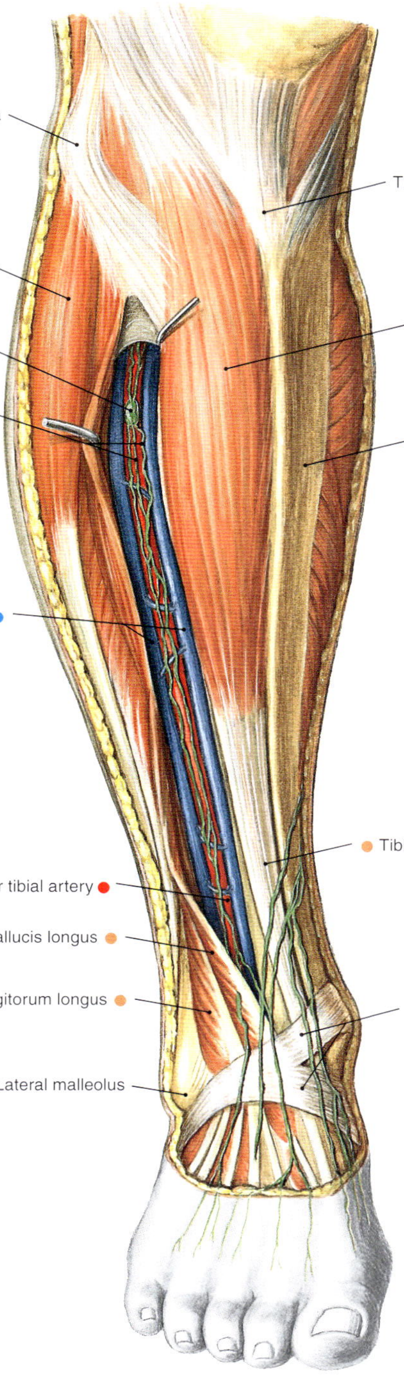

Fig. 1139 Vessels of the anterior region of leg; the extensor muscles spread by retractors.

The superficial lymphatics regularly follow the major epifascial veins and converge along the great saphenous vein to the medial side of the leg. The deep lymphatics are found within the connective tissue sheaths of the deep arteries and veins of the leg.

Arteries and nerves of the leg

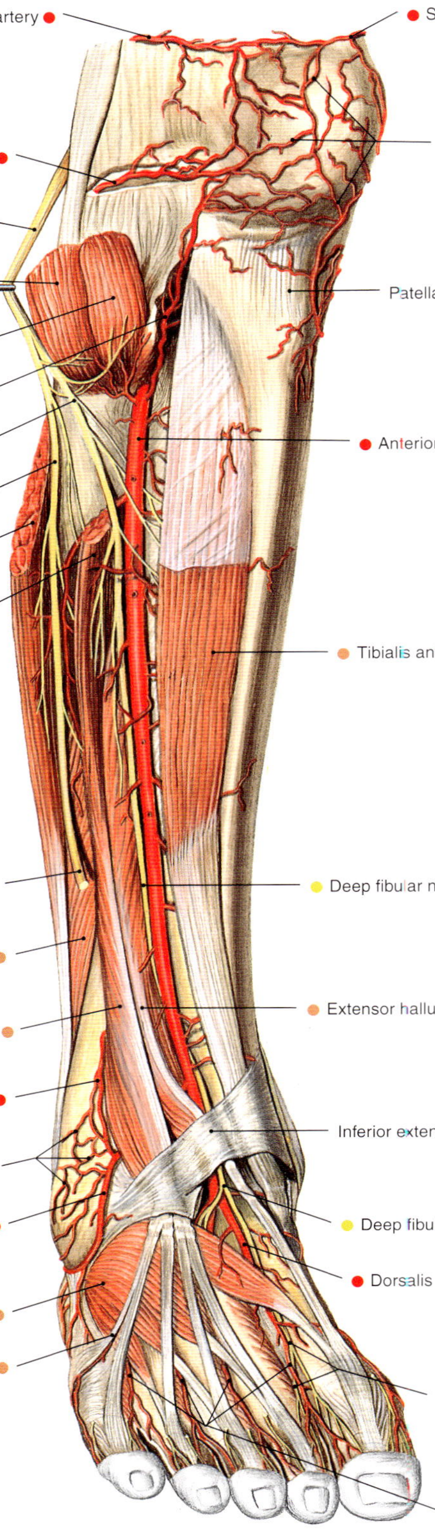

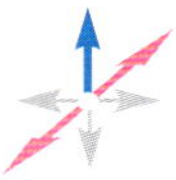

1123
1124
1148
1139

Fig. 1140 Arteries and nerves of the anterior region of leg and the dorsum of foot;
after removal of the deep fascia of leg and dissection of the extensor digitorum longus and fibularis [peroneus] longus muscles.

Arteries and nerves of the popliteal fossa

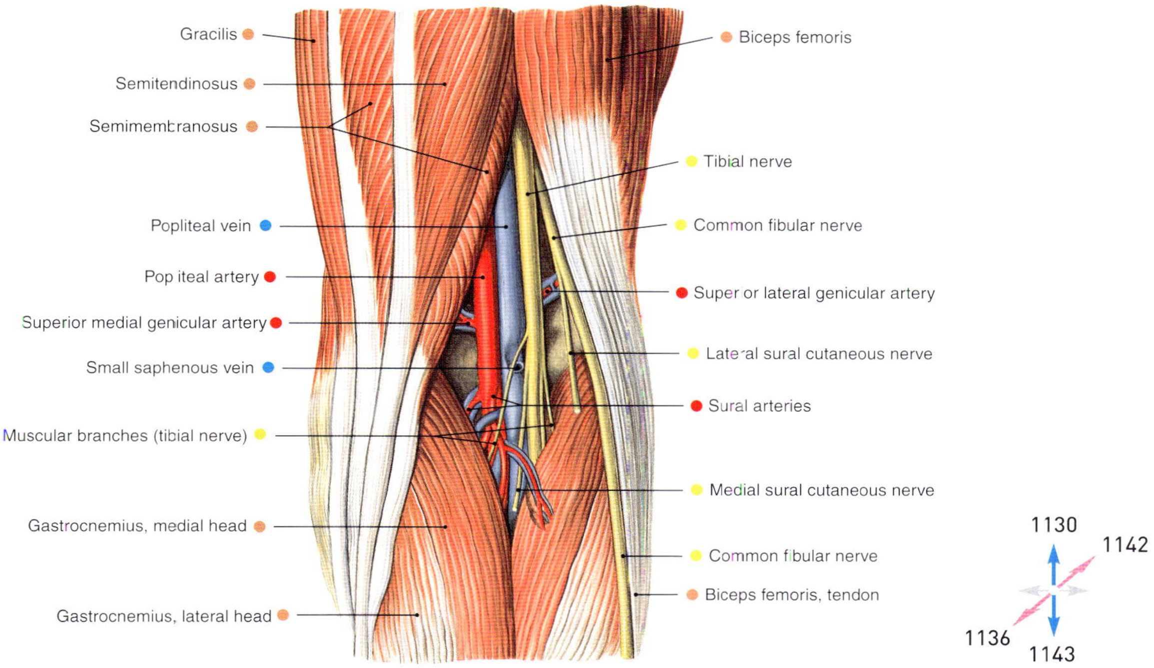

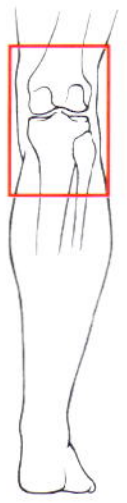

Fig. 1141 Vessels and nerves of the popliteal fossa; after removal of the fascia lata and the deep fascia of leg.

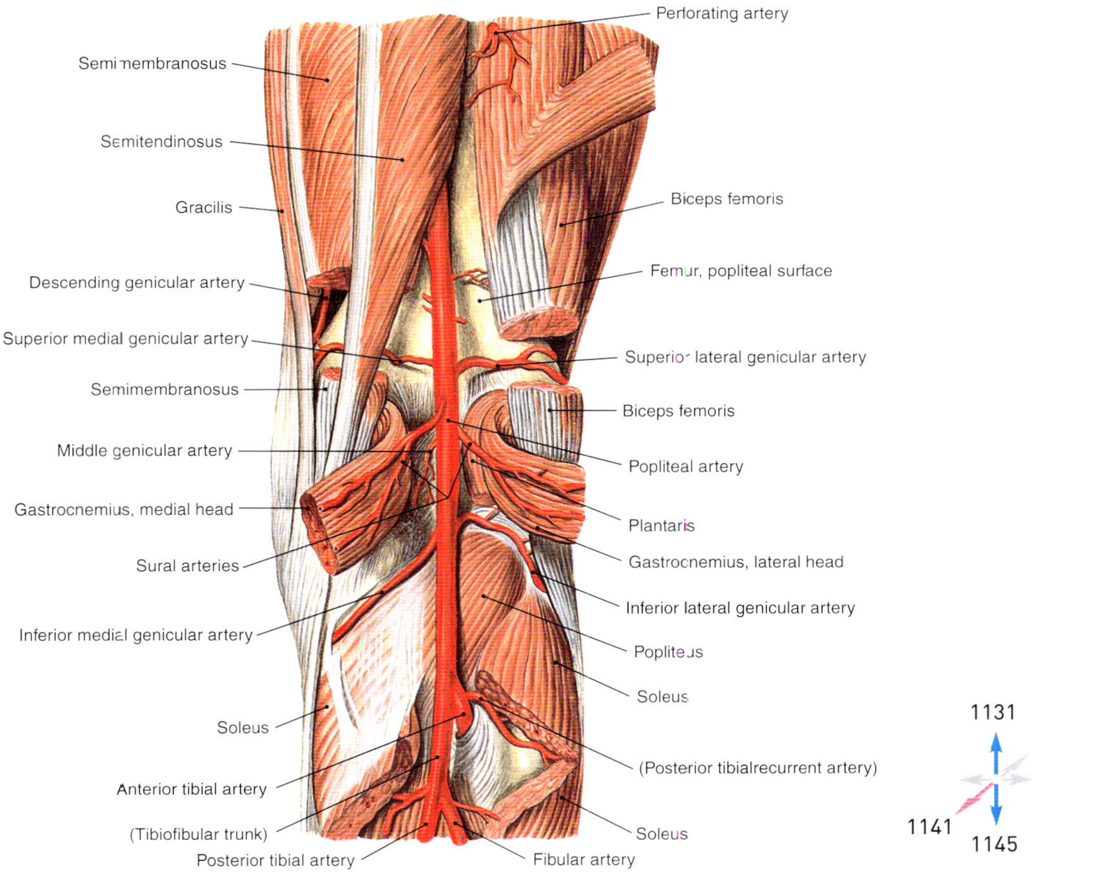

Fig. 1142 Arteries of the popliteal fossa; demonstration of the arterial supply after partial removal of the covering muscles. This branching pattern is found in about 90% of the cases.

Vessels and nerves of the popliteal fossa and the leg

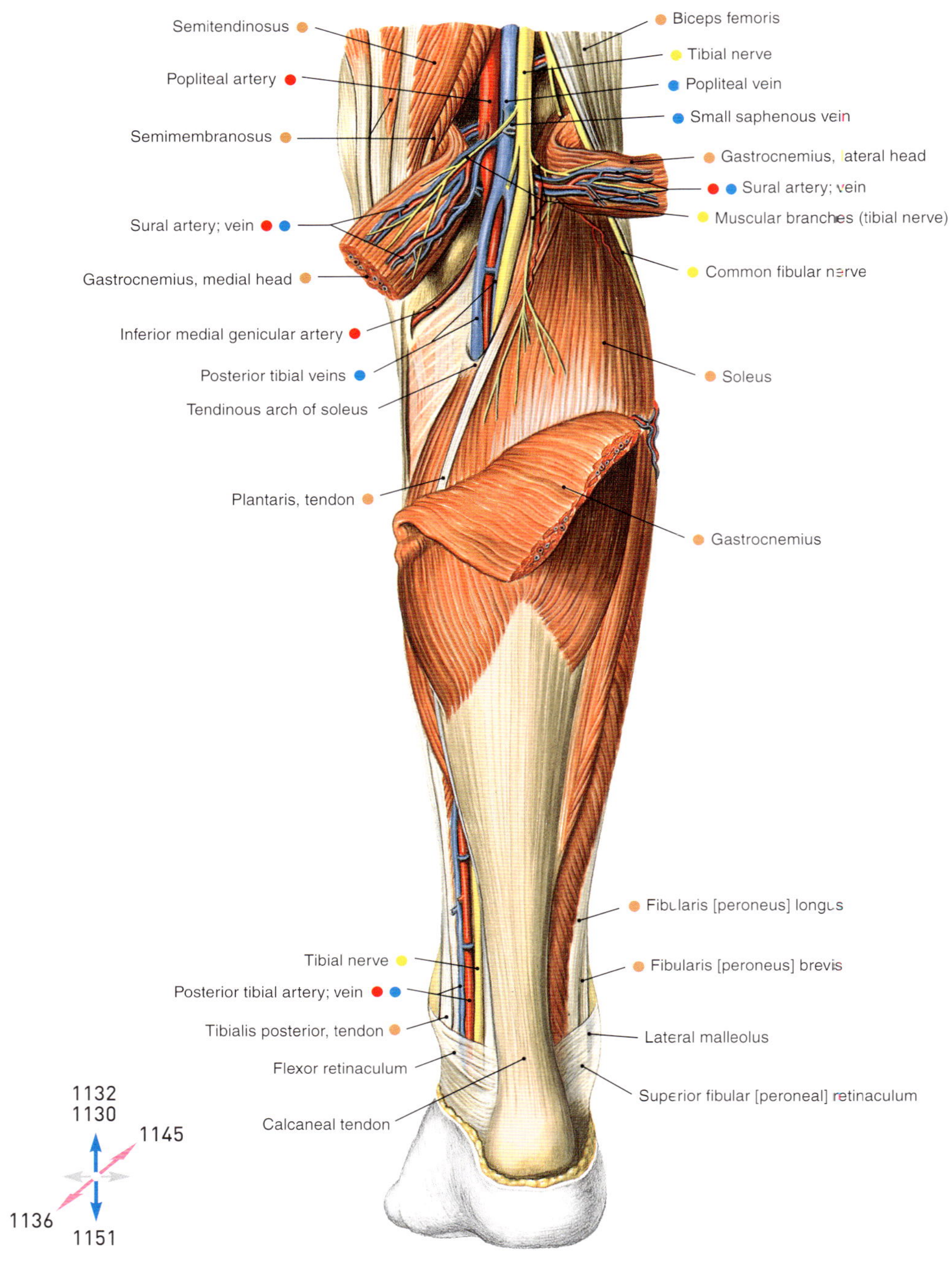

Fig. 1143 Vessels and nerves of the popliteal fossa and the posterior region of leg; after removal of the deep fascia of leg and dissection of the gastrocnemius muscle.

Fig. 1144 a–d Variations in the branching pattern of the popliteal artery.

- **a** Common trunk of the anterior and posterior tibial artery along with the fibular artery.
- **b** The popliteal artery branches off proximally to the superior border of the popliteal muscle.
- **c** Posterior tibial and fibular artery originate from a common proximal trunk.
- **d** The anterior tibial artery passes ventrally to the popliteal muscle.

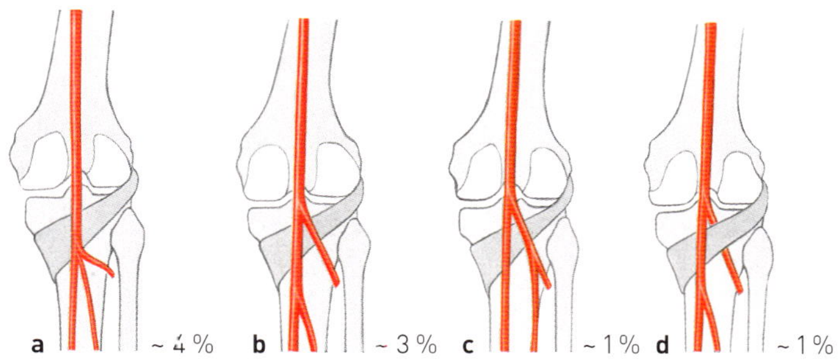

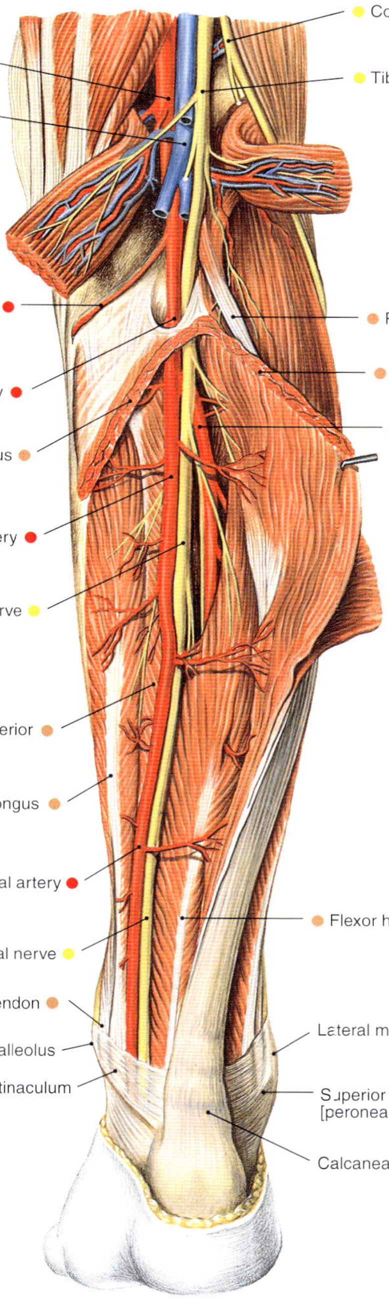

Fig. 1145 Vessels and nerves of the popliteal fossa and the posterior region of leg; deep layer.

1130
1132
1146
1143
1152

Arteries and nerves of the leg

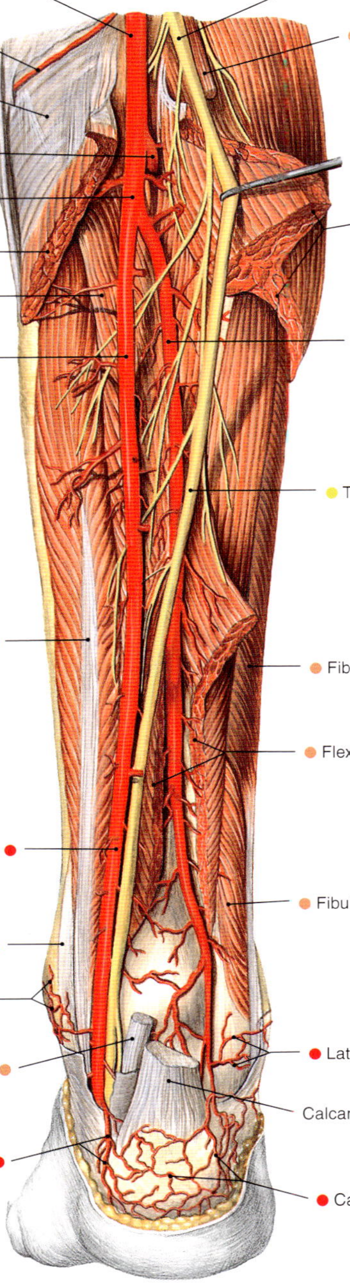

1130
1132
1145
1153

Fig. 1146 Arteries and nerves of the popliteal fossa and the posterior region of leg; deepest layer.

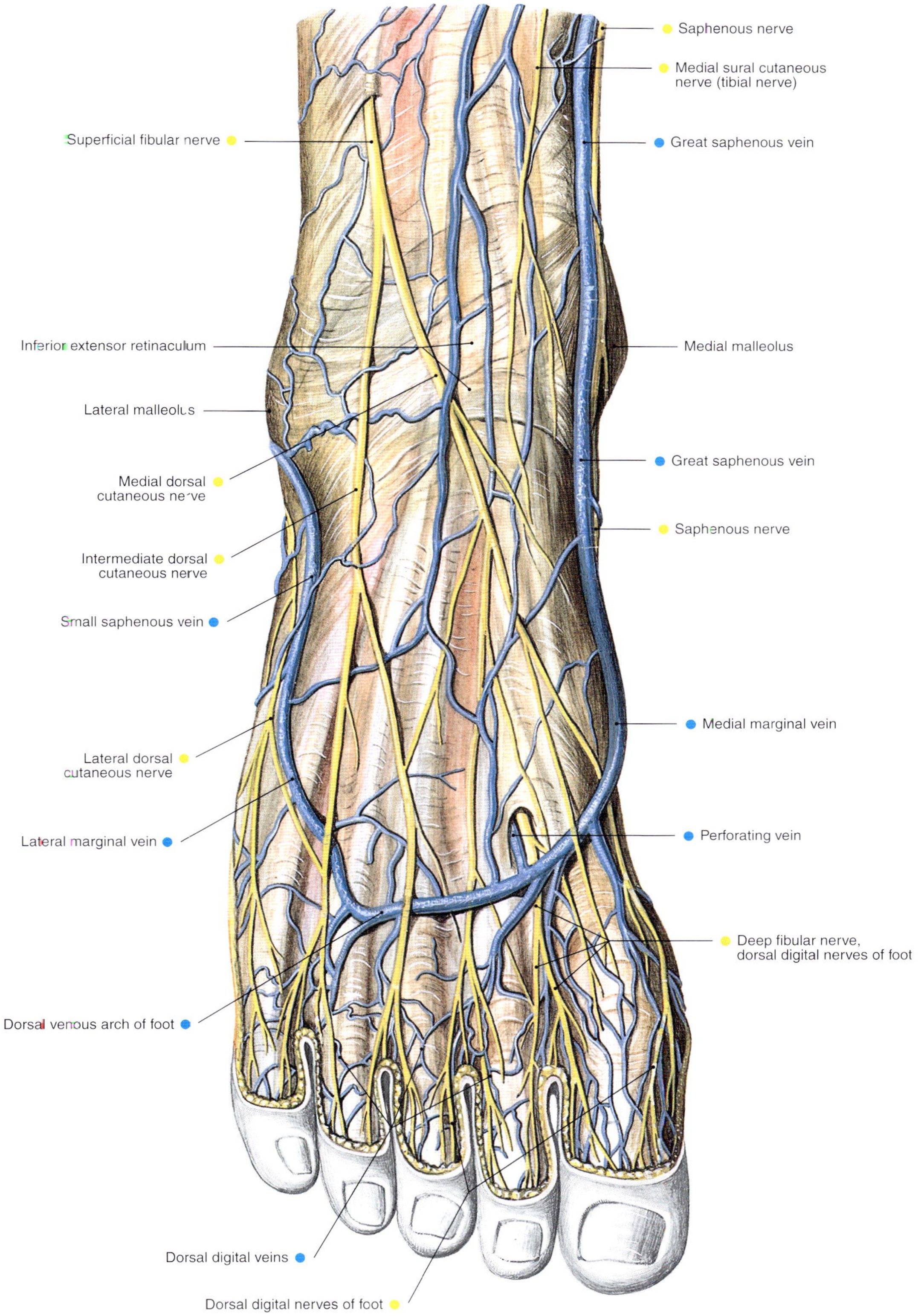

Fig. 1147 Epifascial veins and nerves of the dorsum of foot.

1135
1148

Arteries and nerves of the foot

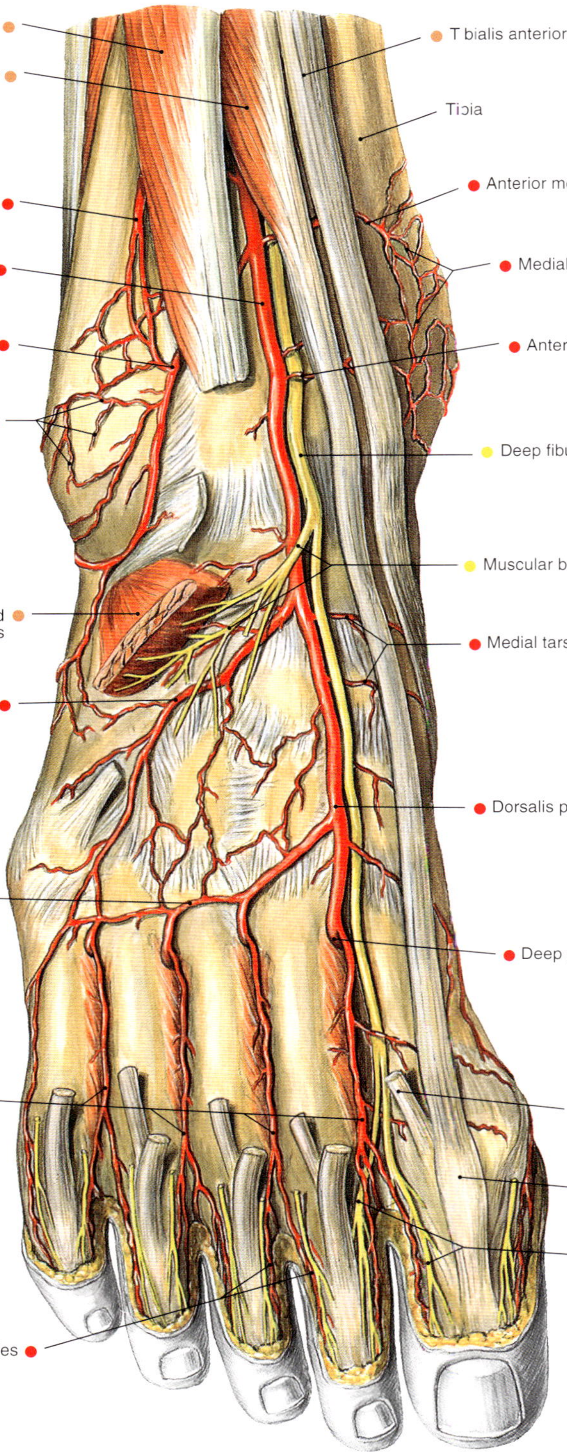

1140
1147

Fig. 1148 Arteries and nerves of the dorsum of foot.

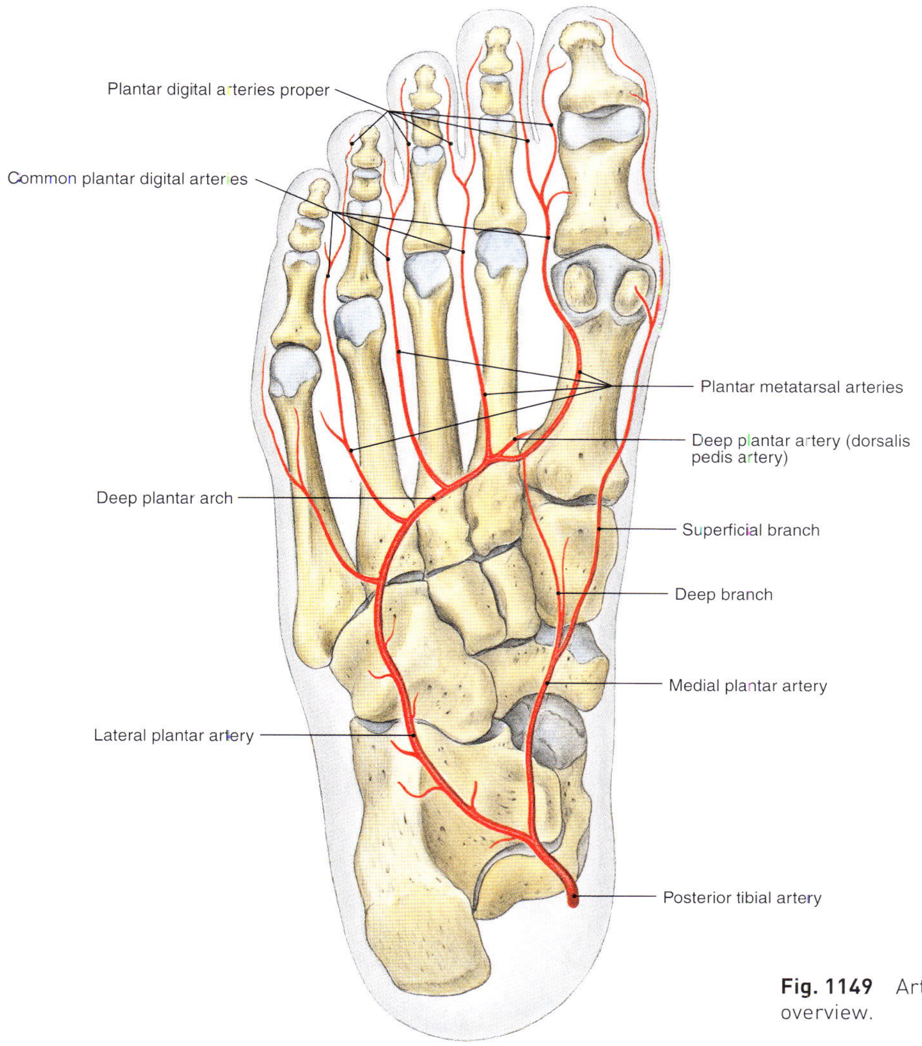

Fig. 1149 Arteries of the sole of foot; overview.

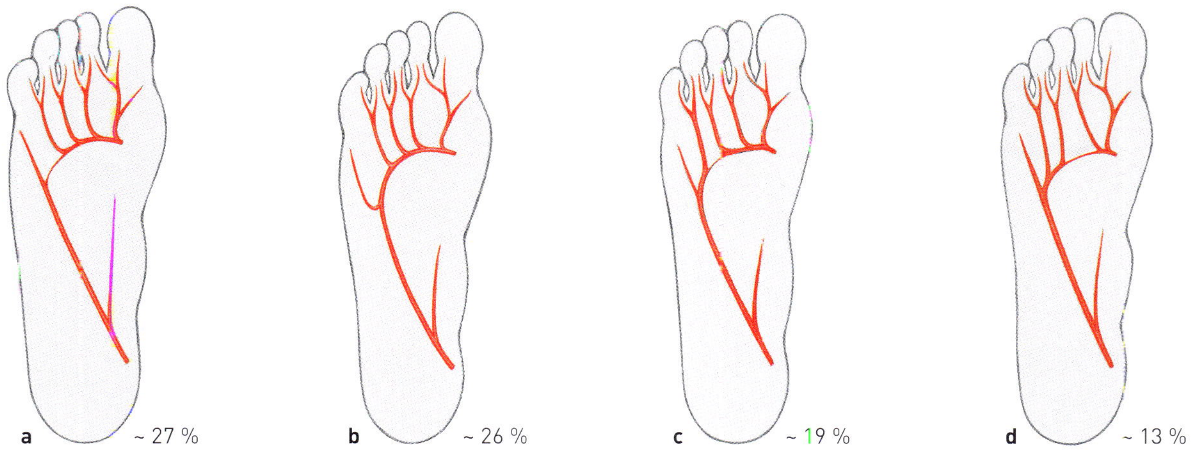

Fig. 1150 a–d Variations in the arterial supply of the sole of foot.
a Dorsalis pedis artery as major supply for the deep plantar arch.
b Posterior tibial artery as major supply for the deep plantar arch.
c The fifth toe and lateral parts of the fourth toe are supplied by the posterior tibial artery, whereas the remaining medially located toes receive their arterial supply through the dorsalis pedis artery.
d The fifth and fourth toe as well as lateral parts of the third toe are supplied by the posterior tibial artery, whereas all remaining medially located toes receive their arterial supply through the dorsalis pedis artery.

Arteries and nerves of the foot

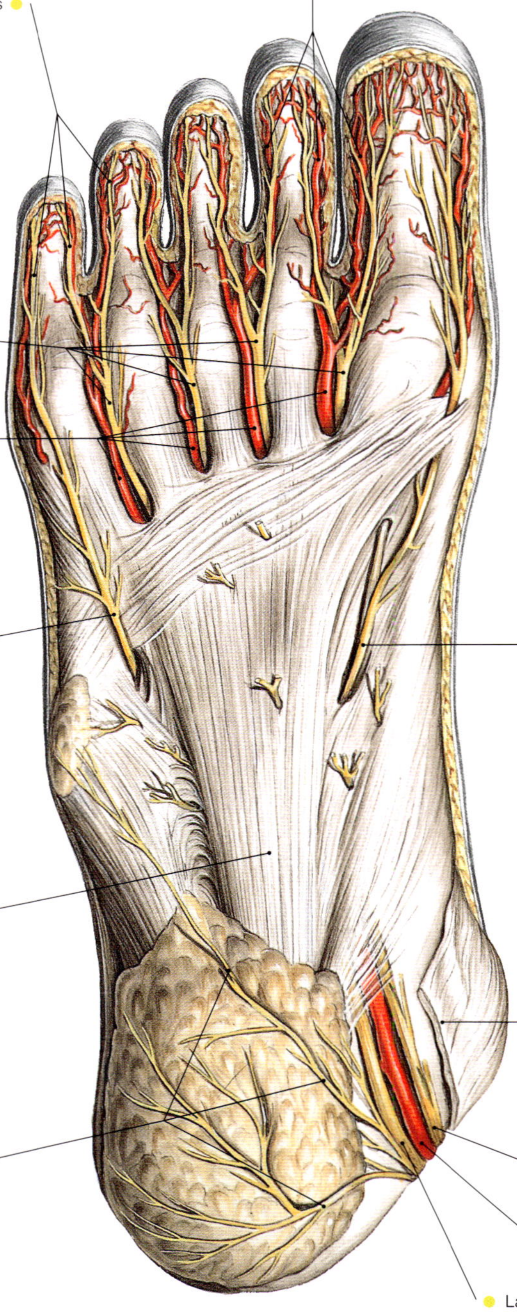

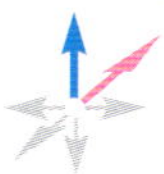

Fig. 1151 Arteries and nerves of the sole of foot.

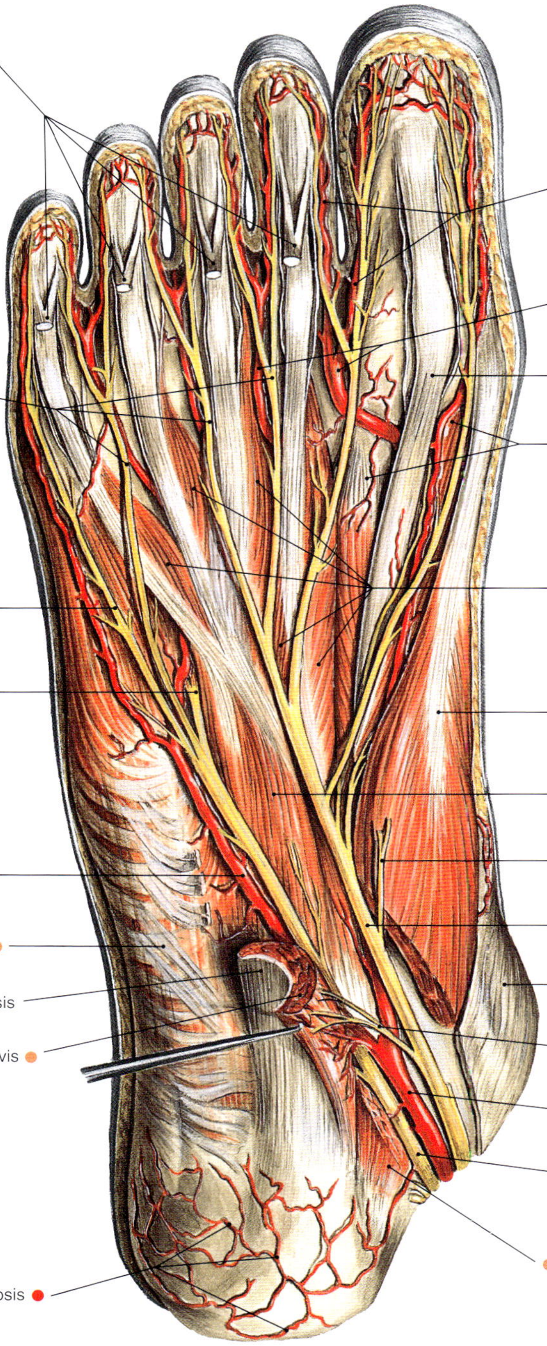

Fig. 1152 Arteries and nerves of the sole of foot deep layer.

* The distal extension of the medial retromalleolar space beneath the abductor hallucis muscle is also known as tarsal tunnel.

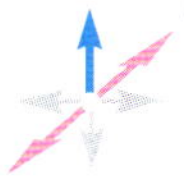

Arteries of the foot

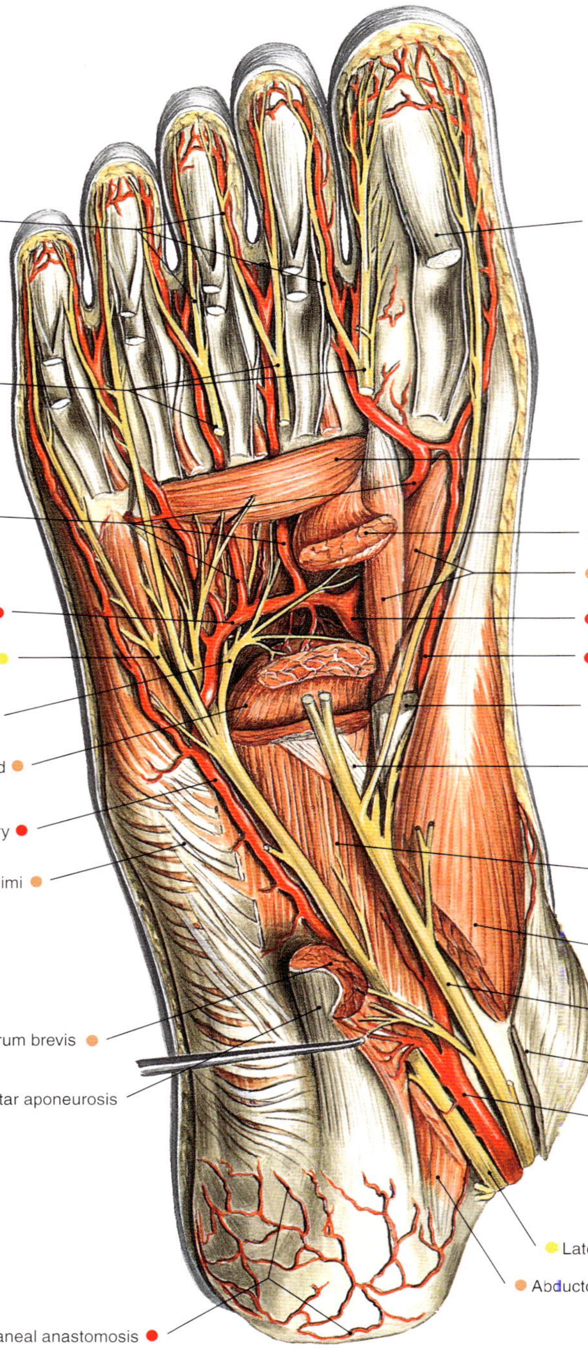

1146
1152

Fig. 1153 Arteries and nerves of the sole of foot; deepest layer.

* Anastomosis with the dorsalis pedis artery

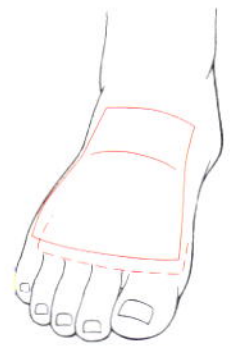

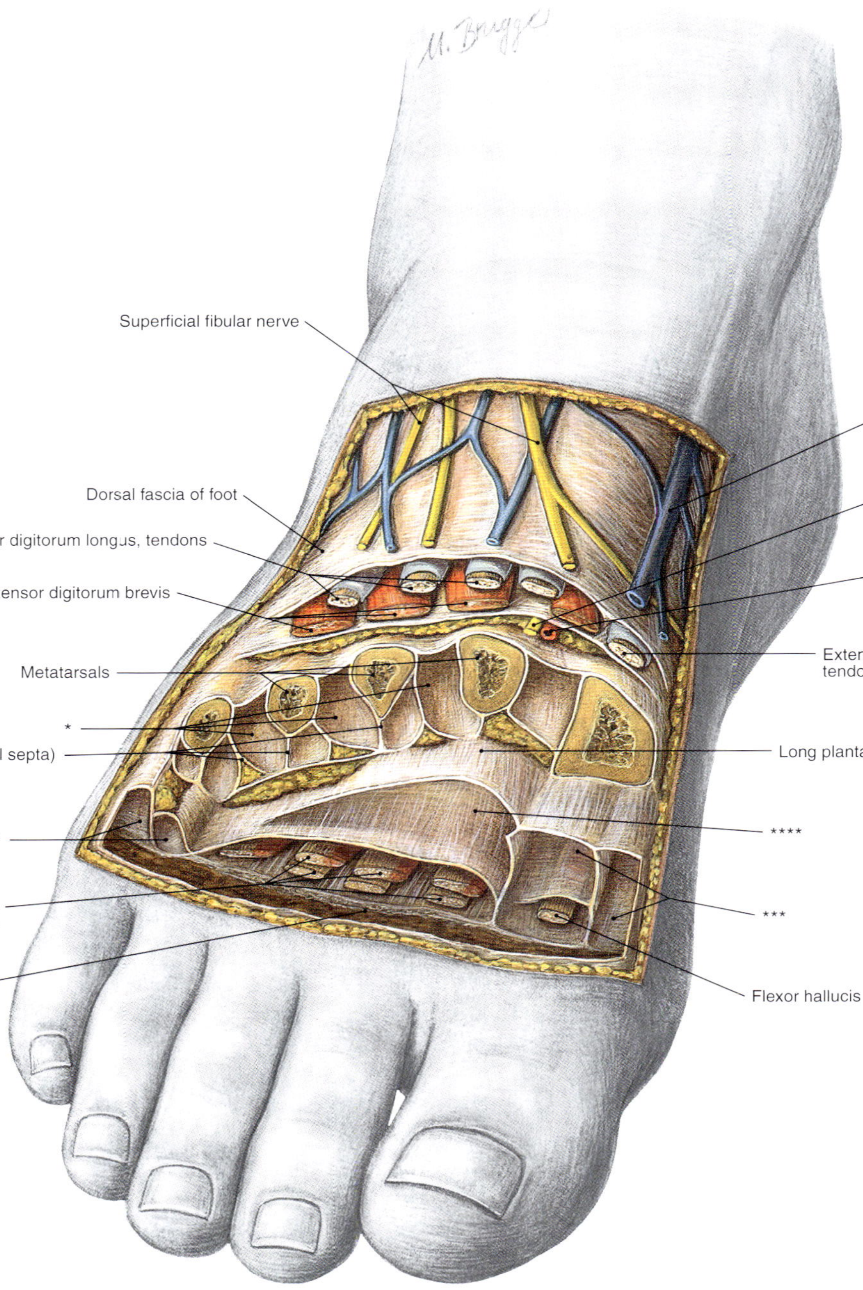

Fig. 1154 Compartments of the foot; stepwise section.

* Space of the interossei muscles
** Lateral compartment
*** Medial compartment
**** Intermediate compartment

Thigh, oblique section

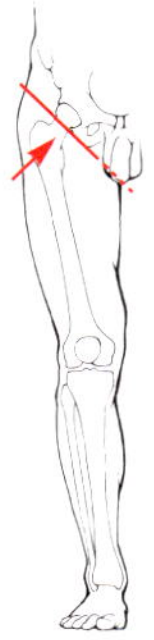

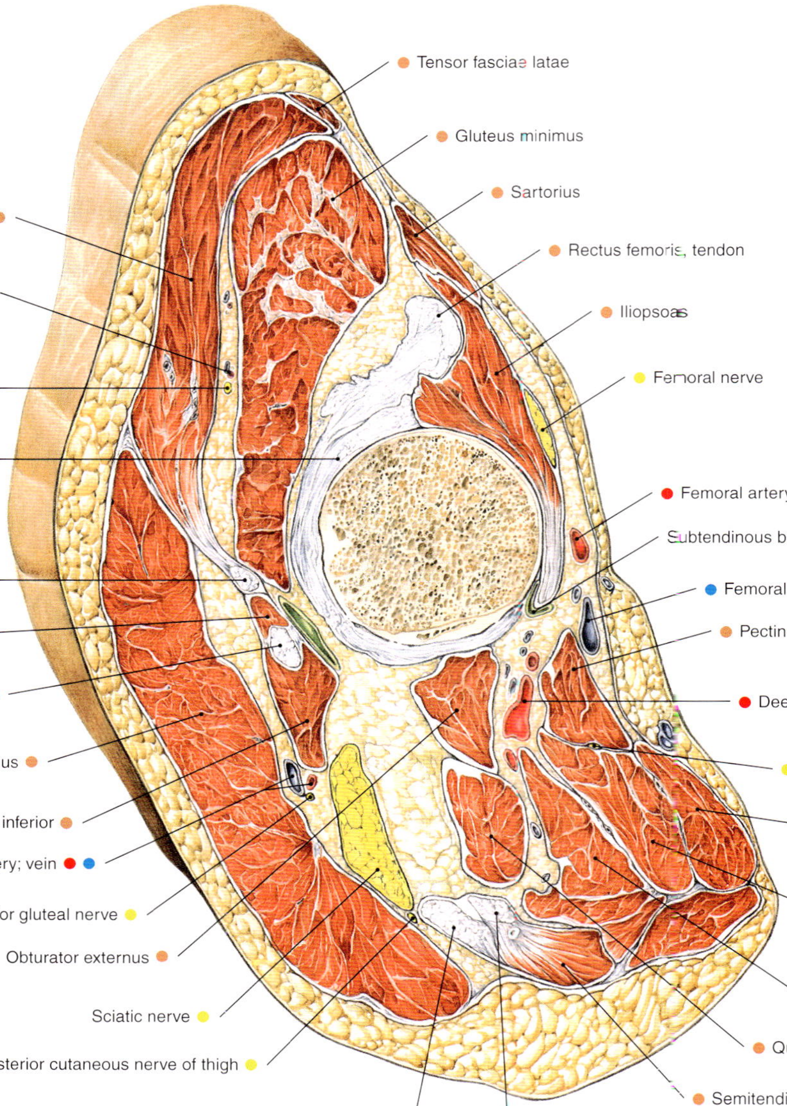

Fig. 1155 Thigh;
oblique section through the hip joint.

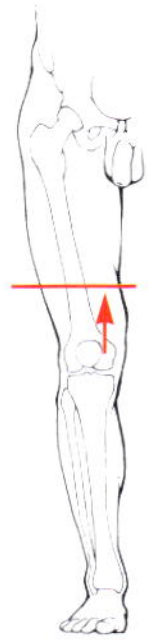

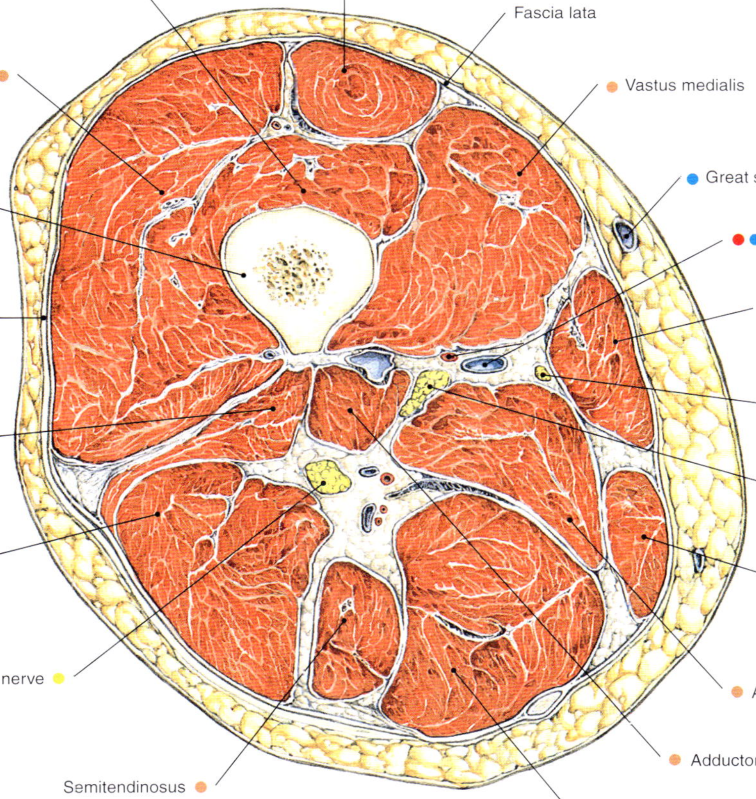

Fig. 1156 Thigh;
cross-section through the middle of the thigh.

Leg, cross section

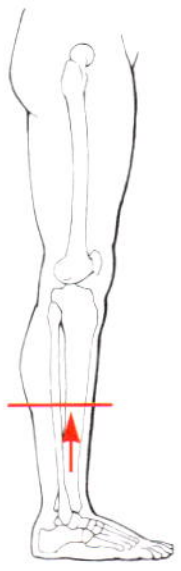

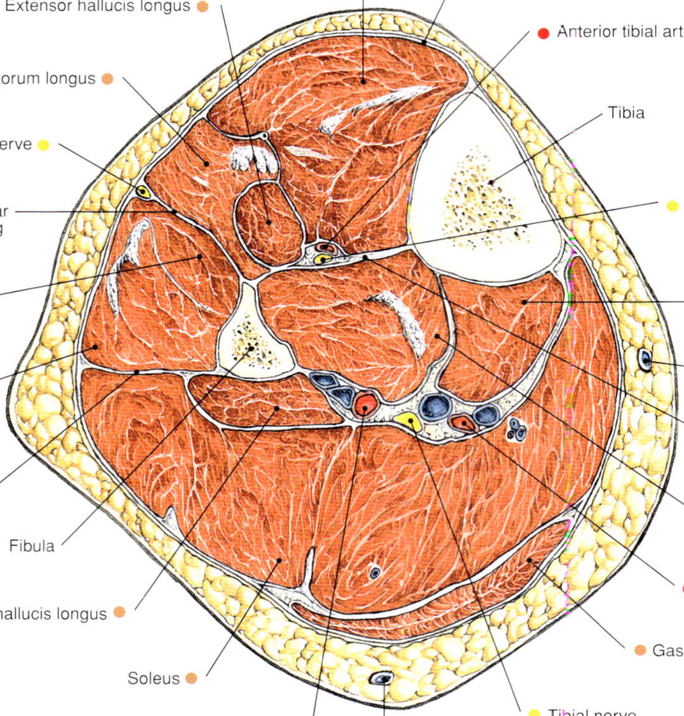

→ 1138

Fig. 1157 Leg;
cross-section through the middle of the leg.

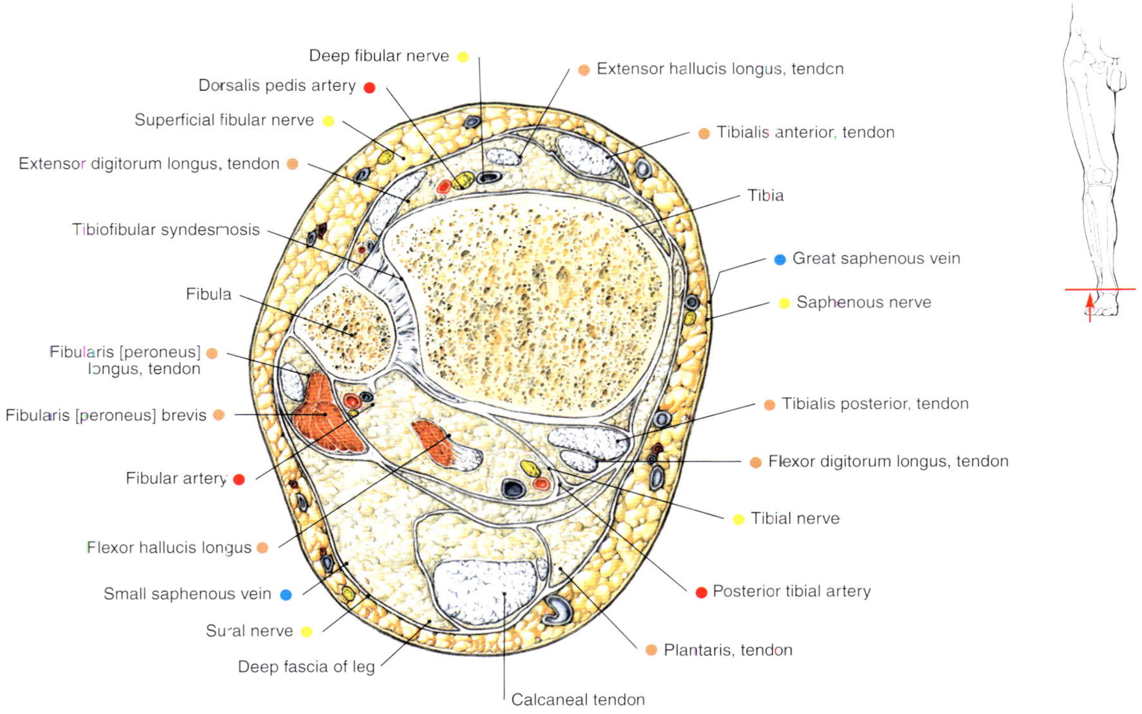

Fig. 1158 Leg;
cross-section just above the ankle joint.

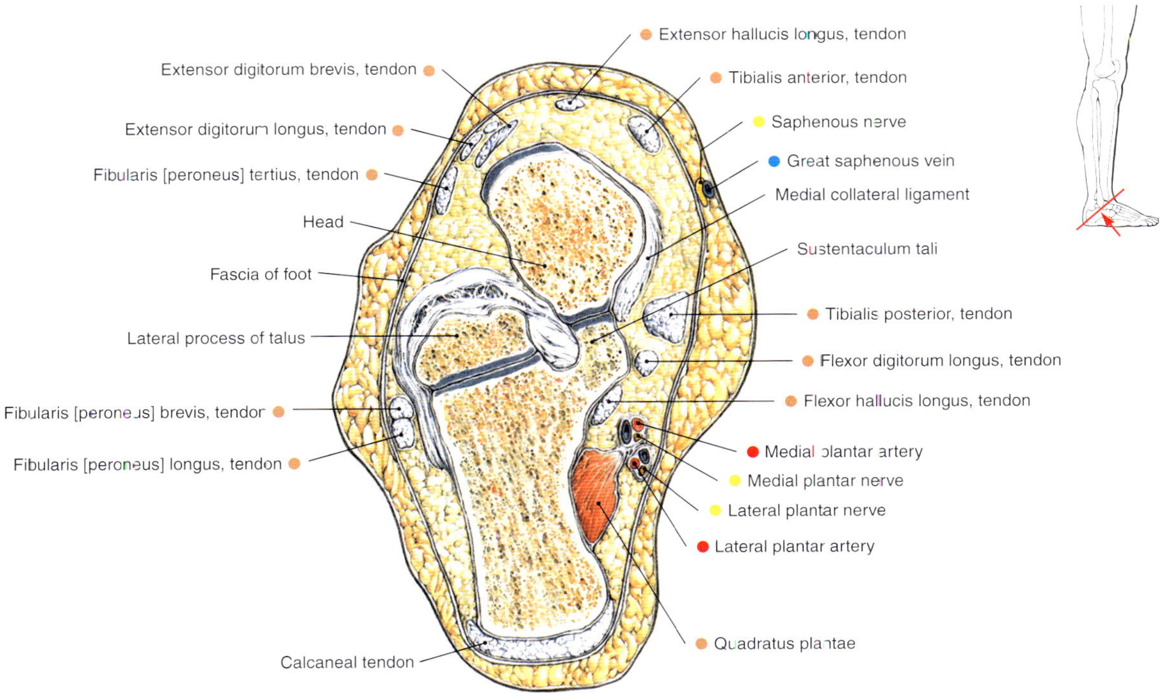

Fig. 1159 Foot;
oblique section through the calcaneus and the head of the talus.

Foot, sagittal sections

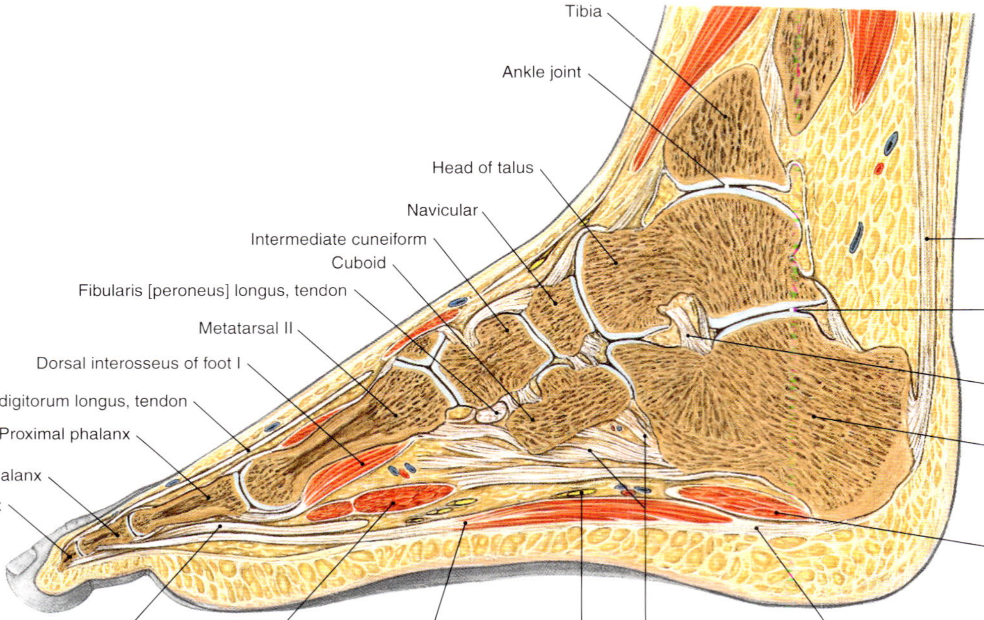

→ 1047, 1048

Fig. 1160 Foot;
sagittal section through the second toe.

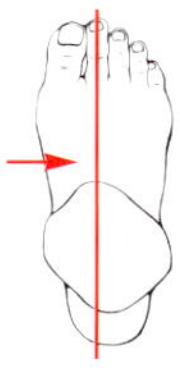

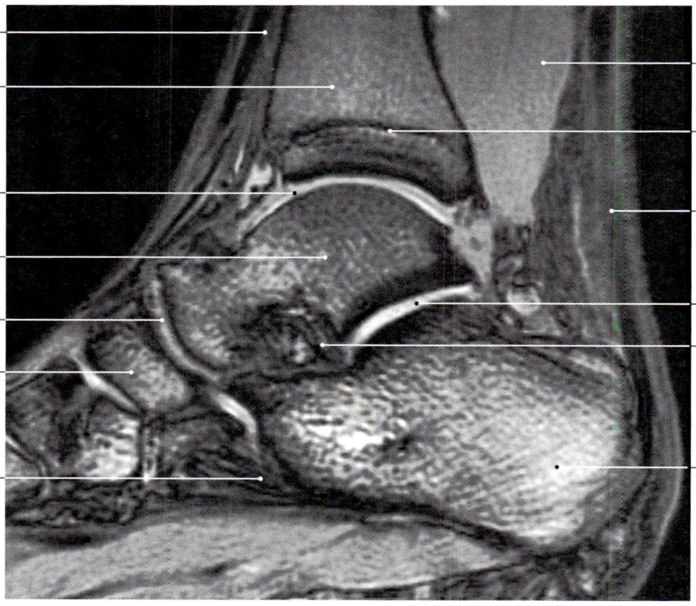

→ 1049, 1050

Fig. 1161 Foot;
magnetic resonance tomography image (MRI); sagittal section.

Foot, cross-section and pedograms

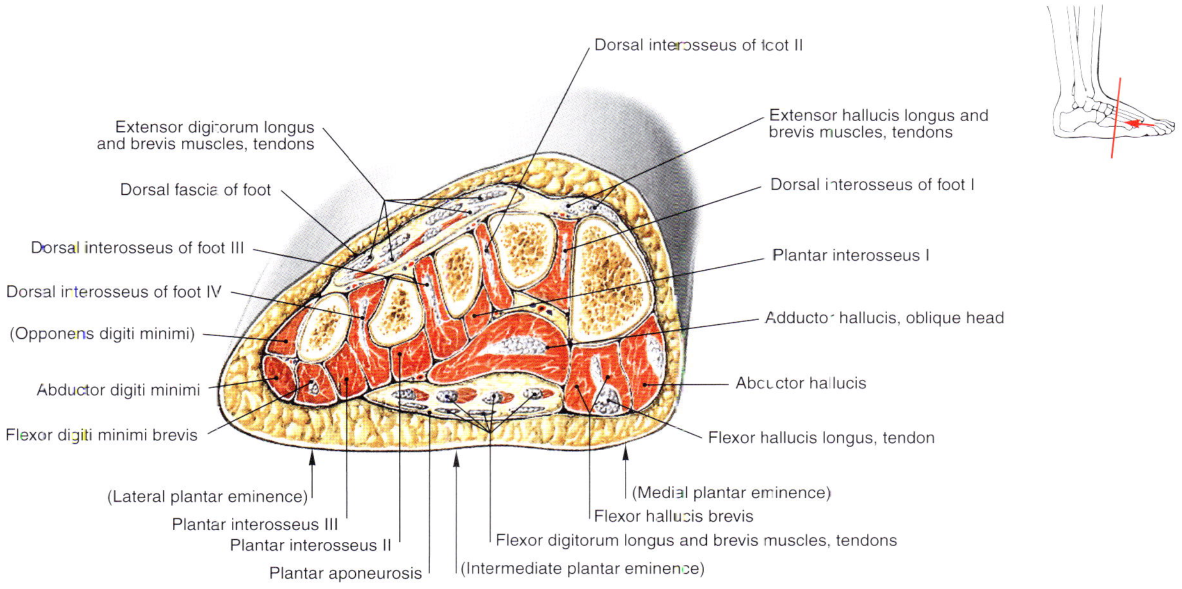

Fig. 1162 Osteofibrous tubes of the foot; frontal section through the metatarsus.

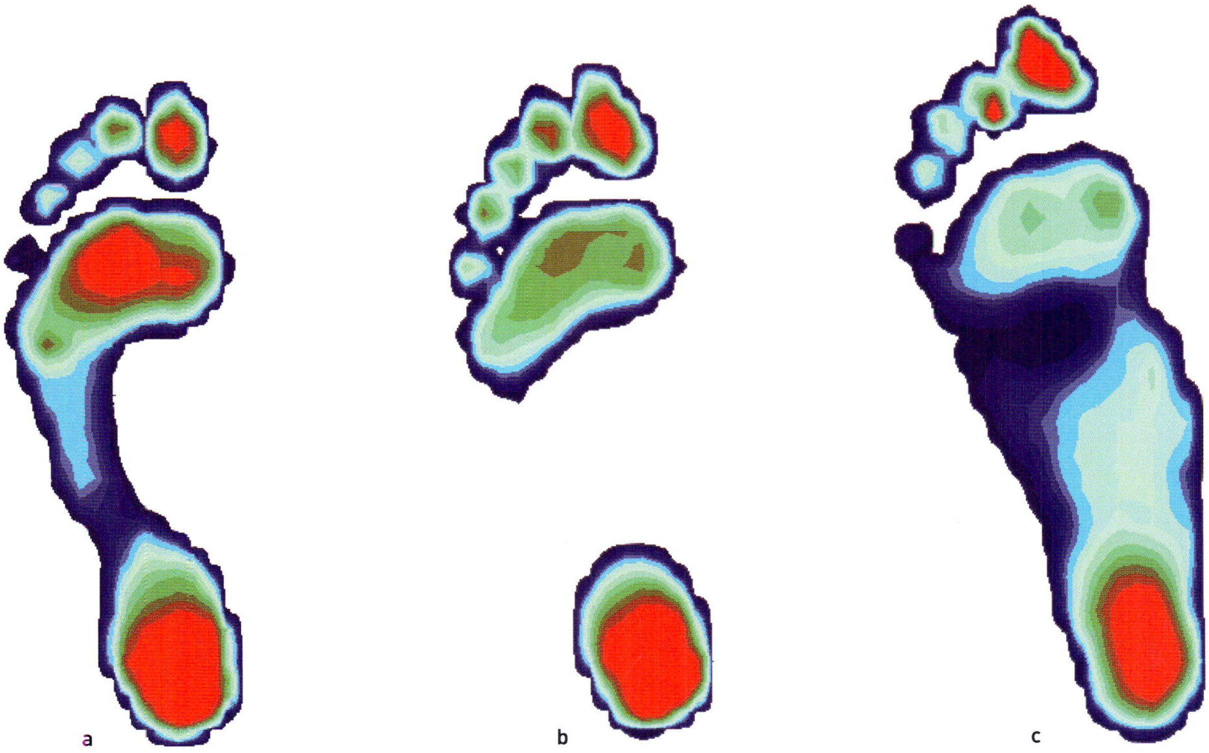

Fig. 1163 Foot prints, pedograms.
a Normal foot
b Pes cavus
c Flat foot

Arteries of the head

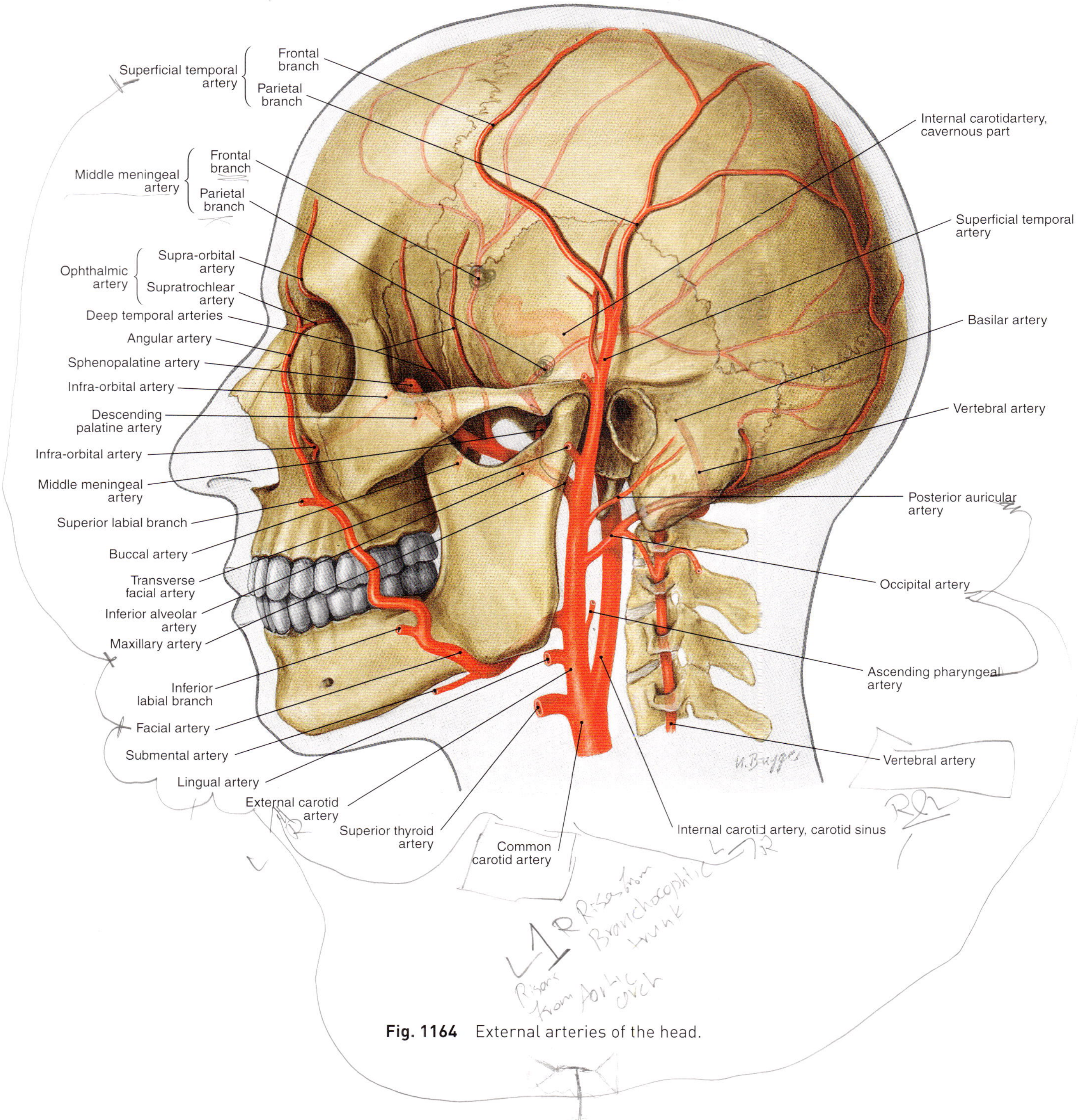

Fig. 1164 External arteries of the head.

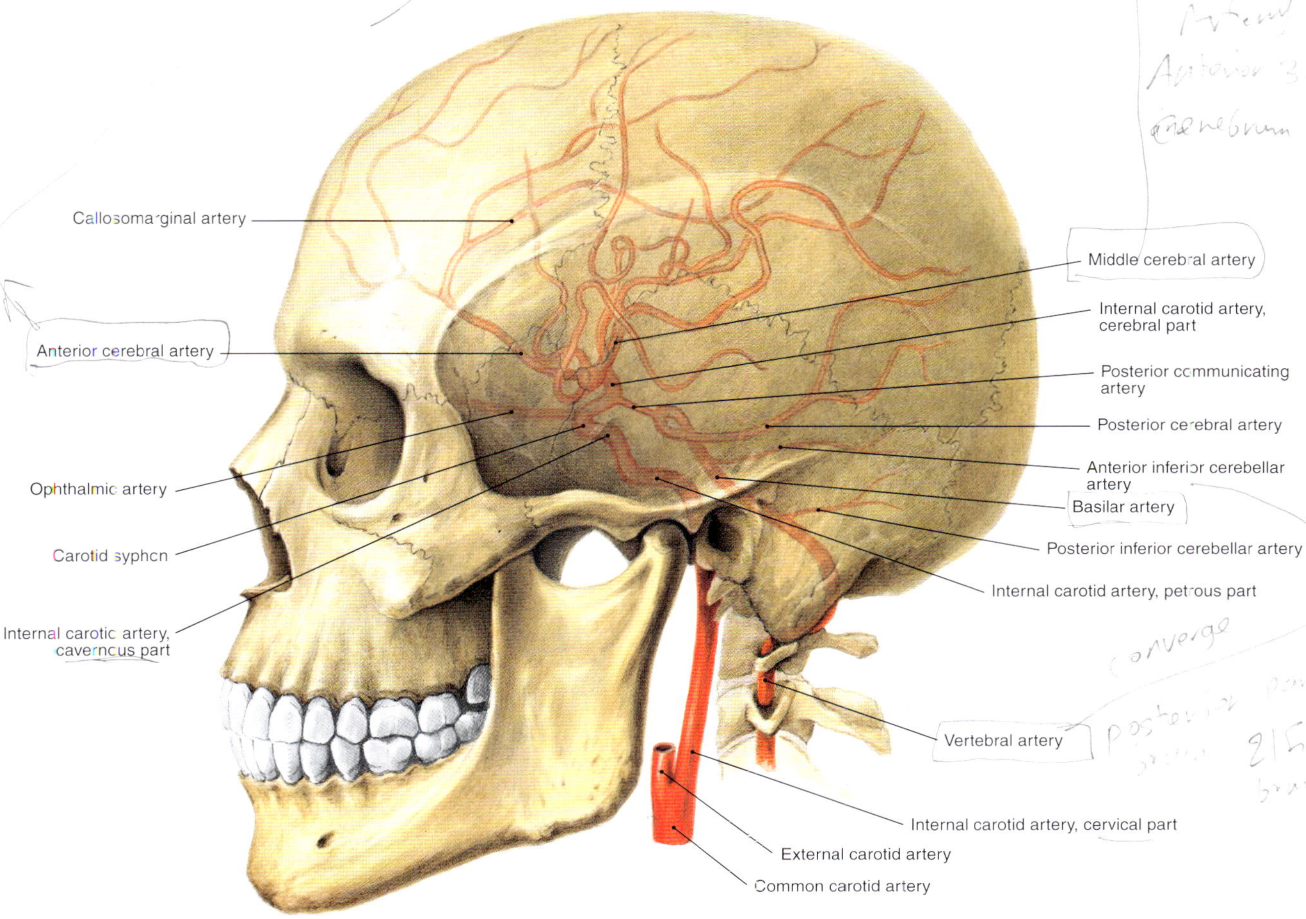

Fig. 1165 Internal arteries of the head.

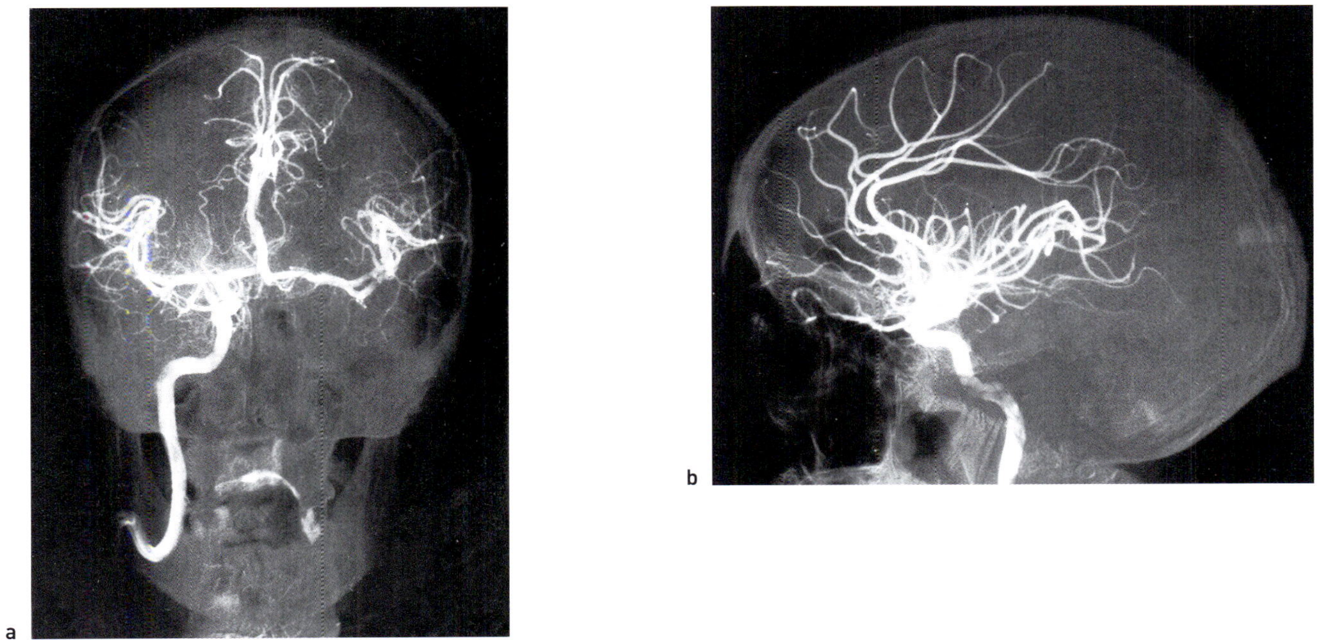

Fig. 1166 a, b Internal carotid artery; radiographs after unilateral injection of a contrast medium (angiograms).

The contrast medium also distributes to the vessels of the contralateral side via the arterial circle.

a AP-radiograph, digital subtraction angiography (DSA)
b Lateral radiograph, digital subtraction angiography (DSA)

Veins of the head

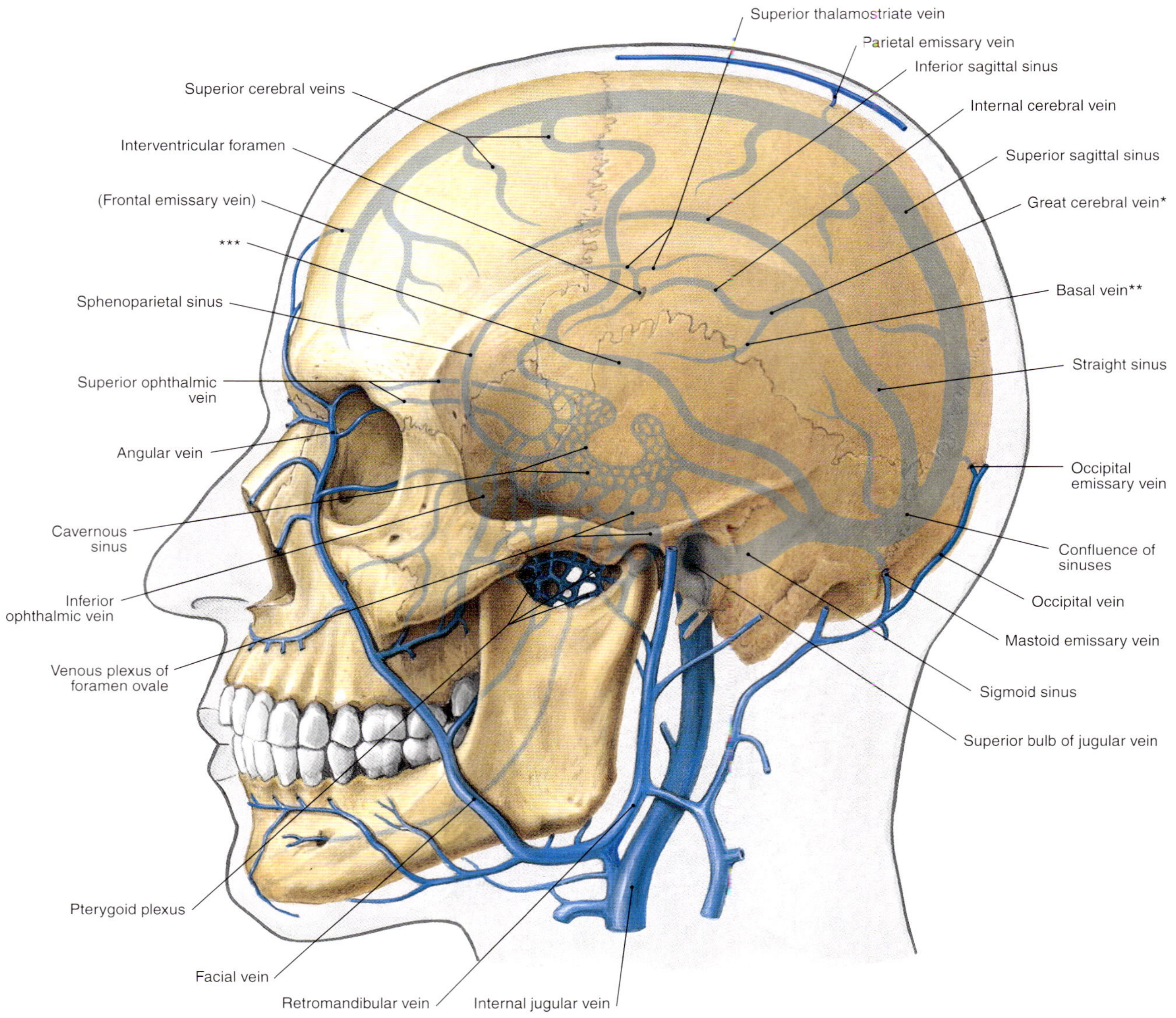

Fig. 1167 Internal and external veins of the head.

* Vein of GALEN
** ROSENTHAL's vein
*** Vein of LABBÉ

Emissary veins – Passages through the skull

Parietal emissary vein – parietal foramen
Mastoid emissary vein – mastoid foramen
Occipital emmissary vein – passage in the region of the external occipital protuberance
Condylar emmissary vein – condylar canal
Venous plexus of hypoglossal canal – hypoglossal canal
Venous plexus of foramen ovale – foramen ovale
Internal carotid venous plexus – carotid canal

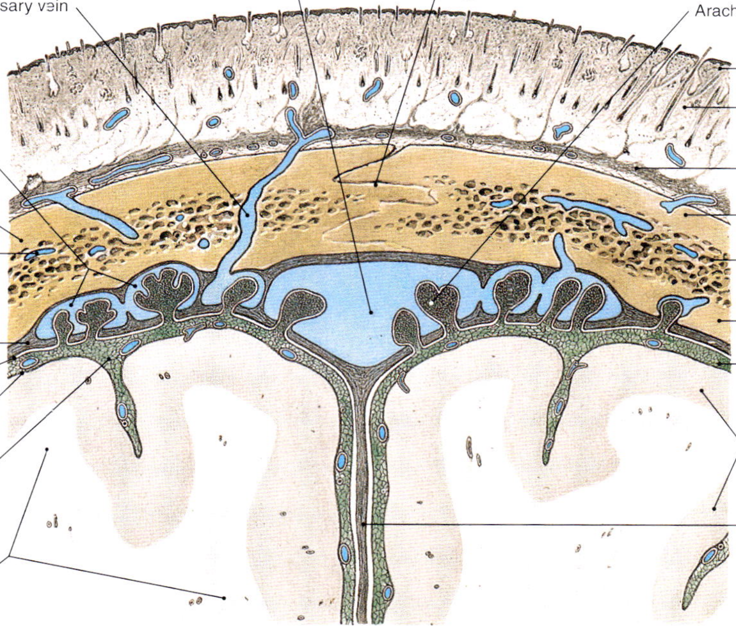

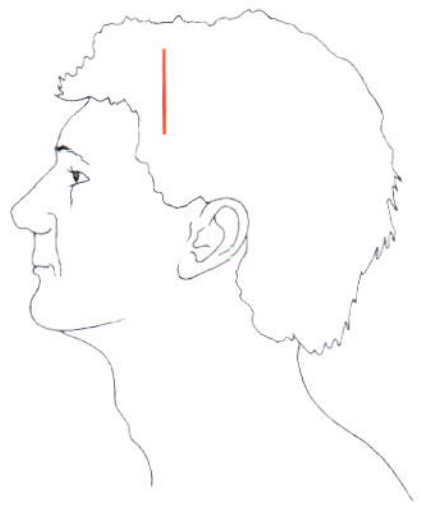

Fig. 1168 Calvaria; meninges and dural venous sinuses.
In the adult, the cerebrospinal fluid is mainly reabsorbed into the venous system through the arachnoid granulations. Additionally, reabsorption occurs through the lymphatic sheaths of small vessels of the cranial pia mater and through the perineural sheaths of the cranial and the spinal nerves.

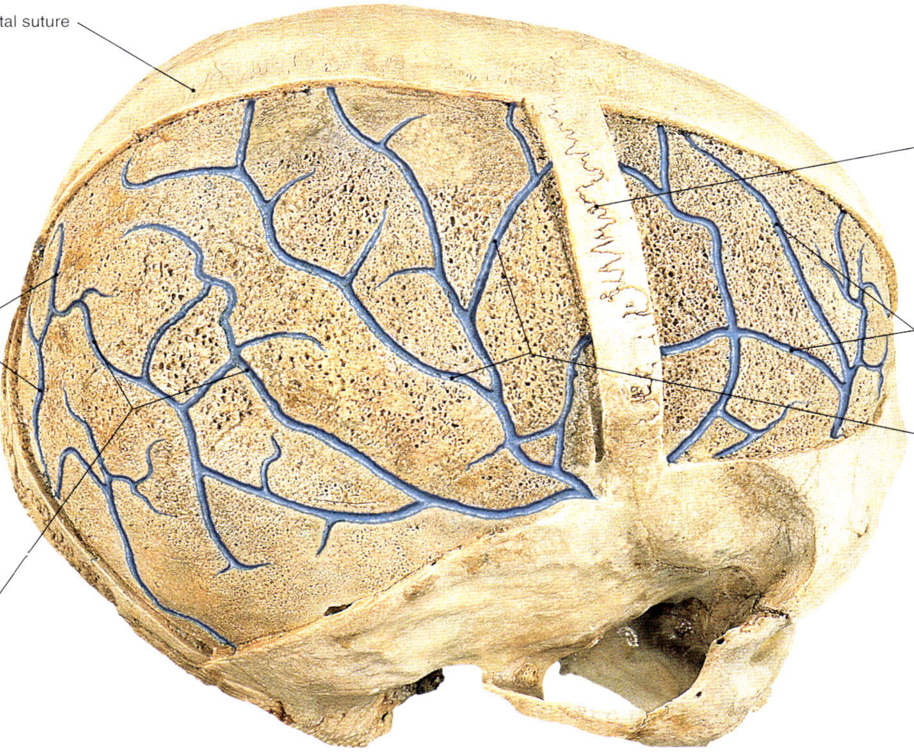

Fig. 1169 Diploic canals and diploic veins of the calvaria; the external table of compact bone has been removed from the calvaria.

Dural venous sinuses

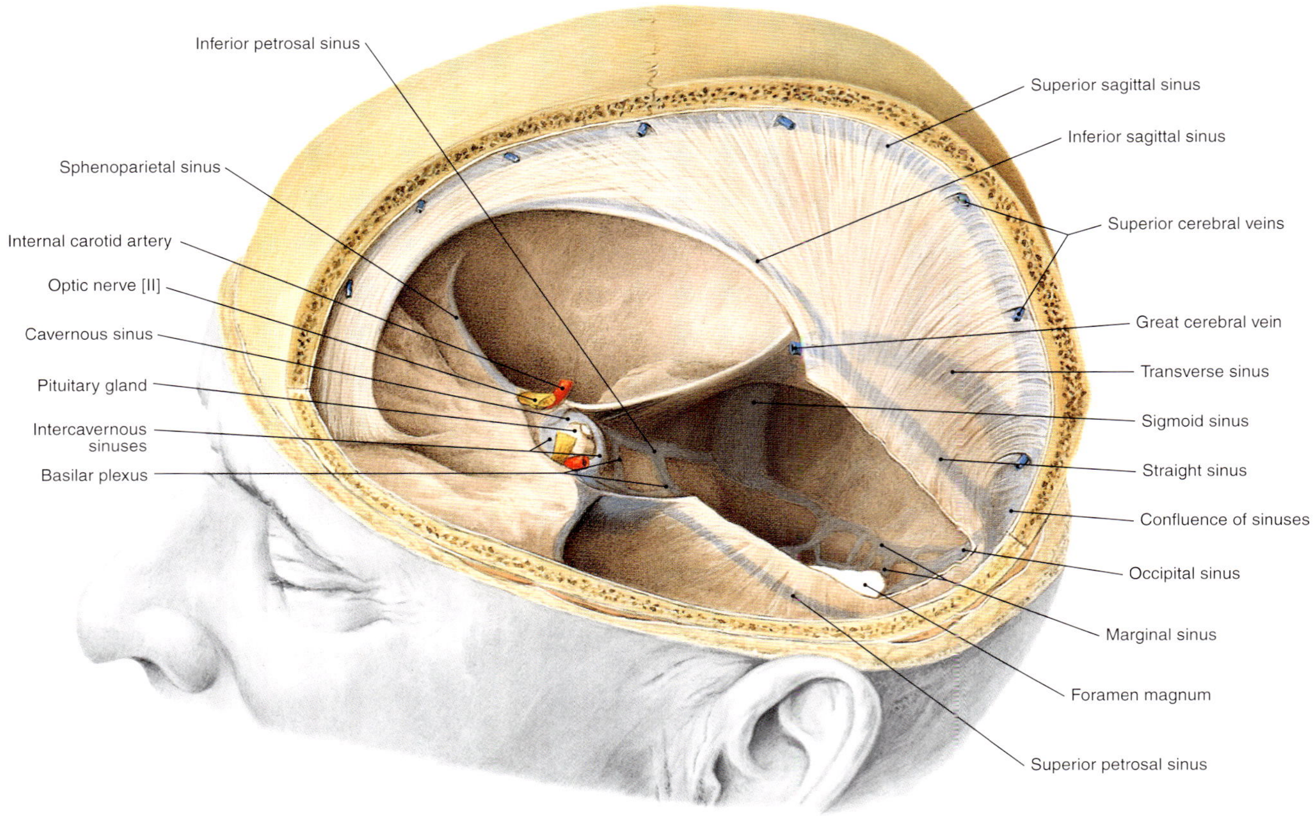

Fig. 1170 Cranial dura mater and dural venous sinuses; after partial removal of the tentorium cerebelli.

Cranial dura mater

The cranial dura mater lines the cranial cavity completely and tightly adheres to the skull bone. The cerebral falx protrudes in the sagittal plane in a sickle-like shape and stretches from the crista galli to the ridge of the tentorium cerebelli, which, in turn, overstretches the posterior cranial fossa and is attached along the transverse sinus and the pyramidal edge. The margins of the tentorial notch envelop the midbrain and taper off into the anterior and posterior clinoid process. The cerebral falx and the tentorium cerebelli divide the cranial cavity into three spaces that are incompletely separated from one another, containing the two cerebral hemispheres and the cerebellum.

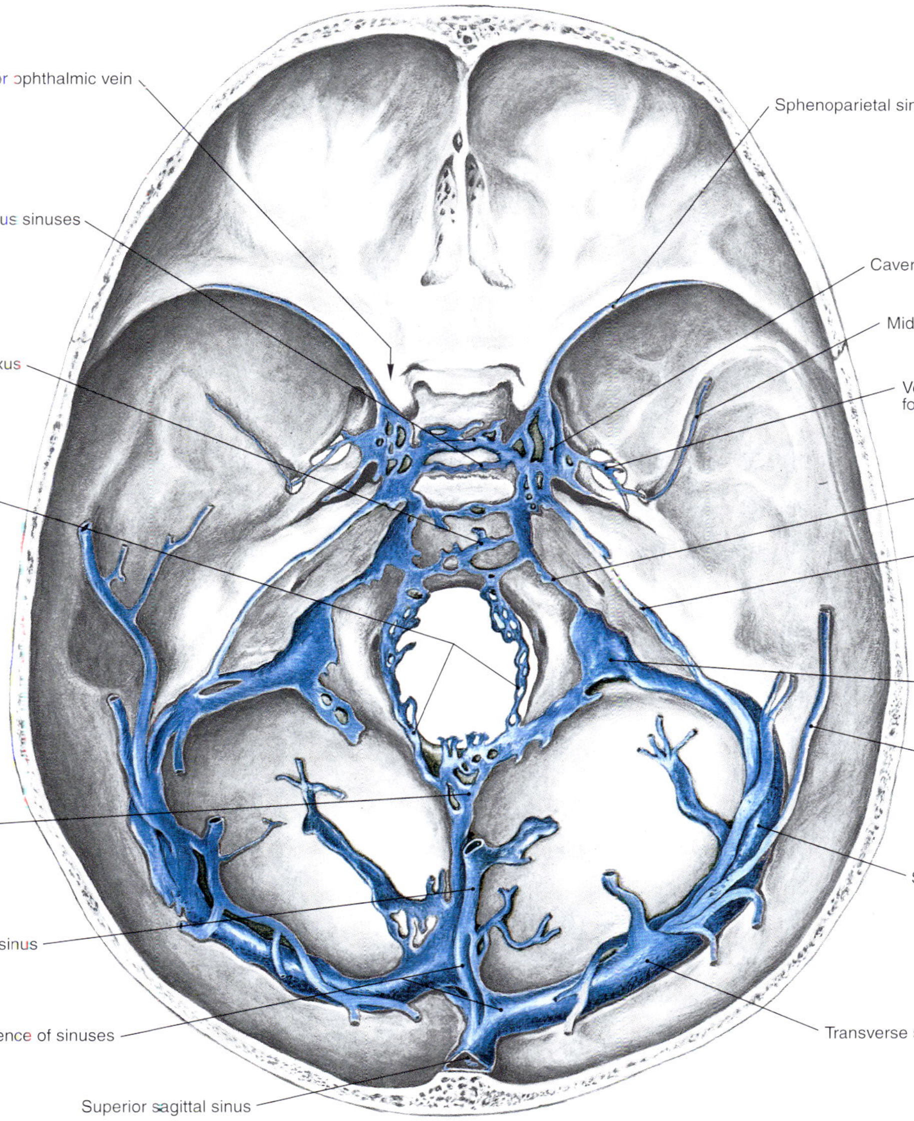

Fig. 1171 Dural venous sinuses; corrosion cast.
The sinuses contain no valves and feature rigid walls.

* Vein of LABBÉ to the superficial middle cerebral veins

Dural venous sinuses

The dural venous sinuses are rigid venous channels without valves draining the venous blood from the brain via so-called bridging veins.
The main drainage from within the skull occurs via the sigmoid sinuses into the internal jugular veins. Additionally, the superior ophthalmic veins and the highly variable emissary veins form a series of smaller, likewise valveless, venous connections between the intra- and extracranial regions.

The two cavernous sinuses assume a central position by being situated in the middle cranial fossa to the right and the left of the sella turcica. They communicate with each other through the intercavernous sinuses and either directly or indirectly with most other sinuses and with the veins of the orbit and the infratemporal fossa.

External surface of the cranial base

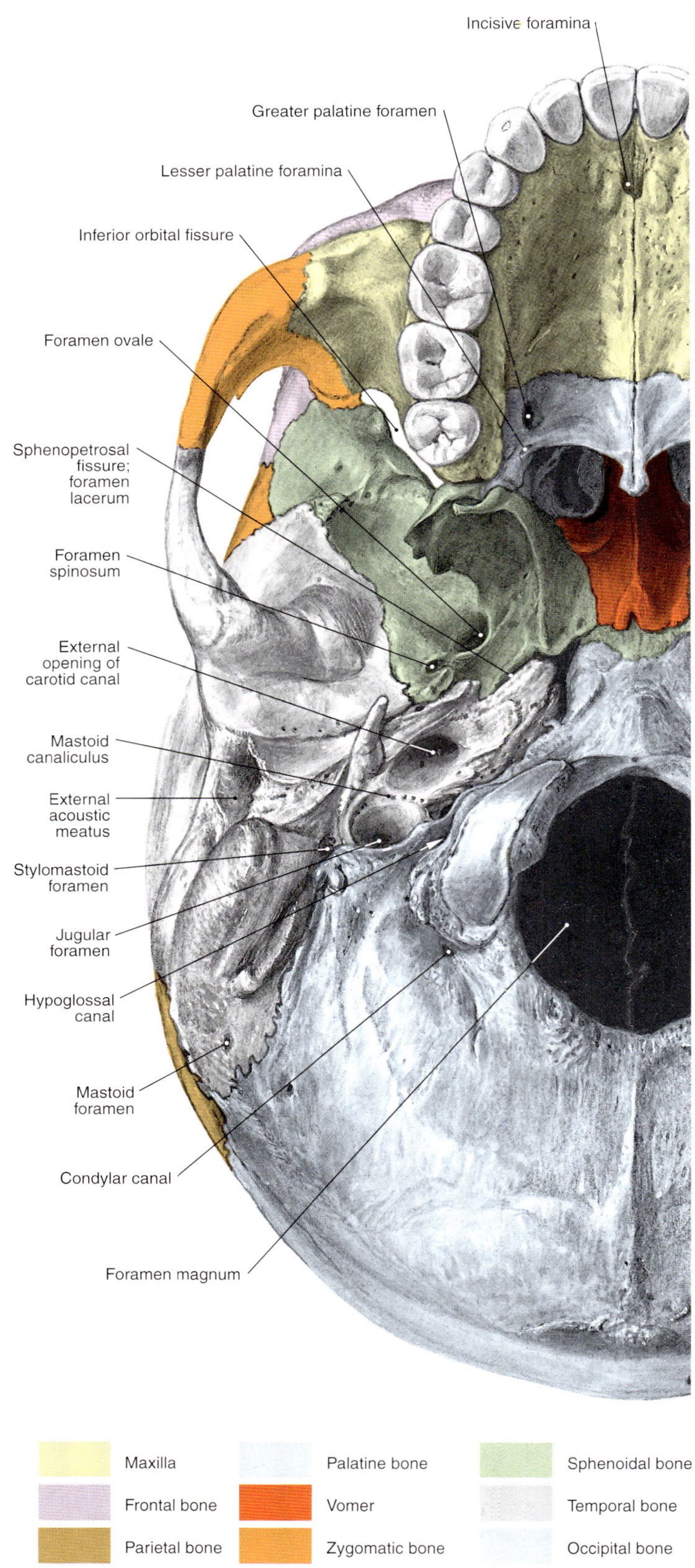

Fig. 1172 External surface of the cranial base and foramina.

Contents of the foramina of the external surface of the cranial base

Incisive foramina
Nasopalatine nerve (maxillary nerve [V/2])

Greater palatine foramen
Greater palatine nerve (maxillary nerve [V/2])
Greater palatine artery (descending palatine artery)

Lesser palatine foramen
Lesser palatine nerves (maxillary nerve [V/2])
Lesser palatine arteries (descending palatine artery)

Inferior orbital fissure
Infraorbital artery (maxillary artery)
Inferior ophthalmic vein
Infraorbital nerve (maxillary nerve [V/2])
Zygomatic nerve (maxillary nerve [V/2])

Foramen rotundum
Maxillary nerve [V/2]

Foramen ovale
Mandibular nerve [V/3]
Venous plexus of foramen ovale

Foramen spinosum
Meningeal branch (mandibular nerve [V/3])
Middle meningeal artery (maxillary artery)

Sphenopetrosal fissure and foramen lacerum
Lesser petrosal nerve (glossopharyngeal nerve [IX])
Greater petrosal nerve (facial nerve [VII])
Deep petrosal nerve (internal carotid plexus)

External opening of carotid canal → carotid canal
Internal carotid artery, petrosal part
Internal carotid venous plexus
Internal carotid plexus (sympathetic trunk, superior cervical ganglion)

Stylomastoid foramen
Facial nerve [VII]

Jugular foramen
Anterior part:
Inferior petrosal sinus
Glossopharyngeal nerve [IX]
Posterior part:
Posterior meningeal artery (ascending pharyngeal artery)
Sigmoid sinus (superior bulb of jugular vein)
Vagus nerve [X]
Meningeal nerve (vagus nerve [X])
Accessory nerve [XI]

Mastoid canalicul
Auricular branch of vagus nerve (vagus nerve [X])

Hypoglossal canal
Hypoglossal nerve [XII]
Venous plexus of hypoglossal canal

Condylar canal
Condylar emissary vein

Foramen magnum
Meninges
Internal vertebral venous plexus (marginal sinus)
Vertebral arteries (subclavian arteries)
Anterior spinal artery (vertebral arteries)
Medulla oblongata/spinal cord
Spinal roots (accessory nerve [XI])

Contents of the foramina of the internal surface of the cranial base

Lamina cribrosa
Olfactory nerves [I]
Anterior ethmoidal artery (ophthalmic artery)

Optic canal
Optic nerve [II]
Ophthalmic artery (internal carotid artery)
Meninges; sheath of optic nerve

Superior orbital fissure
Medial part:
Nasociliary nerve (ophthalmic nerve [V/1])
Oculomotor nerve [III]
Abducent nerve [VI]
Lateral part:
Trochlear nerve [IV]
Common trunk of the:
- frontal nerve (ophthalmic nerve [V/I])
- lacrimal nerve (ophthalmic nerve [V/I])
Orbital branch (middle meningeal artery)
Superior ophthalmic vein

Foramen rotundum
Maxillary nerve [V/2]

Foramen ovale
Mandibular nerve [V/3]
Venous plexus of foramen ovale

Foramen spinosum
Meningeal branch (mandibular nerve [V/3])
Middle meningeal artery (maxillary artery)

Sphenopetrosal fissure and foramen lacerum
Lesser petrosal nerve (glossopharyngeal nerve [IX])
Greater petrosal nerve (facial nerve [VII])
Deep petrosal nerve (internal carotid plexus)

External opening of carotid canal → carotid canal
Internal carotid artery, petrosal part
Internal carotid venous plexus
Internal carotid plexus (sympathetic trunk, superior cervical ganglion)

Pore → internal acoustic meatus
Facial nerve [VII]
Vestibulocochlear nerve [VIII]
Labyrinthine artery (basilar artery)
Labyrinthine veins

Jugular foramen
Anterior part:
Inferior petrosal sinus
Glossopharyngeal nerve [IX]
Posterior part:
Posterior meningeal artery (ascending pharyngeal artery)
Sigmoid sinus (superior bulb of jugular vein)
Vagus nerve [X]
Accessory nerve [XI]
Meningeal nerve (vagus nerve [X])

Hypoglossal canal
Hypoglossal nerve [XII]
Venous plexus of hypoglossal canal

Condylar canal
Condylar emissary vein

Foramen magnum
Meninges
Internal vertebral venous plexus (marginal sinus)
Vertebral arteries (subclavian arteries)
Anterior spinal artery (vertebral arteries)
Medulla oblongata/spinal cord
Spinal roots (accessory nerve [XI])

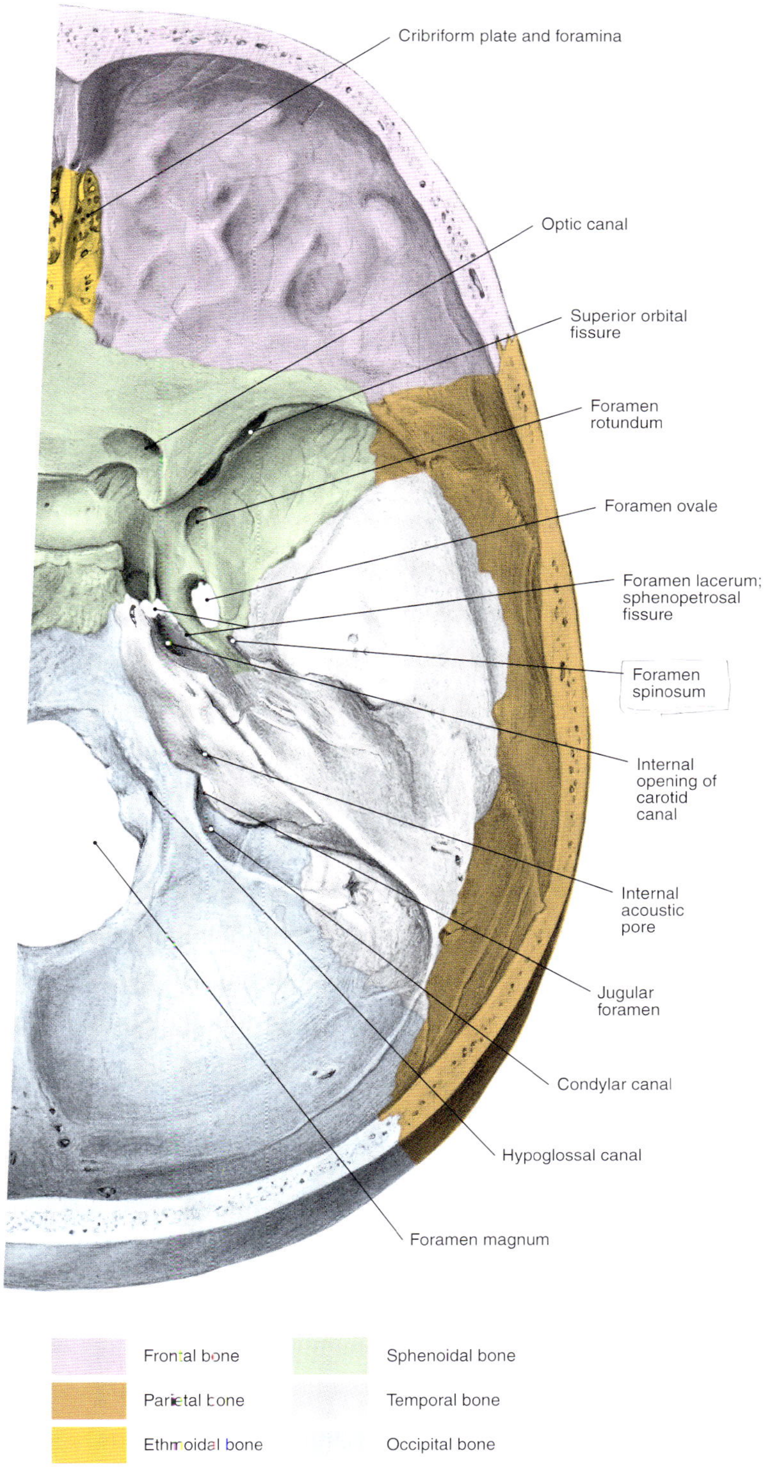

Fig. 1173 Internal surface of the cranial base and foramina.

Cranial nerves, overview

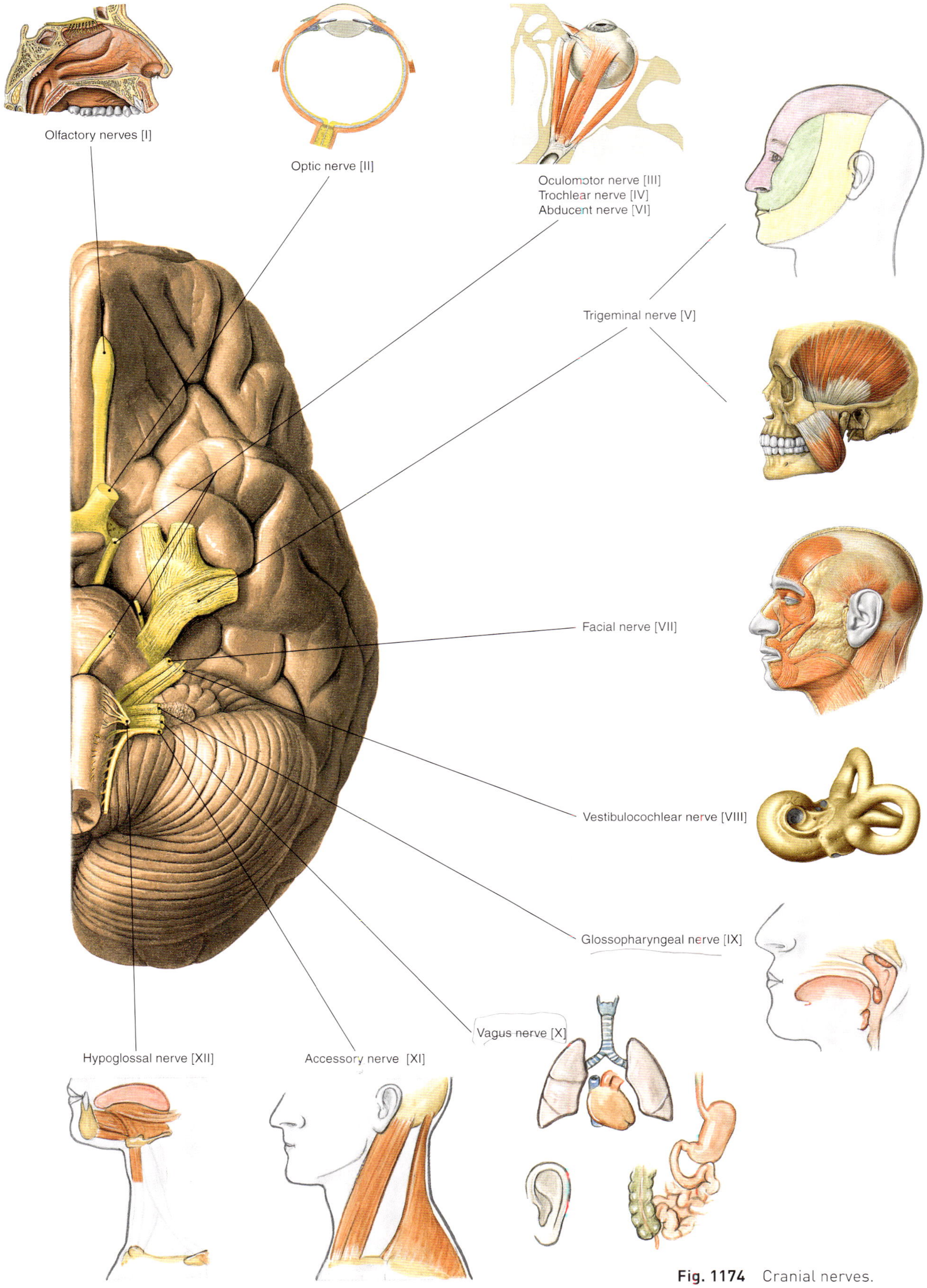

Fig. 1174 Cranial nerves.

→ T 55, T 57

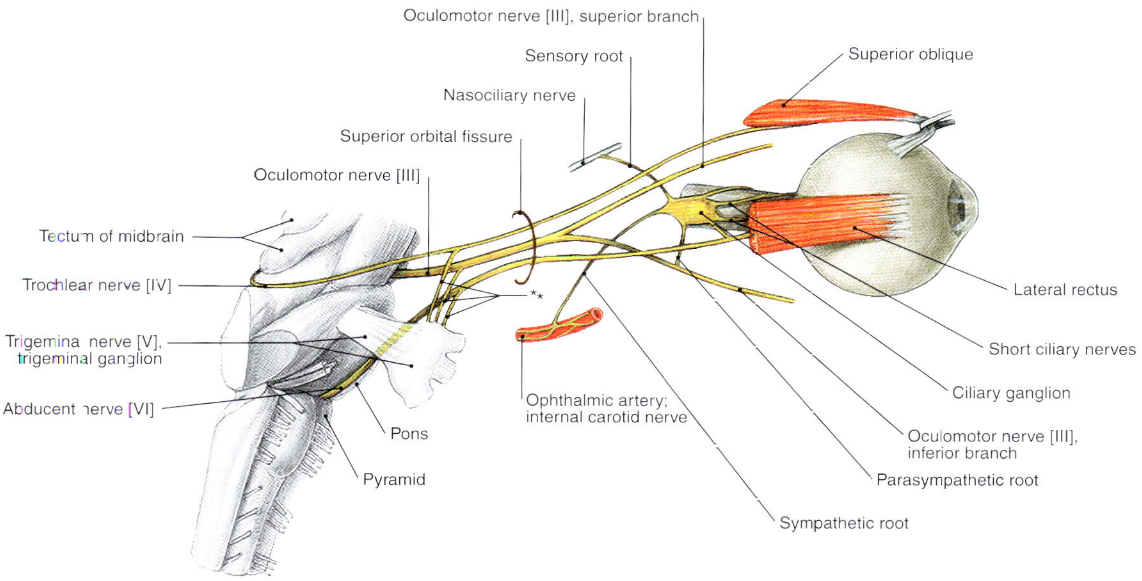

Fig. 1175 Oculomotor nerve [III], trochlear nerve [IV] and abducent nerve [VI]; viewed from the right.

→ T 57 c, d, f

* Connections to the trigeminal ganglion

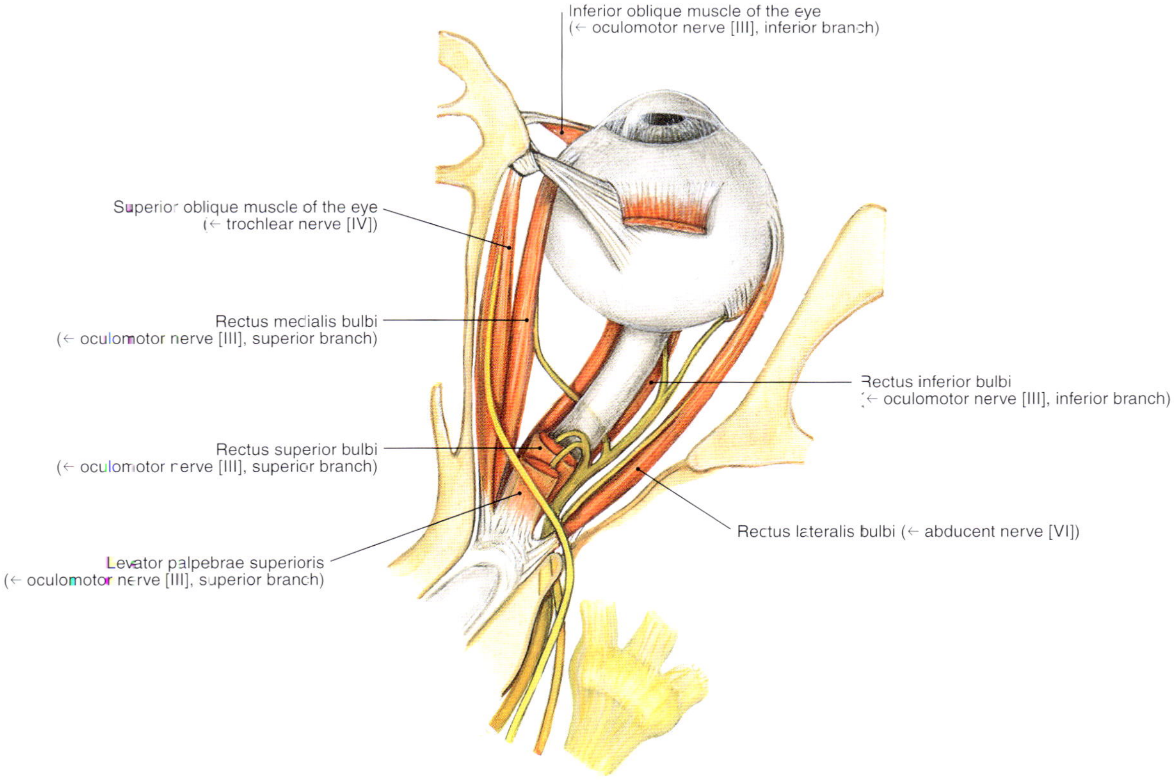

Fig. 1176 Innervation of the ocular muscles; superior view.

Cranial nerves

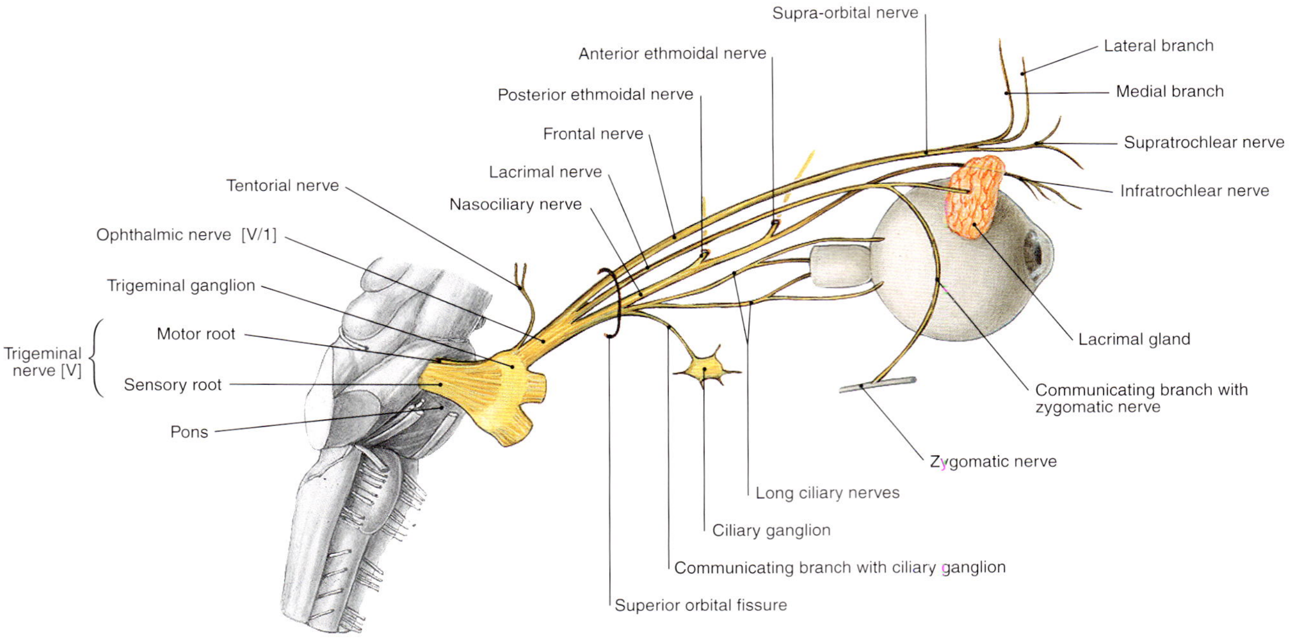

→ T 57 e

Fig. 1177 Ophthalmic nerve [V/1]; viewed from the right.

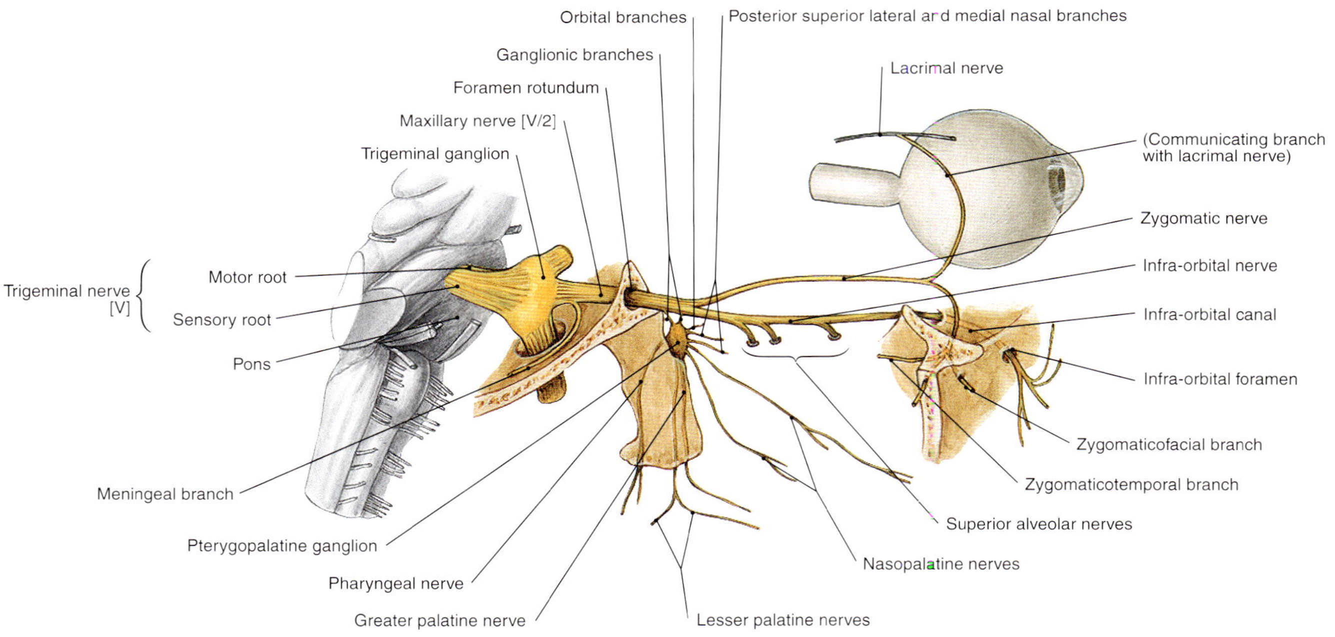

→ T 57 e

Fig. 1178 Maxillary nerve [V/2]; viewed from the right.

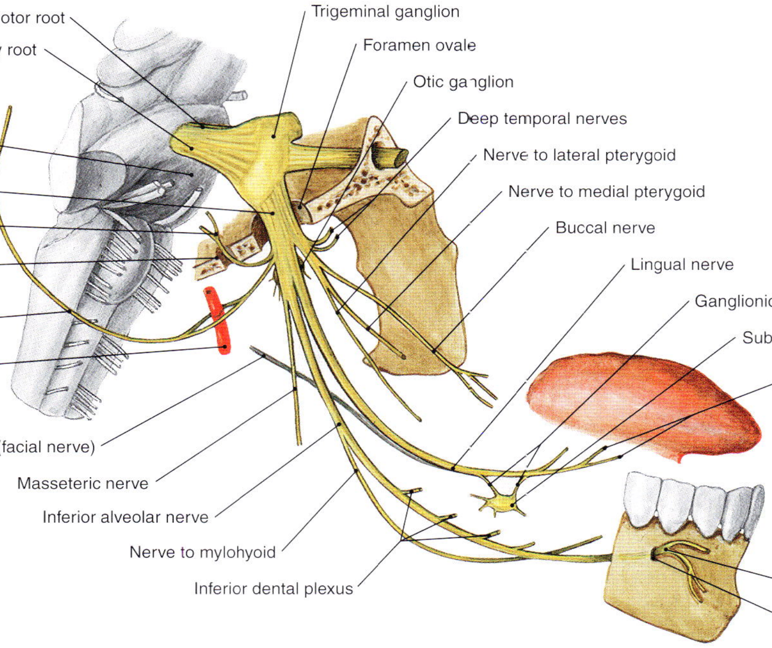

Fig. 1179 Mandibular nerve [V/3]; viewed from the right.

→ T 57 e

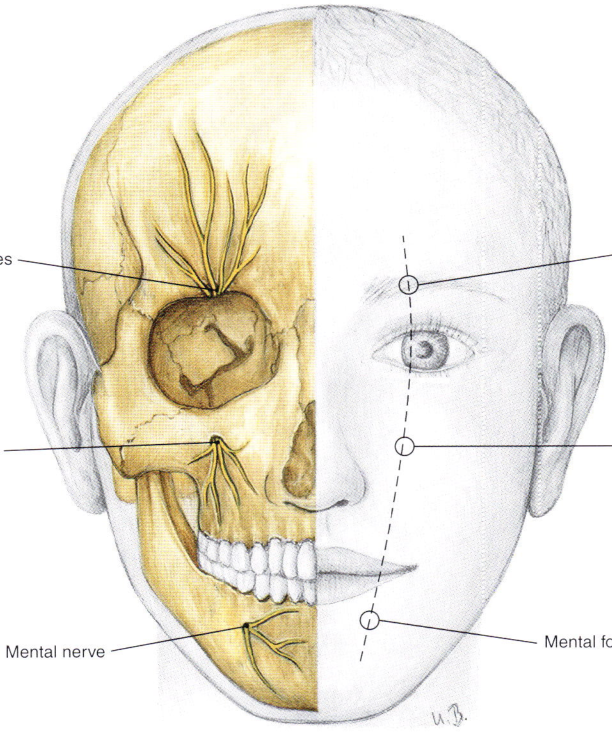

Fig. 1180 Exit points of the cutaneous branches of the trigeminal nerve [V]. Clinically, they are referred to as nerve exit points.

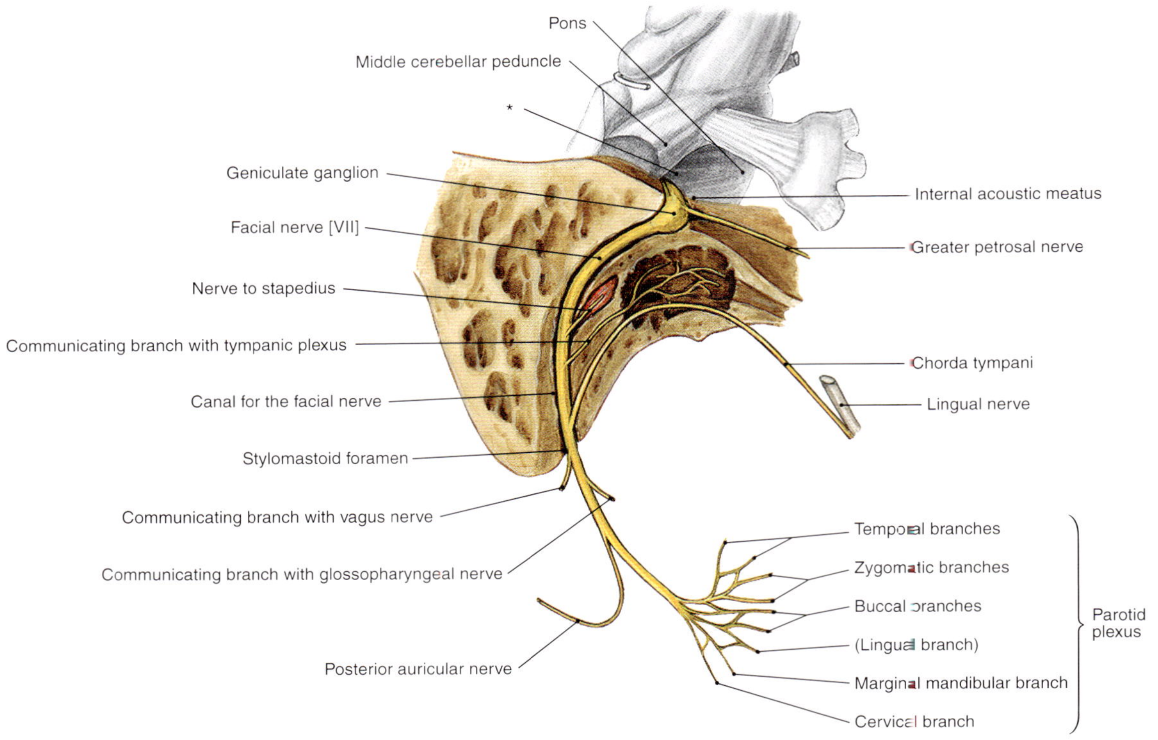

→ T 57 g

Fig. 1181 Facial nerve [VII];
the facial canal and the tympanic cavity have been opened;
viewed from the right.

* Clinical term: cerebellopontine angle

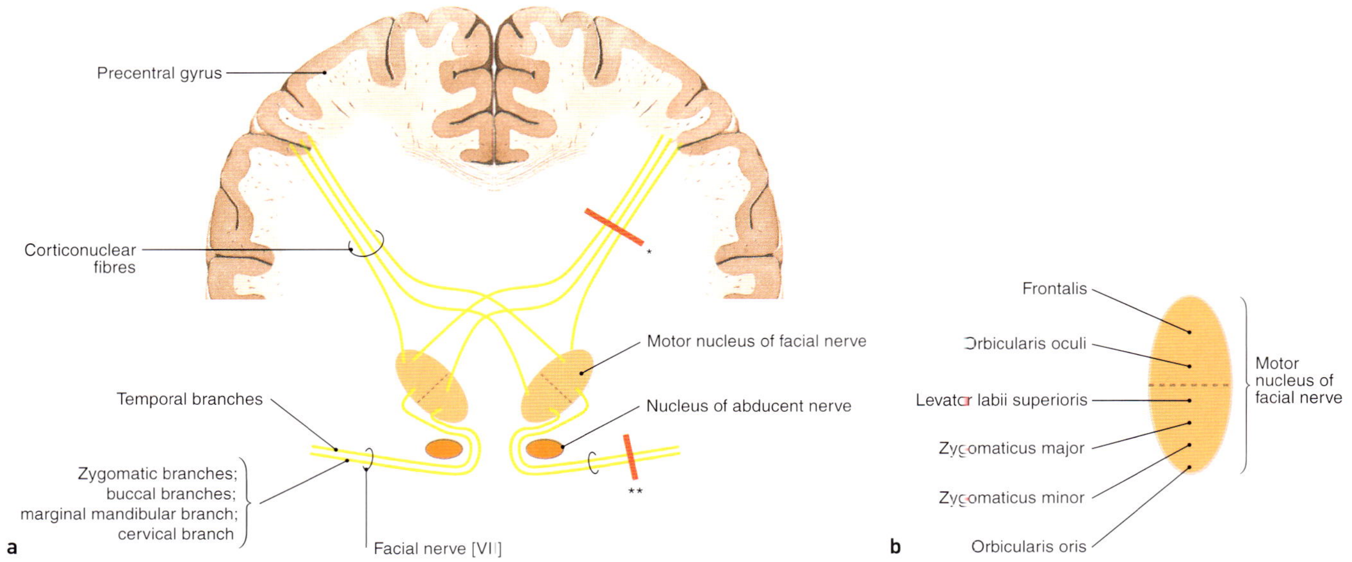

Fig. 1182 a, b Neuronal structure of the motor part of the facial nerve [VII].

a Overview

b Representation of the facial muscles in the motor nucleus of the facial nerve

Though the nuclei of the upper facial muscles receive innervation from both hemispheres, those of the lower facial muscles are only innervated from the contralateral side. Therefore, patients with central palsy (*) are still able to frown the brow and to close the eyelids just sufficiently. However, in patients with peripheral palsy (**) all facial muscles are paralyzed.

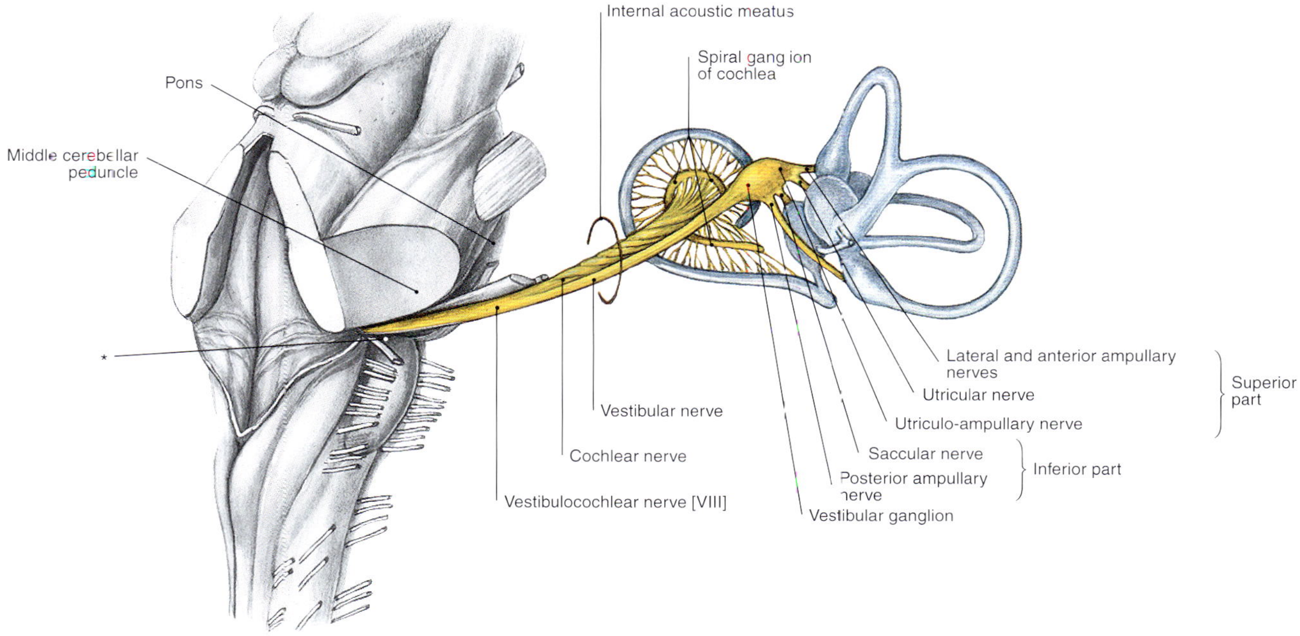

Fig. 1183 Vestibulocochlear nerve [VIII]; the membranous labyrinth is greatly enlarged; posterior view from the right.

* Clinical term: cerebellopontine angle

→ T 57 h

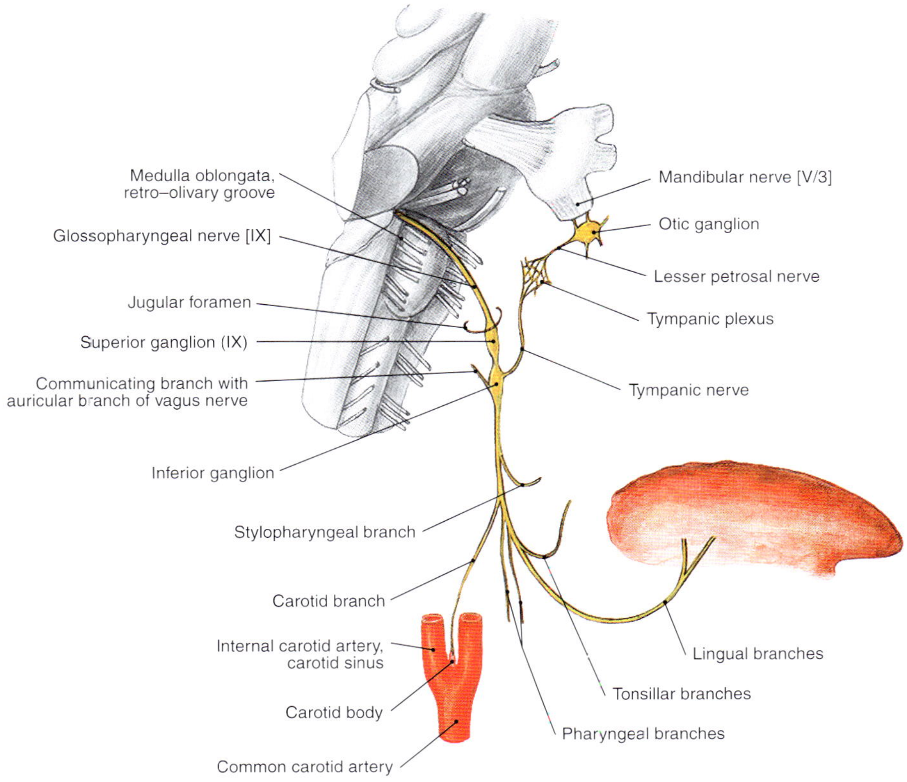

Fig. 1184 Glossopharyngeal nerve [IX]; viewed from the right.

→ T 57 i

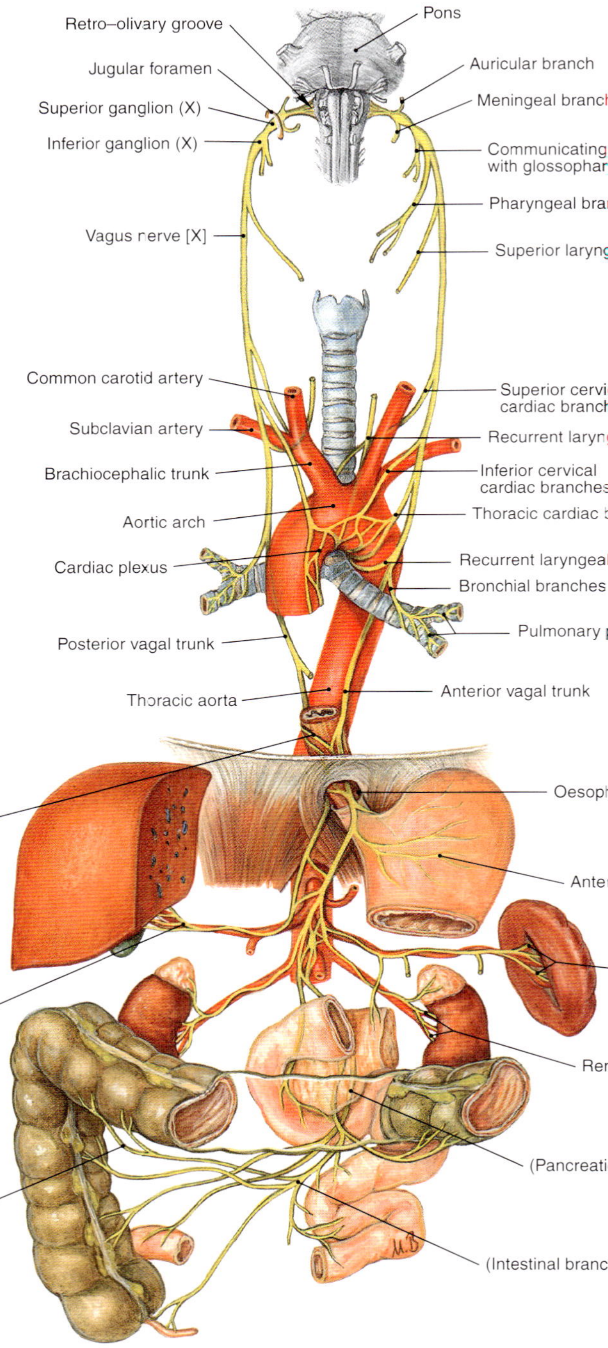

→ T 57 j

Fig. 1185 Vagus nerve [X];
both nerves;
semi-schematic;
anterior view.

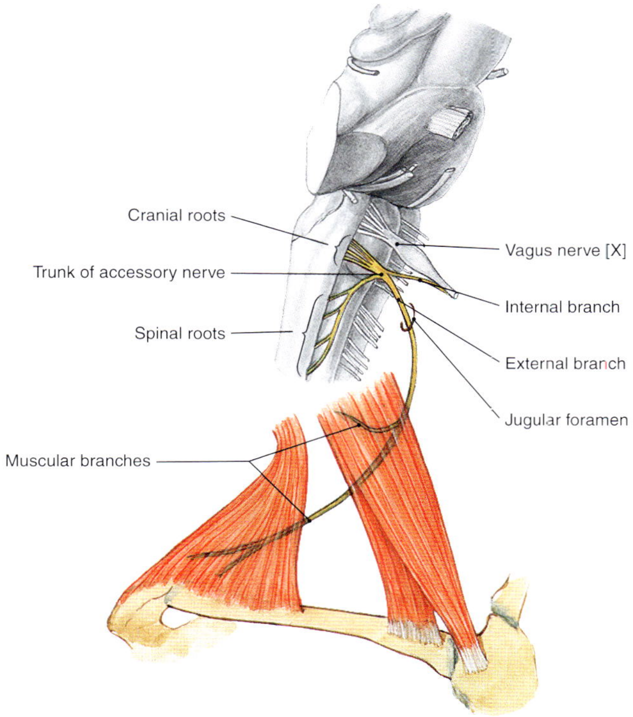

Fig. 1186 Accessory nerve [XI];
viewed from the right.

→ T 57 k

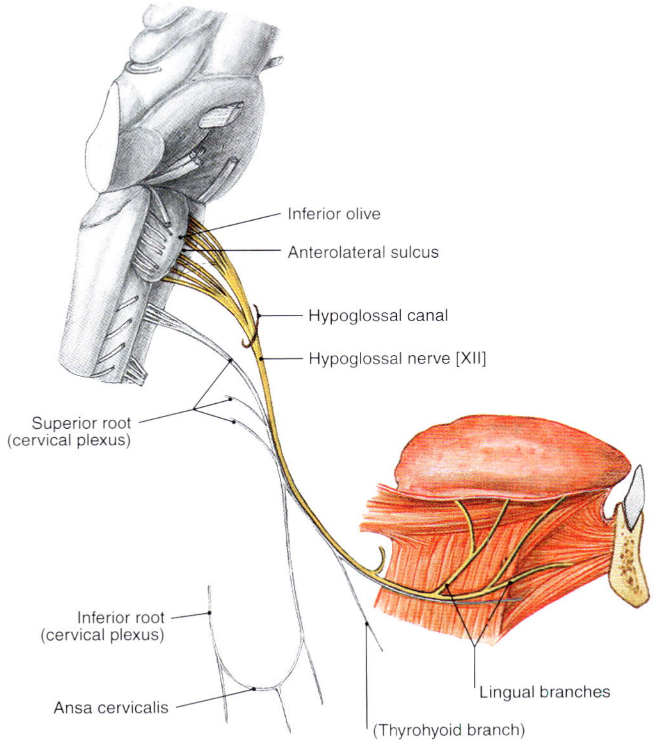

Fig. 1187 Hypoglossal nerve [XII];
viewed from the right.

→ T 57 l

Cranial nerves

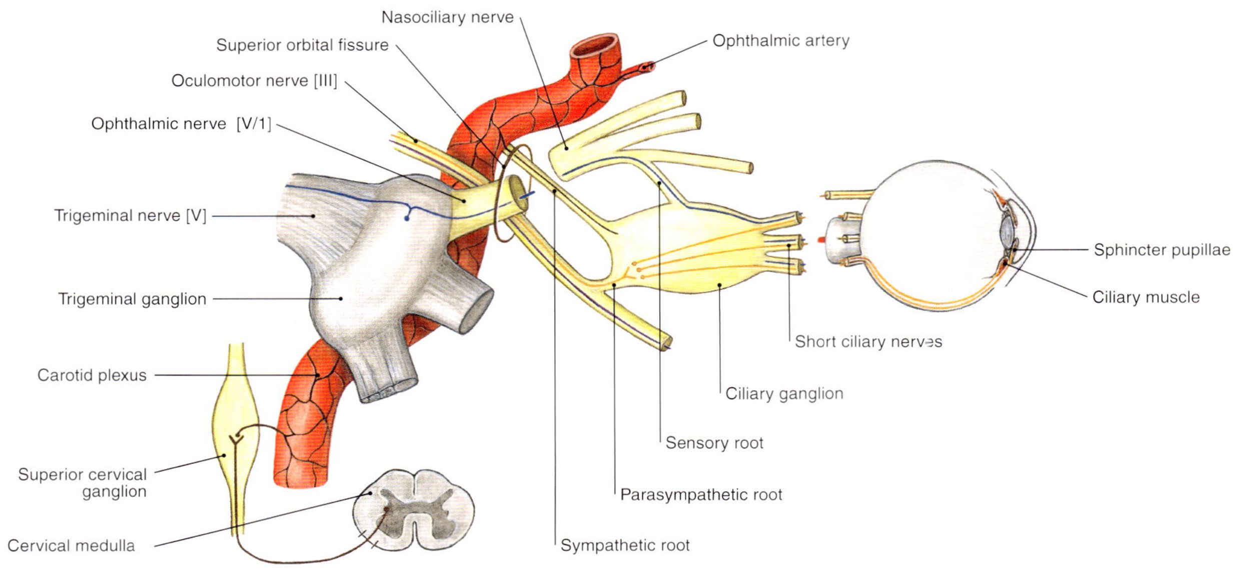

Fig. 1188 Ciliary ganglion; overview.

Nuclear region:
Accessory nucleus of the oculomotor nerve

General visceral-efferent fibres (GVE)
Specific visceral-efferent fibres (SVE)
General and specific visceral-afferent fibres (G/SVA)
General somatic-afferent fibres (GSA)
Sympathetic fibres

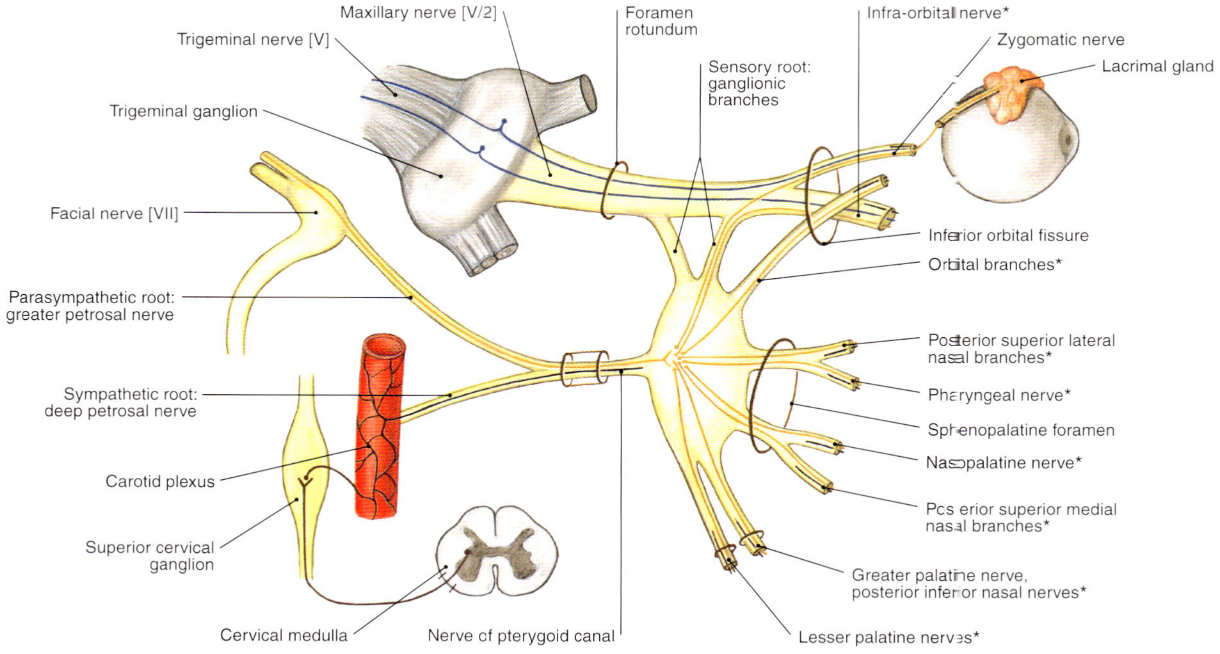

Fig. 1189 Pterygopalatine ganglion; overview.

* Innervation of the glands of the nose and the palate

Nuclear region:
Superior salivatory nucleus

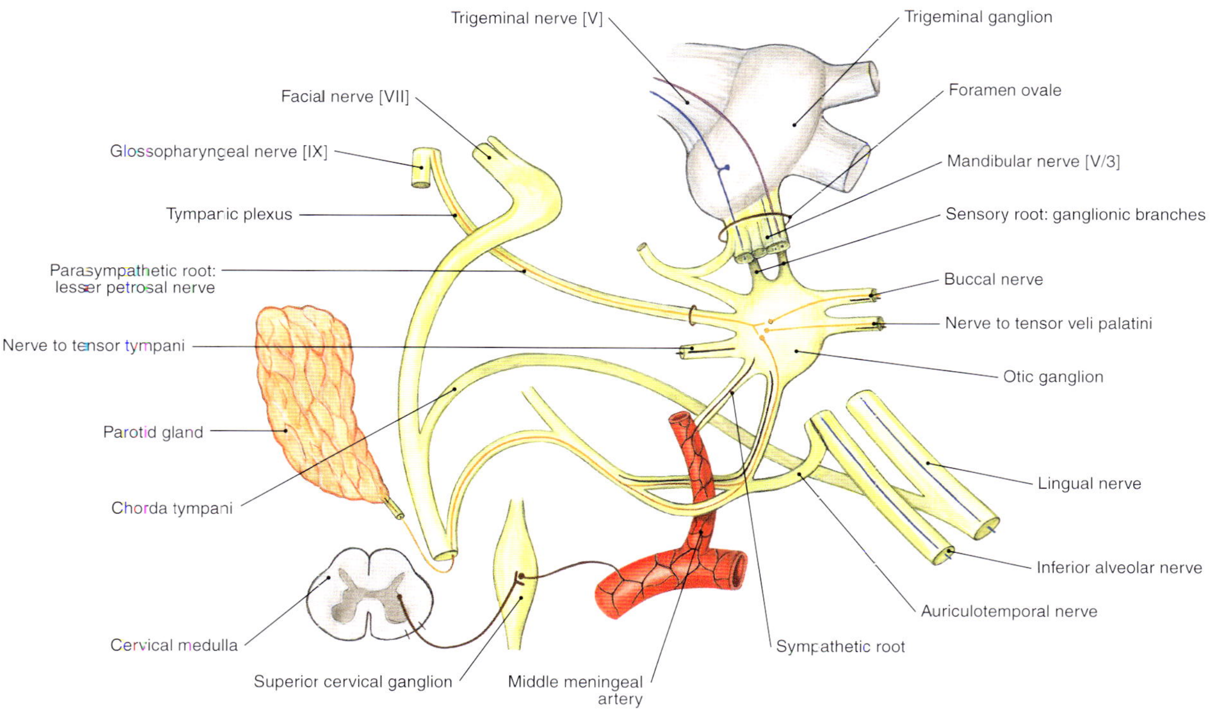

Fig. 1190 Otic ganglion; overview.

Nuclear region:
Inferior salivatory nucleus

- General visceral-efferent fibres (GVE)
- Specific visceral-efferent fibres (SVE)
- General and specific visceral-afferent fibres (G/SVA)
- General somatic-afferent fibres (GSA)
- Sympathetic fibres

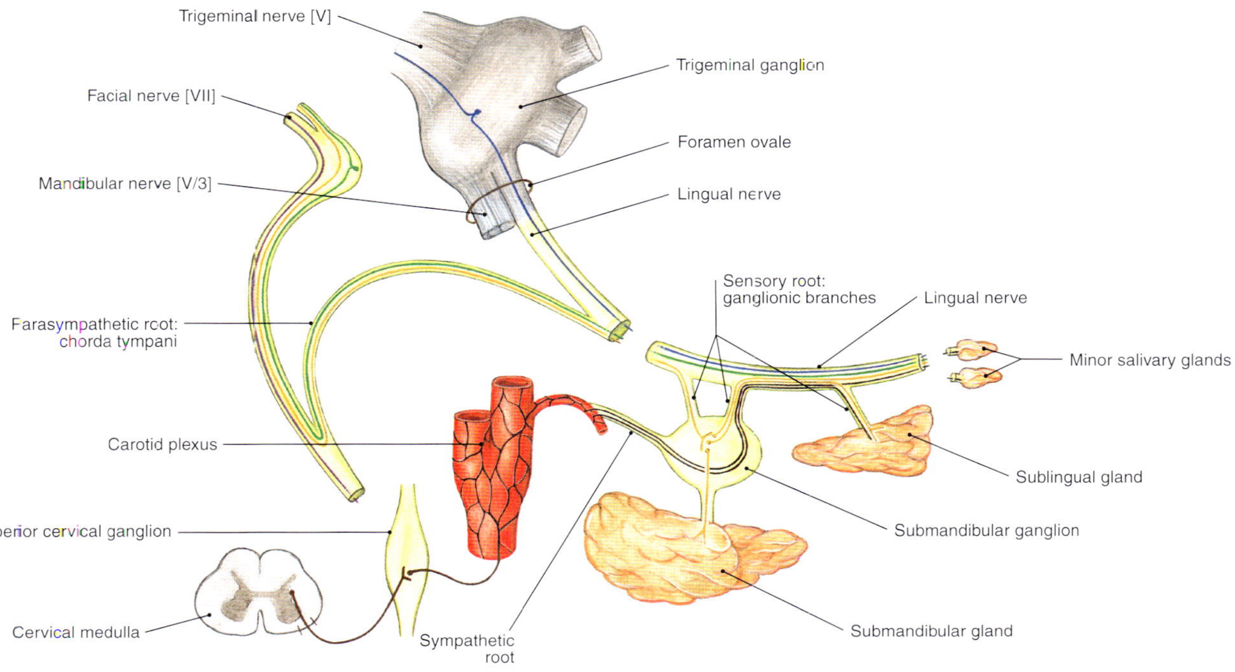

Fig. 1191 Submandibular ganglion; overview.

Nuclear region:
Superior salivatory nucleus

Cranial nerves, topography

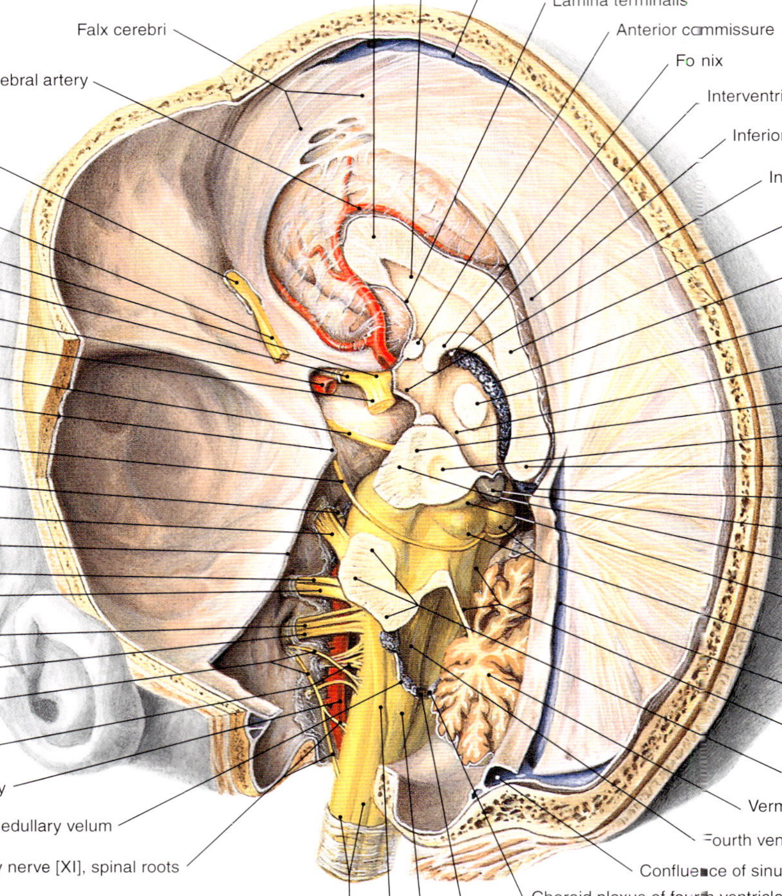

Fig. 1192 Course of the cranial nerves in the subarachnoid space; the left hemisphere of the cerebrum and the cerebellum as well as the tentorium cerebelli have been removed.

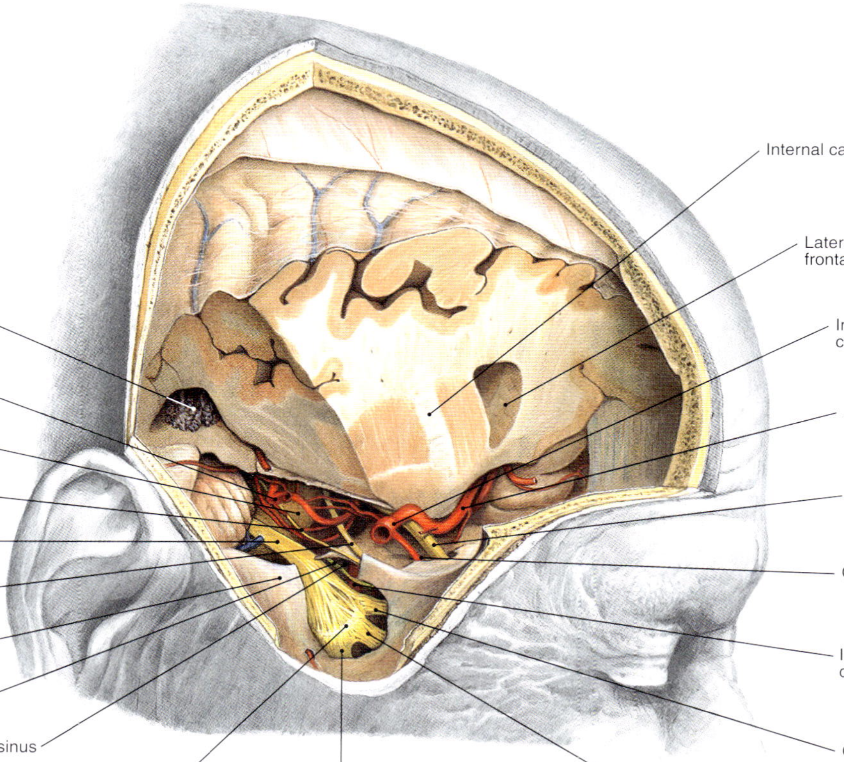

Fig. 1193 Course of the cranial nerves in the middle cranial fossa.

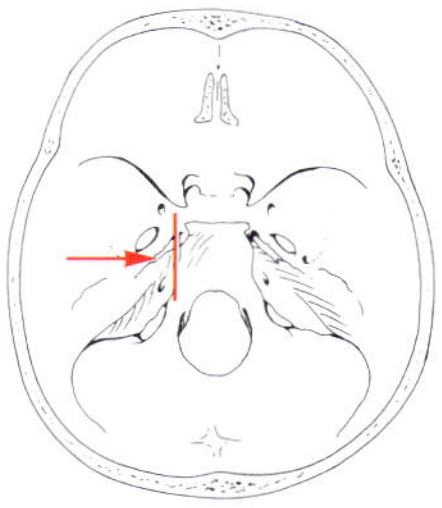

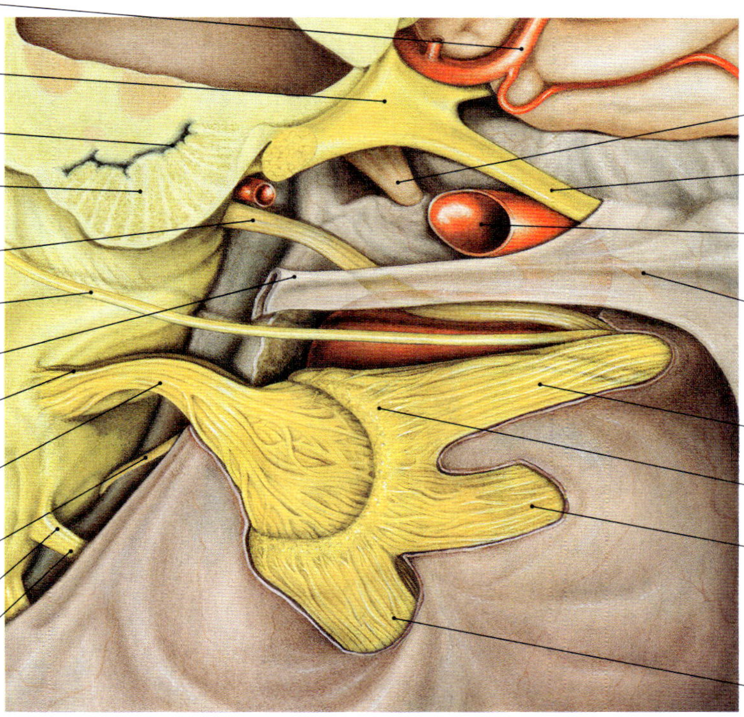

Fig. 1194 Arteries and nerves in the region of the sella turcica and the cavernous sinus.

* Clinical term: GASSERian ganglion

Vessels and nerves of the cranial base

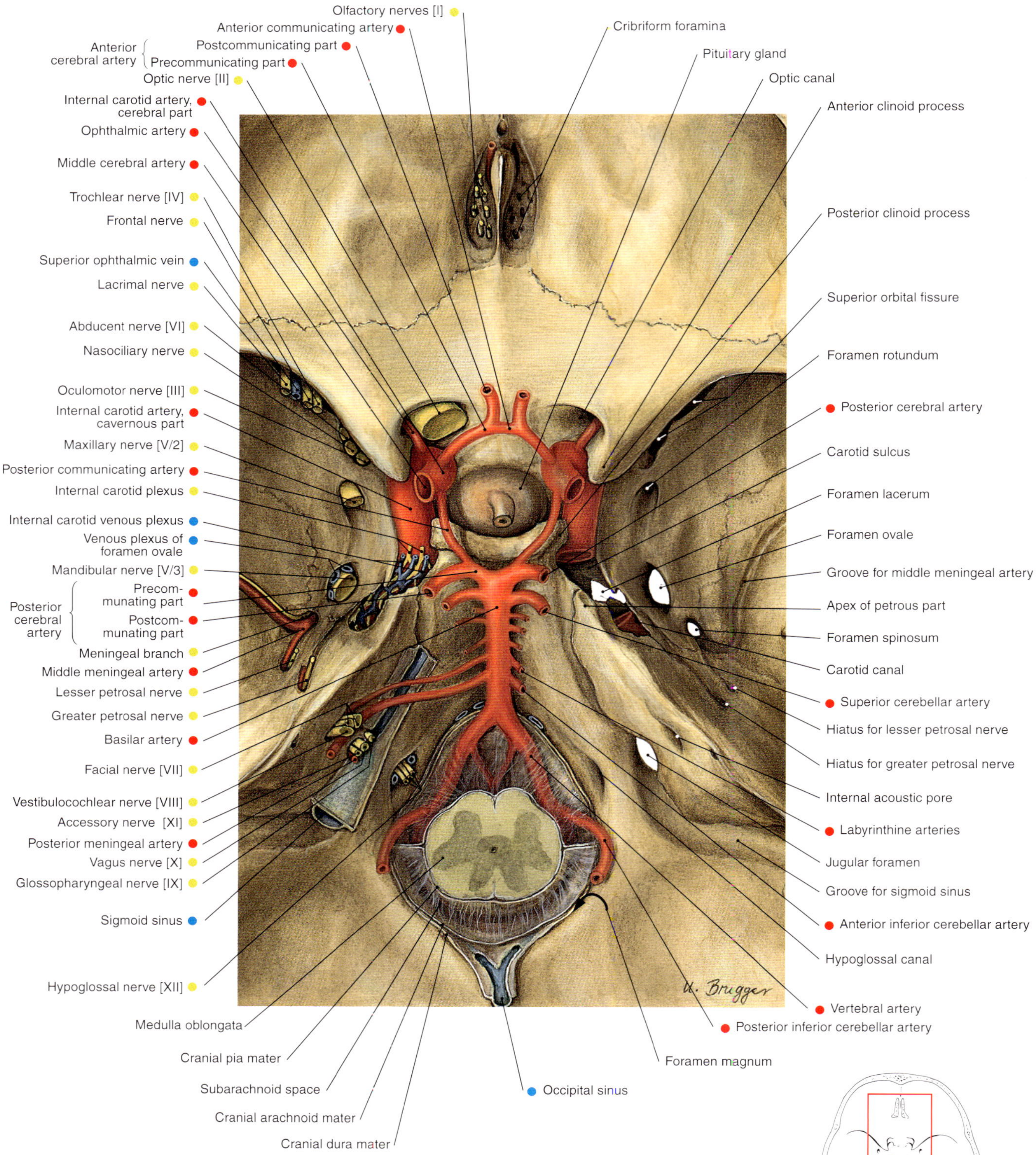

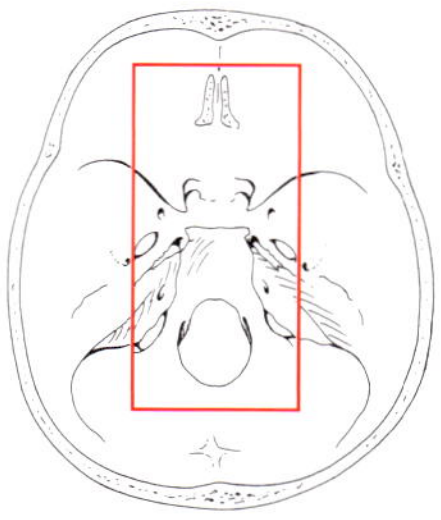

→ 1172, 1173, 1268

Fig. 1195 Passage of vessels and nerves through the internal surface of cranial base and the cerebral arterial circle; superior view.

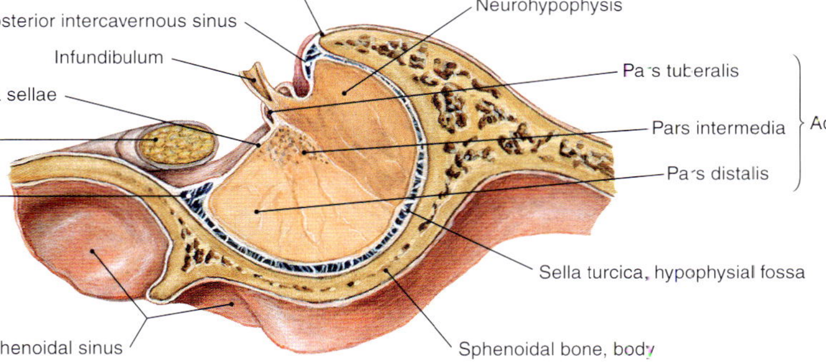

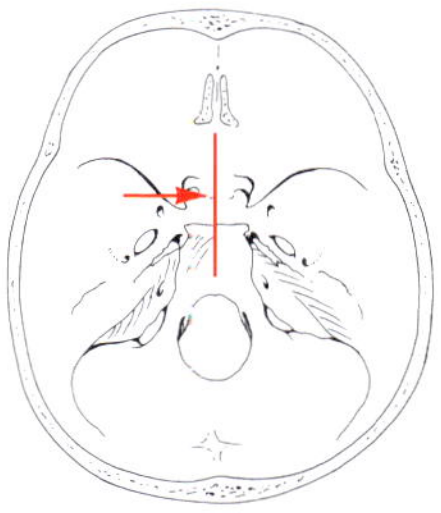

Fig. 1196 Pituitary gland.

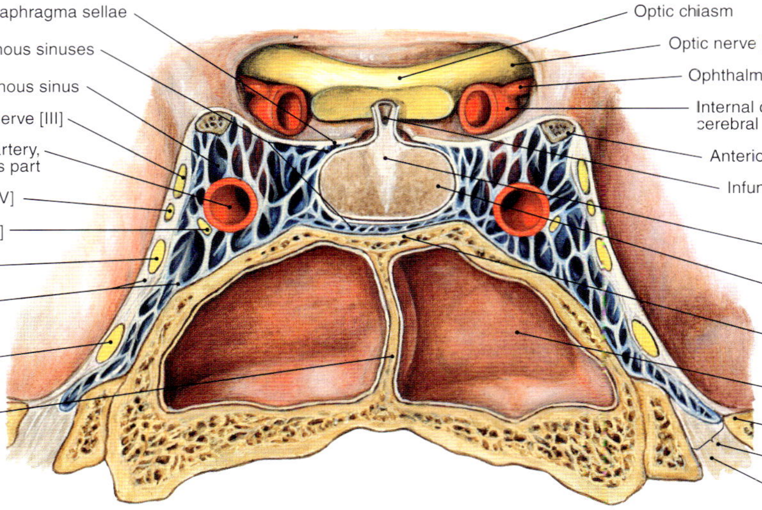

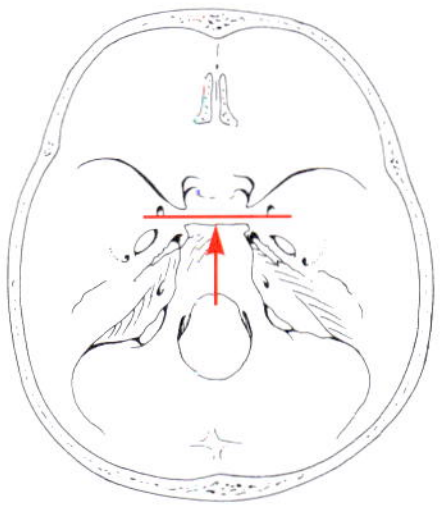

Fig. 1197 Pituitary gland and cavernous sinus.

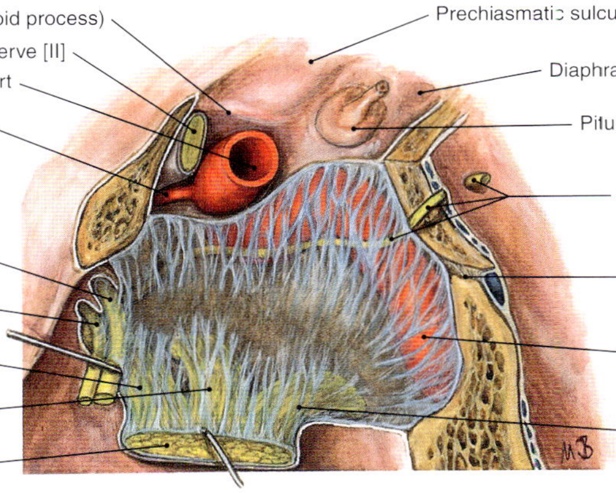

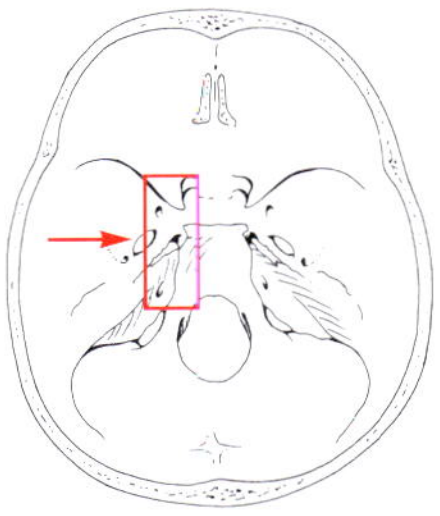

Fig. 1198 Cavernous sinus;
the part of the cranial dura mater forming the lateral wall of the cavernous sinus has been removed;
the trigeminal ganglion has been reflected to the side.

Cranial dura mater and superior sagittal sinus

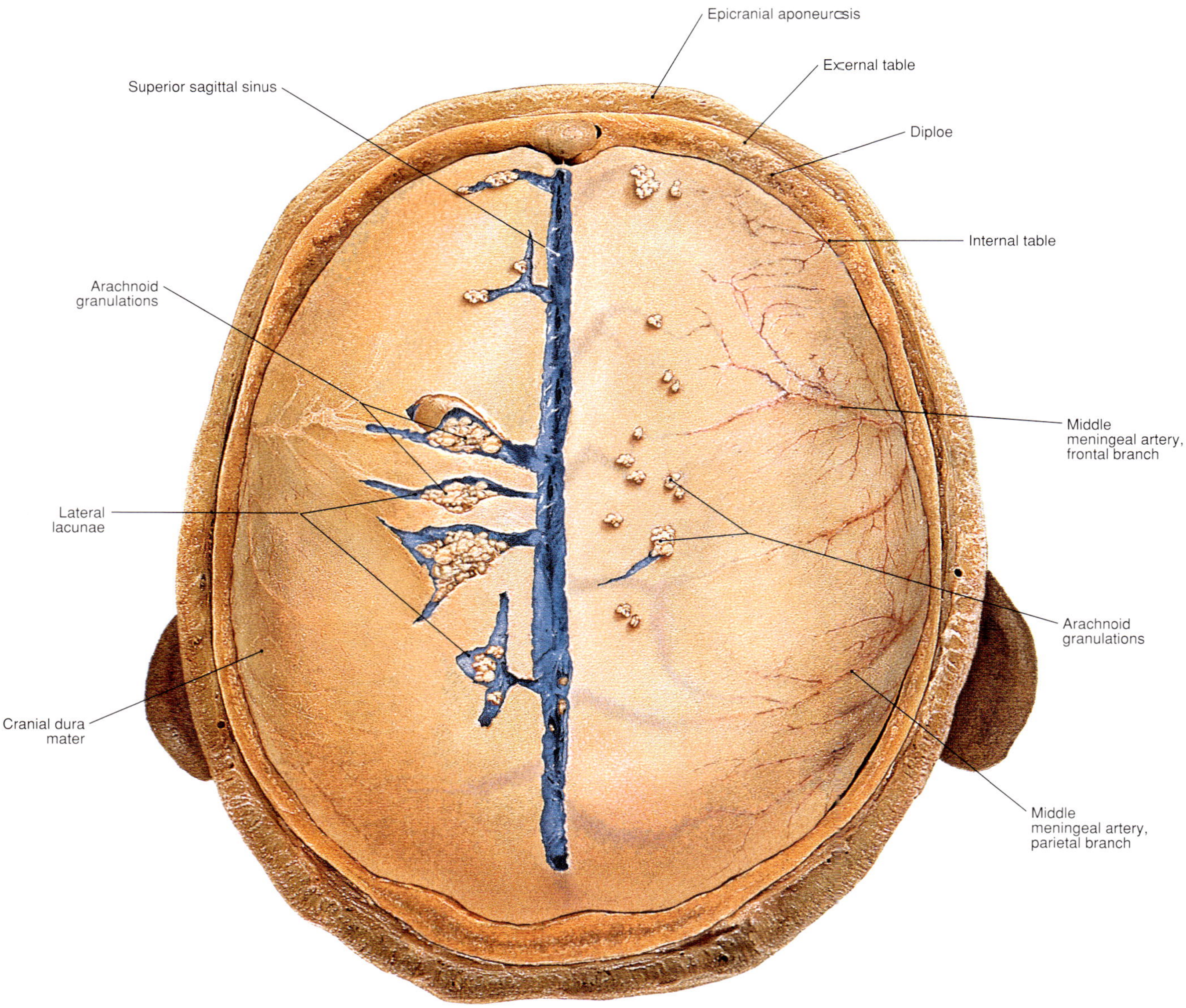

Fig. 1199 Cranial dura mater and superior sagittal sinus with some lateral lacunae.

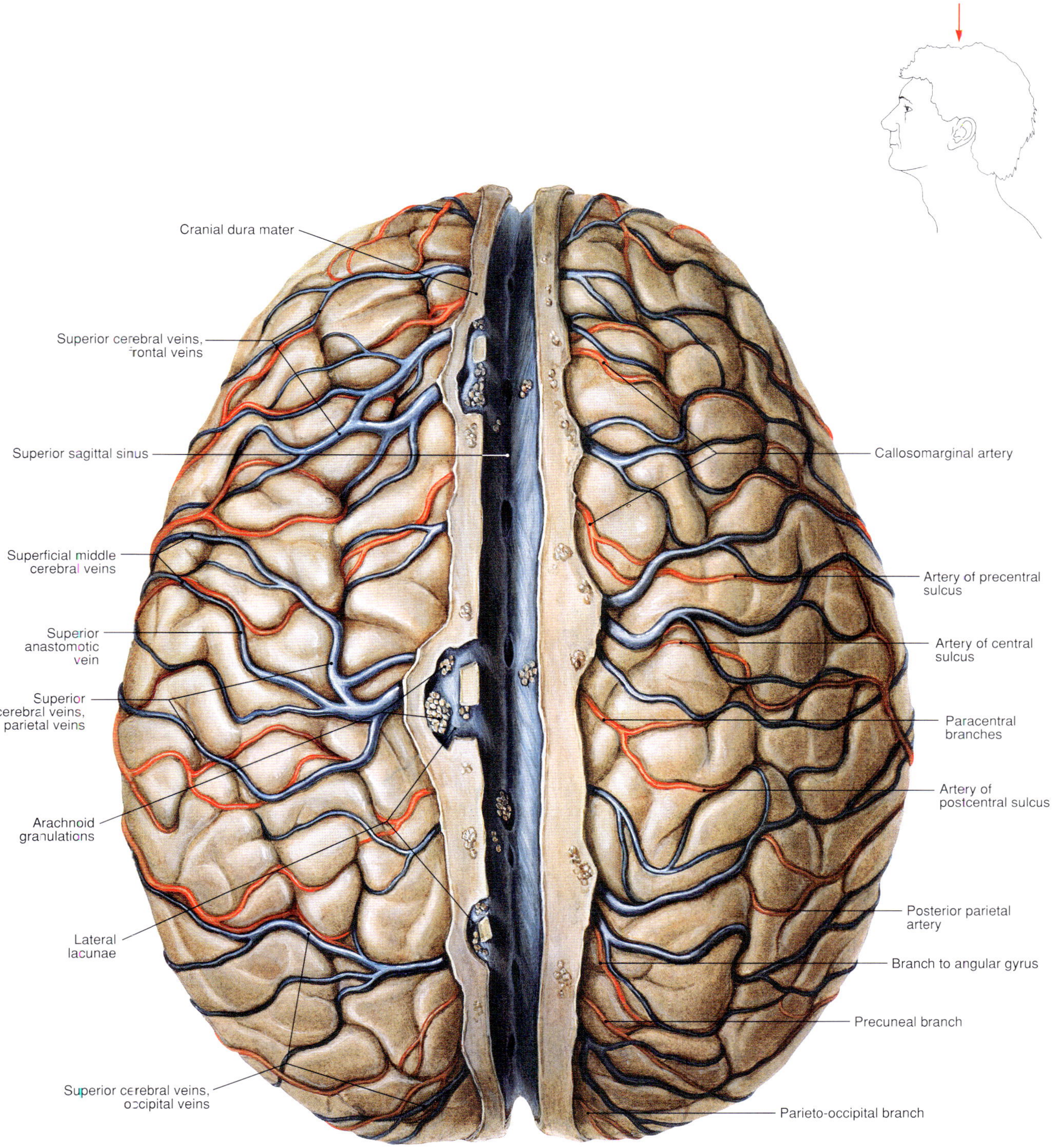

Fig. 1200 Superficial arteries and veins of the brain; the cranial dura mater has been removed and the superior sagittal sinus has been sectioned; after removal of the cranial arachnoid mater.

Cranial arachnoid mater

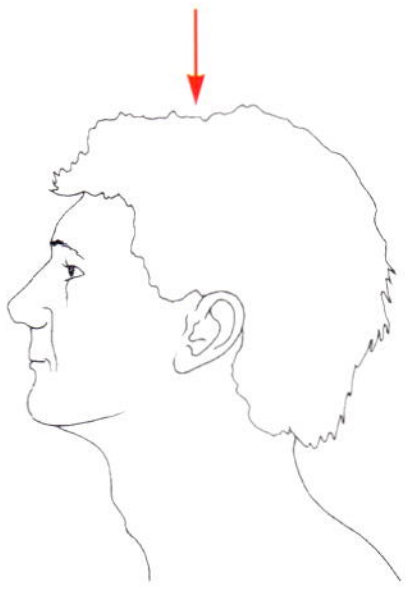

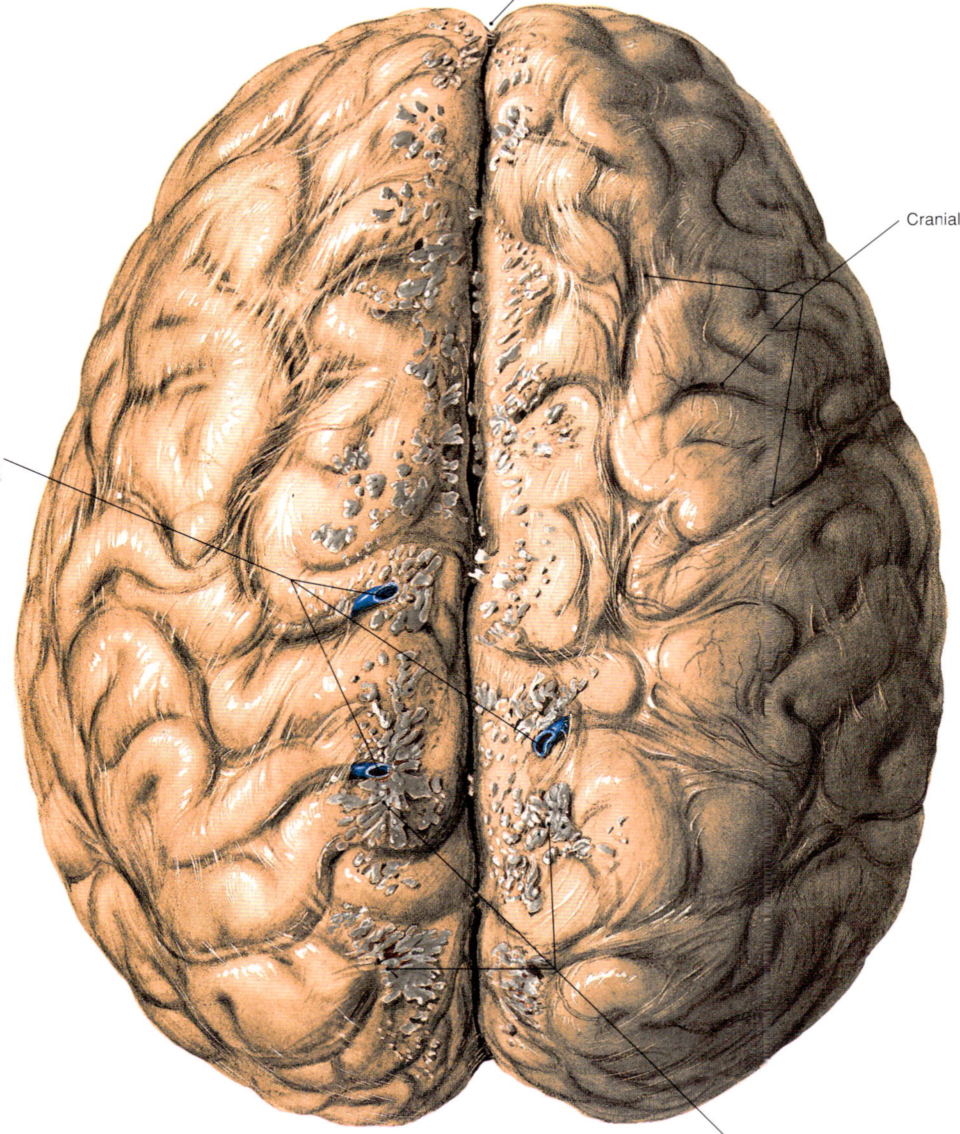

Fig. 1201 Brain with cranial arachnoid mater; superior view.

* Also: PACCHIONIan granulations

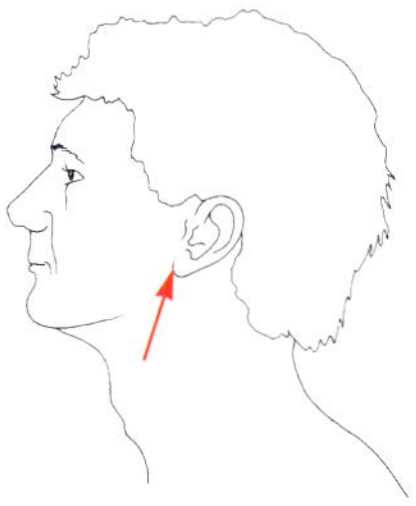

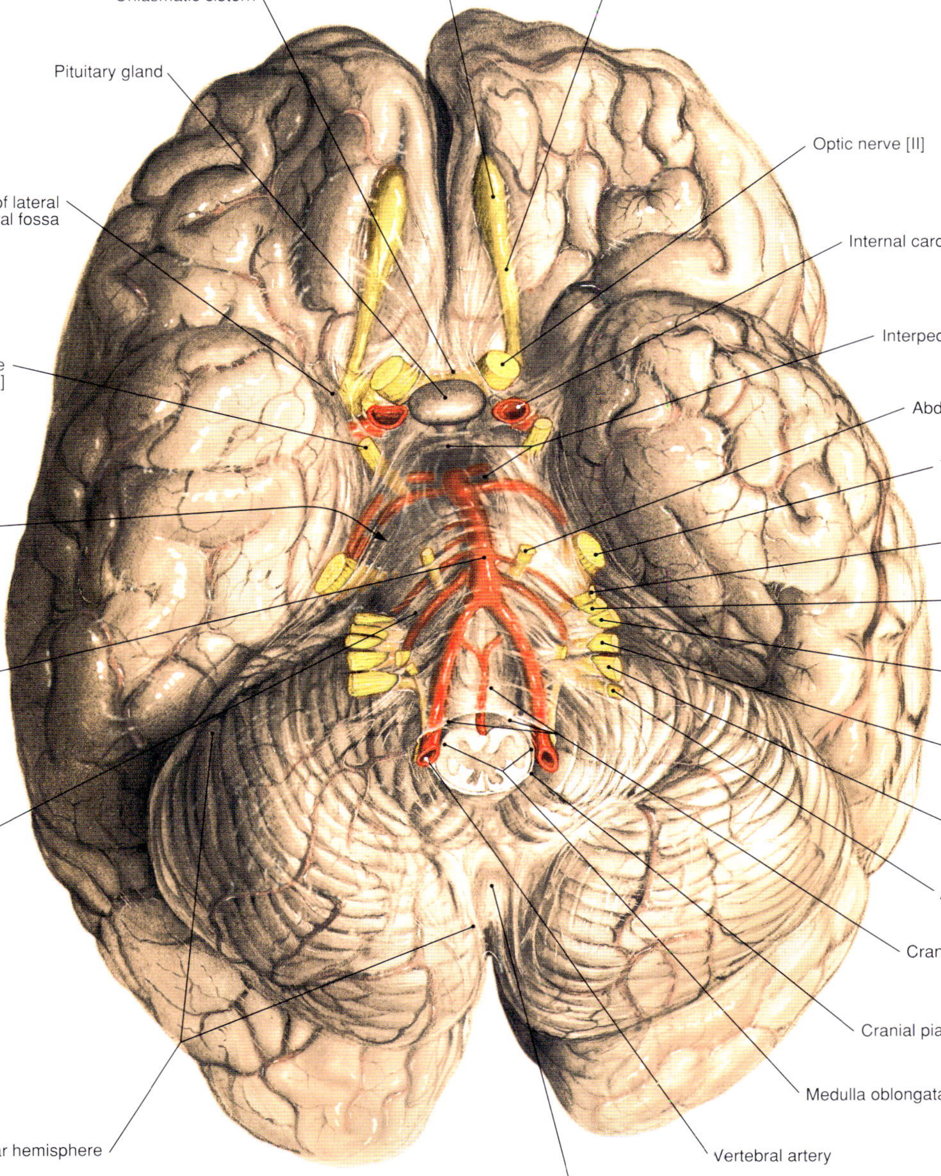

Fig. 1202 Brain with cranial arachnoid mater.

Organisation of the brain

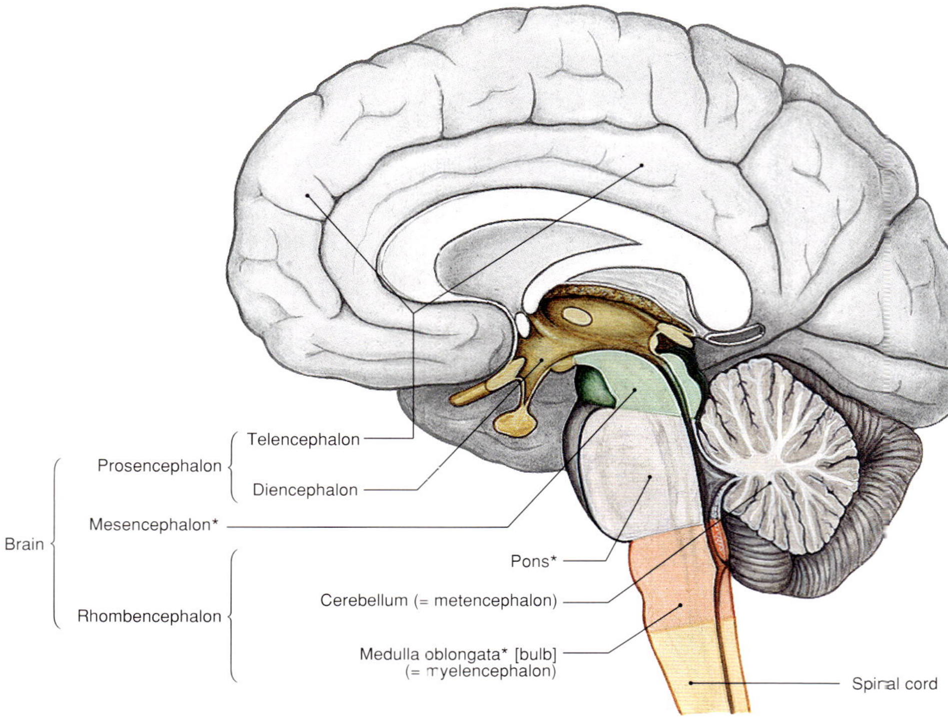

Fig. 1203 Organisation of the central nervous system; median section; schema.
Parts marked with * together form the brainstem.

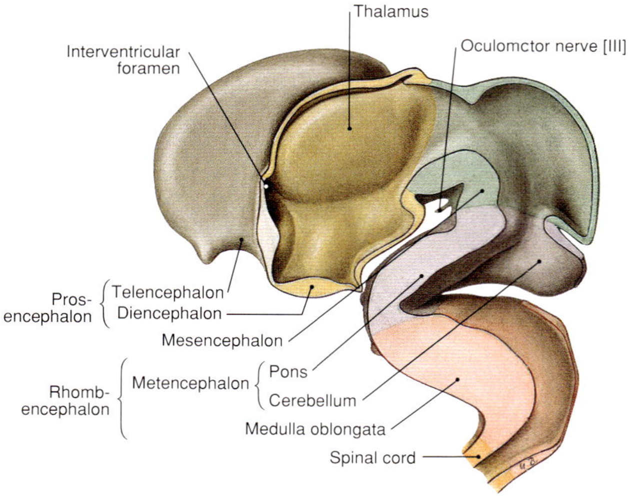

Fig. 1204 Development of the brain; model of the brain of an approx. 2-month-old embryo; median section.

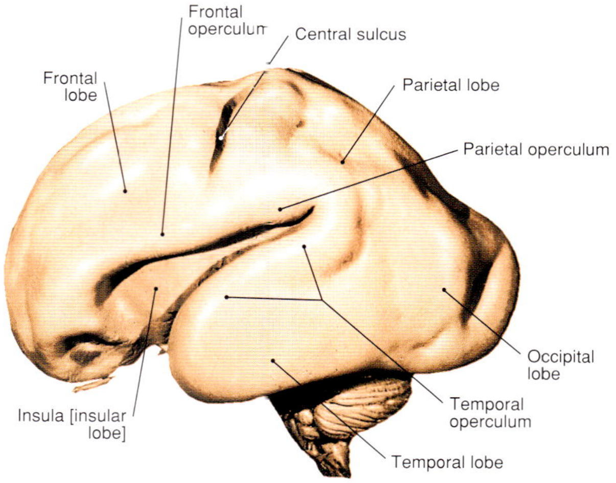

Fig. 1205 Development of the brain; brain of an approx. 4-month-old foetus (crown-rump length 20 cm); viewed from the left.

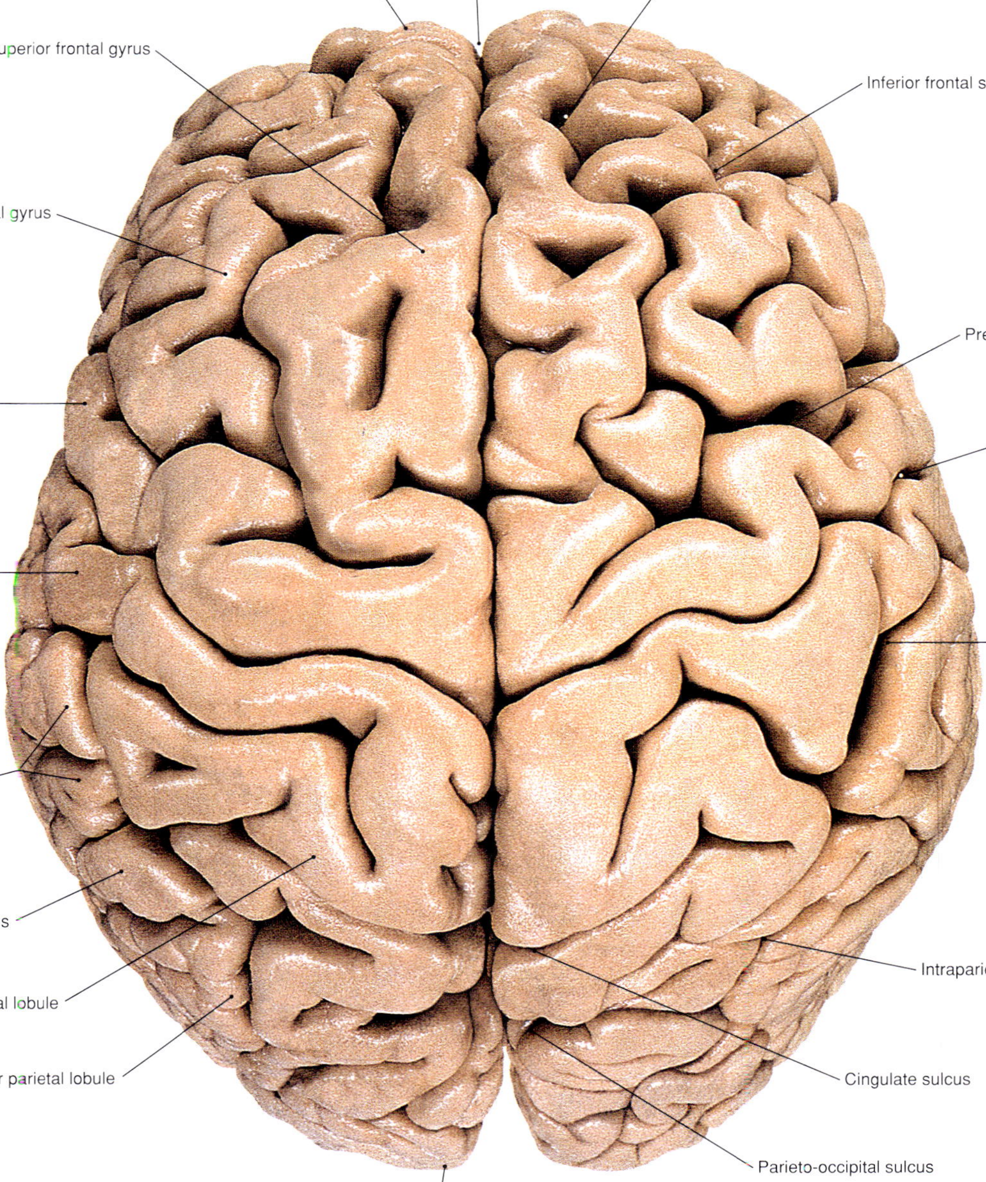

Fig. 1206 Cerebrum;
after removal of the cranial arachnoid mater;
superior view.
Formation of the gyri varies considerably.

Base of the brain

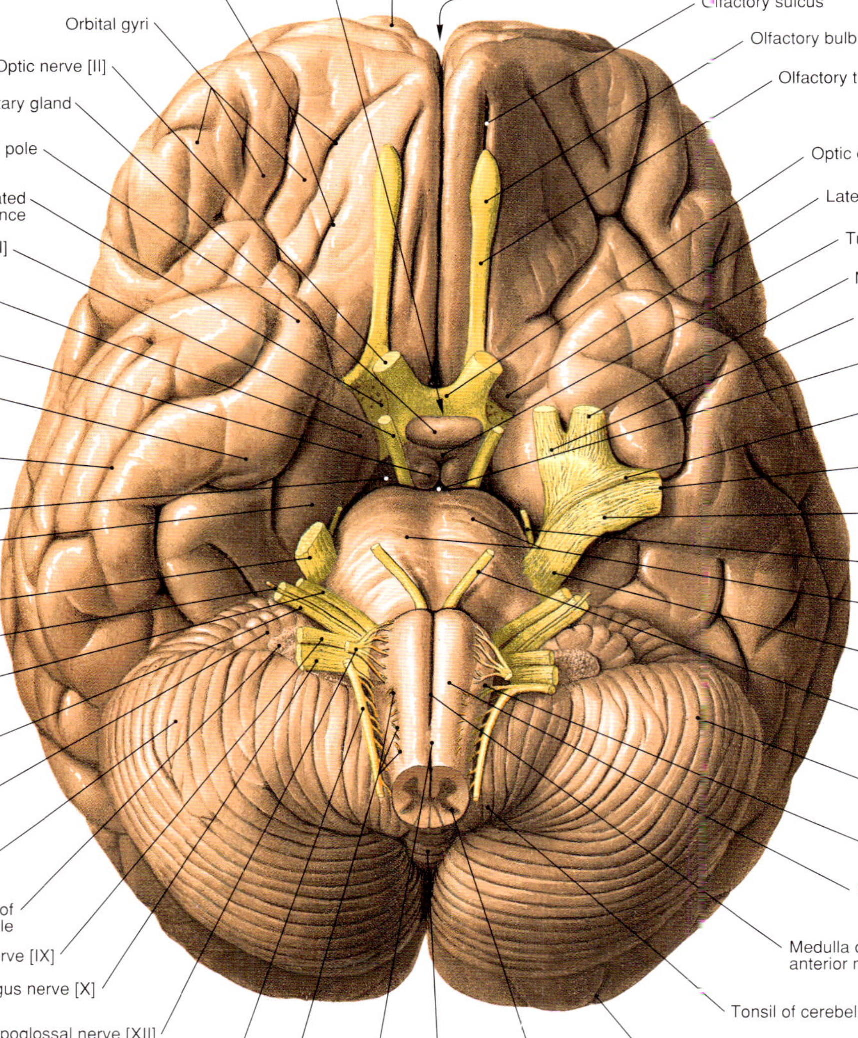

Fig. 1207 Cerebrum;
brainstem with cerebellum as well as cranial nerves;
inferior view.

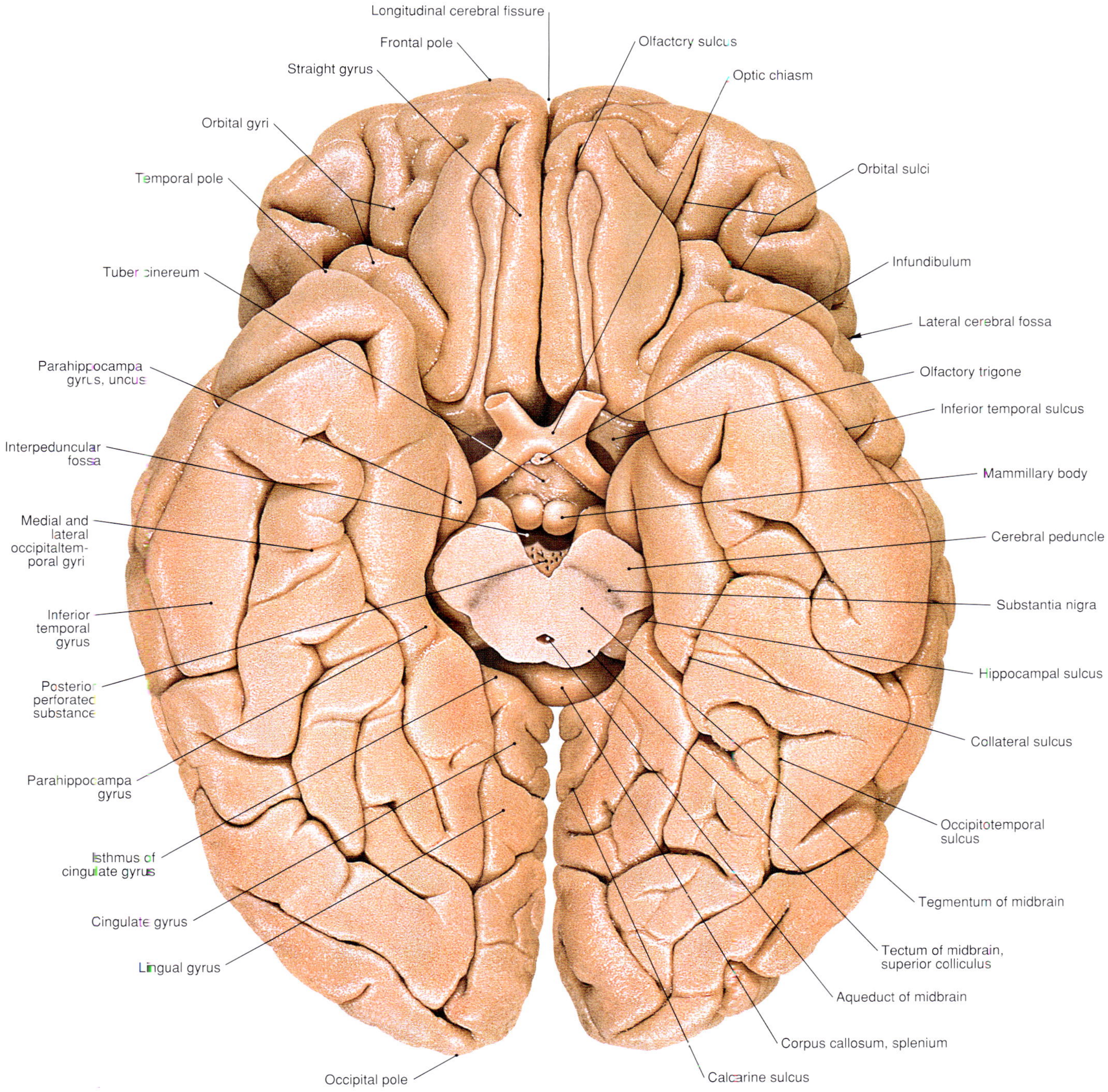

Fig. 1208 Gyri and grooves of the cerebral hemispheres; the midbrain has been sectioned.

Lobes of the telencephalon

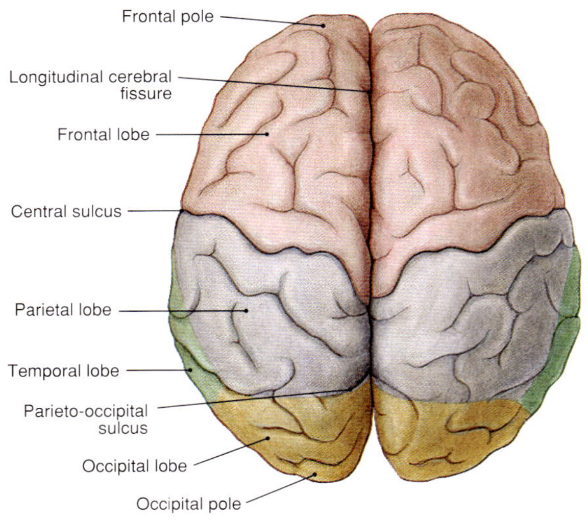

Fig. 1209 Lobes of the cerebrum; superior view.

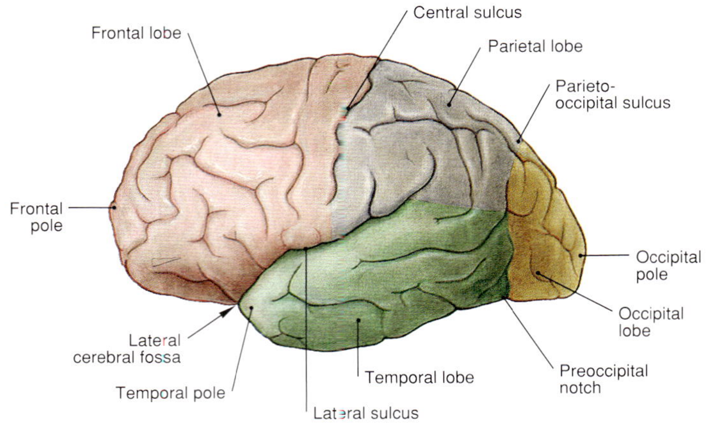

Fig. 1210 Lobes of the cerebrum; viewed from the left.

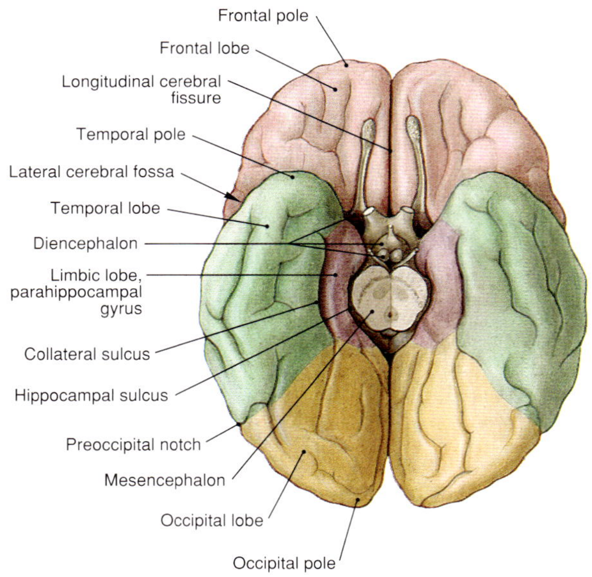

Fig. 1211 Lobes of the cerebrum; inferior view.

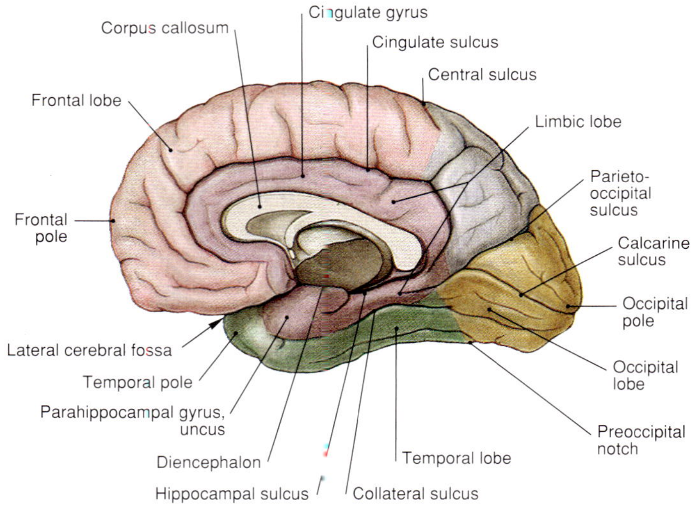

Fig. 1212 Lobes of the cerebrum; medial view.

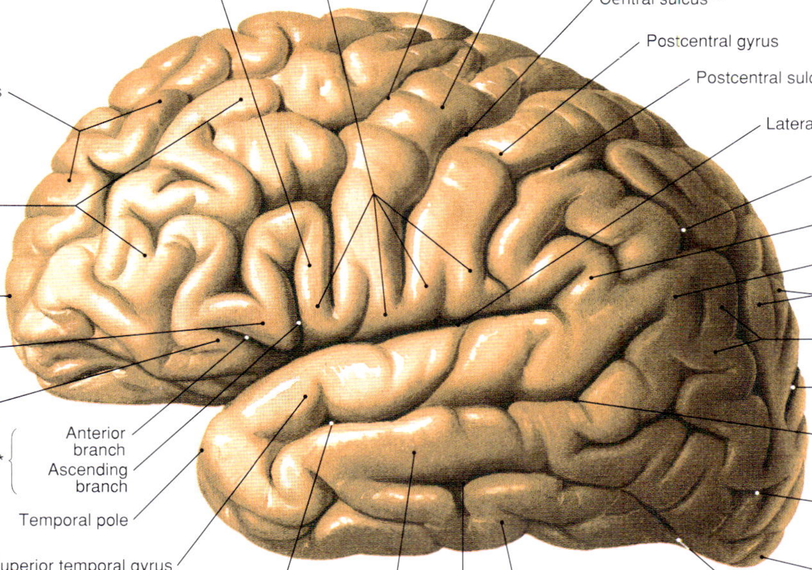

Fig. 1213 Gyri and grooves of the cerebral hemispheres;
viewed from the left.

* Sulcus of SYLVIUS
** Sulcus of ROLANDO

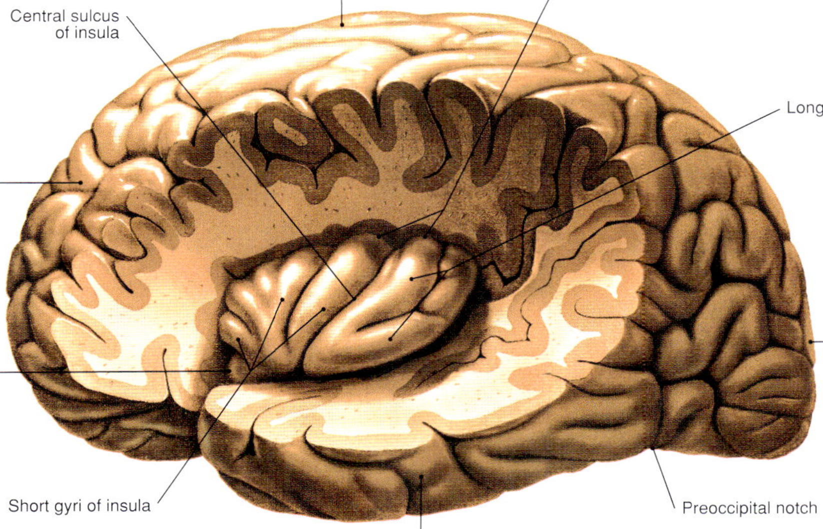

Fig. 1214 Gyri and grooves of the cerebral hemispheres;
exposure of the insula after removal of the frontal, parietal and temporal opercula;
viewed from the left.

Gyri of the cerebral hemispheres

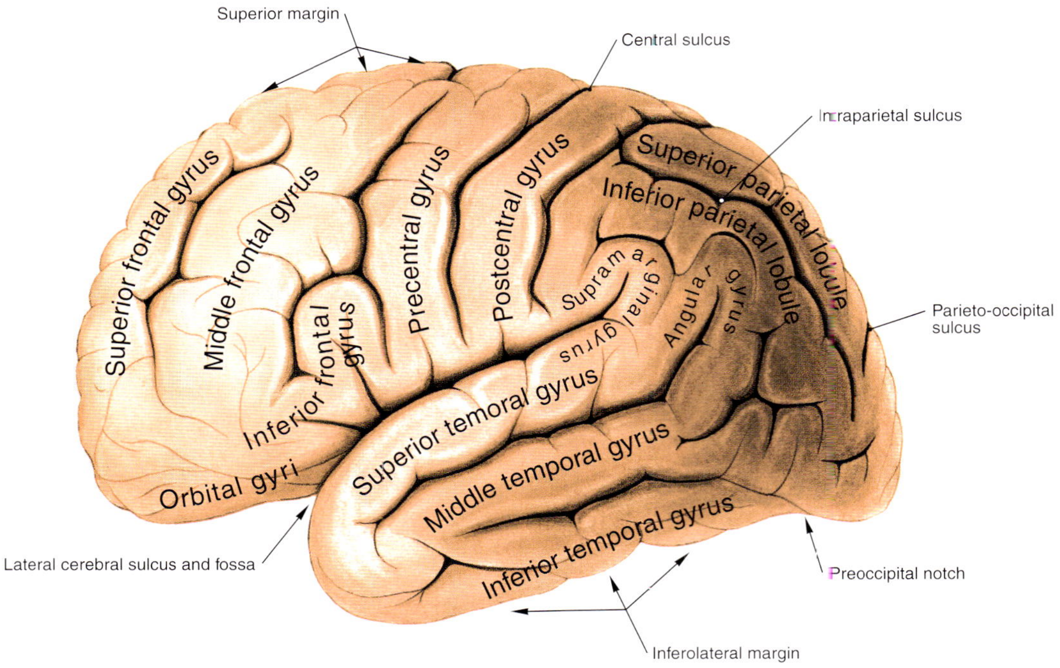

Fig. 1215 Gyri of the cerebral hemispheres; viewed from the left.

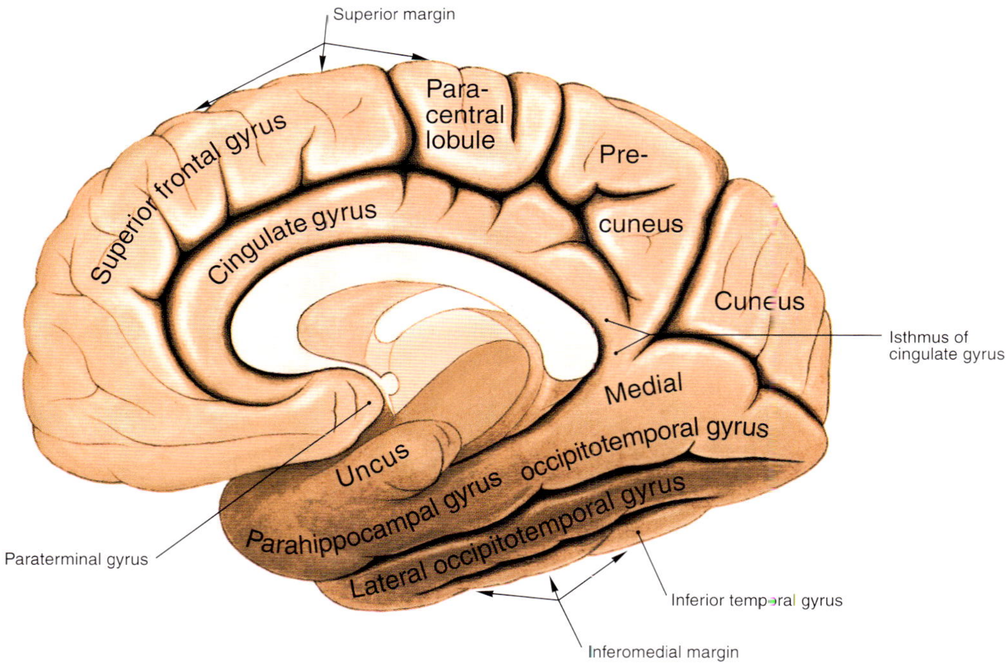

Fig. 1216 Gyri of the cerebral hemispheres; medial view.

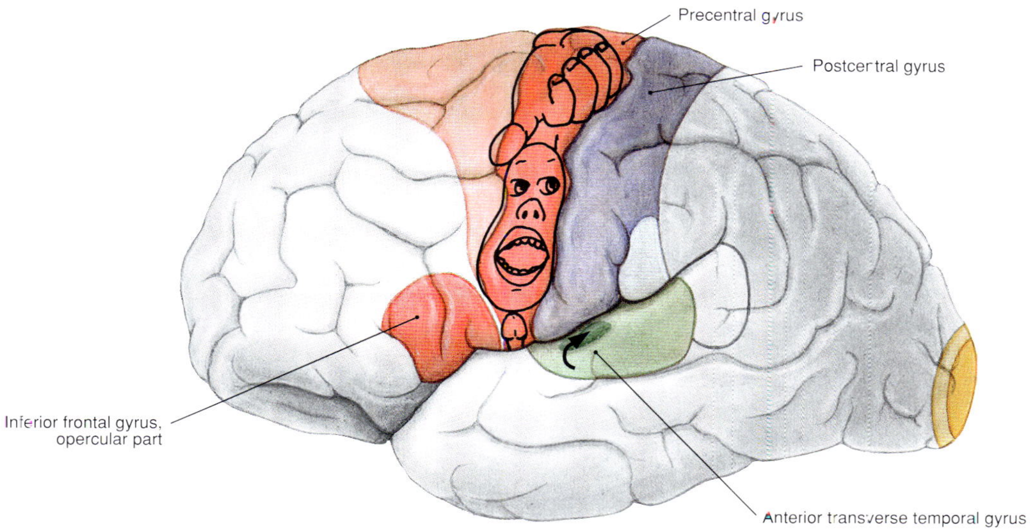

Fig. 1217 Functional cortical areas of the cerebral hemispheres according to FOERSTER; viewed from the left.

The somatotopic organisation is illustrated schematically. The primary receiving area for auditory impulses (☾) extends over the upper edge of the temporal lobe onto its inner surface.

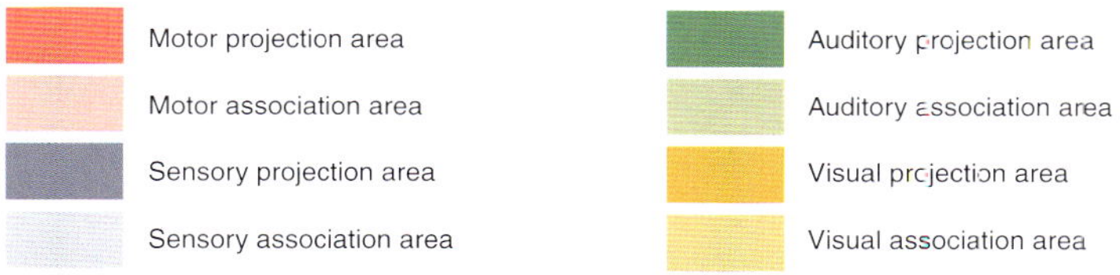

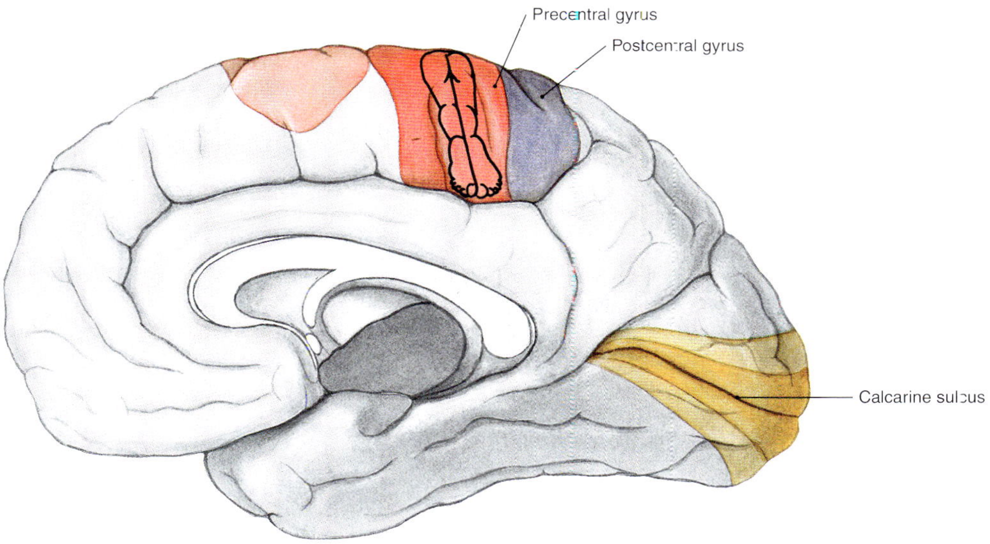

Fig. 1218 Functional cortical areas of the cerebral hemispheres according to FOERSTER; medial view.

The somatotopic organisation is illustrated schematically.

Fornix

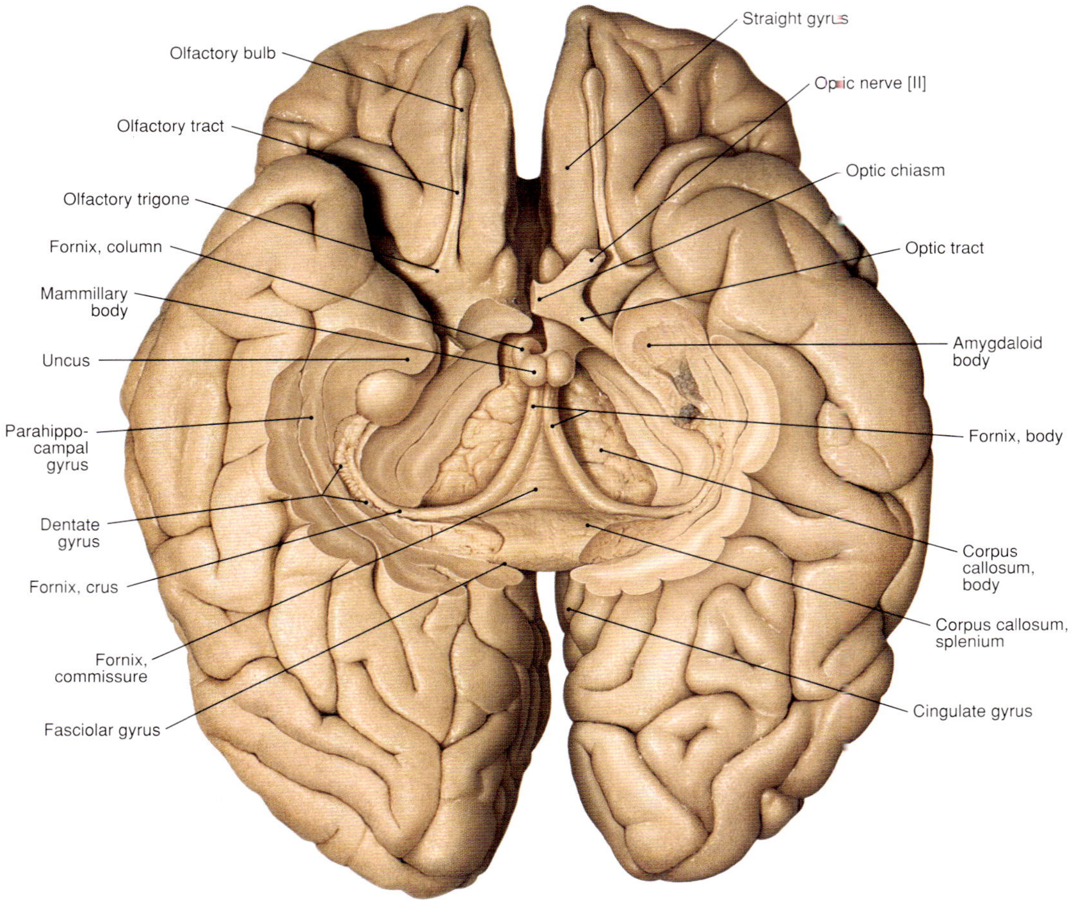

Fig. 1219 Fornix;
after removal of the basal parts of the brain;
inferior view.

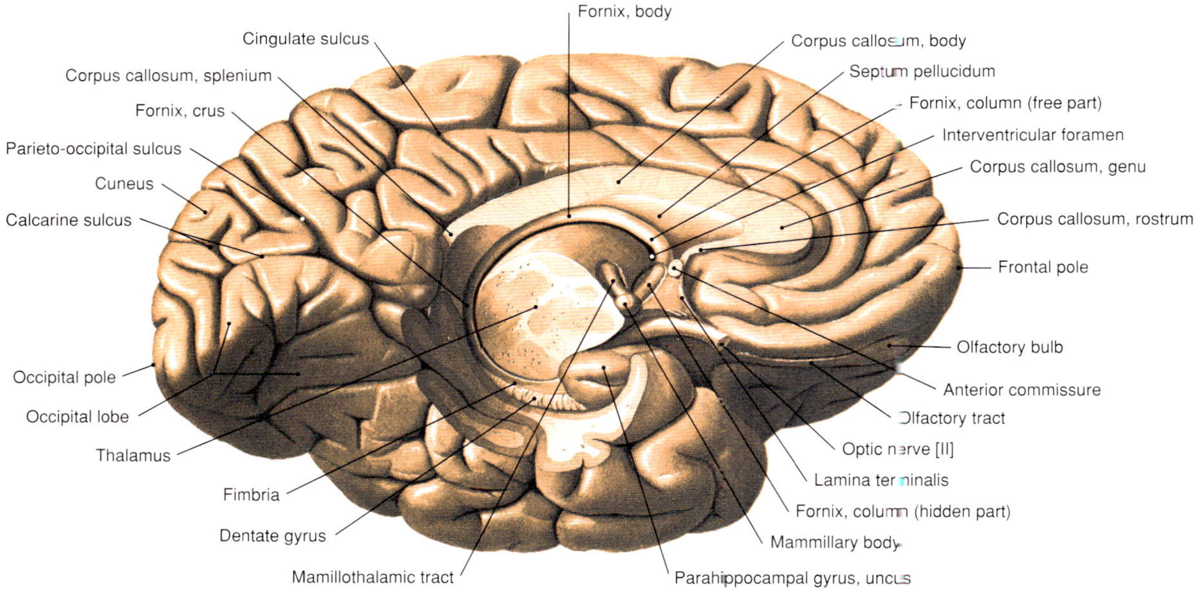

Fig. 1220 Fornix;
inferomedial view.

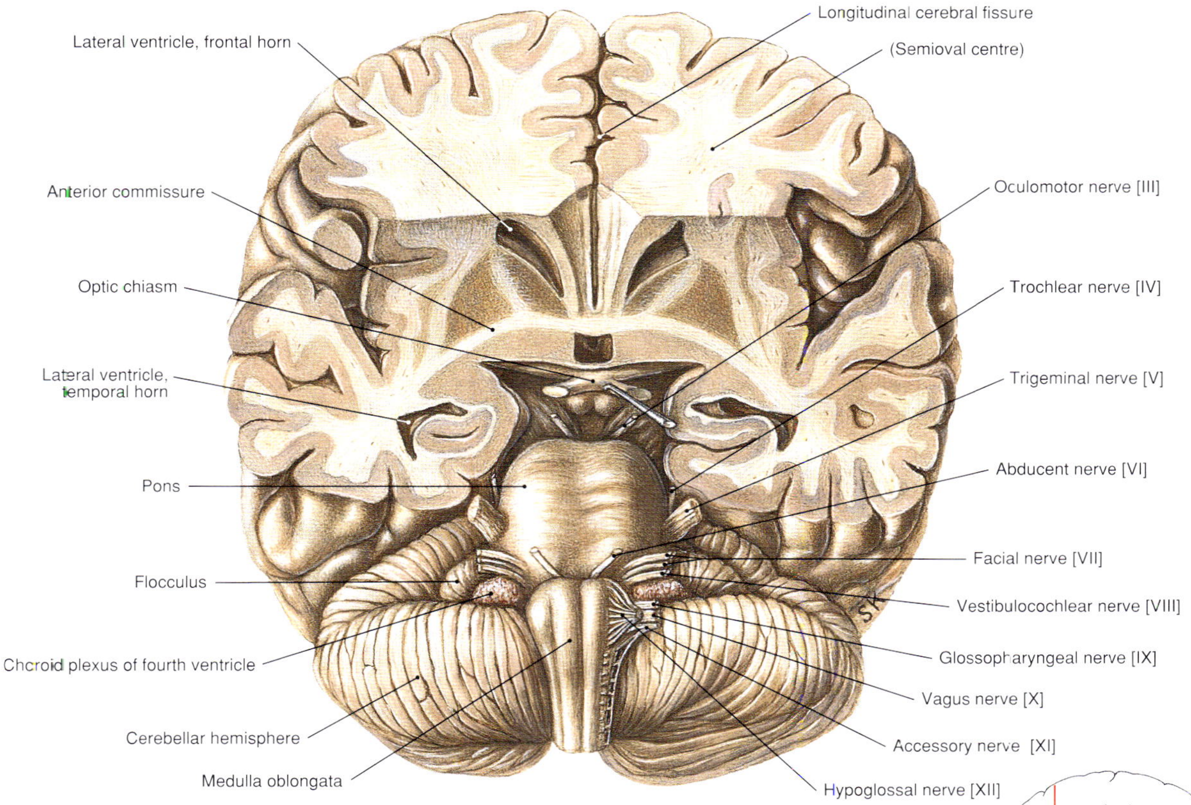

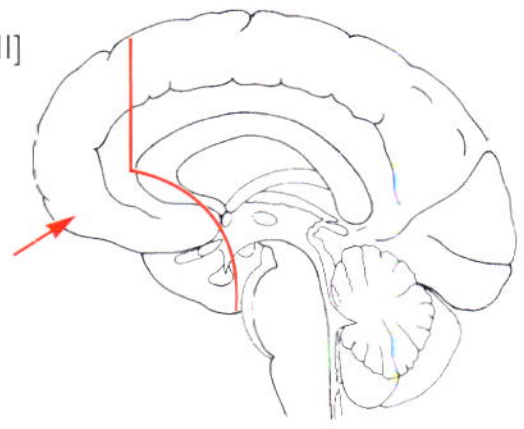

Fig. 1221 Anterior commissure and brainstem; after partial removal of the basal parts of the cerebrum; anterior-inferior view.

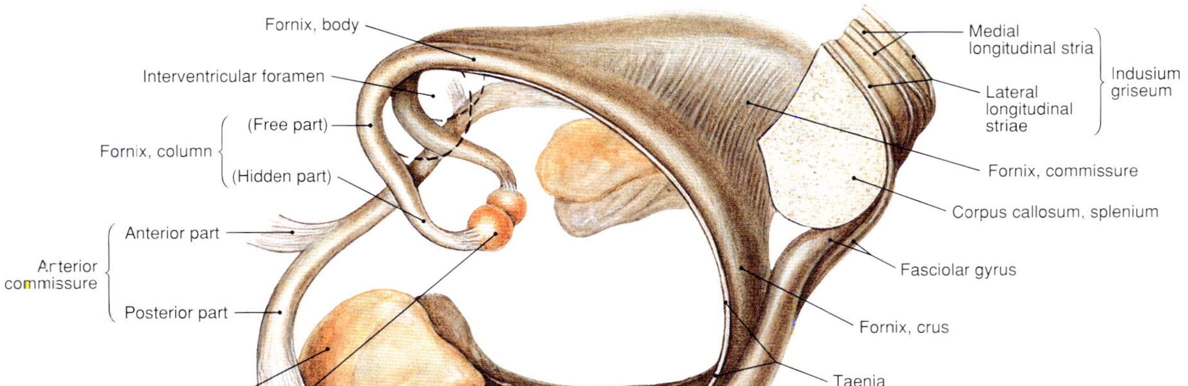

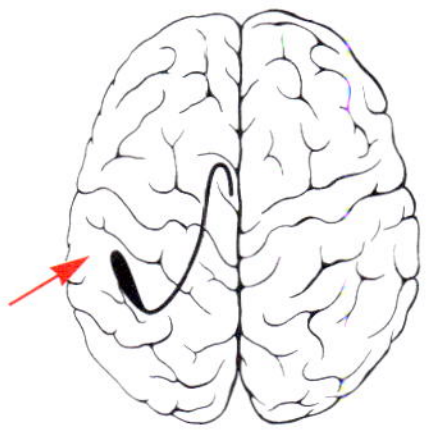

Fig. 1222 Both fornices and anterior commissure; viewed from the left.

Basal ganglia

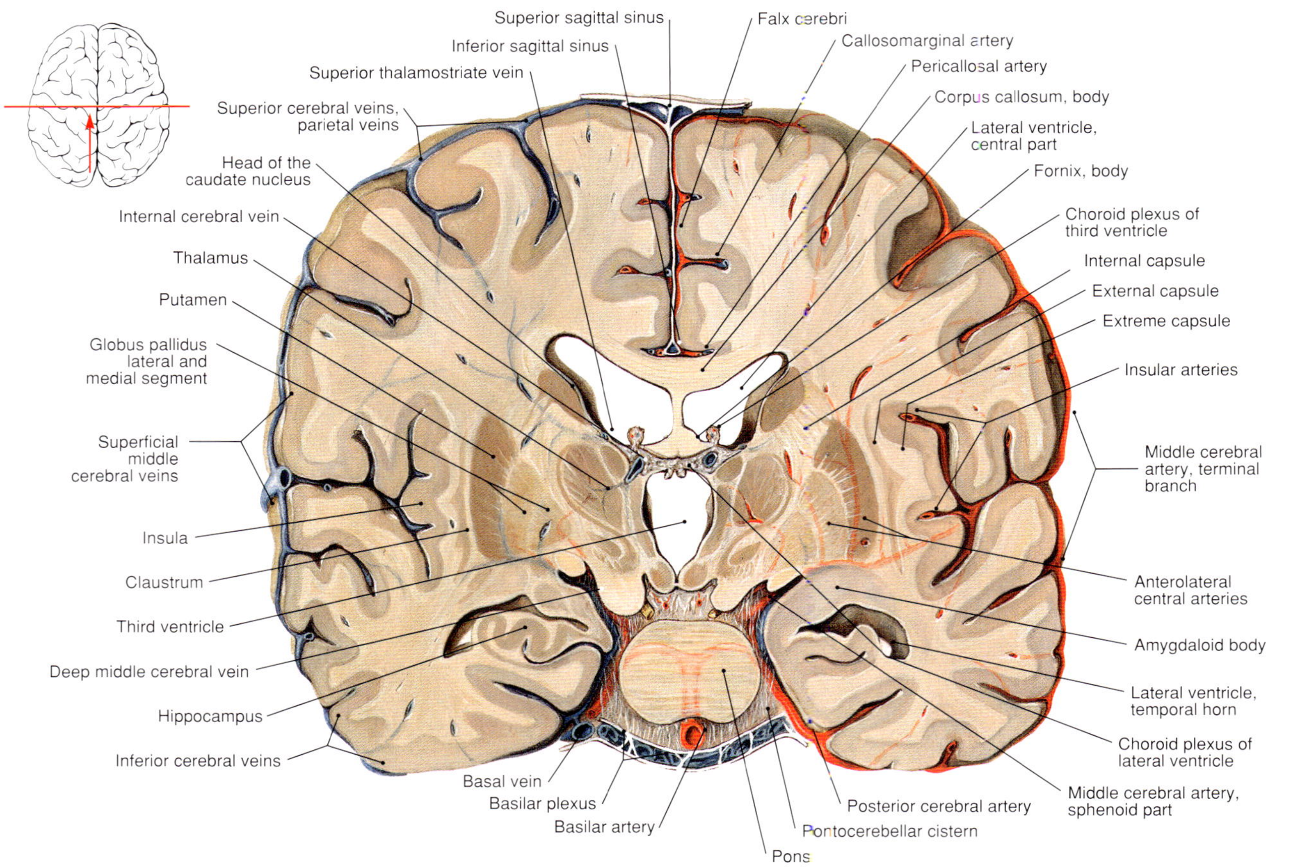

Fig. 1223 Blood supply of the basal ganglia;
frontal section;
the arteries are shown on the right and the veins on the left;
posterior view.

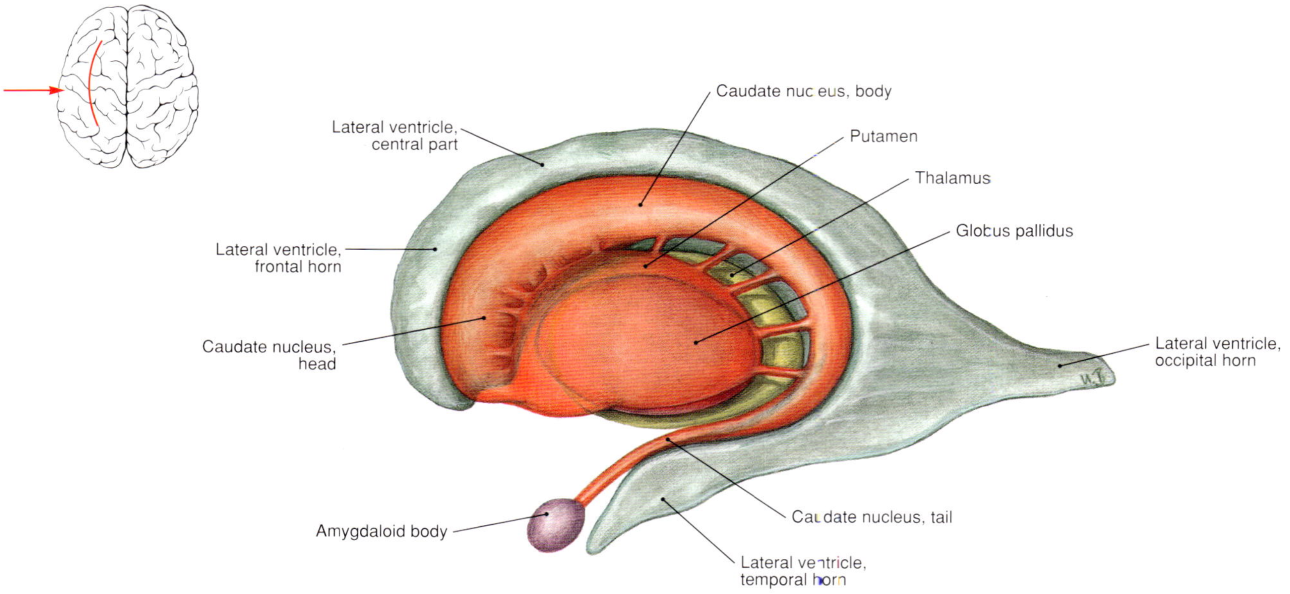

Fig. 1224 Basal ganglia and thalamus;
viewed from the left.

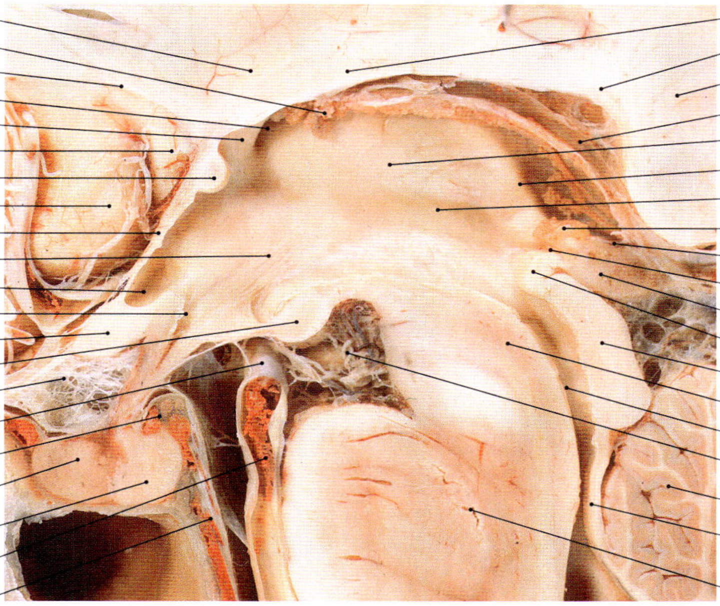

Fig. 1225 Third ventricle;
median section.

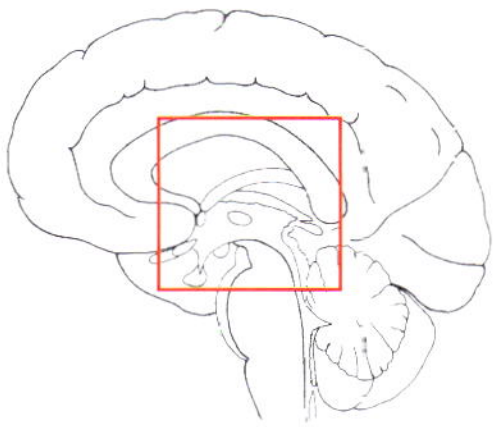

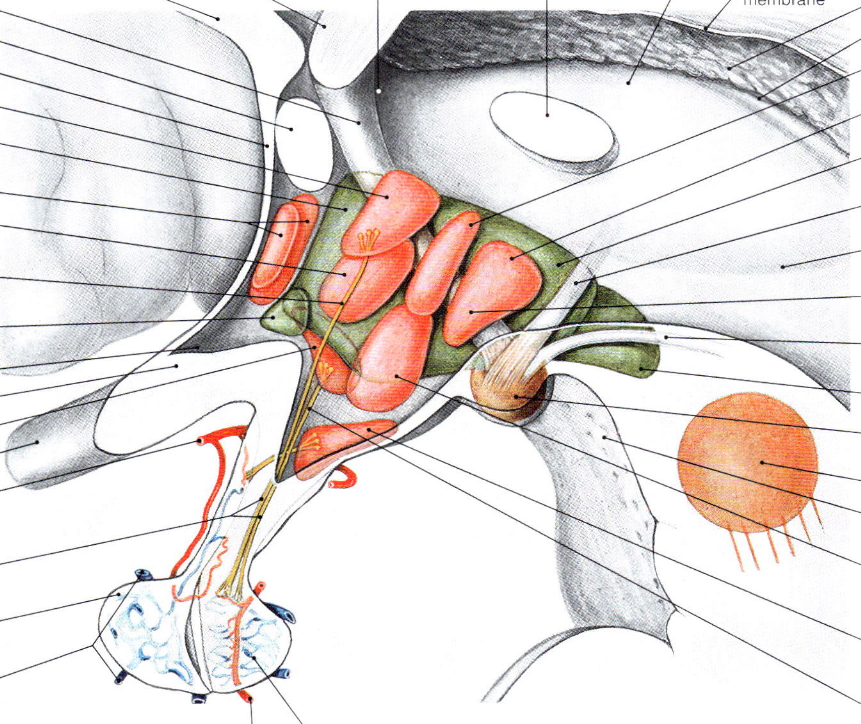

Fig. 1226 Hypothalamus;
overview; nuclei are illustrated translucently;
medial view.

Thalamic nuclei

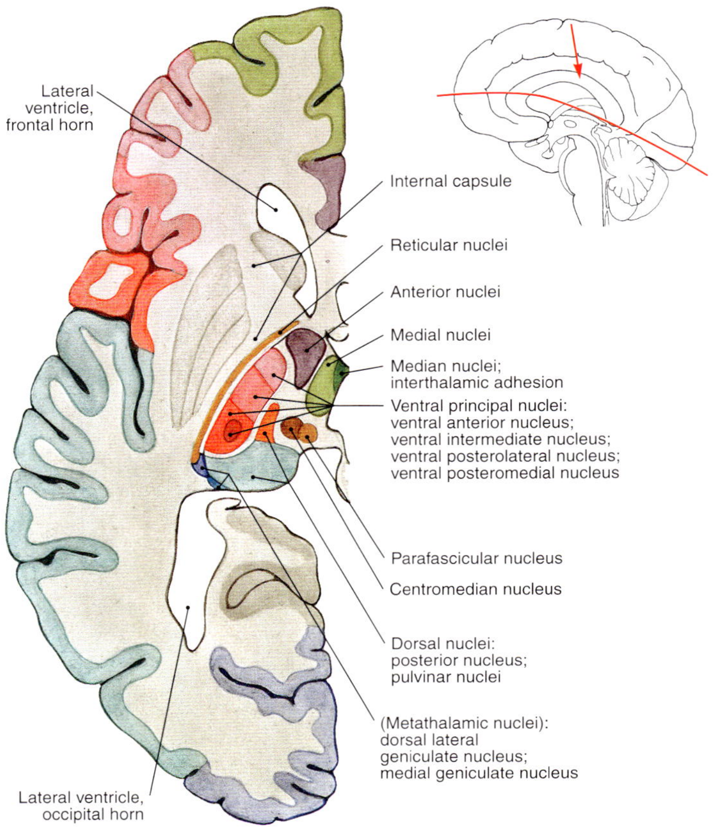

a Horizontal section through the left cerebral hemisphere

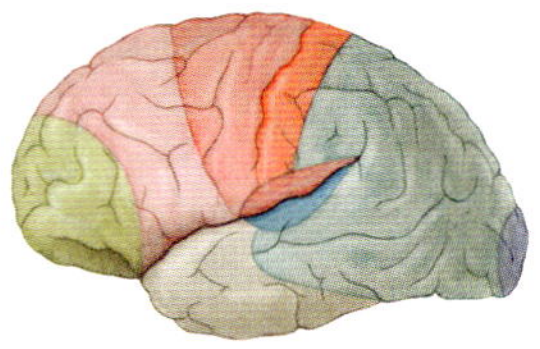

b Left cerebral hemisphere; viewed from the left

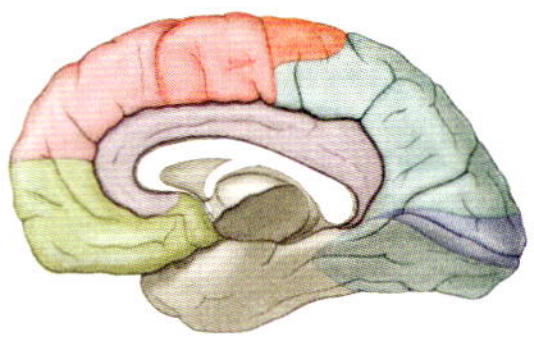

c Right cerebral hemisphere; medial view

Fig. 1227 a–c Nuclei and cortical projections of the thalamus. Corresponding nuclei and cortical projections are indicated by the same colour.

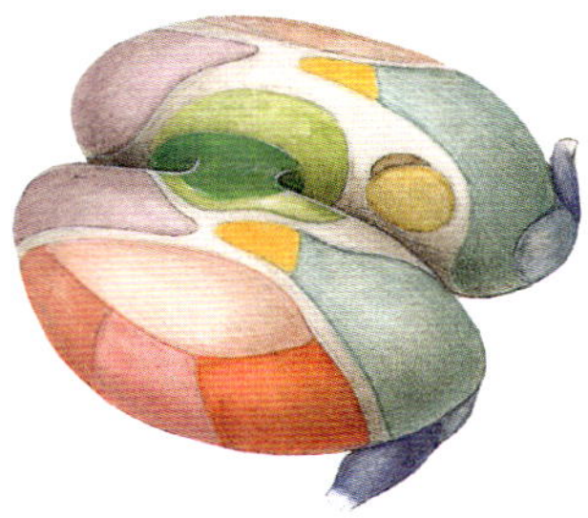

Fig. 1228 Thalamic nuclei; oblique view from posterior. For colour coding see Fig. 1227.

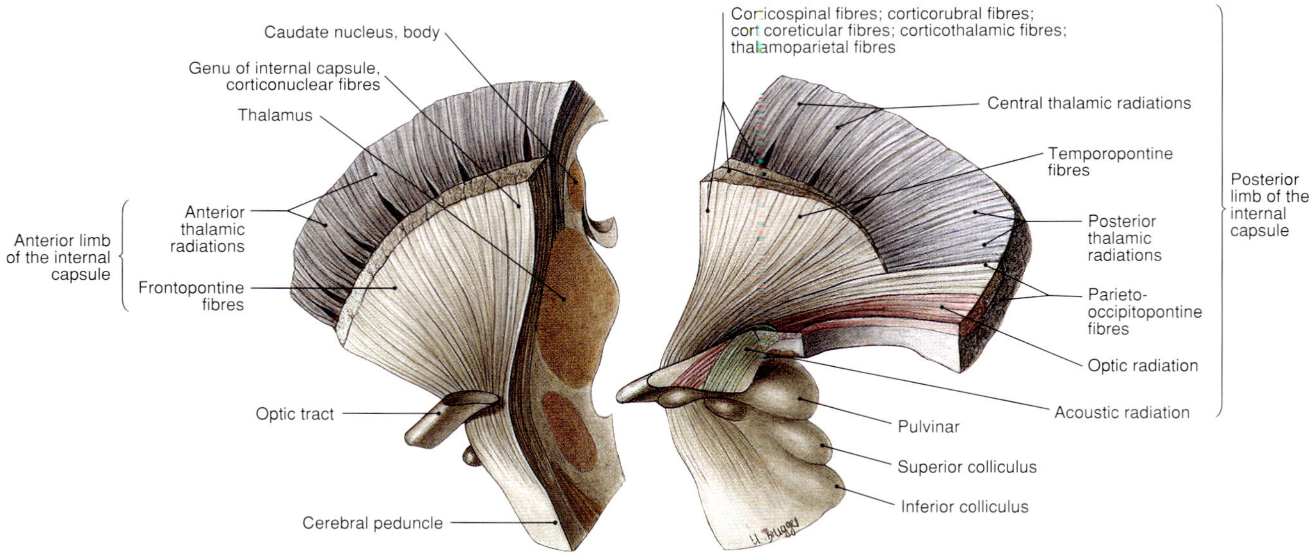

Fig. 1229 Thalamic radiation and internal capsule have been divided by a frontal section; viewed from the left.

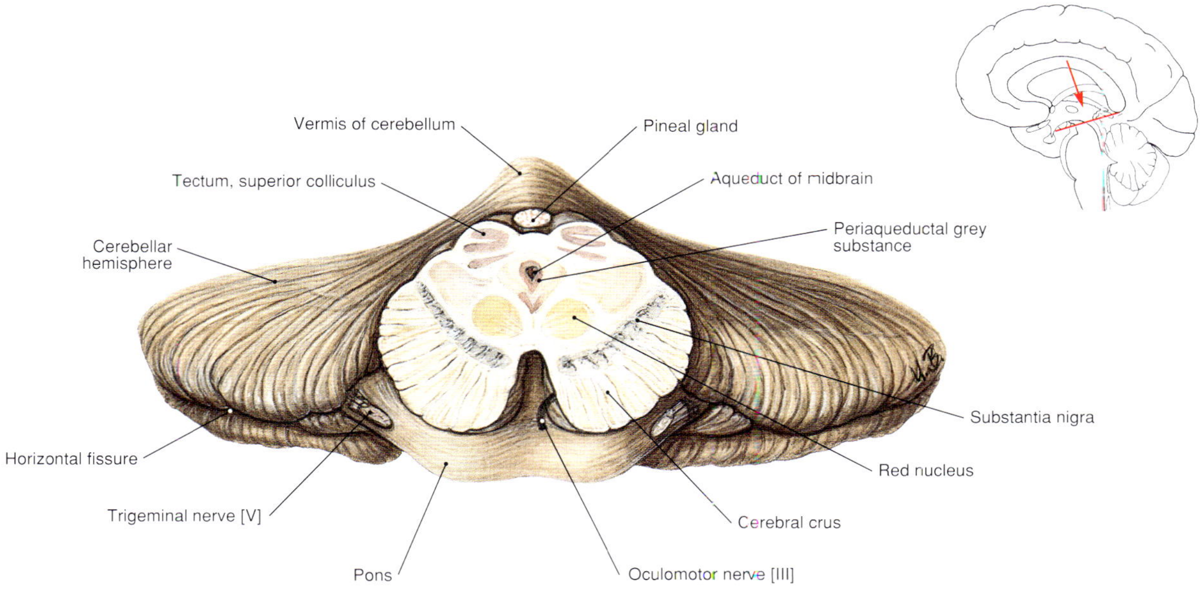

Fig. 1230 Midbrain;
cross-section at the level of the superior colliculi;
anterior view.

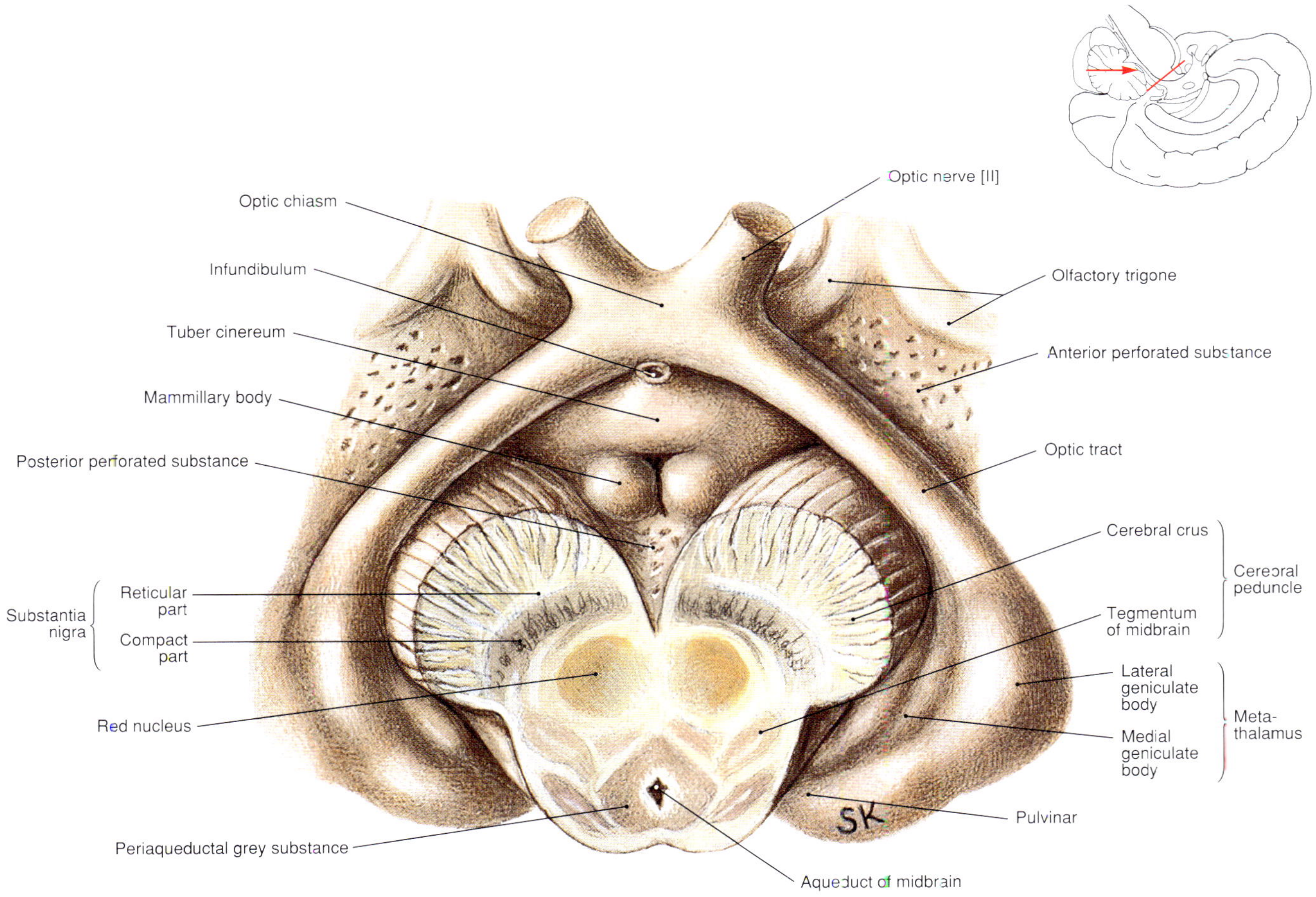

Fig. 1231 Midbrain and diencephalon;
after oblique section of the midbrain;
inferior view.

Midbrain and medulla oblongata

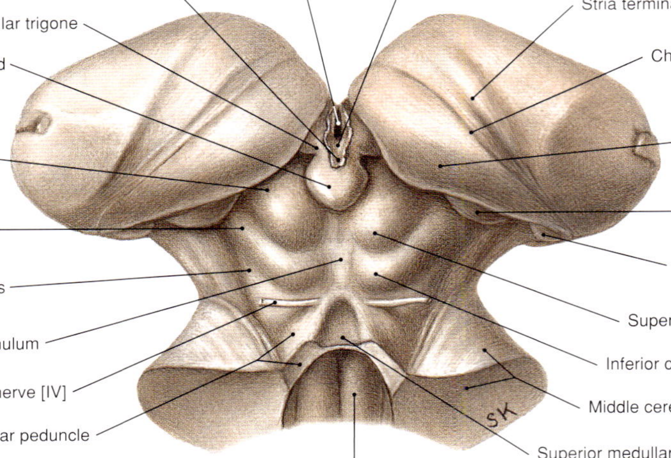

Fig. 1232 Midbrain and pineal gland; posterior-superior view.

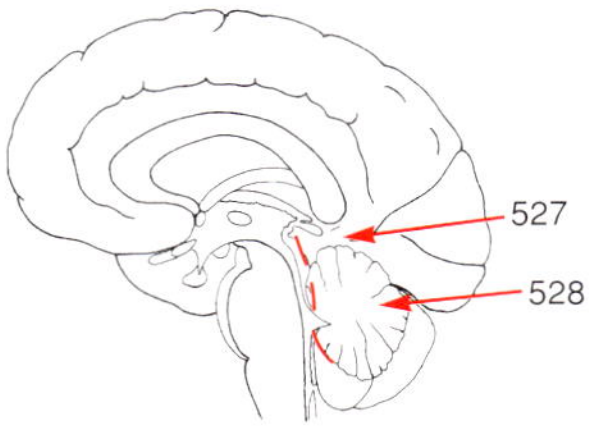

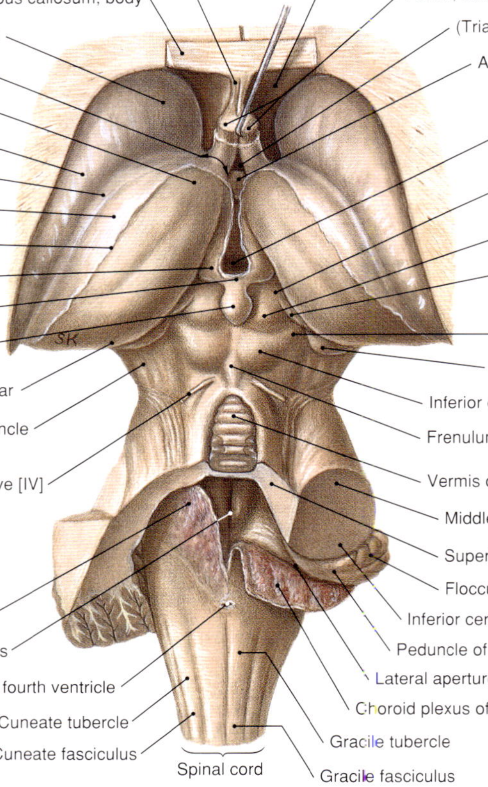

Fig. 1233 Brainstem;
the pons and major parts of the cerebellum have been removed; the tela choroidea of the fourth ventricle has been sectioned in the median plane and reflected to the right; posterior-superior view.

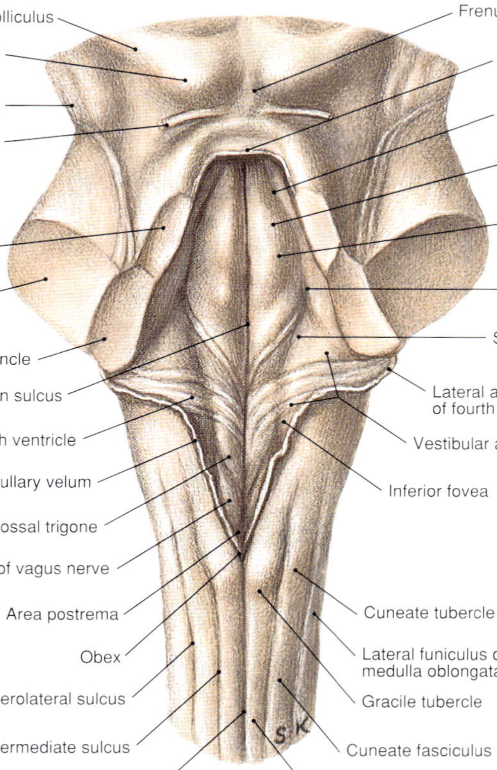

Fig. 1234 Rhomboid fossa;
view on the floor of the fourth ventricle after section of the cerebellar peduncles;
posterior-superior view.

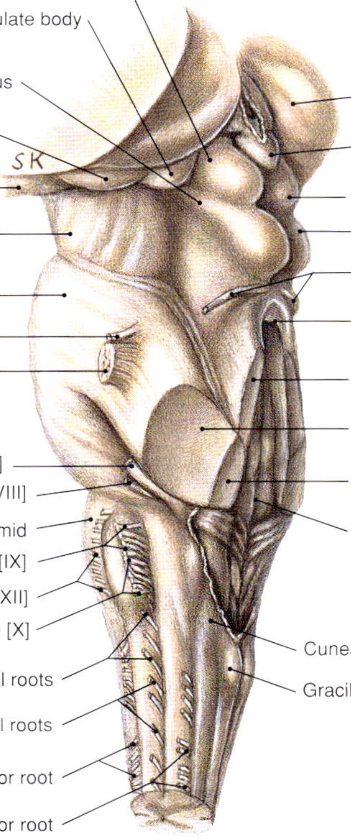

Fig. 1235 Brainstem;
oblique view on the floor of the fourth ventricle after section of the cerebellar peduncles;
lateral view.

Nuclei of the cranial nerves

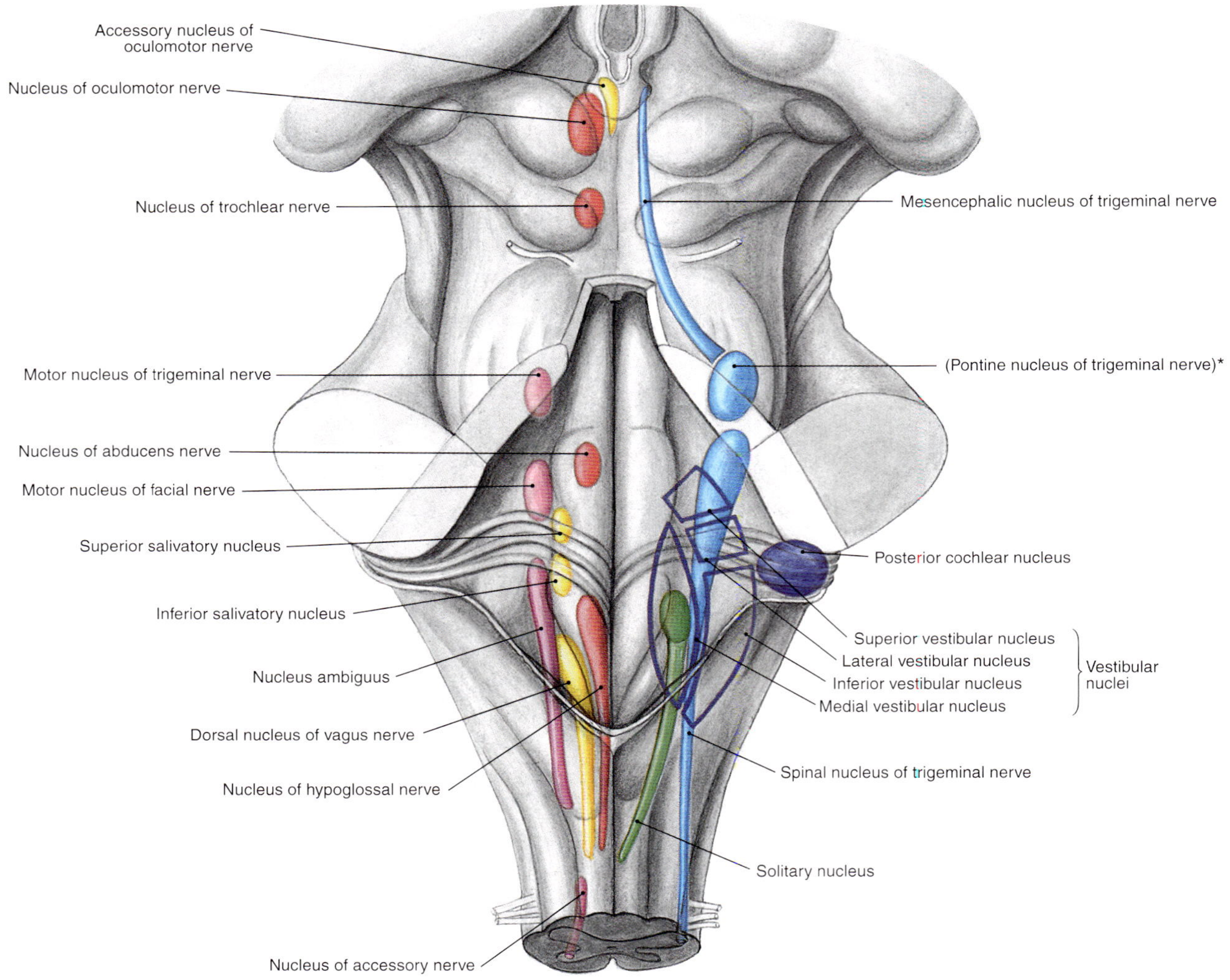

Fig. 1236 Cranial nerves;
topographic overview of the nuclei;
posterior view.

On the left the motor nuclei and on the right the sensory nuclei are shown.

* Clinical term: principal sensory nucleus of the trigeminal nerve

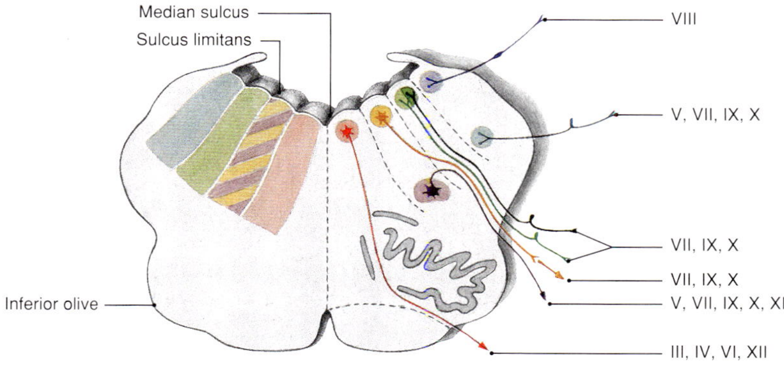

Fig. 1237 Cranial nerves;
schematic cross-section through the rhomboid fossa demonstrating the nuclei.

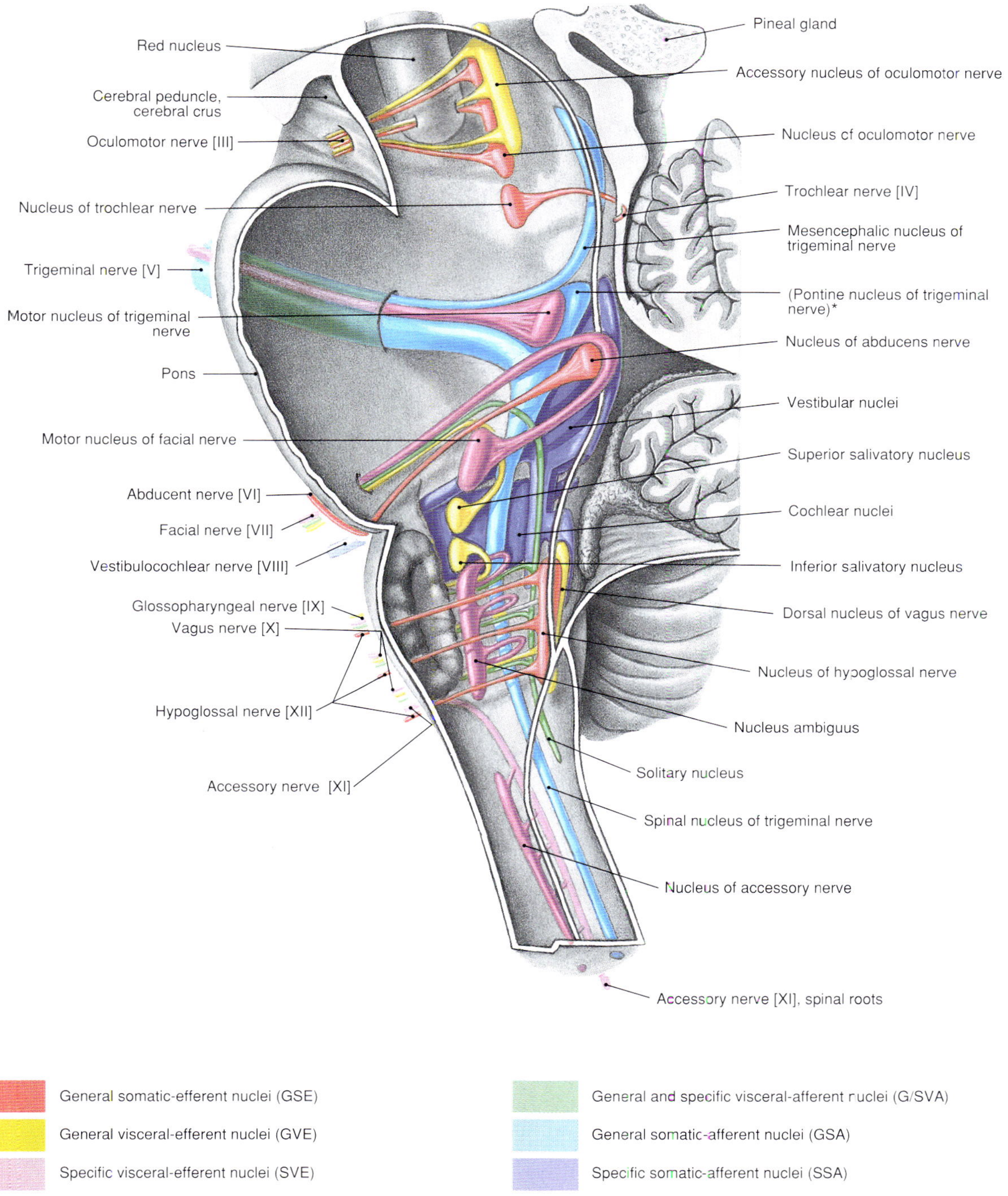

Fig. 1238 Cranial nerves;
topographic overview of the nuclei in the median plane.

* Clinical term: principal sensory nucleus of the trigeminal nerve

Cerebellum

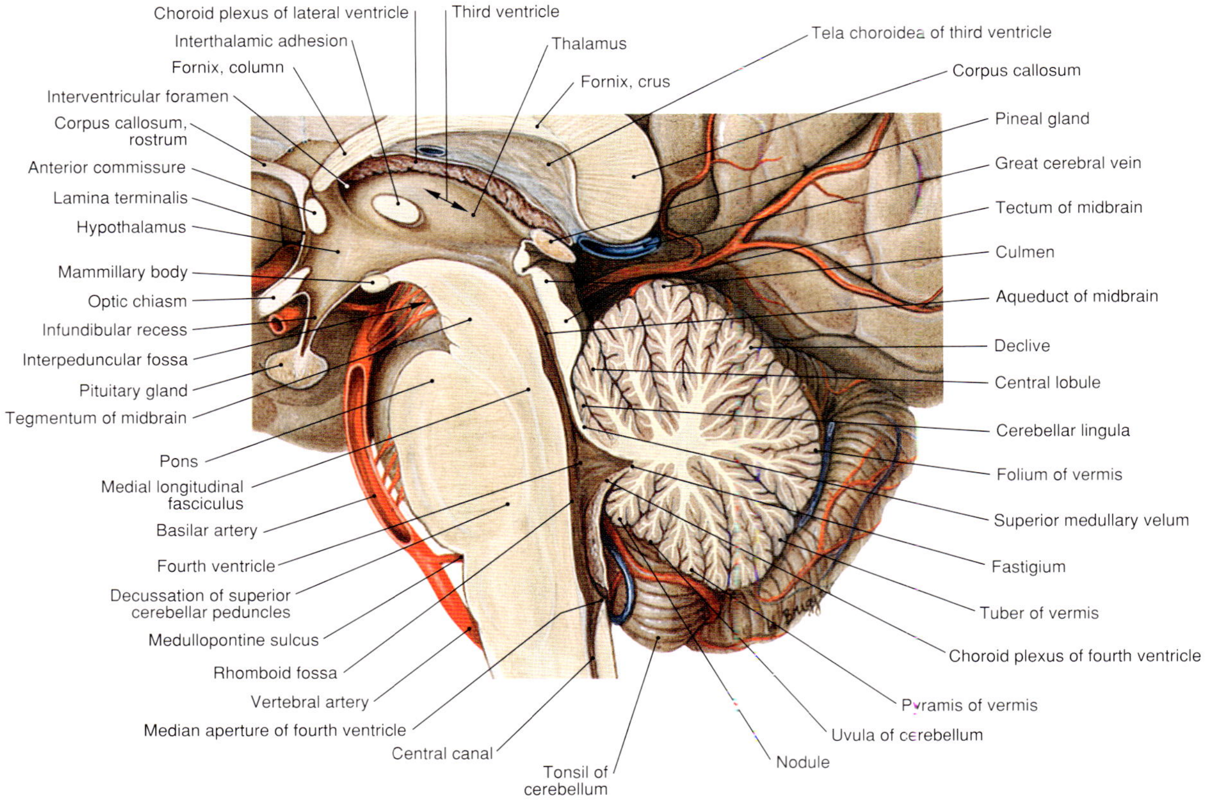

Fig. 1239 Brainstem with the cerebellum and the fourth ventricle; median section.

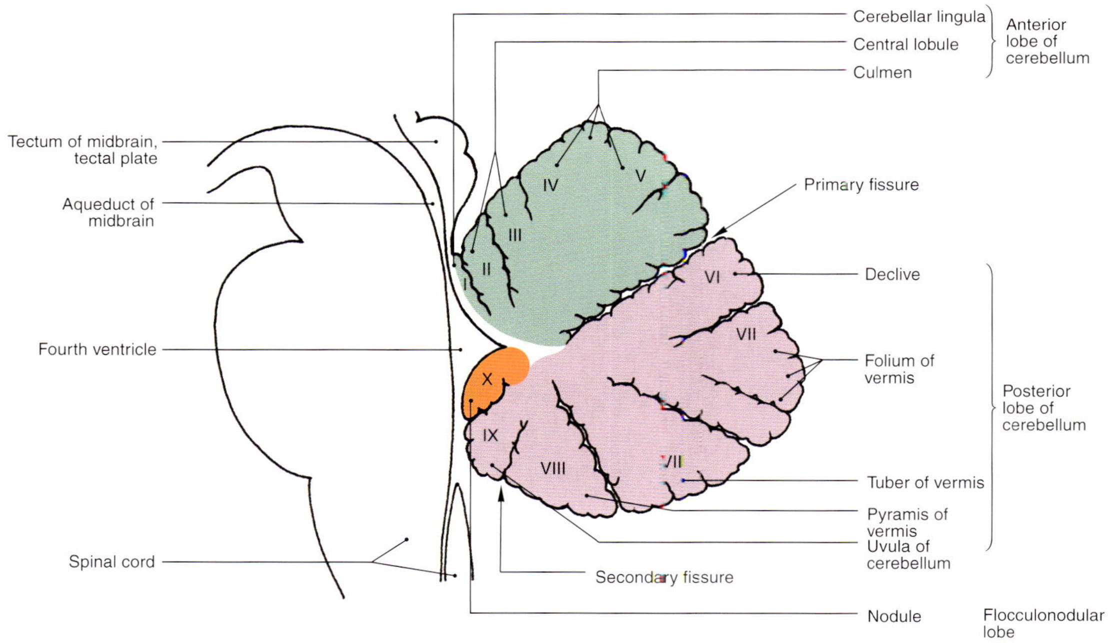

Fig. 1240 Parts of the cerebellar vermis; median section; overview.

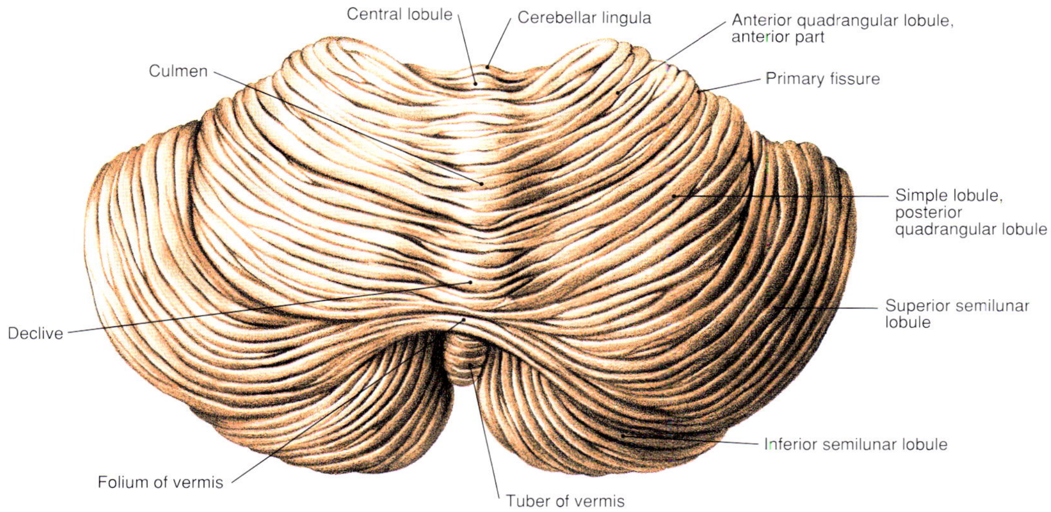

Fig. 1241 Cerebellum;
posterior-superior view.

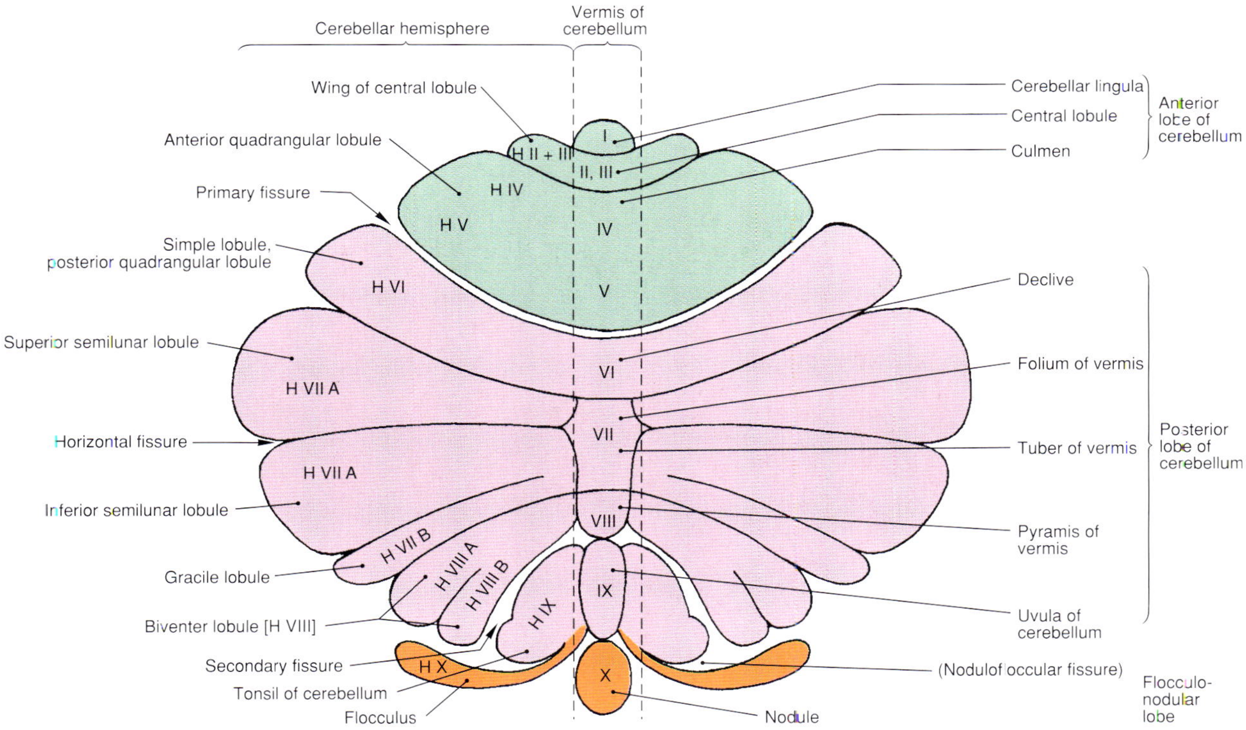

Fig. 1242 Cerebellum;
diagram of the cerebellar cortex outstretched;
overview.

Cerebellum

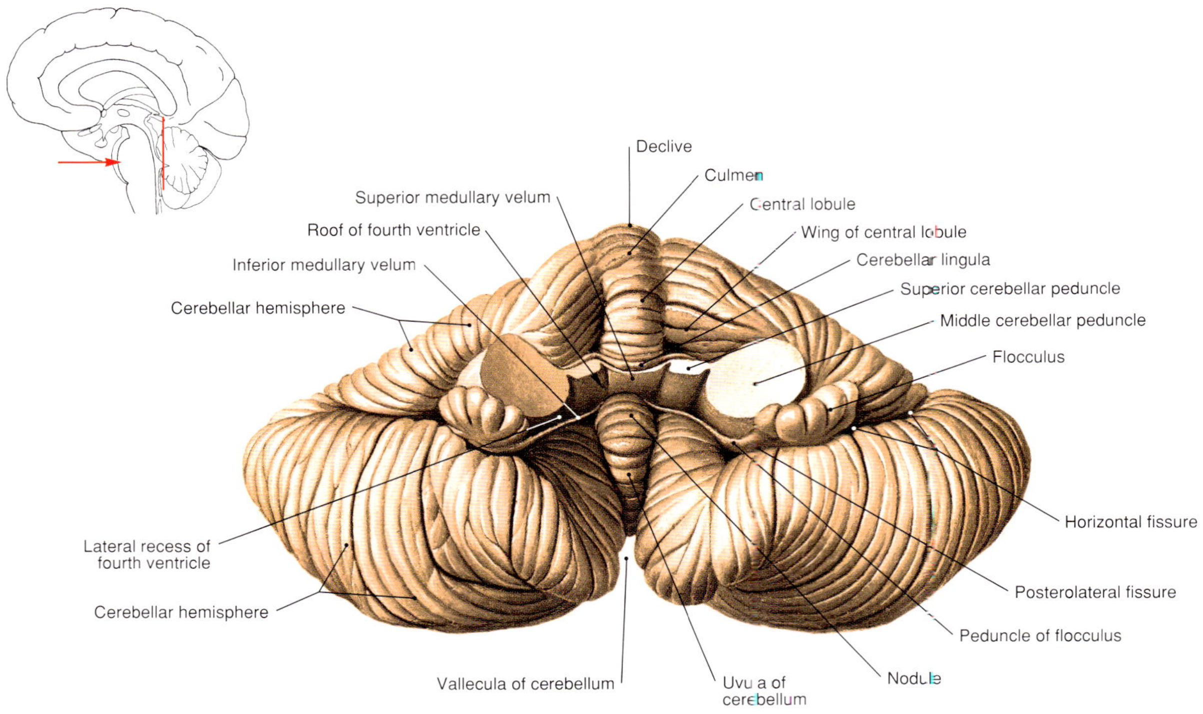

Fig. 1243 Cerebellum;
after section of the cerebellar peduncles;
anterior view.

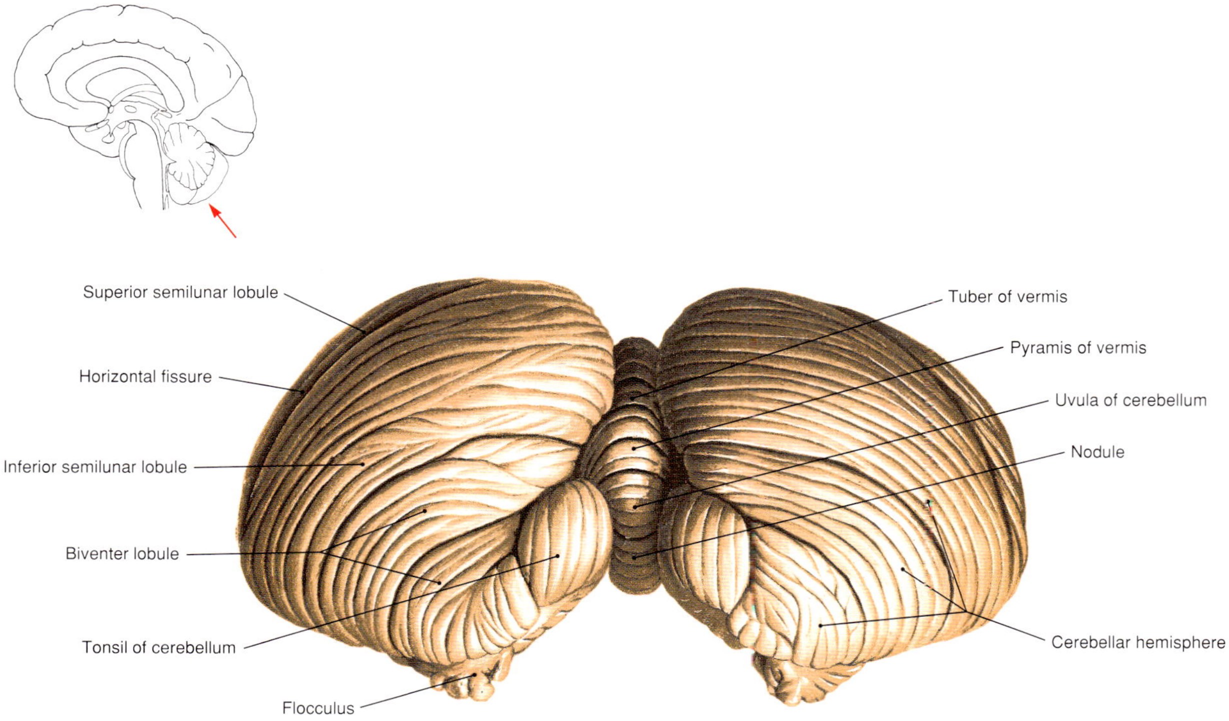

Fig. 1244 Cerebellum;
posterior-inferior view.

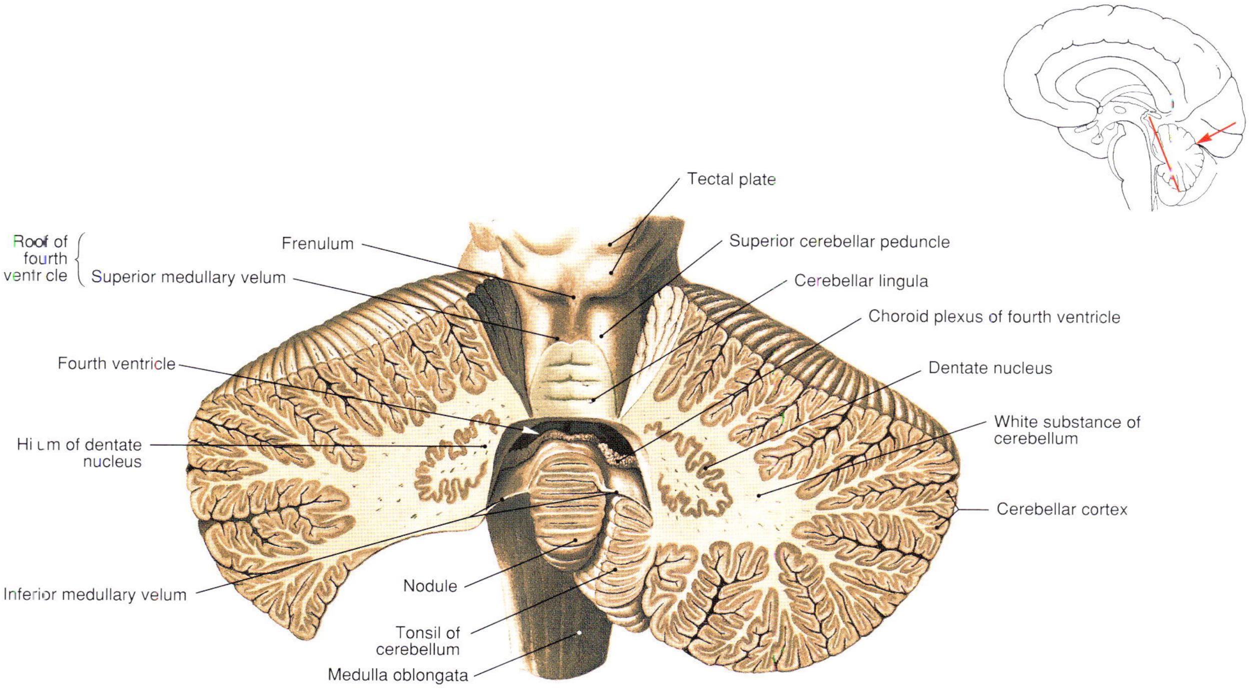

Fig. 1245 Cerebellum;
oblique section;
posterior view.

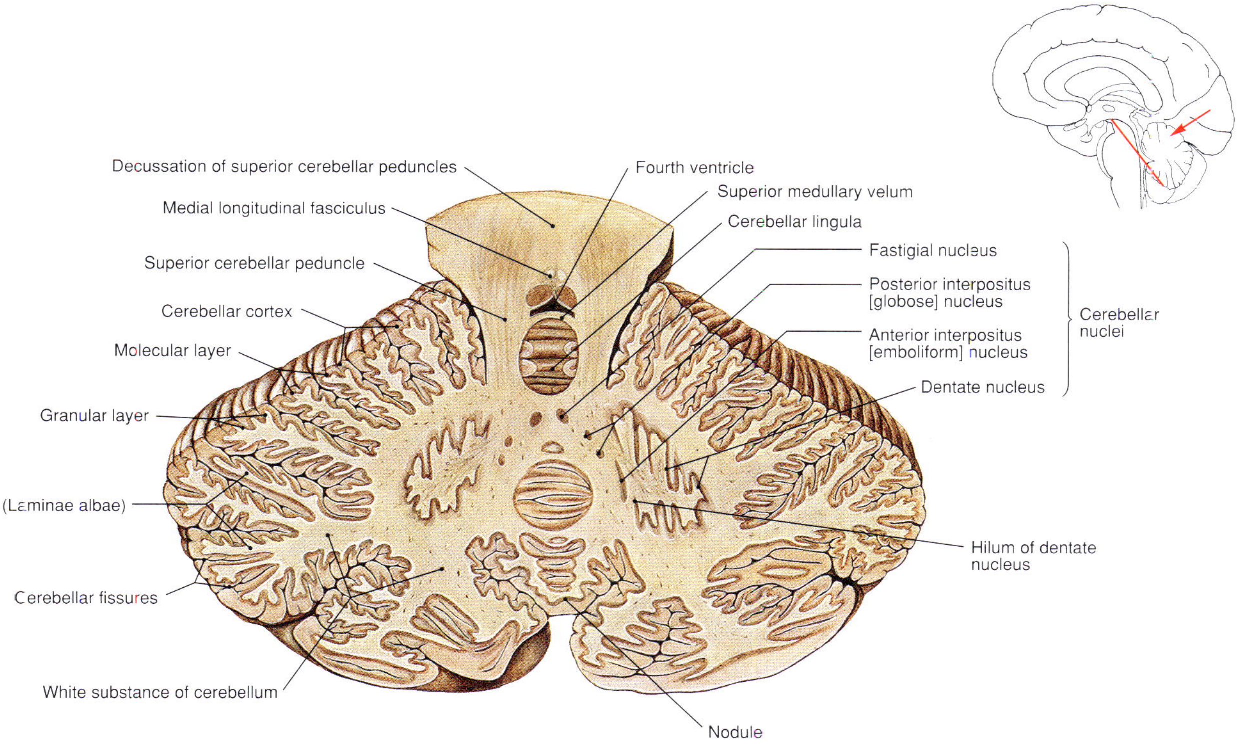

Fig. 1246 Cerebellum;
oblique section through the upper cerebellar peduncles;
posterior view.

Association and commissural tracts

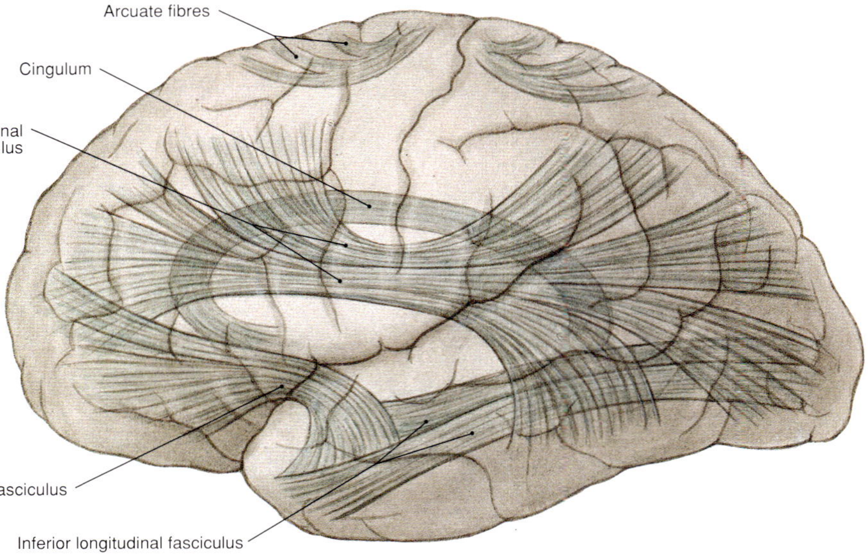

Fig. 1247 Association tracts;
projection onto the cerebral hemisphere;
overview;
viewed from the left.

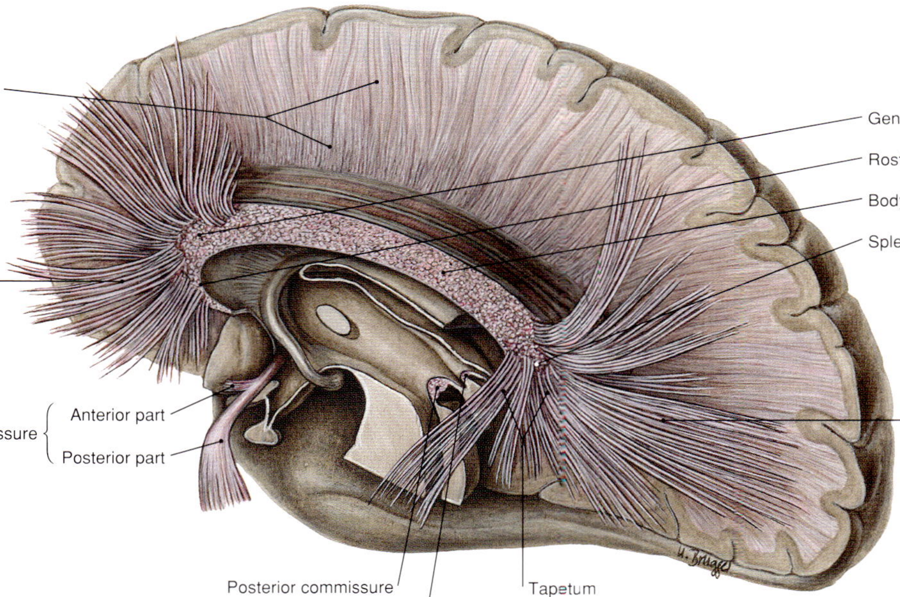

Fig. 1248 Commissural tracts;
topographic overview after extensive removal of the corpus callosum in the paramedian plane;
single fibres of the corpus callosum are shown;
viewed from the left.

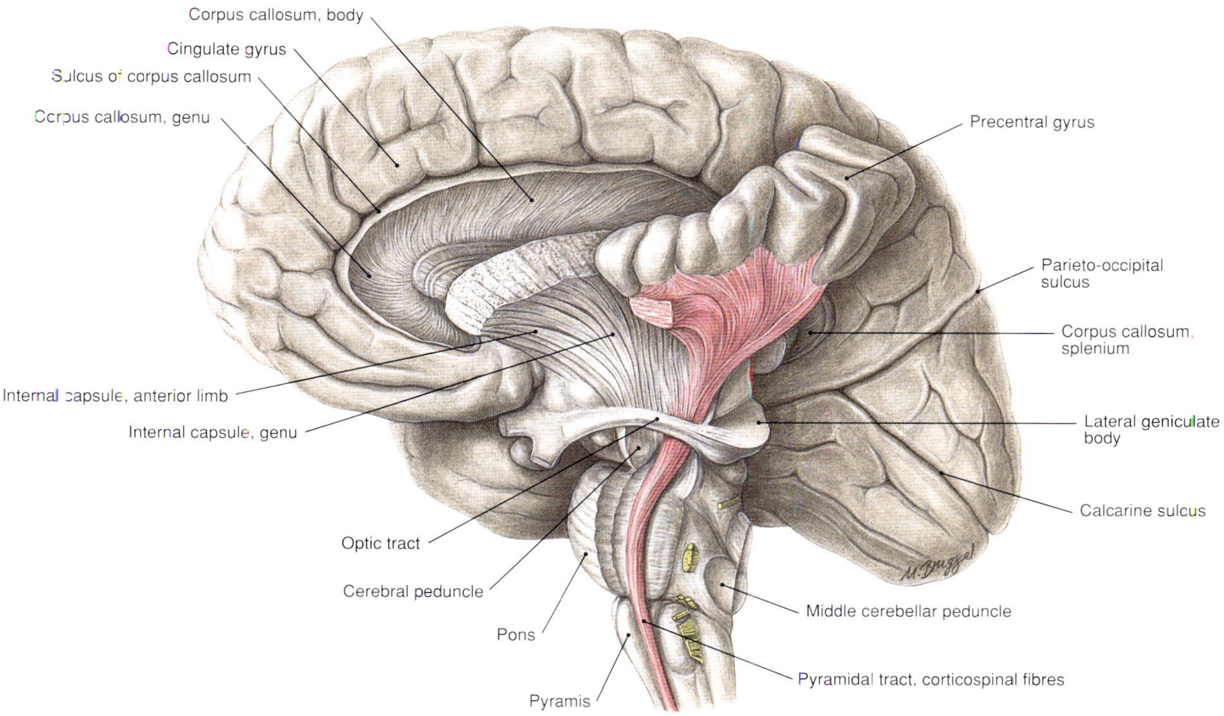

Fig. 1249 Projection tracts;
the internal capsule and the pyramidal tract have been exposed;
viewed from the left.

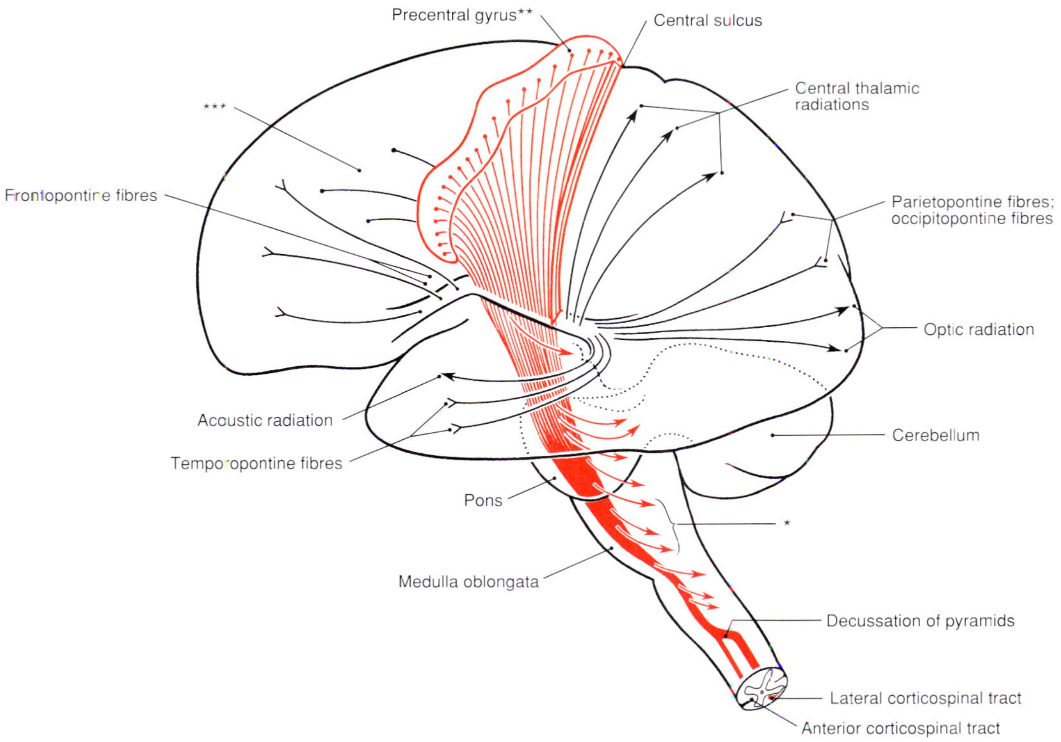

Fig. 1250 Internal capsule and pyramidal tract;
functional overview;
viewed from the left.

* Fibres to the tectal plate and the nuclei of the hindbrain
** Perikarya of the pyramidal tract
*** Perikarya of areas 6 and 8 (premotor cortex)

Internal capsule

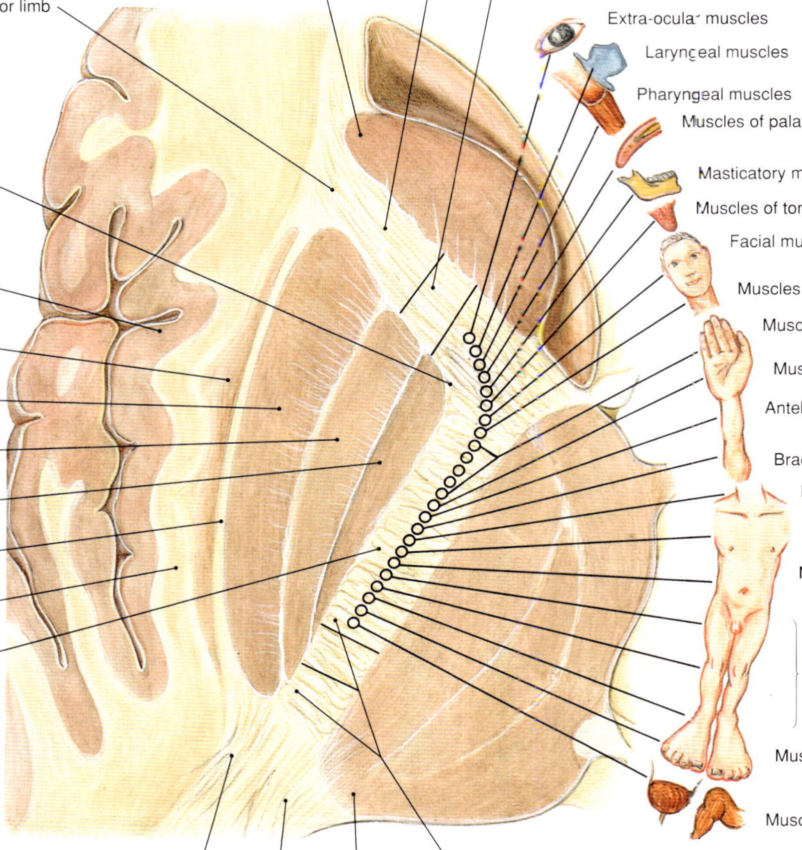

Fig. 1251 Internal capsule; functional organisation.

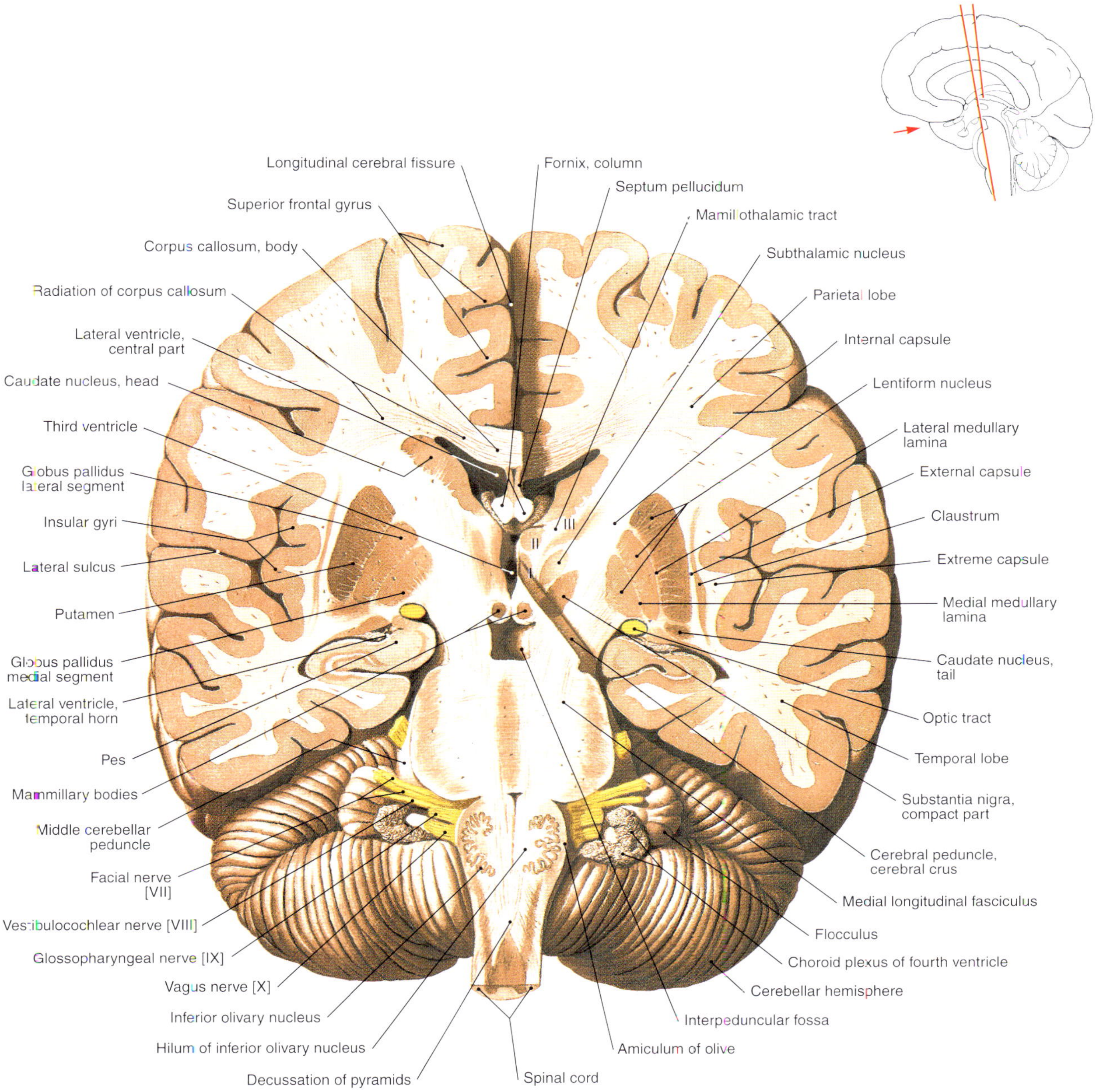

I–III = Thalamic nuclei:
I = Median nuclei
II = Anterior nuclei
III = Ventral principal nuclei

Fig. 1252 Pyramidal tract and basal ganglia;
obliquely staggered section through the posterior limb of the internal capsule, the cerebral peduncles, and the medulla oblongata.

Ventricles, projection

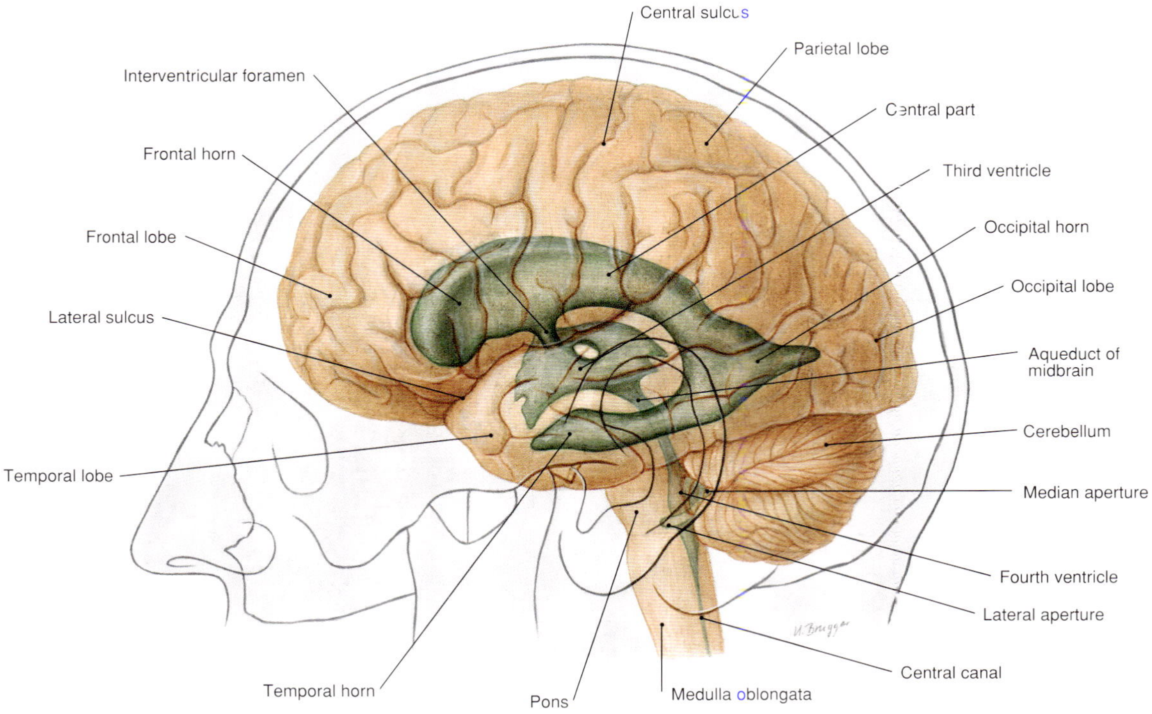

Fig. 1253 Ventricles of the brain.

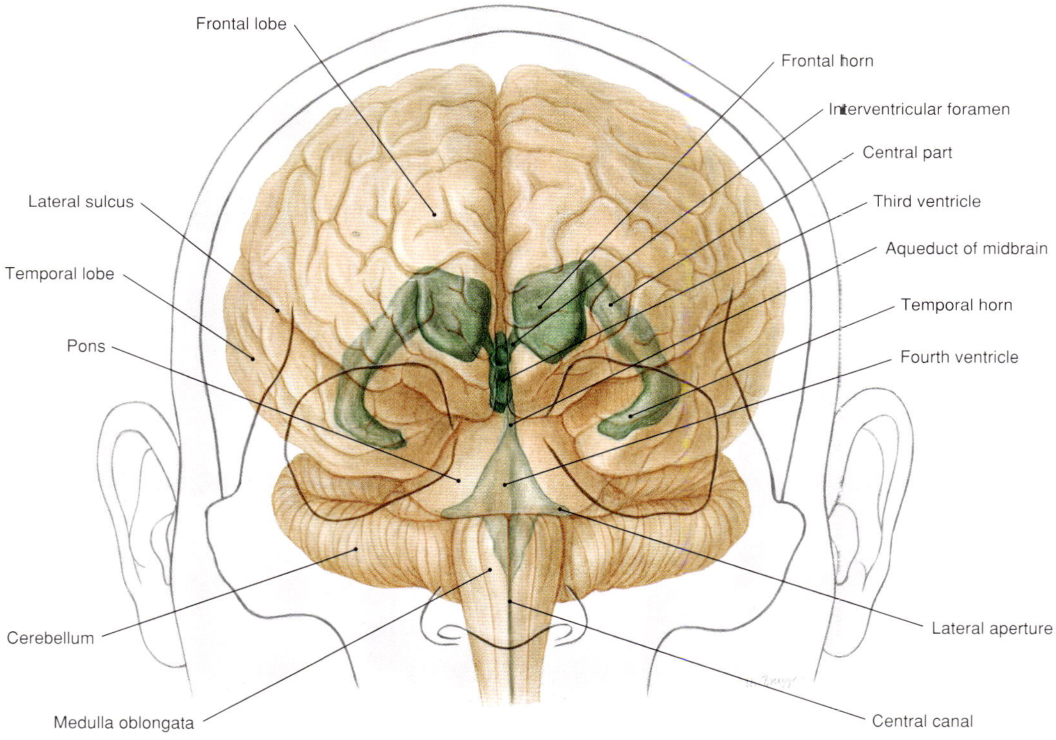

Fig. 1254 Ventricles of the brain; anterior view.

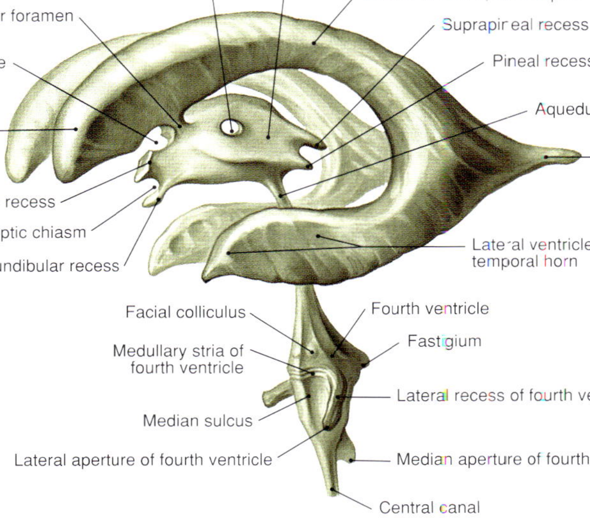

Fig. 1255 Inner liquor spaces;
corrosion cast specimen;
oblique view from the left.

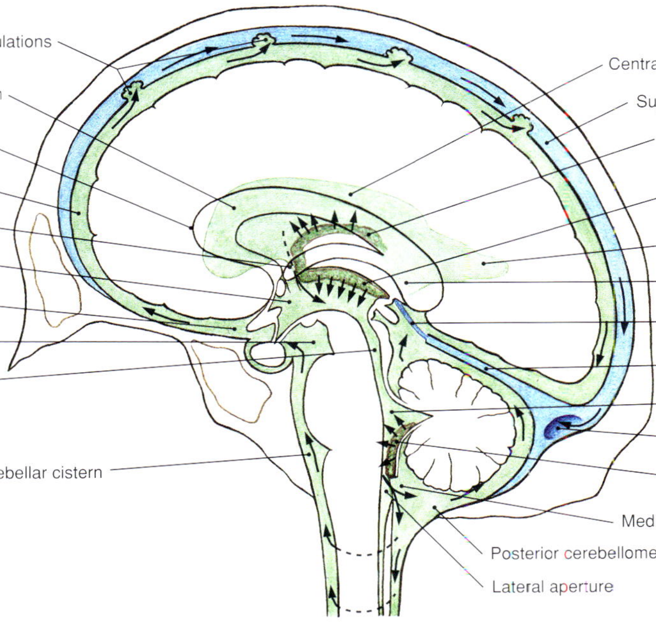

Fig. 1256 Ventricles of the brain and subarachnoid space;
schema of the circulation (arrows) of the cerebrospinal fluid
from the inner to the outer liquor spaces.

* Clinical term: foramen of MONRO
** Clinical term: cerebral aqueduct of SYLVIUS

Brain, topography

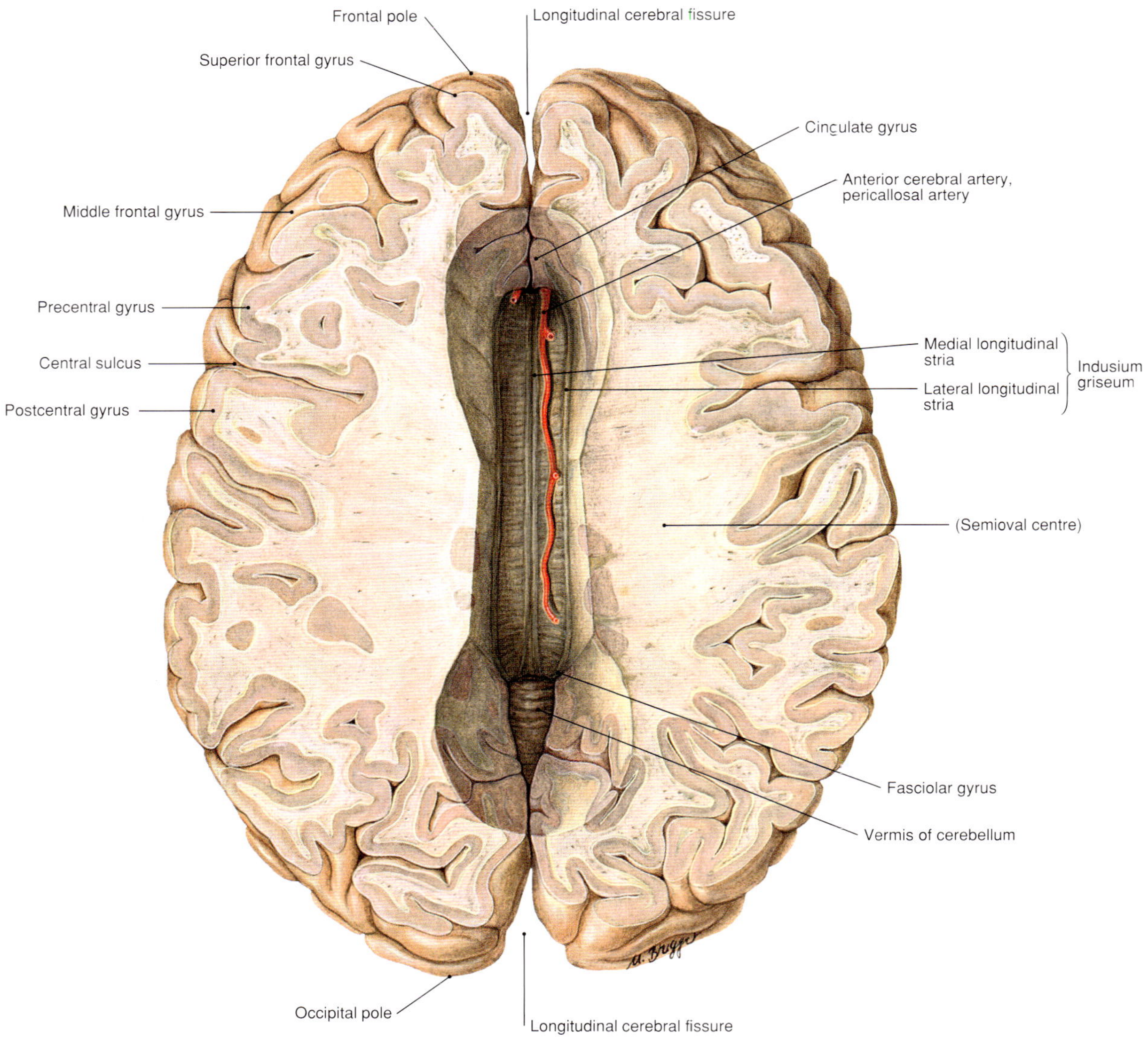

1258

Fig. 1257 Corpus callosum;
after removal of the upper parts of the cerebral hemispheres;
superior view.

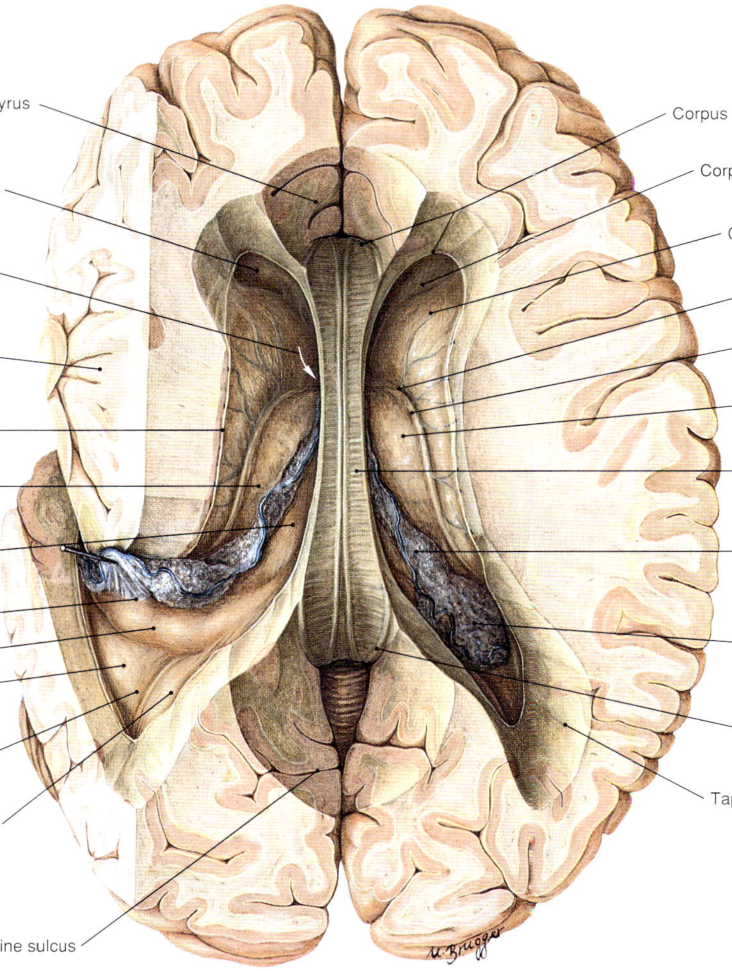

Fig. 1258 Lateral ventricles;
after removal of the upper parts of the cerebral hemispheres;
superior view.

1254
1257

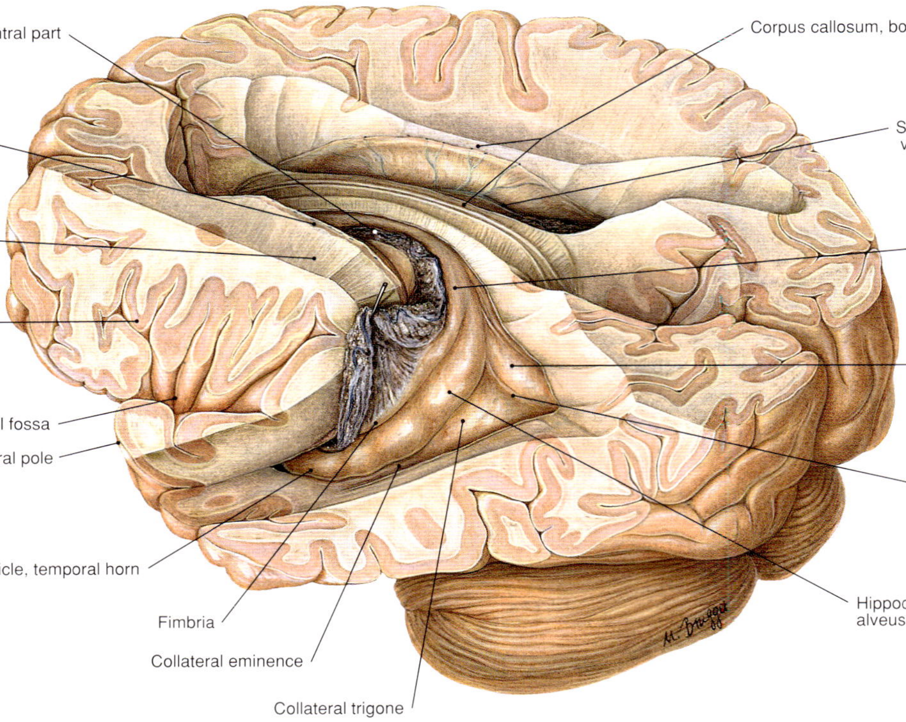

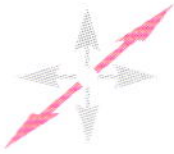

Fig. 1259 Lateral ventricles;
after removal of the upper parts of the cerebral hemispheres;
posterior view from the left.

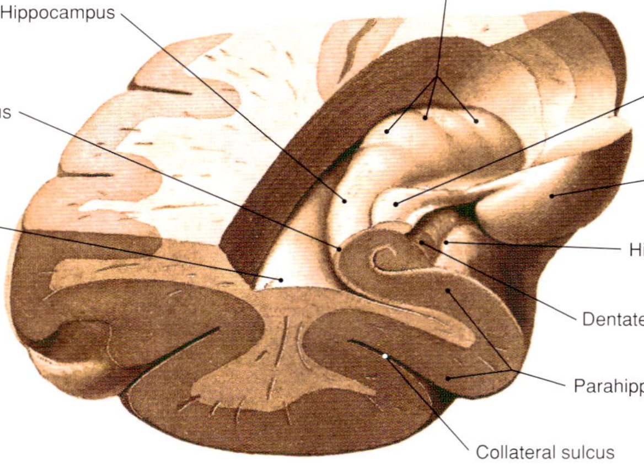

Fig. 1260 Left temporal horn of the lateral ventricle;
frontal section after removal of the temporal wall;
posterior-superior view.

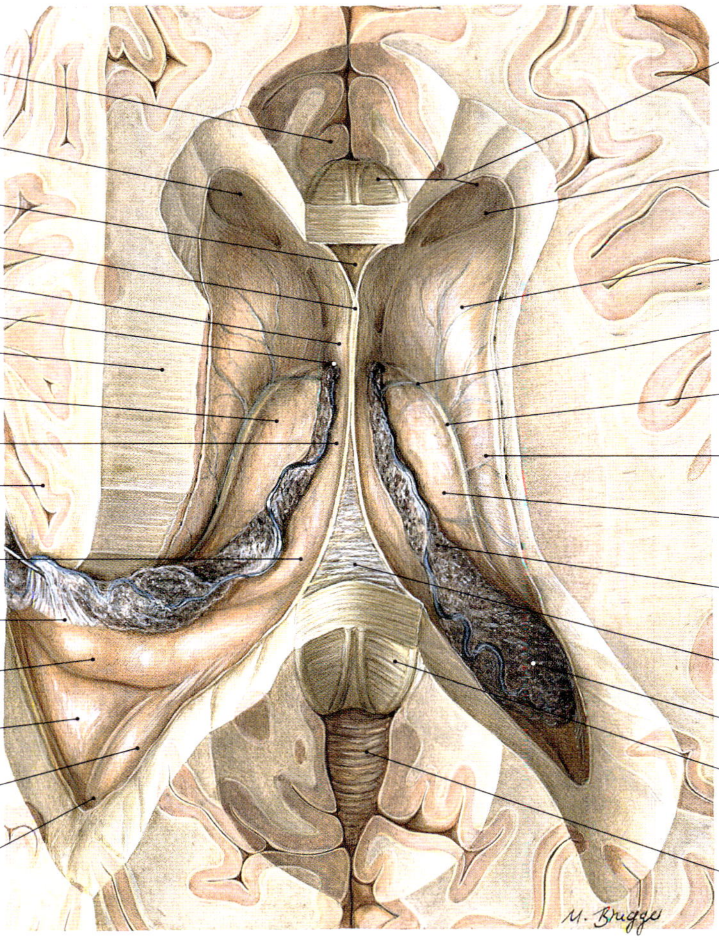

1263
1259

Fig. 1261 Lateral ventricles;
after removal of the upper parts of the cerebral hemispheres and the central part of the corpus callosum; superior view.

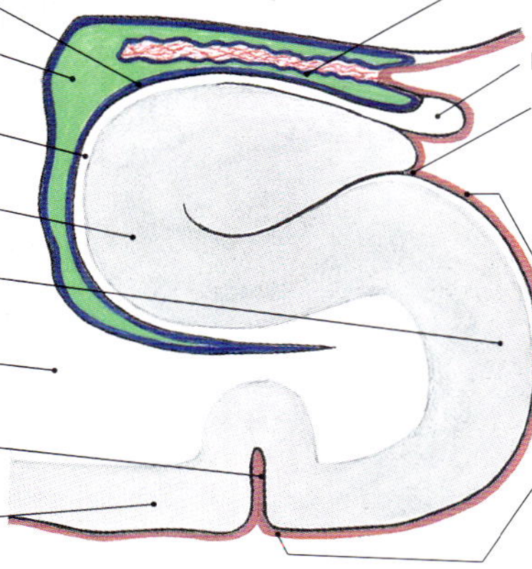

Fig. 1262 Temporal horn of the lateral ventricle;
schematic frontal section.

Brain, topography

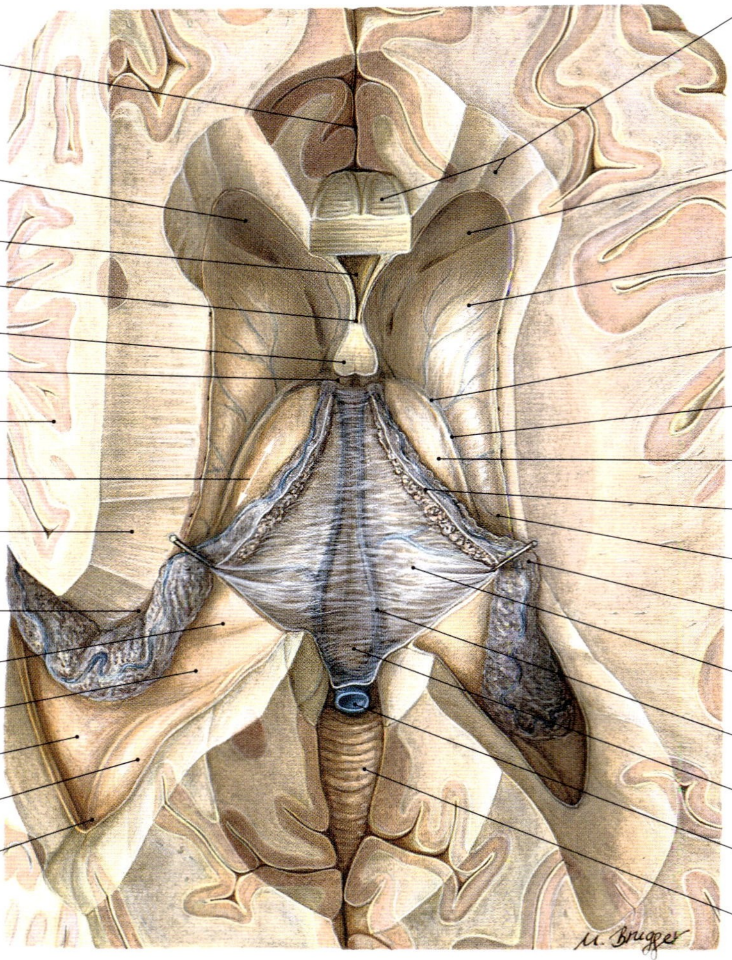

1265
1261

Fig. 1263 Lateral ventricles;
after removal of the central part of the corpus callosum and the columns of the fornix;
superior view.

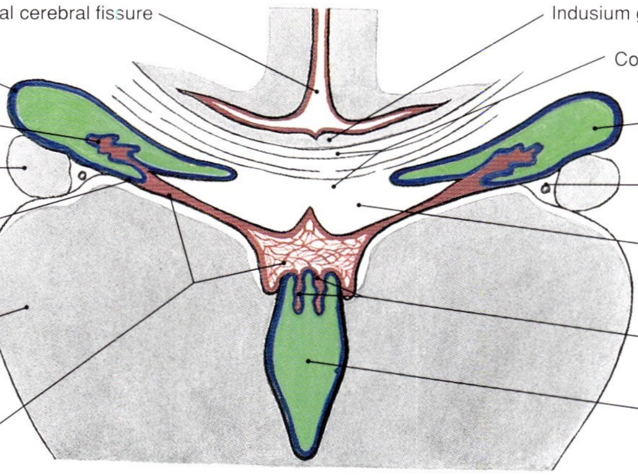

Fig. 1264 Central parts of the lateral ventricles and third ventricle;
schematic frontal section.

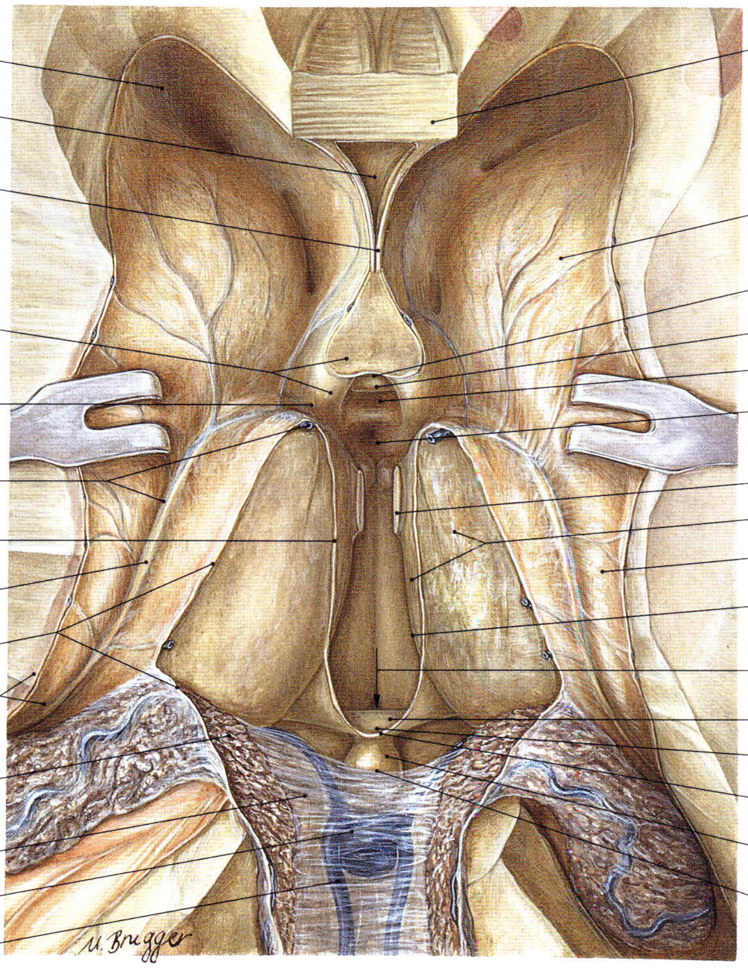

Fig. 1265 Lateral ventricles and third ventricle;
parts of the cerebral hemispheres, the central part of the corpus callosum as well as the fornix and the choroid plexus have been removed, the tela choroidea of the third ventricle has been reflected;
superior view.

1263

* The interthalamic adhesion has been sectioned in the median plane.

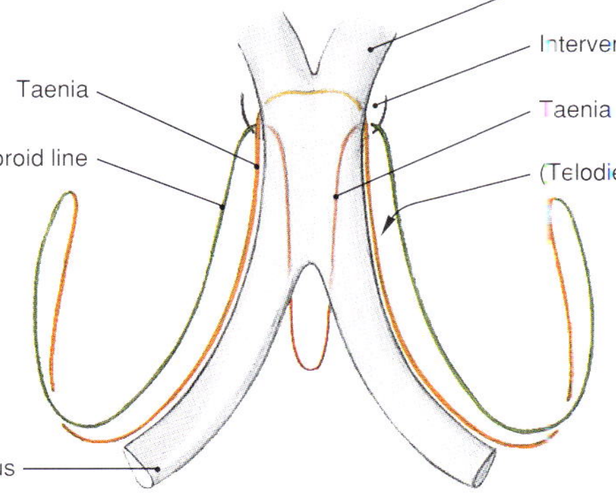

Fig. 1266 Taeniae of the choroid plexus of the cerebrum;
superior view.

Arteries of the base of the brain

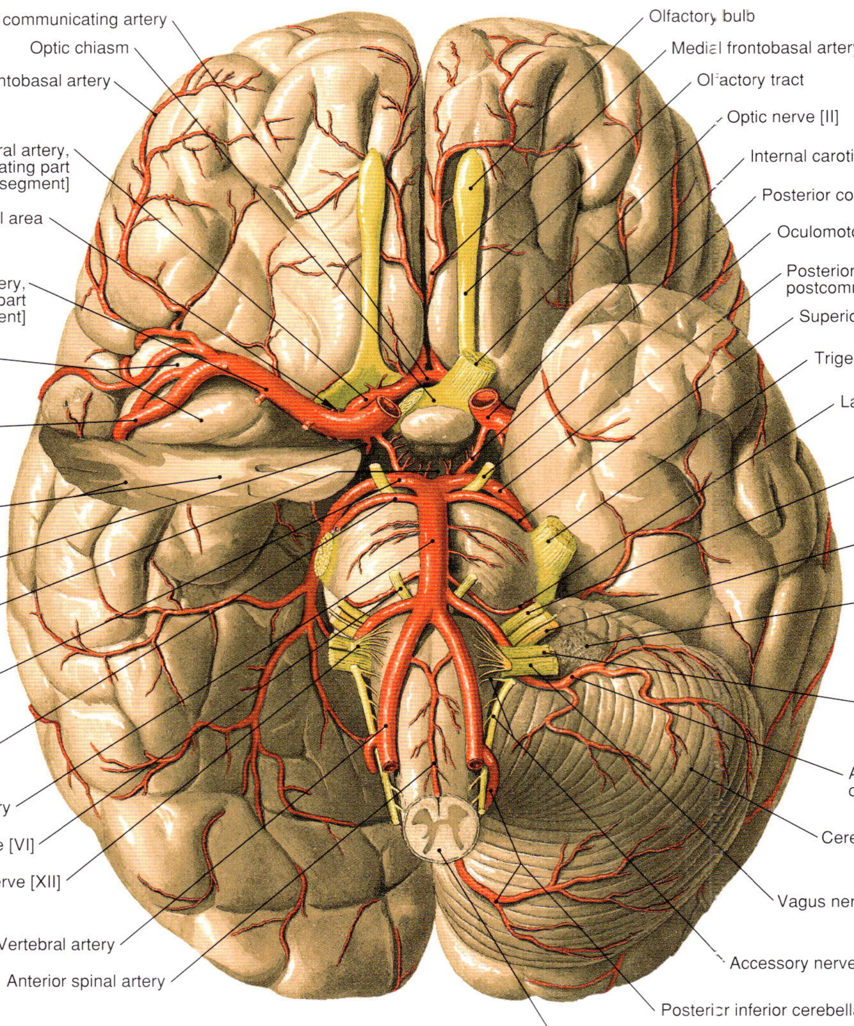

→ 1271, 1272

1195

Fig. 1267 Arteries of the brain.

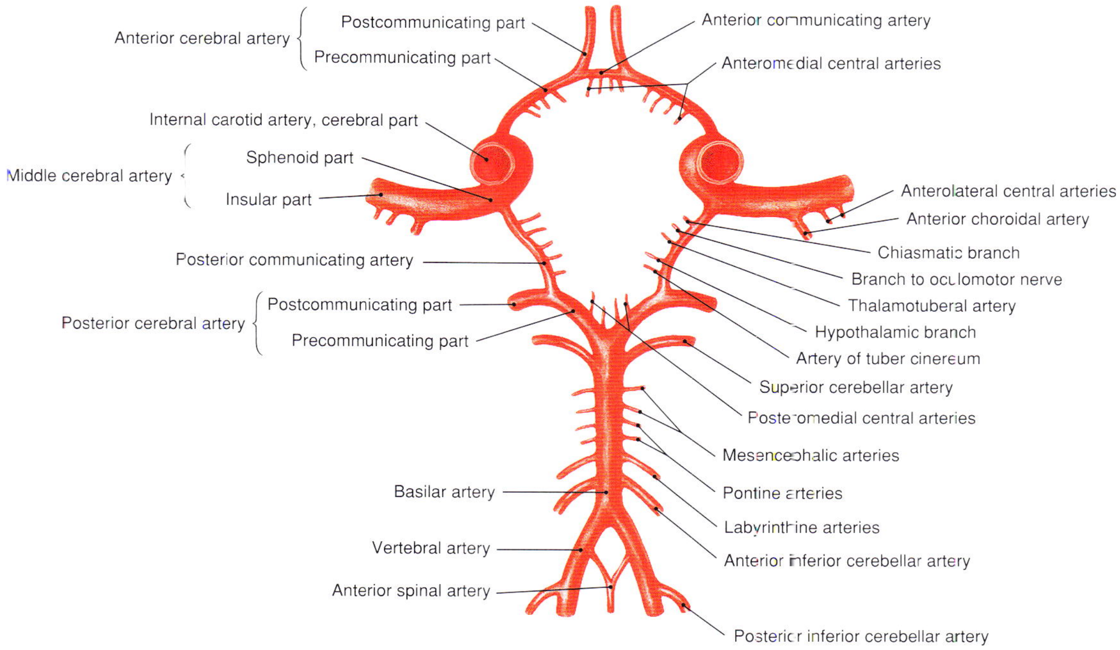

Fig. 1268 Arterial circle of the brain [WILLIS].

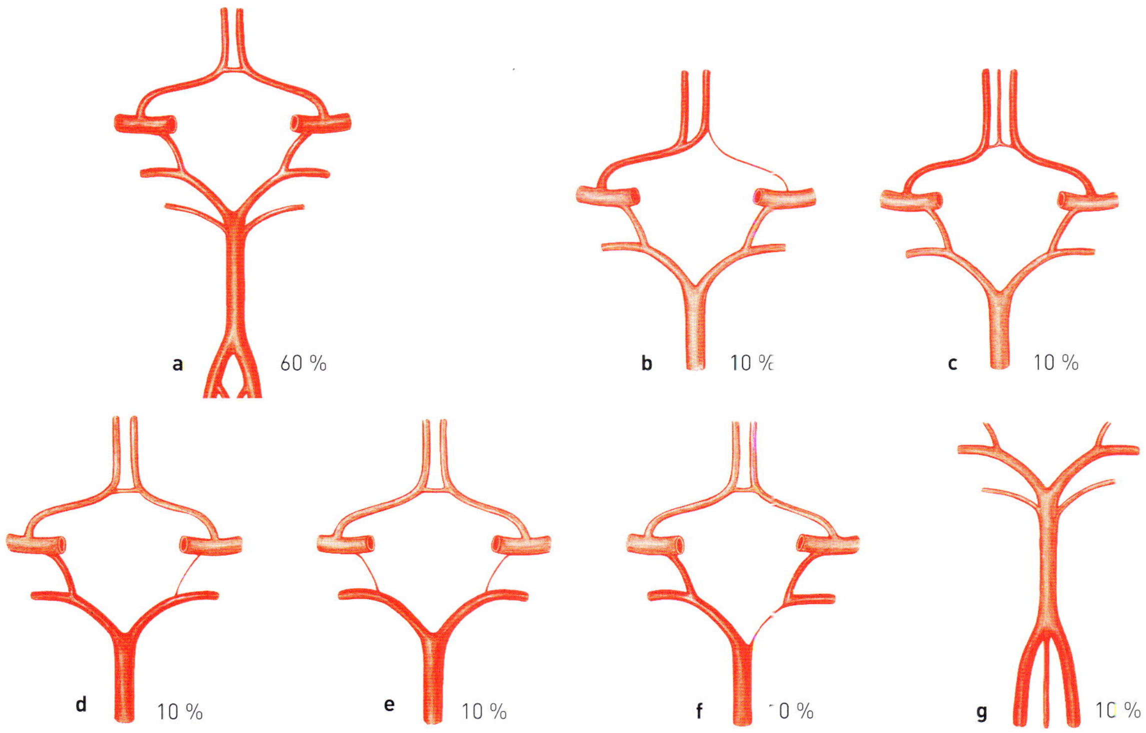

Fig. 1269 a–g Arterial circle of the brain.

a–c Variations of the anterior portion
d–f Variations of the posterior portion
g Very far inferior union of the vertebral arteries

Arteries of the brain

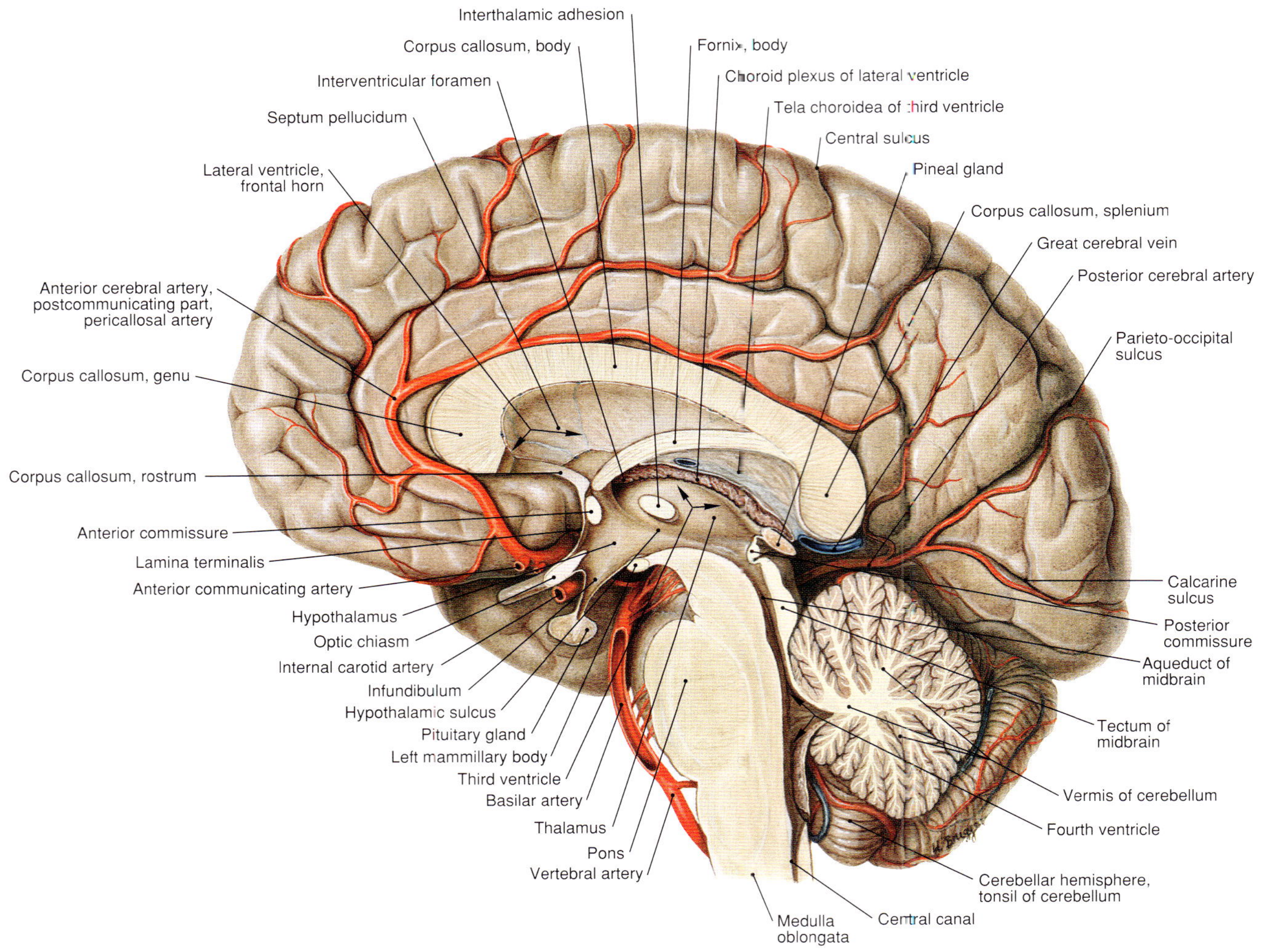

Fig. 1270 Medial surface of the brain; diencephalon and brainstem; staggered median section; viewed from the left.

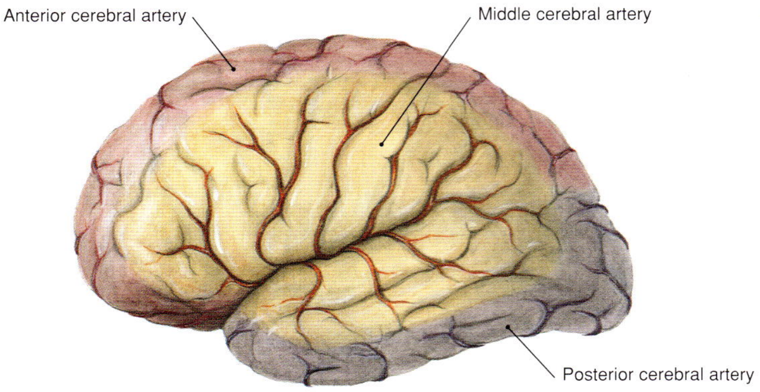

Fig. 1271 Arterial supply of the brain; viewed from the left.

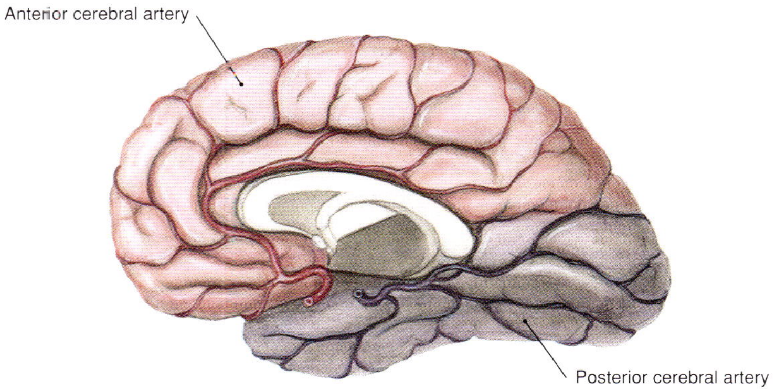

Fig. 1272 Arterial supply of the brain; medial view.

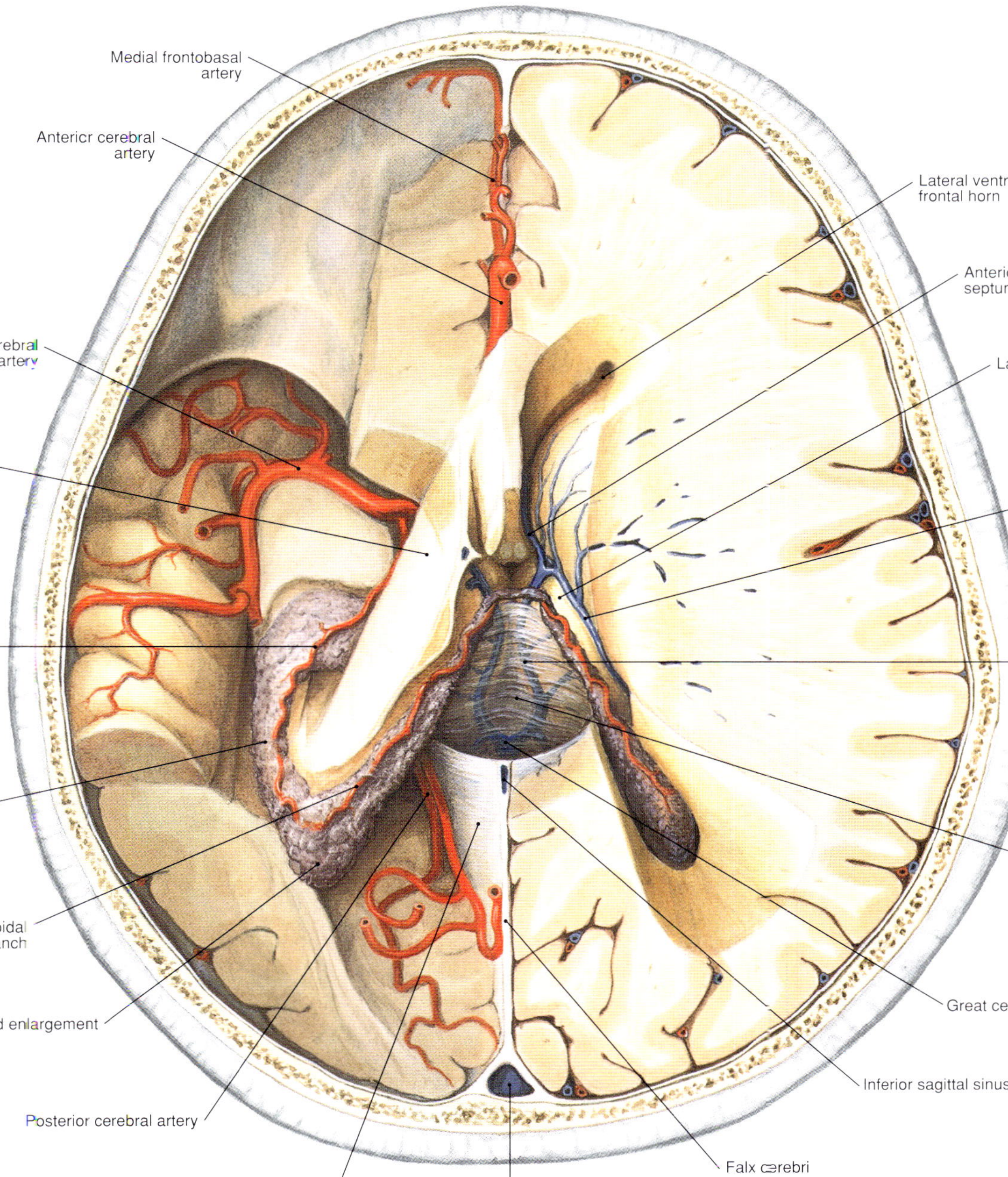

Fig. 1273 Arteries and veins of the brain.

Veins of the brain

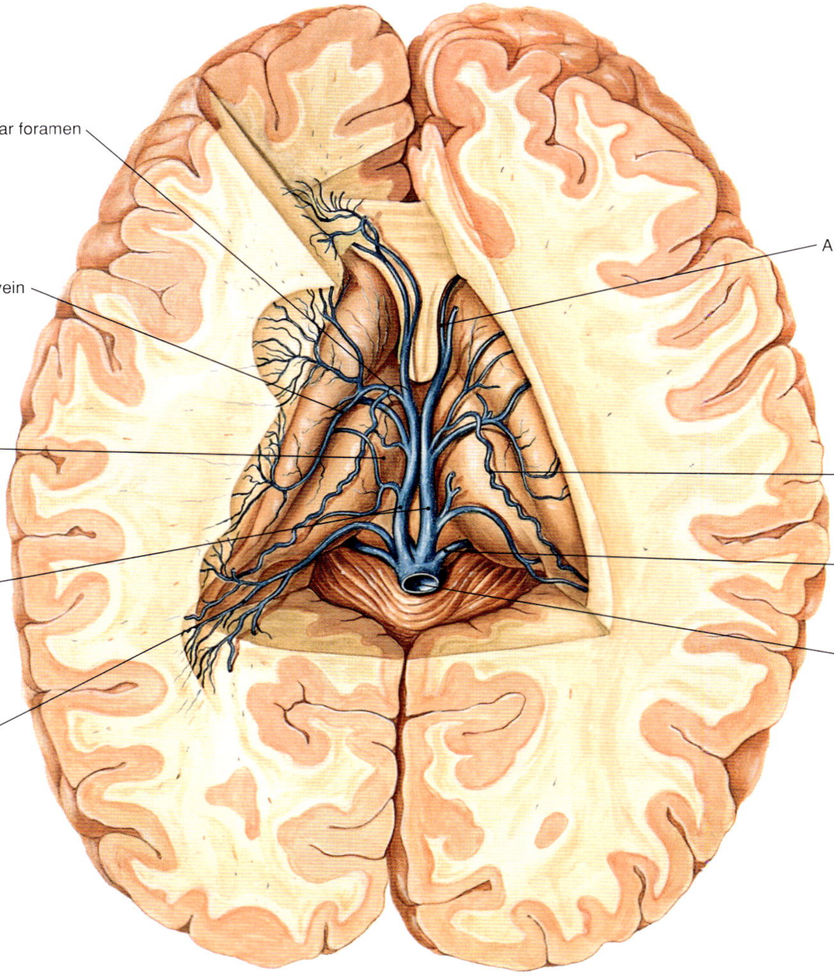

Fig. 1274 Deep veins of the brain.
The internal cerebral veins run within the tela choroidea of the third ventricle.

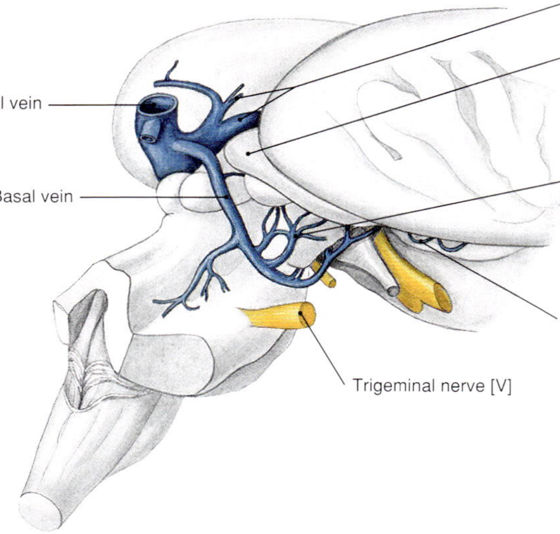

Fig. 1275 Deep veins of the brain; posterior view from the right.

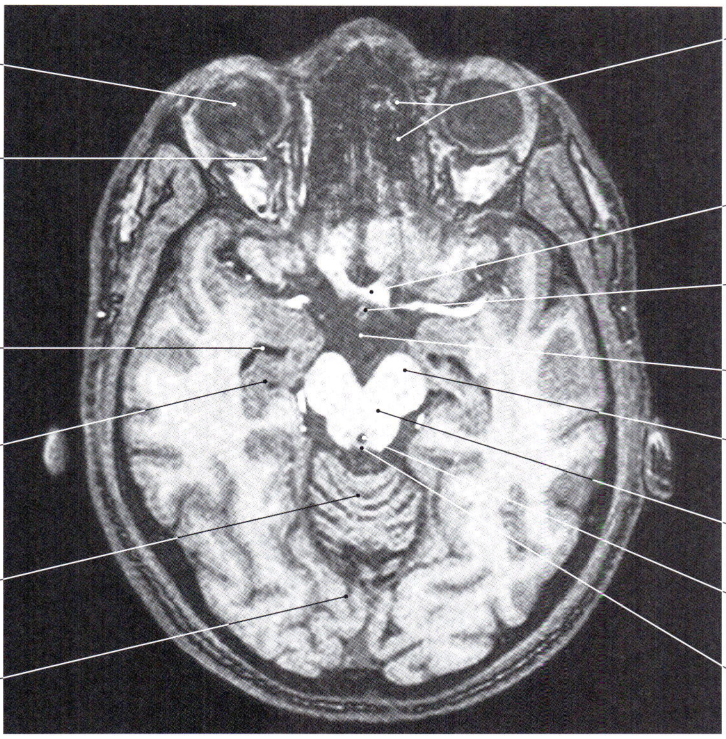

Fig. 1276 Brain;
magnetic resonance tomographic image (MRI);
horizontal section at the level of the midbrain and the temporal horns of the lateral ventricles;
superior view.

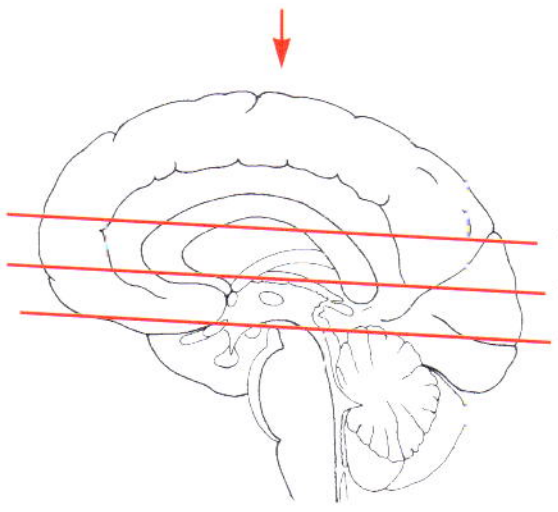

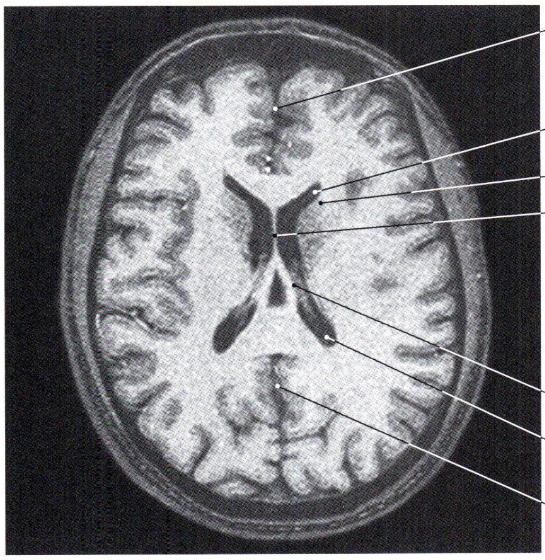

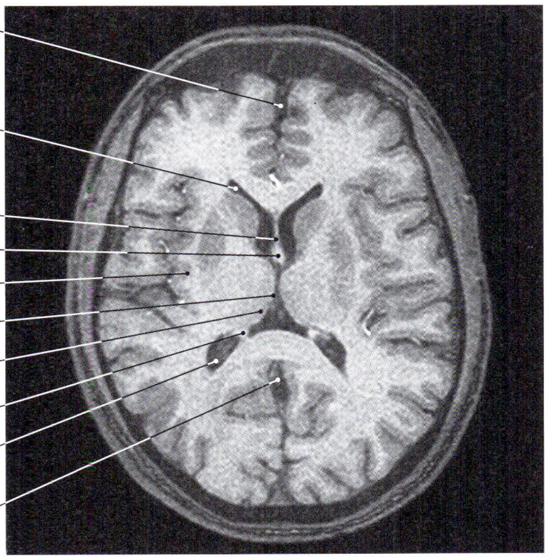

Fig. 1277 Brain;
magnetic resonance tomographic image (MRI);
horizontal section at the level of the central parts of the lateral ventricles;
superior view.

Fig. 1278 Brain;
magnetic resonance tomographic image (MRI);
horizontal section at the level of the third ventricle and the opening of the temporal horns of the lateral ventricles;
superior view.

Brain, sections

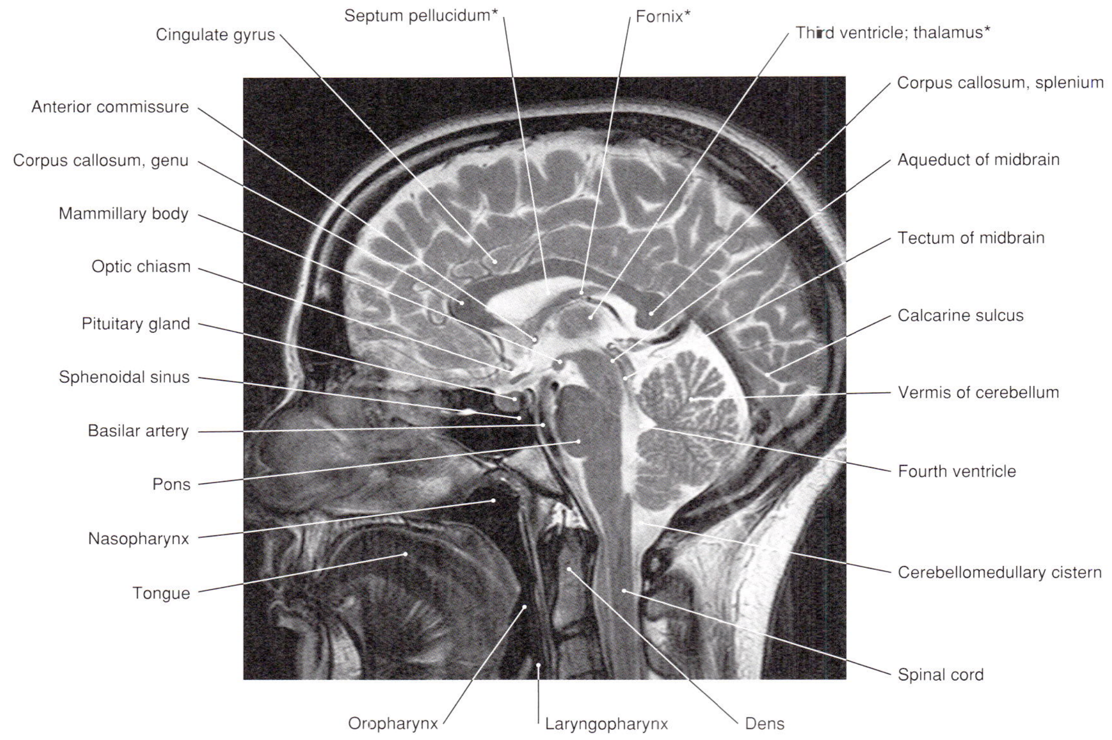

Fig. 1279 Brain;
magnetic resonance tomographic image (MRI);
median section. The structures marked with * appear partly falsified as a consequence of the "partial-volume-effect".

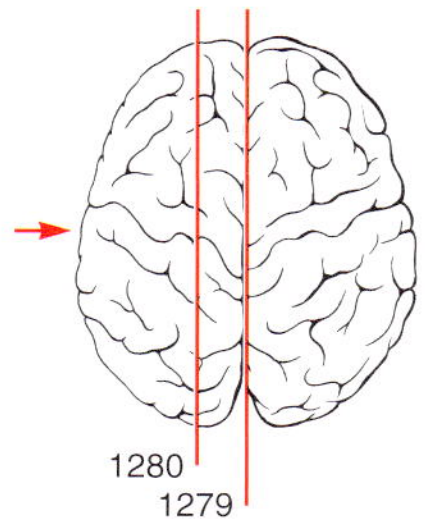

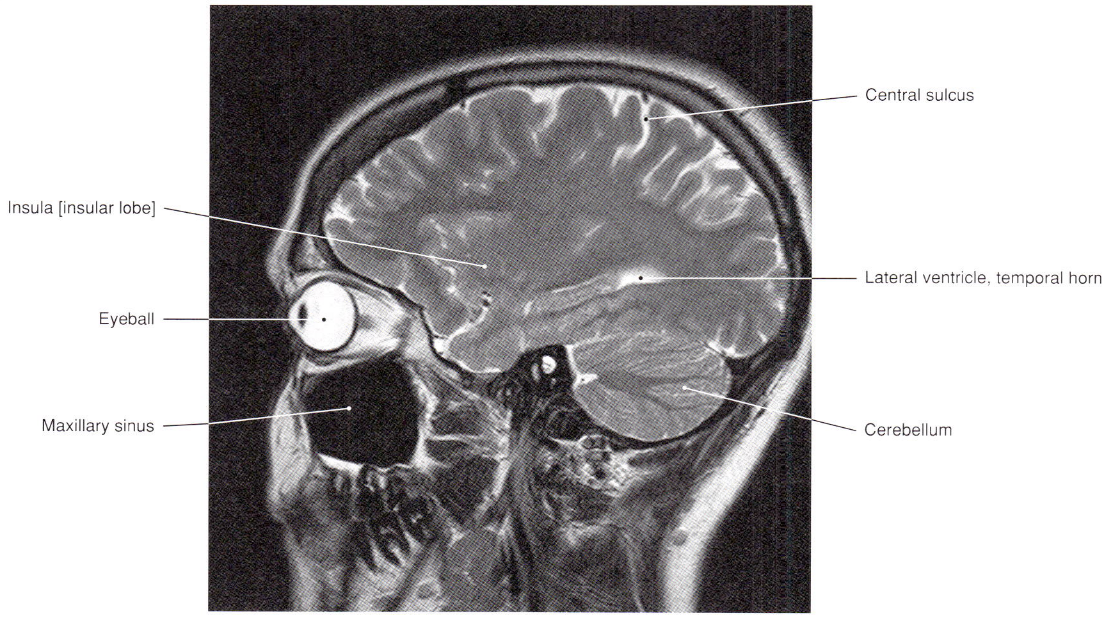

Fig. 1280 Brain;
magnetic resonance tomographic image (MRI);
sagittal section.

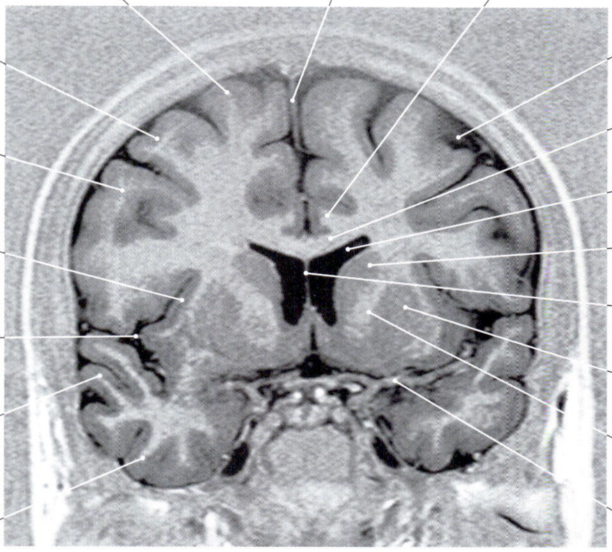

Fig. 1281 Brain;
magnetic resonance tomographic image (MRI);
frontal section.

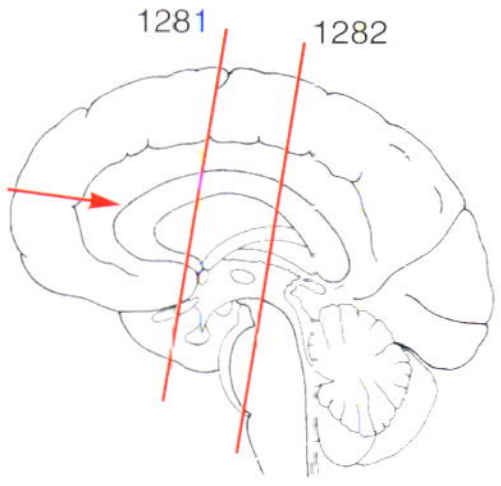

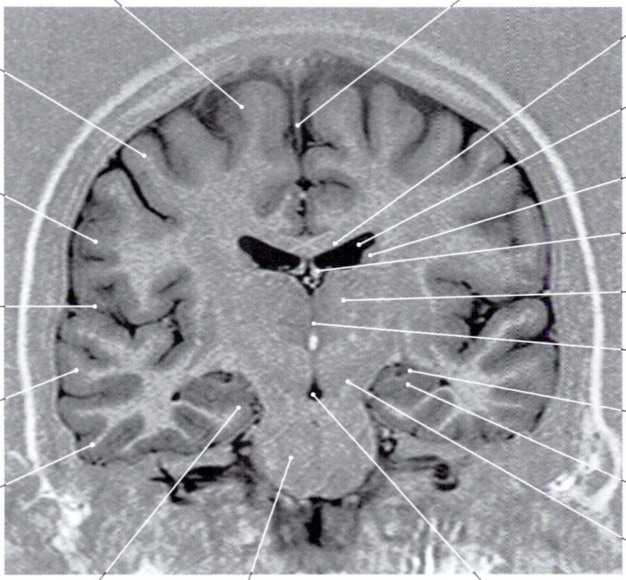

Fig. 1282 Brain;
magnetic resonance tomographic image (MRI);
frontal section.

Brain, frontal sections

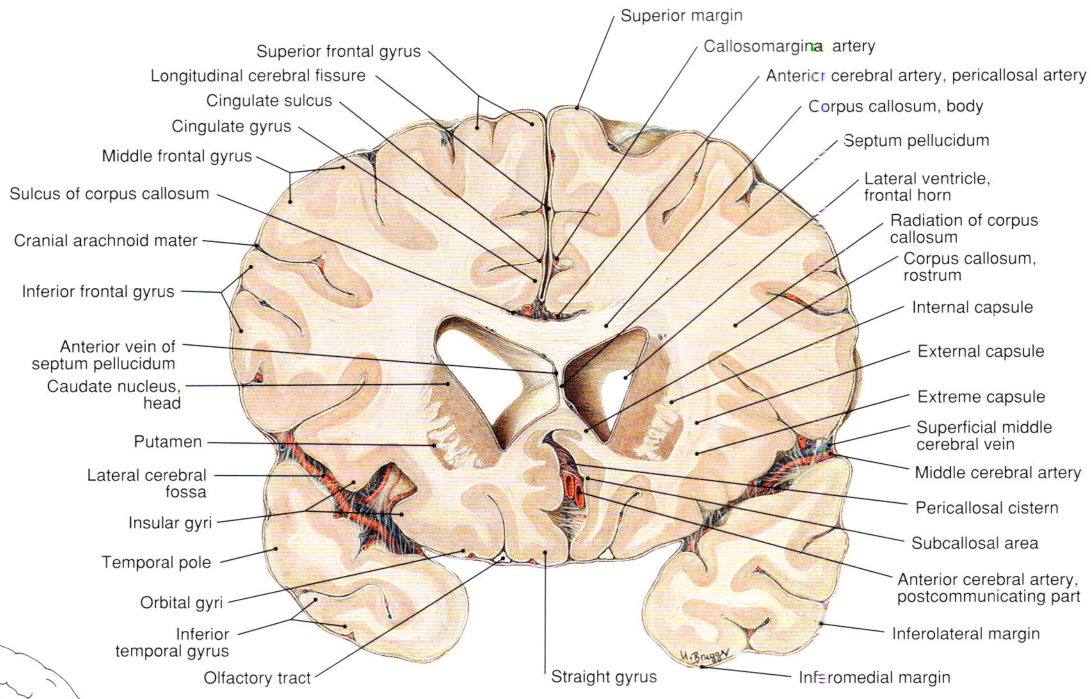

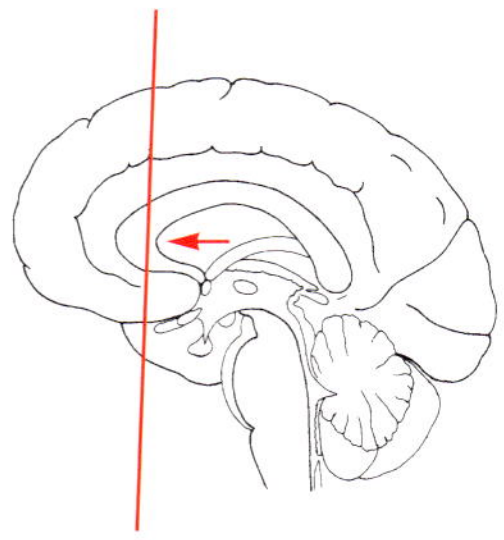

Fig. 1283 Brain;
frontal section at the level of the anterior parts of the frontal horns of the lateral ventricles.

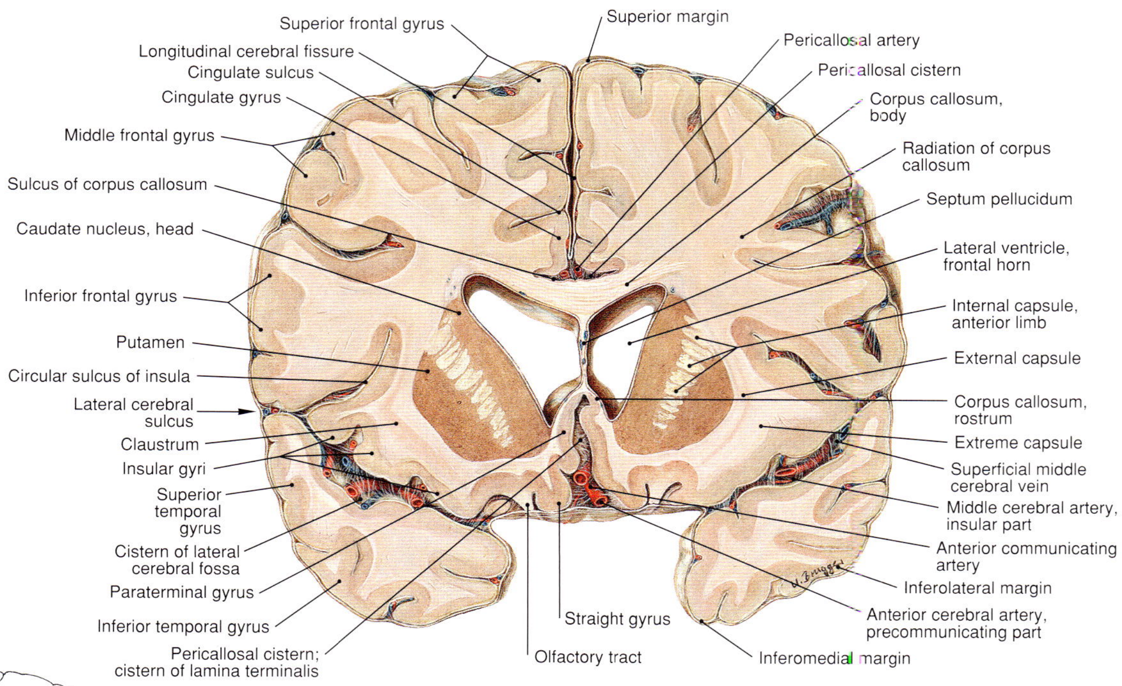

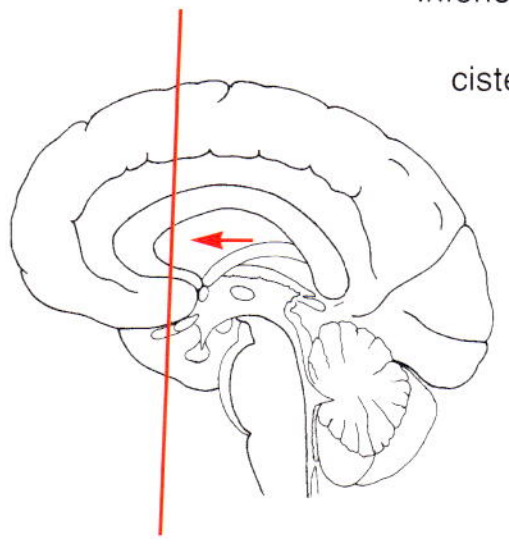

Fig. 1284 Brain;
frontal section at the level of the posterior parts of the frontal horns of the lateral ventricles.

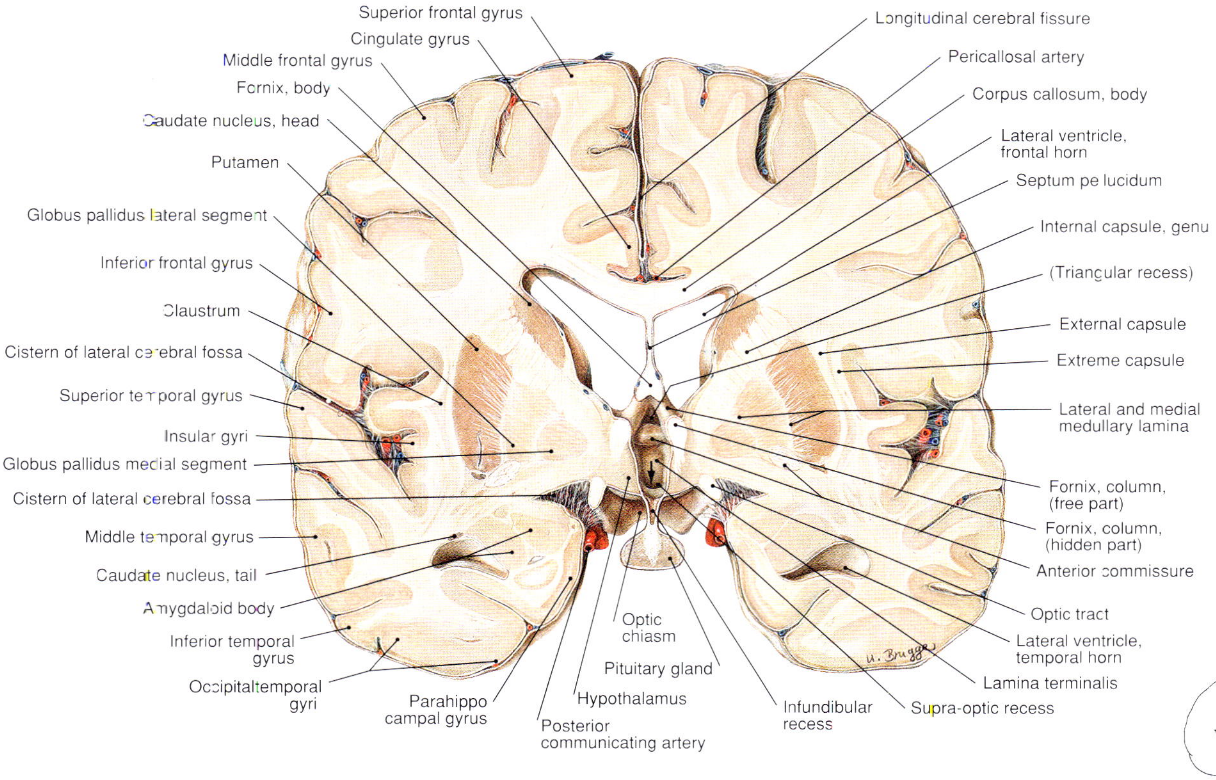

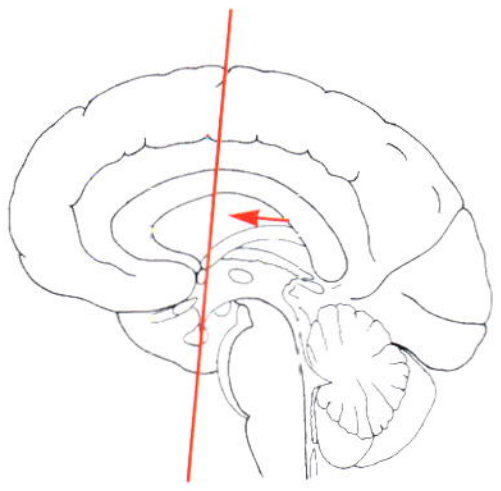

Fig. 1285 Brain;
frontal section at the level of the interventricular foramina.

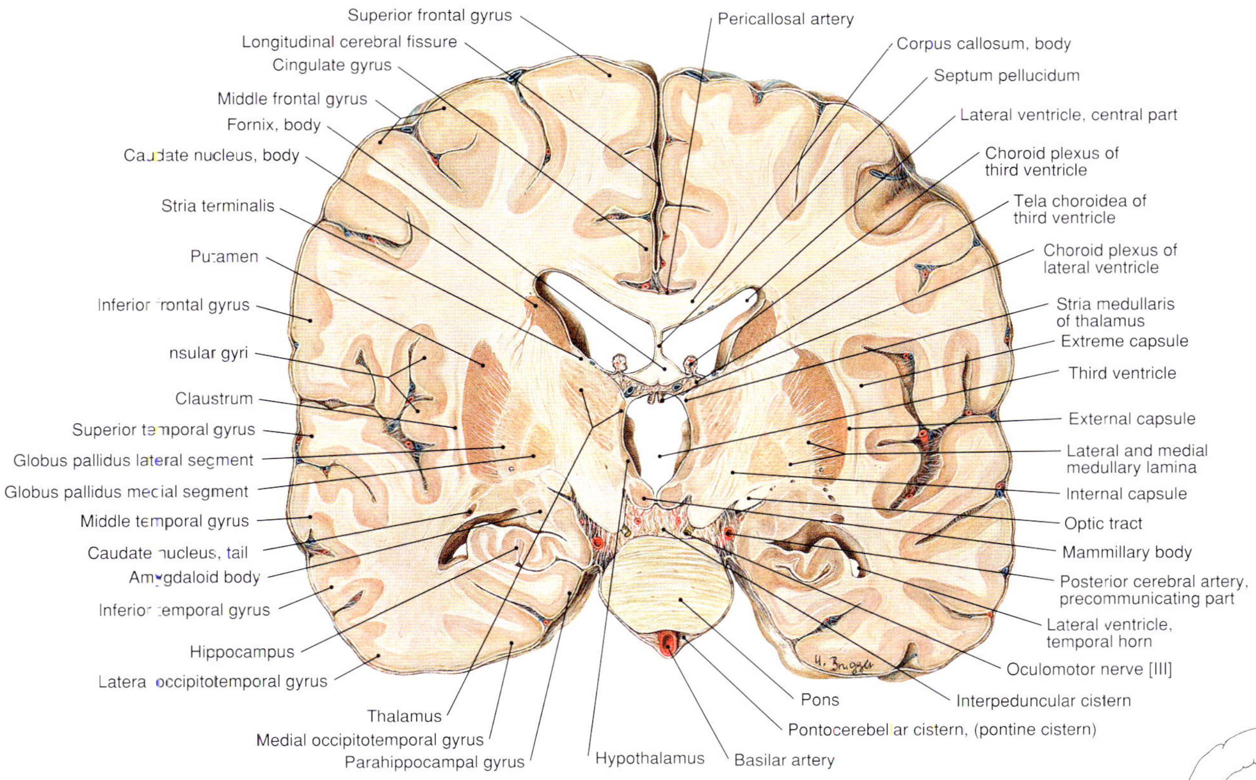

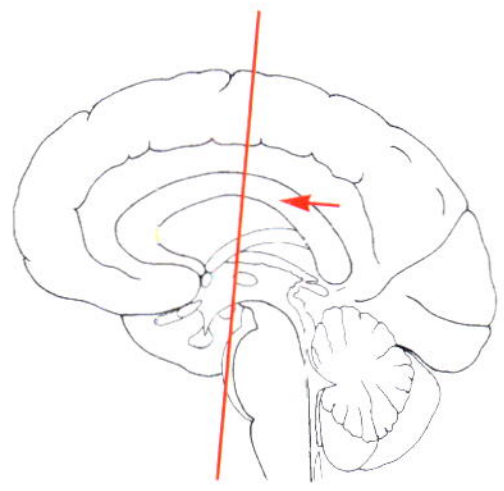

Fig. 1286 Brain;
frontal section at the level of the mamillary bodies.

Brain, frontal sections

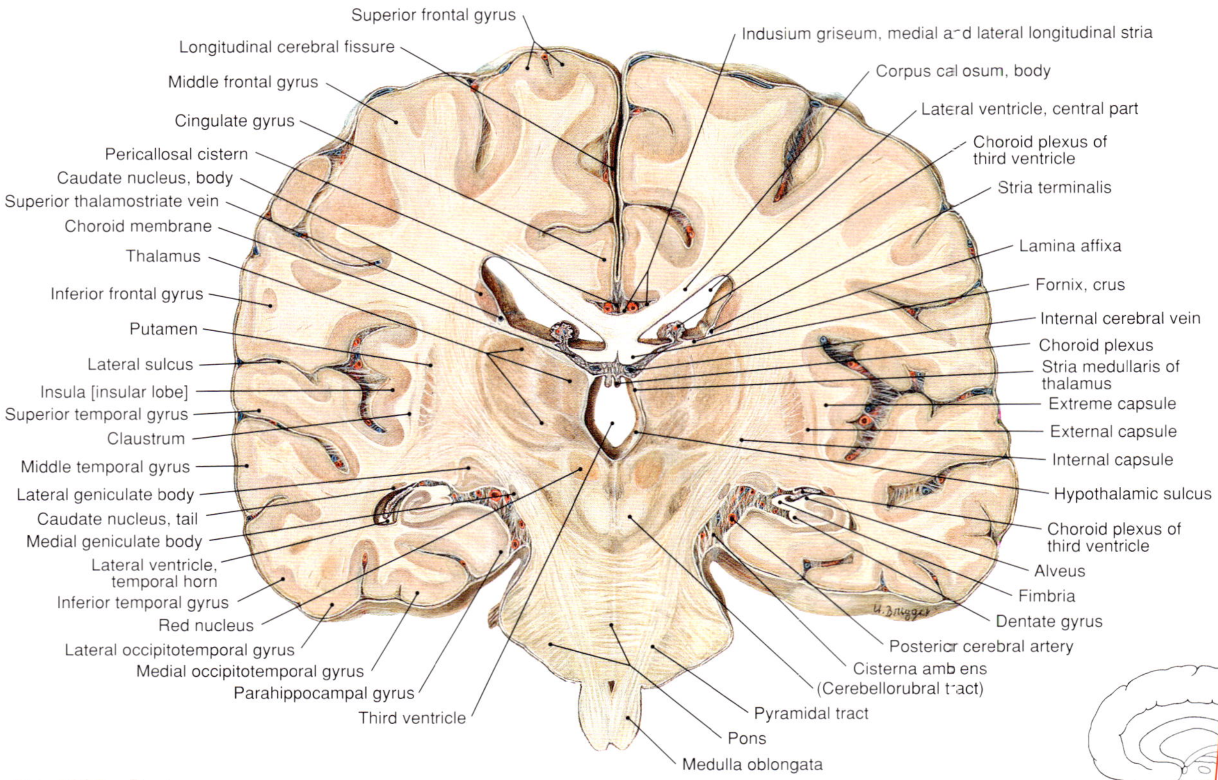

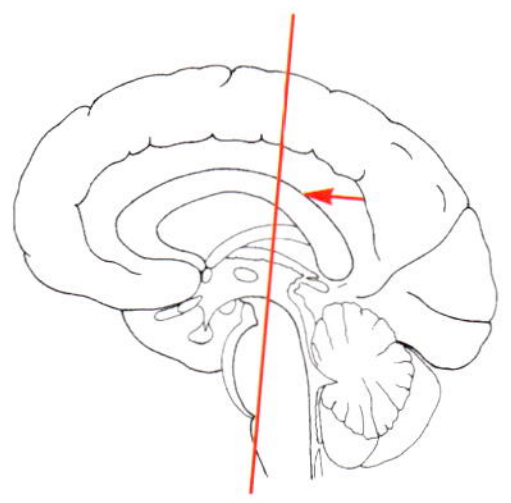

Fig. 1287 Brain;
frontal section at the level of the central part of the third ventricle. Right and left thalamus are frequently connected by the interthalamic adhesion at this level.

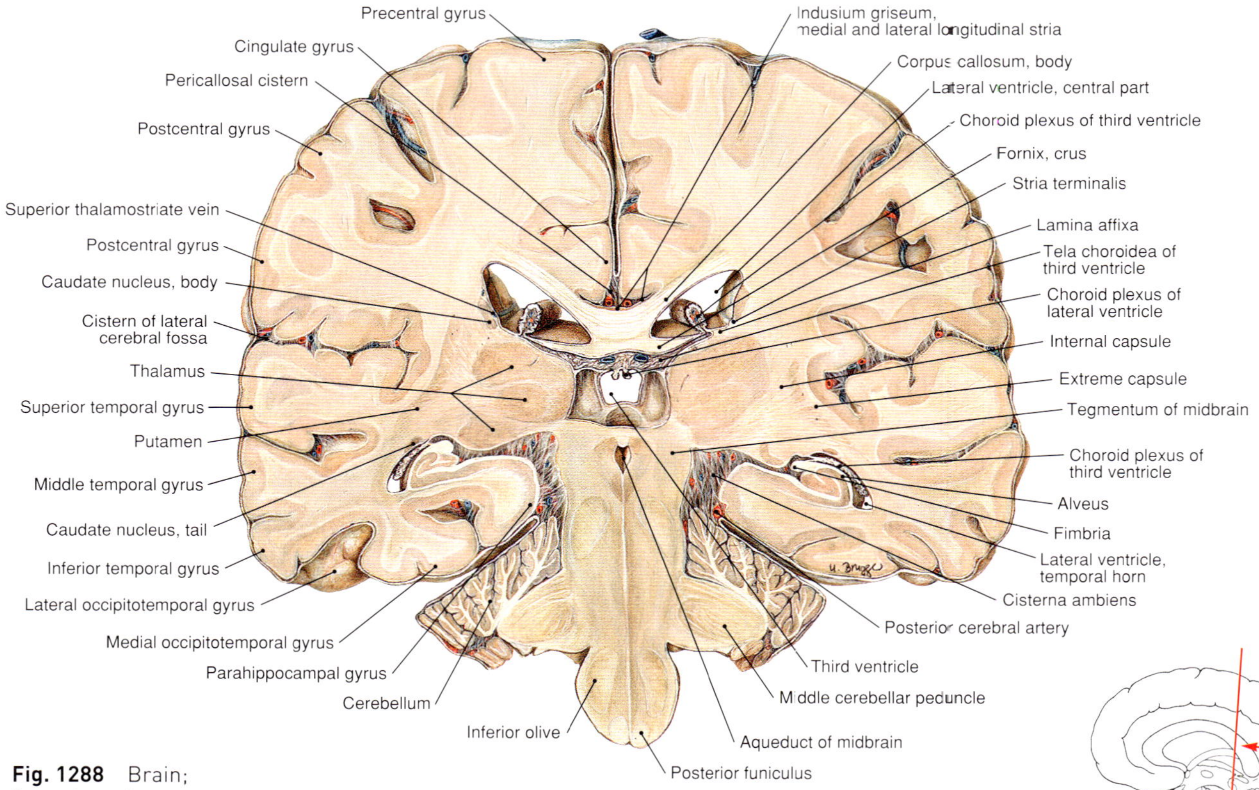

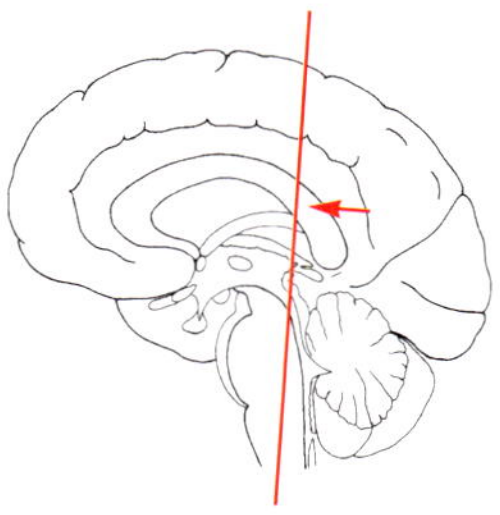

Fig. 1288 Brain;
frontal section at the level of the posterior wall of the third ventricle.

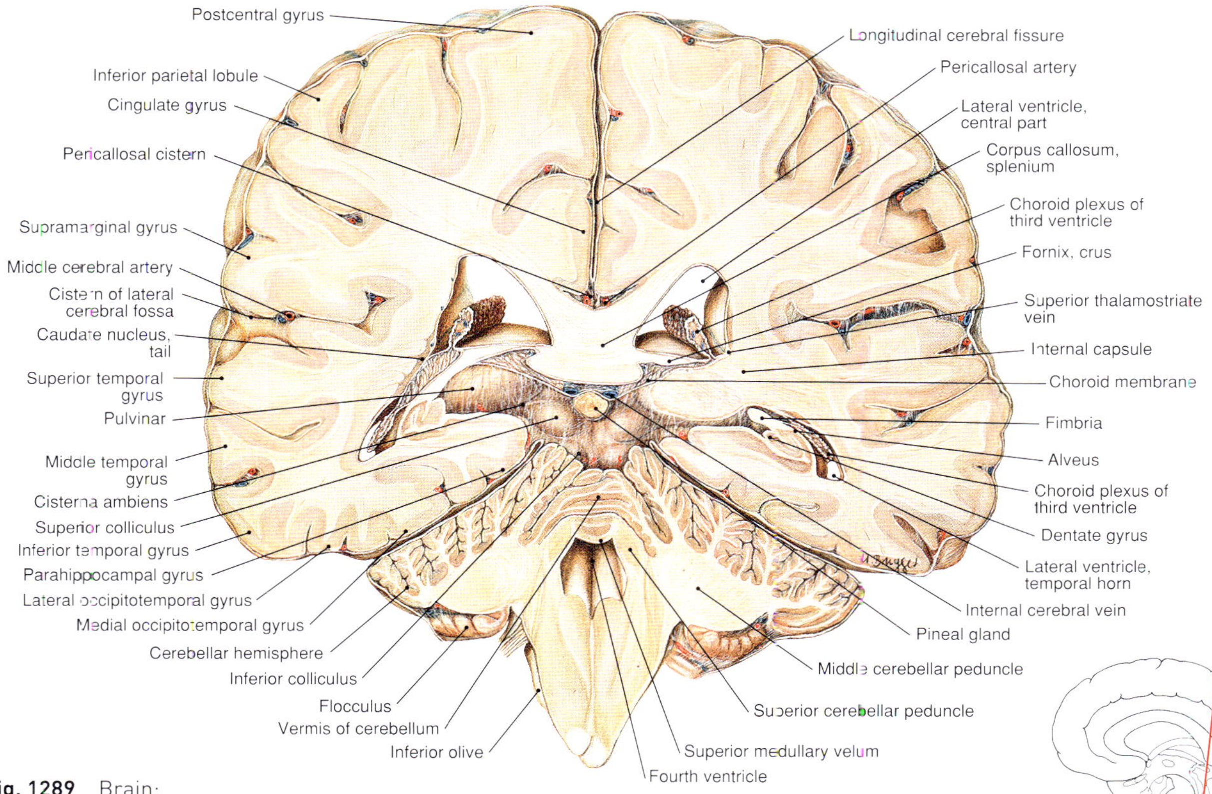

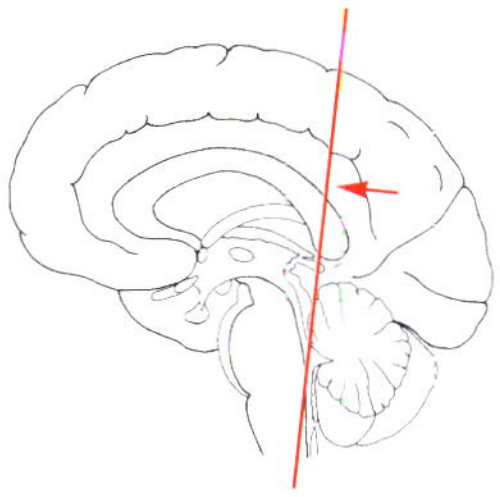

Fig. 1289 Brain;
frontal section at the level of the pineal gland and the fourth ventricle.

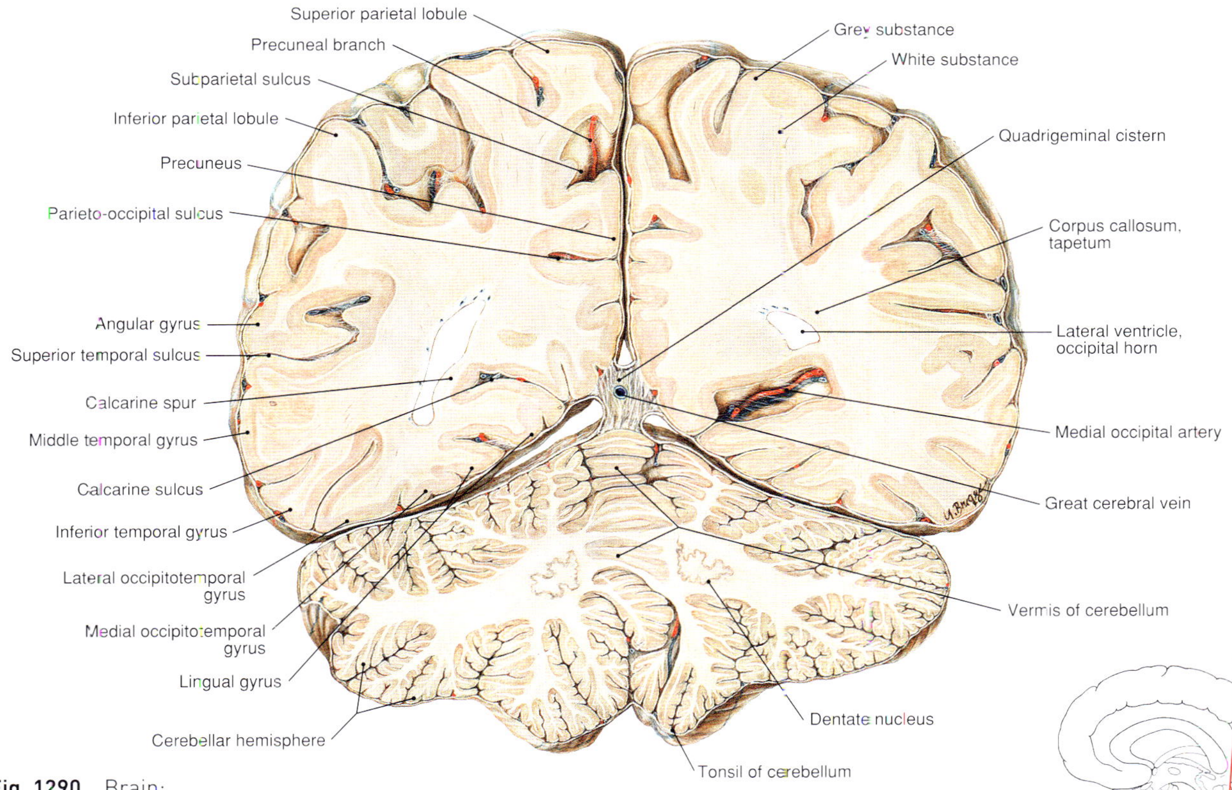

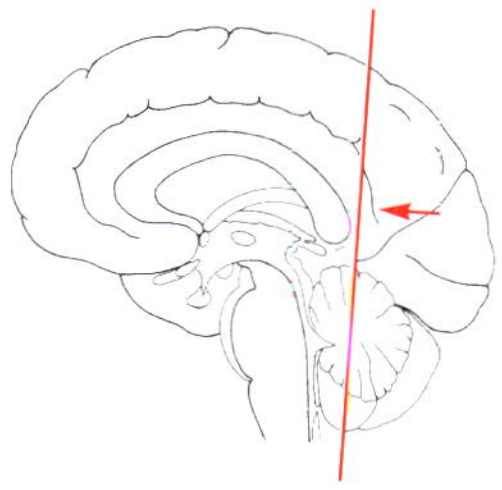

Fig. 1290 Brain;
frontal section at the level of the occipital horns of the lateral ventricles.

Brain, horizontal section

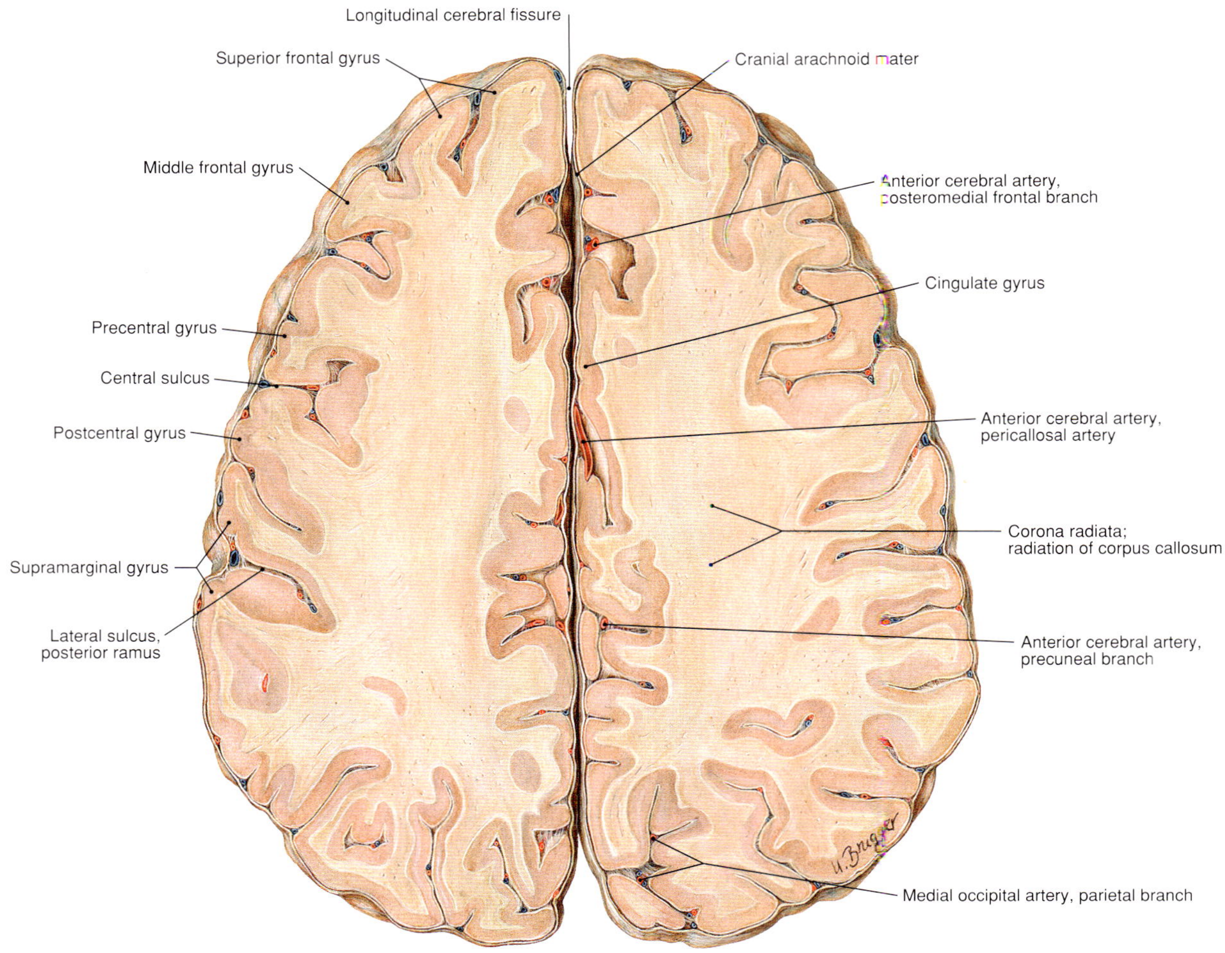

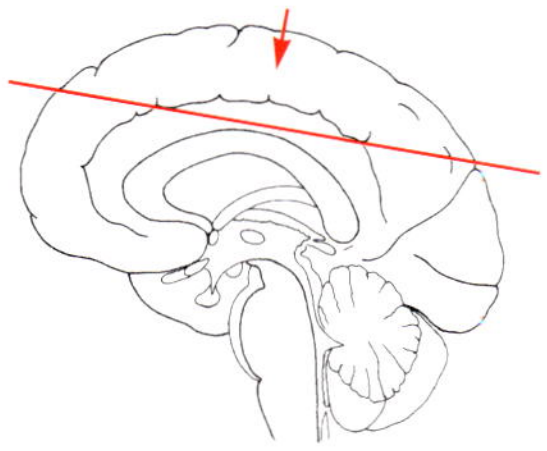

Fig. 1291 Brain;
horizontal section just above the corpus callosum.
In Fig. 1283–1303, the subarachnoid space appears somewhat enlarged, particularly in the region of the hemispheric sulci, due to the fact that these specimens were taken from elderly individuals.

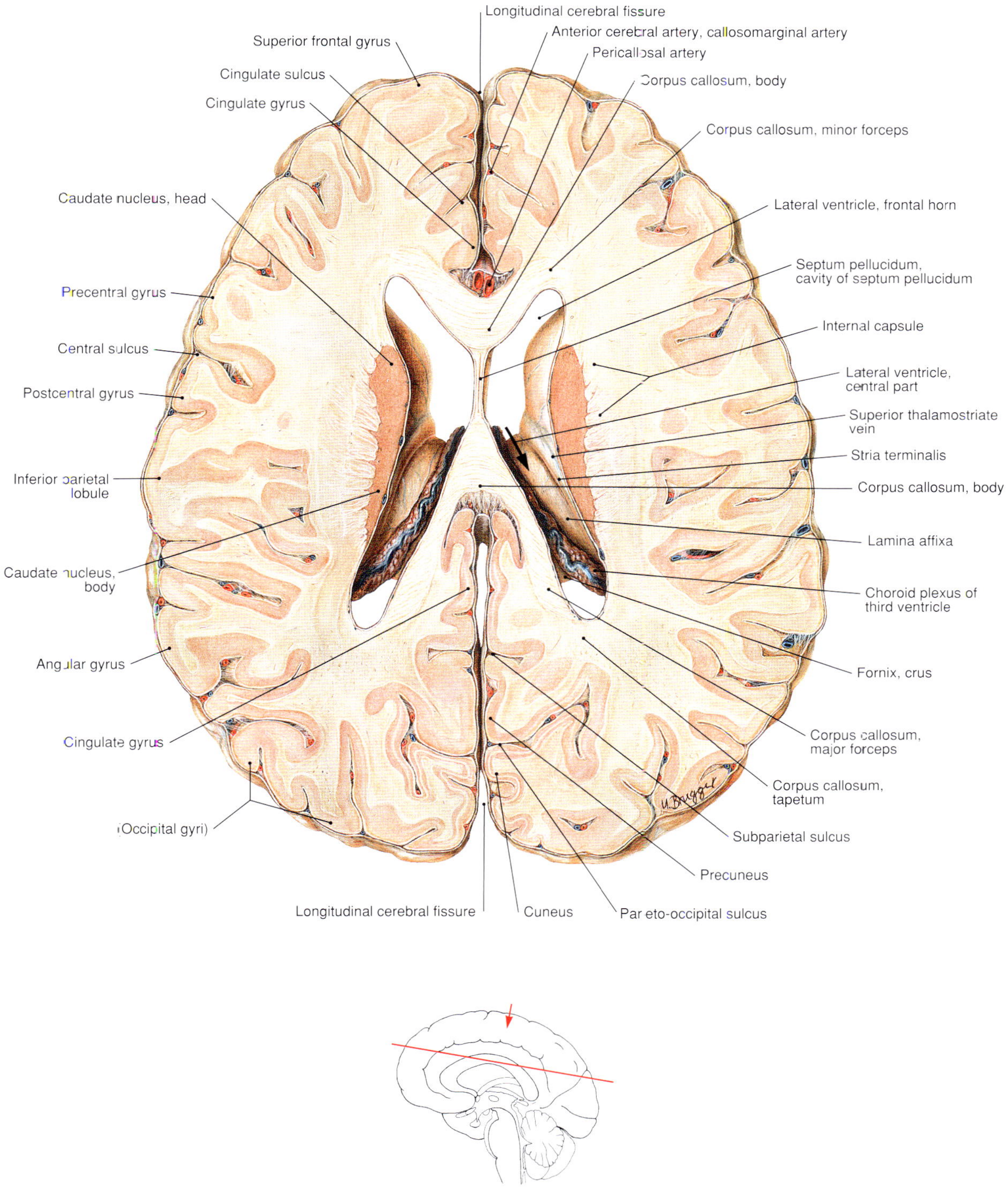

Fig. 1292 Brain;
horizontal section at the level of
the central part of the lateral ventricles.

Brain, horizontal section

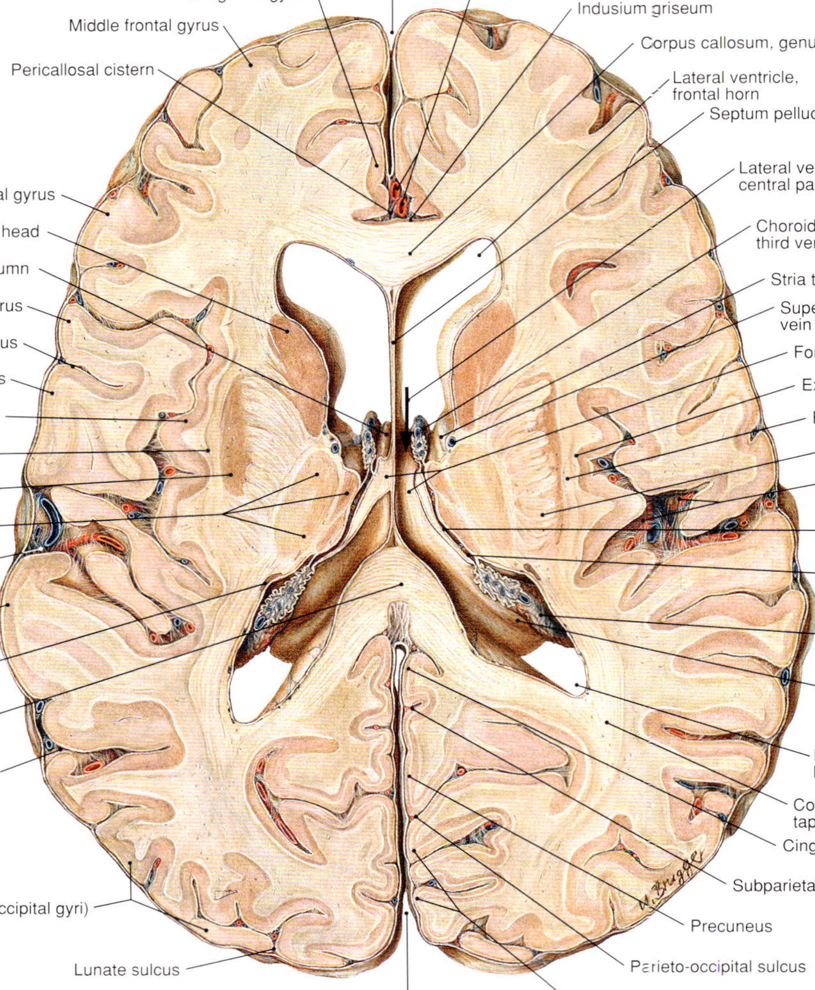

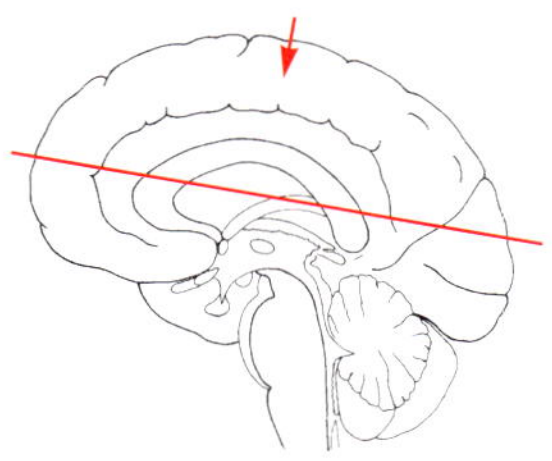

Fig. 1293 Brain;
horizontal section at the level of the floor of the central part of the lateral ventricles.

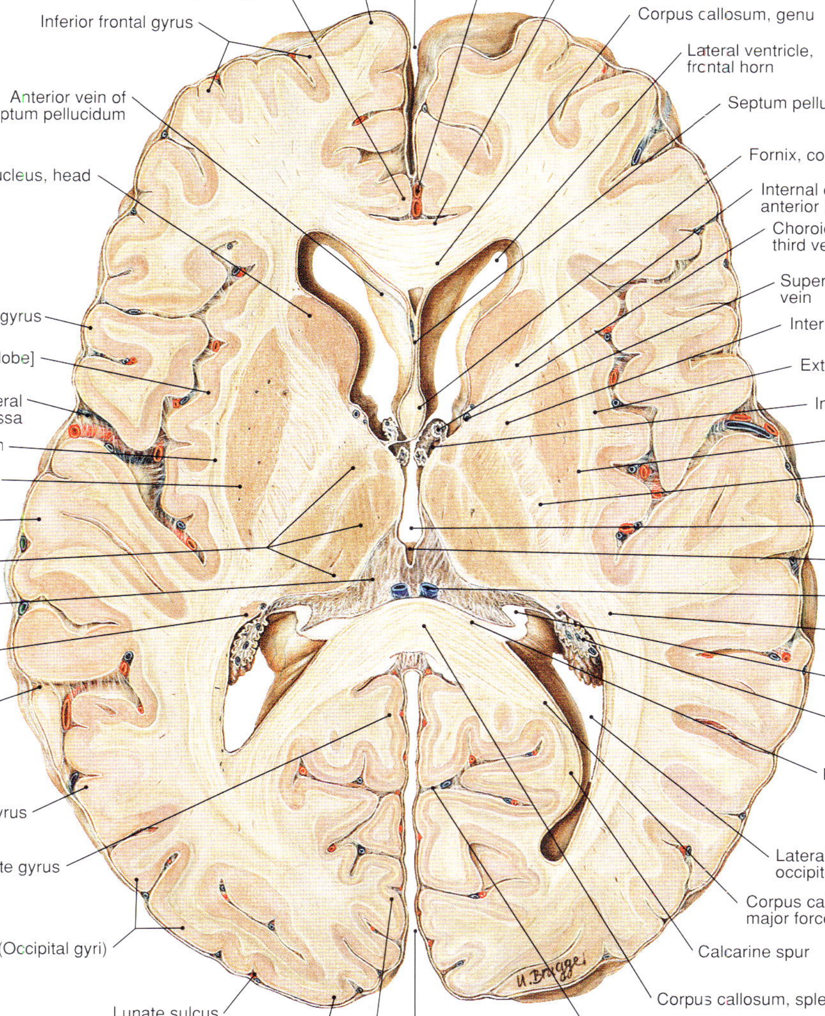

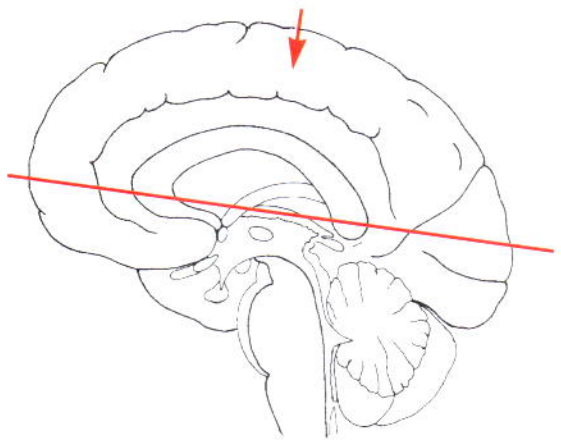

Fig. 1294 Brain;
horizontal section at the level of the upper part of the third ventricle.

Brain, horizontal section

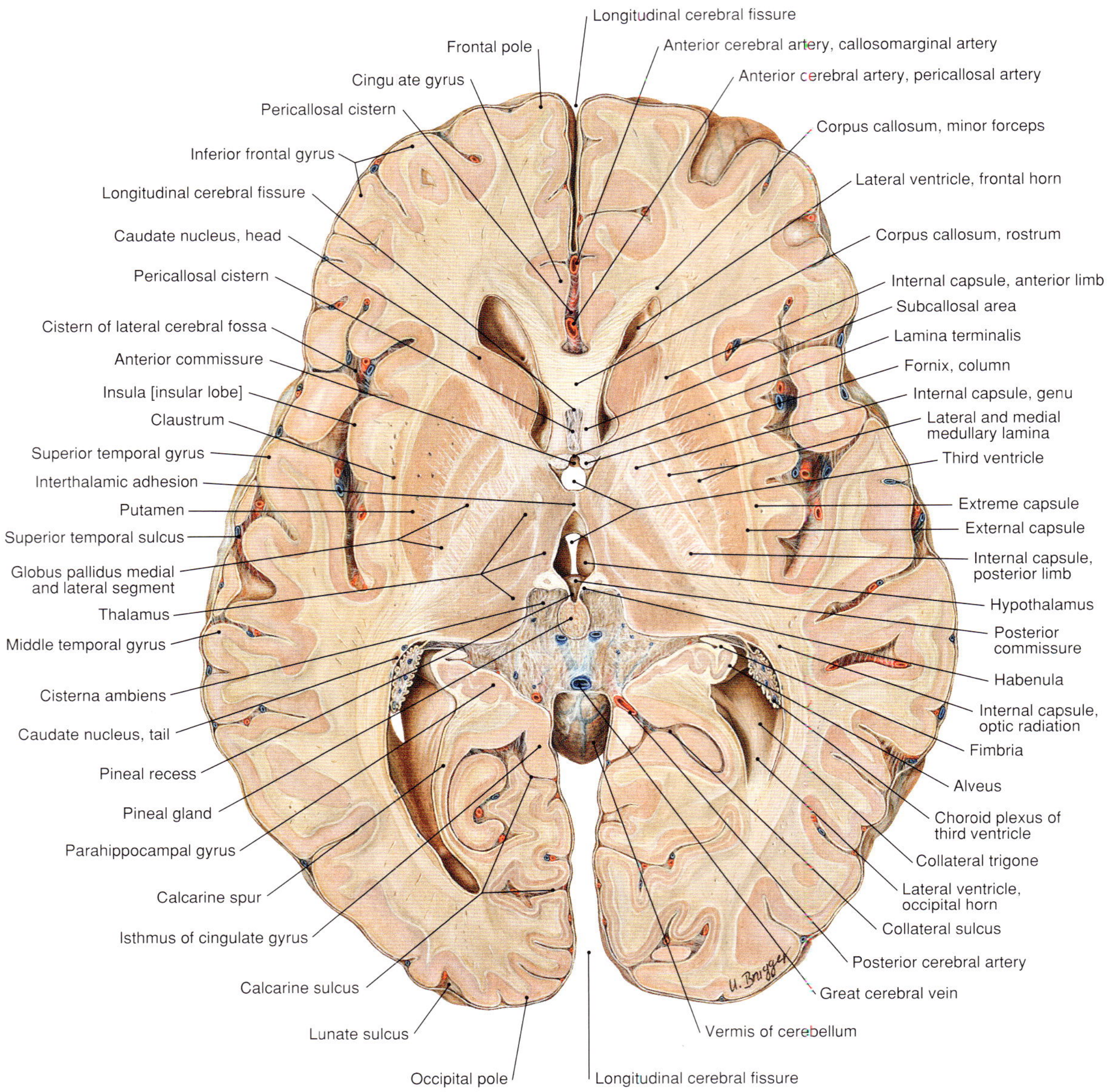

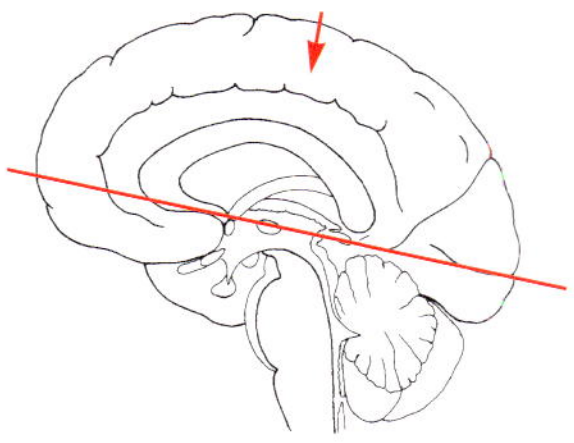

Fig. 1295 Brain;
horizontal section through the centre of the third ventricle at the level of the interthalamic adhesion.

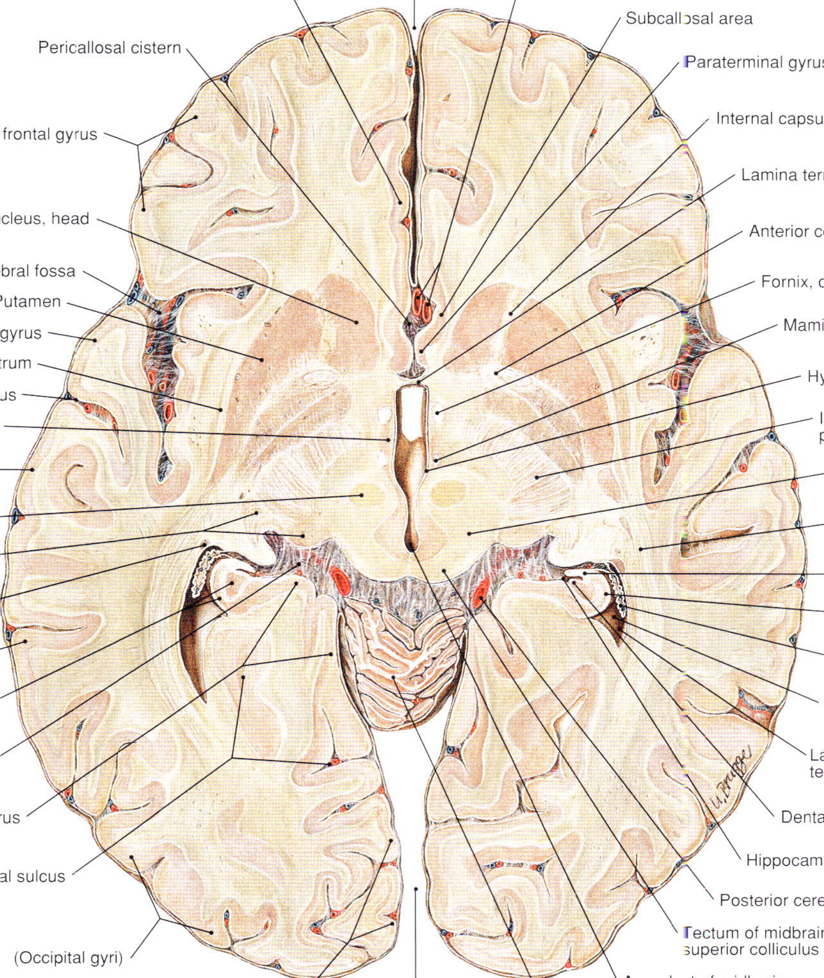

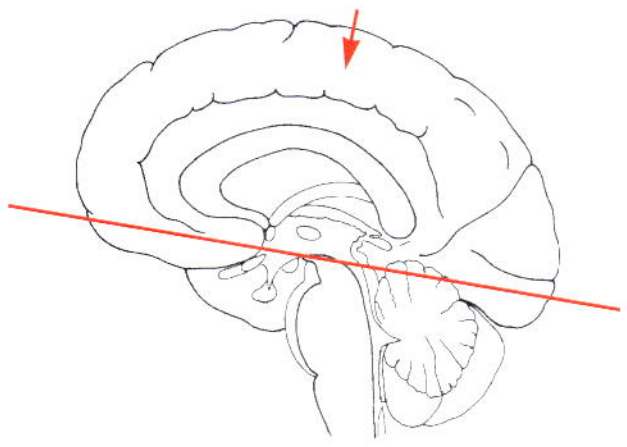

Fig. 1296 Brain;
horizontal section through the third ventricle at the level of the opening of the cerebral aqueduct.

Brain, horizontal section

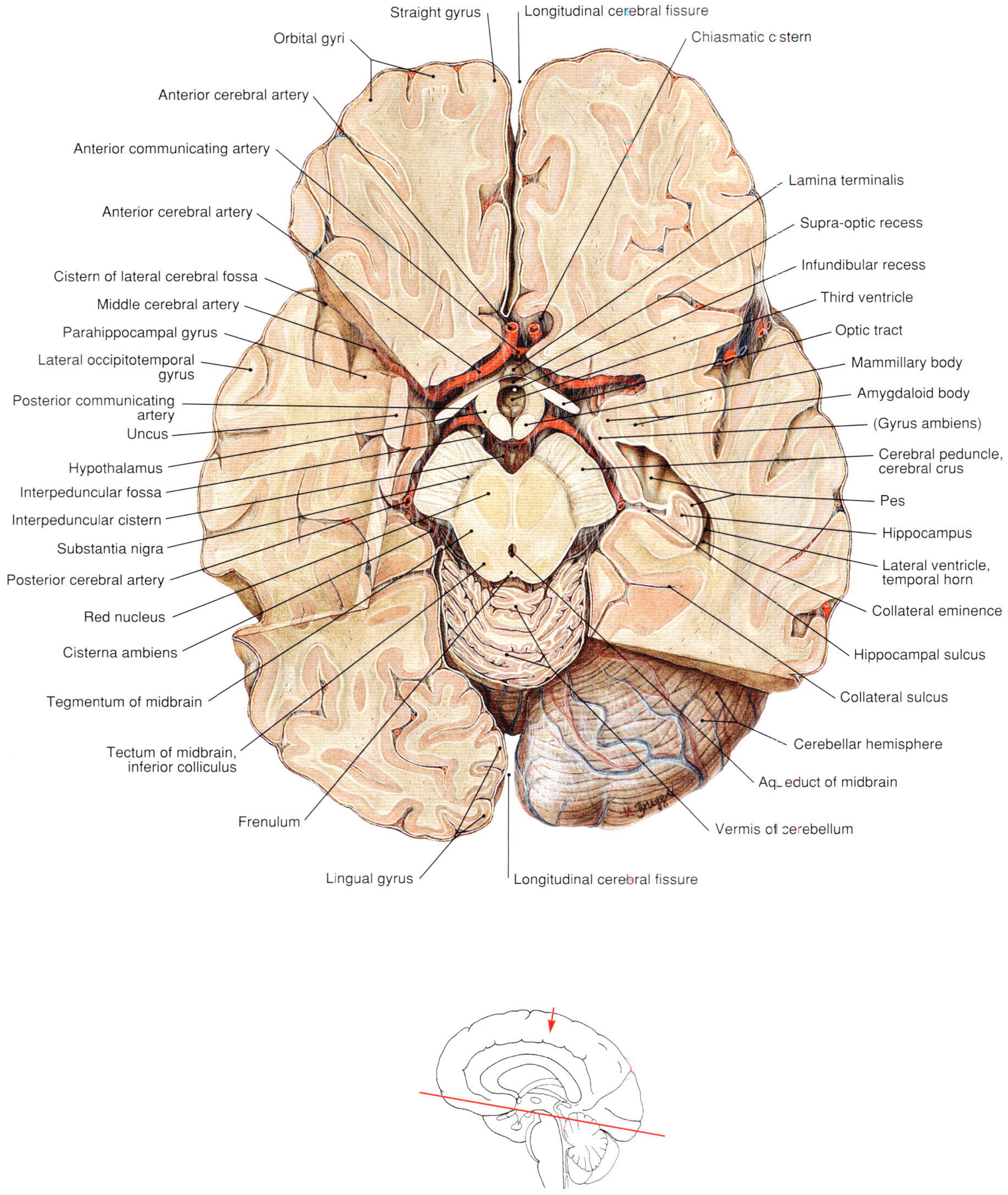

Fig. 1297 Brain;
staggered horizontal section through the floor of the third ventricle at the level of the mamillary bodies.

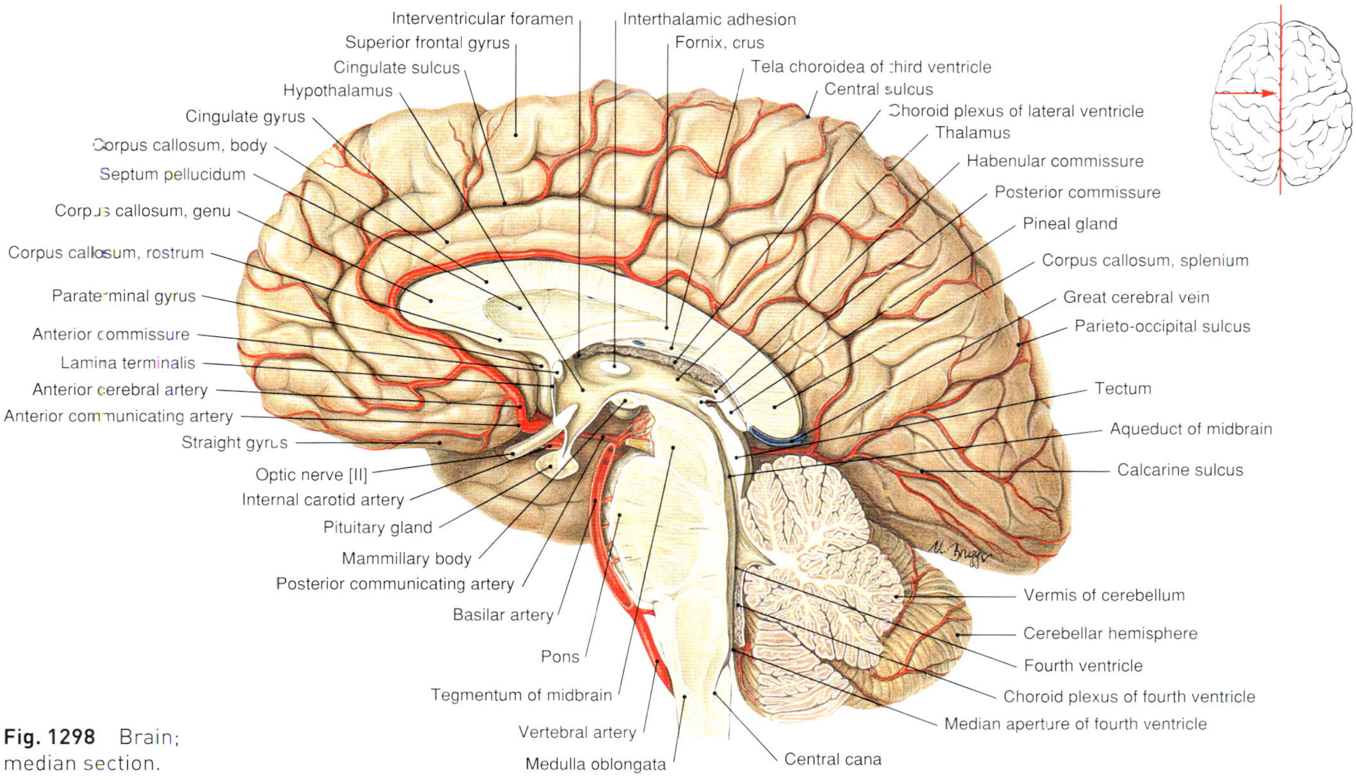

Fig. 1298 Brain; median section.

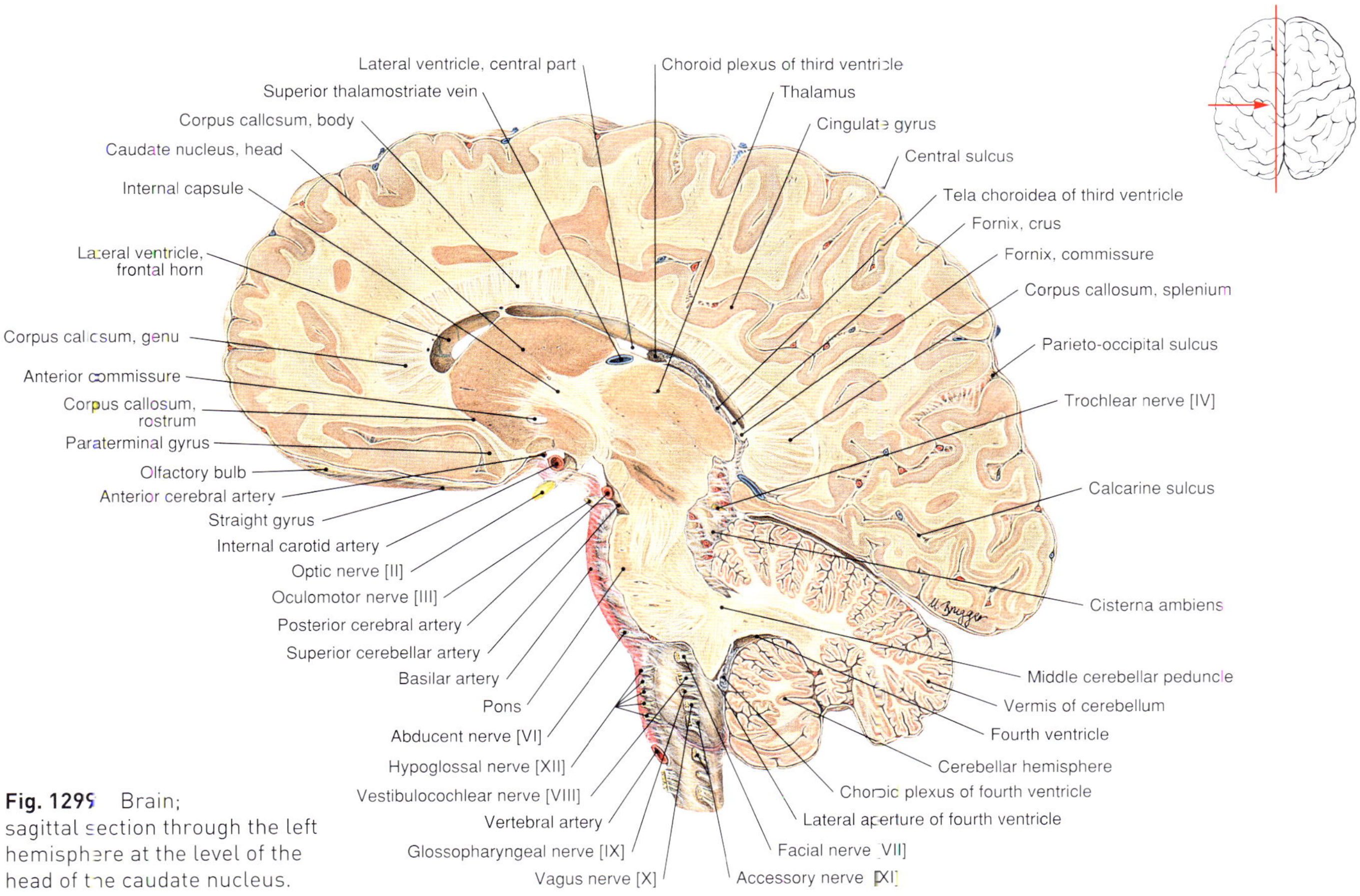

Fig. 1299 Brain; sagittal section through the left hemisphere at the level of the head of the caudate nucleus.

Brain, sagittal sections

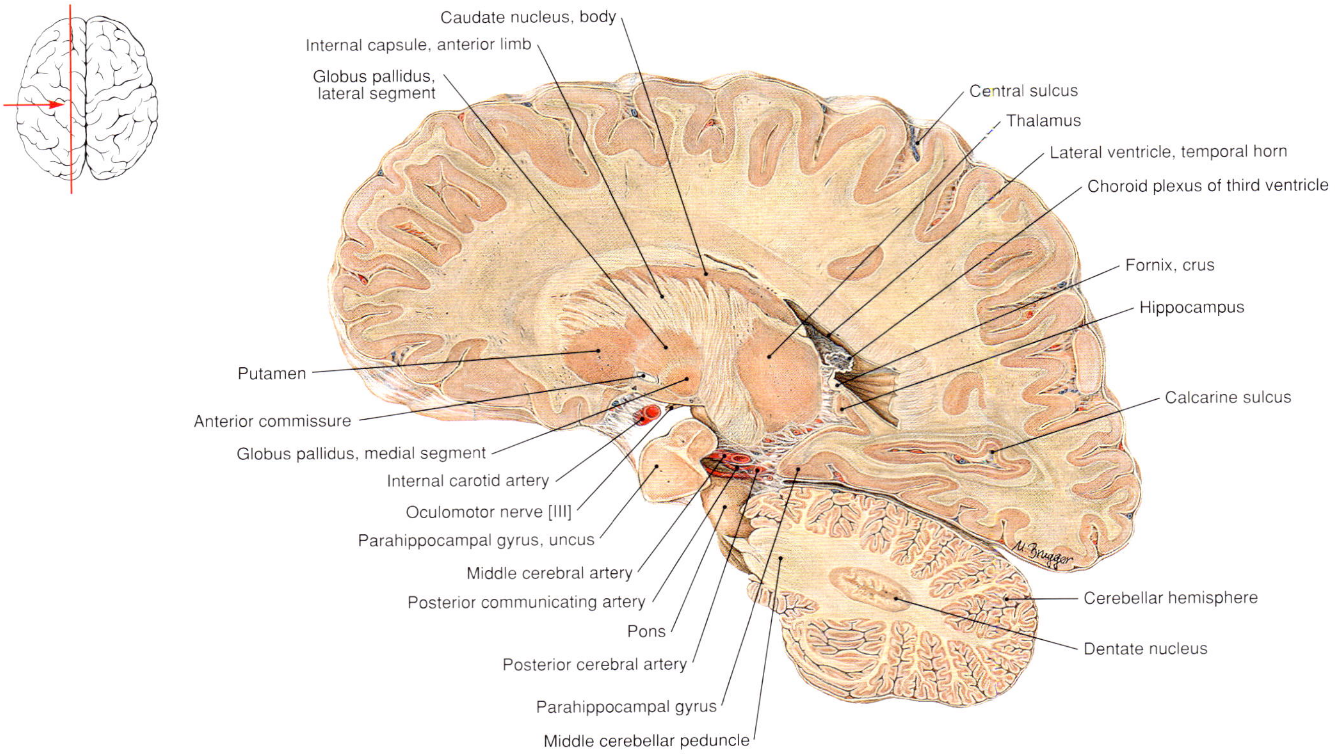

Fig. 1300 Brain;
sagittal section through the left hemisphere
at the level of the body of the caudate nucleus

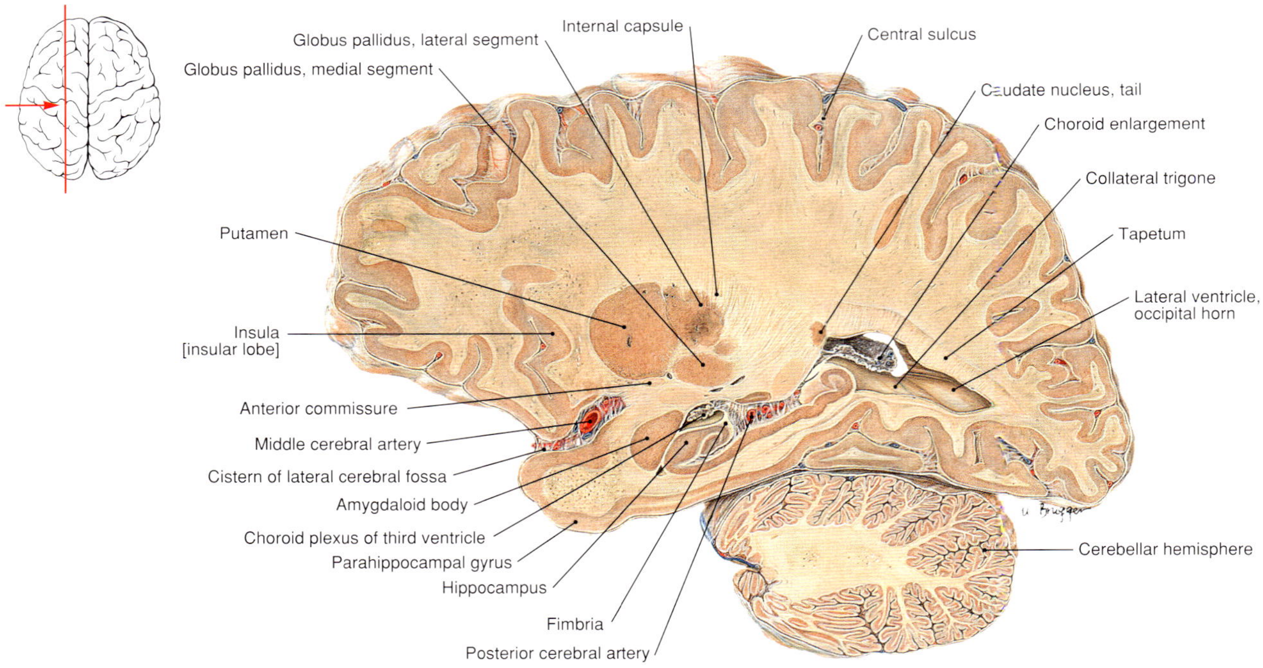

Fig. 1301 Brain;
sagittal section through the left hemisphere
at the level of the amygdaloid body.

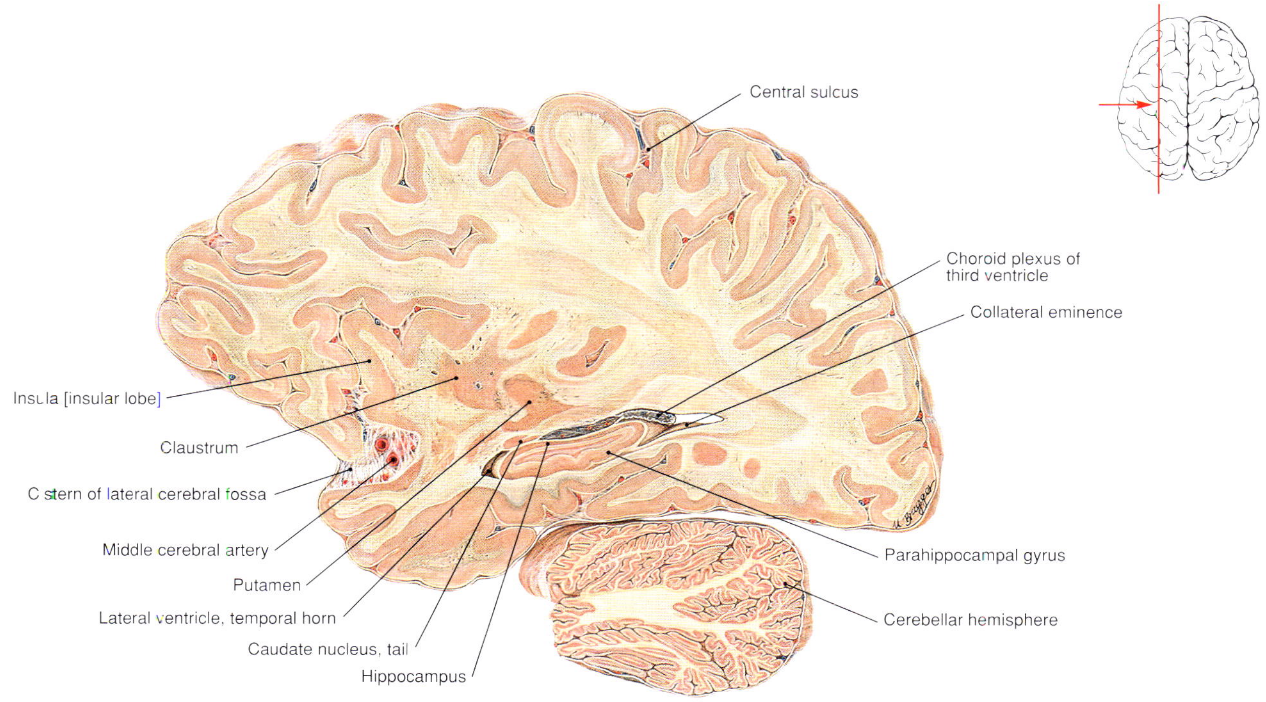

Fig. 1302 Brain;
sagittal section through the left hemisphere
at the level of the apex of the temporal horn.

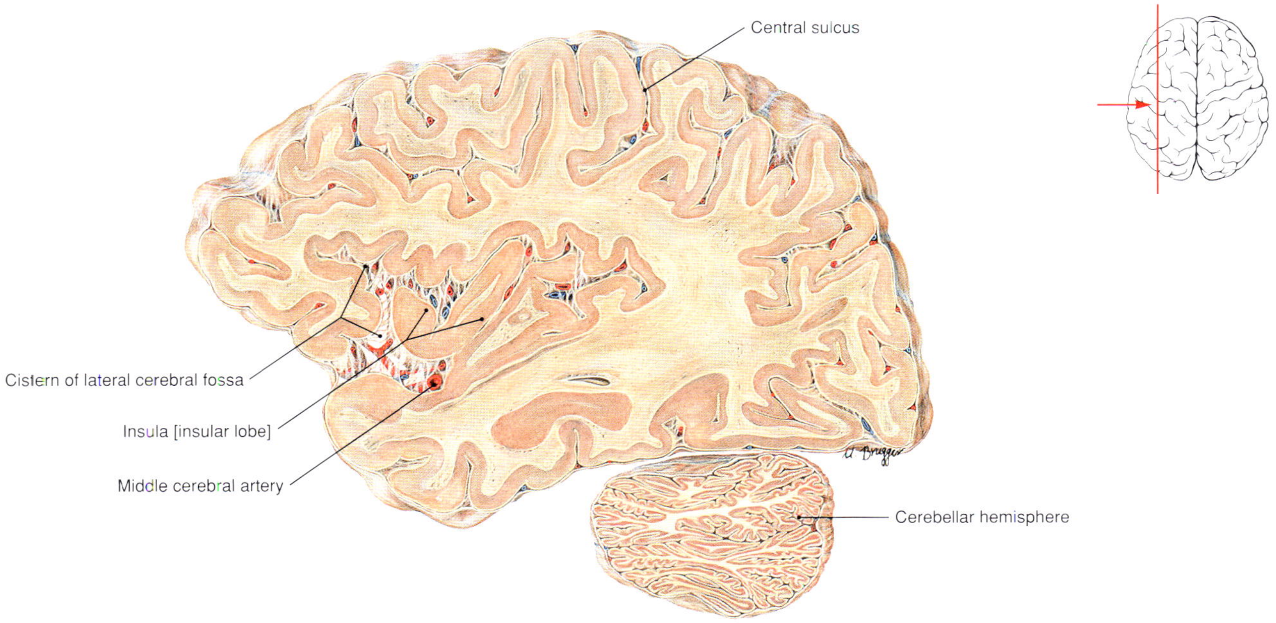

Fig. 1303 Brain;
sagittal section through the left hemisphere
at the level of the insula.

Situs of the spinal cord

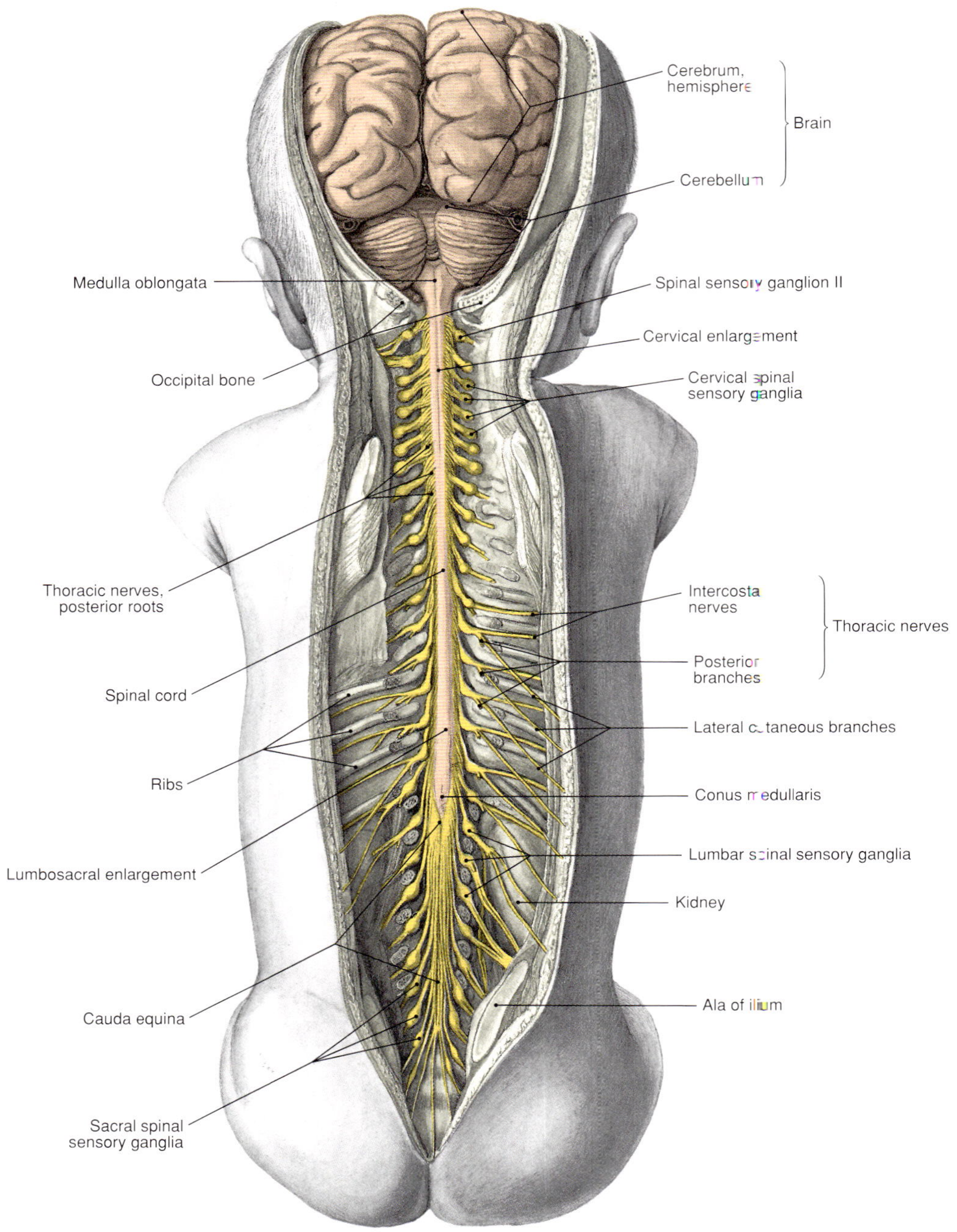

Fig. 1304 Brain; spinal cord and spinal nerves; brain and spinal nerves in a neonate.
In the neonate, the spinal cord extends two vertebral segments further caudally compared to the adult.

Segmental structure of the spinal cord

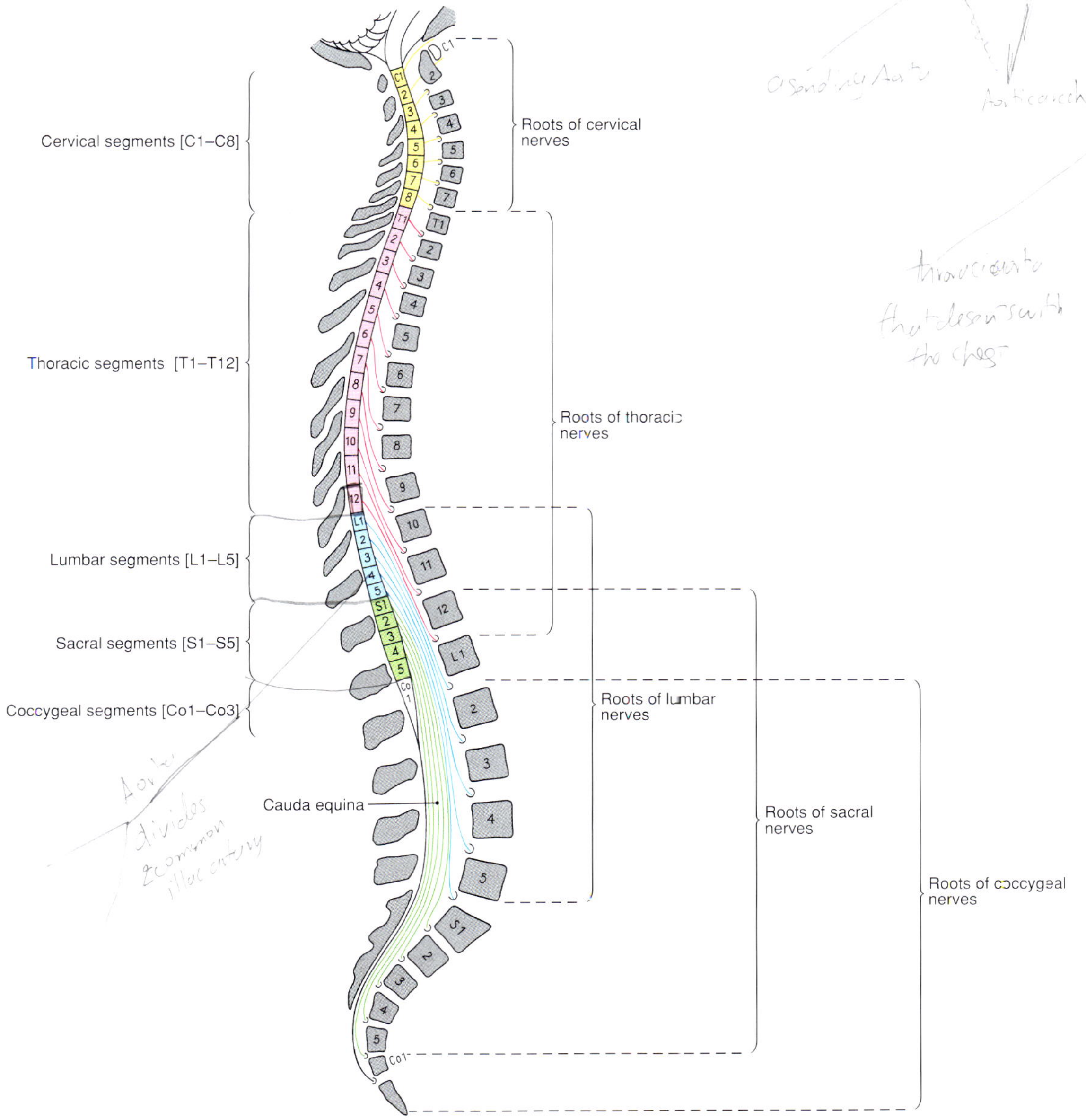

Fig. 1305 Spinal cord segments and spinal nerve roots; schematic median section.
As the spinal cord does not follow the growth of the vertebral column, the course of the spinal roots towards their corresponding segmental intervertebral foramina becomes steeper from cranial to caudal. In the neonate, the spinal cord ends at the level of the spinous process of the fourth lumbar vertebra, whereas in the adult, it extends normally only to the second lumbar vertebra.

Spinal cord

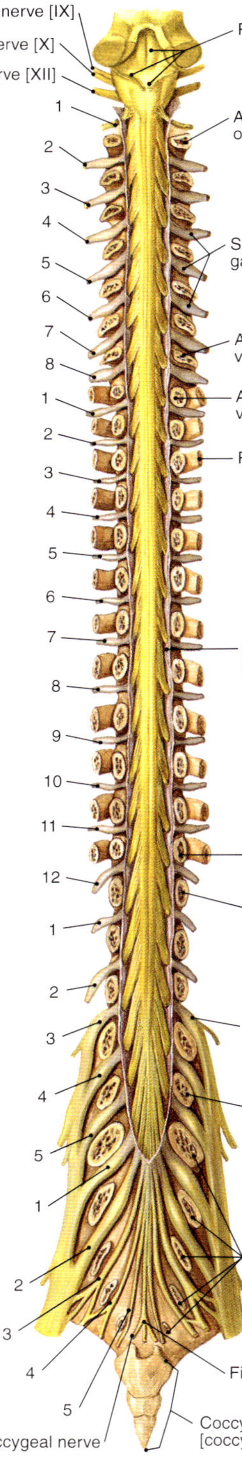

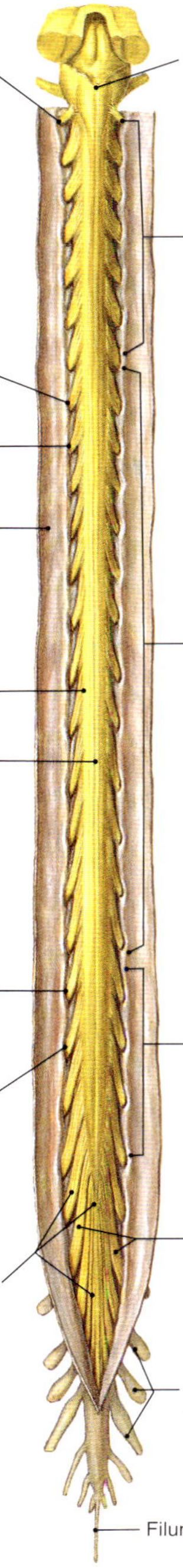

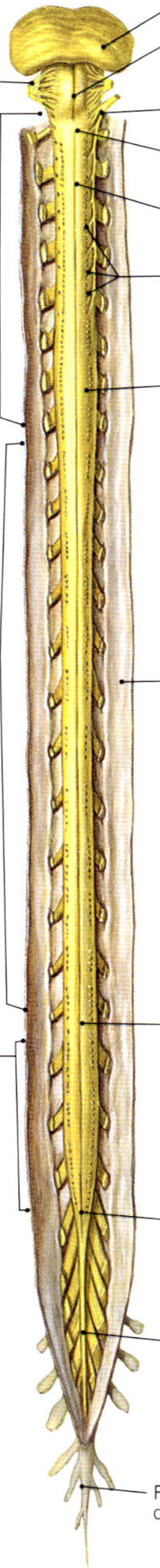

Fig. 1306 Spinal cord and spinal nerves; situs of the spinal cord; dorsal view.
As spinal cord segments are numbered according to the spinal nerves, and the uppermost spinal nerve is counted as the first cervical nerve, there are actually eight cervical segments.

Fig. 1307 Spinal cord and spinal nerves; the spinal dura mater has been opened; dorsal view.

Fig. 1308 Spinal cord and spinal nerves; the spinal dura mater has been opened; ventral view.

Spinal cord

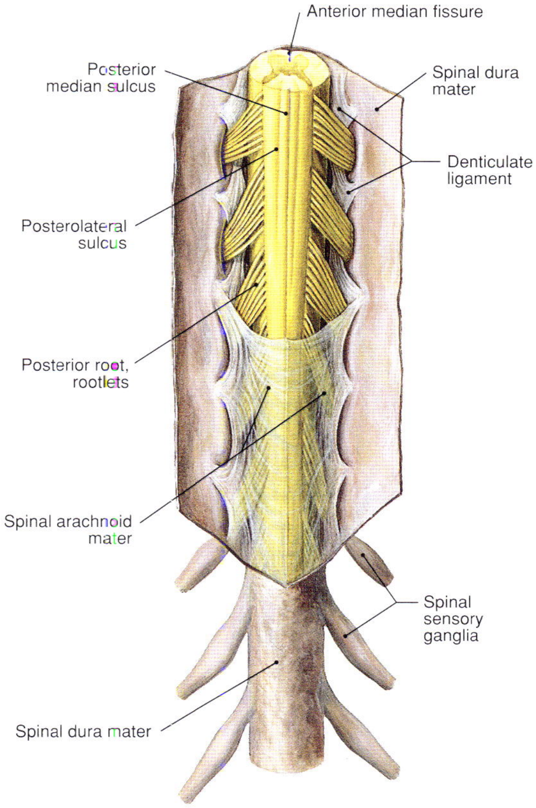

Fig. 1309 Spinal cord and spinal meninges; dorsal view.

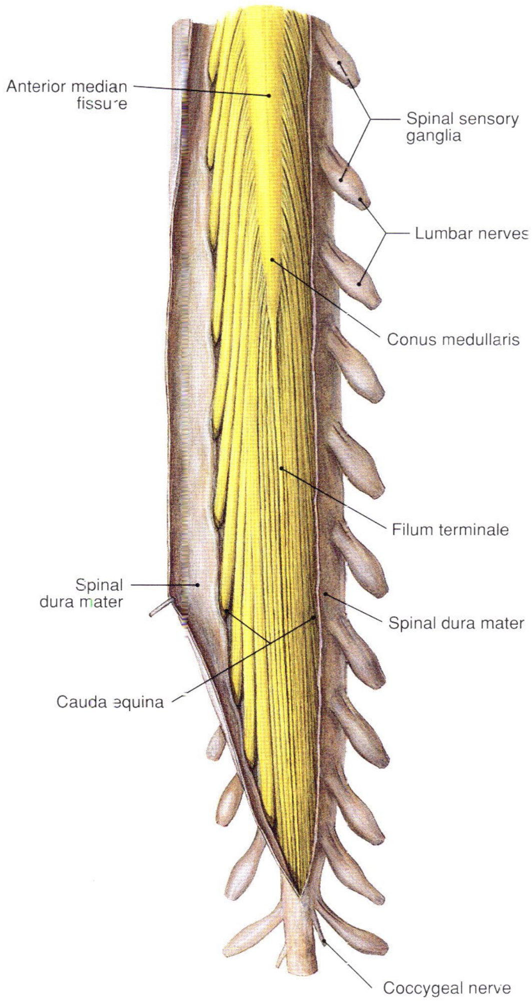

Fig. 1310 Spinal cord; caudal part with the cauda equina; ventral view.

→ 550

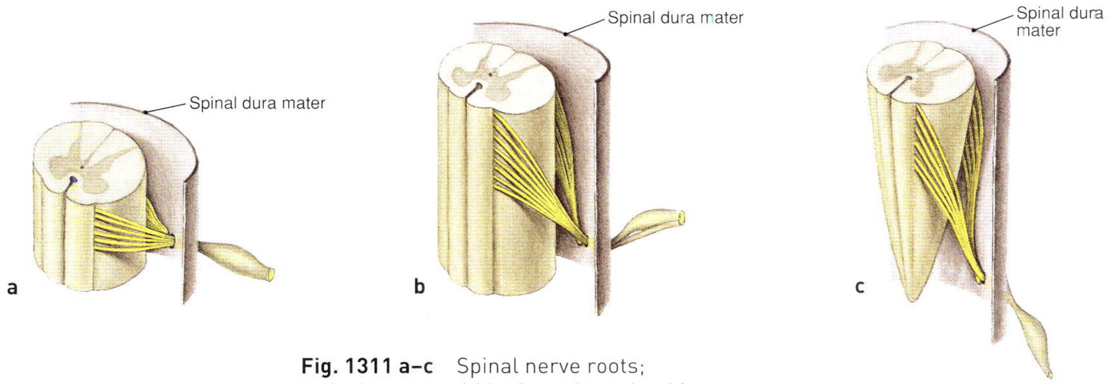

Fig. 1311 a–c Spinal nerve roots; typical course within the subarachnoid space
a Cervical segment
b Thoracic segment
c Lumbar segment

Arteries of the spinal cord

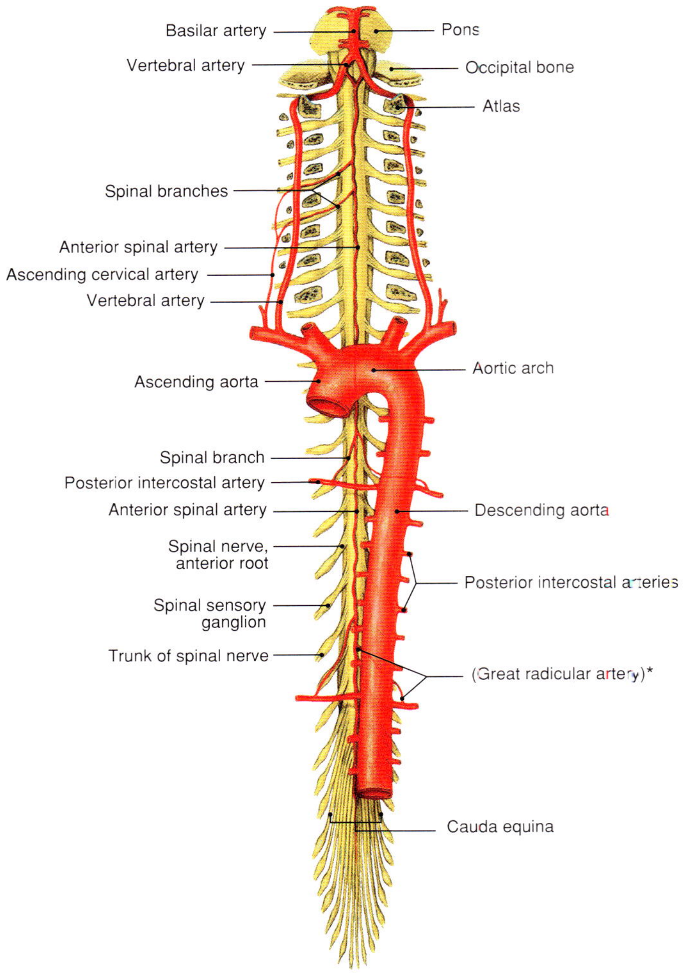

Fig. 1312 Arteries of the spinal cord.

* Clinical term: artery of ADAMKIEWICZ

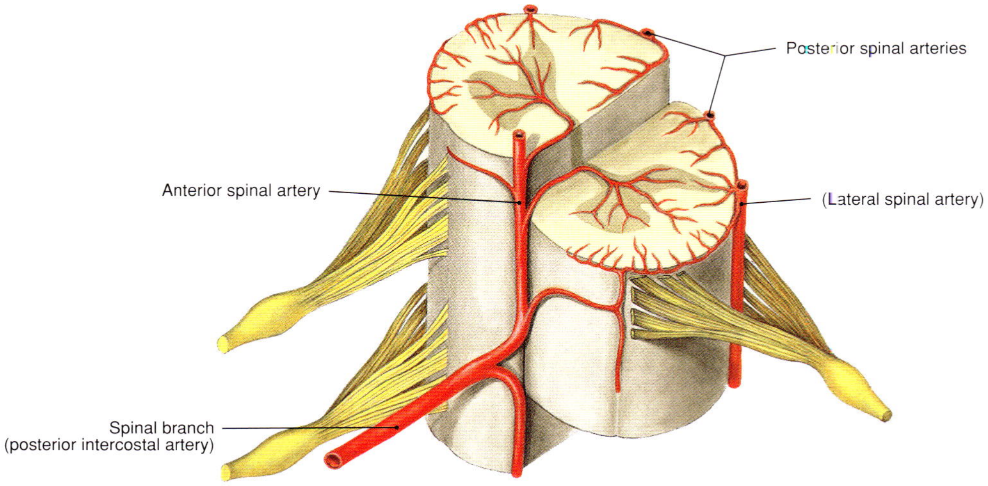

Fig. 1313 Arteries of the spinal cord.

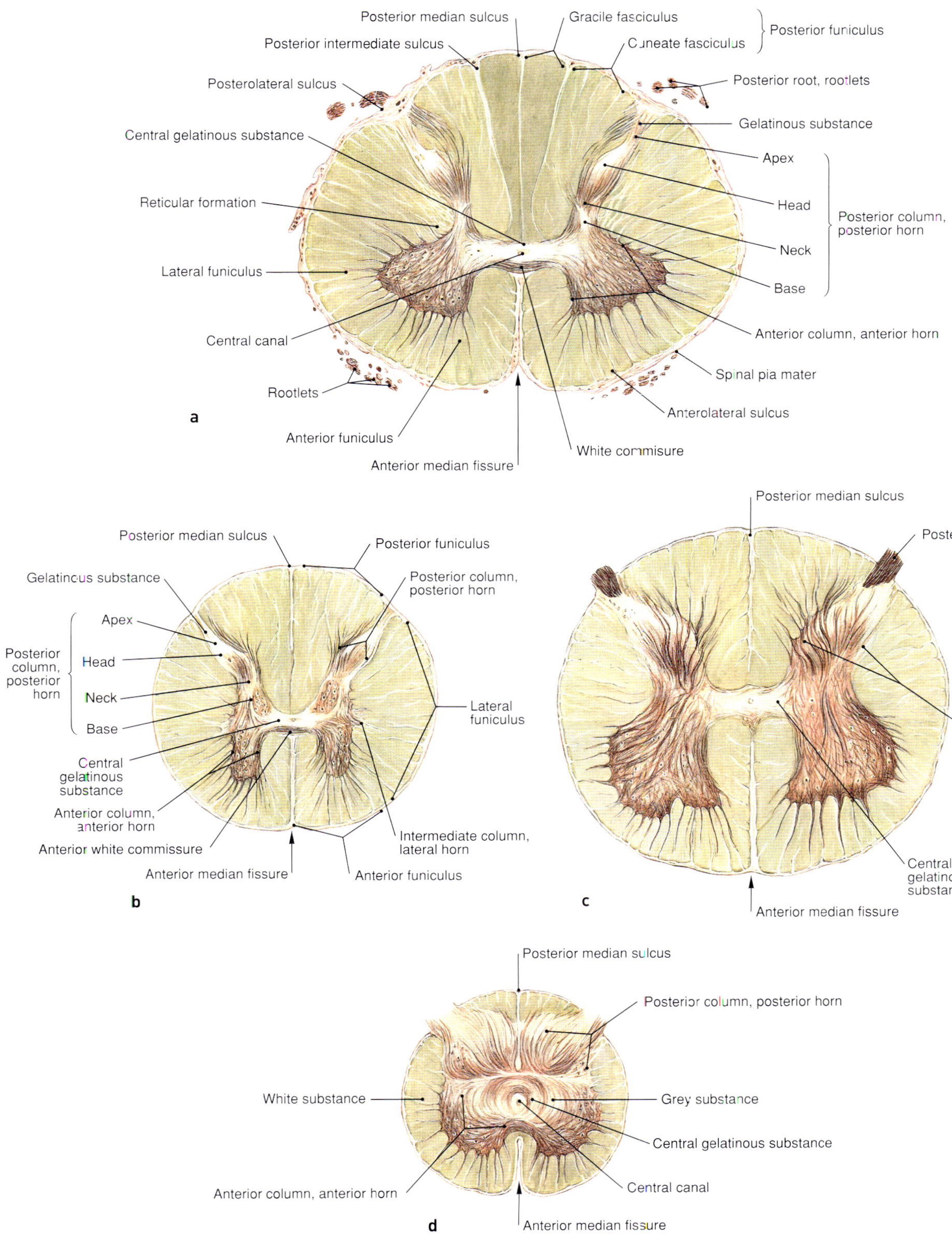

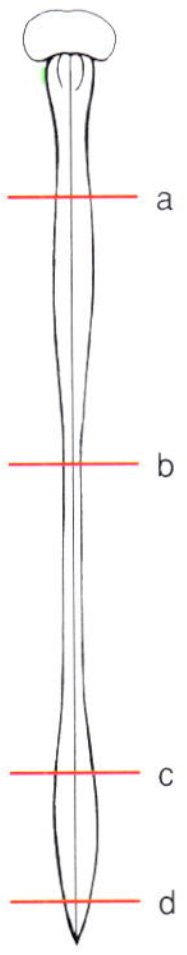

Fig. 1314 a–d Spinal cord;
cross-sections; myelin stain; approx. 500%.
a Cervical part
b Thoracic part
c Lumbar part
d Sacral part

Functional organisation of the spinal cord

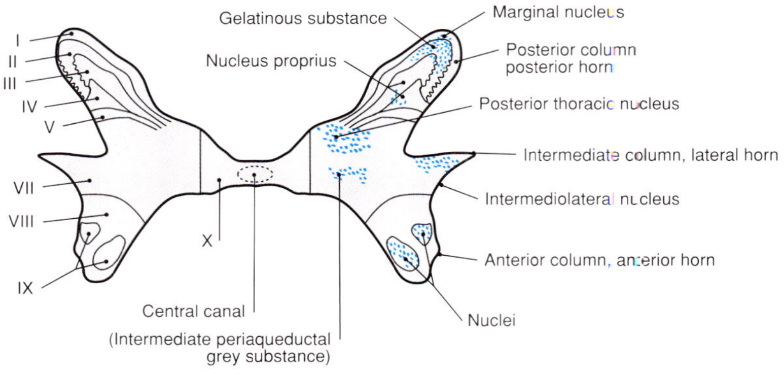

Fig. 1315 Spinal cord;
laminar organisation of the grey matter according to its cytoarchitecture (according to REXED, 1952), exemplified by the tenth thoracic segment (T10).
Formation and number of the laminae vary in different spinal cord segments.

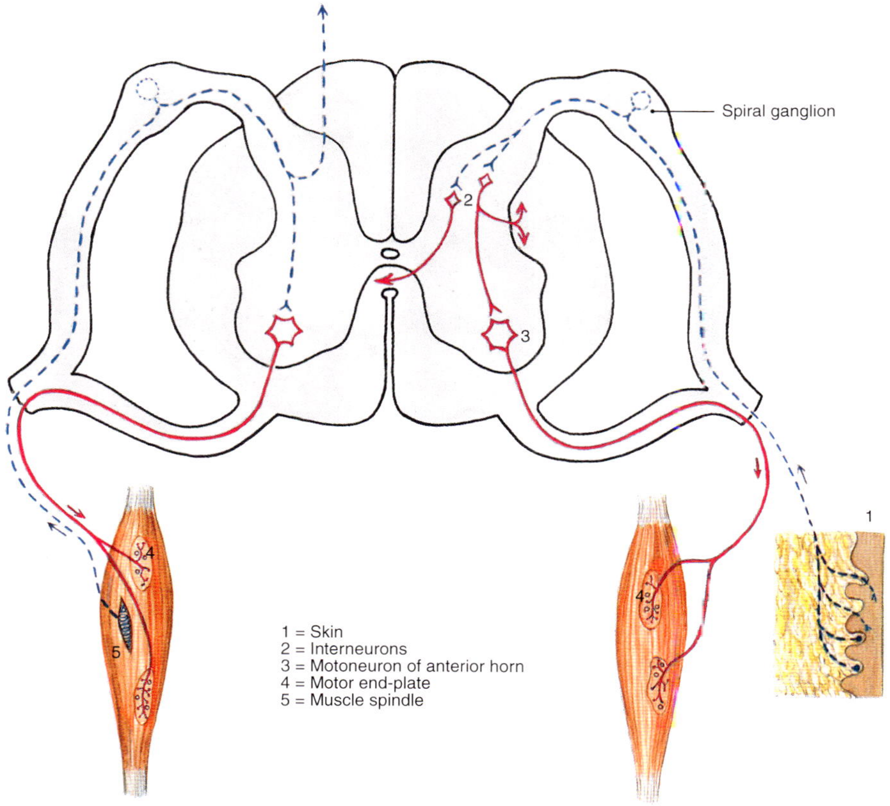

Fig. 1316 Reflexes at the spinal cord;
left: monosynaptic reflex (bineuronal, proprioceptive, myostatic, e.g., patellar tendon reflex, Achilles tendon reflex, etc.);
right: polysynaptic reflex (polyneuronal, e.g., abdominal reflex, cremasteric reflex, plantar reflex, etc.).

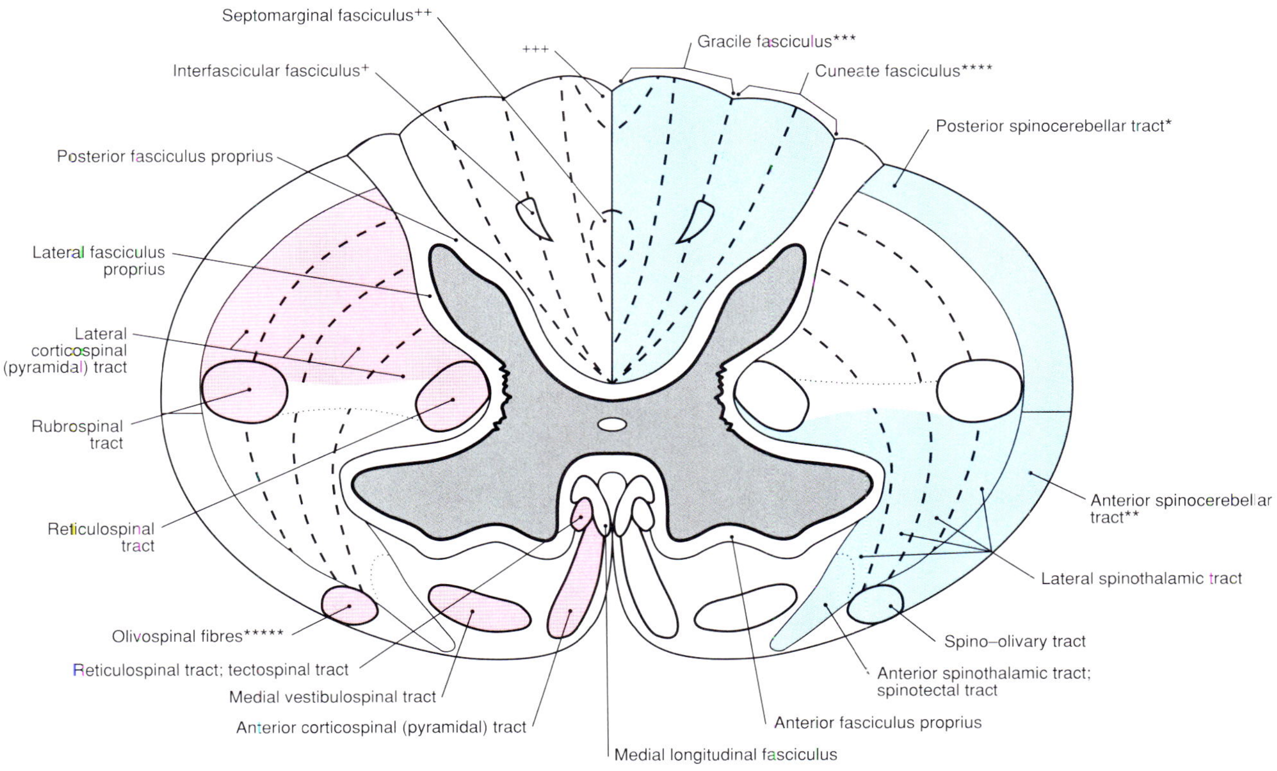

Fig. 1317 Spinal cord;
schematic organisation of the white matter exemplified by a lower cervical segment.
Afferent (= ascending) pathways in blue;
efferent (= descending) pathways in red.

* Clinical term: FLECHSIG's tract
** Clinical term: GOWER's tract
*** Clinical term: GOLL's tract
**** Clinical term: BURDACH's tract
***** The actual existence of these fibres has not definitely been documented.

The regions indicated by +, ++, and +++ designate descending collateral tracts of the posterior fasciculi.

\+ SCHULTZE's comma tract (cervical part)
++ FLECHSIG's oval bundle (thoracic part)
+++ Triangle of PHILIPPE-GOMBAULT (lumbar and sacral parts)

Pathways of the spinal cord

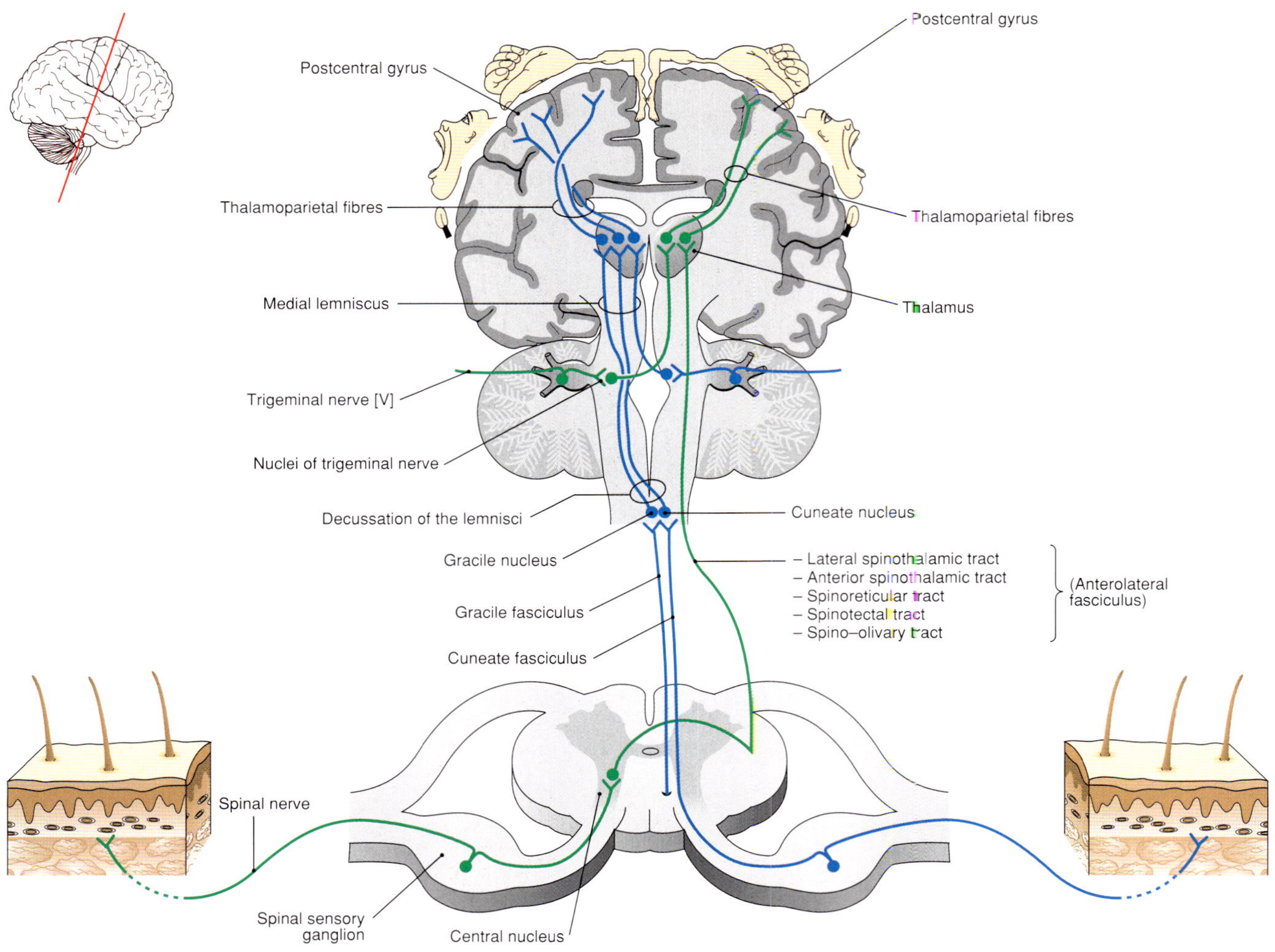

Fig. 1318 Pathways for epicritic (blue) and protopathic (green) sensibility.

Ascending pathways

Pathway for epicritic sensibility (tactile pathway)
(Precise differentiation of pressure and touch)

1. neuron (uncrossed)
   From receptors (exteroceptors) in the skin and the mucosa, as well as the periosteum, the joints and the muscle spindles etc., to the cuneate and gracile nucleus in the medulla oblongata: gracile and cuneate fasciculus (perikarya in the spinal ganglia): descending collaterals (see Fig. 1317).
2. neuron (crossed)
   From the medulla oblongata (cuneate and gracile nucleus) to the thalamus (medial lemniscus, perikarya in the cuneate and gracile nucleus).
3. neuron (uncrossed)
   From the thalamus to the cerebral cortex, particularly to the postcentral gyrus (thalamocortical fibres, perikarya in the thalamus).

Pathway for protopathic sensibility (pain pathway)
(Pain, temperature, general pressure sensation)

1. neuron (uncrossed)
   From receptors (exteroceptors) of the skin and the mucosa etc., to the posterior horn laminae I–V (perikarya in the spinal ganglia).
2. neuron (crossed, some fibres possibly uncrossed)
   From the posterior horn to the thalamus, in the reticular formation and to the midbrain tectum (anterior and lateral spinothalamic tracts, spinoreticular tract, spinotectal tract; perikarya in the posterior column).
3. neuron (uncrossed)
   From the thalamus among others to the cerebral cortex, particularly to the postcentral gyrus (thalamocortical fibres, perikarya in the thalamus).

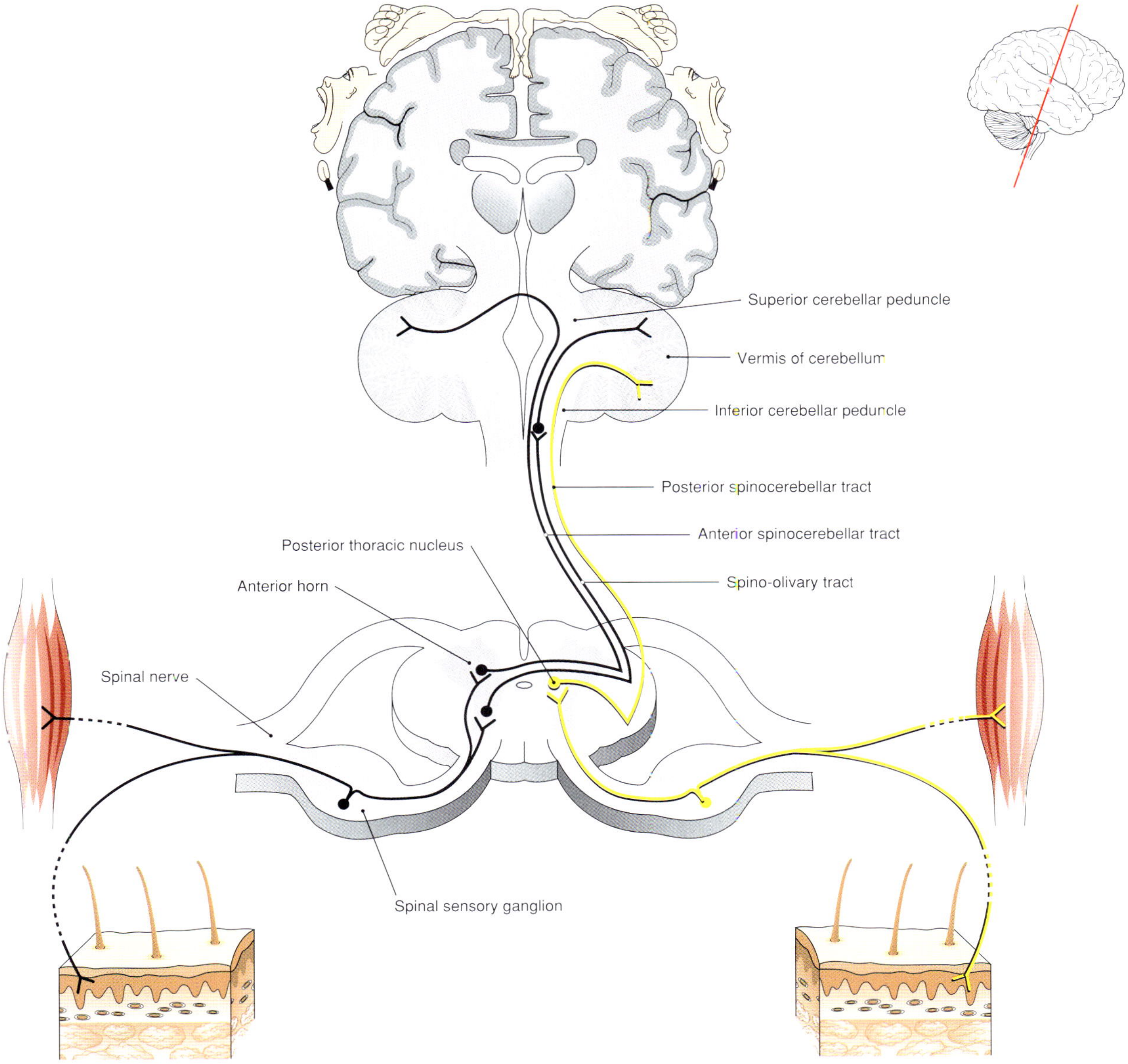

Fig. 1319 Pathways for unconscious deep sensibility.

Ascending pathways

Pathway for unconscious deep sensibility
(Unconscious, but precise spatial differentiation as a prerequisite for movement coordination by the cerebellum)

Via the anterior cerebellar tract

1. neuron (uncrossed)
   From receptors (proprioceptors) in muscles, tendons, and the connective tissue to the nuclei of the intermediate zone and the anterior column (perikarya in the spinal ganglia).
2. neuron (crossed)
   From the anterior horn within the anterior spinocerebellar tract of the anterolateral tract to the cerebellum via the superior cerebellar peduncle (perikarya in the intermediate zone and the anterior horn).

Via the posterior cerebellar tract

1. neuron (uncrossed)
   From end organs (proprioceptors) in muscles, tendons, and the connective tissue to the nuclei of the posterior column and the thoracic nucleus (perikarya in the spinal ganglia).
2. neuron (uncrossed)
   From the posterior horn and the thoracic nucleus within the posterior spinocerebellar tract of the lateral tract to the cerebellum via the inferior cerebellar peduncle (perikarya in the thoracic nucleus and at the base of the posterior column).

Pathways of the spinal cord

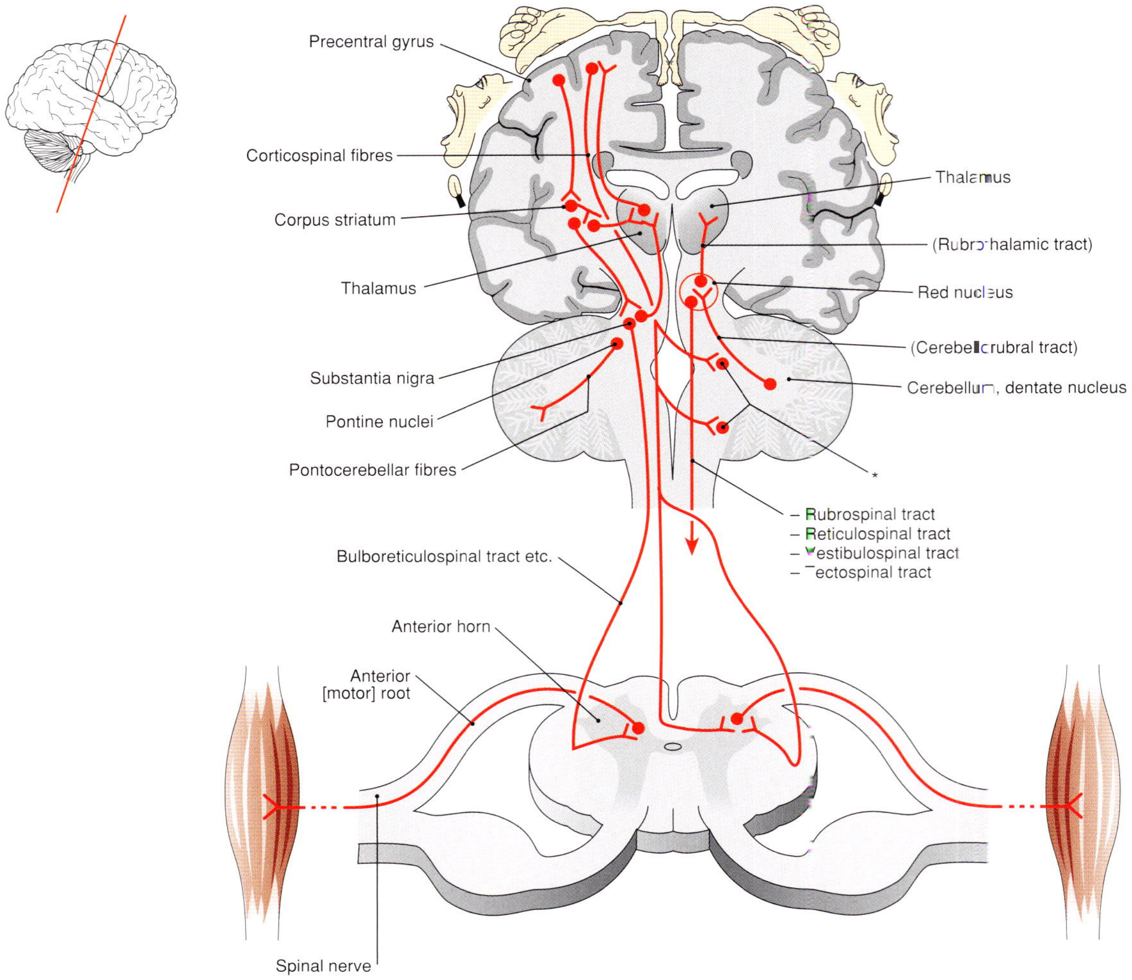

Fig. 1320 Pathways of the motor system.

* Motor nuclei of cranial nerves

Descending pathways

The motor system comprises a large number of nuclear regions and tracts. The "motor final path" are the motoneurons. Despite the extraordinary complexity of these circuits, the traditional organisation will be maintained for didactic reasons.

(So-called) Pyramidal tract

1. (central) neuron (crossed)
   From the cerebral cortex through the internal capsule and the cerebral peduncles to interneurons within the anterior and posterior column (lateral corticospinal tract, anterior corticospinal tract, perikarya in the precentral gyrus). Branching off of fibres to the nuclei of the cranial nerves (corticonuclear fibres and bulbar corticonuclear fibres).
2. (peripheral) neuron (motor end pathway, α-motoneurons)
   From the anterior horn to the motor end plates of the skeletal musculature (motoneurons, perikarya in the anterior horn).

(So-called) Extrapyramidal motor system

1. central neurons (crossed and uncrossed)
   From the cerebral cortex, particularly the precentral gyrus and the adjacent cortical areas including synapses to the basal ganglia, thalamus, subthalamic nucleus, red nucleus, substantia nigra, cerebellum, etc. and feedback loops to the interneurons of the anterior column (rubrospinal tract, medial and lateral vestibulospinal tract, reticulospinal tract, tectospinal tract).
2. peripheral neuron (motor end pathway, α-motoneurons)
   From the anterior horn to the motor end-plates of the skeletal muscles (motoneurons; perikarya in the anterior horn).

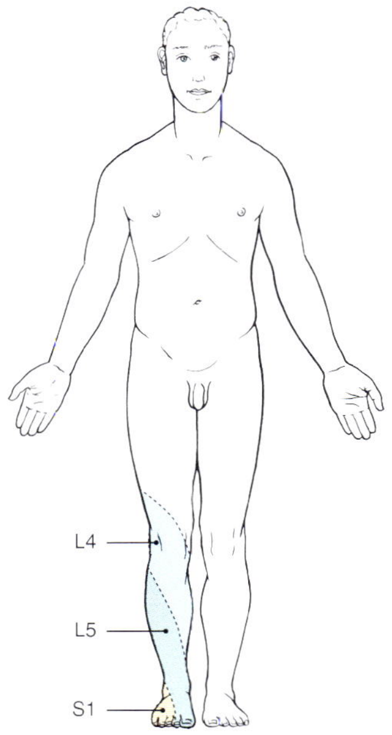

Fig. 1321 Dysfunctional cutaneous innervation due to palsy of certain, frequently affected spinal nerves.

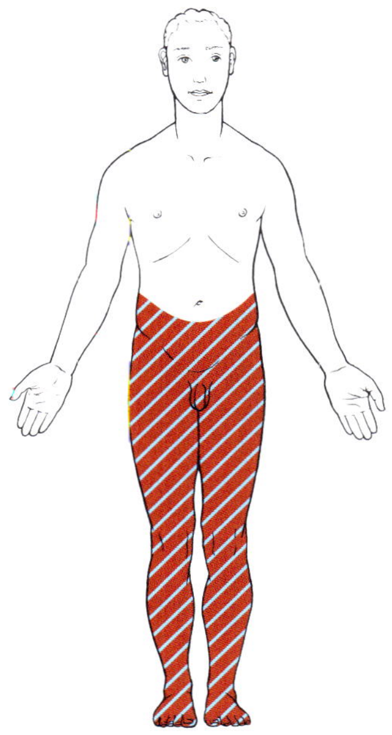

Fig. 1322 Complete paraplegia at the level of the eleventh thoracic segment.
Paralysis of the complete motor and sensory system.

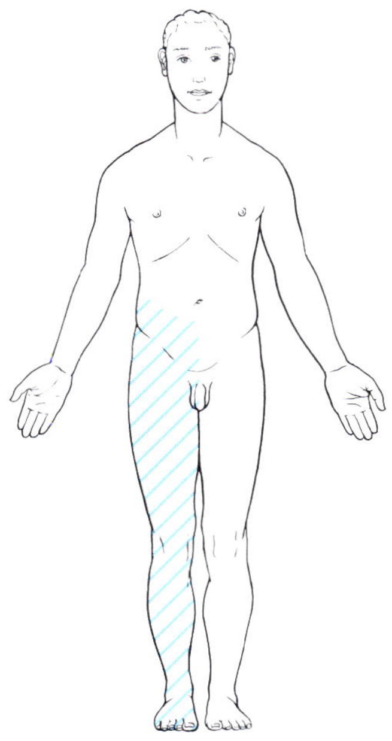

Fig. 1323 Paralysis of the tracts of the right posterior funiculus at the level of the eleventh thoracic segment.
Loss of fine tactile sensation as well as loss of sense of position and vibration (rough touch sensation remains functional).

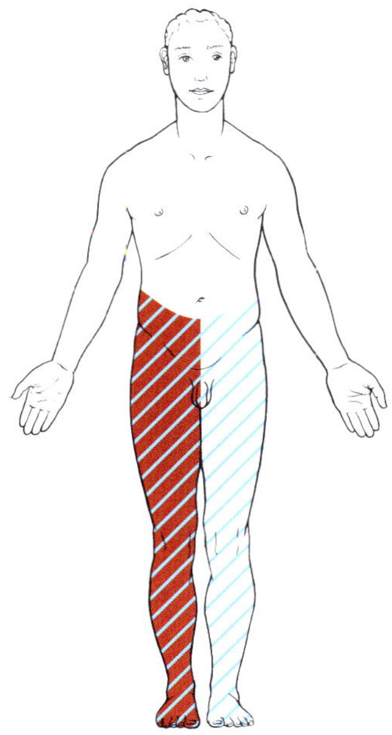

Fig. 1324 Hemiplegia (BROWN-SÉQUARD) due to disruption of the half of the spinal cord on the right side at the level of the eleventh thoracic segment.
On the right side (ipsilaterally): loss of motor function (initially flaccid, later spastic); loss of fine tactile sensation as well as loss of sense of position and vibration (rough touch sensation remains functional).
On the left side (contralaterally): loss of pain and temperature sensation

Eyelids

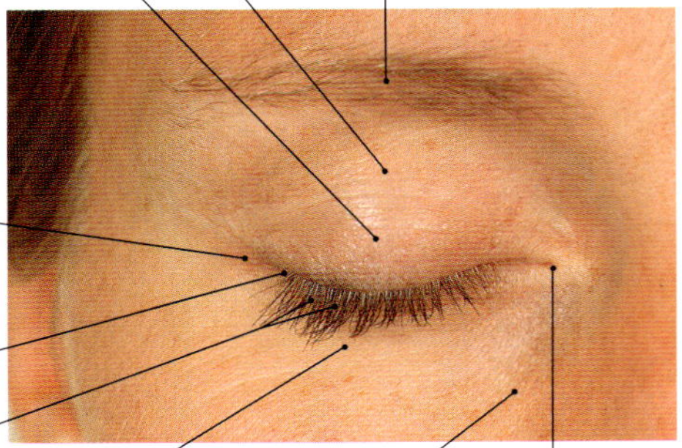

Fig. 1325 Eyelids.

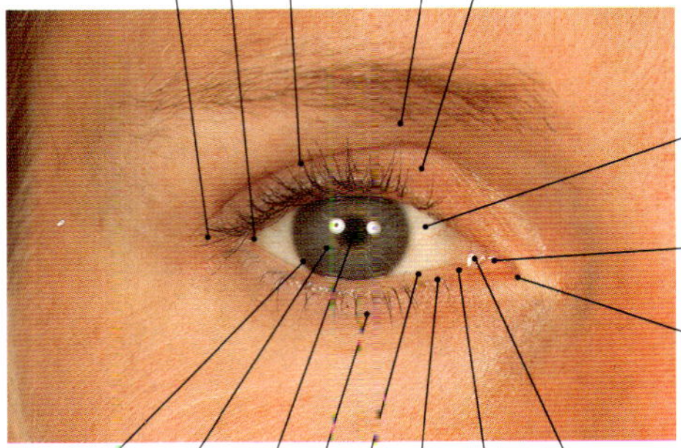

Fig. 1326 Eye and eyelids.

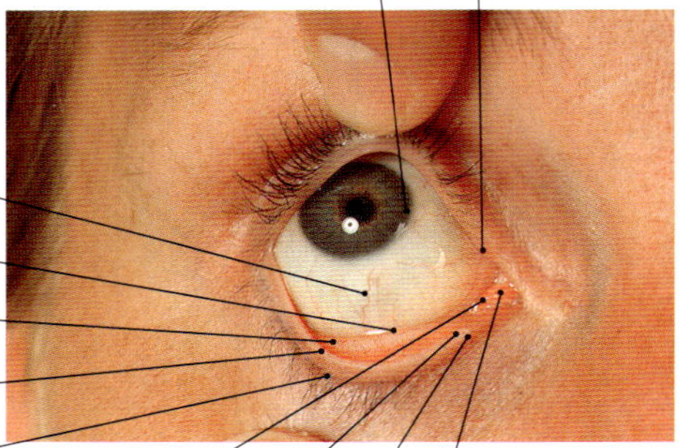

Fig. 1327 Eye and eyelids.

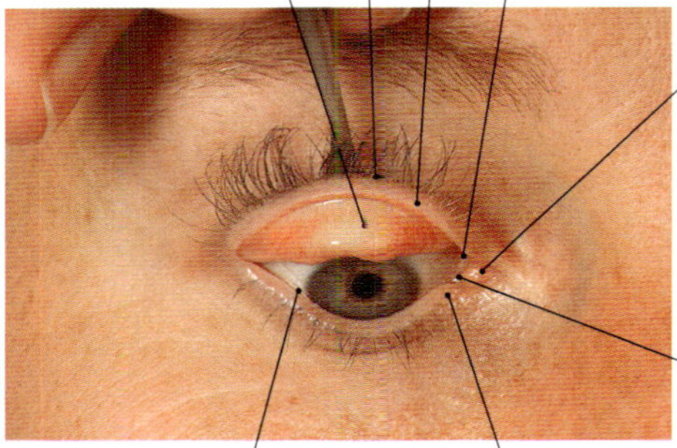

Fig. 1328 Eye and eyelids.
Eversion of the upper eyelid (extropionisation) is hindered by the stiffness of the tarsus, but can be facilitated with the aid of a small hook.

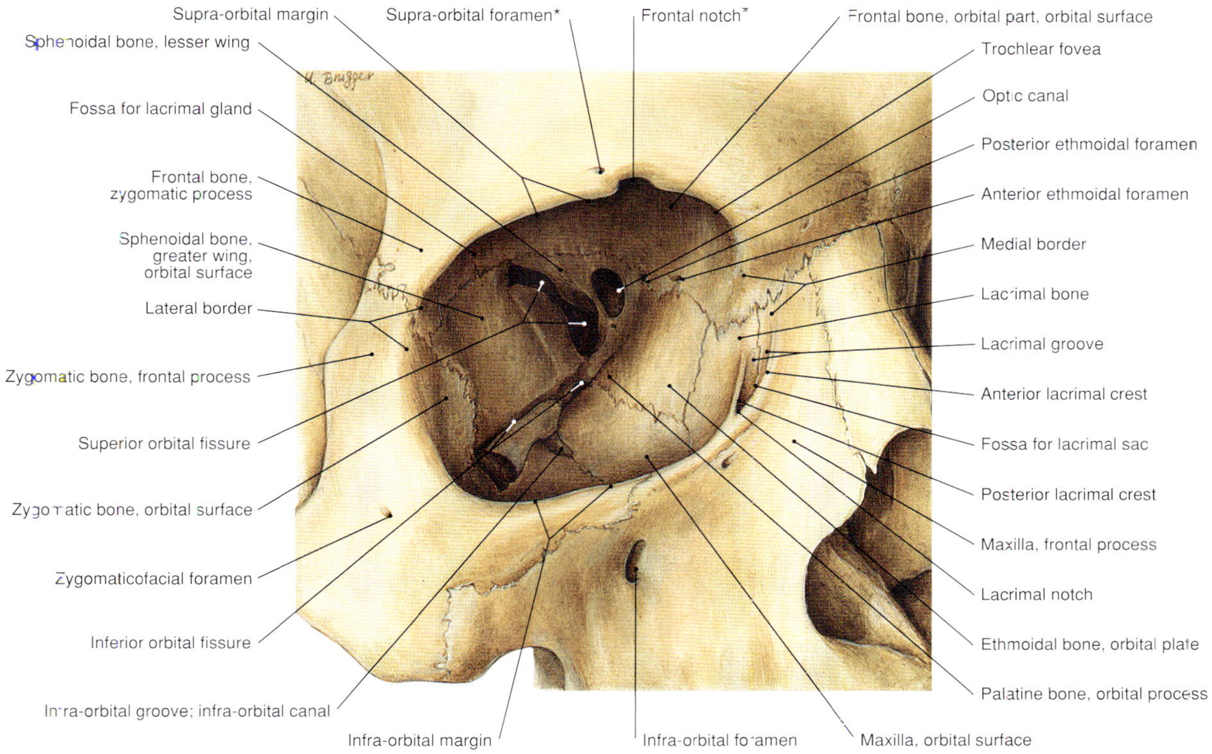

Fig. 1329 Orbit;
oblique view from lateral.

* These structures can be present as foramina or notches.

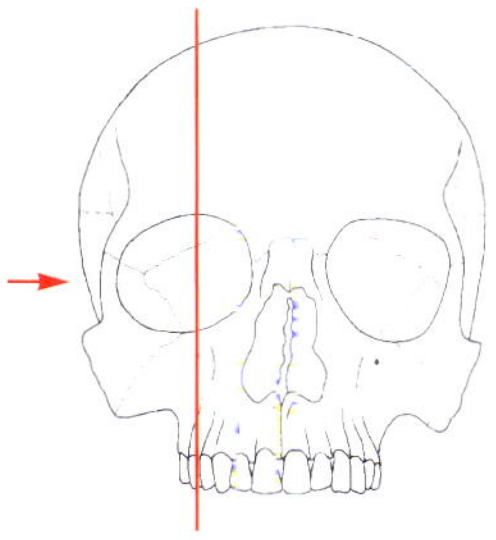

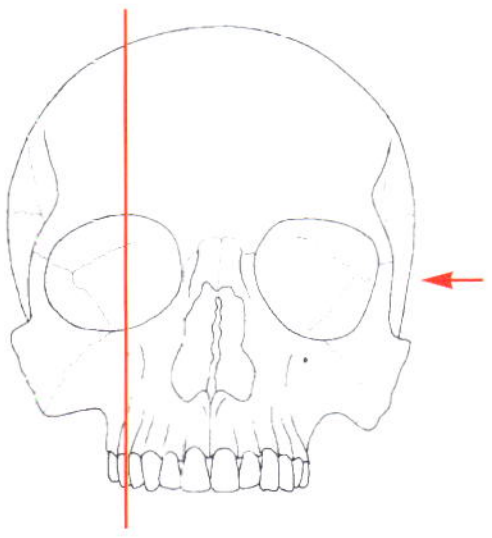

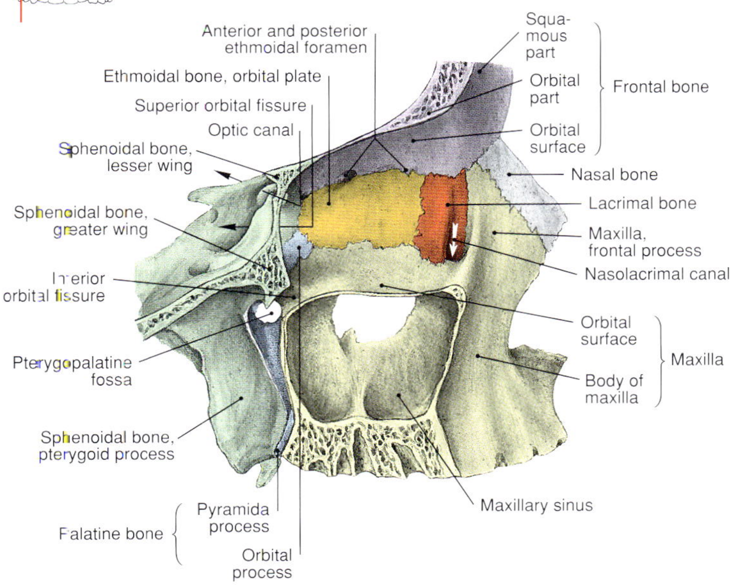

Fig. 1330 Medial wall of the orbit;
lateral view.

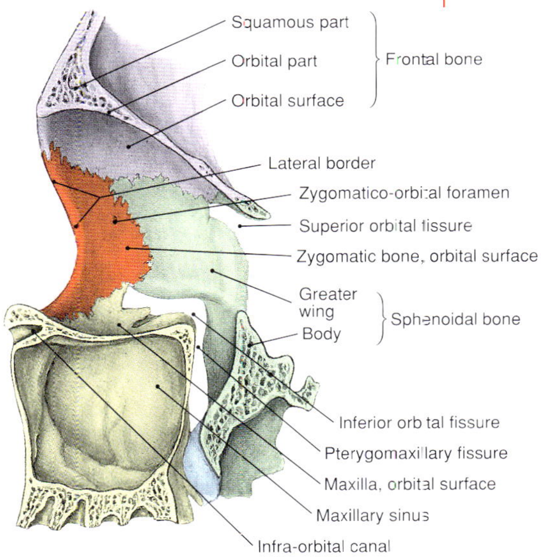

Fig. 1331 Lateral wall of the orbit;
medial view.

Eyelids

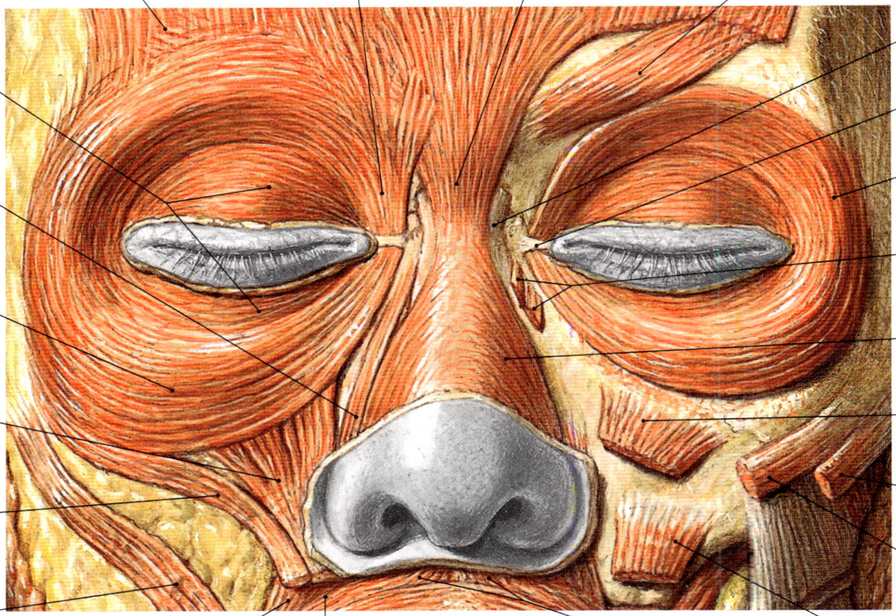

→ 119, 120, T 1 a, c, d, e

Fig. 1332 Facial muscles.

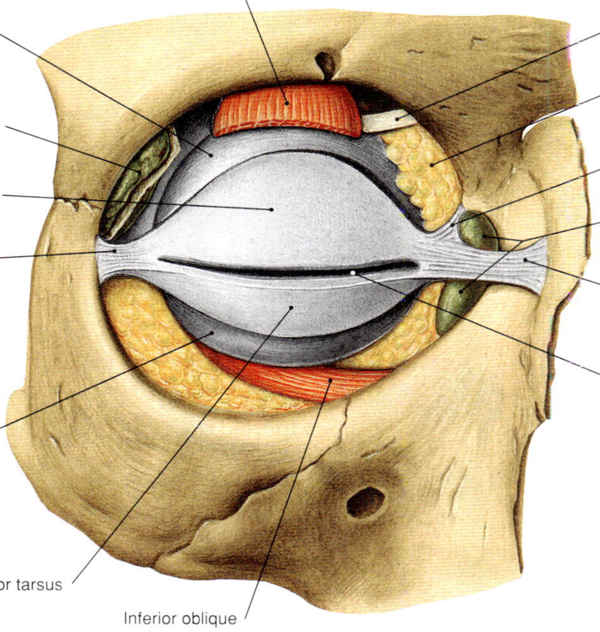

Fig. 1333 Orbital opening with eyelids.

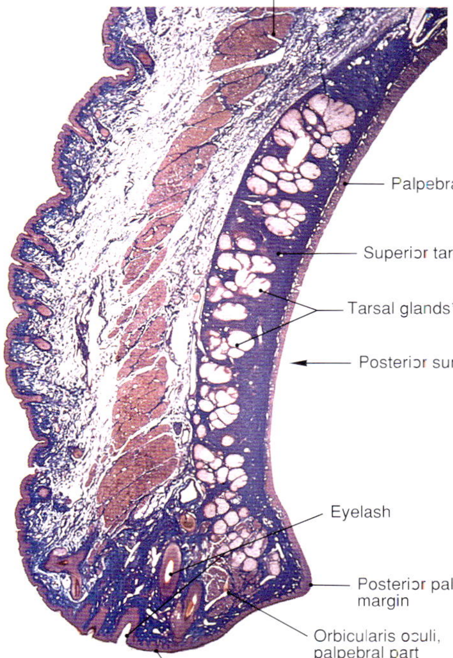

Fig. 1334 Upper eyelid;
photograph of a microscopic specimen;
azan stain;
sagittal section, magnified.

* Clinical term: MEIBOMian glands

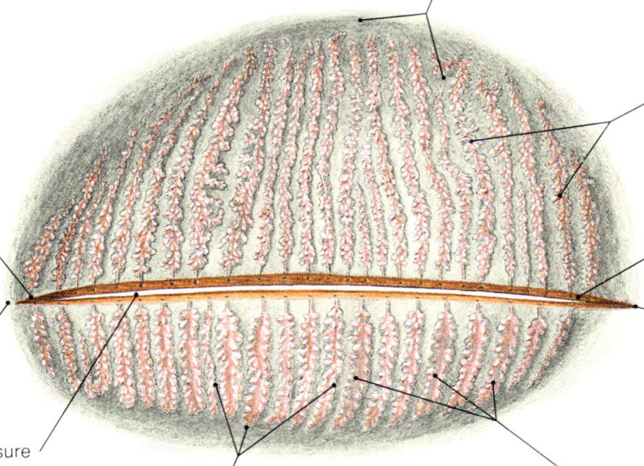

Fig. 1335 Eyelids;
translucent specimen illustrating the excretory ductules of the tarsal glands;
posterior view.

Lacrimal apparatus

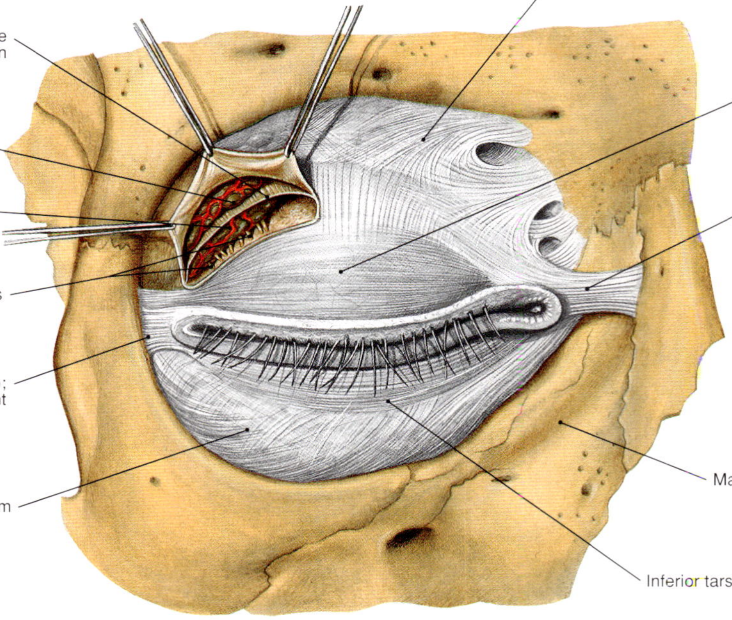

Fig. 1336 Orbital opening with eyelids and lacrimal gland.

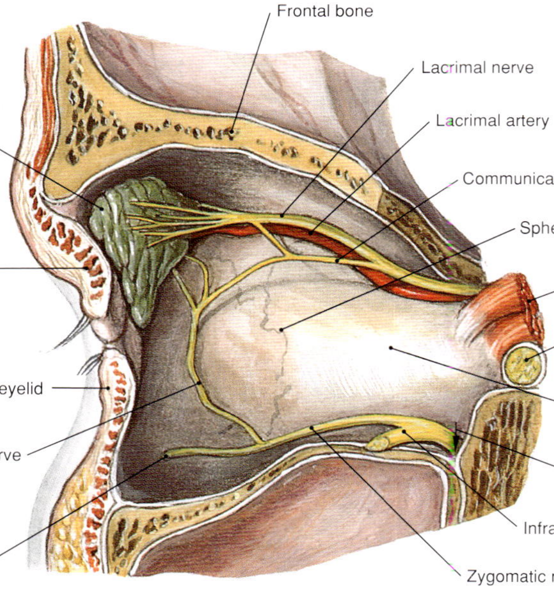

Fig. 1337 Innervation of the lacrimal gland; medial view.

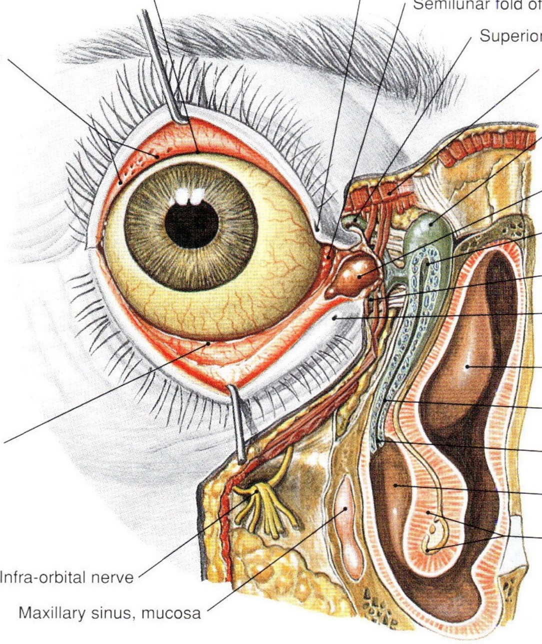

Fig. 1338 Lacrimal apparatus;
the eyelids have been pulled away from the eyeball;
the nasolacrimal duct has been opened up to the inferior nasal meatus.

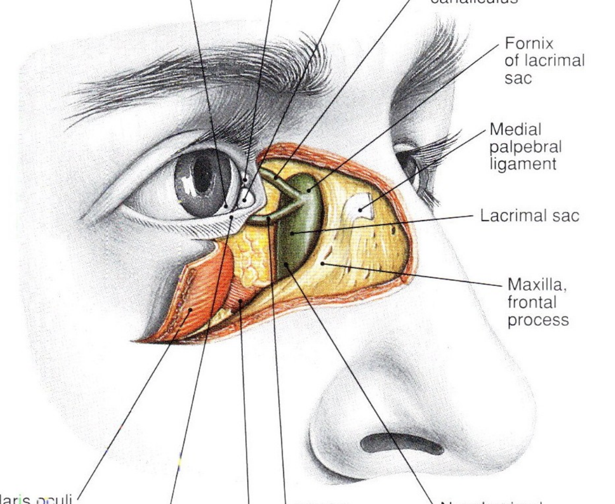

Fig. 1339 Lacrimal apparatus.

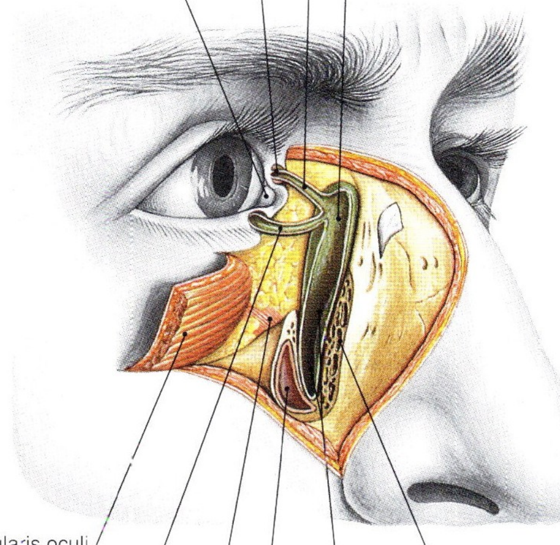

Fig. 1340 Lacrimal apparatus;
the nasolacrimal duct and the nasolacrimal canal have been opened.

Extra-ocular muscles

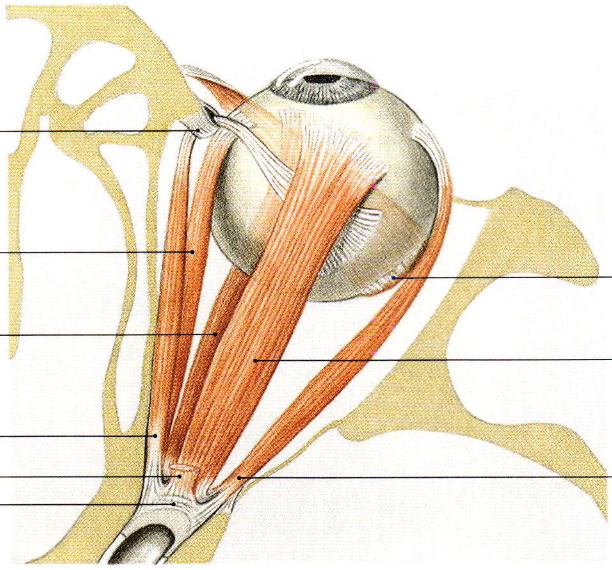

Fig. 1341 Extra-ocular muscles; schema; superior view.

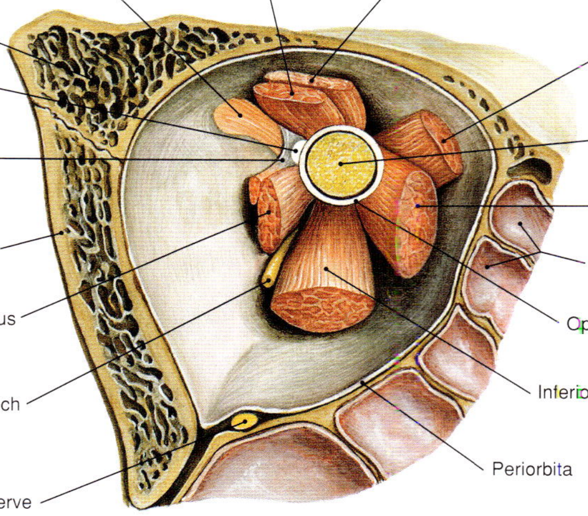

Fig. 1342 Extra-ocular muscles; anterior view.

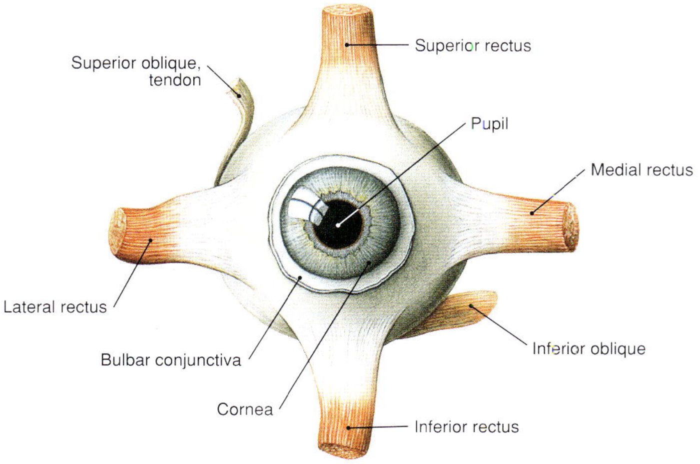

Fig. 1343 Extra-ocular muscles.

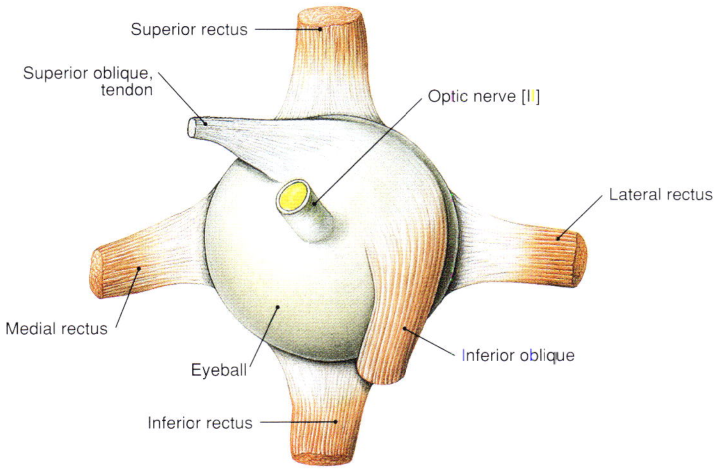

Fig. 1344 Extra-ocular muscles; posterior view.

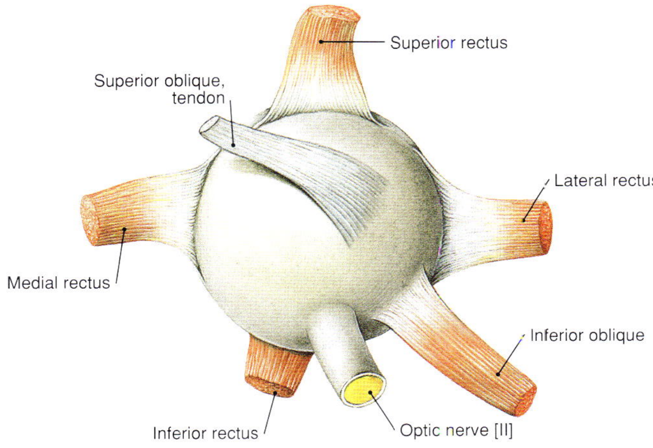

Fig. 1345 Extra-ocular muscles; posterior-superior view.

Extra-ocular muscles

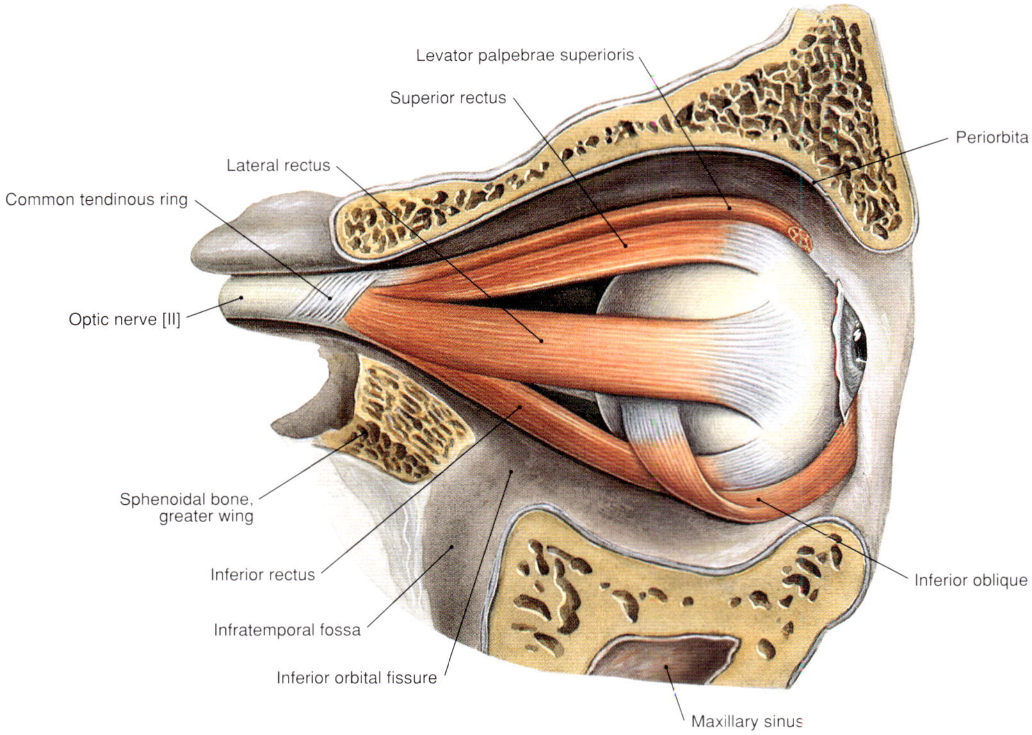

Fig. 1346 Extra-ocular muscles; lateral view.

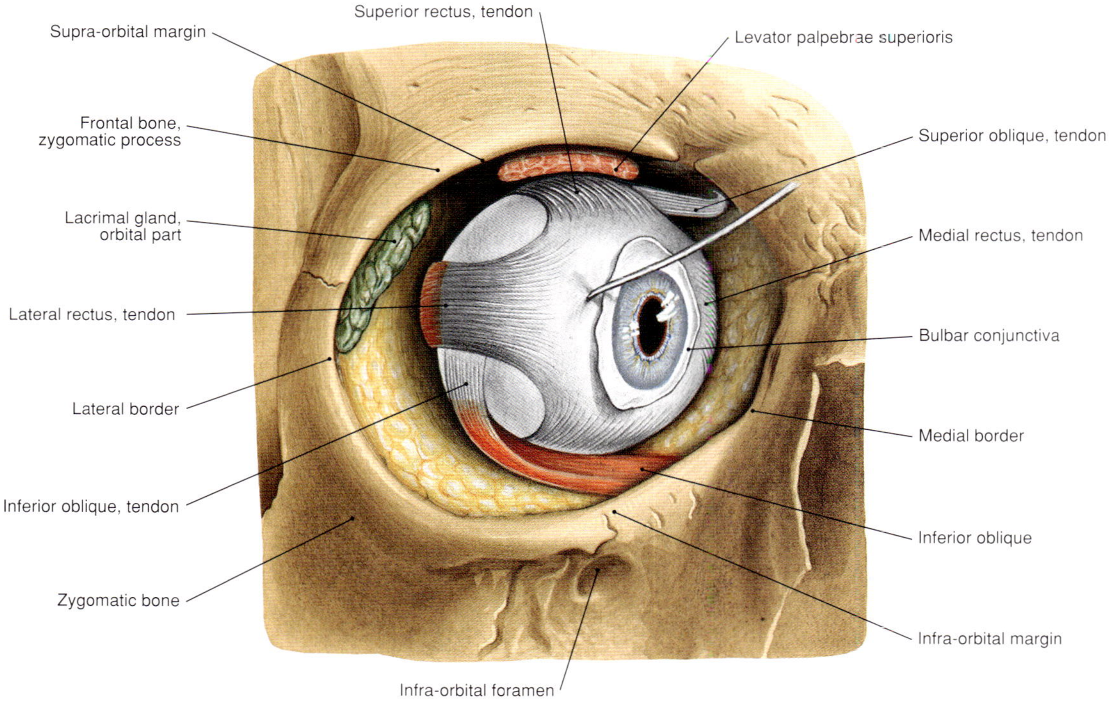

Fig. 1347 Extra-ocular muscles; oblique view from anterior.

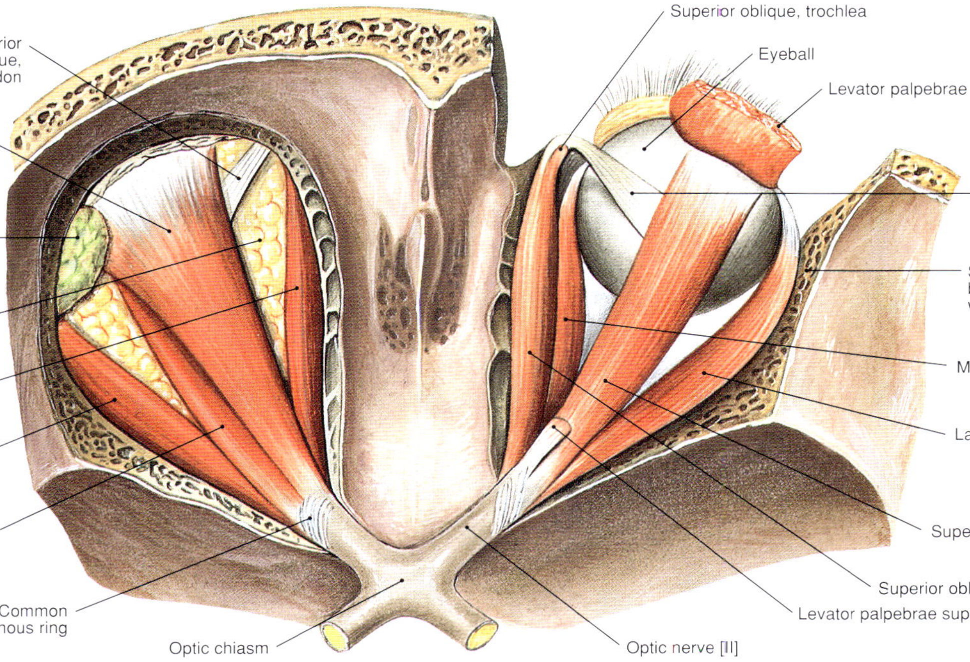

Fig. 1348 Extra-ocular muscles; superior view.

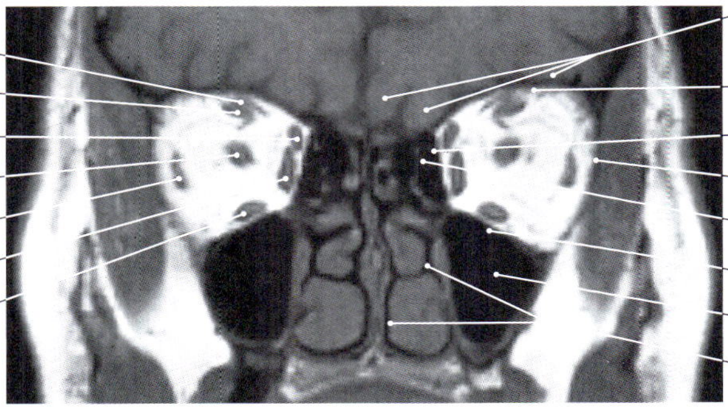

Fig. 1349 Extra-ocular muscles; magnetic resonance tomographic image (MRI); frontal section through the middle of the orbit; anterior view.

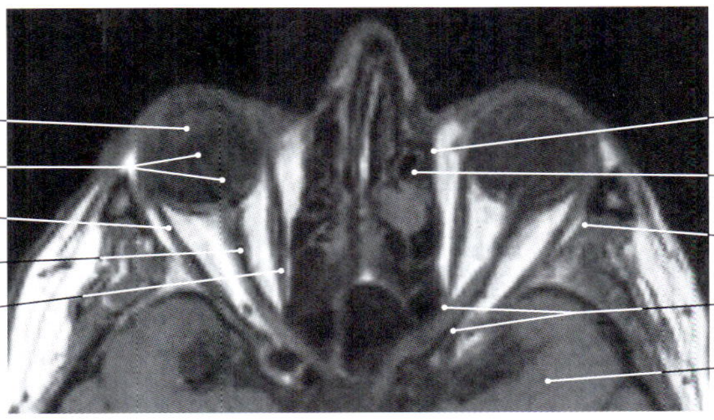

Fig. 1350 Eyeball and extra-ocular muscles; magnetic resonance tomographic image (MRI); horizontal section at the level of the optic nerve; superior view.

Eyeball, structure

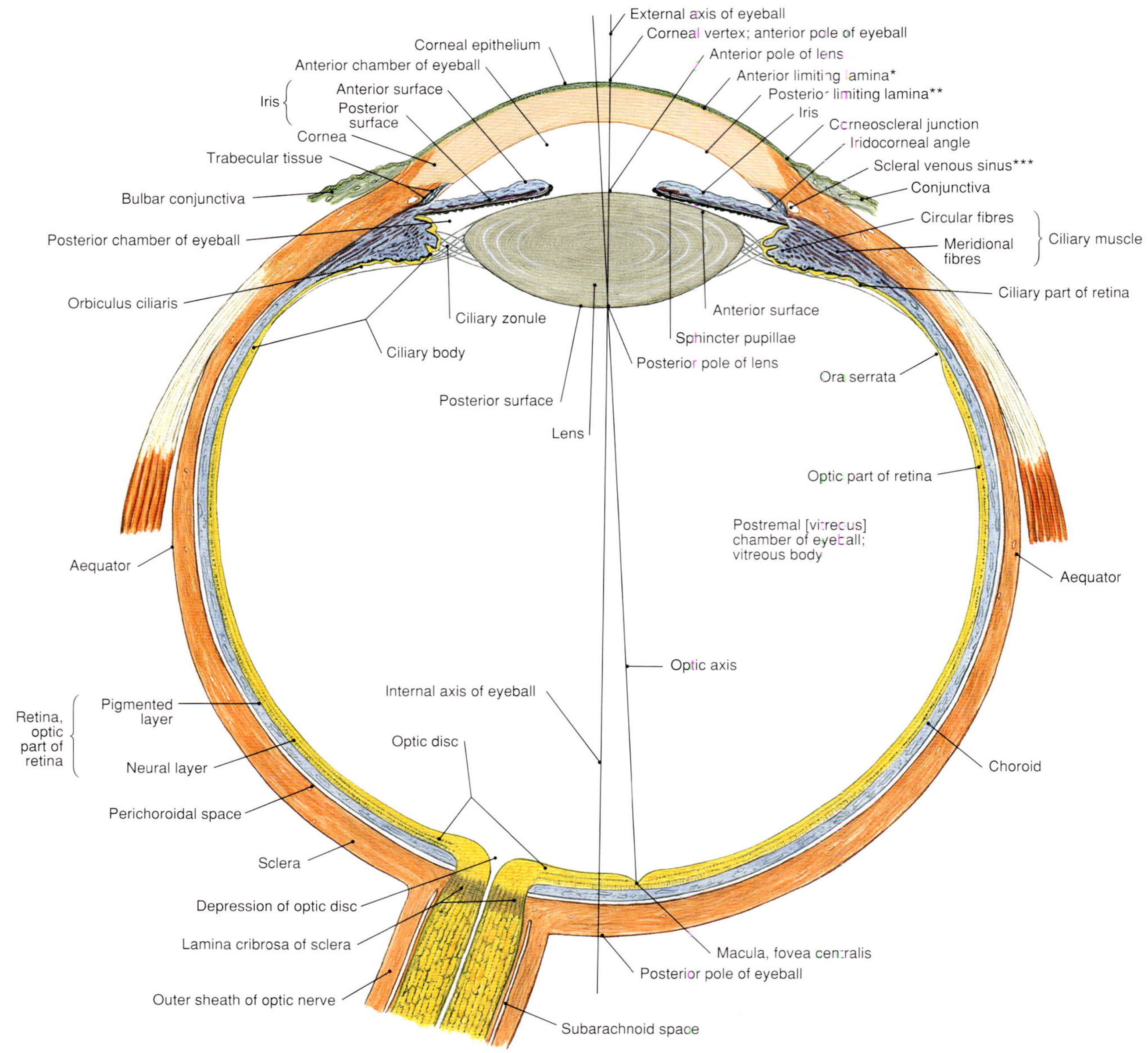

Fig. 1351 Eyeball;
schematic horizontal section at the level of the exit of the optic nerve.

* Clinical term: BOWMAN's membrane
** Clinical term: DESCEMET's membrane
*** Clinical term: canal of SCHLEMM

Dimensions of the eyeball

(Average values according to the anatomic and ophthalmologic literature)

External bulbar axis	24.0 mm
Internal bulbar axis	22.5 mm
Thickness of the cornea	0.5 mm
Depth of the anterior chamber	3.6 mm
Thickness of the lens	3.6 mm
Distance between lens and retina	15.6 mm
Thickness of the retina	0.3 mm
Radius of curvature of the sclera	13.0 mm
Radius of curvature of the cornea	7.8 mm
Power of the entire eye (distance vision)	59 dioptres
Power of the cornea	43 dioptres
Power of the lens (distance vision)	19 dioptres
Interpupillary distance	61–69 mm

Blood vessels of the eyeball

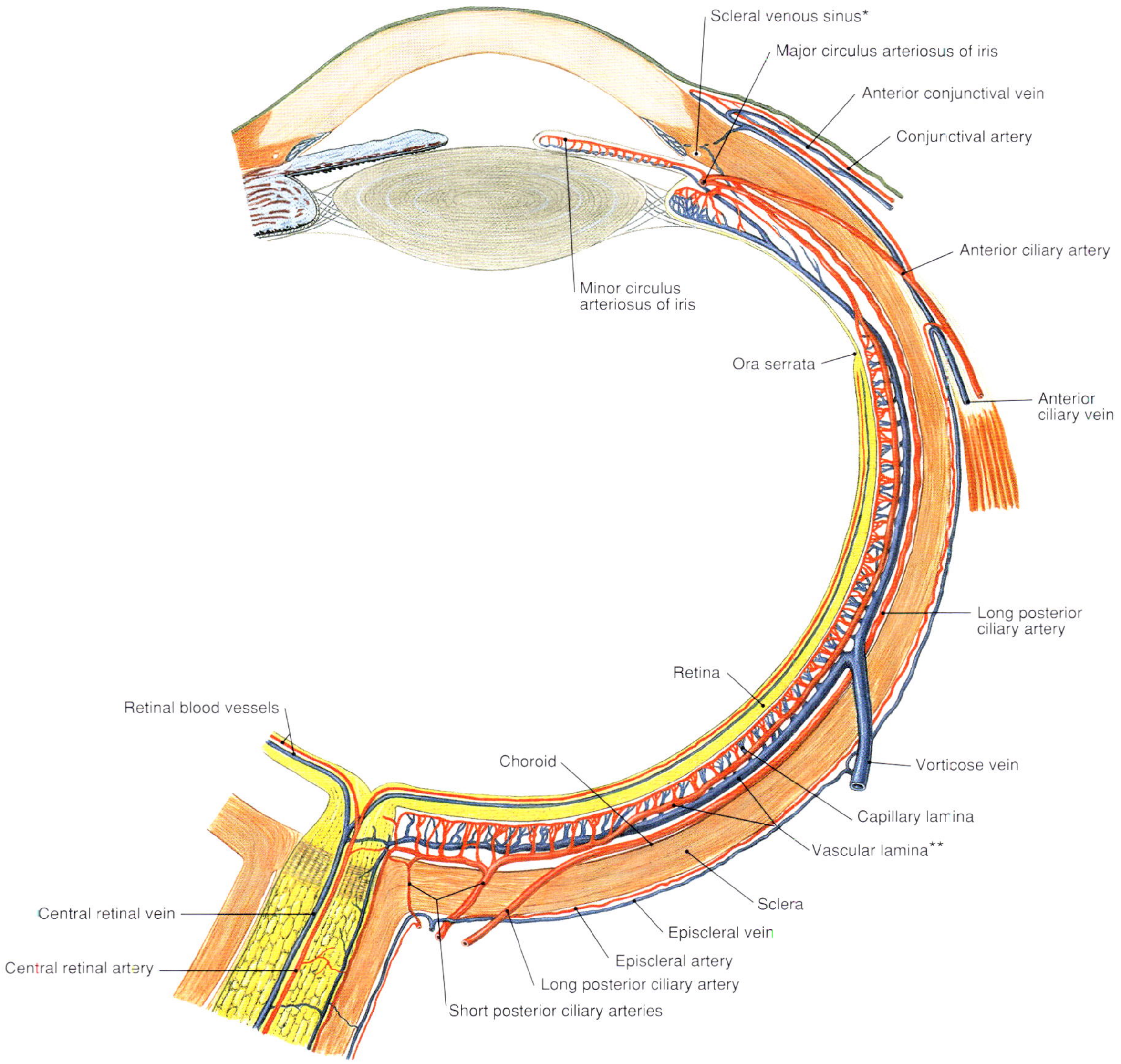

Fig. 1352 Blood vessels of the eyeball.

* Clinical term: canal of SCHLEMM

** Clinical term: uvea

Layers of the eyeball

Fibrous layer of the eyeball
- Cornea (pronounced curvature, translucent)
- Sclera (lesser curvature, opaque; bluish-white in infancy, yellowish-white in senescence)

Vascular layer of the eyeball
- Iris with the central circular opening, the pupil
- Ciliary body with the ciliary muscle, the ciliary process, the ciliary zonule with the zonular fibres and the zonular spaces
- Choroid

Inner layer of the eyeball (retina)
- Nonvisual retina (from the pupillary-iridial margin, to the ora serrata)
  Iridial part of the retina (single-layered, heavily pigmented), ciliary part of the retina (single-layered, unpigmented)
- Optic part of the retina (stratified)
  1. neuron: vision cells (rod cells – brightness; cone cells – colour)
  2. neuron: bipolar ganglion cells within the retina (ganglion of the retina)
  3. neuron: multi-polar ganglion cells (optic ganglion), whose long axons form the optic nerve and continue in the optic tract

Ciliary body and iris

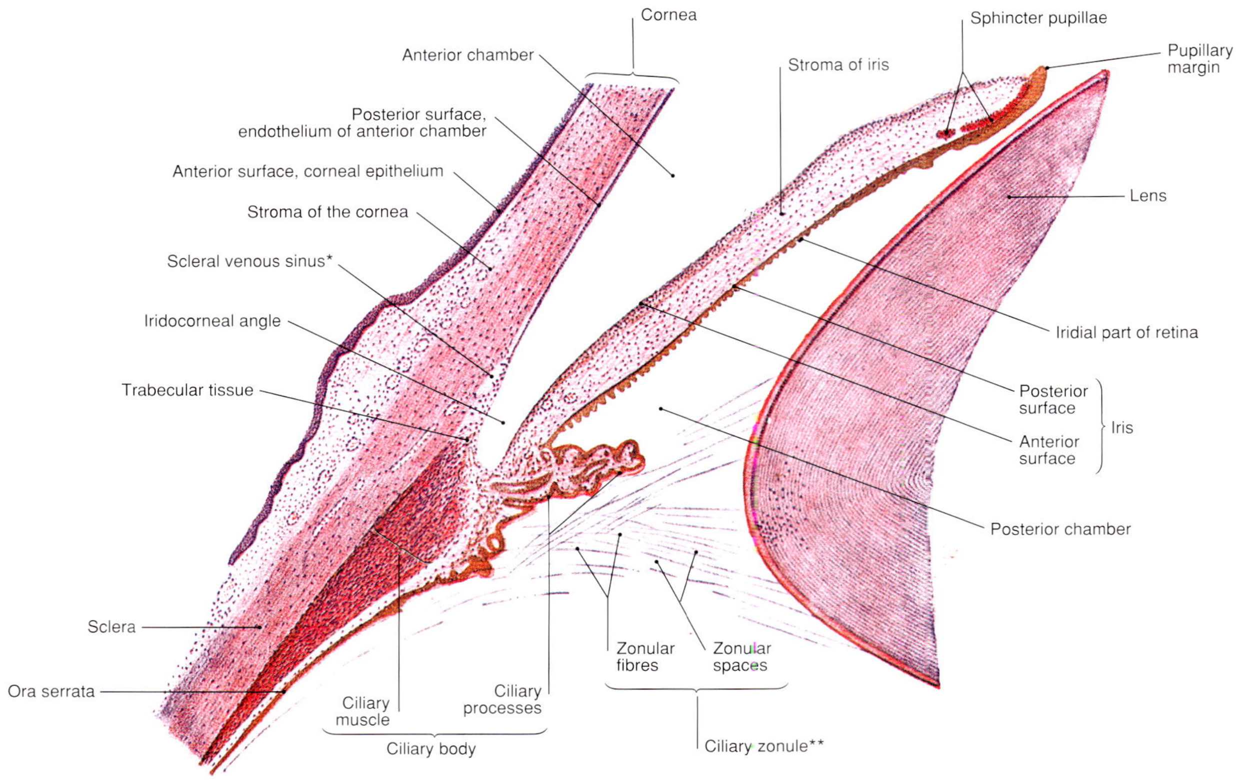

Fig. 1353 Eyeball;
schematic horizontal section at the level of the pupil.

* Clinical term: canal of SCHLEMM
** Clinical term: zonule of ZINN

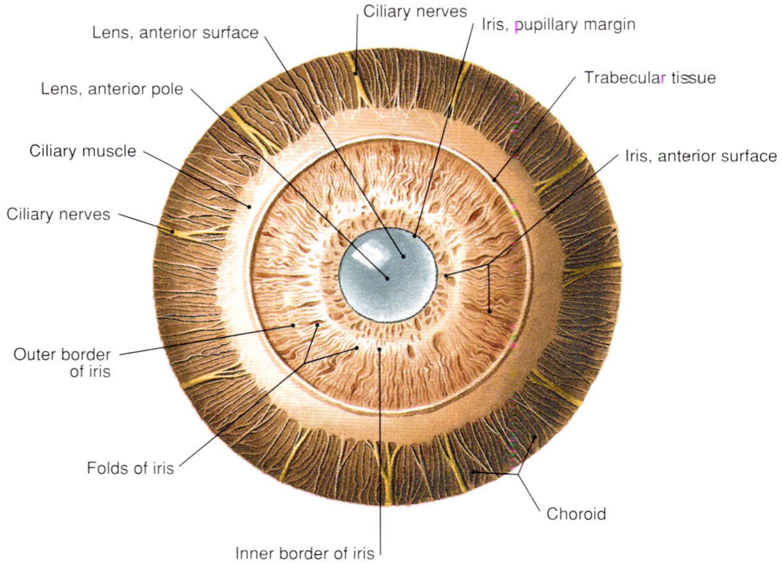

Fig. 1354 Iris and pupil;
after removal of the sclera and cornea;
anterior view.

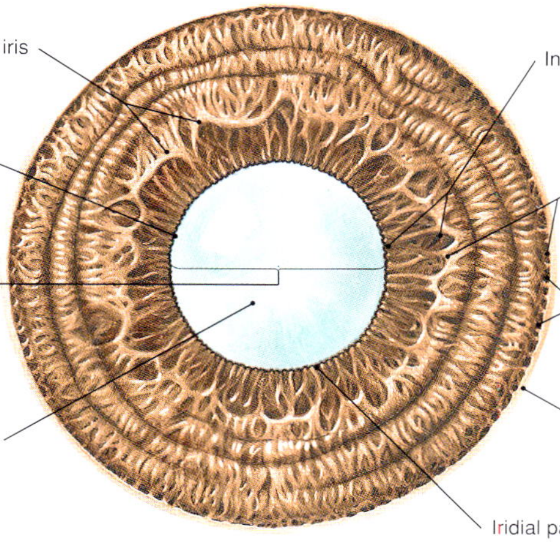

Fig. 1355 Iris;
after removal of the cornea;
anterior view.

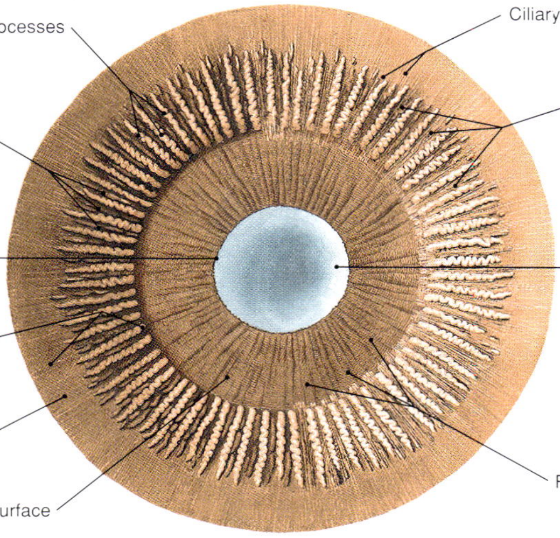

Fig. 1356 Iris;
posterior view.

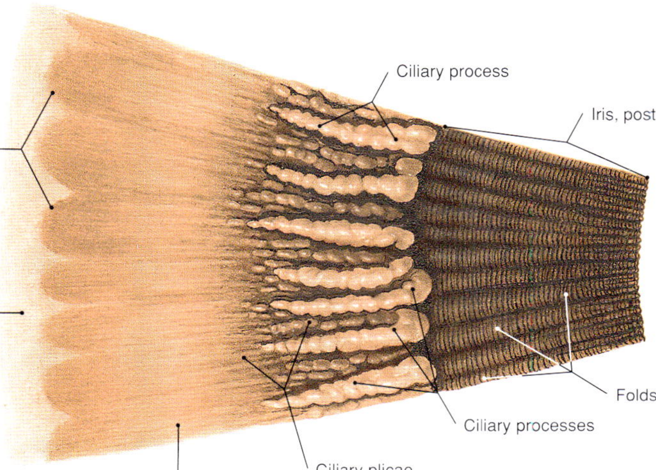

Fig. 1357 Iris;
section of Fig. 1356;
posterior view.

Lens

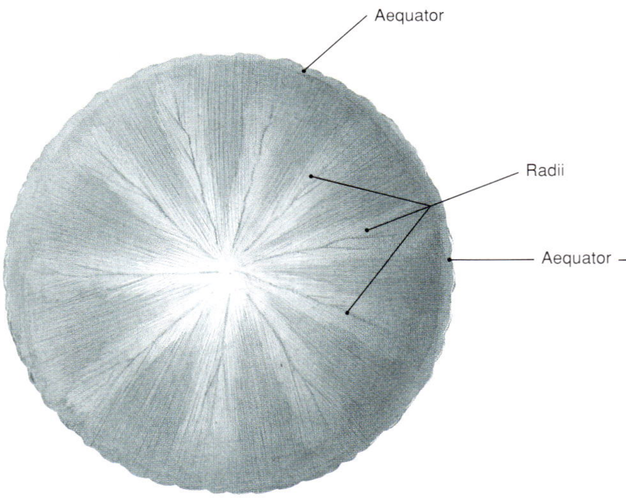

Fig. 1358 Lens;
anterior view.

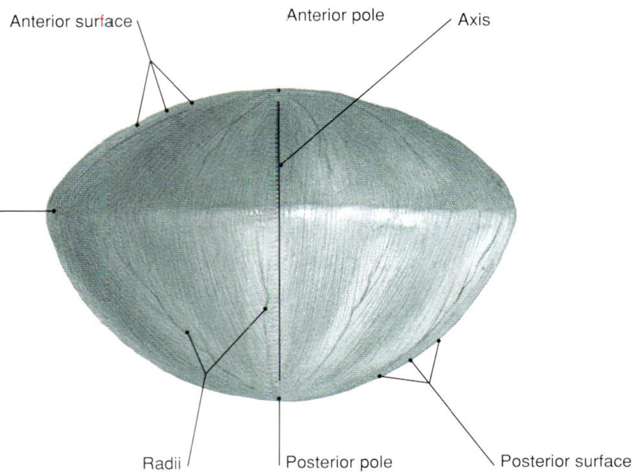

Fig. 1359 Lens;
viewed from the equator.

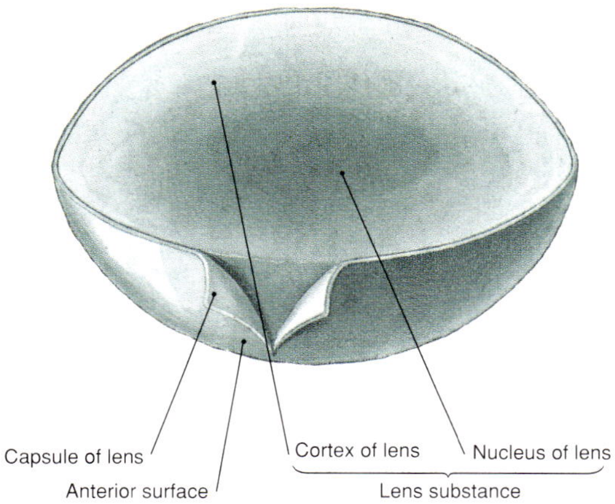

Fig. 1360 Lens;
oblique view from anterior.

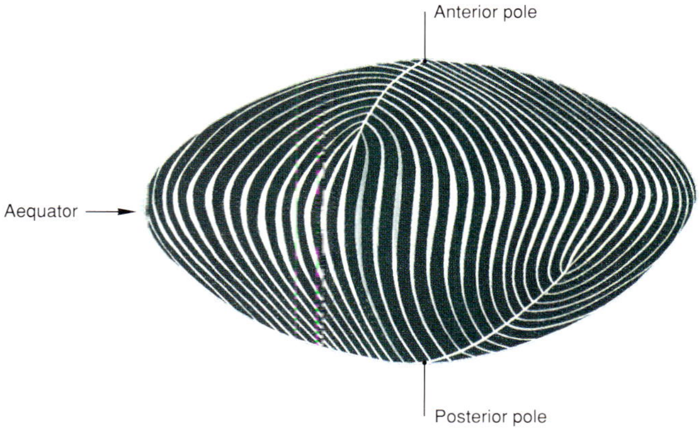

Fig. 1361 Lens;
schema of the lens fibres in a neonate;
viewed from the equator.

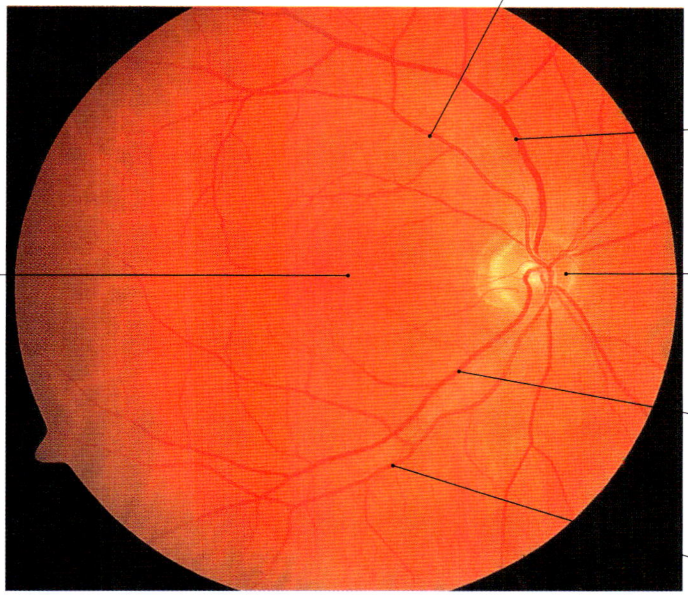

Fig. 1362 Ocular fundus;
ophthalmoscopic picture of the central region;
anterior view.

* Clinical term: yellow spot
** Clinical term: papilla or blind spot

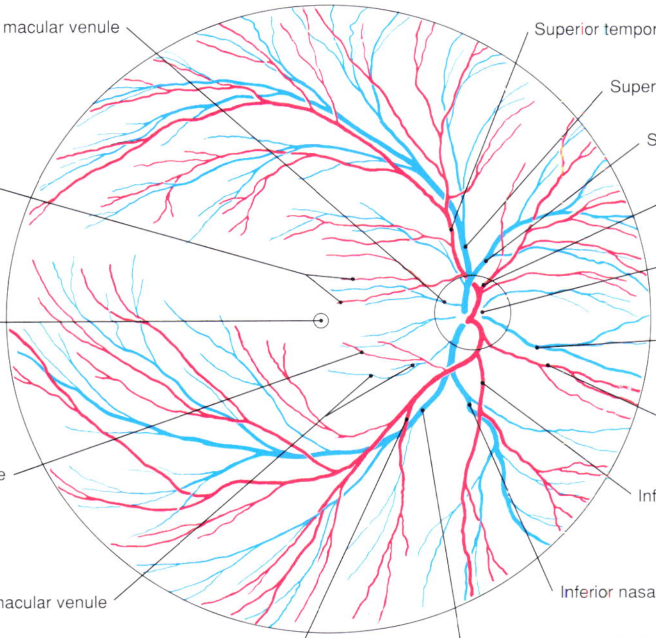

Fig. 1363 Blood vessels of the retina;
schema of the course of the vessels;
anterior view.

Optic nerve

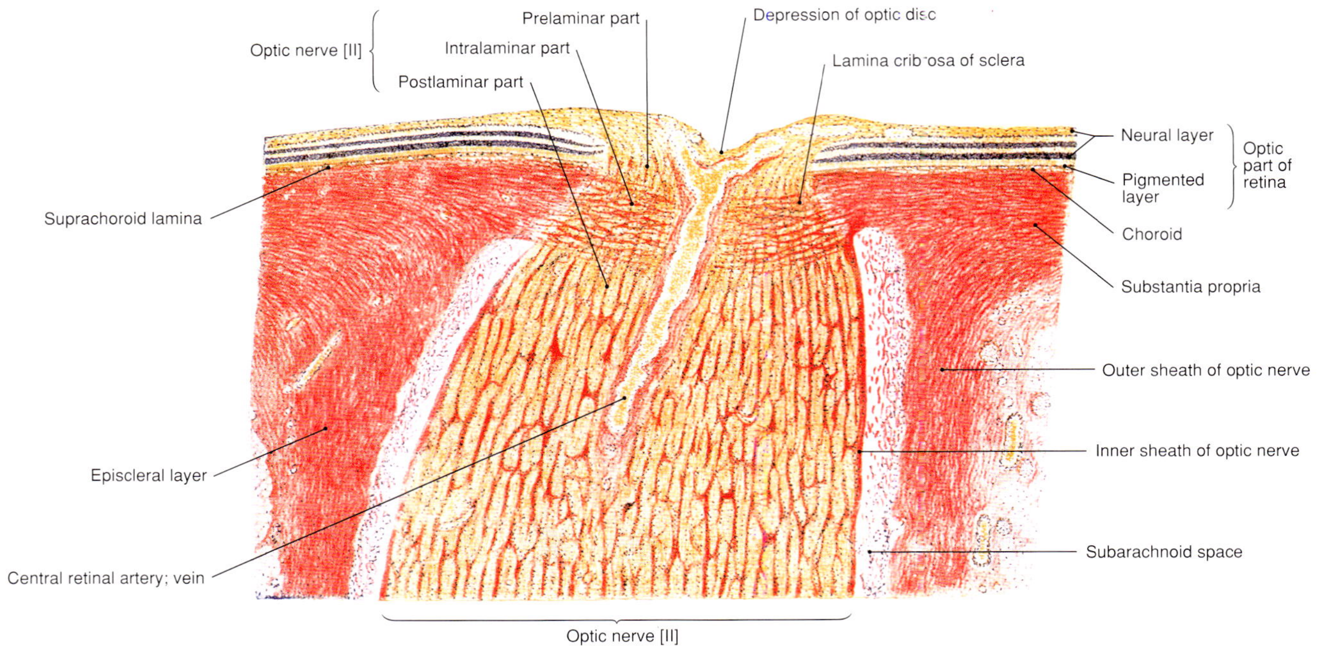

Fig. 1364 Optic nerve [II];
horizontal section at its exit from the eyeball.

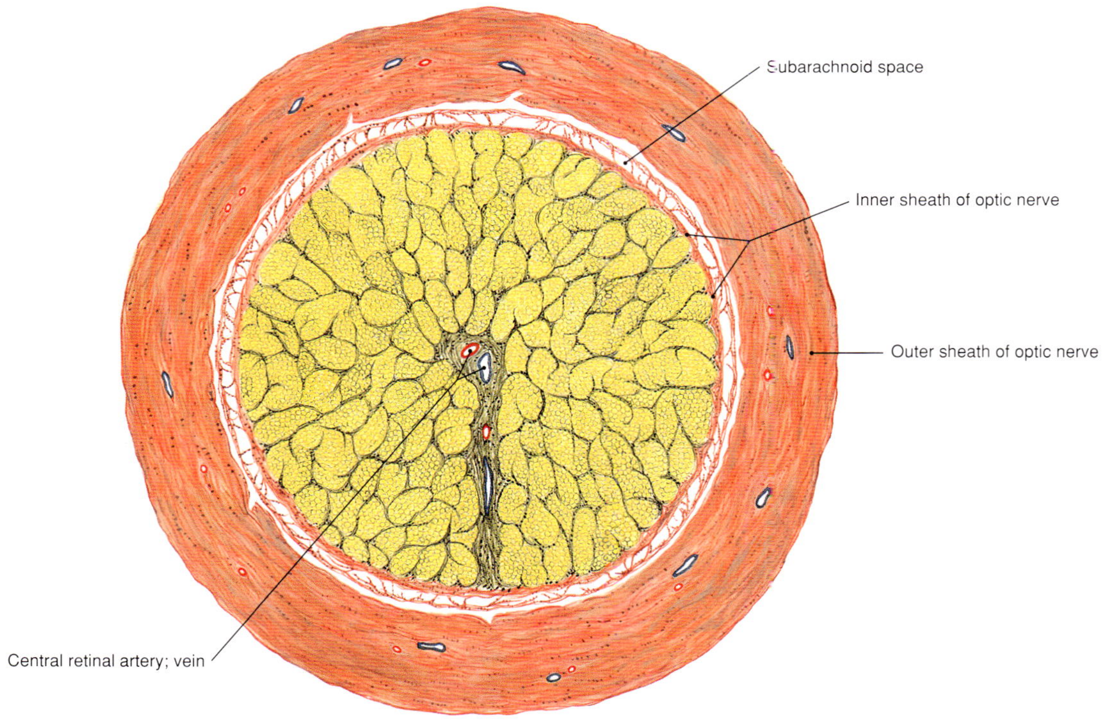

Fig. 1365 Optic nerve [II];
cross-section near the eyeball.

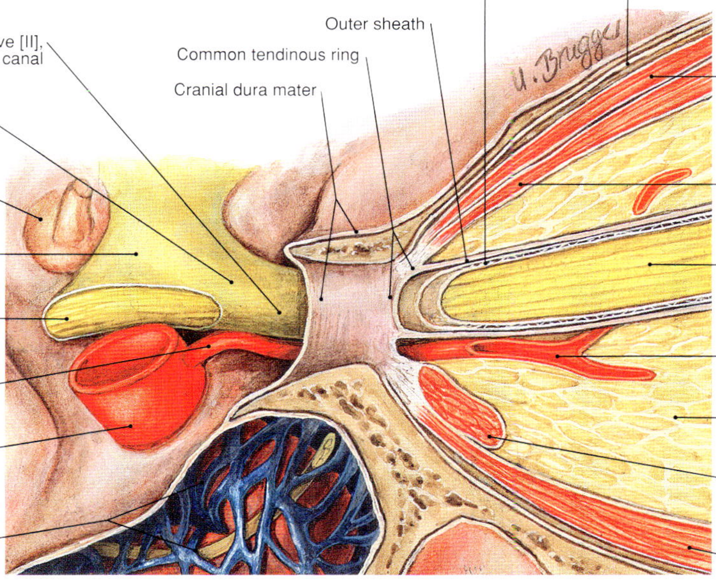

Fig. 1366 Optic nerve [II];
the optic canal has been opened;
viewed from the right.

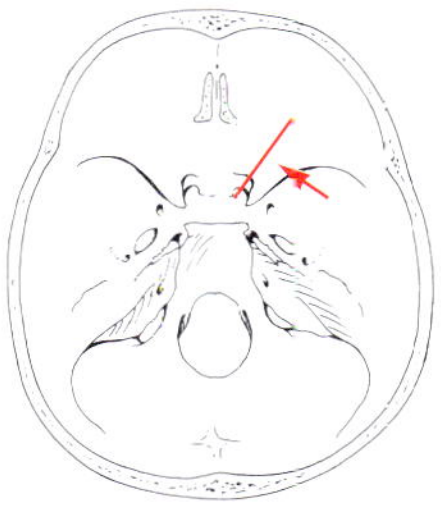

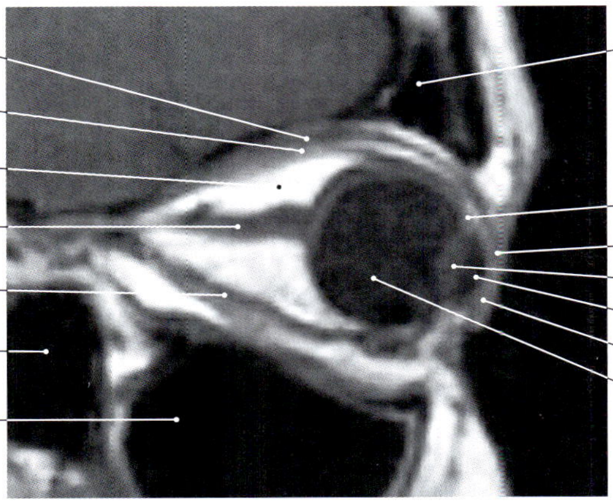

Fig. 1367 Orbit;
magnetic resonance tomographic image (MRI);
vertical section along the optic nerve;
viewed from the right.

→ 1379

Optic pathway and blood vessels

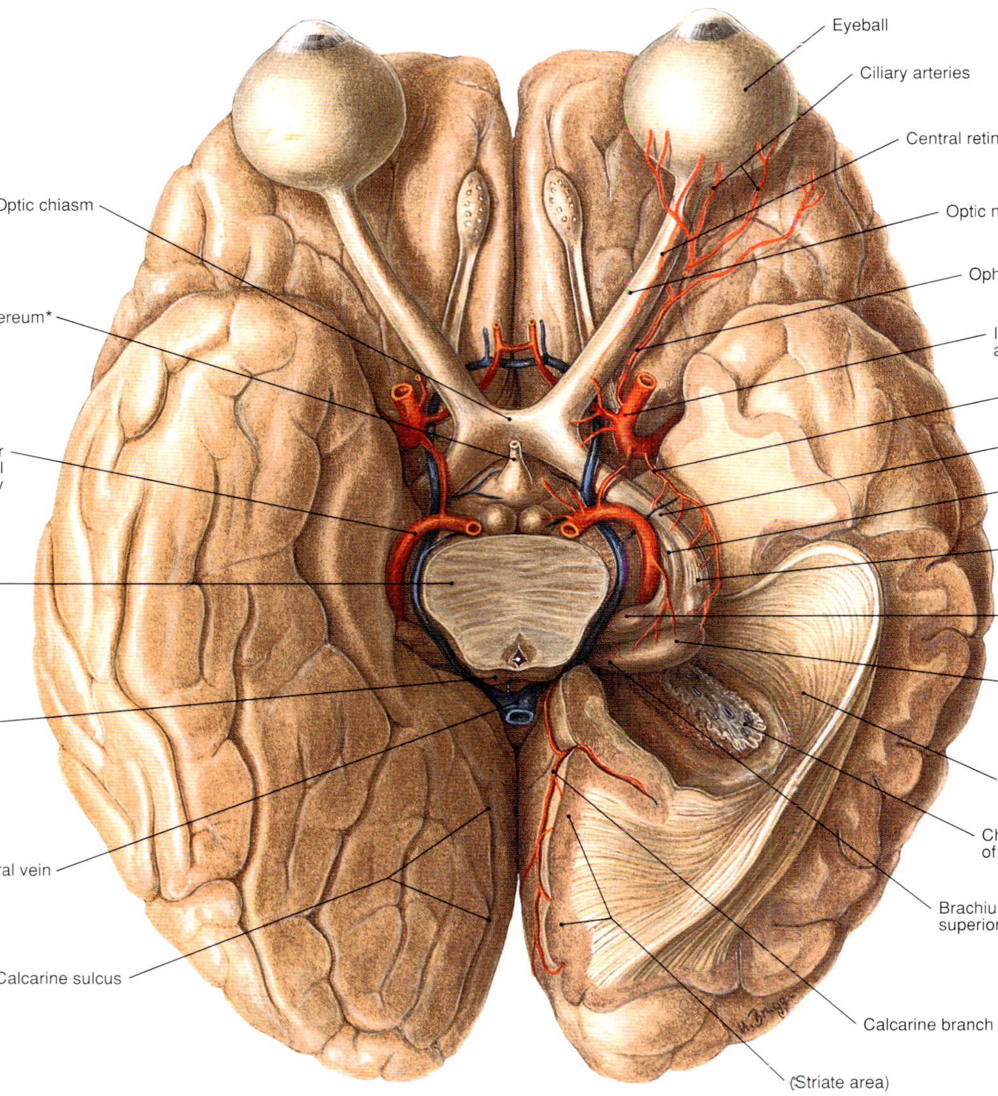

Fig. 1368 Brain and blood supply of the parts of the optic pathway; inferior view.
The pituitary gland has been removed at its infundibulum (*). Due to the close proximity of the pituitary gland and the optic chiasm, pituitary tumours can cause visual disturbances.

Optic pathway

1. neuron: rod cells and cone cells of the retina
2. neuron: bipolar ganglion cells of the retina (perikarya in the retinal ganglion)
3. neuron: multi-polar ganglion cells of the retina (perikarya in the optic ganglion)
   The axons of the optic ganglion cells extend primarily to the lateral geniculate body (lateral root), although several fibres also extend to the pretectal area and the superior colliculus (medial root), as well as to the hypothalamus. They run within the optic nerve to the optic chiasm, where the fibres from the nasal part of the ocular fundus cross to the opposite side. Each optic tract contains fibres, which transmit information from the contralateral half of the visual field.
4. neuron: Its axons travel primarily from the lateral geniculate body to areas 17 and 18 of the cerebral cortex (striate area) in the region surrounding the calcarine sulcus.

Optic pathway

1 Common visual field
1a Visual field of the left eye
1b Visual field of the right eye
2a Projection on the left retina
2b Projection on the right retina

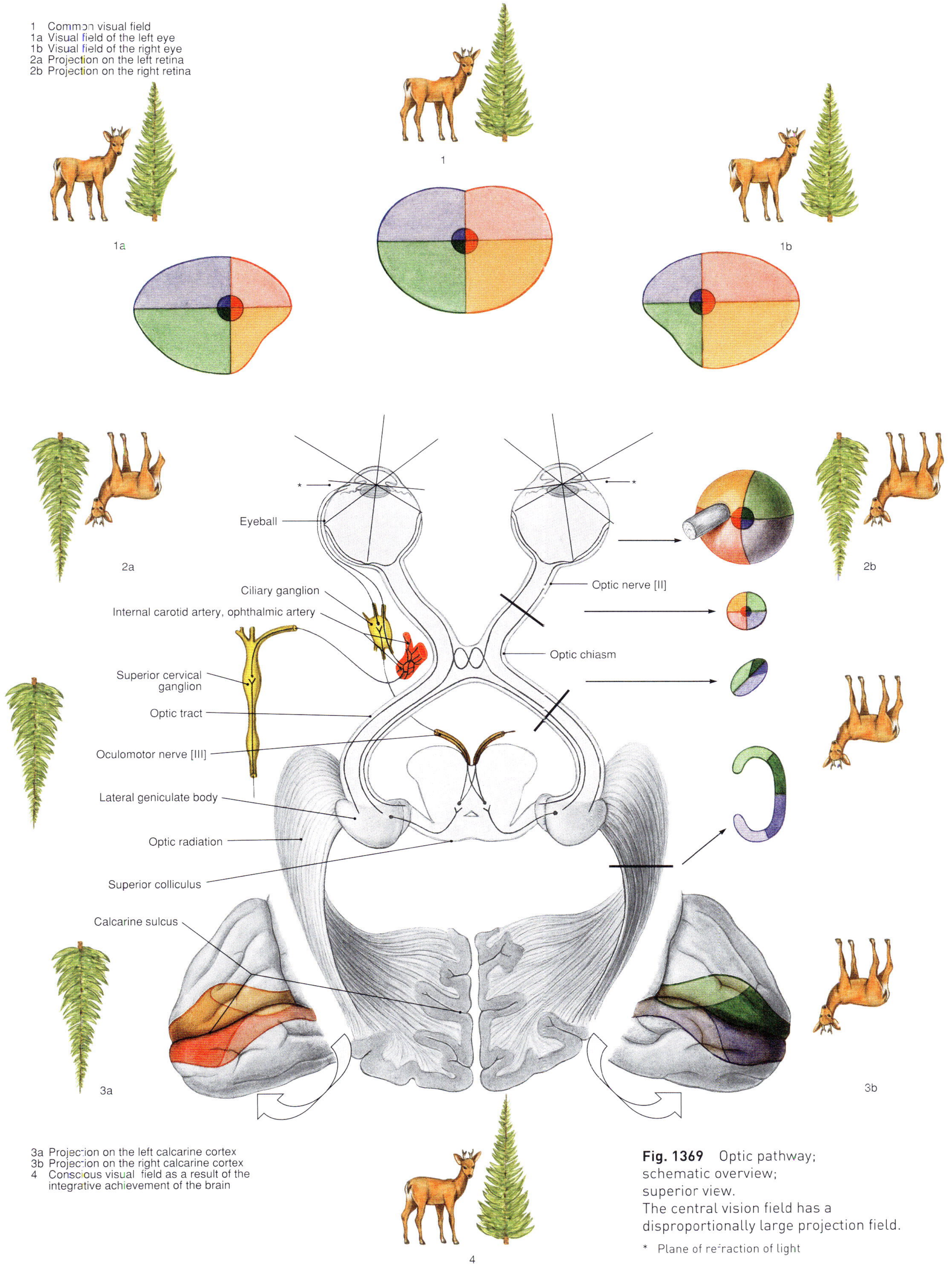

3a Projection on the left calcarine cortex
3b Projection on the right calcarine cortex
4 Conscious visual field as a result of the integrative achievement of the brain

Fig. 1369 Optic pathway; schematic overview; superior view.
The central vision field has a disproportionally large projection field.

* Plane of refraction of light

Orbit, topography

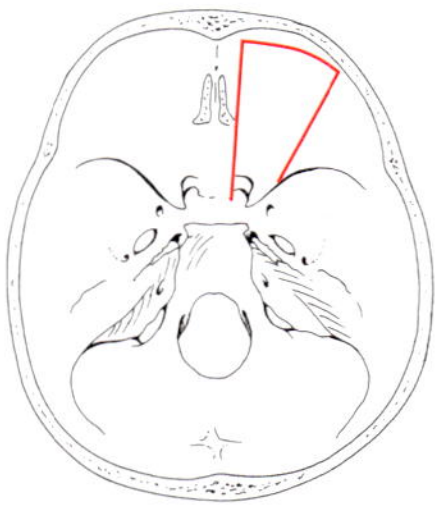

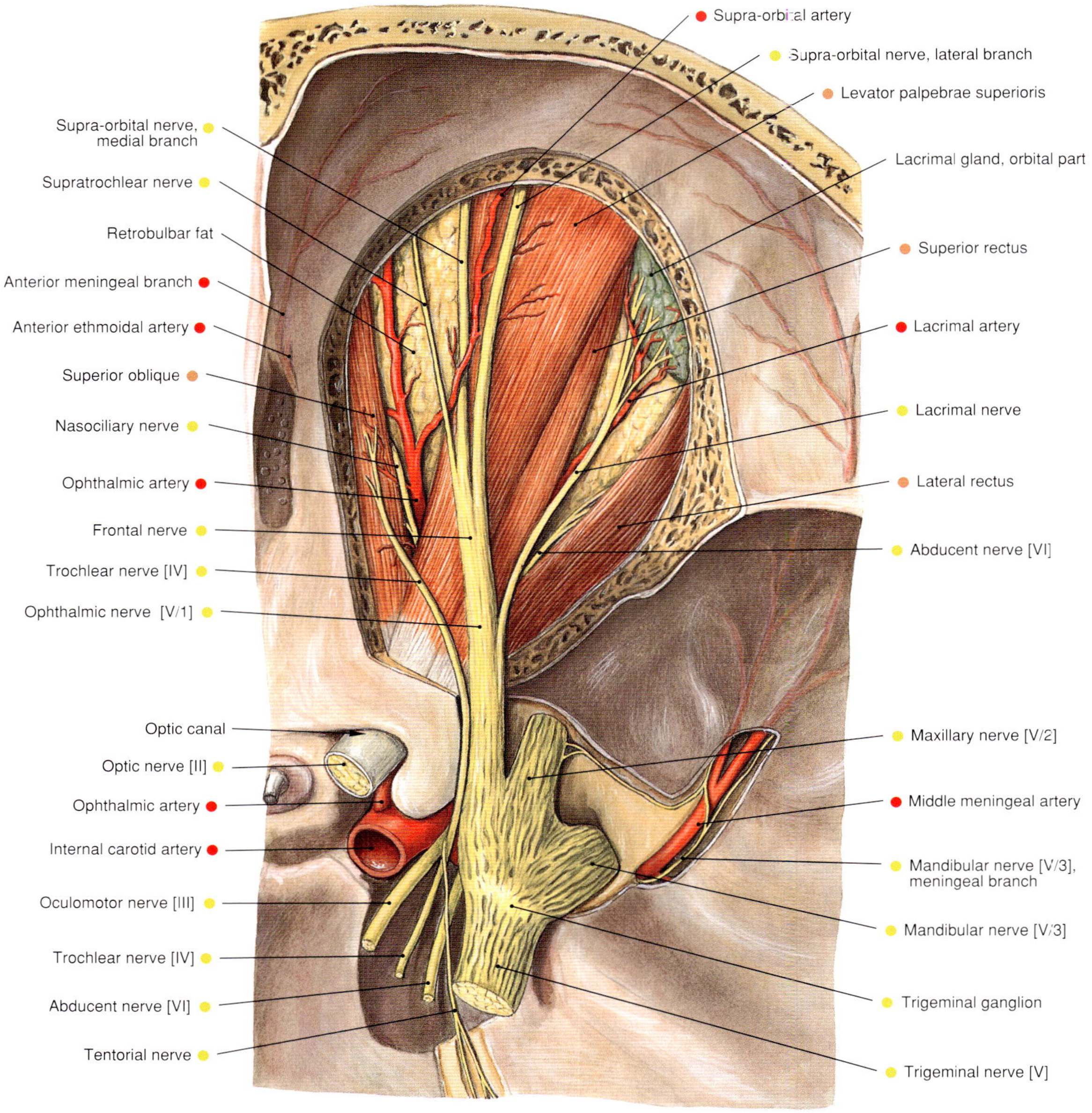

1371

Fig. 1370 Arteries and nerves of the orbit; superior view.

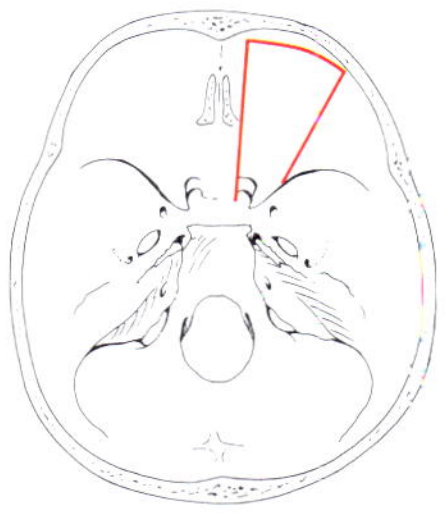

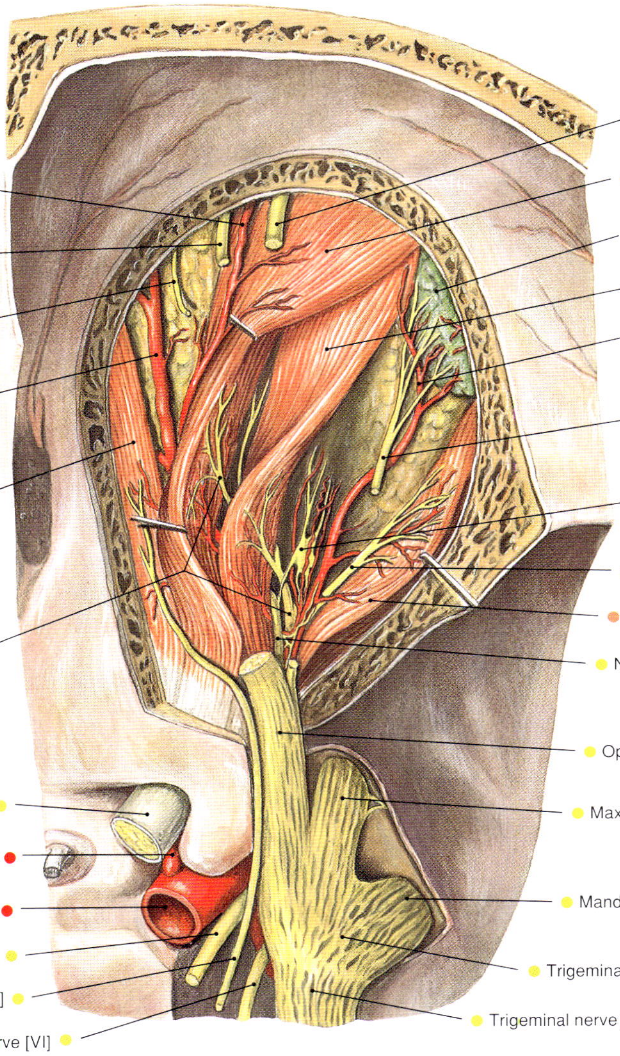

Fig. 1371 Arteries and nerves of the orbit; after removal of the roof of the orbit; superior view.

1372
1370

Orbit, topography

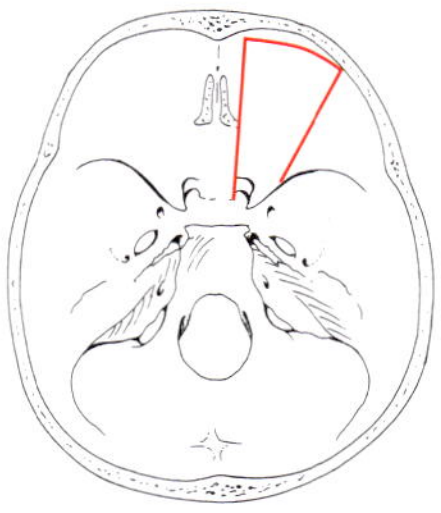

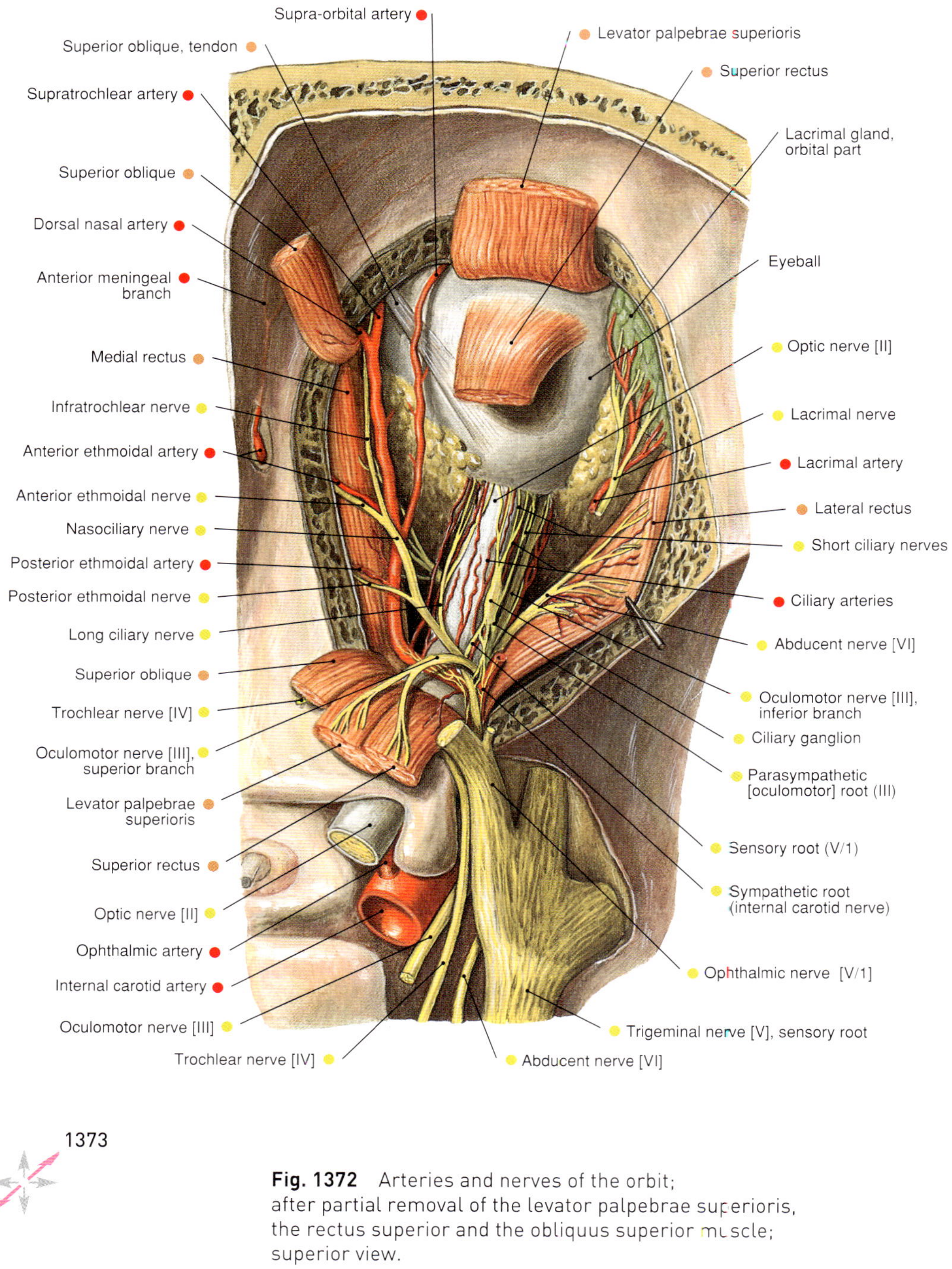

Fig. 1372 Arteries and nerves of the orbit; after partial removal of the levator palpebrae superioris, the rectus superior and the obliquus superior muscle; superior view.

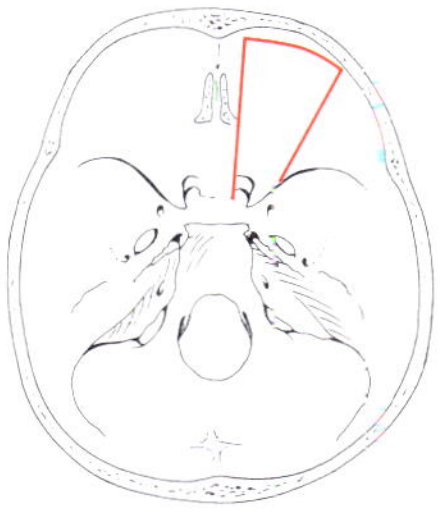

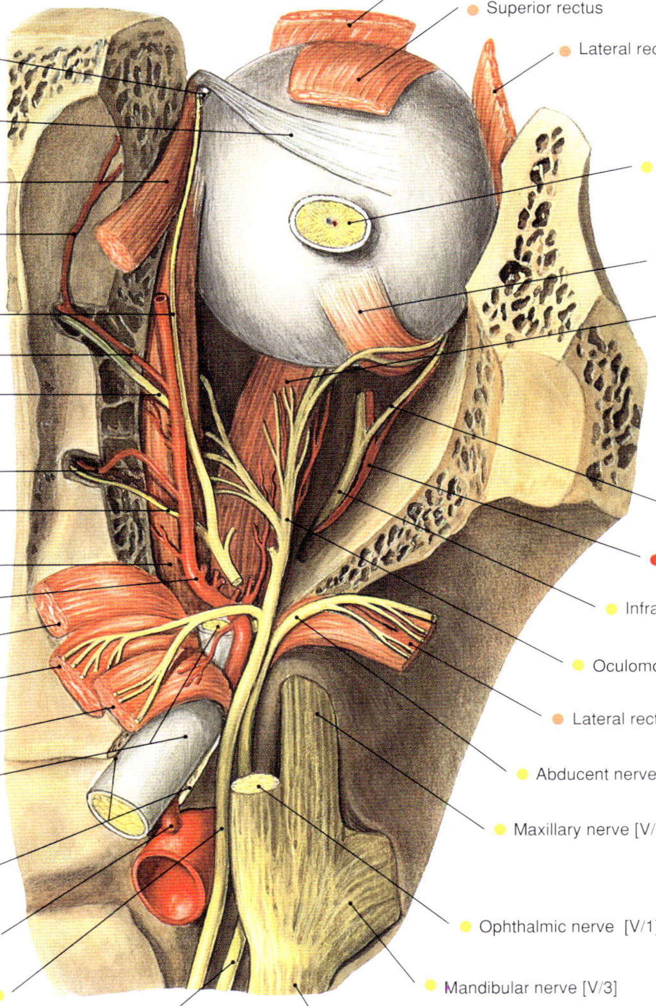

Fig. 1373 Arteries and nerves of the orbit; after removal of the roof of the orbit; superior view.

1372

Blood vessels of the orbit

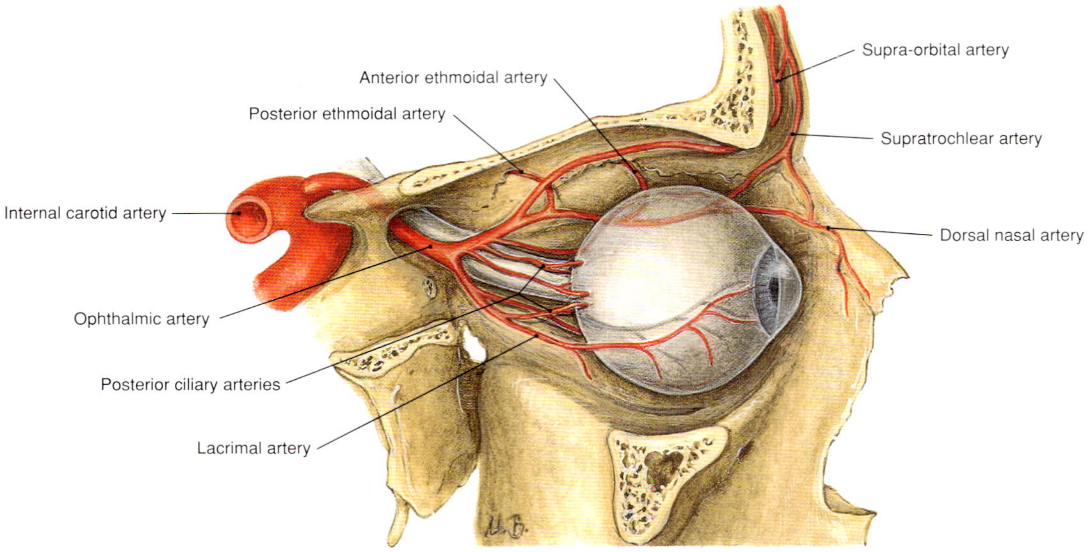

Fig. 1374 Arteries of the orbit; lateral view.

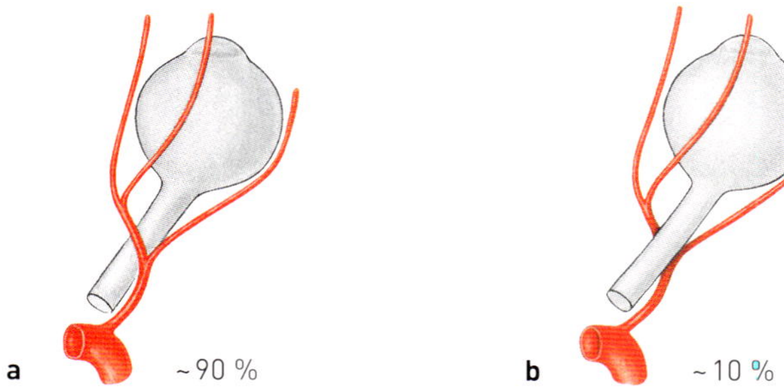

Fig. 1375 a, b Variations of the ophthalmic artery; superior view.

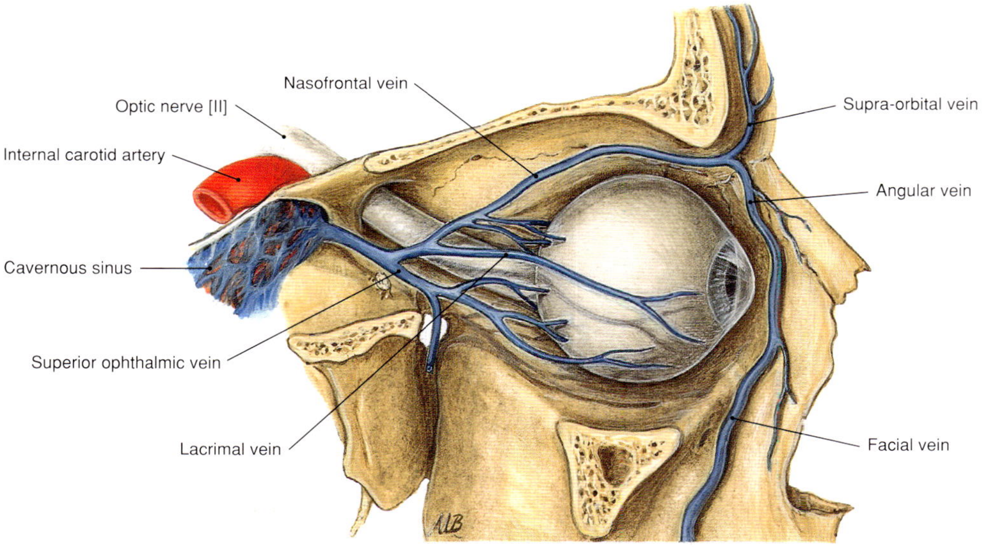

Fig. 1376 Veins of the orbit; lateral view.

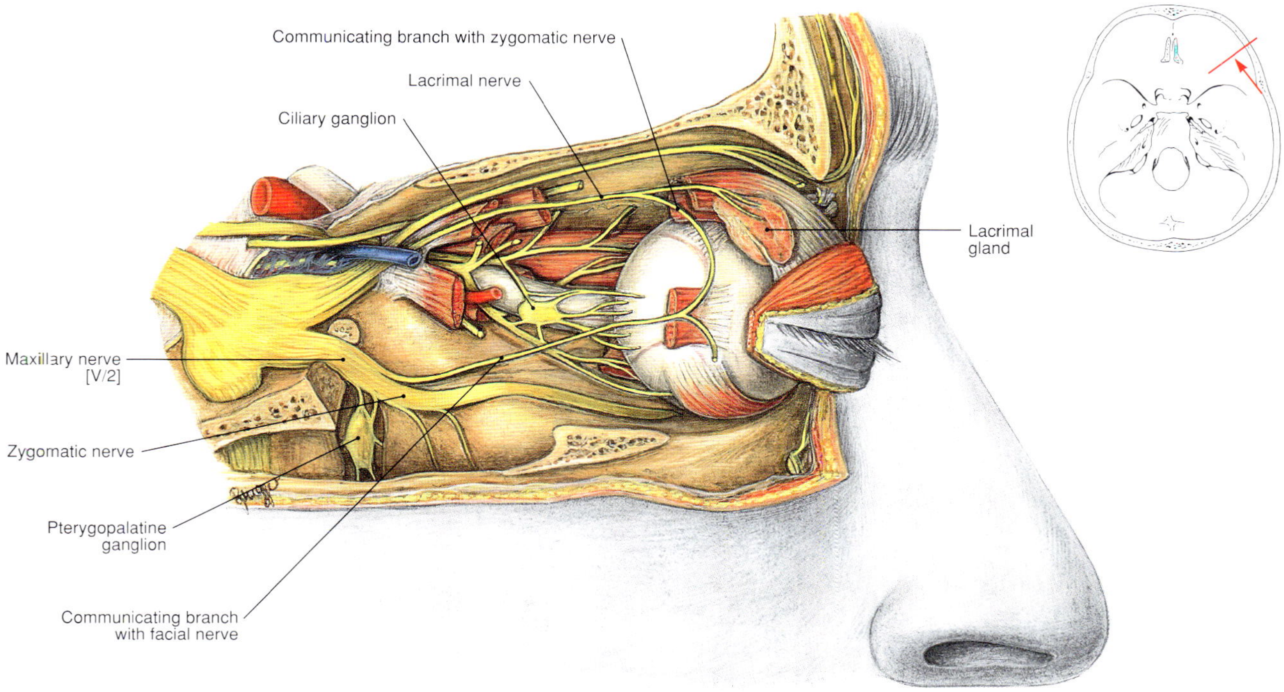

Fig. 1377 Orbit;
viewed from the right.

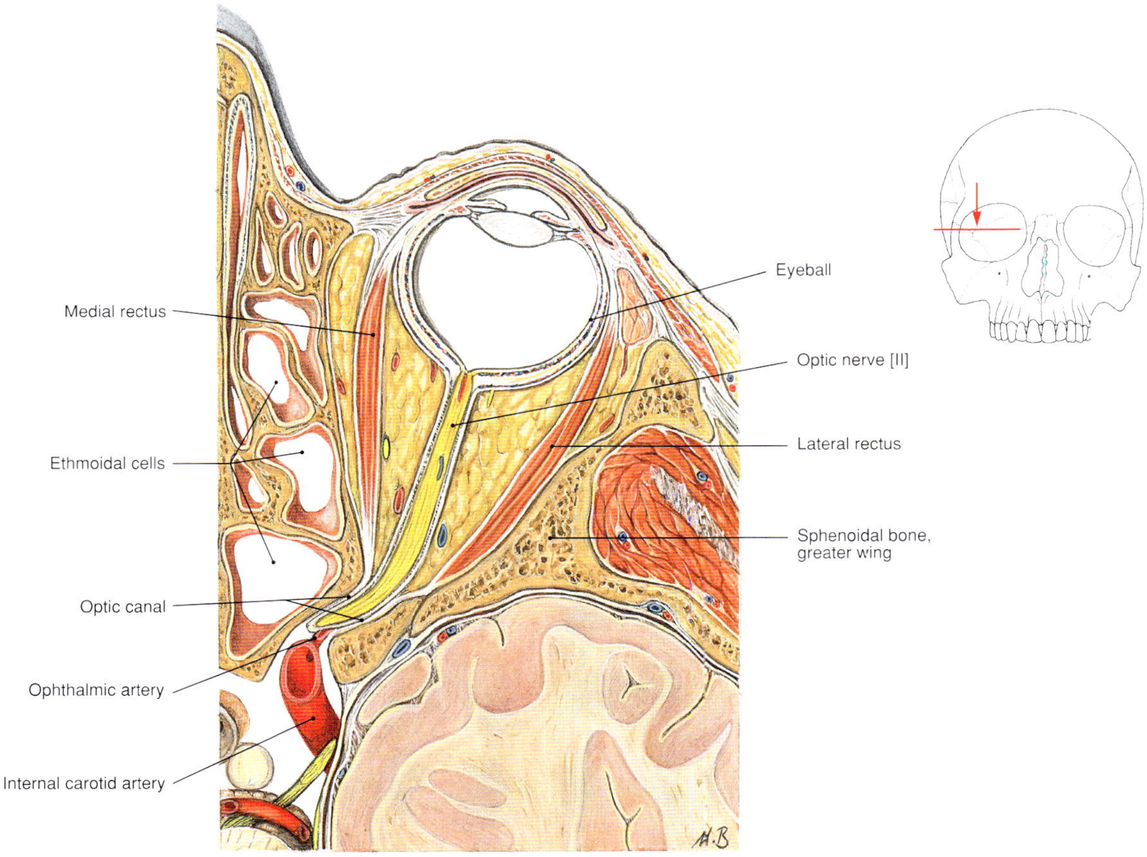

Fig. 1378 Orbit;
horizontal section;
superior view.

Orbit, sections

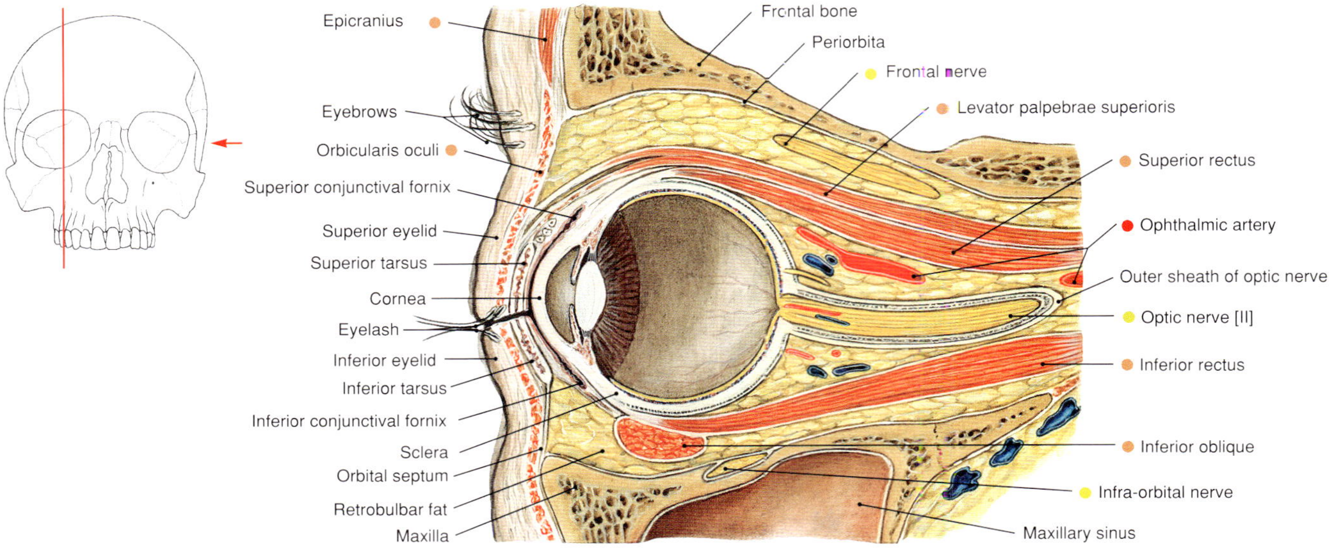

Fig. 1379 Orbit;
vertical section through the eyeball and the optic nerve;
medial view.

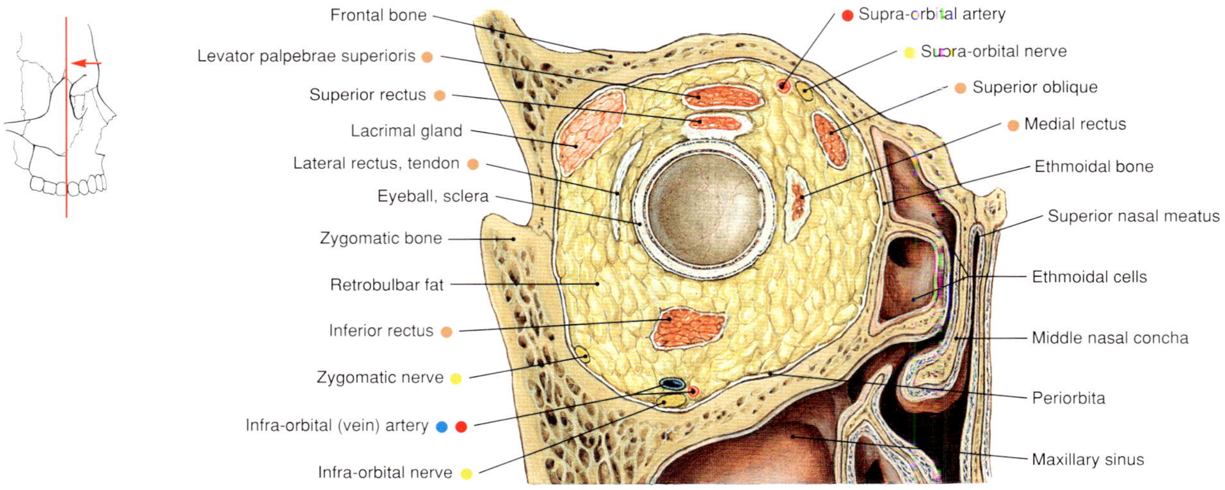

Fig. 1380 Orbit;
frontal section at the level of the posterior part of the eyeball;
anterior view.

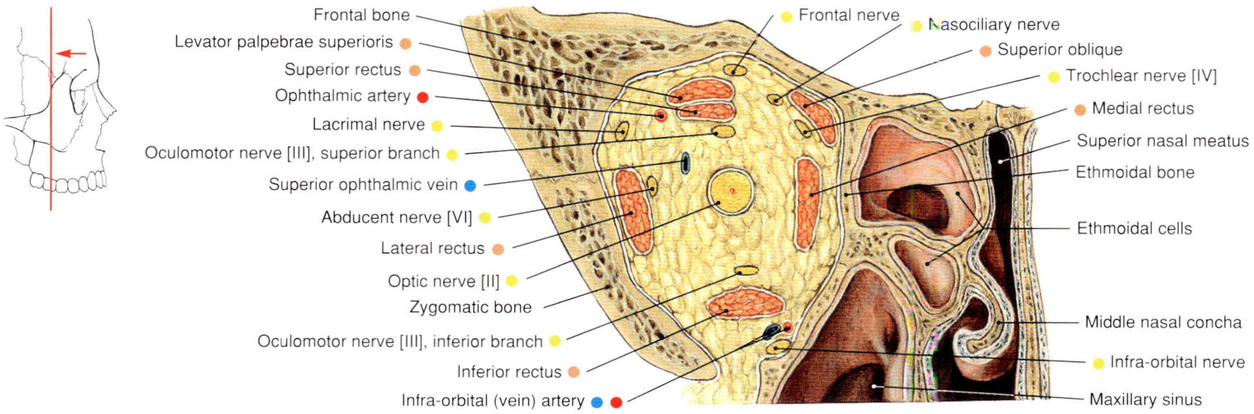

Fig. 1381 Orbit;
frontal section at the level of the middle of the extracranial course of the optic nerve;
anterior view.

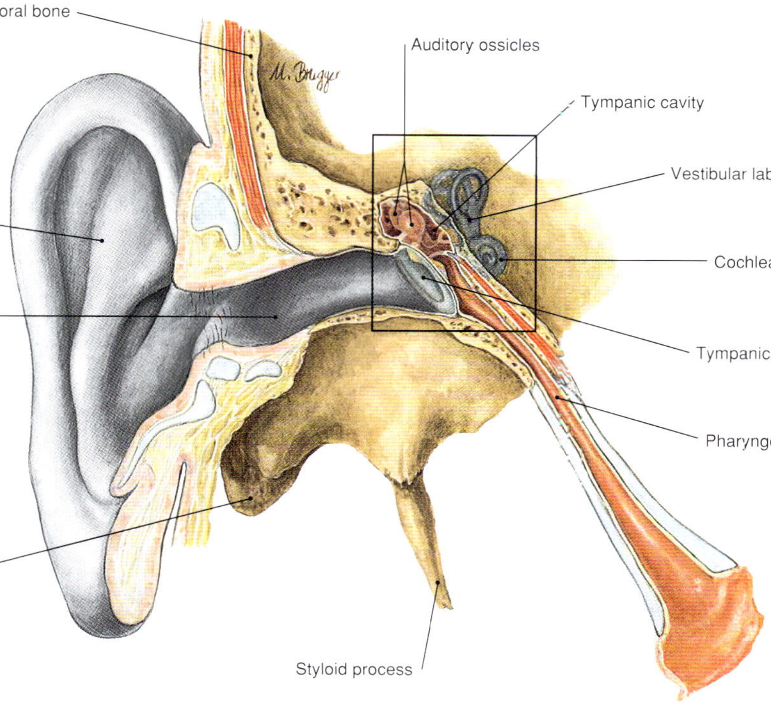

Fig. 1382 Ear.

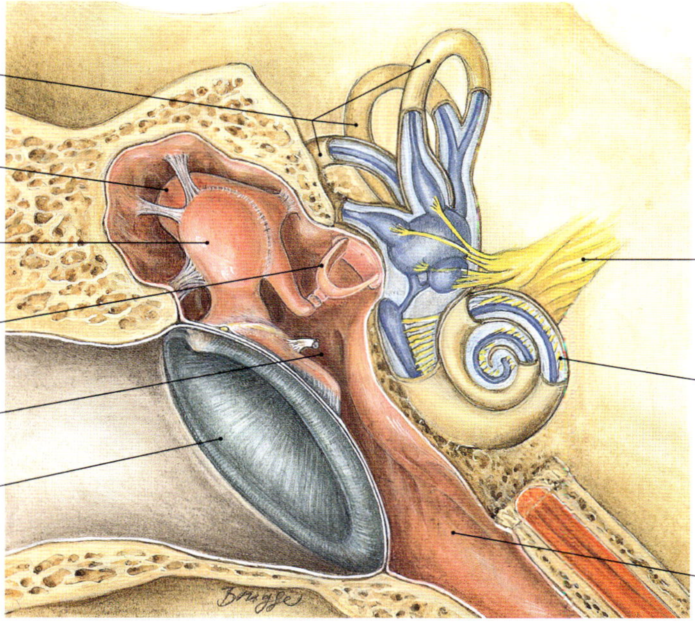

Fig. 1383 Middle and inner ear; section from Fig. 1382; anterior view.

Auricle

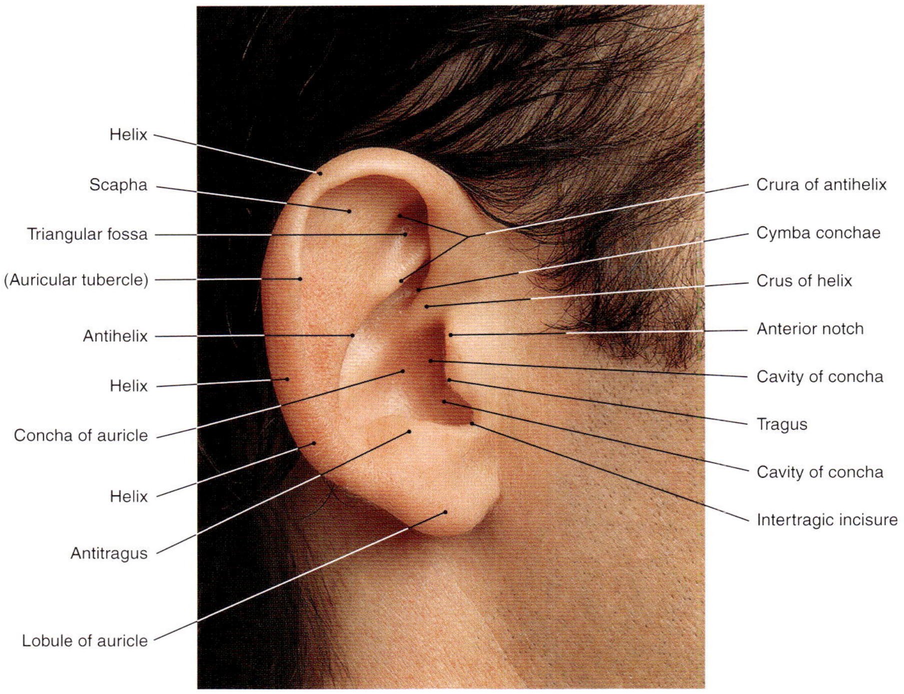

Fig. 1384 Auricle.

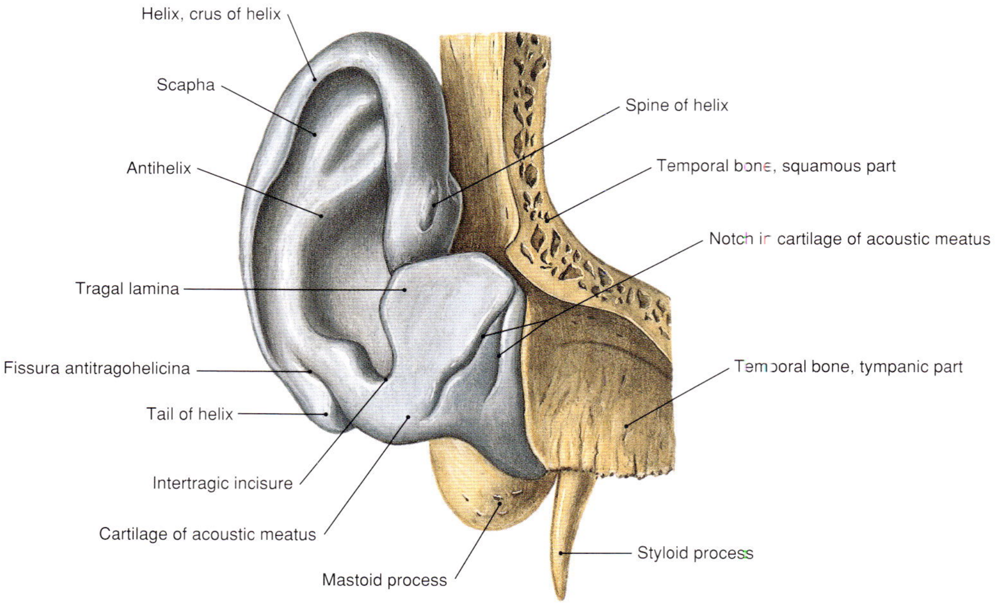

Fig. 1385 Auricular cartilage.

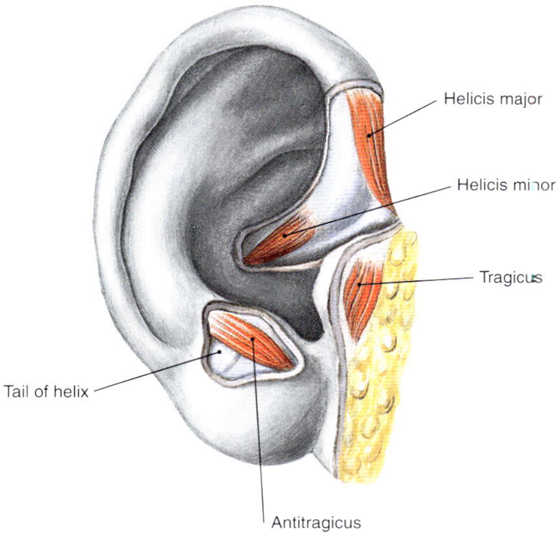

Fig. 1386 Auricular muscles.

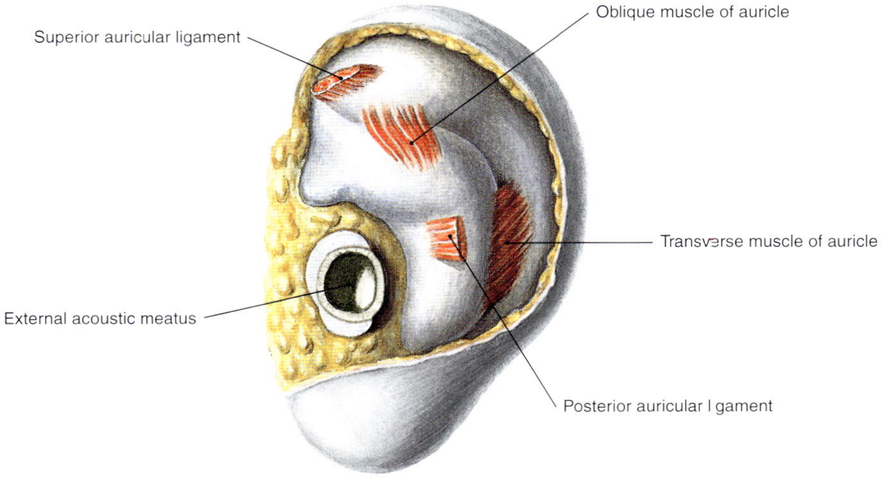

Fig. 1387 Auricular muscles.

External acoustic meatus and tympanic membrane

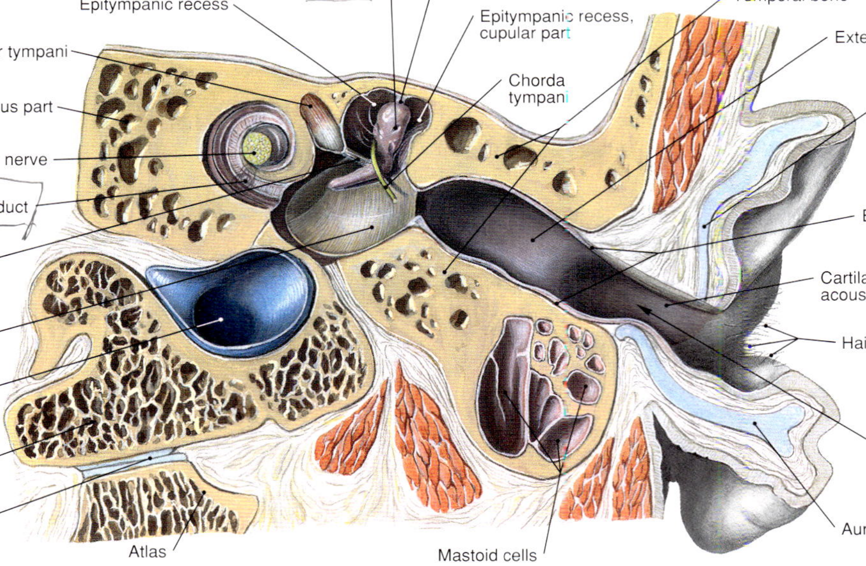

Fig. 1388 External acoustic meatus; tympanic cavity and cochlea; frontal section; posterior view.

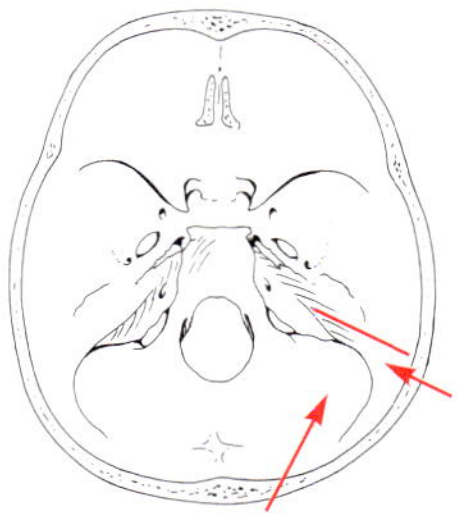

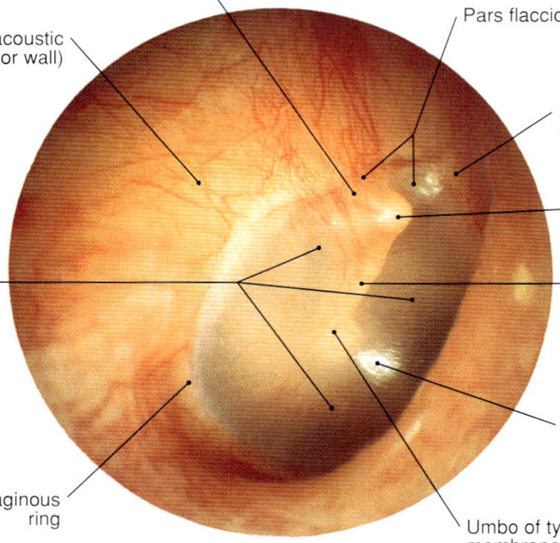

Fig. 1389 Tympanic membrane; otoscopic image; lateral view.

* Clinical term: SHRAPNELL's membrane
** Typically occurring reflection of light

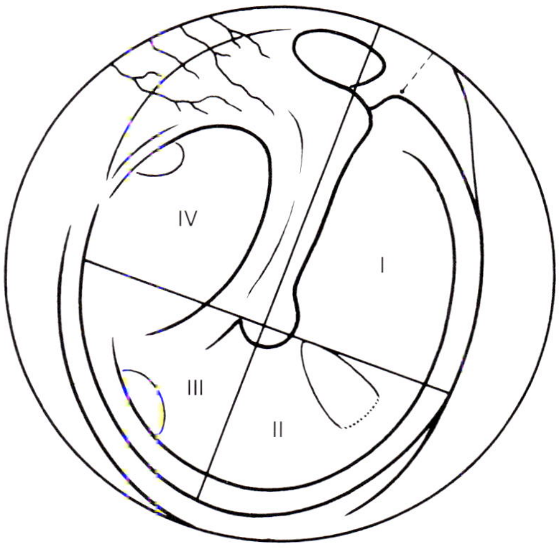

Fig. 1390 Tympanic membrane; quadrant schema; lateral view.

In order to obtain a complete otoscopic overview of the cutaneous surface of the tympanic membrane, the external acoustic meatus must be stretched by pulling the auricle upwards and posteriorly.
To facilitate orientation, the tympanic membrane is usually divided into four quadrants (I–IV).

The longer diameter of the tympanic membrane in the adult is 10–11 mm, the shorter diameter is approx. 9 mm. The light source characteristically produces a triangular reflection of light at the umbo in the region of quadrant II.

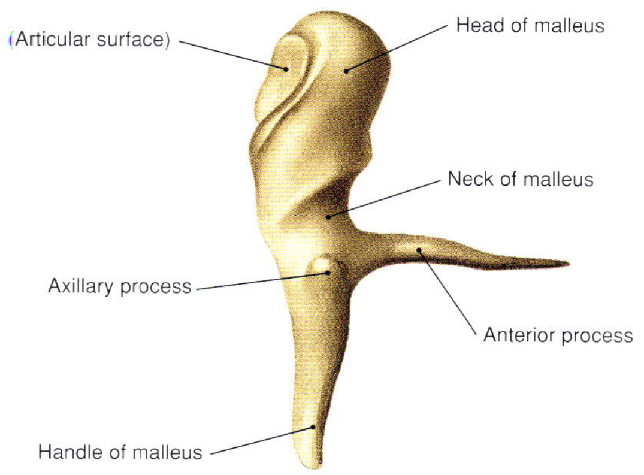

Fig. 1391 Malleus; lateral view.

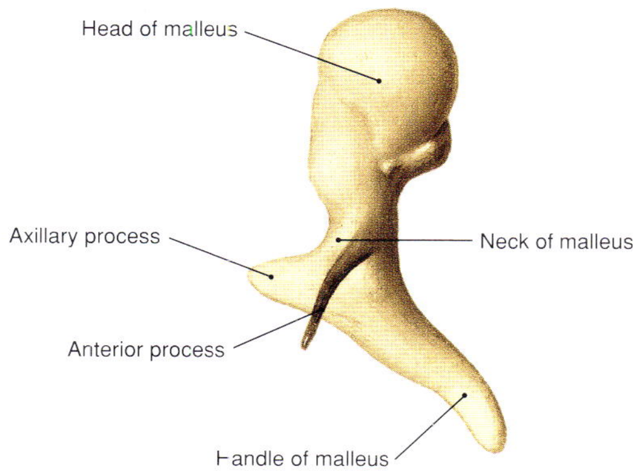

Fig. 1392 Malleus; anterior view.

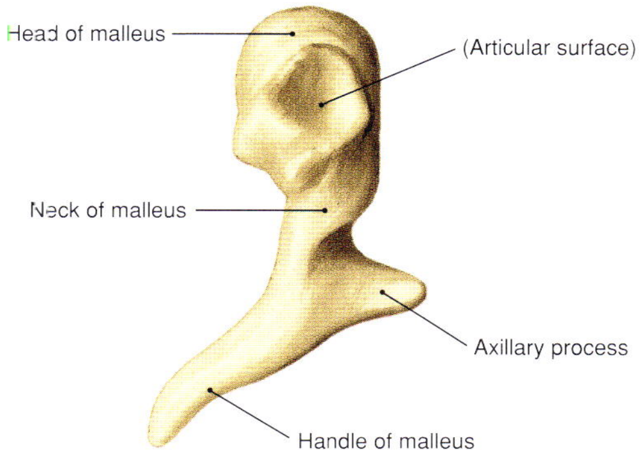

Fig. 1393 Malleus; posterior view.

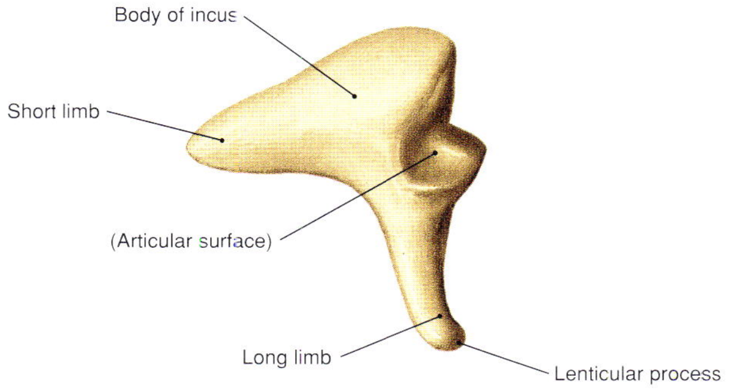

Fig. 1394 Incus; lateral view.

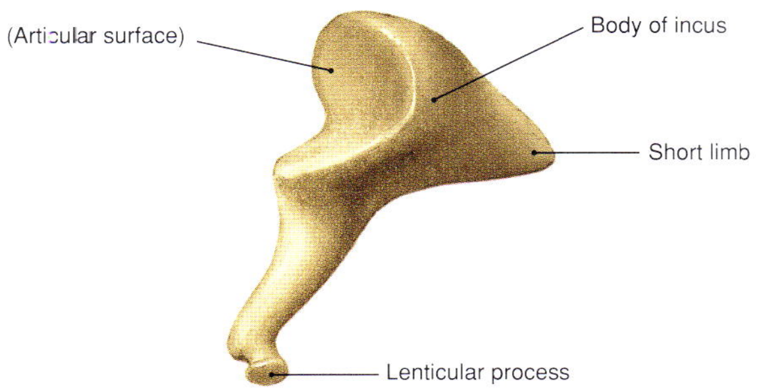

Fig. 1395 Incus; medial view.

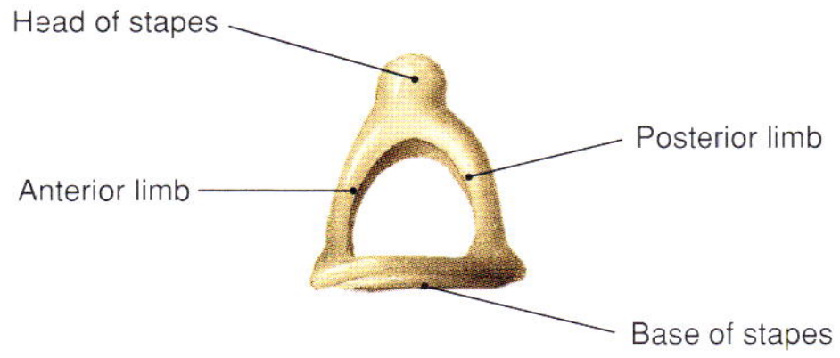

Fig. 1396 Stapes; superior view.

Auditory ossicles

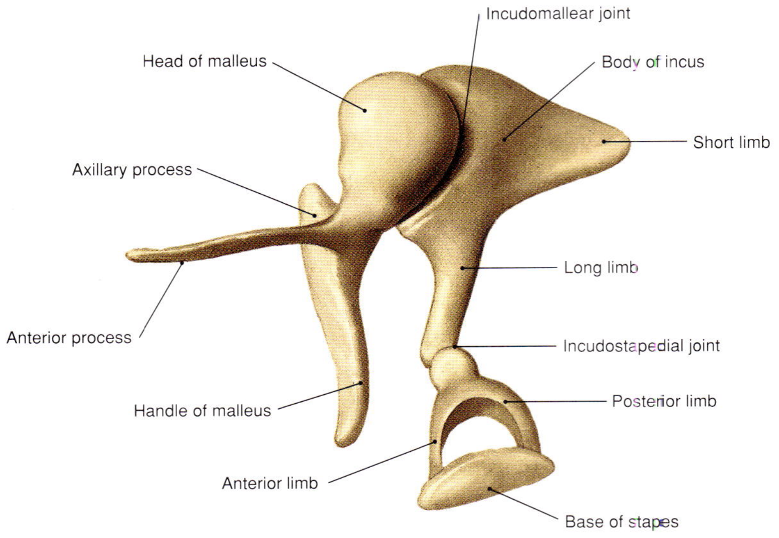

Fig. 1397 Auditory ossicles; superomedial view.

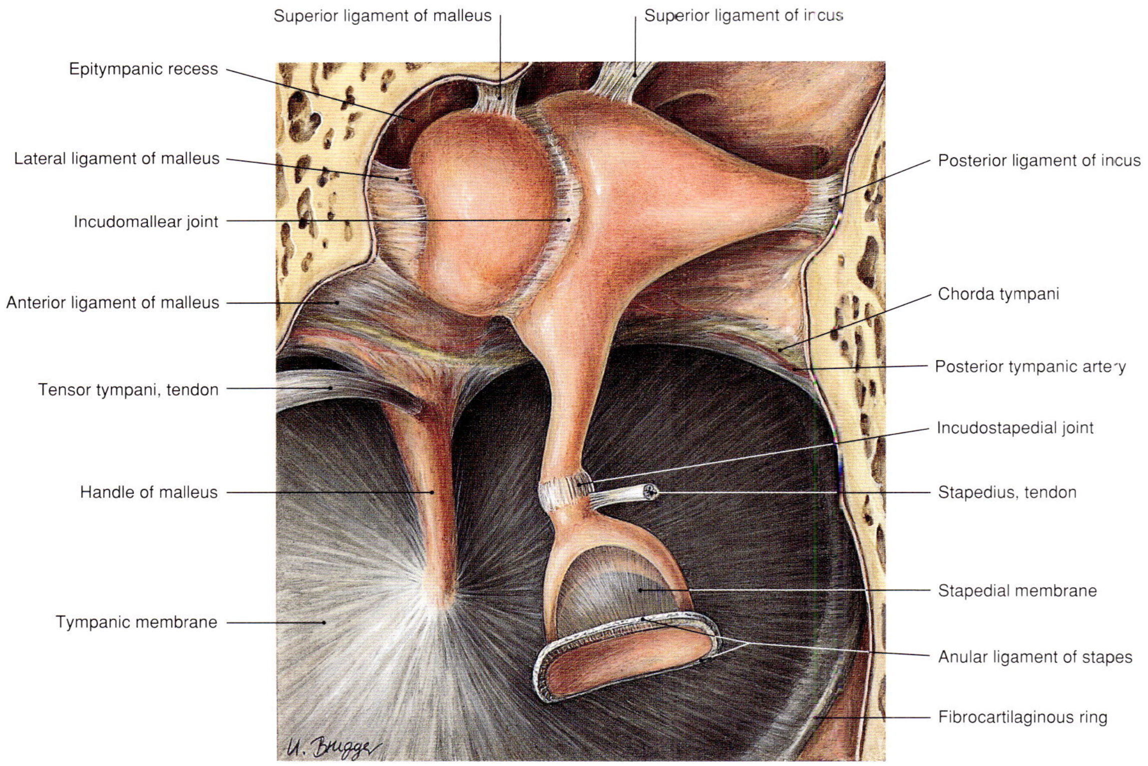

Fig. 1398 Joints and ligaments of the auditory ossicles; covered with mucosa; superomedial view.

Tympanic cavity

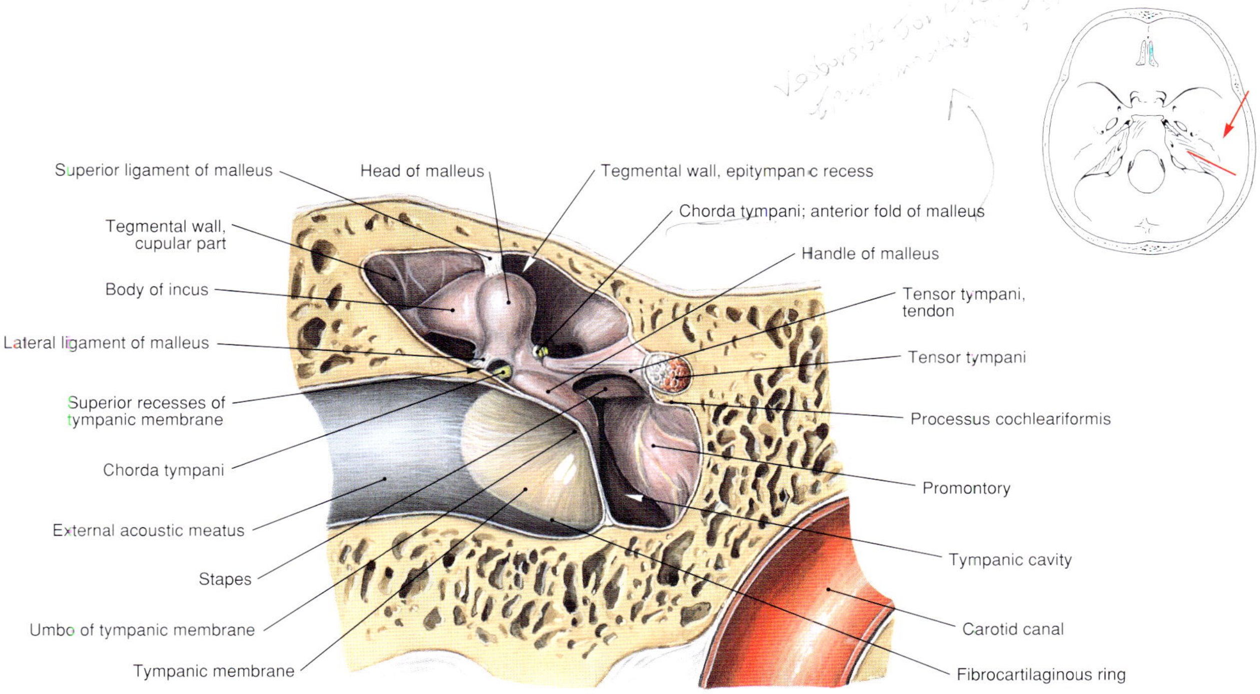

Fig. 1399 Tympanic cavity; frontal section; anterior view.

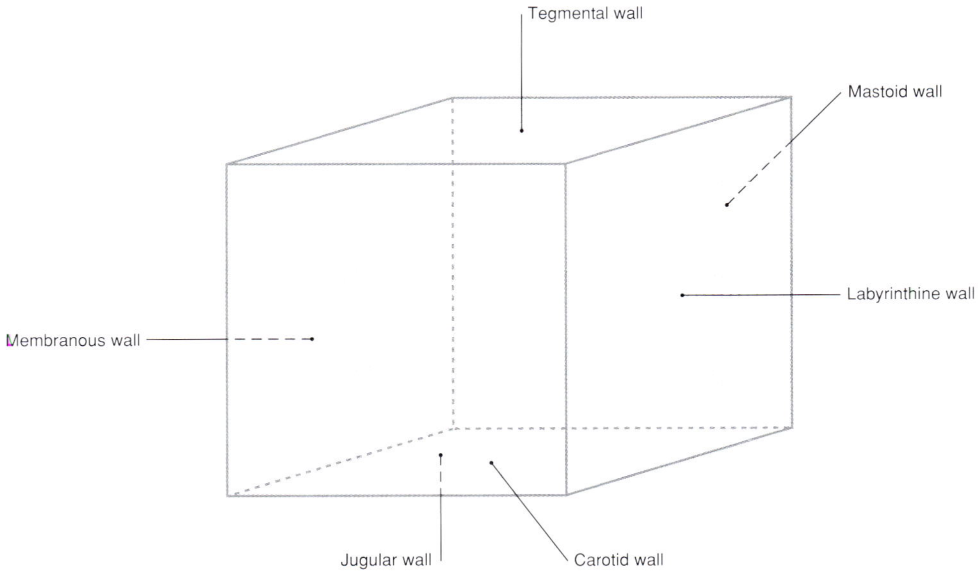

Fig. 1400 Walls of the tympanic cavity; schema for orientation.

Tympanic cavity

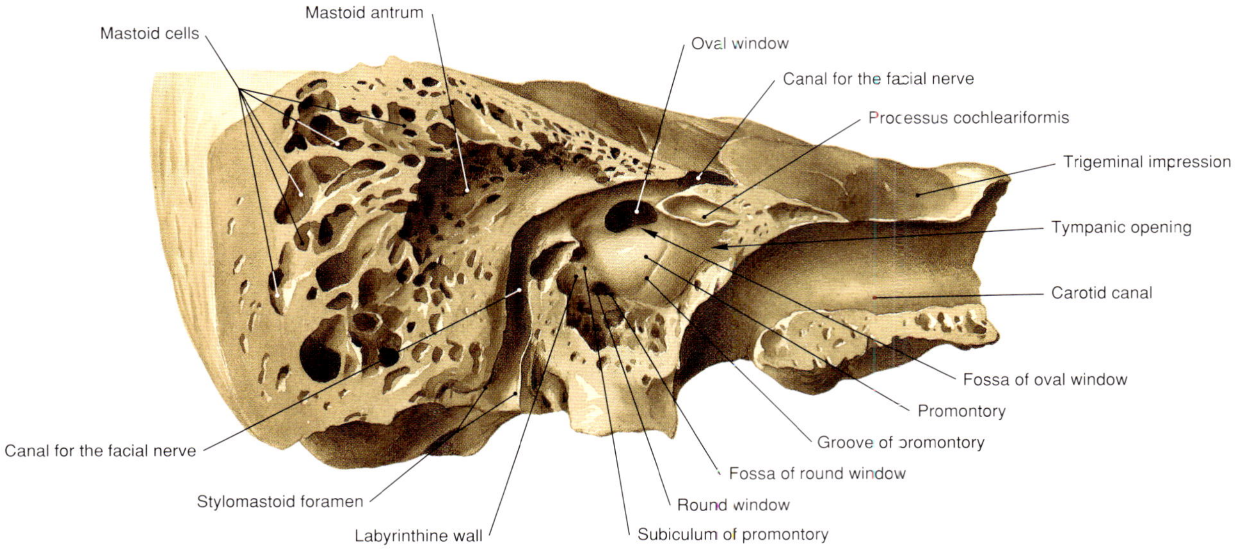

Fig. 1401 Medial wall of the tympanic cavity;
after removal of the lateral wall and the adjacent parts of the anterior and superior wall;
the facial canal and the carotid canal have been opened;
anterolateral view.

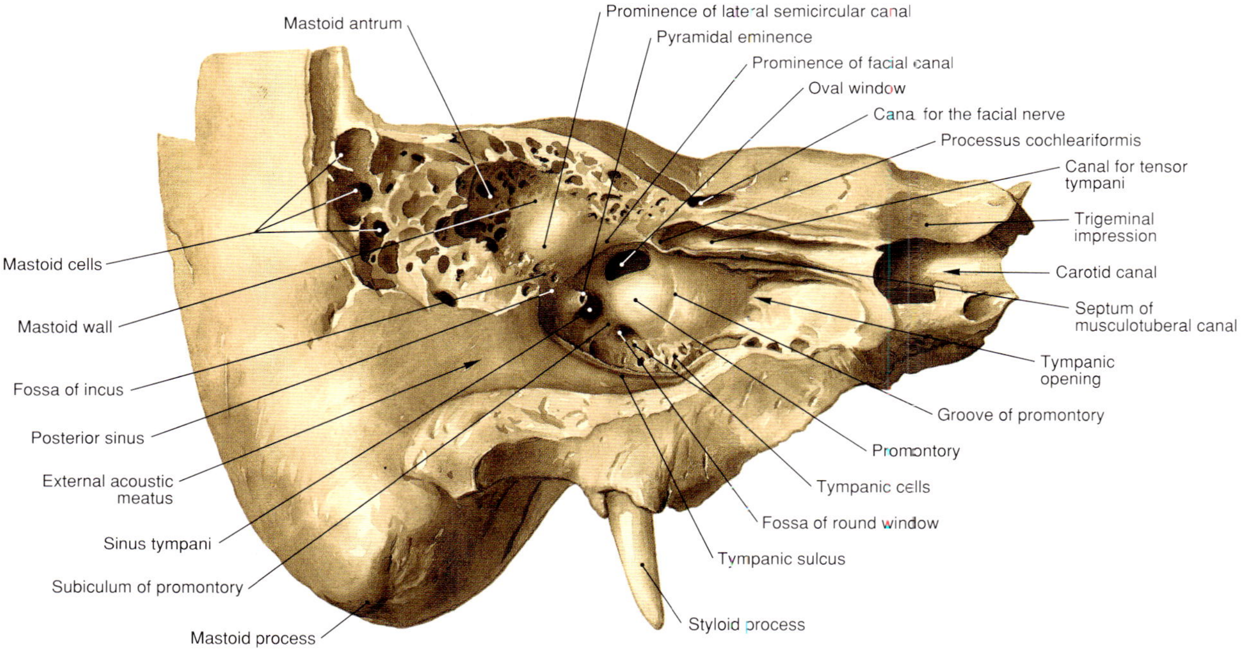

Fig. 1402 Medial wall of the tympanic cavity;
vertical section along the longitudinal axis of the petrous part of the temporal bone;
anterolateral view.

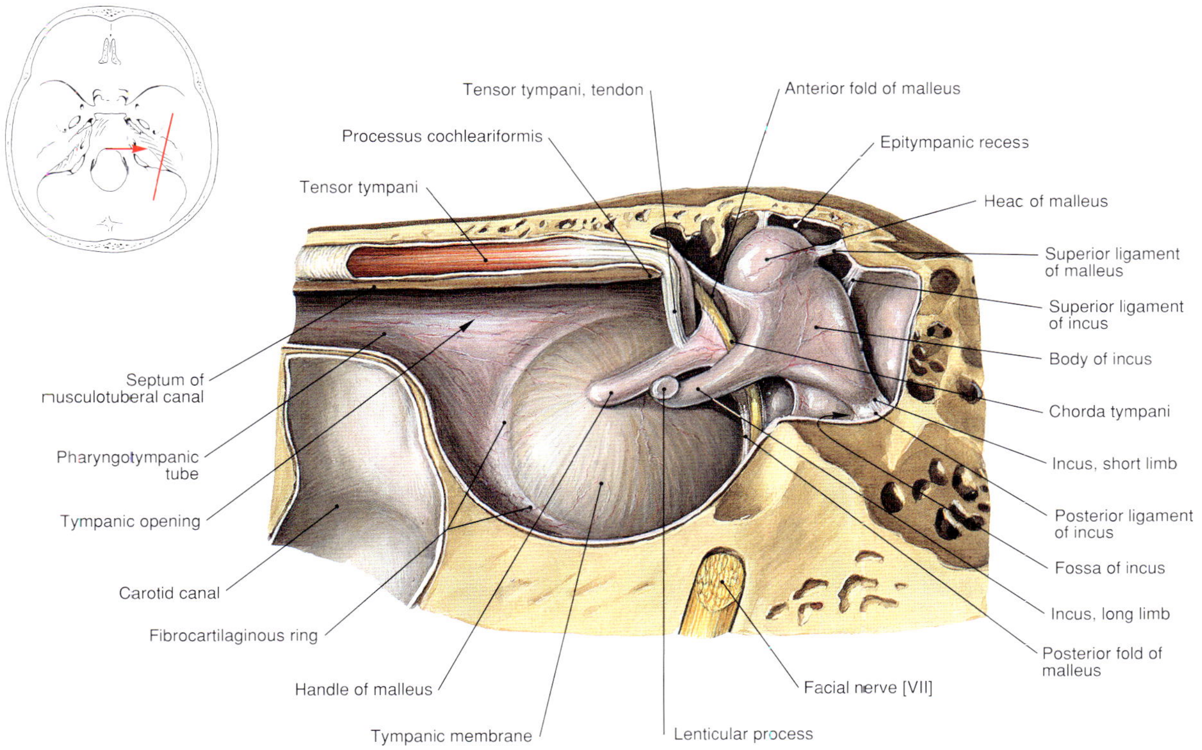

Fig. 1403 Lateral wall of the tympanic cavity; medial view.

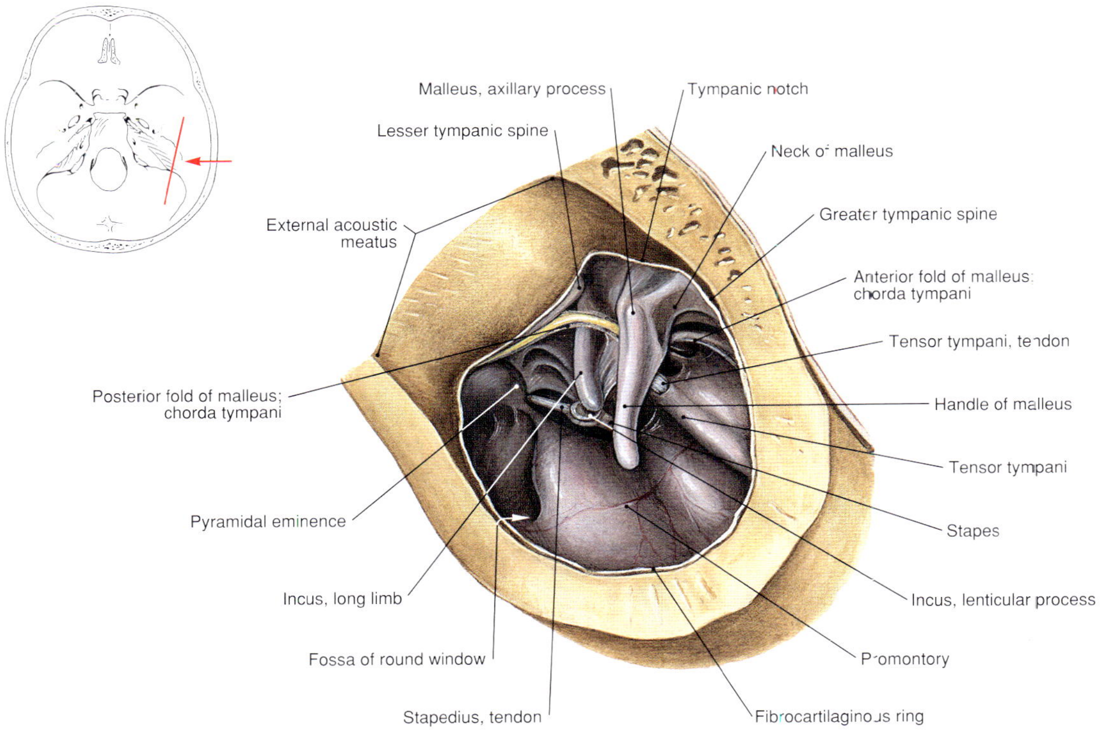

Fig. 1404 Tympanic cavity; after removal of the tympanic membrane; lateral view.

Auditory tube

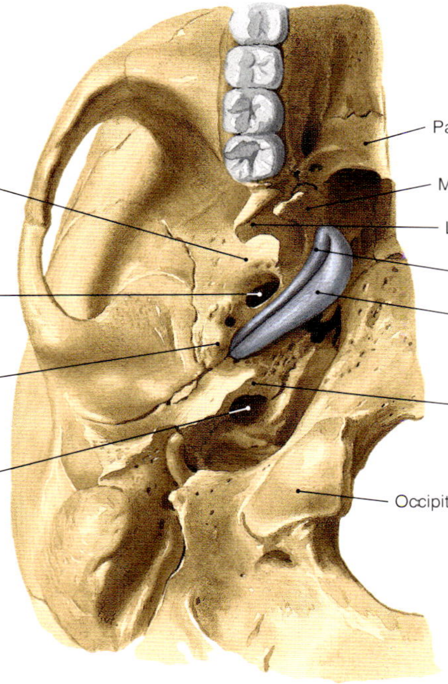

Fig. 1405 Cartilage of the auditory tube; exposed at the base of the skull; inferior view.

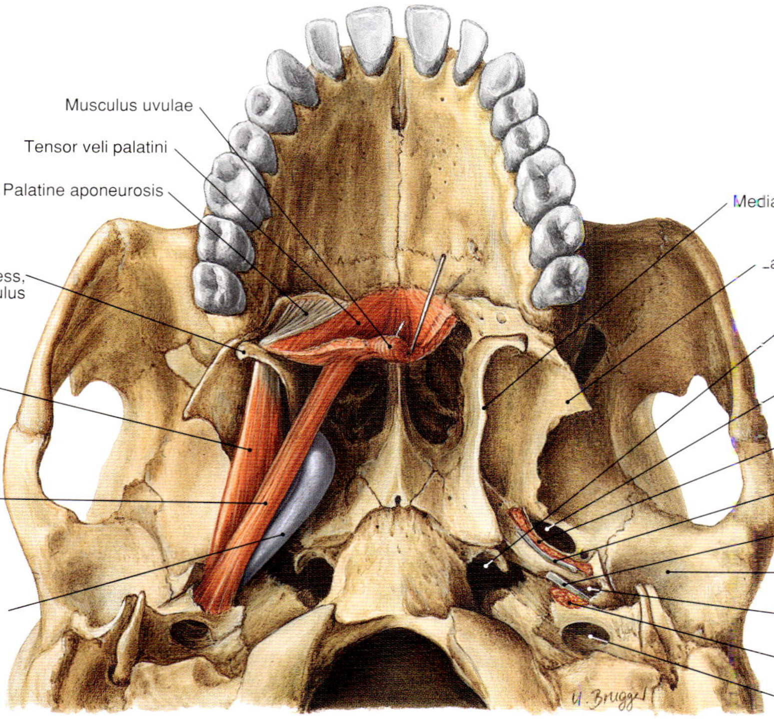

→ 246, 249, T 3

Fig. 1406 Levator and tensor veli palatini muscles and the cartilage of the auditory tube.

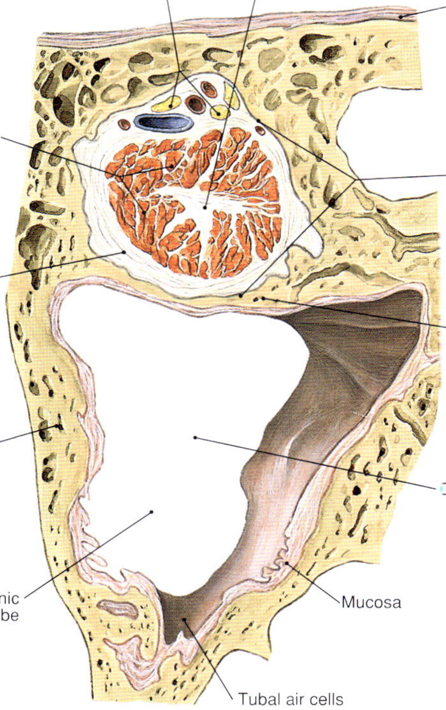

Fig. 1407 Auditory tube;
cross-section at the level of the osseous part;
lateral view.

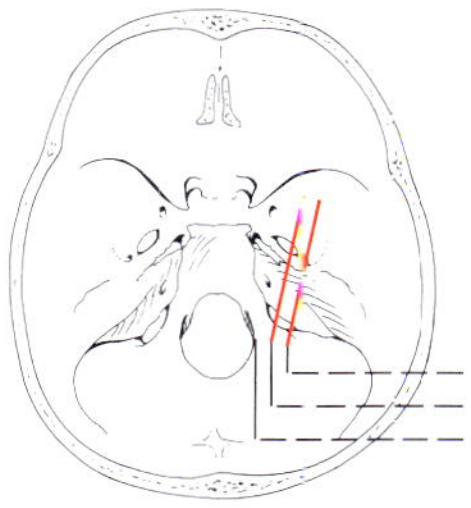

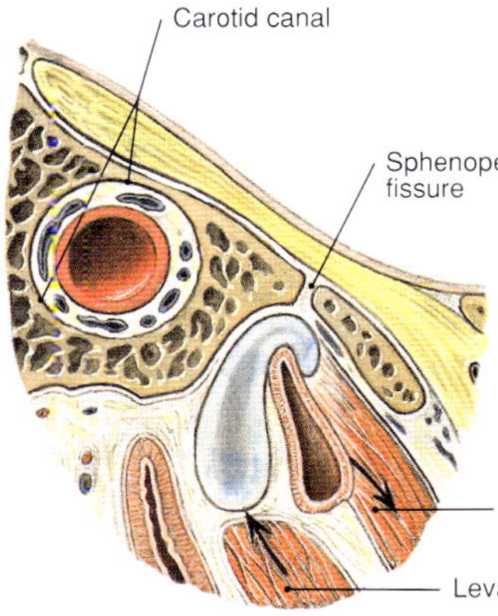

Fig. 1408 Auditory tube;
cross-section at the level of the lateral aspect of the cartilaginous part;
lateral view.

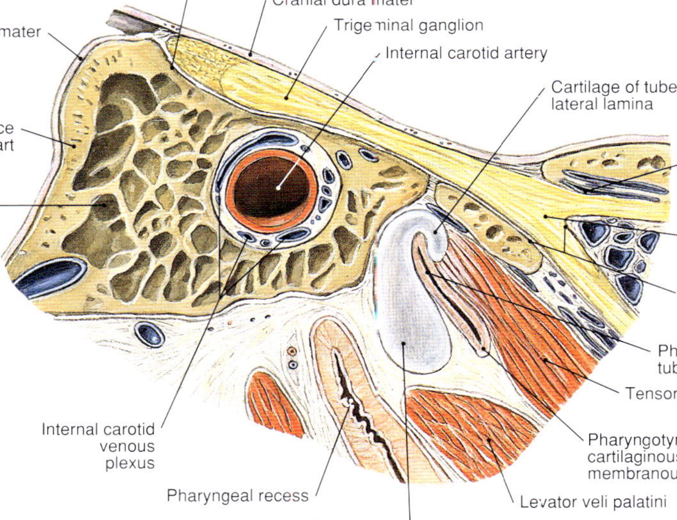

Fig. 1409 Auditory tube;
cross-section at the level of the medial aspect of the cartilaginous part;
lateral view.

Bony labyrinth

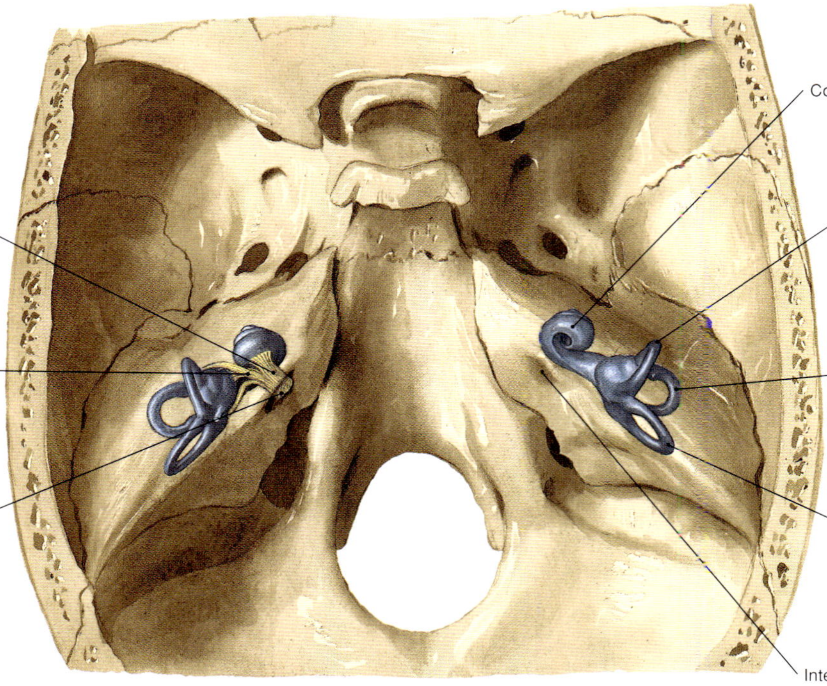

Fig. 1410 Inner ear and vestibulocochlear nerve [VIII]; cast specimen projected onto the petrous part of the temporal bone illustrating its natural position; superior view.

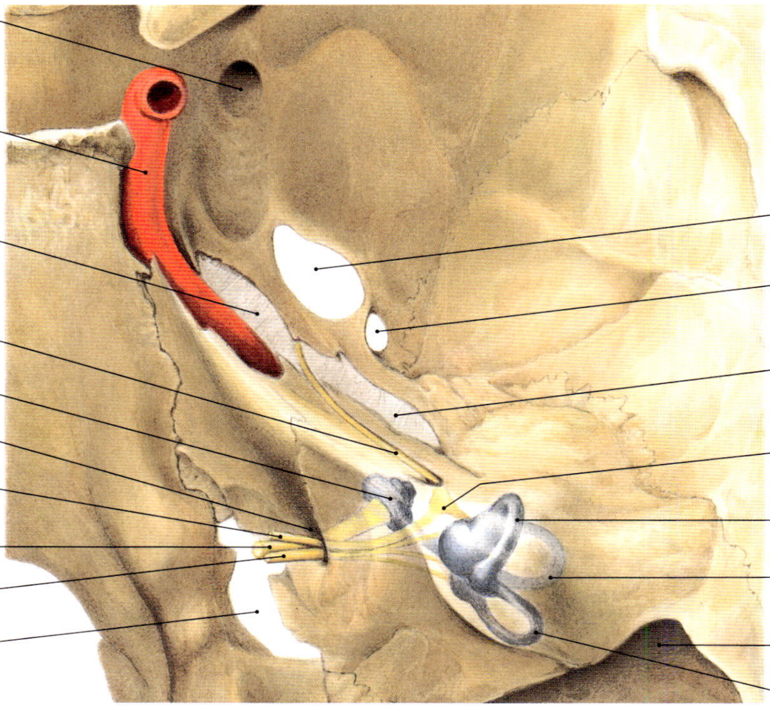

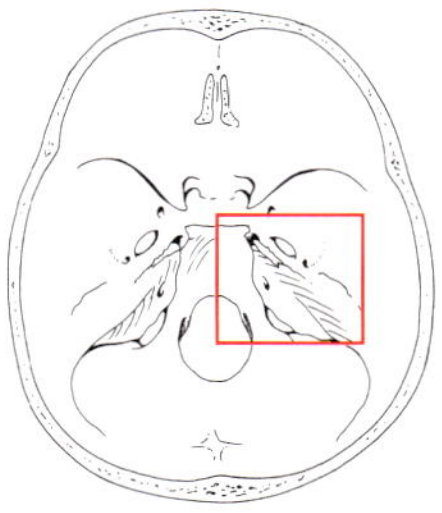

→ 1173

Fig. 1411 Inner ear with the facial nerve and the vestibulocochlear nerve; projected onto the petrous part of the temporal bone; superior view.

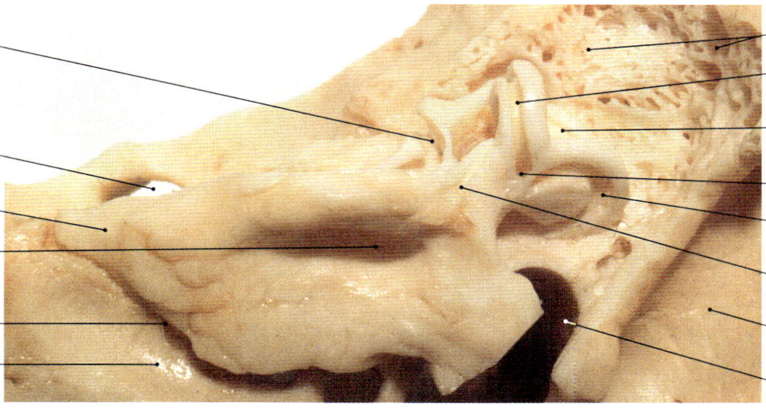

a

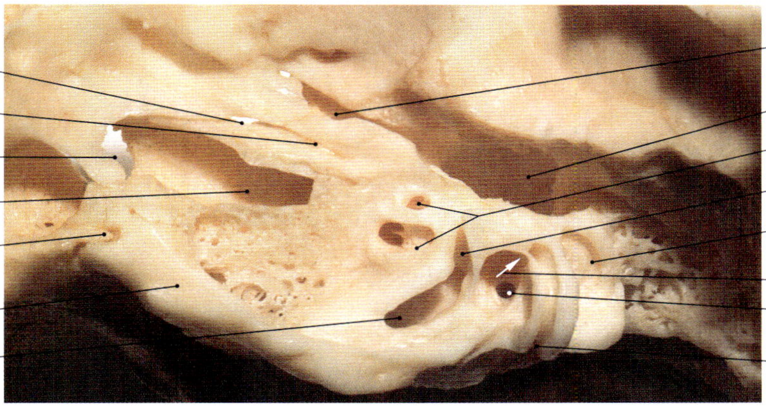

b

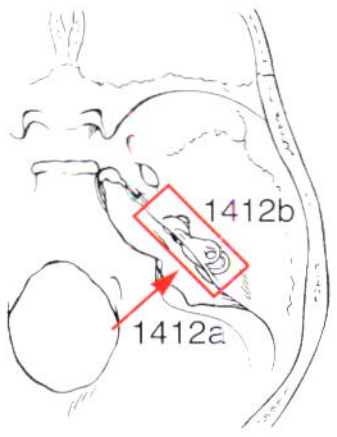

Fig. 1412 a, b Bony labyrinth;
hollowed out of the petrous part of the temporal bone.
a Posterior-superior view
b Superior view

* Opening of the posterior canaliculus

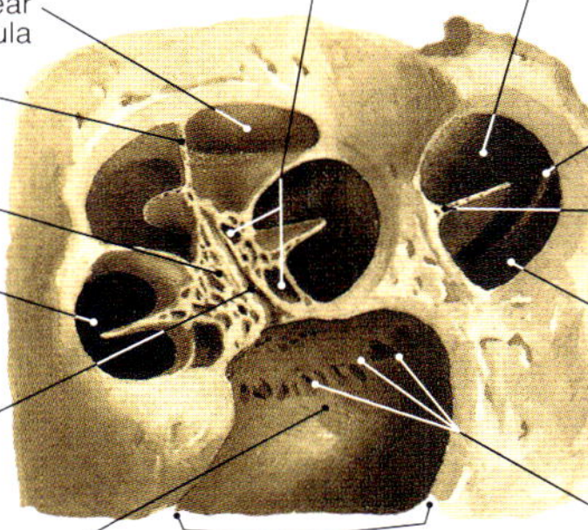

Fig. 1413 Spiral canal of the cochlea; opened along the axis of the modiolus; superior view.

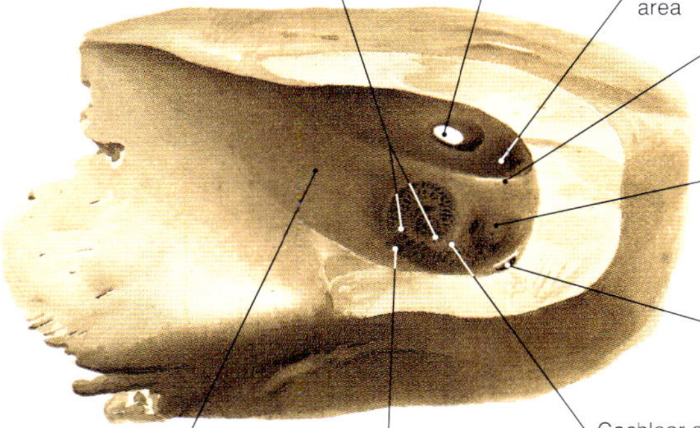

Fig. 1414 Internal acoustic meatus and fundus of the internal acoustic meatus; after partial removal of the posterior wall; medial view.

→ 1173

Bony labyrinth

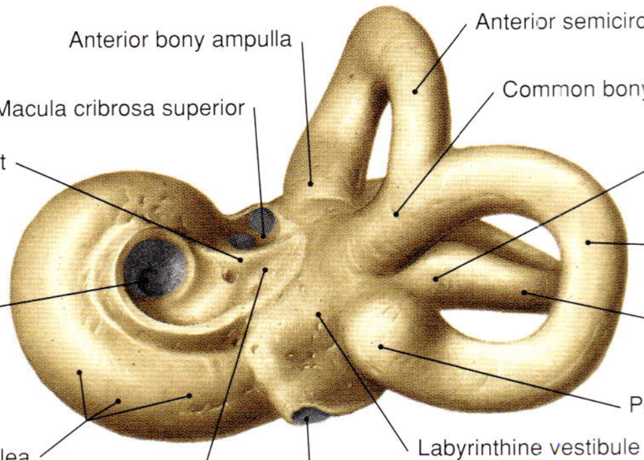

Fig. 1415 Bony labyrinth; the osseous lining of the membranous labyrinth has been hollowed out of the petrous part of the temporal bone; oblique view from posterior.

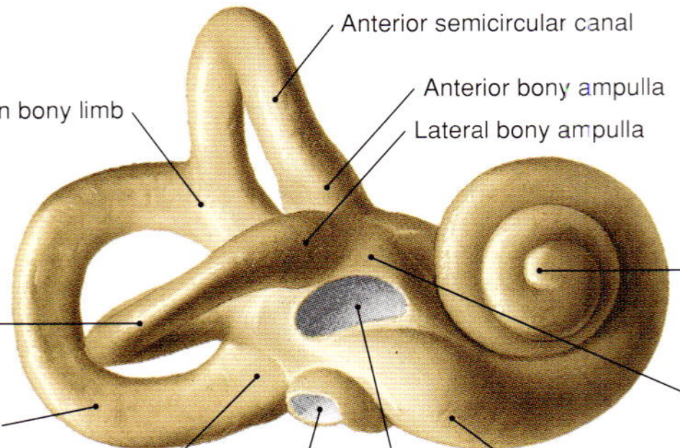

Fig. 1416 Bony labyrinth; the osseous lining of the membranous labyrinth has been hollowed out of the petrous part of the temporal bone; lateral view.

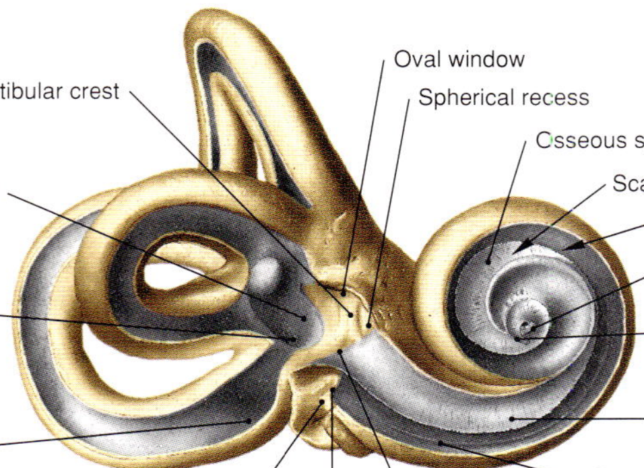

Fig. 1417 Bony labyrinth; cavities have been hollowed out; anterolateral view.

Membranous labyrinth

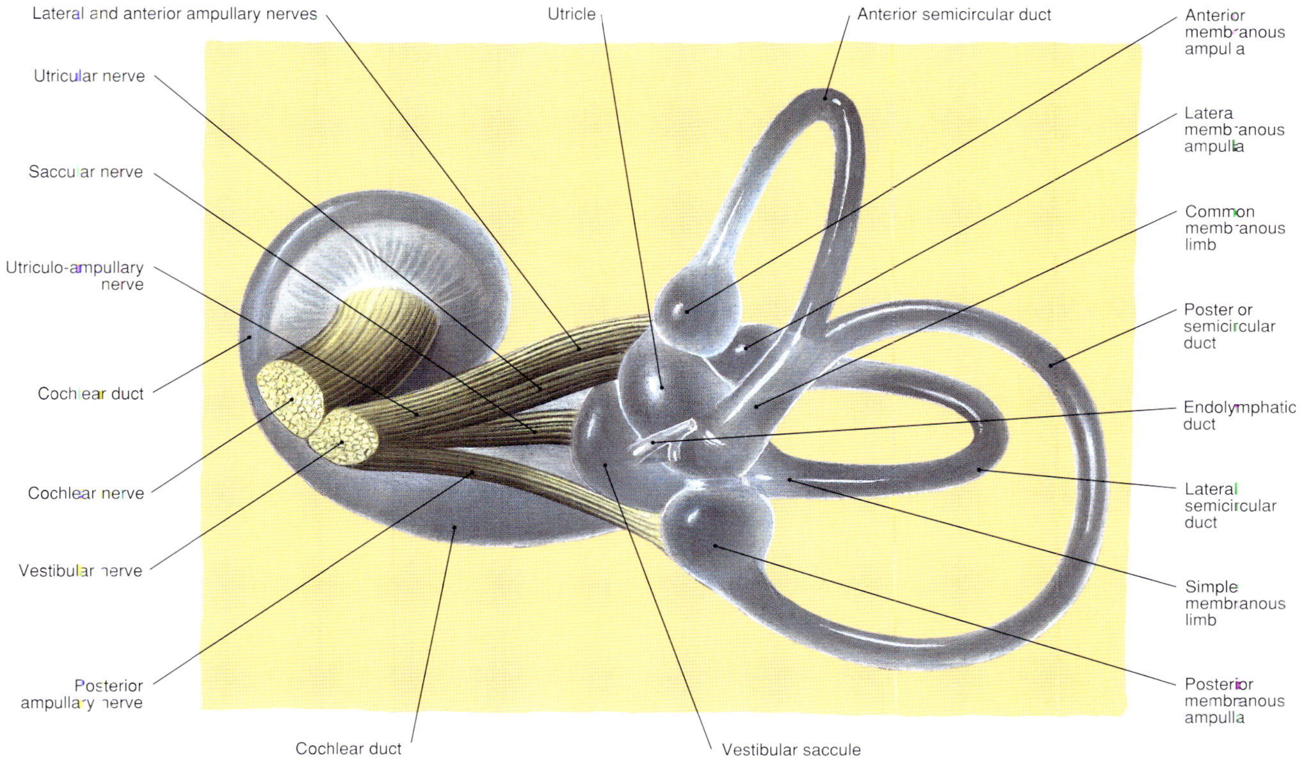

Fig. 1418 Vestibulocochlear nerve and membranous labyrinth; semi-schematic overview; posterior view.

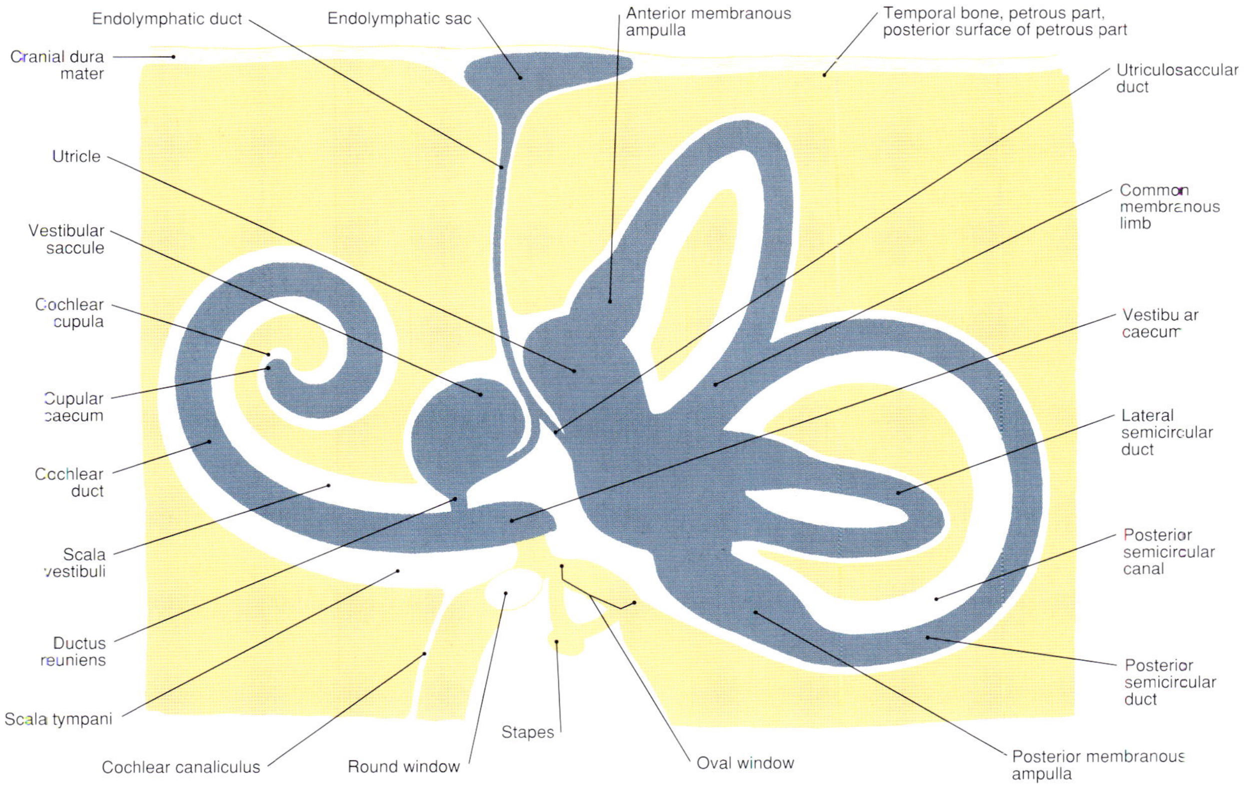

Fig. 1419 Membranous labyrinth; overview.

Cochlea

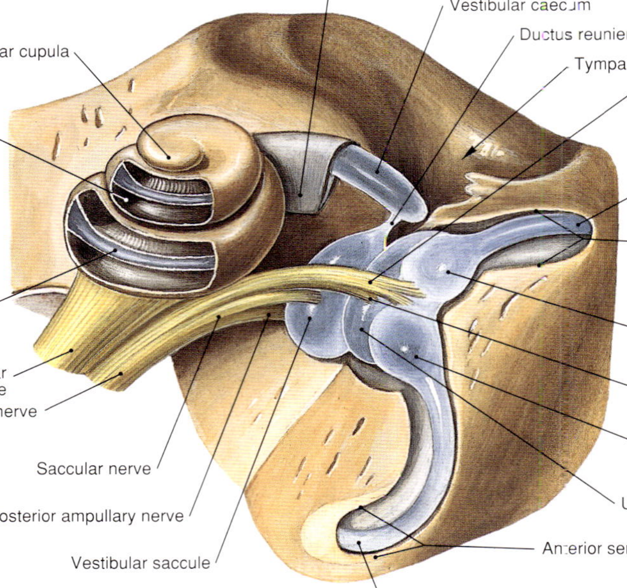

Fig. 1420 Vestibulocochlear nerve and membranous labyrinth; superior view.

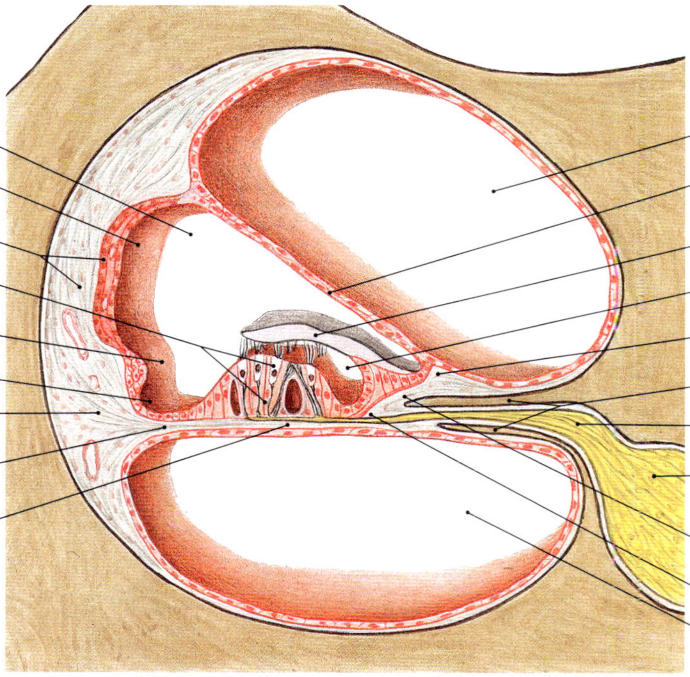

Fig. 1421 Cochlea with the spiral organ.

* Clinical term: organ of CORTI
** Clinical term: REISSNER's membrane

Equilibrium organ, structure

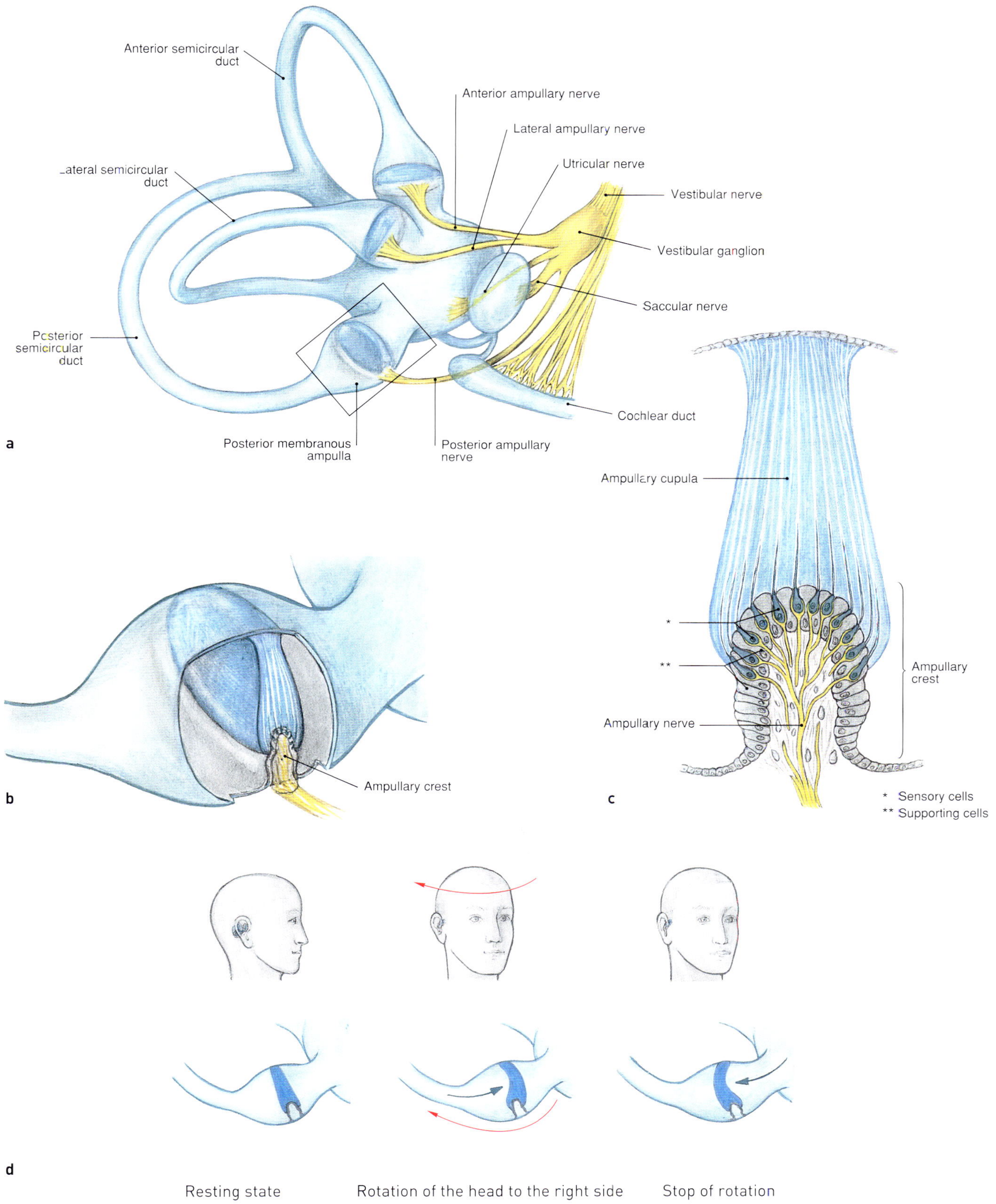

Fig. 1422 a–d Equilibrium organ.
a Anterior view
b Higher magnification of the area indicated in a: the anterior part of the posterior membranous ampulla has been opened.
c Cross-section through the ampullary crest
d Function of the cupula of the lateral semicircular duct, during rotation of the head

Hearing and equilibrium

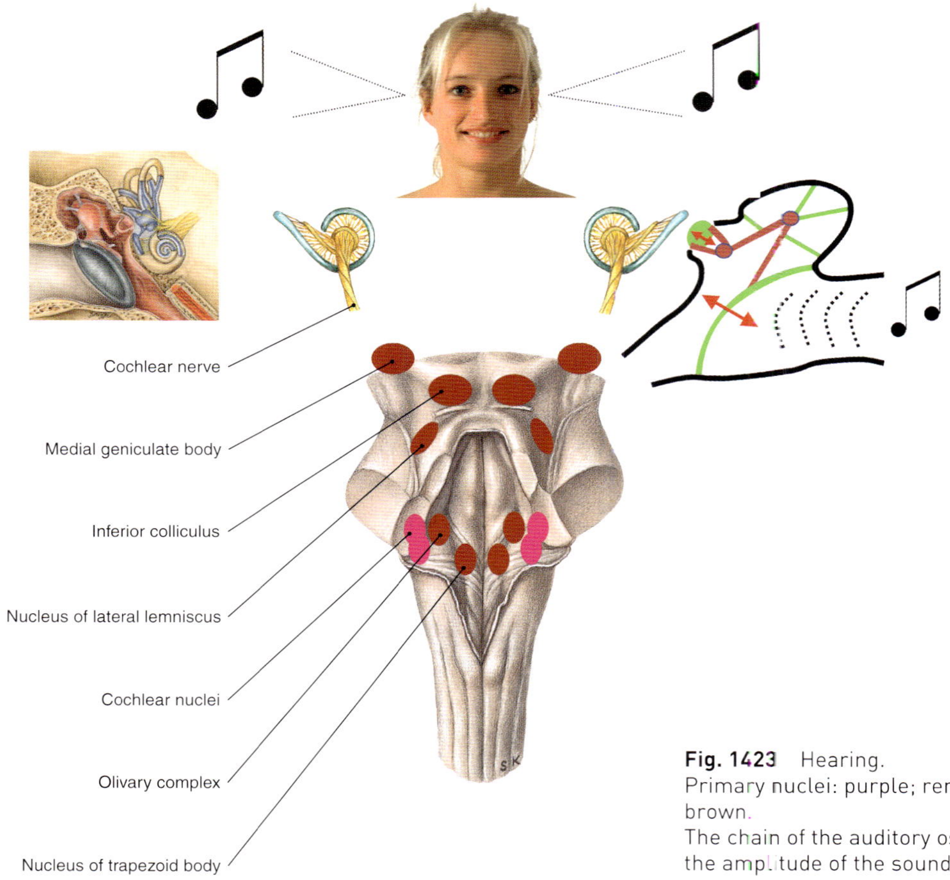

Fig. 1423 Hearing.
Primary nuclei: purple; remaining nuclei: brown.
The chain of the auditory ossicles amplifies the amplitude of the sound waves physically.

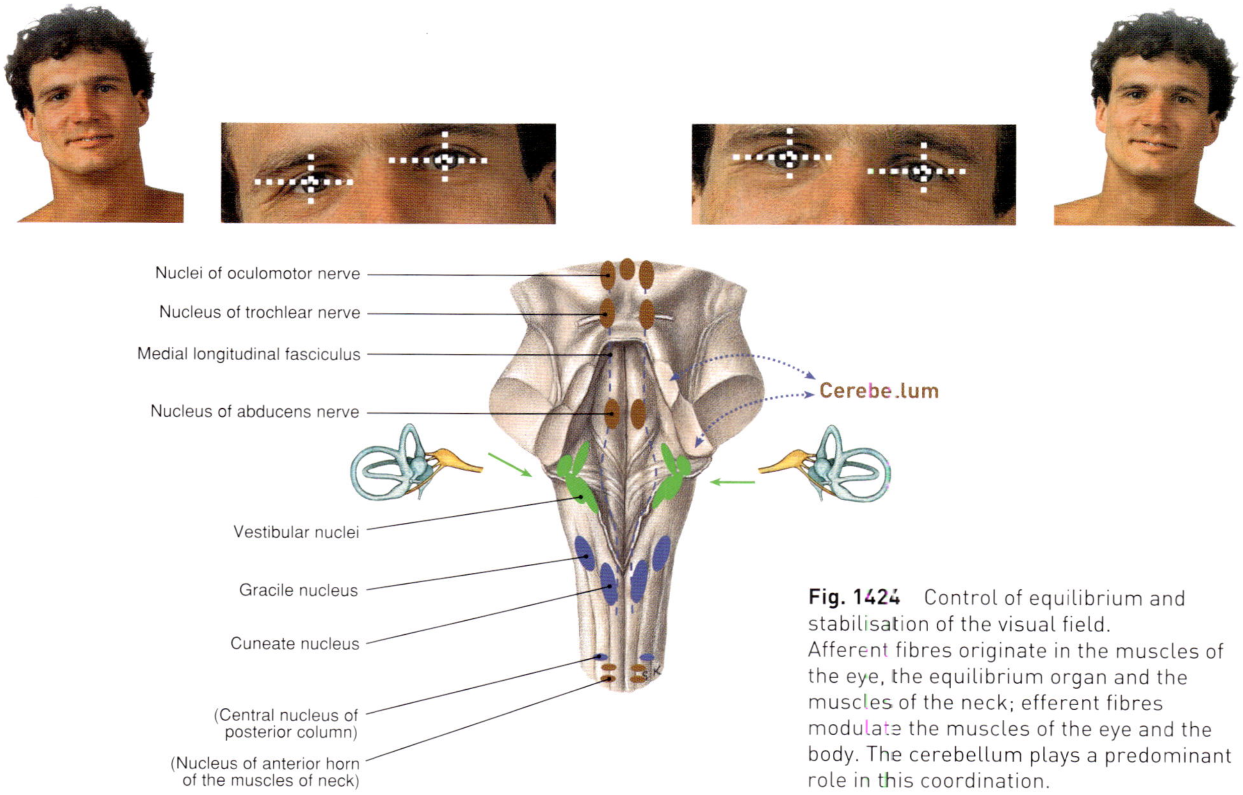

Fig. 1424 Control of equilibrium and stabilisation of the visual field.
Afferent fibres originate in the muscles of the eye, the equilibrium organ and the muscles of the neck; efferent fibres modulate the muscles of the eye and the body. The cerebellum plays a predominant role in this coordination.

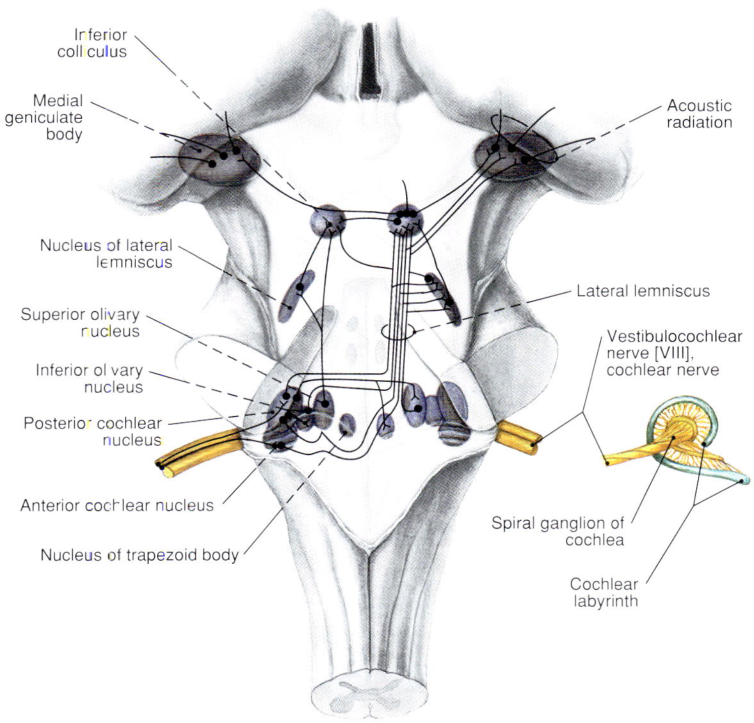

Fig. 1425 Auditory pathway; overview.

Auditory pathway

1. neuron: Bipolar cells in the spiral cochlear ganglion. After exiting the small apertures of the foraminous spiral tract within the internal acoustic meatus, the fibres form the cochlear nerve and unite with the vestibular nerve at the floor of the internal acoustic meatus to form the vestibulocochlear nerve [VIII]. Fibres from the basal cochlear parts traverse to the posterior cochlear nucleus and those from the apical parts terminate in the anterior cochlear nucleus.
2. neuron: Multi-polar ganglion cells of the cochlear nuclei. The fibres from the anterior cochlear nucleus pass mainly within the trapezoid body to the opposite side and form the lateral lemnicus, which provides a connection to the inferior colliculus. A few fibres join the lateral lemniscus of the same side. The axons of the posterior cochlear nucleus cross superficially to the rhomboid fossa and enter the lateral lemniscus of the opposite side.
3. or 4. neuron: From the inferior colliculus connections are made with the medial geniculate body.
4. or 5. neuron: The acoustic radiation connects the medial geniculate body to HESCHL's transverse gyrus and with WERNICKE's centre in the temporal lobe.

Equilibrium pathway

1. neuron: Bipolar cells in the vestibular ganglion. Their neurites pass the inferior and superior vestibular areas to form the vestibular nerve at the floor of the internal acoustic meatus, which together with the cochlear nerve then forms the vestibulocochlear nerve [VIII]. These fibres terminate at the vestibular nuclei in the lateral angle of the floor of the rhomboid fossa.
2. and subsequent neurons: Fibres originating in the lateral vestibular nucleus (DEITERS' nucleus) traverse within the lateral vestibulospinal tract to the anterior column of the spinal cord.
Fibres originating in the superior vestibular nucleus (nucleus of BECHTEREW), the medial vestibular nucleus (SCHWALBE's nucleus) as well as the inferior vestibular nucleus (ROLLER's nucleus) traverse to the cerebellum and connect to the motor nuclei of the cranial nerves III, IV and VI, mostly via the medial longitudinal fasciculus.
The medial vestibular nucleus and the inferior vestibular nucleus send fibres along the medial vestibulospinal tract to the anterior column of the spinal cord.

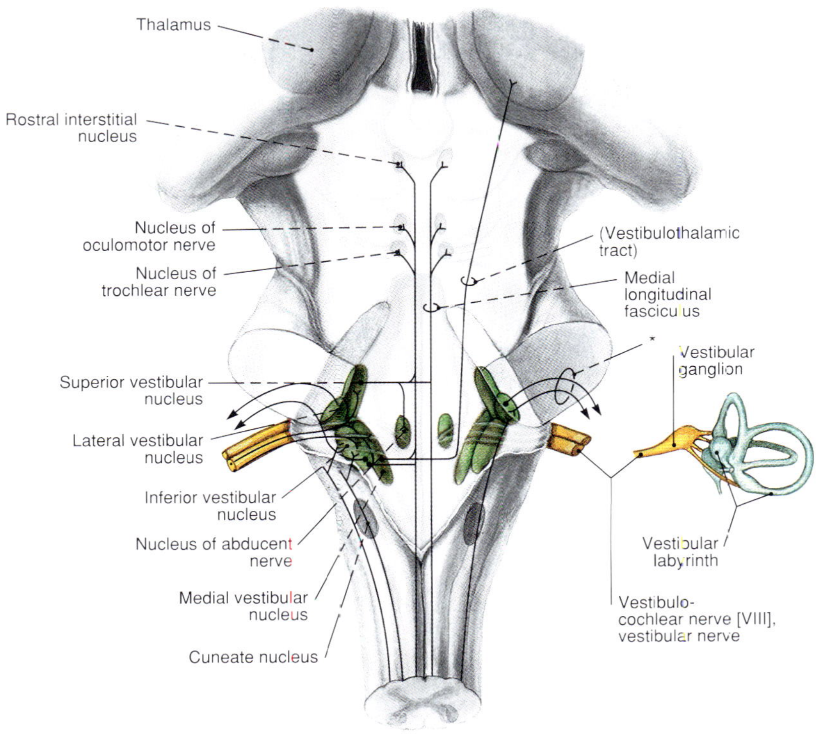

Fig. 1426 Equilibrium pathway; overview.

* Connections to the cerebellum

Nerves in the petrous part of the temporal bone

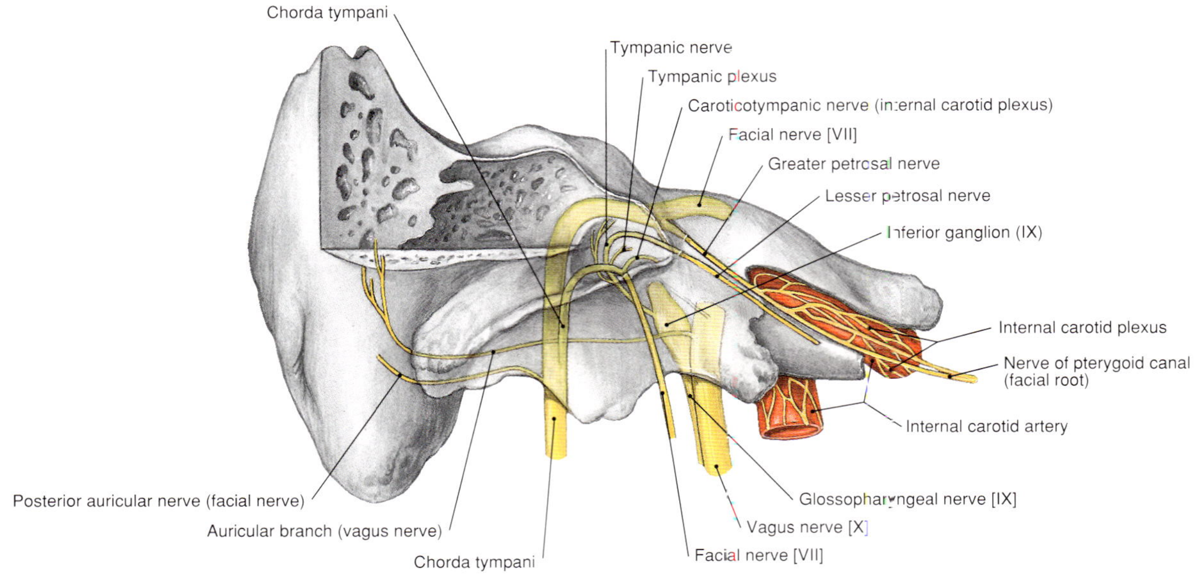

→ 1181

Fig. 1427 Facial nerve;
glossopharyngeal nerve;
and vagus nerve [X];
the petrous part of the temporal bone has been partly sectioned;
the nerves are illustrated translucently;
anterior view.

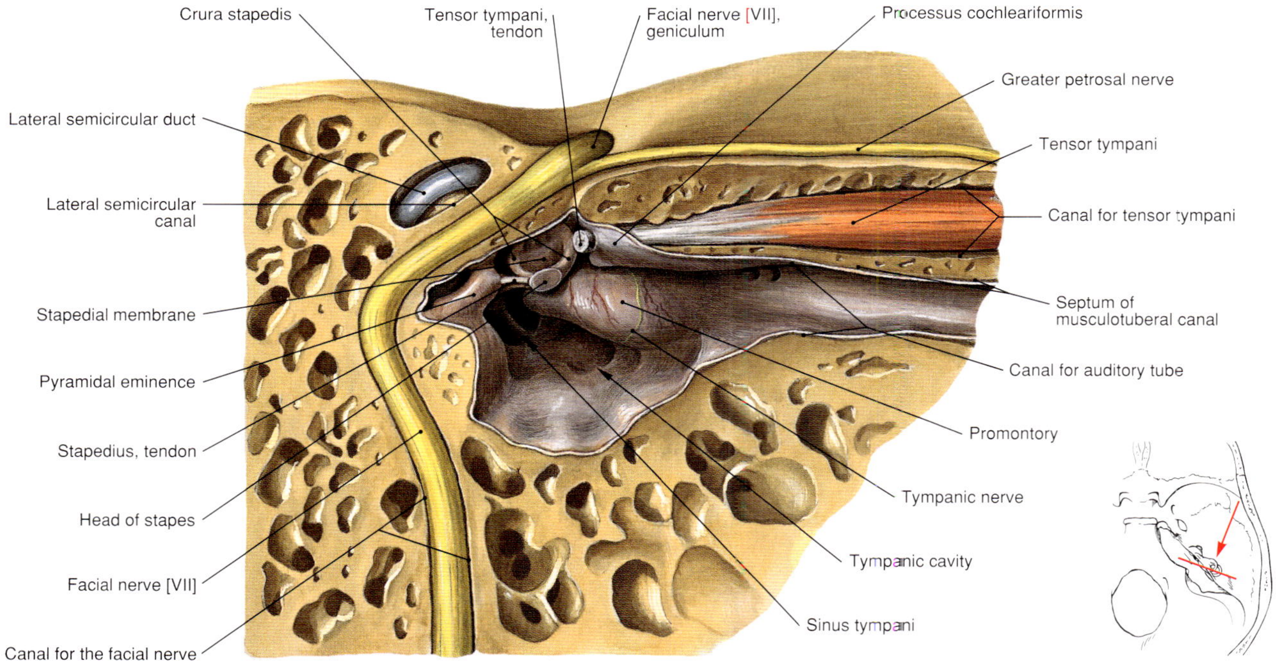

Fig. 1428 Facial nerve and tympanic cavity;
vertical section along the longitudinal axis of the
petrous part of the temporal bone;
the facial canal has been opened;
anterior view.

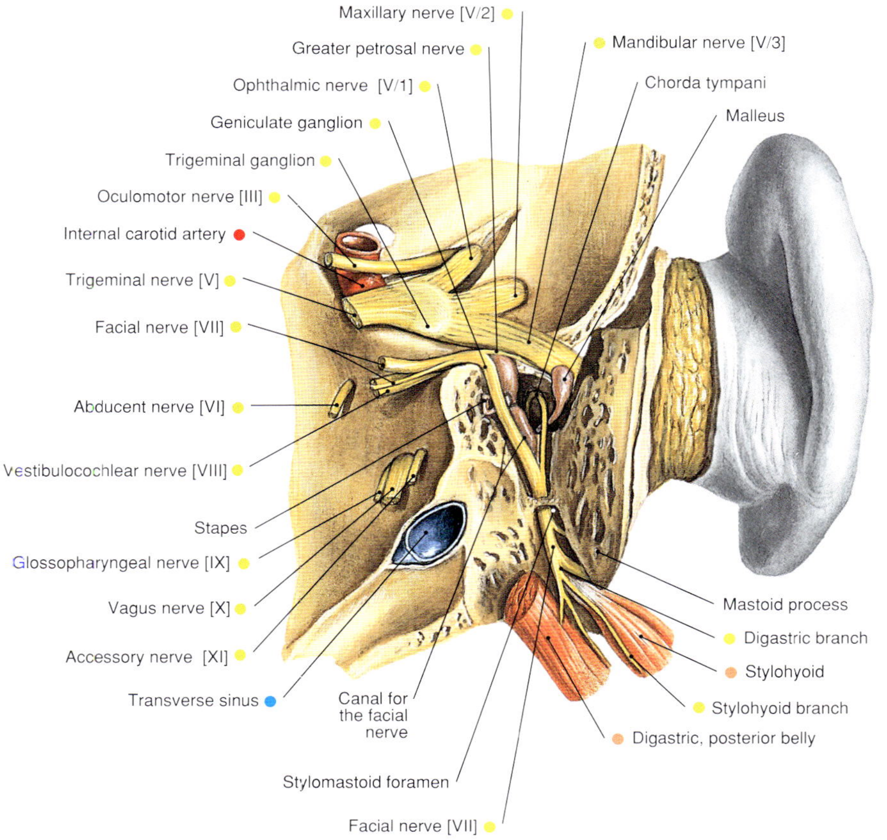

Fig. 1429 Facial nerve within the petrous part of the temporal bone; the petrous part of the temporal bone as well as the facial canal and the tympanic cavity have been partially opened; posterior view.

→ 1181

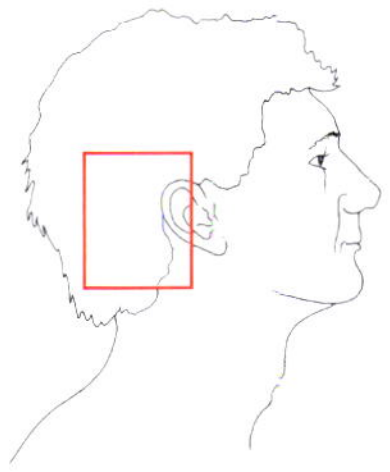

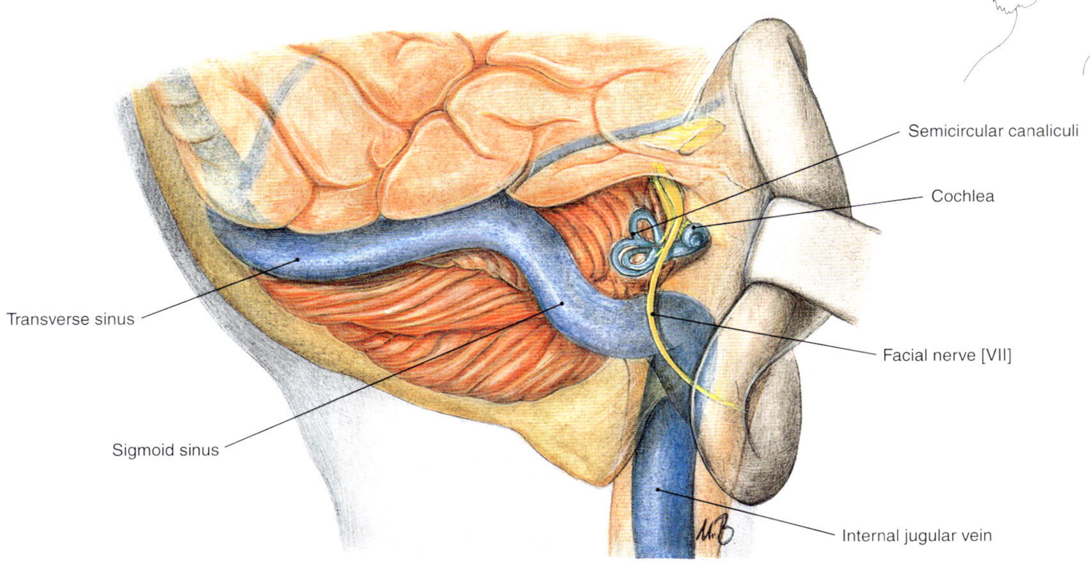

Fig. 1430 Lateral projection of the inner ear.

Petrous part of the temporal bone, imaging

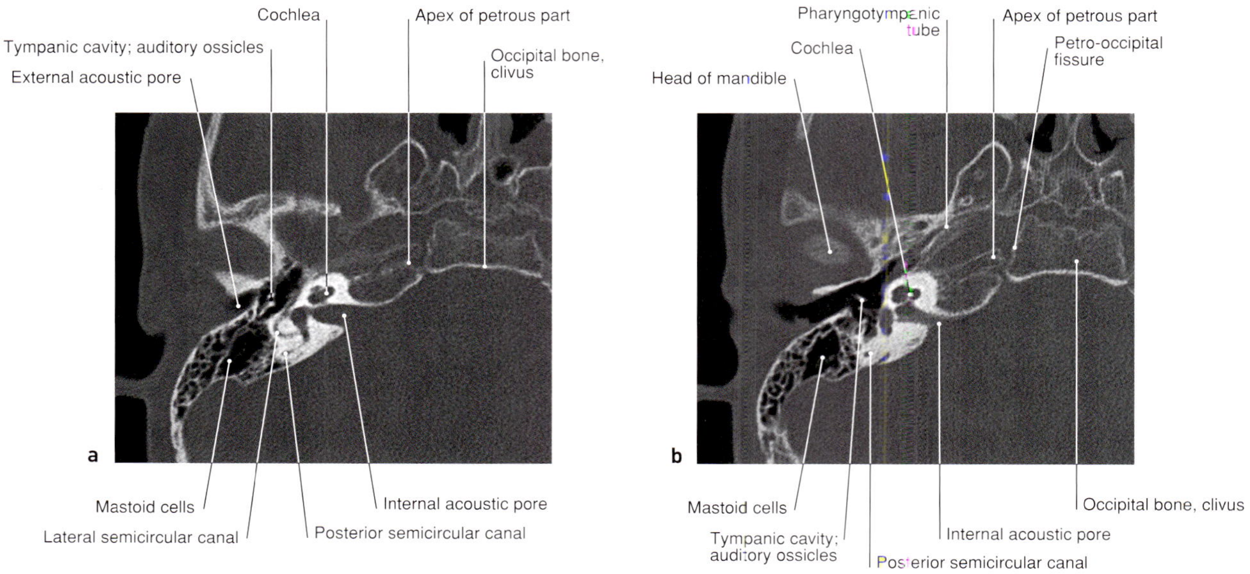

Fig. 1431 a, b Petrous part of the temporal bone,;
high-resolution computed tomographic horizontal sections (HRCT);
inferior view.
a Through the lateral semicircular canal
b Inferior to the lateral semicircular canal

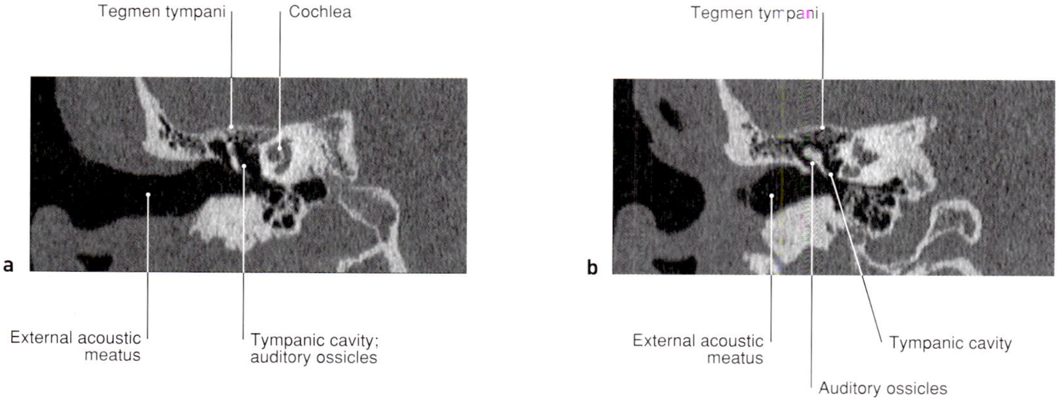

Fig. 1432 a, b Ear;
high-resolution computed tomographic frontal sections (HRCT);
anterior view.
a Through the base of the cochlea
b Through the external acoustic meatus

Index

The numbers refer to the page numbers.
The numbers with "T" refer to the numbers of the tables in the separate booklet.

B

E

F

T

U

X

Y

Z

Tables of Muscles, Joints and Nerves

Contents

Tables of Muscles, Joints and Nerves

1 Facial muscles (Fig. 119-122, 247, 253, 1332)

Only parts of the facial muscles actually originate from bony structures. All of them insert to the skin.

a Forehead, top of the head, temple

Occipitofrontalis
(Together, the occipitofrontalis and the temporoparietalis are referred to as epicranius:)
Facial nerve [VII]

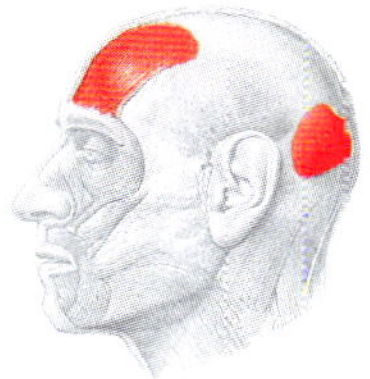

O: Frontal belly: Skin of the eyebrow and the Glabella, forms a common muscular layer with the procerus, corrugator supercilii, depressor supercilii and orbicularis oculi
Occipital belly: Highest nuchal line

I: Epicranial aponeurosis

F: Moves the scalp, creates oblique wrinkle at the forehead

Temporoparietalis
Facial nerve

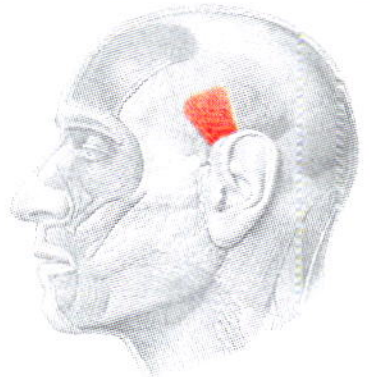

O: Temporal skin, temporal fascia

I: Epicranial aponeurosis

F: Moves the scalp

b Auricle

Auricularis anterior
Facial nerve [VII]

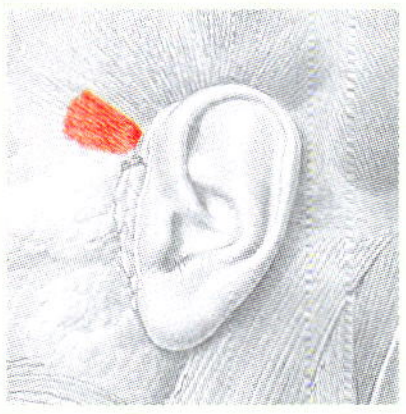

O: Temporal fascia

I: Spine of helix

F: Moves the auricle forwards and upwards

Auricularis superior
Facial nerve [VII]

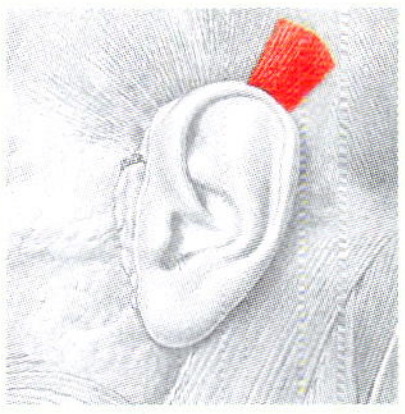

O: Epicranial aponeurosis

I: Dorsocranial part of the auricular root

F: Moves the auricle backwards and upwards

Auricularis posterior
Facial nerve [VII]

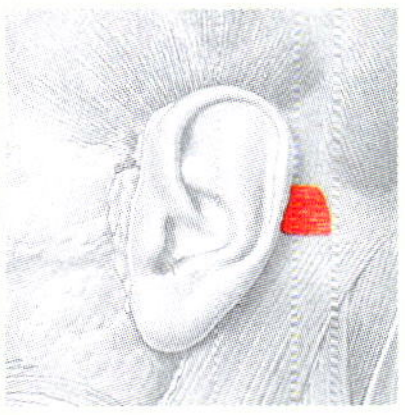

O: Mastoid process, tendon of the sternocleidomastoideus

I: Dorsal part of the auricular root

F: Moves the auricle backwards

1 Facial muscles (continuation)

c Palpebral fissure

Orbicularis oculi (located around the orbital opening in a sphincter-like fashion)
Facial nerve [VII]

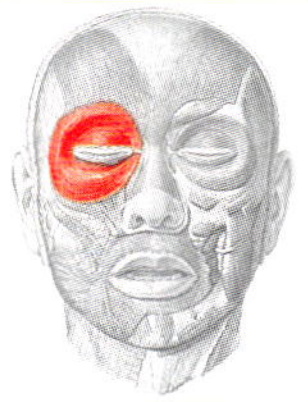

O: Orbital part: Nasal part of the frontal bone, frontal process of the maxilla, lacrimal bone, medial palpebral ligament
Palpebral part: Medial palpebral ligament, lacrimal sac
Lacrimal part: Posterior lacrimal crest of the lacrimal bone, lacrimal sac

I: Orbital part: Lateral palpebral ligament, lateral transition into a circular ring-shaped muscle
Palpebral part: Lateral palpebral ligament
Lacrimal part: Lacrimal canaliculi, edges of the eyelids

F: Closes the eyelids, compresssses the lacrimal sac, moves the eyebrows

Depressor supercilii (branch of the orbital part of the orbicularis oculi)
Facial nerve [VII]

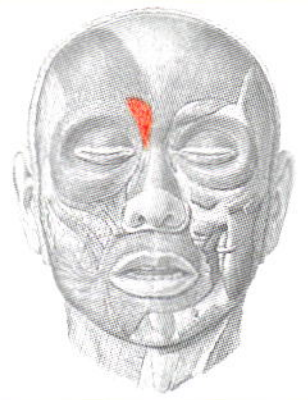

O: Nasal part of the frontal bone, back of the nose

I: Medial third of the skin of the eyebrow

F: Lowers the skin of the forehead and of the eyebrows, creates an oblique wrinkle just above the root of the nose

Corrugator supercilii
Facial nerve [VII]

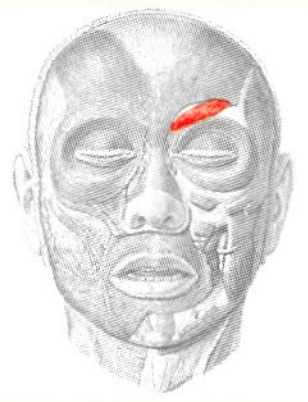

O: Nasal part of the frontal bone

I: Middle (lateral) third of the skin of the eyebrow, epicranial aponeurosis

F: Moves the skin of the forehead and of the eyebrows towards the root of the nose, creates a vertical wrinkle just above-the root of the nose

Procerus
Facial nerve [VII]

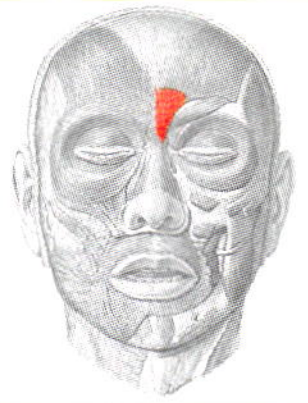

O: Nasal bone, lateral nasal cartilage

I: Skin of the glabella

F: Lowers the skin of the forehead and of the eyebrows

1 Facial muscles (continuation)

d Nose

Nasalis
Facial nerve [VII]

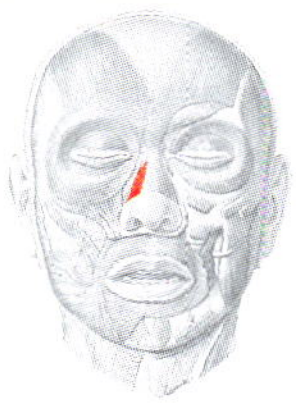

O: Alar part: Alveolar yoke of the lateral incisor tooth
Transverse part: Alveolar yoke of the canine tooth

I: Alar part: Nose wings border of the nostril
Transverse part: Lateral nasal cartilage, tendinous membrane of the back of the nose

F: Moves the nowe wings and thus the nose itself
Alar part: Dilates the nostrils
Transverse part: Narrows the nostrils

Depressor septi nasi
Facial nerve [VII]

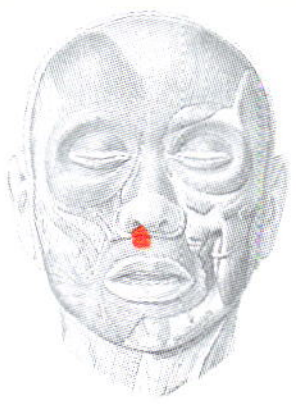

O: Alveolar yoke of the medial incisor tooth

I: Major alar cartilage, septal nasal cartilage

F: Moves the nose wings and thus the nose itself

e Mouth

Orbicularis oris
Facial nerve [VII]

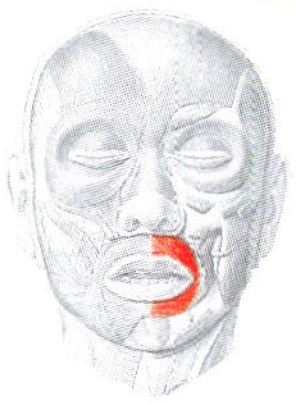

O: Marginal part and **labial part:** Lateral to the angle of mouth

I: Skin of the lips

F: Closes the lips, thereby also moving the nose wings, cheeks and the skin of chin

Buccinator
Facial nerve [VII]

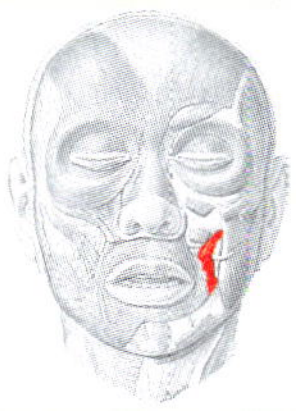

O: Posterior part of the alveolar process of the maxilla, pterygo-mandibular raphe, posterior part of the alveolar process of the mandible

I: Angle of mouth, upper and lower lip

F: Tenses the lips, increases the intraoral pressure (as in blowing and chewing)

Levator labii superioris
Facial nerve [VII]

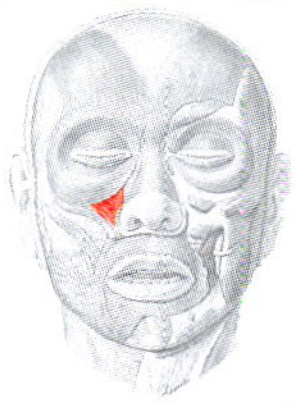

O: Infra-orbital margin and adjacent part of the zygomatic process of the maxilla; originates from the muscle mass of the orbicularis oculi

I: Upper lip

F: Draws the upper lip laterally and upwards

1 Facial muscles (continuation)

Depressor labii inferioris
Facial nerve [VII]

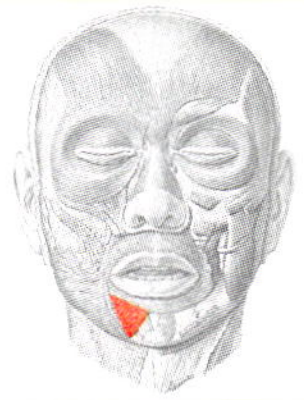

O: Base of mandible medial to the mental foramen

I: Lower lip, chin, deep fibres to the mucosa

F: Draws the lower lip laterally and downwards

Mentalis
Facial nerve [VII]

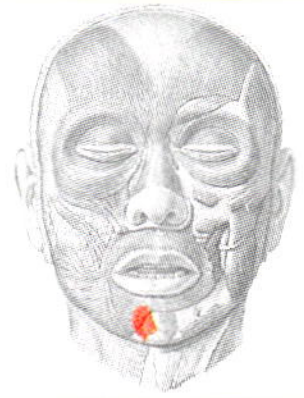

O: Alveolar yoke of the lower, lateral incisor tooth

I: Skin of the chin

F: Creates the chin's dimple, everts the lower lip (together with the orbicularis oris)

Transversus menti
Facial nerve [VII]

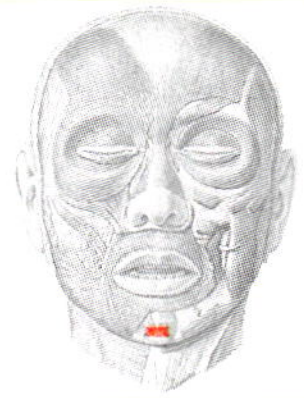

O: Oblique branch from the mentalis

I: Skin of the chin

F: Moves the skin of the chin

Depressor anguli oris
Facial nerve [VII]

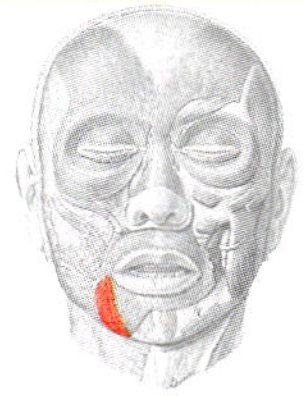

O: Base of mandible, just below the mental foramen

I: Lower lip, cheek lateral to the angle of mouth, upper lip

F: Pulls the angle of mouth downwards

Risorius (frequently a part of the platysma or the depressor anguli oris)
Facial nerve [VII]

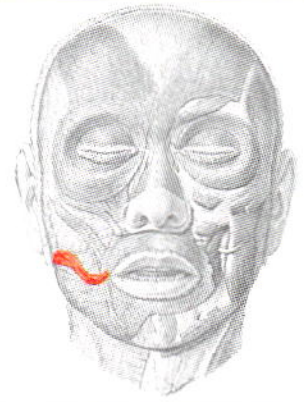

O: Parotid fascia, masseteric fascia

I: Upper lip, angle of mouth

F: Pulls the angle of mouth laterally and upwards, creates the cheek's dimple

1 Facial muscles (continuation)

Levator anguli oris
Facial nerve [VII]

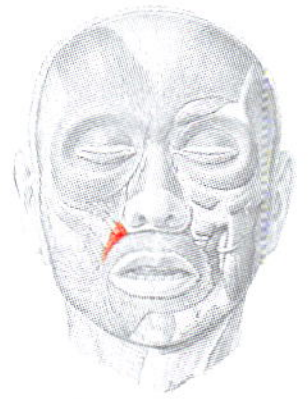

O: Canine fossa of the maxilla

I: Angle of mouth

F: Draws the angle of mouth medially and upwards

Zygomaticus major
Facial nerve [VII]

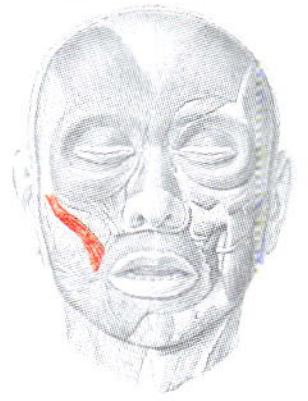

O: Zygomatic bone adjacent to the zygomaticotemporal suture

I: Upper lip, angle of mouth

F: Draws the angle of mouth laterally and upwards

Zygomaticus minor
Facial nerve [VII]

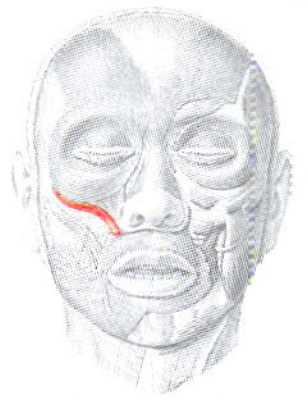

O: Zygomatic bone adjacent to the zygomaticomaxillary suture

I: Upper lip, angle of mouth

F: Moves the lips the nose wings, the cheeks and the skin of the chin, increases the nasolabial sulcus

Levator labii superioris alaeque nasi
Facial nerve [VII]

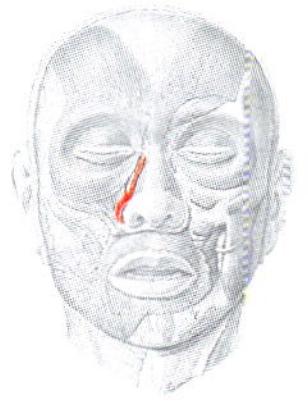

O: Frontal process of the maxilla; originates from the muscle mass of the orbicularis oculi

I: Nose wings, angle of mouth, upper lip, deep fibres: lateral and posterior parts of the nostril

F: Moves the lips, the nose wings, the cheeks and the skin of the chin

f Neck (Fig. 253)

Platysma
Facial nerve [VII]

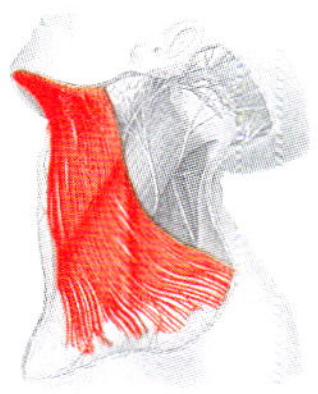

O: Base of mandible, parotid fascia

I: Skin below the clavicle, pectoral fascia

F: Tenses the skin of the neck, creates vertical wrinkles

2 Muscles of the tongue (Fig. 178–180, 186–189)

a Internal muscles of the tongue

Superior longitudinal muscle
Hypoglossal nerve [XIII]

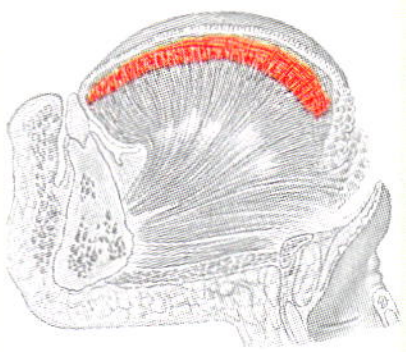

O: Root of tongue

I: Apex of tongue

F: Retracts and broadens the tongue, elevates the apex of the tongue

Interior longitudinal muscle
Hypoglossal nerve [XII]

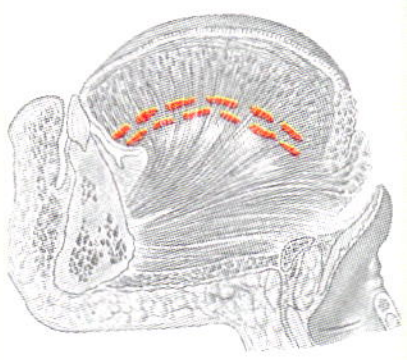

O: Root of tongue

I: Apex of tongue

F: Retracts and broadens the tongue, lowers the apex of the tongue

Transverse muscler
Hypoglossal nerve [XII]

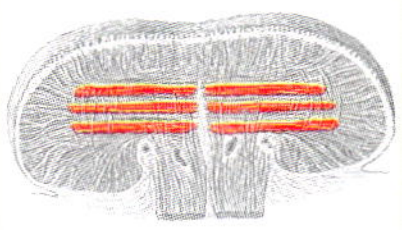

O: Lateral margin of the tongue; lingual septum

I: Lateral margin of the tongue, lingual aponeurosis

F: Narrows the tongue, elongates the tongue together with the vertical muscle

Vertical muscle
Hypoglossal nerve [XII]

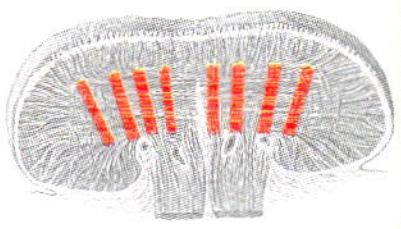

O: Root of tongue; originates from the genioglossus

I: Lingual aponeurosis

F: Broadens the tongue

2 Muscles of the tongue (continuation)

b External muscles of the tongue

Genioglossus
Hypoglossal nerve [XIII]

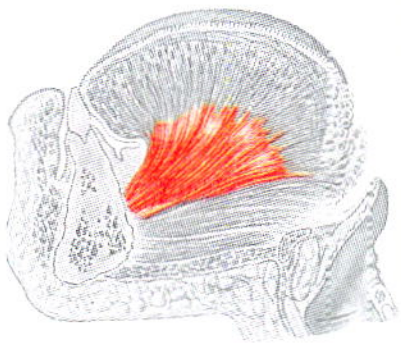

O: Mental spine of the mandible

I: Lingual aponeurosis

F: Protrudes and depresses the tongue

Hyoglossus
Hypoglossal nerve [XII]

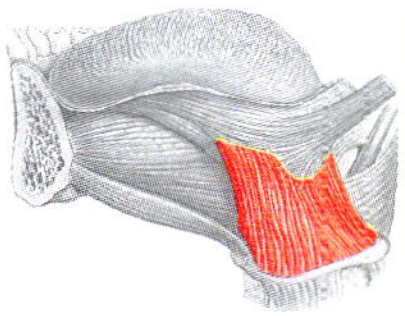

O: Greater horn and body of hyoid bone

I: Lateral parts of the lingual aponeurosis

F: Retracts and depresses the tongue

Chondroglossus (variably formed)
Hypoglossal nerve [XII]

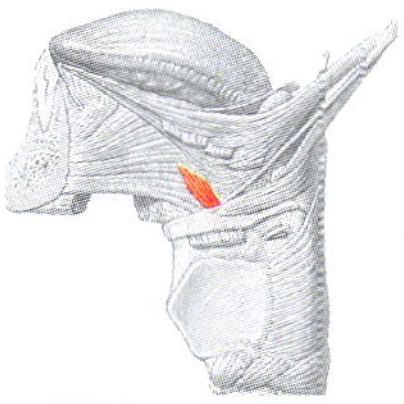

O: Lesser horn of hyoid bone

I: Lateral parts of the lingual aponeurosis

F: Retracts the tongue, depresses the root and the back of the tongue

Styloglossus
Hypoglossal nerve [XII]

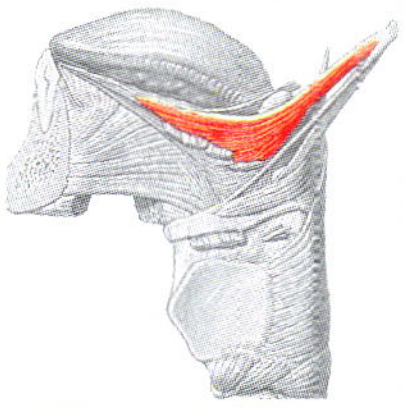

O: Anterior margin of the styloid process of the temporal bone, stylomandibular ligament

I: Enters lateral parts of the tongue from above and behind

F: Retracts and elevates the tongue

3 Muscles of the palate (Fig. 174, 1406)

Levator veli palatini
Pharyngeal branches of the glossopharyngeal nerve [IX] and the vagus nerve [X] (= pharyngeal plexus)

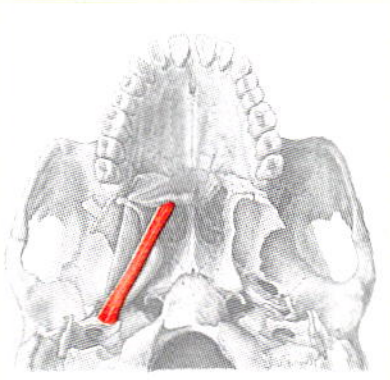

O: Inferior surface of the petrous part of the temporal bone, cartilage of tube

I: Palatine aponeurosis

F: Tenses and elevates the soft palate, expands the lumen of the auditory tube

Tensor veli palatini (surrounds the pterygoid hamulus as hypomochlion)
Nerve to tensor veli palatine of the mandibular nerve [V/3]

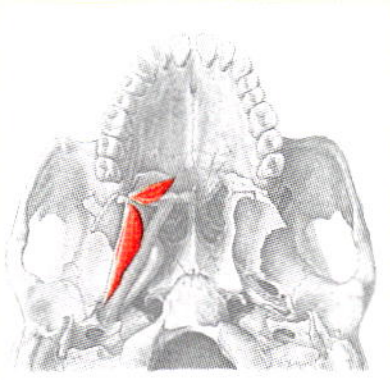

O: Scaphoid fossa at the base of the medial lamina of the pterygoid process. Spine of sphenoid bone, membranous part of the pharyngotympanic tube

I: Palatine aponeurosis

F: Tenses (and elevates) the soft palate,
expands the lumen of the auditory tube

Palatoglossus
Glossopharyngeal nerve [IX]

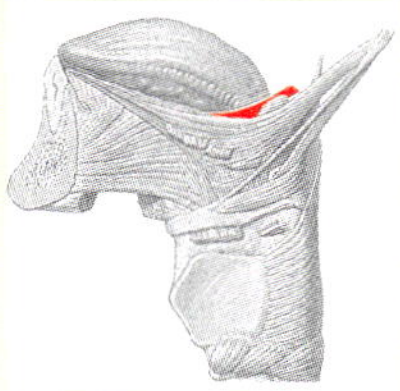

O: Palatine aponeurosis

I: Enters the internal muscles of the tongue, in particular the transverse muscle

F: Depresses the soft palate, elevates the root of the tongue in order to narrow the pharynx

Musculus uvulae (solitary muscle)
Pharyngeal branches of the glossopharyngeal nerve [IX] and the vagus nerve [X] (= pharyngeal plexus)

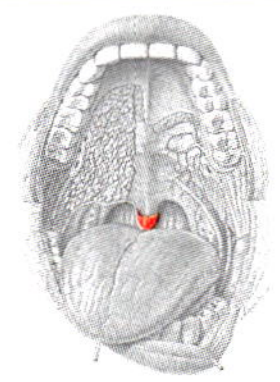

O: Lingual aponeurosis

I: Stroma of the uvula

F: Shortens and thus thickens the uvula

4 Masticatory muscles (Fig. 111, 114–119, 121, 122)

The course of the masseter from the zygomatic arch to the mandibular angle may well be palpated through the skin. When clenching the teeth, the temporalis can be felt in the temporal fossa. The medial pterygoid inserts at the inner surface of the mandibular angle. The lateral pterygoid extends interiorely from the temporomandibular joint.

Temporalis
Deep temporal nerves (mandibular nerve [V/3]

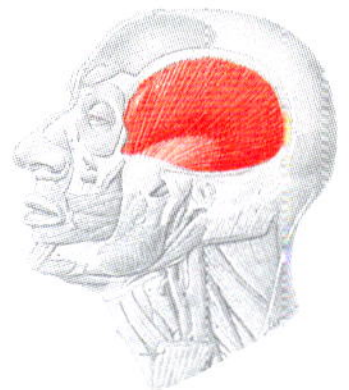

O: Temporal bone below the inferior temporal line, deep layer of the temporal fascia

I: Apex and medial surface of the coronoid process of the mandible

F: Anterior fibres close the jaws, posterior fibres retract the mandible (= retrusion)

Masseter
Masseteric nerve (mandibular nerve [V/3])

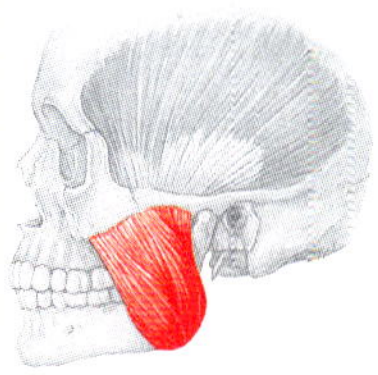

O: Superficial part: Anterior two thirds of the inferior margin of the zygomatic (tendinous) arch
Deep part: Posterior third of the inner surface of the zygomatic arch

I: Superficial part: Angle of mandible, masseteric tuberosity
Deep part: Inferior margin of the mandible

F: Closes the jaws

Medial pterygoid
Nerve to medial pterygoid (mandibular nerve [V/3])

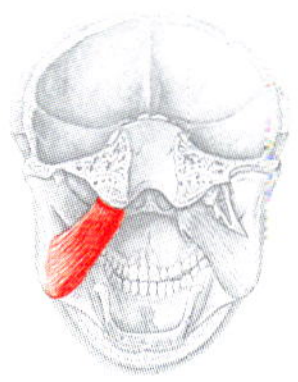

O: Pterygoid fossa, medial surface of the lateral lamina of the pterygoid process, pyramidal process of the palatine bone

I: Inferior margin of the mandible pterygoid tuberosity

F: Closes the jaws

Lateral pterygoid
Nerve to lateral pterygoid (mandibular nerve [V/3])

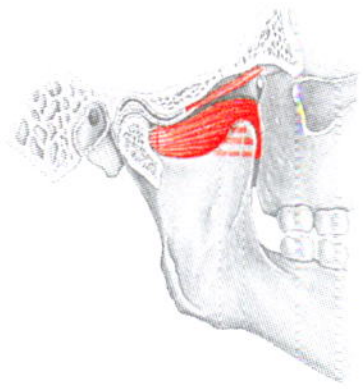

O: Upper head: Outer surface of the lateral lamina of the pterygoid process, maxillary tuberosity (accessory)
Lower head: Temporal surface of the greater wing of the sphenoidal bone

I: Upper head: Disc and capsule of the temporomandibular joint
Lower head: Pterygoid fovea of the condylar process of the mandible

F: Lower head: draws the mandible interiorely (=protrusion)

5 Muscles of the pharynx (Fig. 189, 247, 248, 252)

The pharyngeal muscles are divided into the pharyngeal constrictors (superior, middle anc inferior constrictor) and the pharyngeal levator muscles (stylopharyngeus, salpingopharyngeus and palatopharyngeus).

a Pharyngeal constrictors

Superior constrictor
Pharyngeal branches of the glossopharyngeal nerve [IX] (= pharyngeal plexus)

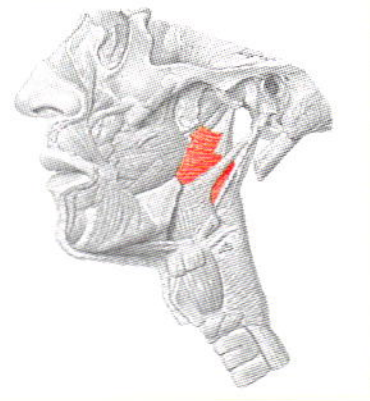

O: Pterygopharyngeal part: posterior margin of the medial lamina of the pterygoid process, hook of pterygoideus
Buccopharyngeal part: Pterygomandibular raphe
Mylopharyngeal part: Mylohoid line of the mandible
Glossopharyngeal part: Transverse muscle

I: Pharyngobasilar membrane, superior third of the pharyngeal raphe

F: Constricts the pharynx, separates the Epipharynx from the Mesopharynx (together with the palatopharyngeus), promotes transport of food into the oesophagus by wave-like contractions (peristaltic wave)

Middle constrictor
Pharyngeal branches of the glossopharyngeal nerve [IX] and the vagus nerve [X] (= pharyngeal plexus)

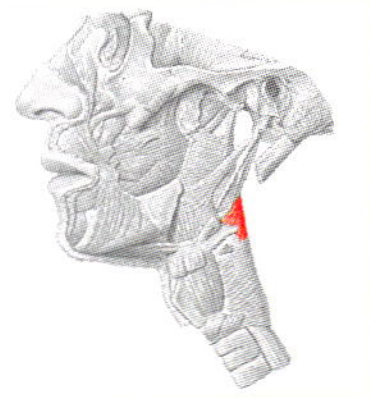

O: Chondropharyngeal part: Lesser horn of hyoid bone
Ceratopharyngeal part: Greater horn of hyoid bone

I: Middle third of the pharyngeal raphe, overlaps the superior constrictor

F: Constricts the pharynx from behind, promotes transport of food into the oesophagus by wave-like contractions (peristaltic wave)

Inferior constrictor
Pharyngeal branches of the vagus nerve [X] (= pharyngeal plexus)

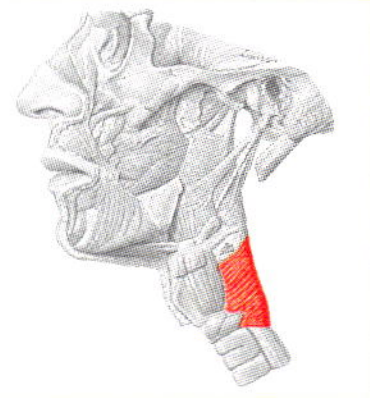

O: Thyropharyngeal part: Outer surface of the thyroid cartilage behind the oblique line
Cricopharyngeal part: Lateral surface of the cricoid cartilage
Tracheopharyngeal part: Lateral surface of the tracheal cartilage I

I: Middle and inferior third of the pharyngeal raphe, overlaps the middle constrictor

F: Constricts the pharynx from behind, promotes transport of food into the oesophagus by wave-like contractions (peristaltic wave)

b Pharyngeal levator muscles

Palatopharyngeus (Functionally, this muscle also belongs to the muscles of the palate.)
Pharyngeal branches of the glossopharyngeal nerve [IX] (= pharyngeal plexus)

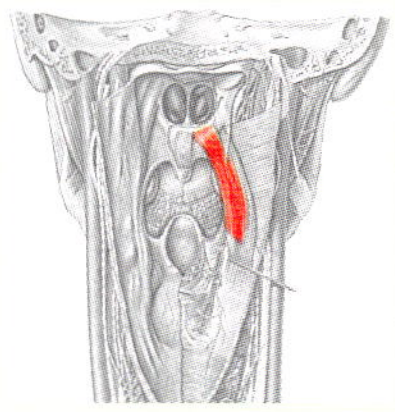

O: Palatine aponeurosis, hook of pterygoideus

I: Thyroid cartilage, inserts into the lateral and the posterior wall of the pharynx

F: Constricts the isthmus of fauces, depresses the soft palate, elevates the pharyngeal wall towards the soft palate

5 Muscles of the pharynx (continuation)

Salpingopharyngeus
Pharyngeal branches of the glossopharyngeal nerve [IX] (= pharyngeal plexus)

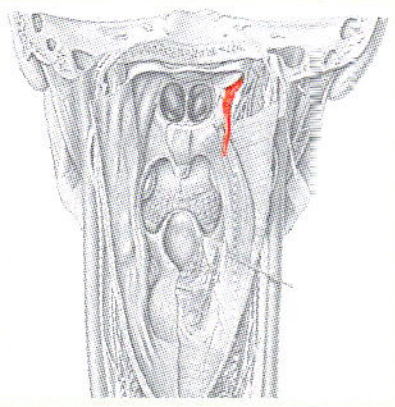

O: Free margin and inferior surface of the cartilage of tube

I: Inserts into the lateral wall of the pharynx

F: Elevates the pharynx

Stylopharyngeus
Stylopharyngeal branch of the glossopharyngeal nerve [IX]

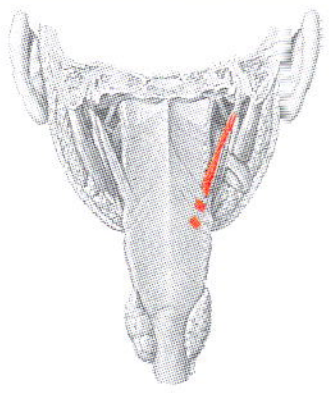

O: Styloid process of the temporal bone

I: Thyroid cartilage, inserts into the lateral wall of the pharynx between the superior constrictor and the middle constrictor

F: Elevates the pharynx

6 Muscles of the larynx (Fig. 224–227)

Cricothyroid (straight part: superficial, oblique part: deep)
External branch of the superior laryngeal nerve of the vagus nerve [X]

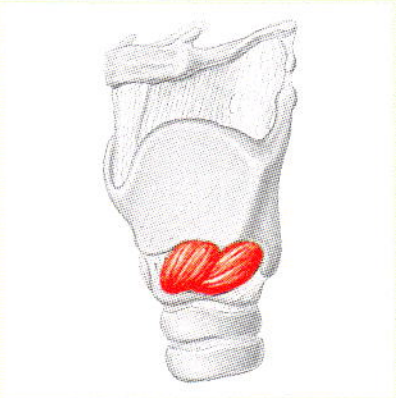

O: Outer surface of the arch of the cricoid cartilage

I: Inferior margin of the lamina of thyroid cartilage

F: Tenses the vocal cords by tilting the cricoid cartilage around a transverse axis

Posterior crico-arytenoid
Recurrent laryngeal nerve of the vagus nerve [X]

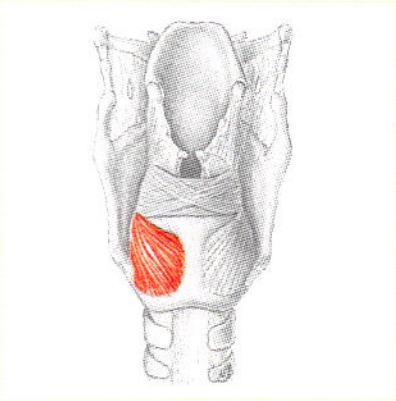

O: Posterior surface of the lamina of the cricoid cartilage

I: Muscular process of the arytenoid cartilage

F: Opens the rima glottidis by rotating the vocal process of the arytenoid cartilage outwards around a longitudinal axis, as well as by tilting the arytenoid cartilage sidewards

Lateral crico-arytenoid
Recurrent laryngeal nerve of the vagus nerve [X]

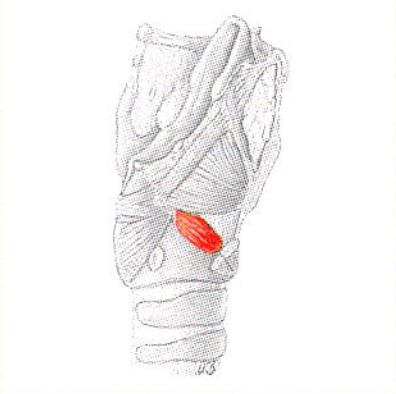

O: Lateral upper martin of the arch of the cricoid cartilage

I: Muscular process of the arytenoid cartilage

F: Closes the intermembranous part of the rima glottidis by rotating the arytenoid cartilage inwards around a longitudinal axis

Transverse arytenoid
Recurrent laryngeal nerve of the vagus nerve [X]

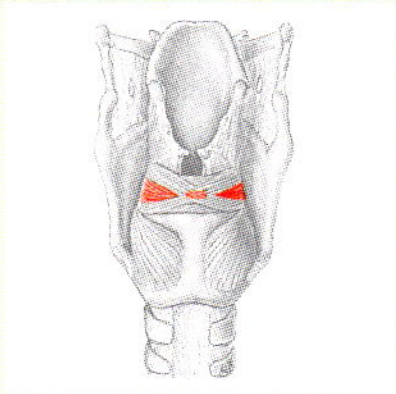

O: Lateral edge and posterior surface of the arytenoid cartilage

I: Lateral edge and posterior surface of the contralateral arytenoid cartilage

F: Closes the intercartilagenous part of the rima glottidis by approximating both arytenoid cartilages

Oblique arytenoid
Recurrent laryngeal nerve of the vagus nerve [X]

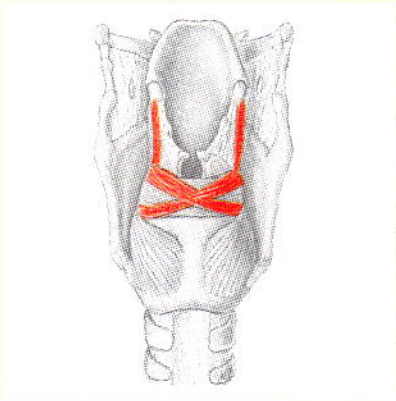

O: Base of the superior surface of the arytenoid cartilage
Ary-epiglottic part: apex of the arytenoid cartilage

I: Apex and posterior surface of the contralateral muscular process
Ary-epiglottic part: lateral margin of the epiglottic cartilage

F: Draws the arytenoid cartilage medially and narrows the intercartilagenous part of the rima glottidis by tilting the arytenoid cartilages inwards

6 Muscles of the larynx (continuation)

Vocalis
Recurrent laryngeal nerve of the vagus nerve [X]

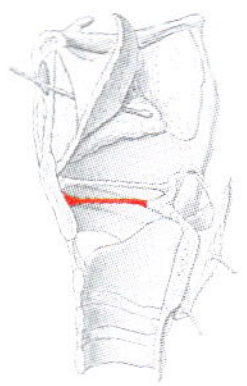

O: Inner surface of the "bow" of the thyroid cartilage

I: Vocal process and oblong fovea of the arytenoid cartilage

F: Tenses the vocal cord and forms the edge of the rima glottidis, regulates the ability of the vocal fold to vibrate

Thyroarytenoid
Recurrent laryngeal nerve of the vagus nerve [X]

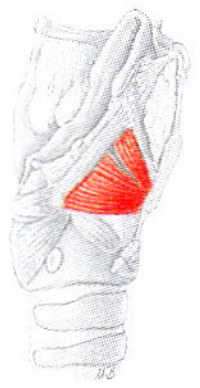

O: Inner surface of the lamina of thyroid cartilage in close proximity to the origin of the vocalis
Thyro-epiglottic part: Inner surface of the lamina of the thyroid cartilage in close proximity to the origin of the thyroarytenoid

I: Muscular process and anterior surface of the arytenoid cartilage
Thyro-epiglottic part: Lateral margin of the epiglottic cartilage

F: Narrows the inter of the rima glottidis by rotating the arytenoid cartilage inwards around a longitudinal axis
Thyro-epiglottic part: Narrows the laryngeal orifice

7 Branches and supplying areas of the cervical plexus (Fig. 253)

	Motor function	Sensory function
Ansa cervicalis Superior root (= anterior root) Inferior root (= posterior root)	Infrahyoid muslces	
Muscular branches	Longus colli Longus capitis Rectus capitis anterior Intertransversarii anteriores cervicis Trapezius Levator scapulae Scalenus medius Geniohyoid	
Branches of the so-called Punctum nervosum		
Great auricular nerve		Skin of the uper neck, the area of the mandibular angle, the anterior and posterior areas surrounding the auricle, and most of the auricle itself
Transverse cervical nerve		Skin of the upper anterior neck
Lesser occipital nerve		Skin of the occipital region
Medial, intermediate, lateral supraclavicular nerves		A strip of skin below the clavicle
Phrenic nerve	Diaphragm	Parietal pleura, pericard, peritoneum

8 Lateral muscle of the neck (Fig. 204, 208)

The sternocleidomastoid develops from the same embryonic anlage as the trapezius (same innervation). It traverses obliquely from the mastoid process in an anterior mediocaudal direction and is integrated in the investing layer of the cervical fascia

Sternocleidomastoid
Accessory nerve [XII]; cervical plexus

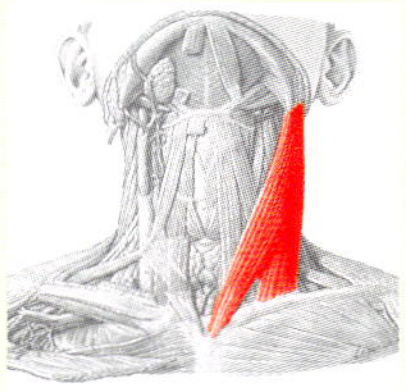

O: Sternal head: With a long tendon from the ventral surface of the Sternum
Clavicular head: With a short tendon from the sternal third of the clavicle

I: Posterior area of the mastoid process,
lateral margin of the superior nuchal line

F: Unilateral innervation: rotates the head contralaterally,
bilateral innervation: elevates the head and draws the head anteriorly, flexes the caudal cervical vertebrae and stretches both the cranial cervical vertebrae as well as the cranio-cervical joints

9 Suprahyoid muscles (Fig. 183–187, 204, 208)

The suprahyoid muscles form the floor of the oral cavity and function as antagonists to the infrahyoid muscles. The anterior belly of the digastric is located most superficially. The next layer consists of the mylohyoid, which forms a broad plate. The geniohyoid is located adjacently to the interior surface of the mylohyoid as a round strand. The posterior belly of the digastic and the stylohyoid are located dorsally.

Mylohyoid (The right and the left muscle together, secure the floor of the mouth in a plate-like shape.)
Nerve to the mylohyoid (mandibular nerve [V/3])

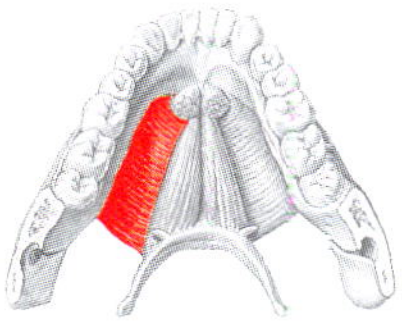

O: With a short tendon from the mylohyoid line of the mandible

I: Mylohyoid raphe, upper margin of the body of hyoid bone

F: Elevates the floor of the mouth and the tongue (as in swallowing), depresses the mandible, also elevates the hyoid bone, forms the muscular support for the tongue

Digastric (Posterior and anterior belly are connected by an intertendon attached to the lesser horn of the hyoid bone. Posterior belly: from the origin to the intertendon; anterior belly: from the intertendon to the insertion.)
Anterior belly: *nerve to mylohyoid (mandibular nerve [V/3]);*
posterior belly: *digastric branch (facial nerve [VII])*

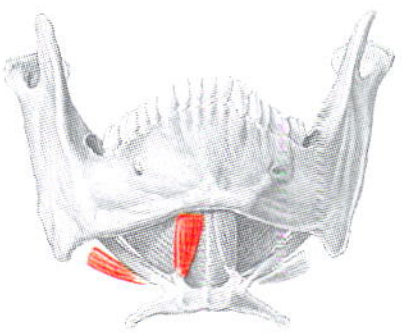

O: Mastoid notch of the temporal bone

I: Digastric fossa of the mandible

F: Supports the mylohyoid

Stylohyoid
Stylohyoid branch (facial nerve [VII])

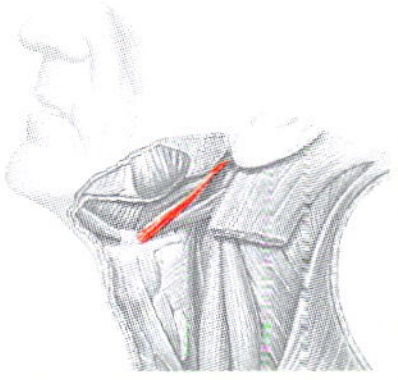

O: Styloid process of the temporal bone

I: Lateral margin of the body of hyoid bone with two parts surrounding the intertendon of the digastric

F: Draws the hyoid bone dorsocranially

Geniohyoid (The right and the left muscle are closely juxtaposed, only separated by a thin septum of connective tissue.)
Ventral branches from C1–C2

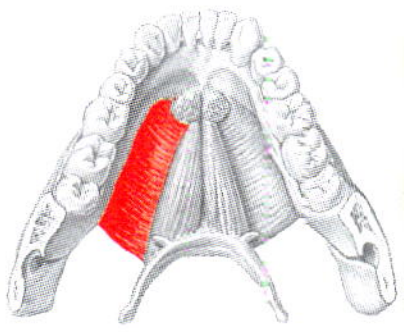

O: With a short tendon from the mental spine of the mandible

I: Anterior surface of the body of hyoid bone

F: Supports the mylohyoid in elevating the tongue, depresses the mandible, elevates the hyoid bone

10 Infrahyoid muscles (Fig. 183, 204, 208)

The infrahyoid musles function as antagonists to the suprahyoid muscles.
The sternohyoid is located superficially and is followed below by the sternohyoid and the thyrohyoid. The omohyoid stretches most laterally.

Sternohyoid
Ansa cervicalis (cervical plexus)

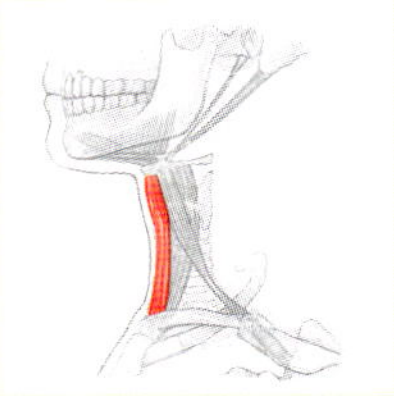

O: Cranial margin of the costal cartilage I, inner surface of the manubrium of sternum and the capsule of the sternoclavicular joint

I: Inferior margin of the body of hyoid bone

F: Draws the hyoid bone caudally

Sternohyoid
Ansa cervicalis (cervical plexus)

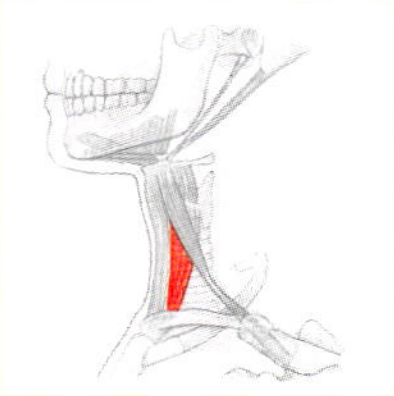

O: Inner surface of the costal cartilage I, inner surface of the manubrium of sternum caudal to the sternohyoid

I: Outer surface, oblique line of the lamina of the thyroid cartilage

F: Depresses the larynx, regulates the position of the larynx between the hyoid bone and the sternum together with the thyrohyoid

Thyrohyoid
Ansa cervicalis (cervical plexus)

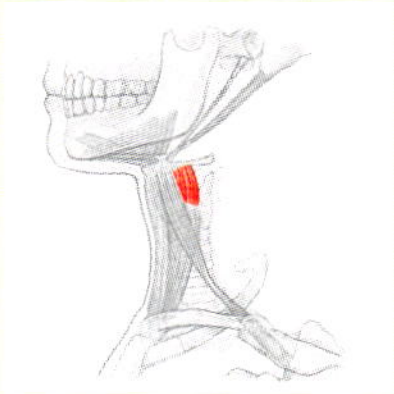

O: Outer surface, oblique line of the lamina of the thyroid cartilage

I: Lateral third of the body and the root of the greater horn of the hyoid bone

F: Approximates the hyoid bone and the larynx, regulates the position of the larynx between the hyoid bone and the sternum together with the sternothyroid

Omohyoid (Interior and superior belly are connected by an intertendon, which is attached to the carotid sheath)
Ansa cervicalis (cervical plexus)

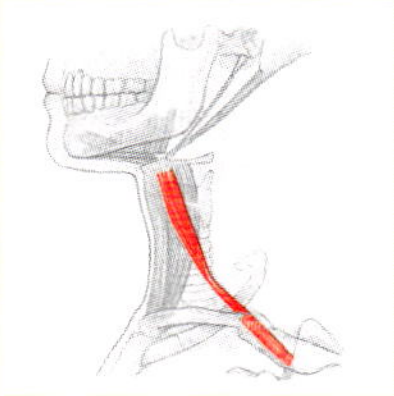

O: Inferoir belly: Superior border of the scapula medial to the suprascapular notch

I: Superior belly: Caudal margin of the lateral outer surface of the body of hyoid bone

F: Tenses the cervical fascia due to its attachment to the carotid sheath, prevents the collapse of the internal jugular vein

11 Scalenus muscles (Fig. 204, 208, 209, 573)

The three scalenus muscles, scalenus anterior, scalenus medius and scalenus posterior, traverse to the upper ribs and form a three sided muscle layer laterally to the cervical part of the vertebral column.

Scalenus anterior
Direct branches of the cervical plexus and the brachial plexus

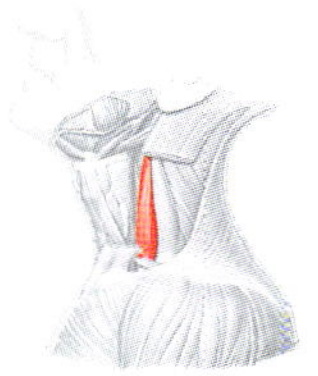

O: Anterior tubercles of the transverse processes of the 3. (4.)–6. cervical vertrebra

I: With a short tendon at the scalene tubercle of the 1. rib

F: Vertebral column:
flexes the cervical part of the vertebral column laterally
Thorax:
elevates the first rib, thereby elevating the thorax
(muscle of inspiration)

Scalenus medius
Direct branches of the cervical plexus and the brachial plexus

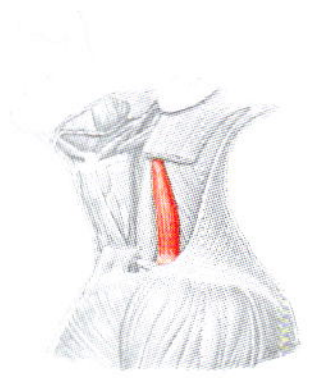

O: Tubercles of the transverse processes of the 3.–7. cervical vertebra

I: With a short tendon at the 1. rib, just behind the groove for subclavian artery

F: Vertebral column:
flexes the cervical part of the vertebral column laterally
Thorax:
elevates the first rib, thereby elevating the thorax
(muscle of inspiration)

Scalenus posterior
Direct branches of the cervical plexus and the brachial plexus

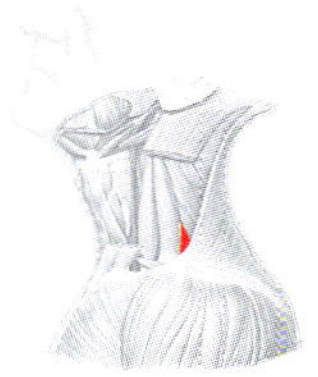

O: Posterior tubercles of the transverse processes of the 5. and 6. cervical vertebra

I: With a short and flat tendon at the upper margin of the 2. (3.) rib

F: Vertebral column:
flexes the cervical part of the vertebral column laterally
Thorax:
elevates the first rib, thereby elevating the thorax
(muscle of inspiration)

12 Prevertebral muscles (Fig. 209, 573)

The prevertebral muscles are located to the both sides of the bodies of the cervical and upper thoracic vertebrae, and are ensheathed by the prevertebral layer of the cervical fascia. The anterolateral part of the atlas and axis are connected by the short rectus capitis anterior.

Rectus capitis anterior
Ventral branches of the cervical plexus

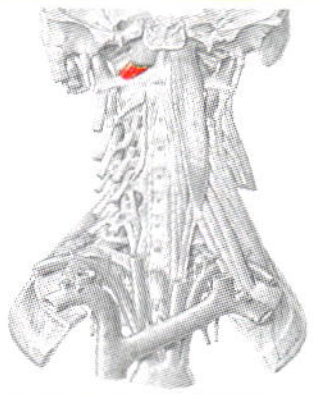

O: Transverse process and lateral mass of the atlas

I: Basilar part of the occipital bone

F: Flexes the head lateroventrally, (rotates the head ipsilaterally)

Longus capitis
Direct branches of the cervical plexus

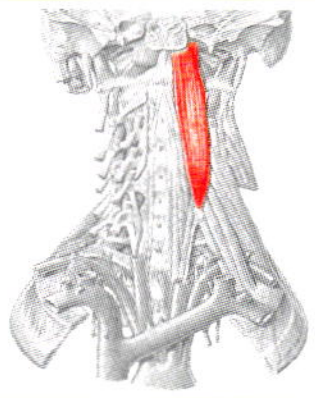

O: Anterior tubercles of the transverse processes of the 3.–6. cervical vertreba

I: Outer surface of the basilar part of the occipital bone

F: Flexes the head ventrally, (rotates the head ipsilaterally)

Longus colli
Direct branches of the cervical plexus

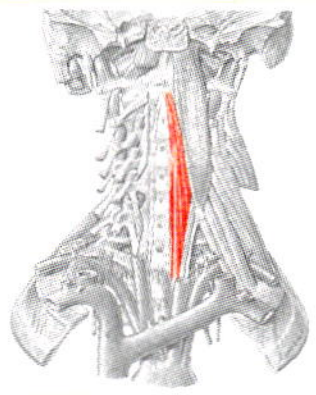

O: Bodies of the 5. cervical – 3. thoracic vertebra, anterior tubercles of the transverse processes of the 2.–5. cervical vertebra

I: Transverse processes of the 5.–7. cervical vertebra, bodies of the 2.–4. cervical vertebra, anterior tubercle of the atlas

F: Flexes the head ventrally, (rotates the head ipsilaterally)

13 Muscles of the thoratic wall (Fig. 571–577)

The pectoralis major moulds the surface anatomy of the anterior upper thoracic wall. The pectoralis minor is situated just below. Together with the subclavius, these muscles belong to the group of the ventral muscles of the shoulder (see Tab. 26).
The external and internal intercostal muscles fill the intercostal space. The subcostales and the transversus thoracis are located at the inner surface of the thoracic wall. Sometimes a superficially located sternalis can be found.

Sternalis (inconstant muscle, in approx. 5% of the cases located on the pectoral fascia)
Branches of the pectoral nerves (brachial plexus, supraclavicular part) of intercostal nerves (thoracic nerves)

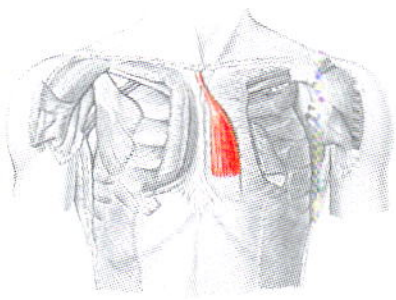

O: Edge of the manubrium of sternum

I: Inserts into the rectus sheath

F: Contracts the pectoral skin

External intercostal muscles
Intercostal nerves (thoracic nerves)

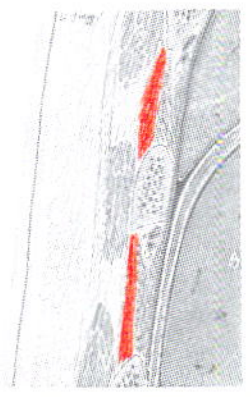

O: Inferior margin of the 1.–11. rib from the tubercle to the junction between cartilage and bone

I: Superior margin of the corresponding lower rib

F: Elevate the ribs, reinforce the intercostal space in deep inspiration

Internal intercostal muscles (Interiorly, the posterior intercostal vessels and the intercostal nerve delineate the innermost intercostal muscles.)
Intercostal nerves (thoracic nerves)

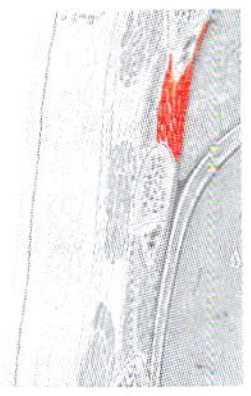

O: Superior margin of the 2.–12. rib from the sternal end of the costal cartilage to the angle

I: Inferior margin of the corresponding upper rib

F: Depress the ribs, reinforce the intercostal space in deep expiration

Subcostales (inconstant muscles)
Intercostal nerves (thoracic nerves)

O: Superior margin of the lower ribs between the tubercle and angle

I: Inferior margin of the lower ribs, always skipping one rib

F: Reinforce the thoric wall, depress the ribs in deep expiration

Transversus thoracis (inconstant muscles)
Intercostal nerves (thoracic nerves)

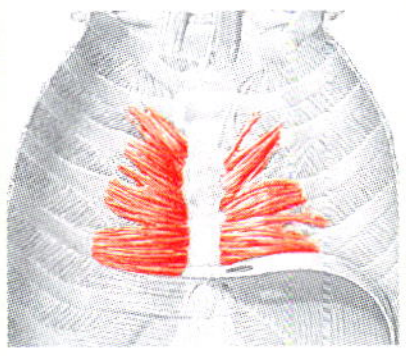

O: Body of sternum, dorsolateral margin of the xiphoid process, costal cartilage of the (6.) 7. rib

I: Costal cartilage of the 2.–6. rib close to the junction between cartilage and bone

F: Reinforces the thoracic wall in deep expiration

14 Ventral muscles of the abdominal wall (Fig. 575–578, 601)

The ventral muscles of the abdominal wall, the rectus abdominis and the pyramidalis, are located within the rectus sheath.

Rectus abdominis
Intercostal nerves (thoracic nerves); less frequently ventral branches of the upper lumbar nerves

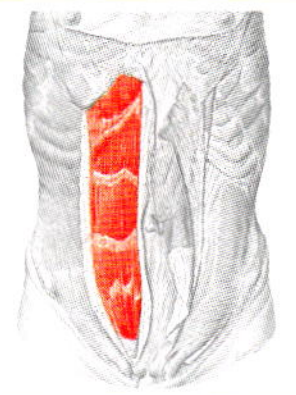

O: Outer surface of the costal cartilage of the 5.–7. rib, xiphoid process, costoxiphoid ligaments

I: Pubic crest of the hip bone, pubic symphysis

F: Flexes the trunk, compresses the abdomen, expiration

Pyramidalis (inconstant muscles)
Caudal intercostal nerves (thoracic nerves)

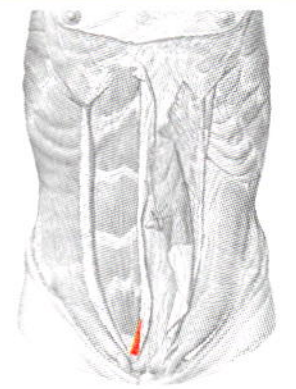

O: Pubic crest of the hip bone, pubic symphysis ventral to the rectus abdominis

I: Linea alba

F: "Tenses" the linea alba

15 Lateral muscles of the abdominal wall (Fig. 569–571, 575–578, 583, 601)

Together the external oblique, the internal oblique and the transversus abdominis are referred to as lateral muscles of the abdominal wall. Their tendinous layers together form the rectus sheath. In the male, parts of the internal oblique and the transversus abdominis branch off to form the cremaster.

External Oblique
Caudal intercostal nerves (thoracic nerves); iliohypogastric nerve; ilio-inguinal nerve (lumbar plexus)

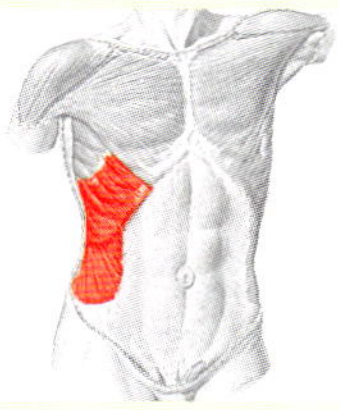

O: Outer surface of the 5.–12. rib, indented by fleshy digitations with the serratus anterior

I: Outer lip of the iliac crest, inguinal ligament, pubic tubercle, pubic crest, linea alba, participates in the formation of the anterior layer of the rectus sheath

F: Unilateral innervation: rotates the thorax contralaterally, flexes the vertebral column ipsilaterally, bilateral innervation: flexes the trunk, compresses the abdomen, expiration

Internal Oblique (In the male, the most caudal fibres branch off as cremaster and traverse into the spermatic cord.)
Caudal intercostal nerves (thoracic nerves); iliohypogastric nerve; ilio-inguinal nerve (lumbar plexus)

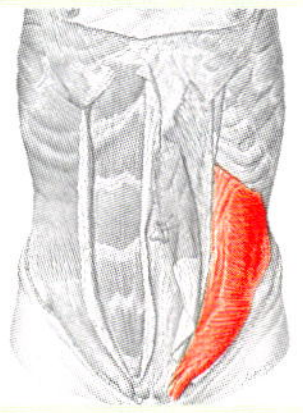

O: Superficial layer of the thoracolumbar fascia, intermediate zone of the iliac crest, lateral two thirds of the inguinal ligament

I: Inferior margin of the costal cartilage of the (9.) 10.–12. rib, linea alba, superior to the arcuate line the muscle participates in the formation of both layers of the rectus sheath, whereas inferior to it all fibres insert into the anterior layer only

F: Unilateral innervation: rotates the thorax ipsilaterally, flexes the vertebral column ipsilaterally, bilateral innervation: flexes the trunk, compresses the abdomen, expiration, cremaster elevates the testis

15 Lateral muscles of the abdominal wall (continuation)

Transversus abdominis (In the male, the most caudal fibres branch off as cremaster and traverse into the spermatic cord.)
Candal intercostal nerves (thoracic nerves); iliohypogastric nerve; ilio-inguinal nerve (lumbar plexus); genitofemoral nerve

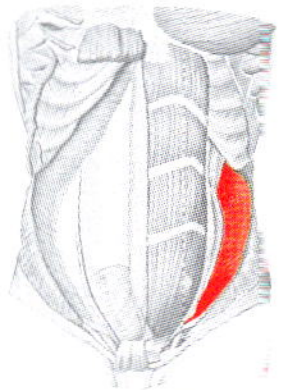

O: Inner surface of the costal cartilage of the (5., 6.) 7.–12. rib, costal processes of the lumbar vertebrae via the deep layer of the thoracolumbar fascia, inner lip of the iliac crest, lateral third of the inguinal ligament

I: Linea alba, superior to the arcuate line the muscle participates in the formation of the posterior layer of the rectus sheath, whereas inferior to it all fibres insert into the anterior layer

F: Compresses the abdomen, expiration, cremaster elevates the testis

16 Dorsal muscles of the abdominal wall (Fig. 583, 601)

The quadratus lumborum constitutes the muscular fundament of the posterior abdominal wall. Medially, this muscle is juxtaposed to the psoas major (see Tab. 42

Quadratus lumborum
Intercostal nerve (thoracic nerve [T12]); muscular branches (lumbar plexus)

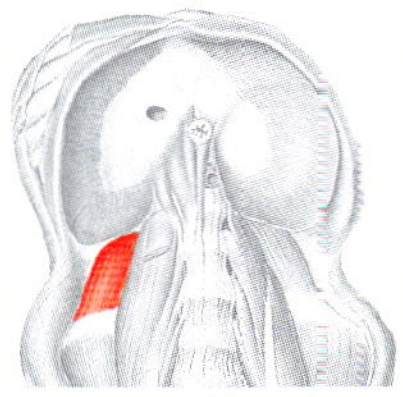

O: Posterior third of the inner lip of the iliac crest iliolumbar ligament

I: Medial part of the 12. rib, costal process of the 4.–1. lumbar vertebra

F: Draws the ribs downwards in expiration, flexes the vertebral column ipsilaterally

17 Trunk – shoulder girdle muscles (Fig. 527, 528, 569, 570, 575, 576)

The dorsal muscles of this group, the trapezius, levator scapulae, rhomboid major and rhomboid minor, belong to the superficial layer according to their position. However, according to their origin and innervation they are referred to as immigrated muscles of the back. The serratus anterior is located at the lateral thoracic wall and traverses dorsally underneath the scapula.
The pectoralis minor and the subclavius originate from the anterior thoracic wall. They are discussed in the section of the ventral muscles of the shoulder (see Tab. 26).

Trapezius (At the origin between the middle and lower thoracic vertebrae and at the spine of scapula, a characteristically shaped aponeurosis is found.)
Accessory nerve [XI] and branches of the cervical plexus

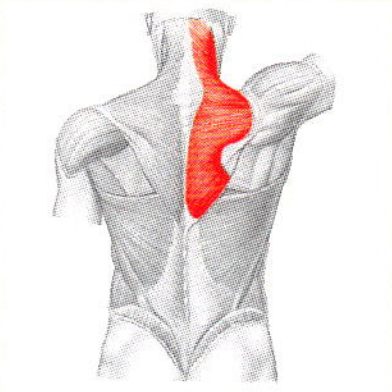

O: Descending part: Squamous part of occipital bone between the highest nuchal line and the superior nuchal line, spinous processes of the upper cervical vertebrae via the ligamentum nuchae
Transverse part: Spinous processes of the lower cervical and upper thoracic vertebrae
Ascending part: Spinous processes of the middle and lower thoracic vertebrae

I: Descending part: Acromial third of the clavicle
Transverse part: Acromion
Ascending part: Spine of scapula

F: Shoulder girdle:
Descending part: prevents the drop of the shoulder girdle and the arm, elevates the scapula and rotates the inferior angle outwards together with the serratus anterior to allow for the arm to be raised over the horizontal, rotates the head contralaterally when shoulders are fixed, extends the cervical part of the vertebral column when both sides are innervated
Transverse part: draws the scapula medially
Ascending part: depresses the scapula and rotates it caudally
Vertebral column:
upon bilateral innervation, flattens the kyphosis of the thoracic part of the vertebral column

Levator scapulae
Direct branches of the cervical plexus and dorsal scapular nerve (brachial plexus, supraclavicular part)

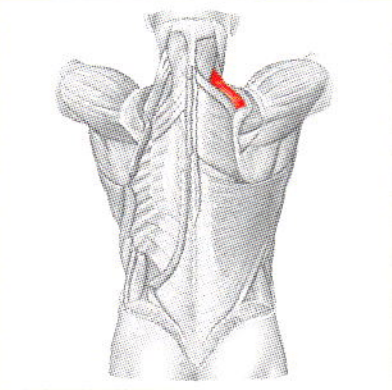

O: Posterior tubercules of the transverse processes of the 1.–4. cervical vertebra

I: Superior angle and adjacent parts of the scapula

F: Shoulder girdle:
elevates the scapula and rotates it cranially
Vertebral column:
extends the cervical part of the vertebral column when shoulders are fixed

Rhomboid minor
Dorsal scapular nerve (brachial plexus, supraclavicular part)

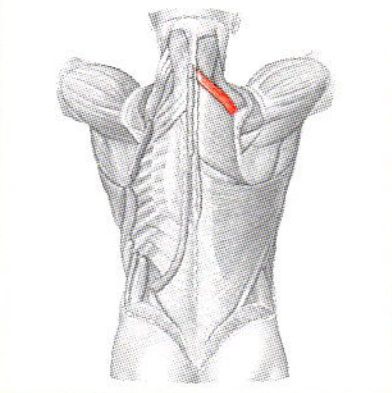

O: Spinous process of the 6. and 7. cervical vertebra

I: Medial border of the scapula cranially to the spine of scapula

F: Draws the scapula medially and upwards,
holds the scapula to the trunk together with the serratus anterior

Rhomboid major
Dorsal scapular nerve (brachial plexus, supraclavicular part)

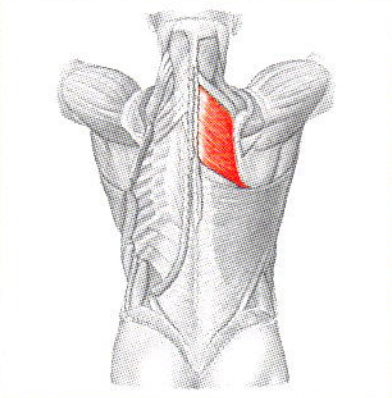

O: Spinous process of the four upper thoracic vertebrae

I: Medial border of the scapula caudally to the spine of scapula

F: Draws the scapula medially and upwards,
holds the scapula to the trunk together with the serratus anterior

17 Trunk – shoulder girdle muscles (continuation)

Serratus anterior (Palsy of the serratus anterior or the rhomboid muscles results in winged scapula)
Long thoracic nerve (brachial plexus, supraclavicular part)

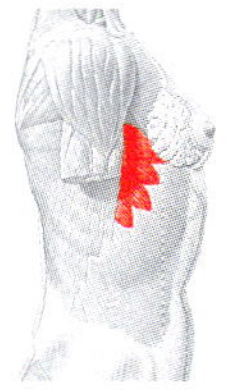

O: Superior part: 1. and 2. rib (reasonably convergent)
Medial part: 2.–4. rib (divergent)
Inferior part: 5.–(8.) 9. rib (strongly convergent), incented with the origin of the external oblique

I: Superior part: Superior angle of the scapula
Medial part: Medial border of the scapula
Inferior part: Inferior angle of the scapula

F: Shoulder girdle:
draws the scapula medially,
presses the scapula onto the thorax together with the thomboid muscles.
Superior part: elevates the scapula
Medial part: depresses the scapula
Inferior part: depresses the scapula and rotates the inferior angle outwards to allow for the arm to be raised over the horizontal together with the trapezius
Thorax:
elevates the ribs when scapula is fixed

18 Trunk – arm muscles (Fig. 527, 528, 569, 570)

The latissimus dorsi and the pectoralis major belong to this group. Both muscles originate from the trunk and traverse to the arm.
Due to the position of its muscular belly, and the fact that it also migrated to the back from ventrally, the latissimus dorsi is grouped with the superficial muscles of the back.
The pectoralis major originates from the thoracic wall and, accordingly, is discussed with the ventral muscles of the shoulder (see Tab. 26).

Latissimus dorsi (subtendinous bursa of latissimus dorsi at the contact area with the teres major)
Thoracodorsal nerve (brachial plexus, supraclavicular part)

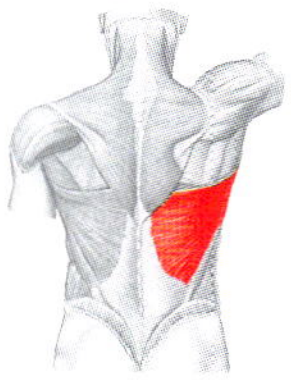

O: Spinous process of the six lower thoracic and lumbar vertebrae (via thoracolumbar fascia), dorsal surface of the sacrum, dorsal third of the outer lip of the iliac crest, (9.) 10.–12. rib, frequently with an additional indentation from the inferior angle of the scapula

I: With a flat tendon surrounding the teres major at the crest of lesser tubercle

F: Shoulder joint:
adduction,
medial rotation,
retroversion
Shoulder girdle:
draws the scapula and the arm medially and downwards

19 Spinocostal muscles (Fig. 528)

The spinocostal muscles, serratus posterior superior and serratus posterior inferior, are slim muscles with minor functional relevance, located in the depth of the muscles of the back on top of the autochthonous muscles of the back.

Serratus posterior superior
Ventral branches of the cervical nerve [C8] and the thoracic nerves [T1–T4]

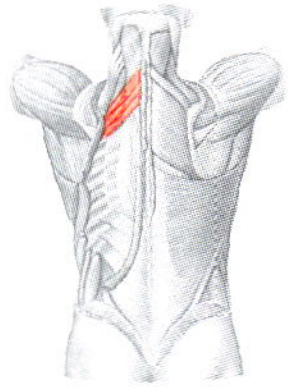

O: Spinous process of the 6., 7. cervical and the 1., 2. thoracic vertebra

I: 1.–4. rib laterally to the angle

F: Elevates the 1.–4. rib (inspiration)

Serratus posterior inferior
Ventral branches of the thoracic nerves [T9–T12]

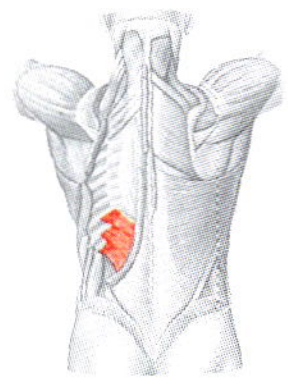

O: Spinous process of the 11., 12. thoracic and 1., 2. lumbar vertebra

I: Caudal margin of the 9.–12. rib

F: Draws the 9.–12. rib downwards (expiration),
with its possible antagonism to the diaphragm, it may also support forced inspiration

20 Autochthonous muscles of the back (Fig. 529, 532–538, 601)

a Autochthonous lateral muscle of the back (Fig. 529, 532, 534, 537, 601)

The lateral tract of the autochthonous muscles of the back covers the medial tract in the neck and lumbar region and is therefore also referred to as superficial part of the autochthonous muscles of the back. The following muscles with longitudinal fibres belong to this tract: iliocostalis, longissimus, intertransversarii. The oblique splenic muscles diverge cranially (spinotransveral). The levatores costarum traverse obliquely with laterocaudal direction to the ribs.

Iliocostalis lumborum
Posterior branches of the lumbar nerves

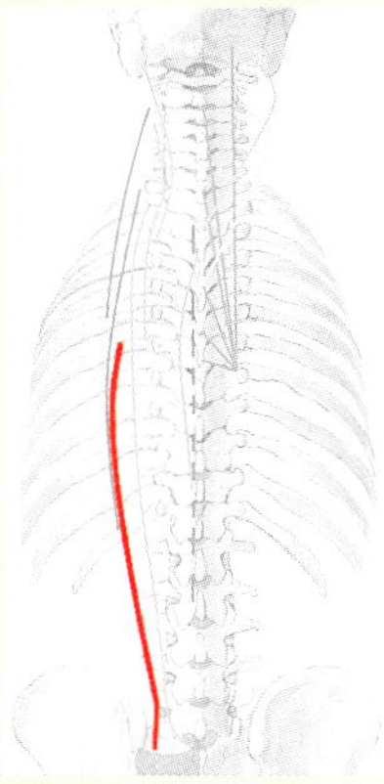

O: Together with the longissimus thoracis from: spinous process of the lumbar vertebrae, dorsal surface of the sacrum, dorsal third of the iliac crest, thoracolumbar fascia

I: Angle of the 12.–5. rib

F: Unilateral innervation: lateral flexion,
bilateral innervation: extension

Iliocostalis thoracis
Posterior branches of the thoracic nerves

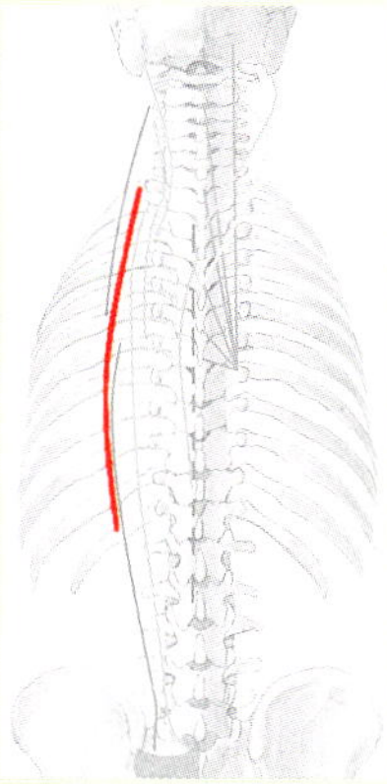

O: 12.–7. rib medially to the angle

I: Angle of the (6.) 7.–1. rib

F: Unilateral innervation: lateral flexion,
bilateral innervation: extension

Iliocostalis cervicis
Posterior branches of the cervical nerves

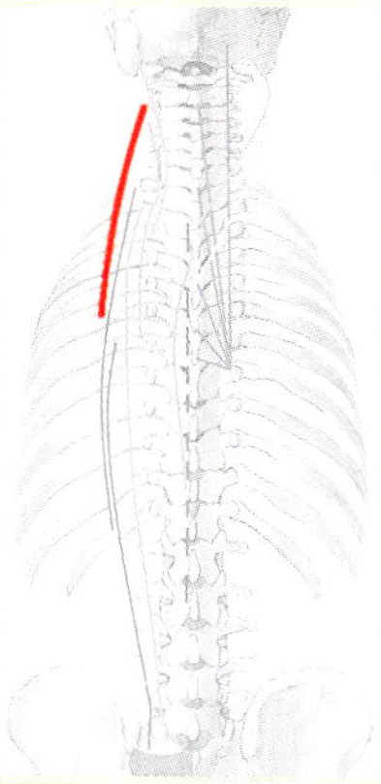

O: 7.–4. (3.) rib medially to the angle

I: Posterior tubercle of the transverse process of the 6.–(4.) 3. cervical vertebra

F: Unilateral innervation: lateral flexion,
bilateral innervation: extension

20 Autochthonous muscles of the back (continuation)

Longissimus thoracis (It is closely attached to the longissimus cervicis and the spinalis.)
Posterior branches of the spinal nerves

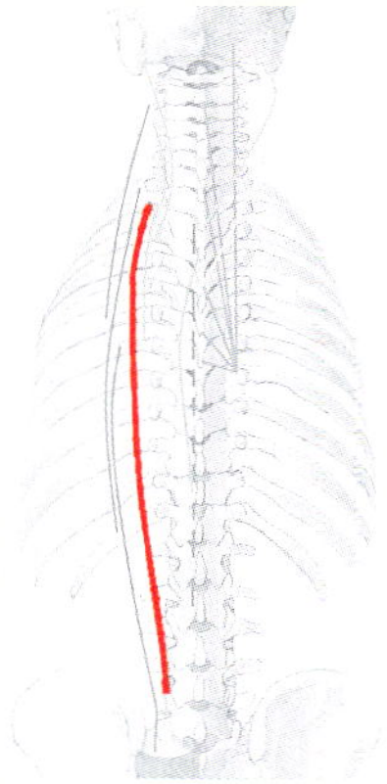

O: Together with the iliocostalis lumborum from: spinous processes of the lumbar vertebrae, dorsal surface of the sacrum, frequently from the mamillary process of the 2. and the 1. lumbar vertebrae, as well as from the transverse process of the 12.–6. thoracic vertebrae

I: Medial part: Mamillary process of the 5. lumbar vertebra, accessory process of the 4.–1. lumbar vertebra, transverse processes of the thoracic vertebrae
Lateral part: Costal process of the 4.–1. lumbar vertebra, deep layer of the thoracolumbar fascia, 12.–2. rib medially to the angle

F: Unilateral innervation: lateral flexion,
bilateral innervation: extension

Longissimus cervicis
Posterior branches of the spinal nerves

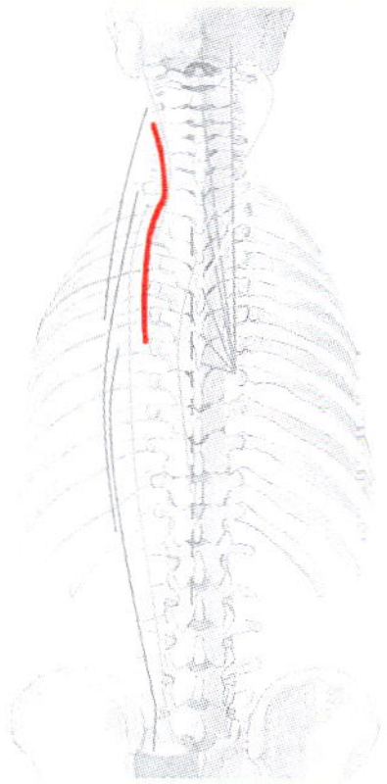

O: Transverse process of the 6.–1. thoracic and 7.–3. cervical vertebra

I: Posterior tubercle of the transverse process of the 5.–2. cervical vertebra

F: Unilateral innervation: lateral flexion,
bilateral innervation: extension

Longissimus capitis
Posterior branches of the spinal nerves

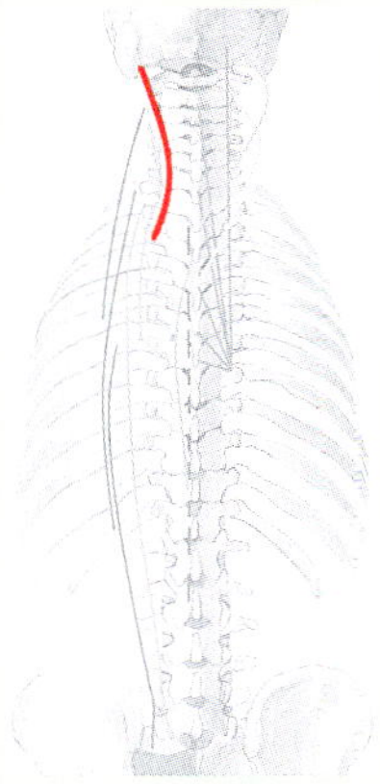

O: Transverse process of the 3. thoracic – 3. cervical vertebra

I: Posterior margin of the mastoid process

F: Unilateral innervation: lateral flexion,
bilateral innervation: extension

20 Autochthonous muscles of the back (continuation)

Intertransversarii laterales lumborum (Strictly speaking, these muscles are of ventral descent and can therefore not be referred to as autochthonous muscle of the back) *Posterior and anterior branches of the spinal nerves*

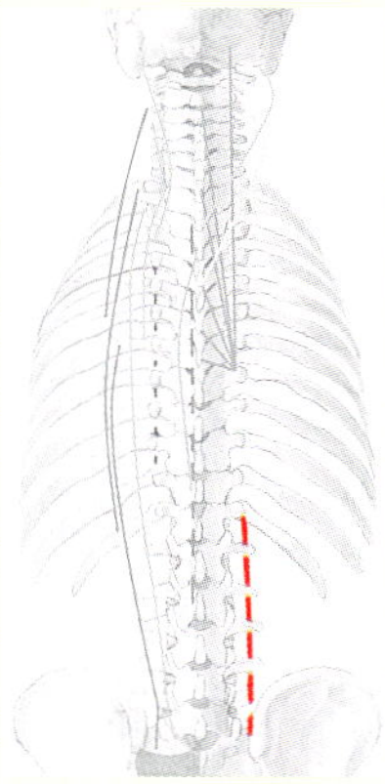

O: Iliac tuberosity, costal process and accessory process of the 5.–1. lumbar vertebra, transverse process of the 12. thoracic vertebra

I: Costal process of the 5.–1. lumbar vertebra, iliac tuberosity

F: Unilateral innervation: lateral flexion,
bilateral innervation: extension

Intertransversarii mediales lumborum
Posterior and anterior branches of the spinal nerves

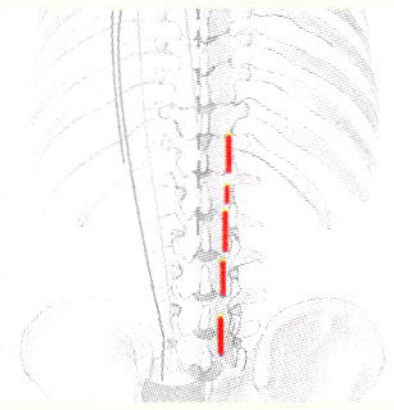

O: Accessory process of the 4.–1. lumbar vertebra

I: Mamillary process of the 5.–2. lumbar vertebra

F: Unilateral innervation: lateral flexion,
bilateral innervation: extension

Intertransversarii thoracis
Posterior and anterior branches of the spinal nerves

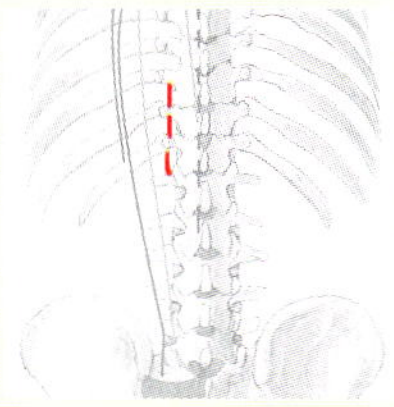

O: Transverse process of the 12.–10. thoracic vertebra

I: Accessory process and mamillary process of the 1. lumbar vertebra up to the transverse process of the 11. thoracic vertebra

F: Unilateral innervation: lateral flexion,
bilateral innervation: extension

Intertransversarii posterios cervicis (Strictly speaking, these muscles are of ventral descent and can therefore not be referred to as autochthonous muscle of the back) *Posterior and anterior branches of the spinal nerves*

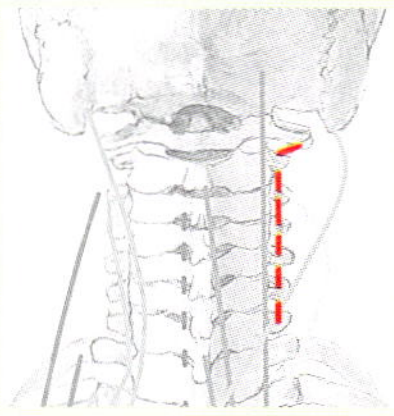

O: Posterior tubercle of the transverse process of the 6.–1. cervical vertebra

I: Posterior tubercle of the transverse process of the 7.–2. cervical vertebra

F: Unilateral innervation: lateral flexion,
bilateral innervation: extension

Intertransversarii anterios cervicis (Strictly speaking, these muscles are of ventral descent and can therefore not be referred to as autochthonous muscle of the back) *Posterior and anterior branches of the spinal nerves*

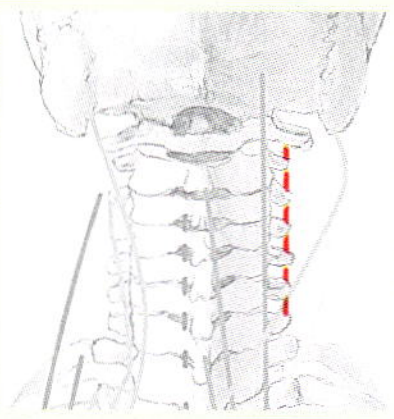

O: Anterior tubercle of the transverse process of the 6.–1. cervical vertebra

I: Anterior tubercle of the transverse process of the 7.–2. cervical vertebra

F: Unilateral innervation: lateral flexion,
bilateral innervation: extension

20 Autochthonous muscles of the back (continuation)

Splenius cervicis
Posterior branches of the cervical nerves

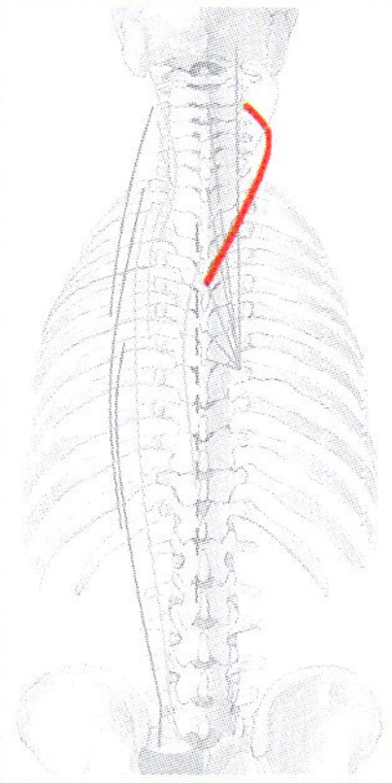

O: Spinous process of the 3. thoracic – 6. cervical vertebra, supraspinous ligament

I: Posterior tubercle of the transverse process of the (3.) 2.–1. cervical vertebra

F: Unilateral innervation: lateral flexion, rotates the cervical part of the vertebral column and the head ipsilaterally, bilateral innervation: extends the cervical part of the vertebral column

Splenius capitis
Posterior branches of the cervical nerves

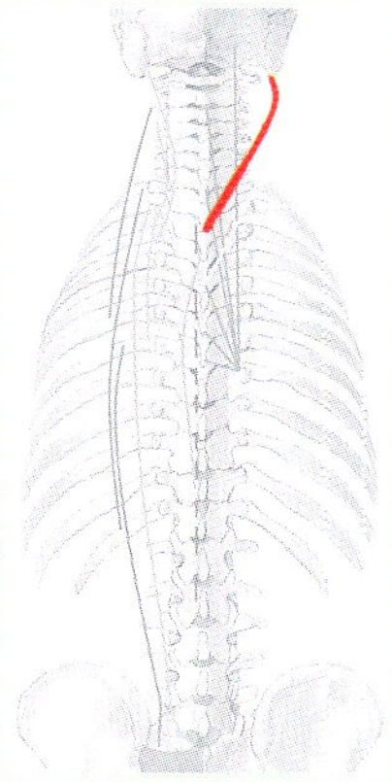

O: Spinous process of the 3.–7. cervical vertebra, ligamentum nuchae

I: Mastoid process (superior nuchal line)

F: Unilateral innervation: lateral flexion, rotates the cervical part of the vertebral column and the head ipsilaterally, bilateral innervation: extends the cervical part of the vertebral column

Levatores costarum (The levatores costarum longi skip one rib, whereas the levatores costarum breves traverse to the adjacent caudal rib. There are no levatores costarum longi in the mid-thoracic part.)
Posterior branches of the cervical nerve [C8] and the thoracic nerves [T1–T10]

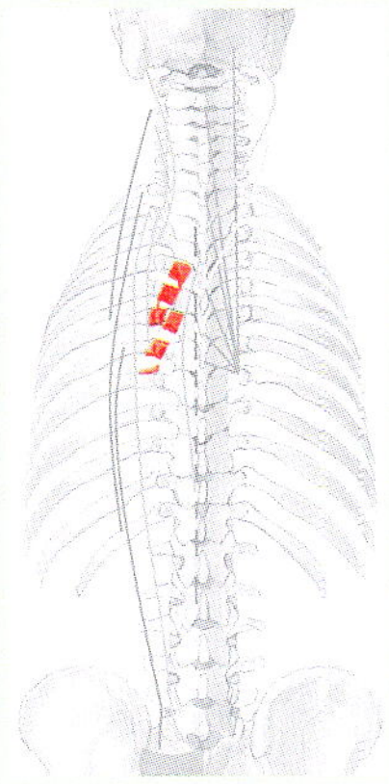

O: Transverse process of the 11. thoracic – 7. cervical vertebra

I: 12.–1. rib laterally to the angle

F: Elevate the ribs, lateral flexion and rotation of the vertebral column

20 Autochthonous muscles of the back (continuation)

b Autochthonous medial muscle of the back (Fig. 529, 532–535, 537, 601)

The medial tract of the autochthonous muscles is located below the lateral tract in the neck and lumbar region and is therefore also referred to as deep part of the autochtonous muscles of the back. The following muscles with longitudinal fibres belong to this tract: The interspinales and the spinalis. The rotatores, the mulfidi and the semispinalis traverse obliquely converging mediocranially (transversospinal).

Interspinales lumborum
Posterior branches of the spinal nerves

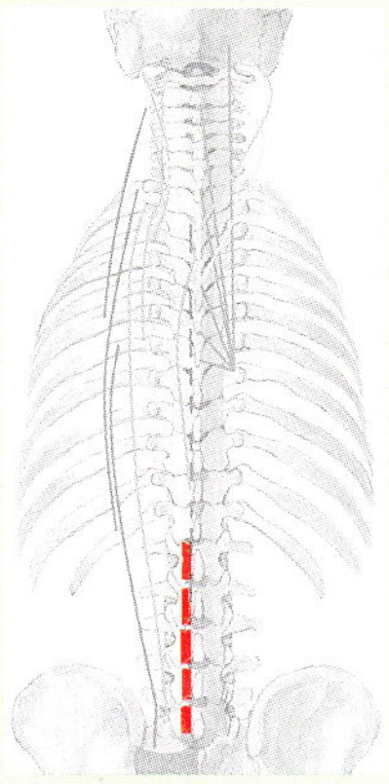

O: Spinous process of the 5.–1. lumbar vertebra

I: Upper margin of the median sacral crest, spinous process of the 5.–2. lumbar vertebra

F: Segmental extension

Interspinales thoracis
Posterior branches of the spinal nerves

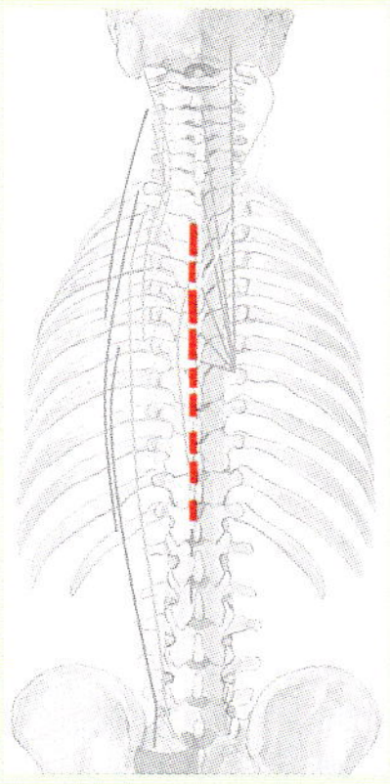

O: Spinous process of the (12.) 11.–2. (1.) thoracic vertebra

I: Spinous process of the (1. lumbar) 12.–3. (2.) thoracic vertebra

F: Segmental extension

Interspinales cervicis
Posterior branches of the spinal nerves

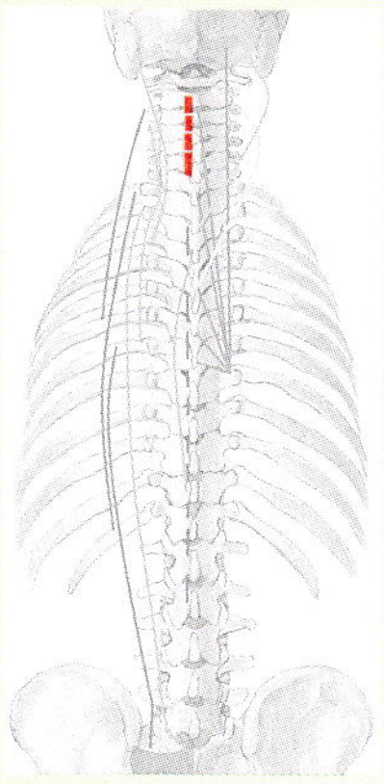

O: Spinous process of the 7.–2. cervical vertebra

I: Spinous process of the 1. thoracic – 3. cervical vertebra

F: Segmental extension

20 Autochthonous muscles of the back (continuation)

Spinalis thoracis (The muscle is tightly attached to the longissimus thoracis at its origin, and to the multifidi at its insertion.)
Posterior branches of the spinal nerves

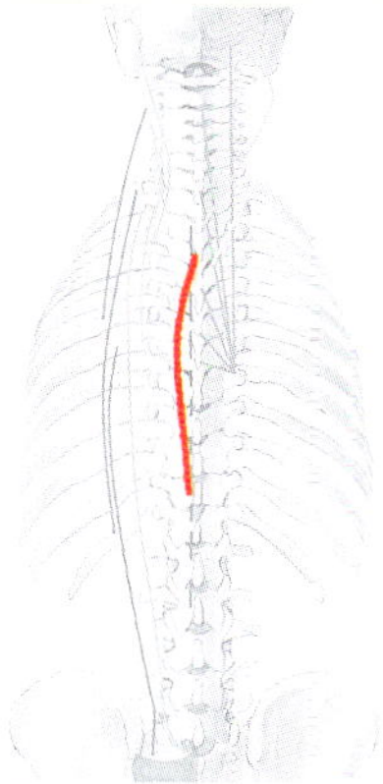

O: Spinous process of the (3.) 2., 1. lumbar and the 12.–10. thoracic vertebra

I: Spinous process of the (10.) 9.–2. thoracic vertebra

F: Unilateral innervation: lateral flexion,
bilateral innervation: extension

Spinalis cervicis
Posterior branches of the spinal nerves

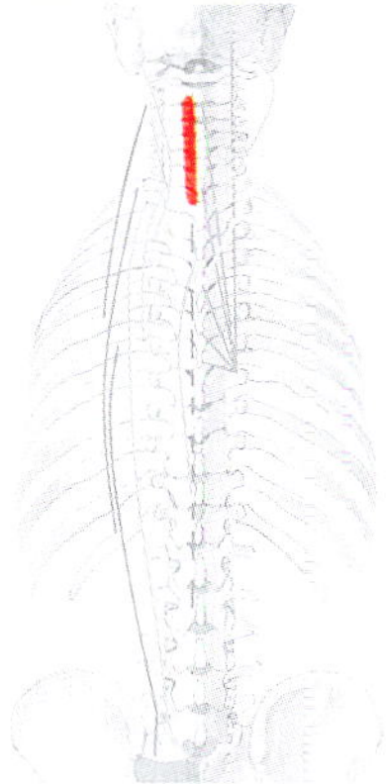

O: Spinous process of the (4.) 3.–1. thoracic and the 7.–6. cervical vertebra

I: Spinous process of the (6.) 5.–2. cervical vertebra

F: Unilateral innervation: lateral flexion,
bilateral innervation: extension

Spinalis capitis (inconstant muscle, tightly attached to the semispinalis capitis at its insertion)
Posterior branches of the spinal nerves

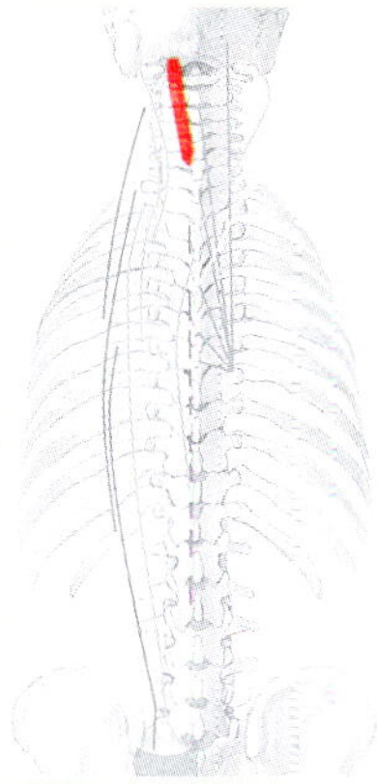

O: Spinous process of the 3.–1. thoracic and the 7.–6. cervical vertebra

I: Squamous part of occipital bone between the highest nuchal line and the superior nuchal line adjacent to the external occipital protuberance

F: Unilateral innervation: lateral flexion,
bilateral innervation: extension

20 Autochthonous muscles of the back (continuation)

Rotatores (They are subdivided into rotatores cervicis, rotatores thoracis and the inconstant rotatores lumborum.
The rotatores breves traverse to the adjacent upper vertebra, whereas the rotatores longi extend to the second next vertebra.)
Posterior branches of the spinal nerves

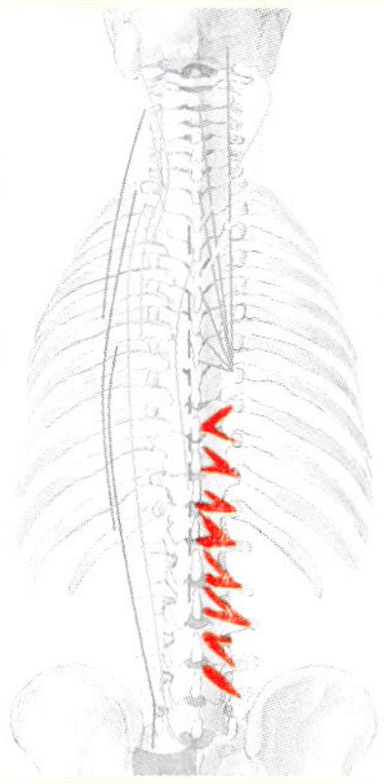

O: Mamillary processes of the lumbar vertebrae, transverse processes of the thoracic vertebrae, inferior articular processes of the cervical vertebrae

I: Root of the spinous process of the 3.–1. lumbar, 12.–1. thoracic and 7.–2. cervical vertebra

F: Unilateral innervation: segmental lateral flexion, rotation,
bilateral innervation: segmental extension

Multifidi (They are particularly well developed in the lumbar part of the vertebral column and skip two to four vertebrae.)
Posterior branches of the spinal nerves

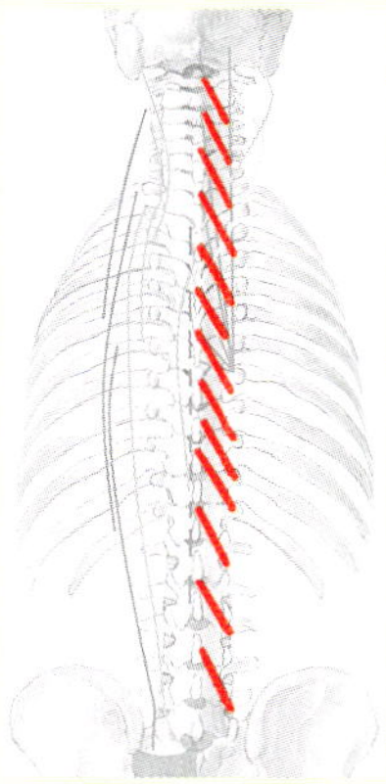

O: Dorsal surface of the sacrum, posterior sacro-iliac ligament, dorsal part of the iliac crest, mamillary processes of the lumbar vertebrae, transverse processes of the thoracic vertebrae, inferior articular process of the 7.–4. cervical vertebra

I: Spinous process of the 5.–1. lumbar vertebra, 12.–1. thoracic and 7.–2. cervical vertebra

F: Unilateral innervation: segmental lateral flexion, rotation,
bilateral innervation: segmental extension

Semispinalis thoracis (Its fibres skip five to seven vertebrae.)
Posterior branches of the spinal nerves

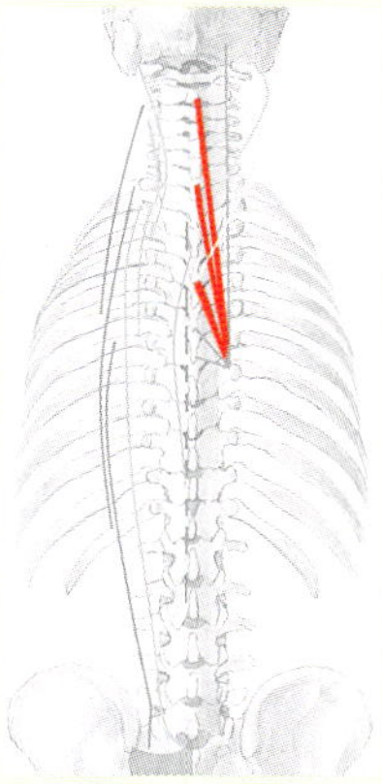

O: Transverse process of the (12.) 11.–7. (6.) thoracic vertebra

I: Spinous process of the (4.) 3. thoracic–6. cervical vertebra

F: Unilateral innervation: rotates the vertebral column and the head contralaterally,
bilateral innervation: extension

20 Autochthonous muscles of the back (continuation)

Semispinalis cervicis *Posterior branches of the spinal nerves*

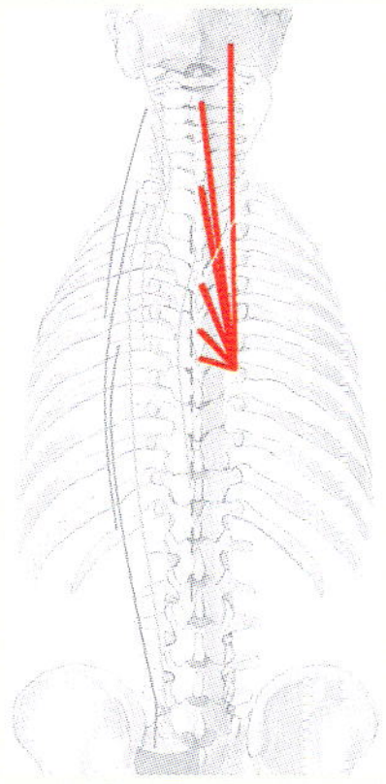

O: Transverse process of the (7.) 6. thoracic–7. cervical vertebra

I: Spinous process of the 6.–3. cervical vertebra

F: Unilateral innervation: rotates the vertebral column and the head contralaterally,
lateral flexion
bilateral innervation: extension

Semispinalis capitis *Posterior branches of the spinal nerves*

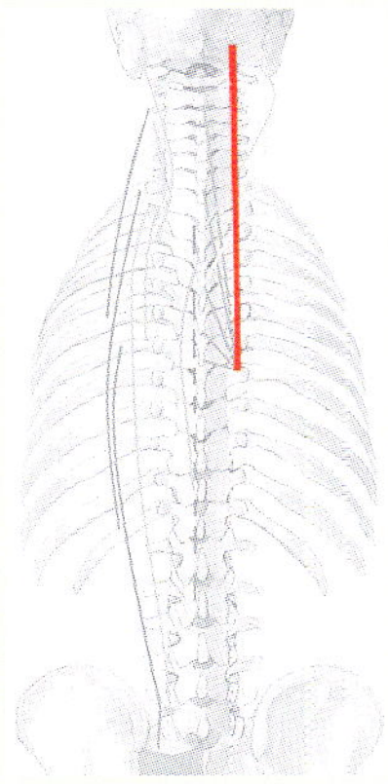

O: Transverse process of the (8.) 7. thoracic–3. cervical vertebra

I: Squamous part of occipital bone between the highest nuchal line and the superior nuchal line, medial area

F: Unilateral innervation: rotates the vertebral column and the head contralaterally,
lateral flexion
bilateral innervation: extension

c Autochthonous deep muscles of the neck (Fig. 532, 533, 535, 536, 538)

The recti capitis posterior minor et major and the obliqui capitis superior and inferior belong to the medial tract of the autochthonous muscles of the back, whereas the rectus capitis lateralis belongs to the lateral tract.

Rectus capitis posterior major *Suboccipital nerve (dorsal branch of the cervical nerve [C1])*

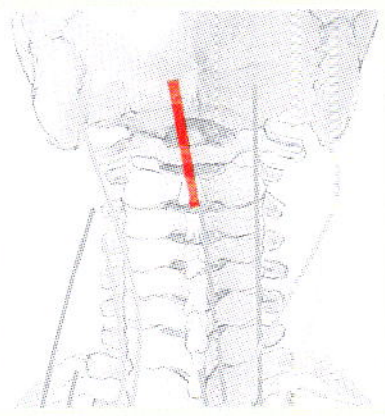

O: Spinous process of the axis

I: Middle third of the inferior nuchal line

F: Unilateral innervation: rotates and flexes the head ipsilaterally,
bilateral innervation: participates in the fine tuning of the position and the movement in the craniocervical joints, extension

Rectus capitis posterior minor *Suboccipital nerve (dorsal branch of the cervical nerve [C1])*

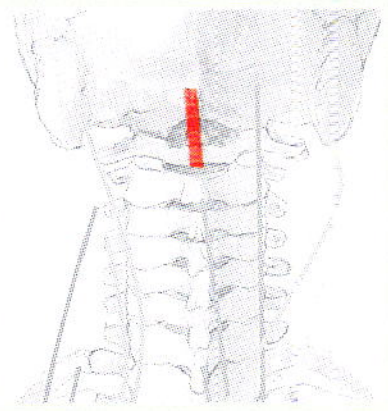

O: Posterior tubercle of the posterior arch of the atlas

I: Medial third of the inferior nuchal line

F: Unilateral innervation: flexes the head ipsilaterally,
bilateral innervation: participates in the fine tuning of the position and the movement in the craniocervical joints, extension

20 Autochthonous muscles of the back (continuation)

Obliquus capitis superior
Suboccipital nerve (dorsal branch of the cervical nerve [C1])

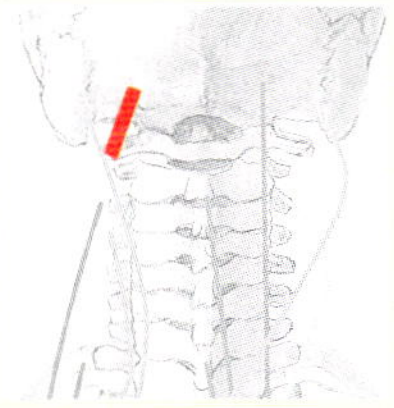

O: Posterior tubercle of the transverse process of the atlas

I: Lateral third of the inferior nuchal line

F: Unilateral innervation: flexes the head ipsilaterally, bilateral innervation: participates in the fine tuning of the position and the movement in the craniocervical joints, extension

Obliquus capitis inferior
Suboccipital nerve (dorsal branch of the cervical nerve [C1])

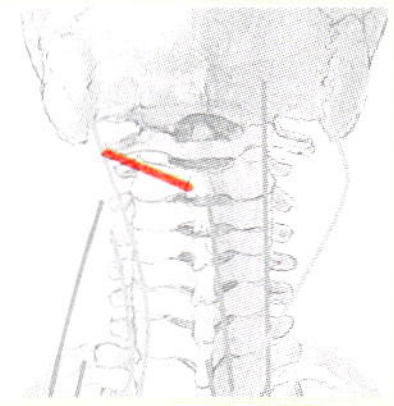

O: Spinous process of the axis

I: Posterior margin of the transverse process of the atlas

F: Unilateral innervation: rotates the atlas (and the head) ipsilaterally, bilateral innervation: participates in the fine tuning of the position and the movement in the craniocervical joints, extension

Rectus capitis lateralis
Vertical branches of the cervical nerve [C1]

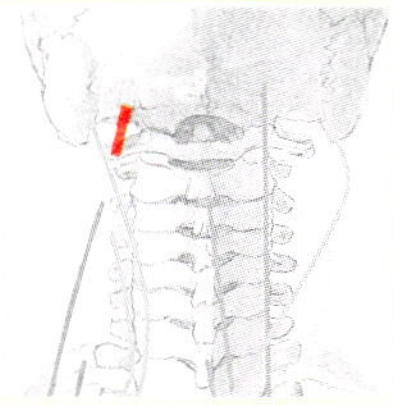

O: Anterior margin of the transverse process of the atlas

I: Jugular process of the occipital bone

F: Unilateral innervation: flexes the head ipsilaterally, bilateral innervation: participates in the fine tuning of the position and the movement in the craniocervical joints

21 Diaphragm (Fig. 578, 538–585)

The diaphragm divides the thoracic and the abdominal cavity. Its "domes" form the floor of the right and left pleural cavity. The lumbar part delineates the retroperitoneal space dorsally and constitutes a part of the dorsal abdominal wall.

Diaphragm
Phrenic nerve (cervical plexus)

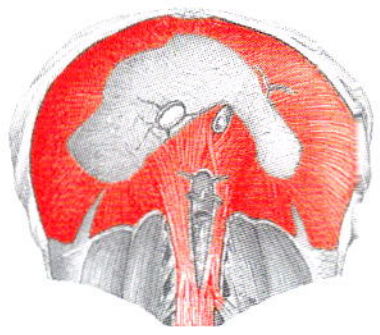

O: Sternal part: Inner surface of the xiphoid process, rectus sheath
Costal part: Inner surface of the costal cartilage of the 12.–6. rib, serrated with indentations of the transversus abdominis
Lumbar part, right crus:
- medial part: body of the 3.–1. lumbar vertebra, intervertebral discs
- lateral part: medial arcuate ligament (psoas arcade) and lateral arcuate ligament (quadratus arcade)

Lumbar part, left crus:
- medial part: body of the 4.–1. lumbar vertebra, intervertebral discs
- lateral part: medial arcuate ligament (psoas arcade) and lateral arcuate ligament (quadratus arcade)

I: All parts merge in the central tendon

F: Diaphragmatic breathing (inspiration), compresses the abdomen

Passages and weak points in the diaphragm

Name	Location	Structures
Aortic hiatus	Lumbar part, between right/left crus and vertebral column	Aorta; thoracic duct
Oesophageal hiatus	Lumbar part, left crus near the midline	Oesophagus; vagal nerves; left phrenicoabdominal branch
Caval opening	Central tendon	Inferior vena cava; right phrenic nerve; right phrenicoabdominal branch
Sternocostal triangle [LARREY's cleft]	Between costal part and lumbar part	Artery; superior epigastric vein
Lumbocostal triangle	Between sternal part and costal part	
Unnamed	Lumbar part, right/left crus, (medial part)	Greater and lesser splanchnic nerve; azygos vein; hemi-azygos vein
Unnamed	Lumbar part, between (medial part) and lateral part	Sympathetic trunk
Unnamed	Central tendon	Left phrenic nerve, left phrenico-abdominal branch

22 Pelvic and urogenital diaphragm (Fig. 901–908, 1065)

Two partially overlapping muscle layers form the floor of the pelvic cavity. The levator ani, the ischiococcygeus and the external anal sphincter form the pelvic diaphragm.
The urogenital diaphragm stretches a triangular plate between both lower rami of the pubic bone. Its fibres are transversally orientated and support the urogenital hiatus. Among others the deep transverse perineal muscle, the urethral sphincter (together they are referred to as compressor urethrae) and the superficial transverse perineal muscle belong to the urogenital diaphragm.
In the male, the urogenital diaphragm is only passed by the urethra, whereas in the female, both the vagina and the urethra pass through.

a Pelvic diaphragm

Levator ani (It consists of the pubococcygeus and the iliococcygeus. The fibres of the levator prostatae, pubovaginalis and puborectalis originate from the pubococcygeus.)
Branches of the sacral nerve [S3 and S4]

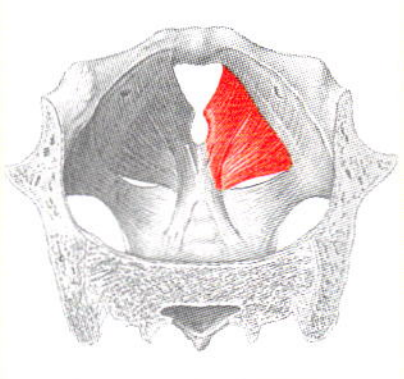

O: Pubococcygeus: Inner surface of the pubic bone near the symphysis, anterior two thirds of the tendinous arch of levator ani, ischiadic spine
Iliococcygeus: Posterior third of the tendinous arch of levator ani

I: Perineal body (prerectal fibres), in the male the fascia of the prostrate (levator prostatae), in the female the wall of the vagina (pubovaginalis) radiates into the external anal sphincter, forms a loop with the contralateral fibres just behind the anus (puborectalis), anococcygeal body, coccyx

F: Spans around the rectum from posterior,
supports the external anal sphincter to close the rectum,
the medial free margin forms the urogenital hiatus, which allows the urethra in the male and both the urethra and the vagina in the female to pass through

Ischiococcygeus
Branches of the sacral nerve [S4 and S5]

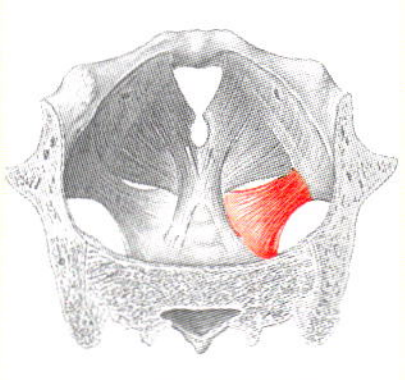

O: Inner surface of the ischiadic spine, predominantly attached to the sacrospinous ligament

I: Lateral margin of the lower segments of the sacrum, coccyx

F: Supports the pelvic diaphragm

External anal sphincter (muscular loop with a ring-like shape up to the levator ani)
Pudendal nerve (sacral plexus)

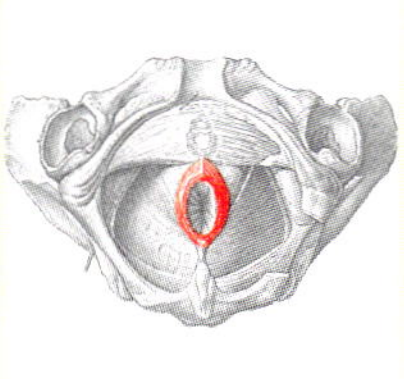

O: Subcutanous part: Dermis and subculaneous tissues surrounding the anus
Superficial part: Perineal body
Deep part: Ring-like muscle

I: Dermis and subcutaneous tissues surrounding the anus, anococcygeal ligament

F: Closure of the anus

22 Pelvic and urogenital diaphragm (continuation)

b Urogenital diaphragm

Deep transverse perineal muscle (It is a triangular supportive muscular layer interwoven with connective tissue with openings for the urethra in the male and for both the urethra and the vagina in the female. It spans obliquely over the pubic arch and subpubic angle, respectively, and is supplemented by the inferior pubic ligament and the deep transverse perineal ligament.)
Pudendal nerve (sacral plexus)

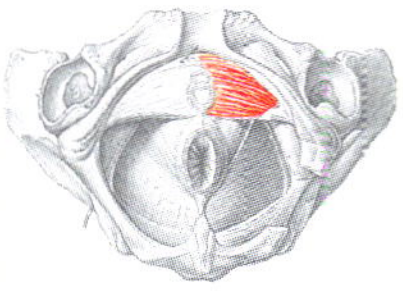

O: Inferior pubic ramus, ramus of ischium, connective tissue envelop of the internal pudendal vessels

I: Perineal body fasciae of the prostate and the vaginal wall

F: Supports the urogenital hiatus, seals the urethra (and the urinary bladder)

Urethral sphincter (muscular traction enveloping the membranous urethra in a ring-like fashion)
Pudendal nerve (sacral plexus)

see Fig. 1174, 1175

O: Ring-like muscle, transverse perineal ligament, fibres from the deep transverse perineal muscle

I: Connective tissue surrounding the urethra (membranous part), contralateral deep transverse perineal muscle, vaginal wall (sphincter urethrovaginalis)

F: Supports the urogenital hiatus, part of the continence organ of the urinary bladder, seals the urinary bladder during ejaculation

Superficial transverse perineal muscle (inconstant muscle)
Pudendal nerve (sacral plexus)

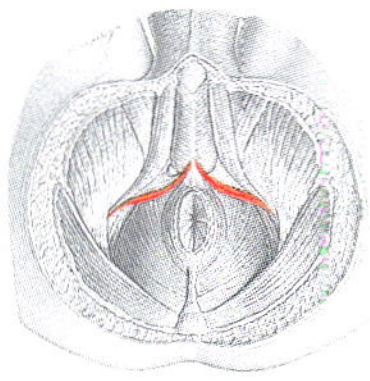

O: Superficial division of the deep transverse perineal muscle, ischial tuberosity

I: Perineal body

F: Supports the deep transverse perineal muscle

Ischiocavernosus
Pudendal nerve (sacral plexus)

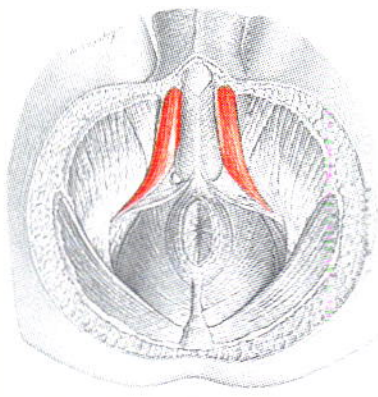

O: Ramus of ischium

I: Tunica albuginea corporum cavernosorum

F: Fixes the crura of penis in the male, and the crura of clitoris in the female to the inferior pubic ramus, as well as to the ramus of the ischium and the urogenital diaphragm, supports the ejaculation and the orgasm, respectively

Bulbospongiosus (spans around the bulb of penis in the male, and around the bulb of vestibule in the female)
Pudendal nerve (sacral plexus)

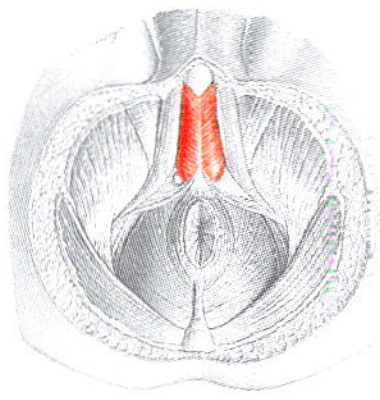

O: Perineal body, in the male additional origin from the raphe of penis at the lower surface of the corpus spongiosum penis

I: In the male, it inserts laterally to the corpus spongiosum penis into the inferior urogenital fascia and the back of the penis; in the female, the fibres are attached to the corpus cavernosum clitoridis and the inferior fascia of urogenital diaphragm

F: In the male, it fixes the bulb of penis to the urogenital diaphragm, and is involved in the ejaculation; in the female, it fixes the bulb of vestibule to the urogenital diaphragm and supports the orgasm

23 Joints of the upper limb (Fig. 276)

a Joints of the shoulder girdle

Name of the joint	Type of the joint	Movements
Sternoclavicular joint	Irregular joint surface functionally: spheroideal joint (distinct feature: articular disc)	Rotation along a sagittal axis (as in raising the shoulder), rotation along a longitudinal axis (as in protraction and retraction of the shoulder), rotation along the longitudinal axis of the clavicle (as in swinging the arm)
Acromioclavicular joint	Plane joint, functionally: spheroideal joint (distinct feature: variable, frequently incomplete articular disc)	Rotation along a sagittal axis (as in raising the shoulder), rotation along a transverse axis (as in swinging the arm), rotation along a longitudinal axis (as in protraction and retraction of the shoulder)

b Joints of the free part of the upper limb

Name of the joint	Type of the joint	Movements
Shoulder joint	Spheroideal joint	Protraction (flexion, anteversion) Retraction (extension, retroversion) Abduction Adduction Medial rotation Lateral rotation (Circumduction: combining flexion, abduction, extension, adduction)
Elbow joint,		
a) Humero-ulnar joint	Hinge joint	Flexion Extension
b) Humeroradial joint	Spheroideal joint (with functional restriction: no abduction)	Flexion Extension Rotation
c) Proximal radio-ulnar joint	Pivot joint	Pronation and supination of the hand
Distal radio-ulnar joint	Pivot joint	
Wrist joints		
a) Wrist joint	Ellipsoid joint	Lateral movements of the hand (ulnar and radial abduction)
b) Midcarpal joint	Hinge joint	Flexion Extension
Carpometacarpal joint of the thumb	Sellar joint	Abduction Adduction Opposition Reposition
Carpometacarpal joints (II–V)	Plane joints	Various distinct movements
Metacarpophalangeal joints	Spheroideal joints (with functional restrictions)	Flexion Extension Abduction* Adduction* (*with regard to the middle finger)
Interphalangeael joints of the fingers	Hinge joints	Flexion Extension

23 Joints of the upper limb (continuatioin)

c Planes and axes of the movements of the joints of the upper limb

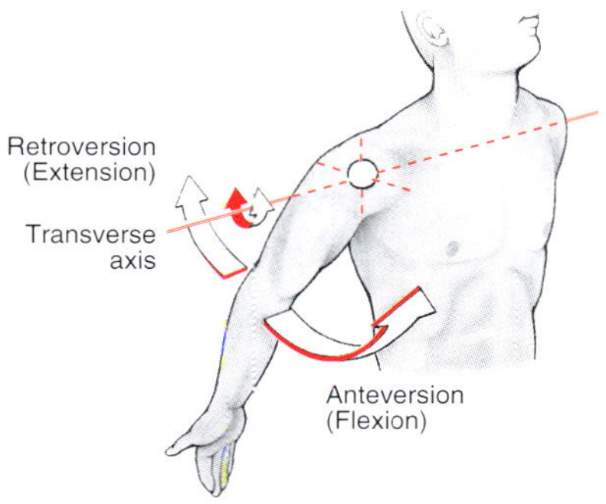

Fig. 1 Shoulder joint;
movements in the sagittal plane.

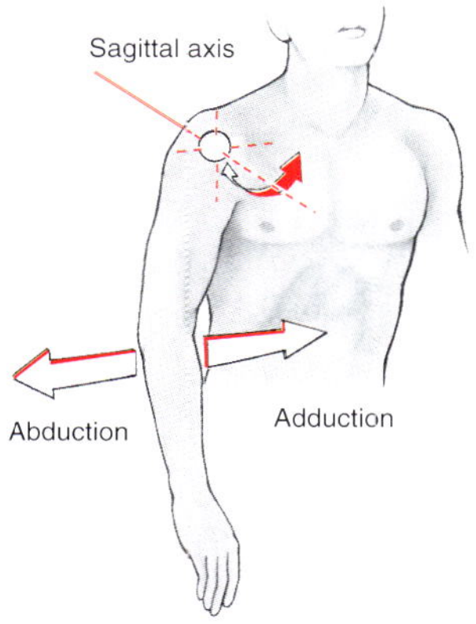

Fig. 2 Shoulder joint;
movements in the frontal plane.

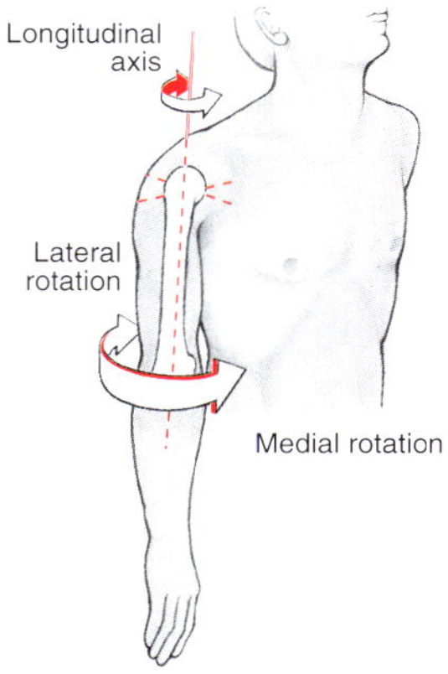

Fig. 3 Shoulder joint;
movements in the transverse plane.

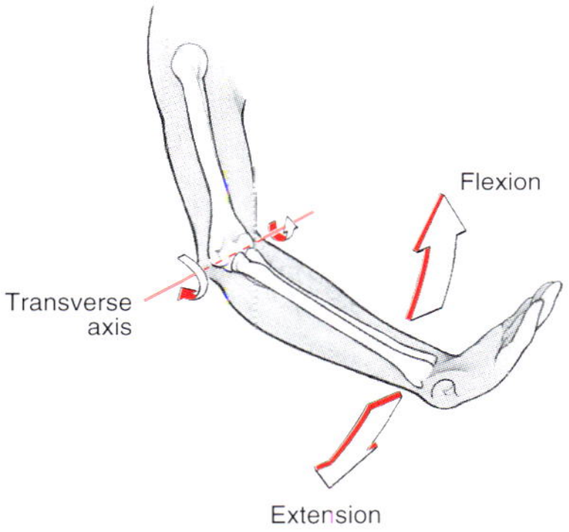

Fig. 4 Elbow joint;
movements in the sagittal plane.

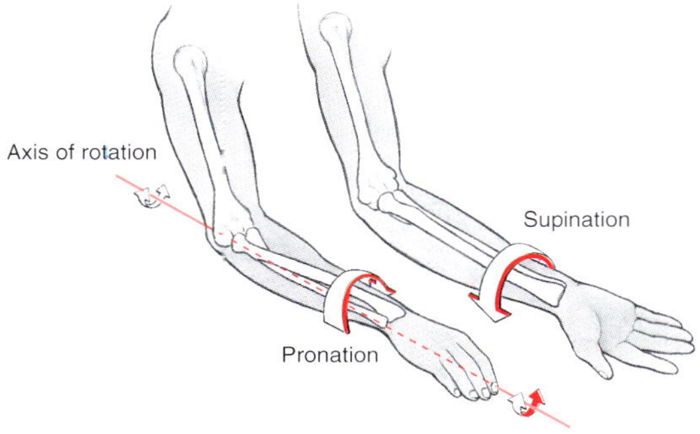

Fig. 5 Elbow joint;
pronation and supination of the hand.

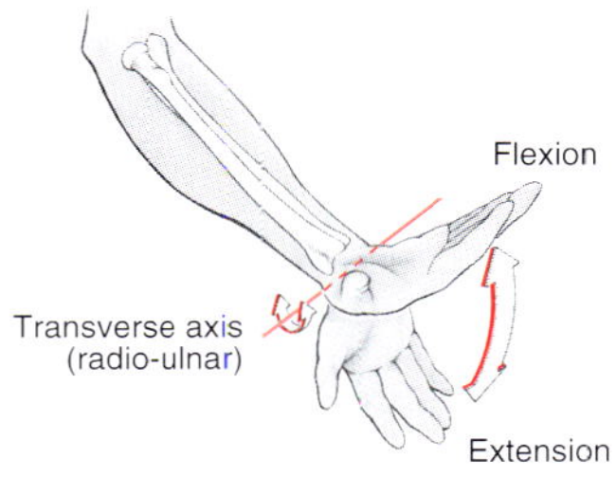

Fig. 6 Wrist joint;
movements in the sagittal plane

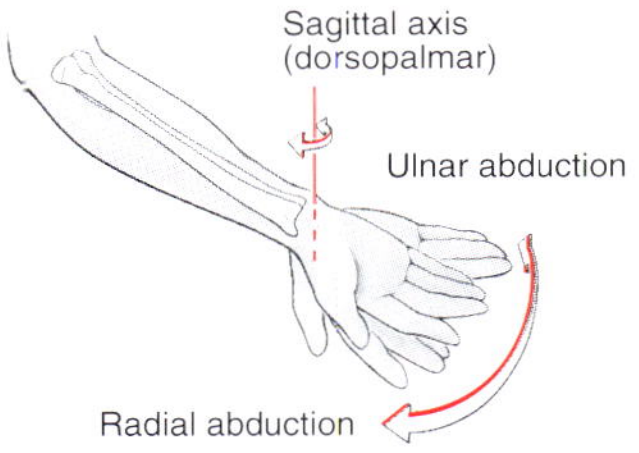

Fig. 7 Wrist joint;
movements in the frontal plane.

With regard to the wrist joints, palmar flexion is also referred to as flexion and dorsal flexion as extension.

24 Branches and supplying areas of the brachial plexus (Fig. 386–395, 397, 398, 400, 401, 403, 404)

	Motor function	Sensory function
Brachial plexus [C5] C4–T1 [T2]		
Dorsal scapular nerve [C3] C4, C5	Levator scapulae, rhomboid muscles	
Suprascapular nerve C4–C6	Supraspinatus, infraspinatus	
Subscapular nerve C5–C7	Subscapularis (teres major)	
Subclavian nerve [C4] C5, C6	Subclavius	
Long thoracic nerve C5–C7 [C8]	Serratus anterior	
Pectoral nerves C8–T1	Pectoralis major, pectoralis minor	
Thoracodorsal nerve C6–C8	Latissimus dorsi, teres major	
Muscular branches	Longus colli, longus capitis	
Musculocutaneous nerve C5–C7	Coracobrachialis, biceps brachii, brachialis	Skin of radiopalmar side of the forearm
Median nerve C6–T1	Pronator teres, flexor carpi radialis, palmaris longus, flexor digitorum superficialis, flexor pollicis longus, flexor digitorum profundus (radial portion), pronator quadratus, flexor pollicis brevis (superficial head), opponens pollicis, lumbricals I, II	Skin of the radial part of the palm ($3^1/_2$ fingers), skin of the dorsal side of the distal phalanx ($3^1/_2$ fingers)
Ulnar nerve C6–T1	Flexor carpi ulnaris, flexor digitorum profundus (ulnar portion), palmaris brevis, flexor digiti minimi, opponens digiti minimi, abductor digiti minimi, flexor pollicis brevis (deep head), adductor pollicis, lumbricals III, IV, interossei	Skin of the ulnar side of the hand (palmar: $1^1/_2$ fingers, dorsal $2\,^1/_2$ fingers), skin of the dorsal side of the distal phalanx ($1^1/_2$ fingers)
Medial cutaneous nerve of arm C8–T1 [T2]		Skin of the mediopalmar side of the arm
Medial cutaneous nerve of forearm C8–T1		Skin of the ulnopalmar side of the forearm
Axillary nerve C5–C7	Deltoid, teres minor	Skin of the shoulder
Radial nerve C5–T1	Triceps brachii, anconeus, brachioradialis, extensor carpi radialis longus, extensor carpi radialis brevis, supinator, extensor digitorum, extensor pollicis longus, abductor pollicis longus, extensor pollicis brevis, extensor indicis, extensor carpi ulnaris	Skin of the dorsal side of the arm, forearm and hand ($2^1/_2$ radial fingers with the exception of the distal phalanges)

25 Segmental innervation of the muscles of the upper limb, muscles of diagnostic importance

(According to MUMENTHALER and SCHLIACK; the indicator muscle of each sement is printed in bold.)

Supraspinatus	C4–C5	Abductor pollicis longus	C6–C8
Teres minor	C4–C5	Extensor pollicis brevis	C7–T1
Deltoid: C5	C5–C6	Extensor pollicis longus	C6–C8
Infraspinatus	C4–C6	Extensor digitorum	C6–C8
Subscapularis	C5–C6	Extensor indicis	C6–C8
Teres major	C5–C7	Extensor carpi ulnaris	C6–C8
Biceps brachii: C6	C5–C6	Extensor digiti minimi	C6–C8
Brachialis	C5–C6	Flexor digitorum superficialis	C7–T1
Coracobrachialis	C5–C7	Flexor digitorum profundus	C7–T1
Triceps brachii: C7	C6–C8	Flexor carpi ulnaris	C7–T1
Brachioradialis	C5–C6	Abductor pollicis brevis	C7–T1
Extensor carpi radialis longus	C5–C7	Flexor pollicis brevis	C7–T1
Extensor carpi radialis brevis	C5–C7	Opponens pollicis	C6–C7
Supinator	C5–C6	Flexor digiti minimi	C7–T1
Pronator teres	C6–C7	Adductor pollicis	C8–T1
Flexor carpi radialis	C6–C7	**Abductor digiti minimi: C8**	C8–T1
Flexor pollicis longus	C6–C8	**Interossei: C8**	C8–T1

26 Ventral muscles of the shoulder (Fig. 338, 340, 341, 343, 344, 569–571)

The pectoralis major spans from the trunk to the upper limb and moulds the surface anatomy of the anterior upper thoracic wall. Below, the pectoralis minor can be found, which together with the subclavius belongs to the muscles spanning from the trunk to the shoulder girdle. Only the subscapularis is located in direct contact to the shoulder joint, spanning from the anterior surface of the scapula to the humerus.

Pectoralis major (Its fibres converge laterally into a broad, flat tendon shaped like a bag with its opening to the top.)
Medial and lateral pectoral nerves (brachial plexus, infra-/supraclavicular part)

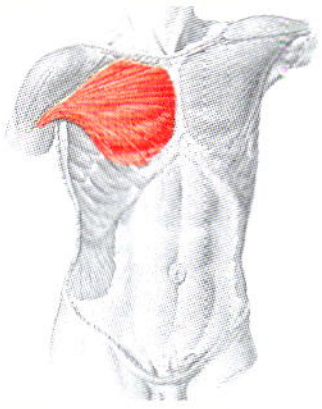

O: Clavicular part: Sternal half of the clavicle
Sternocostal part: Manubrium and body of sternum, costal cartilage of the 1.–7. rib
Abdominal part: Anterior layer of the rectus sheath

I: Crest of greater tubercle of the humerus

F: Shoulder joint:
adduction, particularly effective when the arm is elevated,
medial rotation,
clavicular part: anteversion
Shoulder girdle:
depression,
anteversion
Thorax:
elevates the sternum and the upper ribs when the shoulders are fixed (supports inspiration)

Pectoralis minor
Medial and lateral pectoral nerves (brachial plexus, infra-/supraclavicular part)

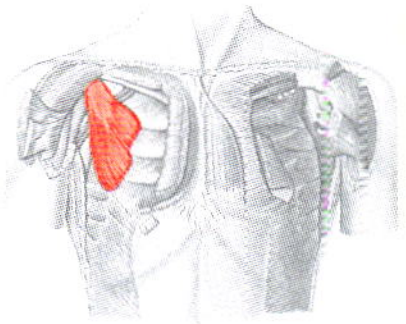

O: (2.) 3.–5. rib close to the junction between cartilage and bone

I: Tip of the coracoid process

F: Shoulder girdle:
depression
Thorax:
elevates the sternum and the upper ribs (supports inspiration)

Subclavius (The fascia of the subclavius is attached to the adventitia of the subclavian vein, thus preventing collapse of its lumen.)
Subclavian nerve (brachial plexus, supraclavicular part)

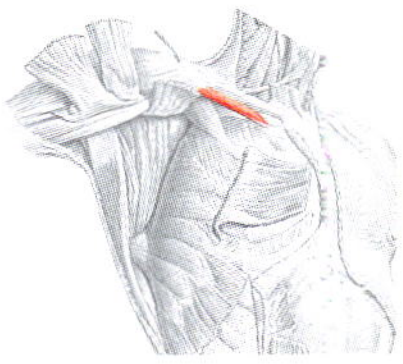

O: Junction between cartilage and bone of the 1. rib

I: Lateral third of the clavicle

F: Shoulder girdle:
depression (with low effectiveness),
antagonizes laterally-directed traction on the clavicle

26 Ventral muscles of the shoulder (continuation)

Subscapularis (The subtendinous bussa of subscapularis lies below the muscle close to its insertion.)
Subscapular nerves (brachial plexus, infraclavicular part)

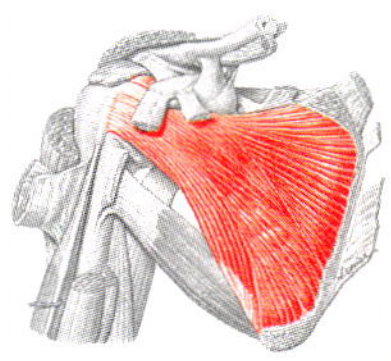

O: Subscapular fossa

I: Lesser tubercle and adjacent part of the crest of lesser tubercle

F: Shoulder joint:
medial rotation,
abduction in the scapular plane (cranial portion),
adduction in the scapular plane (caudal portion)

27 Latral muscles of the shoulder (Fig. 337, 340–345)

The deltoid plays a major role in determining the surface contour of the shoulder. Divided by the subdeltoid bursa, the tendon of the supraspinatus is located directly below the deltoid.

Deltoid
Axillary nerve (brachial plexus, infraclavicular part)

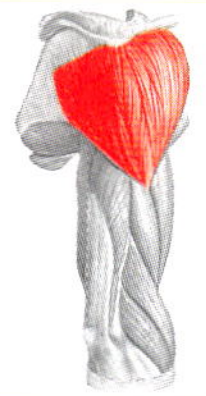

O: Clavicular part: acrominal third of the clavicle
Acromial part: Acromion
Spinal part: lower margin of the spine of scapula

I: Deltoid tuberosity

F: Shoulder joint:
Clavicular part: adduction (from about 60° increasing abduction),
medial rotation,
anteversion
Acromial part: abduction up to the horizontal plane
Spinal part: adduction (from about 60° increasing abduction),
lateral rotation,
retroversion
All parts: carry the weight of the arm

Supraspinatus
Suprascapular nerve (brachial plexus, supraclavicular part)

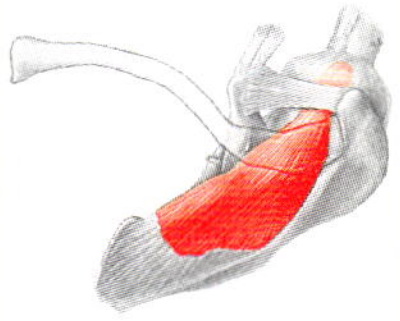

O: Supraspinous fossa, supraspinous fascia

I: Proximal facet of the greater tubercle

F: Shoulder joint:
abduction in the scapular plane up to the horizontal plane,
lateral rotation

28 Dorsal muscles of the shoulder (Fig. 339–341, 343, 344)

The infraspinatus is located most cranially. More caudally are the teres minor and the teres major.
The latissimus dorsi comes from the back (see Tab. 18, trunk-arm muscles) and runs along with the teres major.

Infraspinatus
Suprascapular nerve (brachial plexus, supraclavicular part)

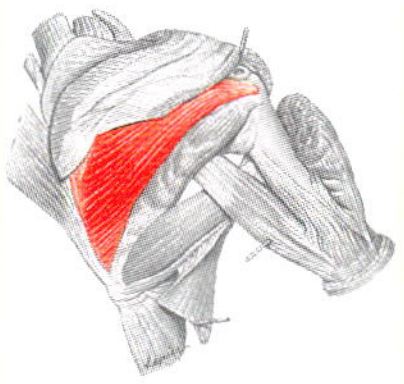

O: Caudal margin of the spine of scapula, infraspinous fossa, infraspinous fascia

I: Middle facet of the greater tubercle

F: Shoulder joint:
cranial portion: lateral rotation, abduction in the scapular plane
caudal portion: lateral rotation, adduction in the scapular plane

28 Dorsal muscles of the shoulder (continuation)

Teres minor *Axillary nerve (brachial plexus, infraclavicular part)*

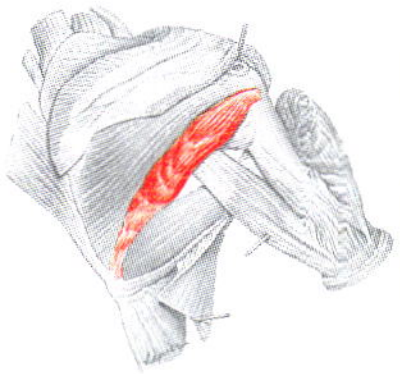

O: Caudal portion of the infraspinous fossa, medial third of the lateral border

I: Distal posterior facet of the greater tubercle

F: Shoulder joint: lateral rotation, adduction in the scapular plane

Teres major (At the insertion, the teres major and latissimus dorsi are separated by the subtendinous bursa of latissimus dorsi.)
Suprascapular nerves or thoracodorsal nerve (brachial plexus, infraclavicular part)

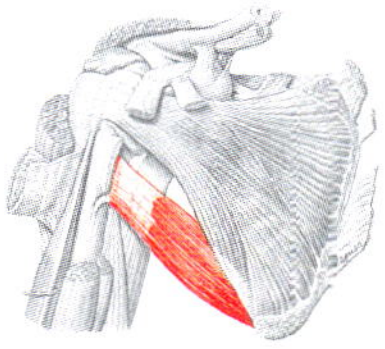

O: Lateral border, inferior angle

I: Crest of lesser tubercle medially to the latissimus dorsi

F: Shoulder joint: medial rotation, adduction in the scapular plane

29 Ventral muscles of the arm (Fig. 343, 344, 347–350)

The biceps brachii determines the surface anatomy of the ventral arm. The coracobrachialis is directly attached to the short head of the biceps brachii. The brachialis is located most deeply.

Biceps brachii (The tendon of the long head traverses directly the shoulder joint. The bicipitoradial bursa is located at its insertion at the radial tuberosity.)
Musculocutaneous nerve (brachial plexus, infraclavicular part)

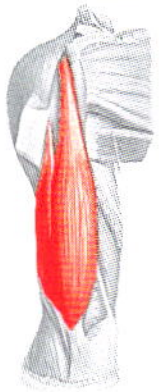

O: **Long head:** Supraglenoid tubercle, glenoid labrum
Short head: Tip of the coracoid process lateral to the coracobrachialis

I: Radial tuberosity via the bicipital aponeurosis at the antebrachial fascia

F: Shoulder joint:
Long head: abduction, anteversion, medial rotation
Short head: adduction, anteversion, medial rotation
Both parts: carry the weight of the arm
Elbow joint: flexion, supination

Coracobrachialis (Normally this muscle is penetrated by the musculocutaneous nerve.)
Musculocutaneous nerve (brachial plexus, infraclavicular part)

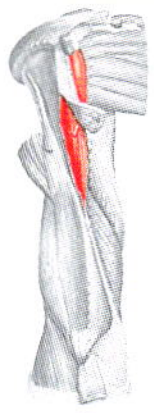

O: Tip of the coracoid process medial to the short head of the biceps brachii

I: Anterior surface of the humerus mediodistal to the crest of lesser tubercle

F: Shoulder joint: medial rotation, adduction, anteversion

Brachialis *Musculocutaneous nerve (brachial plexus, infraclavicular part)*

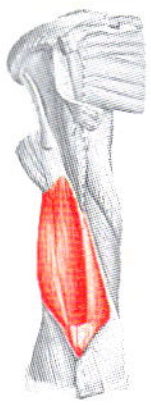

O: Anterior surface of the humerus distal to the deltoid tuberosity

I: Tuberosity of ulna

F: Elbow joint: flexion

30 **Dorsal muscles of the arm** (Fig. 342–344, 346, 351)

The three heads of the triceps brachii determine the surface anatomy of the dorsal arm. The anconeus can be considered as a continuation of the medial head of the triceps brachii to the forearm.

Triceps brachii (The fibres of the long head traverse in longitudinal direction, and those of the medial head and the lateral head in an oblique direction; a common broad aponeurosis is found at the insertion.)
Radial nerve (brachial plexus, infraclavicular part)

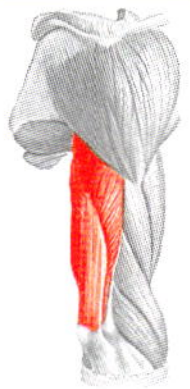	**O: Long head:** Infraglenoid tubercle, lower margin of the glenoid labrum **Medial head:** Posterior surface of the humerus mediodistal to the radial groove, medial intermuscular septum of arm **Lateral head:** Posterior surface of the humerus lateroproximal to the radial groove, proximal two thirds of the lateral intermuscular septum of arm	**I:** Olecranon	**F:** Shoulder joint: **Long head:** adduction, support of the weight of the arm Elbow joint: extension

Anconeus (It is closely positioned to the medial head of the triceps brachii.)
Radial nerve (brachial plexus, infraclavicular part)

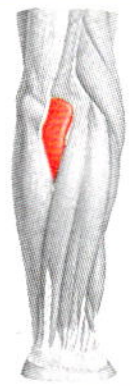	**O:** Lateral epicondyle of the humerus, capsule of the elbow joint, radial collateral ligament	**I:** Posterior surface of the ulna just distal to the olecranon	**F:** Elbow joint: extension

31 Superficial ventral muscles of the forearm (Fig. 352, 353, 355–359, 373)

The group of the superficial ventral muscles of the forearm consists of the following muscles in the order from radial to ulnar: pronator teres, flexor carpi radialis, palmaris longus, flexor digitorum superficialis and flexor carpi ulnaris.

Pronator teres
Median nerve (brachial plexus, infraclavicular part)

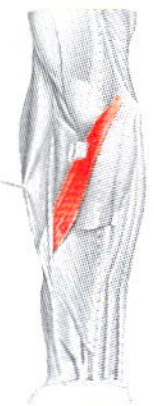

O: Humeral head: Medial epicondyle of the humerus, medial intermuscular septum of arm
Ulnar head: Medial surface of the ulna distal to the coronoid process

I: Middle third of the lateral surface of the radius

F: Elbow joint:
Humeral head: pronation, flexion
Ulnar head: pronation

Flexor carpi radialis
Median nerve (brachial plexus, infraclavicular part)

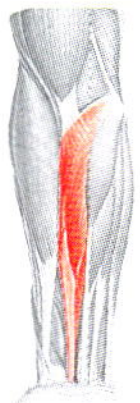

O: Medial epicondyle of the humerus, antebrachial fascia

I: Palmar surface of the base of the metacarpal II (frequently also III)

F: Elbow joint:
flexion,
pronation
Wrist joint:
palmar flexion,
radial abduction

Palmaris longus (inconstant muscle.)
Median nerve (brachial plexus, infraclavicular part)

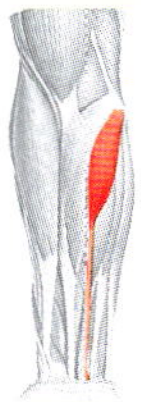

O: Medial epicondyle of the humerus, antebrachial fascia

I: Palmar aponeurosis

F: Elbow joint:
flexion,
Wrist joint:
palmar flexion,
tension of the palmar aponeurosis

Flexor digitorum superficialis (The tendons of this muscle are perforated by the tendons of the flexor digitorum profundus just before their insertion.)
Median nerve (brachial plexus, infraclavicular part)

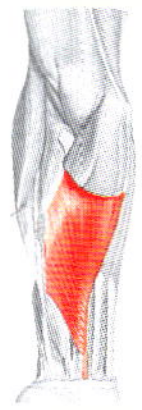

O: Humero-ulnar head: Medial epicondyle of the humerus, coronoid process
Radial head: Anterior surface of the radius distal to the pronator teres

I: With four long tendons at the base of the middle phalanx of the 2.–5. finger

F: Elbow joint:
flexion
Wrist joint:
palmar flexion,
ulnar abduction
Metacarpophalangeal joints (II–V):
flexion,
adduction
Proximal finger joints (II–V):
flexion

Flexor carpi ulnaris
Ulnar nerve (brachial plexus, infraclavicular part)

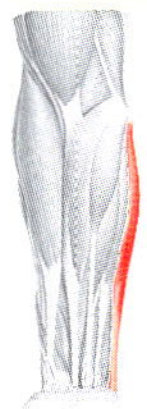

O: Humeral head: Medial epicondyle of the humerus, medial intermuscular septum of arm
Ulnar head: Olecranon, upper two thirds of the posterior border of the ulna, antebrachial fascia

I: Via the pisiform and the pisometacarpal ligament and pisohamate ligament at the base of metacarpal V and the hamate

F: Elbow joint:
flexion,
Wrist joint:
palmar flexion,
ulnar abduction

32 Deep ventral muscles of the forearm (Fig. 352, 354, 355, 359, 360, 370, 371, 374)

The flexor digitorum profundus is located medially with the flexor policis longus being located laterally. The pronator quadratus covers the distal quarter of the bones of the forearm

Flexor digitorum profundus
Ulnar nerve for the ulnar portion, anterior interosseous nerve of the median nerve for the radial portion (brachial plexus, infraclavicular part)

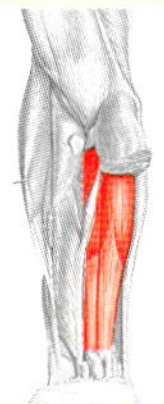

O: Proximal two thirds of the anterior surface of the ulna, interosseous membrane

I: Base of the distal phalanx of the 2.–5. finger

F: Wrist joint: palmar flexion
Metacarpophalangeal joints (II–V): flexion, (adduction)
Finger joints (II–V): flexion

Flexor pollicis longus
Anterior interosseous nerve of the median nerve (brachial plexus, infraclavicular part)

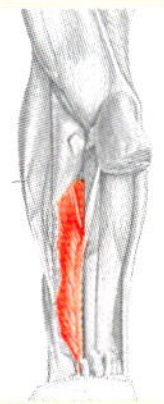

O: Anterior surface of the radius distal to the radial tuberosity

I: Base of the distal phalanx of the thumb

F: Wrist joint: palmar flexion
Carpometacarpal joint of the thumb: adduction, opposition
Thumb joints: flexion

Pronator quadratus
Anterior interosseous nerve (median nerve, brachial plexus, infraclavicular part)

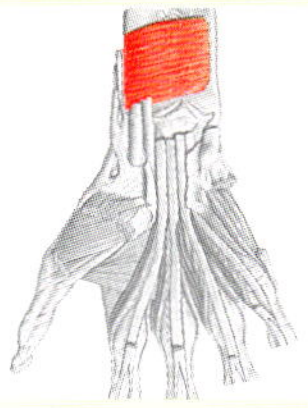

O: Distal quarter of the anterior border of the ulna

I: Anterior border and surface of the radius

F: Radioulnar joints: pronation

33 Lateral (radial) muscle of the forearm (Fig. 352, 362, 366, 370, 371)

The group of the radial muscles of the forearm consists of the following muscles in the order from lateral to medial: brachioradialis, extensor carpi radialis longus and extensor carpi radialis brevis.

Brachioradialis

Radial nerve (brachial plexus, infraclavicular part)

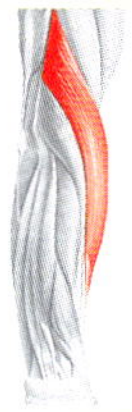

O: Lateral border of the humerus, lateral intermuscular septum of arm

I: Styloid process of the radius

F: Elbow joint:
flexion (particularly strong when forearm is in semipronated position),
pronation or supination (from the corresponding extreme position to an intermediate one)

Extensor carpi radialis longus

Radial nerve (brachial plexus, infraclavicular part)

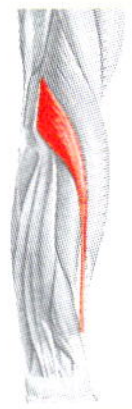

O: Distal end of the lateral border of the humerus, lateral epicondyle of the humerus, lateral intermuscular septum of arm

I: Dorsal surface of the base of metacarpal II

F: Elbow joint:
flexion,
pronation or supination (from the corresponding extreme position to an intermediate one)
Wrist joint:
dorsal flexion,
radial abduction

Extensor carpi radialis brevis

Radial nerve (brachial plexus, infraclavicular part)

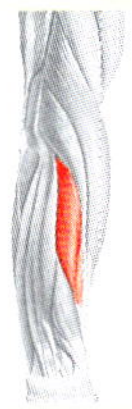

O: Lateral epicondyle of the humerus, anular ligament of radius

I: Dorsal surface of the base of metacarpal III

F: Elbow joint:
flexion,
pronation or supination (from the corresponding extreme position to an intermediate one)
Wrist joint:
dorsal flexion,
radial abduction

34 Superficial dorsal muscles of the forearm (Fig. 361, 363, 367, 368, 379)

The group of the superficial dorsal muscles of the forearm consists of the following muscles in the order from radial to ulnar: extensor digitorum, extensor digiti minimi and extensor carpi ulnaris.

Extensor digitorum

Deep branch of the radial nerve (brachial plexus, infraclavicular part)

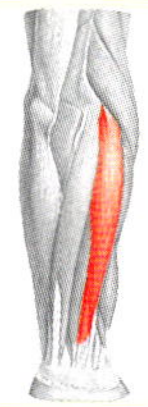

	O: Lateral epicondyle of the humerus, radial collateral ligament and anular ligament of radius, antebrachial fascia	**I:** So-called dorsal aponeuroses of the 2.–5. finger	**F:** Elbow joint: extension Wrist joint: dorsal flexion Metacarpophalangeal (II–V)/ finger joints (II–V): extension

Extensor digiti minimi

Deep branch of the radial nerve (brachial plexus, infraclavicular part)

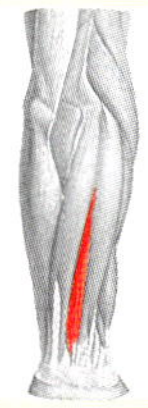

	O: Lateral epicondyle of the humerus, radial collateral ligament and anular ligament of radius, antebrachial fascia	**I:** So-called dorsal aponeurosis of the 5. finger	**F:** Elbow joint: extension Wrist joint: dorsal flexion, ulnar abduction Metacarpophalangeal (V)/ finger joints (V): extension

Extensor carpi ulnaris (This muscle is frequently separated from the extensor digitorum and the extensor digiti minimi by a distinct intermuscular septum.)

Deep branch of the radial nerve (brachial plexus, infraclavicular part)

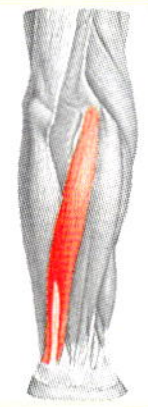

	O: Humeral head: Lateral epicondyle of the humerus, radial collateral ligament **Ulnar head:** Proximal two thirds of the posterior surface of the ulna, antebrachial fascia	**I:** Dorsal surface of the base of metacarpal V	**F:** Elbow joint: extension Wrist joint: dorsal flexion, ulnar abduction

35 Deep dorsal muscles of the forearm (Fig. 356, 361, 364, 365, 368–371, 379)

The supinator enwraps the upper third of the radius laterally. Distally, the extensor pollicis longus, the extensor indicis, the abductor pollicis longus and the extensor pollicis brevis follow from lateral to medial.

Supinator (This muscle is perforated by the deep branch of the radial nerve in a longitudinal direction. A small tendinous arch frames the opening of the supinator canal.)
Deep branch of the radial nerve (brachial plexus, infraclavicular part)

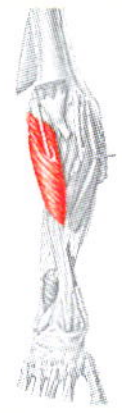

O: Lateral epicondyle of the humerus, supinator crest of the ulna, radial collateral ligament and anular ligament of radius

I: Anterior surface of the radius between the radial tuberosity and the insertion of the pronator teres

F: Radioulnar joints:
supination

Extensor pollicis longus
Deep branch of the radial nerve (brachial plexus, infraclavicular part)

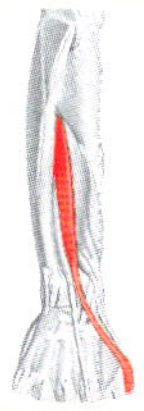

O: Distal quarter of the posterior surface of the ulna, interosseous membrane

I: Distal phalanx of the thumb

F: Wrist joint:
dorsal flexion,
radial abduction
Carpometacarpal joint of the thumb:
adduction,
reposition
Metacarpophalangeal joint of the thumb and thumb joint:
extension

Extensor indicis
Deep branch of the radial nerve (brachial plexus, infraclavicular part)

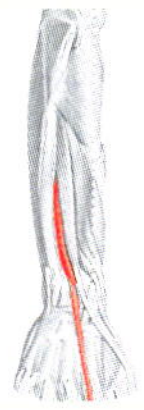

O: Distal quarter of the posterior surface of the ulna, interosseous membrane

I: So-called dorsal aponeurosis of the index finger

F: Wrist joint:
dorsal flexion,
radial abduction
Metacarpophalangeal joint (II):
extension,
adduction
Finger joints (II):
extension

Abductor pollicis longus
Deep branch of the radial nerve (brachial plexus, infraclavicular part)

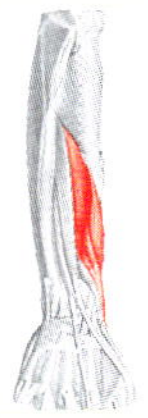

O: Posterior surface of the ulna, interosseous membrane, posterior surface of the radius

I: Base of metacarpal I

F: Radioulnar joints:
supination
Wrist joint:
dorsal flexion,
radial abduction
Carpometacarpal joint of the thumb:
extension,
reposition

Extensor pollicis brevis
Deep branch of the radial nerve (brachial plexus, infraclavicular part)

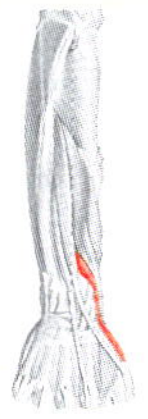

O: Posterior surface of the radius, interosseous membrane

I: Base of the proximal phalanx of the thumb

F: Wrist joint:
palmar flexion,
radial abduction
Carpometacarpal joint of the thumb:
abduction, reposition
Metacarpophalangeal joint of the thumb:
extension

36 Muscles of the thenar eminence (Fig. 372–374, 377, 378)

From superficial to deep the abductor pollicis brevis, the flexor pollicis brevis, the opponens pollicis and the adductor pollicis form the tenar eminence.

Abductor pollicis brevis
Median nerve (brachial plexus, infraclavicular part)

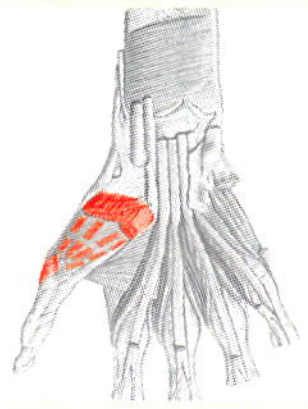

O: Flexor retinaculum, tubercle of scaphoid

I: Radial sesamoid bone of the metacarpophalangeal joint of the thumb, radial margin of the base of the proximal phalanx of the thumb, inserts into the dorsal aponeurosis of the thumb

F: Carpometacarpal joint of the thumb: abduction, opposition
Metacarpophalangeal joint of the thumb: flexion

Flexor pollicis brevis
Superficial head: median nerve; deep head: deep branch of the ulnar nerve (brachial plexus, infraclavicular part)

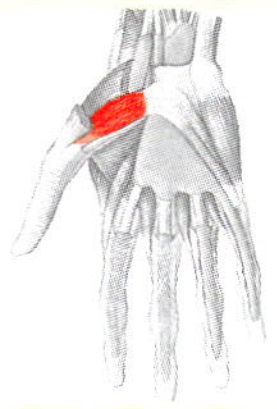

O: Superficial head: flexor retinaculum
Deep head: Capitate, trapezium, trapezoid, base of metacarpal I

I: Radial sesamoid bone of the metacarpophalangeal joint of the thumb, radial margin of the base of the proximal phalanx of the thumb, inserts into the dorsal aponeurosis of the thumb

F: Carpometacarpal joint of the thumb: opposition, abduction
Metacarpophalangeal joint of the thumb: flexion

Opponens pollicis
Median nerve and ulnar nerve (brachial plexus, infraclavicular part)

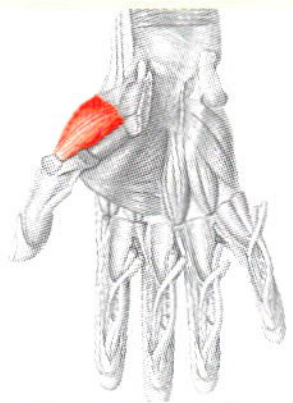

O: Flexor retinaculum, tubercle of trapezium

I: Entire radial margin of metacarpal I

F: Carpometacarpal joint of the thumb: opposition, abduction

Adductor pollicis
Deep branch of the ulnar nerve (brachial plexus, infraclavicular part)

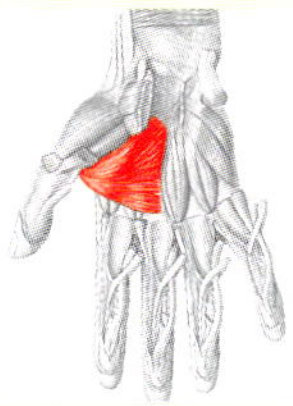

O: Oblique head: Capitate, base of metacarpal II, radiate carpal ligament
Transverse head: palmar surface of metacarpal III

I: Ulnar sesamoid bone of the metacarpophalangeal joint of the thumb, ulnar margin of the base of the proximal phalanx of the thumb, inserts into the dorsal aponeurosis of the thumb

F: Carpometacarpal joint of the thumb: abduction, opposition
Metacarpophalangeal joint of the thumb: flexion

37 Muscles of the palm (Fig. 372–374, 377–379, 382–384)

The muscles of the palm comprise a heterogeneous group. The lumbricals are tightly connected to the tendons of the flexor digitorum profundus. The palmar interossei and the dorsal interossei fill the spaces between the metacarpals.

Lumbricals I–IV
Median nerve (I, II); ulnar nerve (III, IV) (brachial plexus, infraclavicular part)

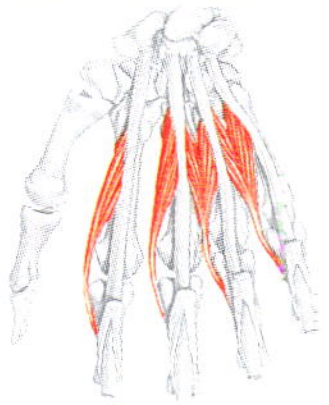

O: Radial side of the tendons I and II, as well as the facing sides of the tendons II–IV of the flexor digitorum profundus

I: Insert radially into the dorsal aponeurosis of the fingers II–V

F: Metacarpophalangeal joints (II–V): flexion, radial abduction
Finger joints (II–V): extension

Palmar interossei I–III
Ulnar nerve (brachial plexus, infraclavicular part)

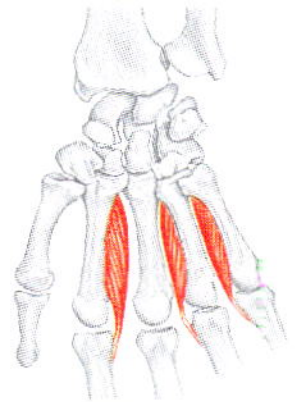

O: Ulnar side of metacarpal II, radial side of metacarpals IV and V

I: Radiate into the dorsal aponeurosis of the fingers II, IV and V

F: Metacarpophalangeal joints (II, IV, V): flexion, adduction (with respect to the axis of the middle finger)
Finger joints (II, IV, V): extension

Dorsal interossei I–IV (double headed)
Ulnar nerve (brachial plexus, infraclavicular part)

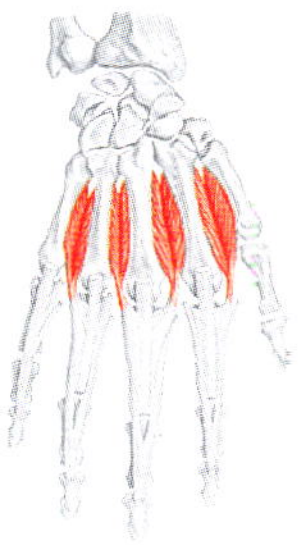

O: Facing sides of the metacarpals I–V

I: Radiate into the dorsal aponeurosis of the fingers II–IV

F: Metacarpophalangeal joints (II–IV): flexion, abduction (with respect to the axis of the middle finger)
Finger joints (II–IV): extension

38 Muscles of the hypothenar eminence (Fig. 372–374, 377)

From lateral to medial, the hypothenar eminence consists of the abductor digiti minimi, the flexor digiti minimi brevis and the opponens digiti minimi. The palmaris brevis also belongs to this group as a skin muscle.

Palmaris brevis (consists of several separated bundles)
Superficial branch of the ulnar nerve (brachial plexus, infraclavicular part)

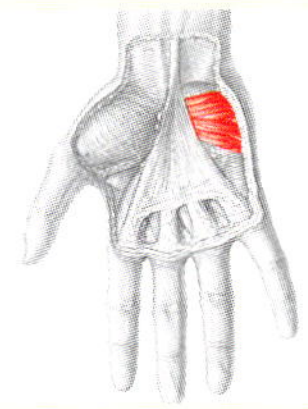

O: Medial margin of the palmar aponeurosis, rarely trapezium

I: Skin of the hypothenar emince

F: Tenses the skin at the hypothenar eminence

Abductor digiti minimi
Deep branch of the ulnar nerve (brachial plexus, infraclavicular part)

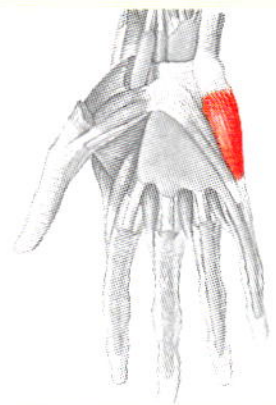

O: Pisiform, pisohamate ligament, flexor retinaculum

I: Ulnar margin of the proximal phalanx, dorsal aponeurosis of the 5. finger

F: Carpometacarpal joint (V): opposition
Metacarpophalangeal joint (V): abduction, flexion
Finger joints (V): extension

Flexor digiti minimi brevis (inconstant muscle)
Deep branch of the ulnar nerve (brachial plexus, infraclavicular part)

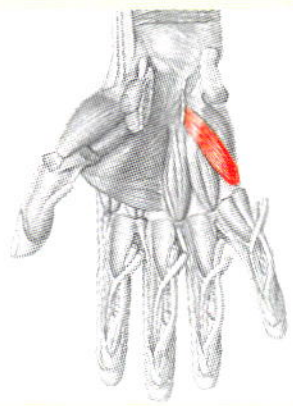

O: Flexor retinaculum, hook of hamate

I: Base of the proximal phalanx of the 5. finger, dorsal aponeurosis of the 5. finger

F: Carpometacarpal joint (V): opposition
Metacarpophalangeal joint (V): flexion, abduction
Finger joints (V): extension

Opponens digiti minimi
Deep branch of the ulnar nerve (brachial plexus, infraclavicular part)

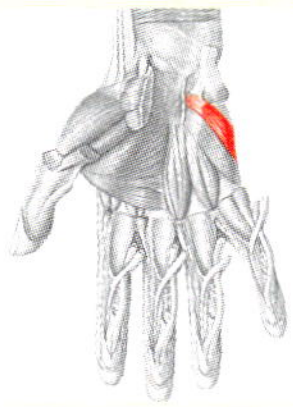

O: Flexor retinaculum, hook of hamate

I: Ulnar surface of metacarpal V

F: Carpometacarpal joint (V): opposition

39 Joints of the lower limb (Fig. 949)

a Joints of the pelvic girdle

Name of the joint	Type of the joint	Movements
Sacroiliac joint	Rigid joint, Amphiarthrosis	
Anterior sacro-iliac ligaments Posterior sacro-iliac ligaments Interosseus sacro-iliac ligaments Sacrotuberous ligament Sacrospinous ligament	Syndesmoses, fibrous joints	Limited displacement and rotation (only a few millimetres); as a consequence of the deformation of the pelvis during gait or weight-bearing
Pubic symphysics	Cartilaginous joint, synchondrosis with interpubic disc	
Superior pubic ligament Inferior pubic ligament		

b Joints of the free part of the lower limb

Name of the joint	Type of the joint	Movements
Hip joint	Spheroideal joint	Flexion (anteversion) extension (retroversion) adduction abduction medial and lateral rotation
Knee joint	Pivot-hinge joint, Trochoginglymus	Flexion extension medial and lateral rotation (only in flexed position)
Superior tibiofibular joint	Rigid joint, Amphiarthrosis	Limited displacements in transverse and vertical direction, limited rotation
Inferior tibiofibular joint	Syndesmosis, fibrous joint	Support of the malleolar brace, which diverges slightly during dorsal extension in the ankle joint
Ankle joint	Hinge joint, Ginglymus	Plantar flexion dorsal flexion
Talotarsal joint a) Talocalcaneonavicular joint (= anterior part) b) Subtalar joint (= posterior part)	Compound spheroidal and conoid joint Spheroideal joint Conoid joint	Lifting of the medial (supination) and lateral (pronation) margin of the foot
Transverse tarsal joint (CHOPART's joint) a) Talocalcaneonavicular joint b) Calcaneocuboid joint	Rigid joints, Amphiarthroses	Minimal plantar and dorsal movements and rotation support of the longitudinal arch of the foot
Intertarsal joints a) Cuneonavicular joint b) Intercuneiform joints c) Cuneocuboid joint	Rigid joints, Amphiarthroses	Minimal movements in the deformations of the foot during adjustment to the ground
Tarsometatarsal joints (LISFRANC's joint)	Rigid joints, Amphiarthroses	Minimal plantar and dorsal movements and rotation of the forefoot
Intermetatarsal joints	Rigid joints, Amphiarthroses	Minimal movements during rotation of the forefoot
Metatarsophalangeal joints	Functionally limited spheroideal joints	Flexion, extension abduction, adduction
Interphalangeal joints	Hinge joints, Ginglymi	Flexion extension of the toes

39 Joints of the lower limb (continuatioin)

c Planes and axes of the movements of the joints of the lower limb

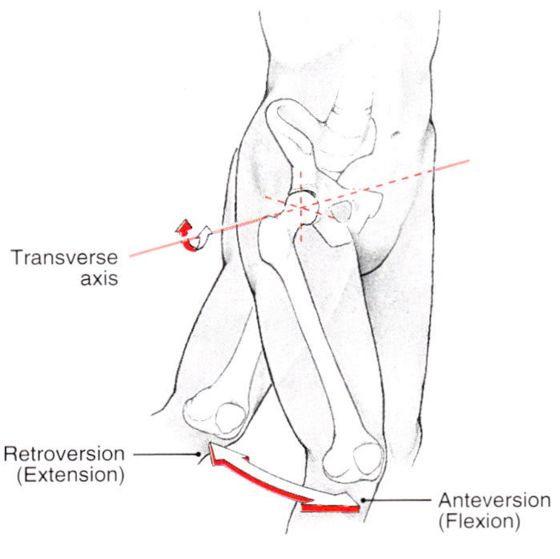

Fig. 8 Hip joint;
movement in the sagittal plane.

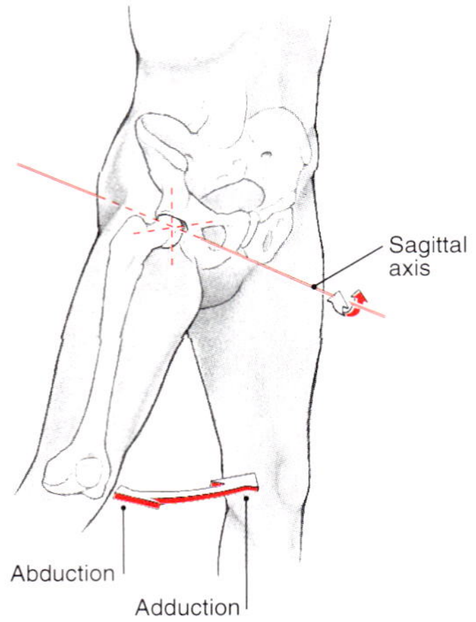

Fig. 9 Hip joint;
movement in the frontal plane

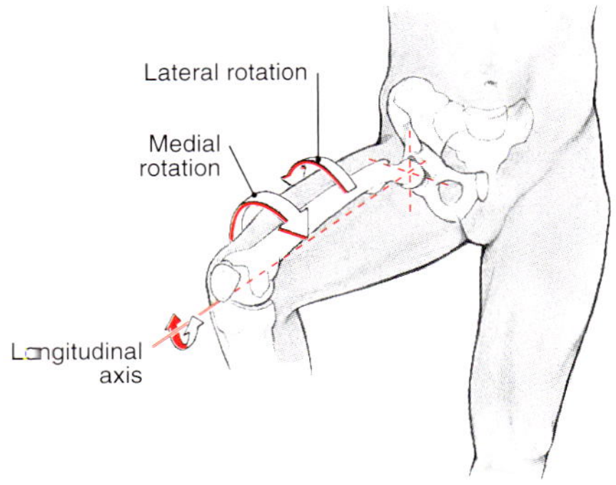

Fig. 10 Hip joint;
movement in the transverse plane.

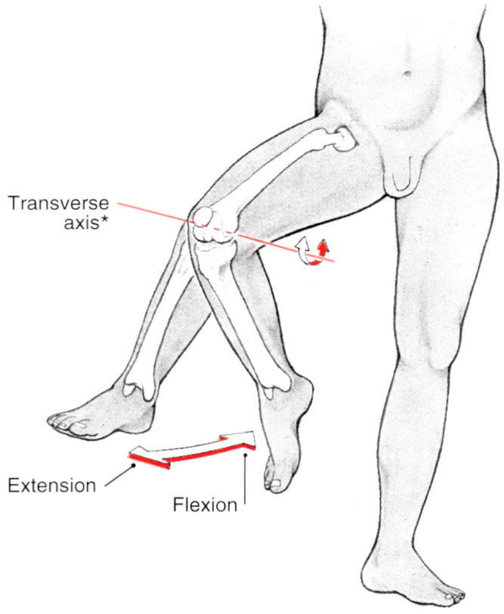

Fig. 11 Knee joint;
movement in the sagittal plane.

* As a consequence of the asymmetric curvature of the femoral condyles this axis, in particular, changes during the movement (inconstant axis)

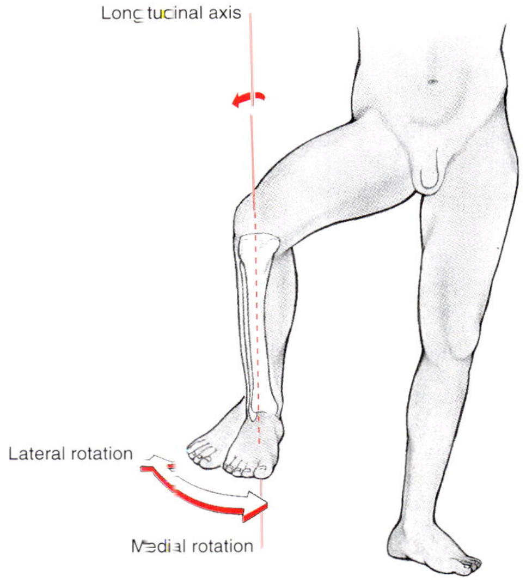

Fig. 12 Knee joint;
movement in the transverse plane.

39 Joints of the lower limb (continuatioin)

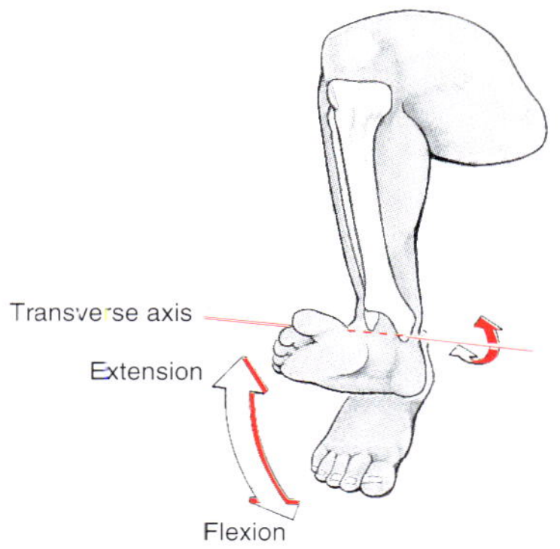

Fig. 4 Ankle joint
movement in the sagittal plane.
Flexion and extension take place almos exclusively in the ankle joint.

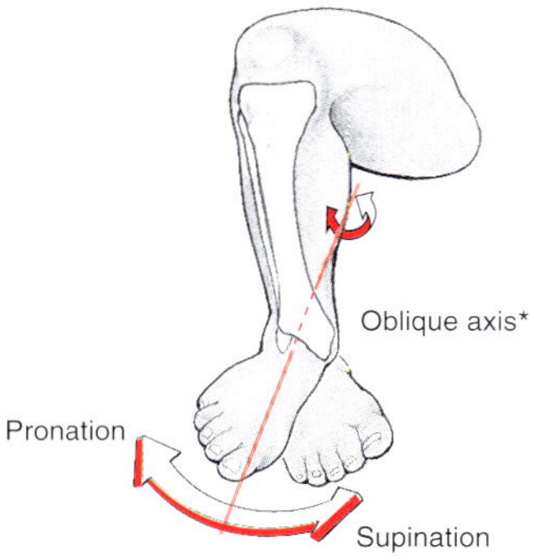

Fig. 14 Talotarsal joint;
supination and pronation movements of the foot.
In extreme plantar flexion, pronation is also referred to as lateral abduction, and supination as medial abduction.
* The axis runs from the inner part of the neck of the talus in a posterior and inferior direction to the lateral process of the calcaneal tuberosity and is actually steeper as illustrated in this figure for didactial reasons.

In the ankle joint, plantar flexion is also referred to as flexion, and dorsal flexion as extension.

40 Branches and supplying areas of the lumbosacral plexus (Fig. 595, 1105–1108)

	Motor function	Sensory function
Lumbar plexus, [T12] L1–L3 [L4]		
Iliohypogastric nerve [iliopubic nerve] T12, L1	Rectus abdominis, external oblique, internal oblique, transversus abdominis, pyramidalis, cremaster	
Lateral cutaneous branch		Skin covering the hip
Anterior cutaneous branch		Skin above the iliac crest, the inguinal ligament and the mons pubis
Ilio-inguinal nerve [T12] L1 [L2]	Rectus abdominis, external oblique, internal oblique, transversus abdominis, pyramidalis, cremaster	
Anterior scrotal nerves/ Anterior labial nerves		Skin of the inguinal region, the root of the penis, and the scrotum and the labia majora, respectively
Genitofemoral nerve L1, L2		
Genital branch		Scrotal coats (including the dartos fascia)
Femoral branch		Skin at the saphenous opening
Lateral cutaneous nerve of thigh L2, L3		Skin of the lateral and anterior side of the thigh up to the knee
Obturator nerve L2–L4		
Anterior branch	Pectineus, adductor brevis, adductor longus, gracilis	Capsule of the hip joint
Cutaneous branch		Skin of the medial side of the thigh superior to the knee
Posterior branch	Obturator externus	Capsule of the hip joint, periosteum of the posterior side of the femur
Muscular branches	adductor magnus, (adductor brevis) adductor minimus	
Accessory obturator nerve L3, L4	Pectineus	Capsule of the hip joint
Femoral nerve L2–L4	Iliopsoas, pectineus, sartorius, quadriceps femoris	Capsule of the hip joint
Muscular branches		
Anterior cutaneous branches		Skin of the anterior and medial side of the thigh up to the knee, periosteum of the anterior side of the femur
Saphenous nerve		
Infrapatellar branch		Skin of the anterior and medial side of the knee and the medial side of the leg as well as the foot
Medial cutaneous nerve of leg		
Sacral plexus [L4] L5–S3 [S4]		
Nerve to obturator internus L5–S2	Obturatorius internus	
Nerve to piriformis	Piriformis	
Nerve to quadratus femoris L5–S1 [S2]	Quadratus femoris	
Superior gluteal nerve L4–S1	Gluteus medius and gluteus minimus, tensor fasciae latae	
Inferior gluteal nerve L5–S2	Gluteus maximus	
Posterior cutaneous nerve of thigh S1–S3		Skin of the posterior side of the thigh and the proximal leg
Inferior clunial nerves		Skin of the gluteal region
Perineal nerves		Perineum, scrotal skin or skin of the labia majora, resp.
Sciatic nerve L4–S3	Ischiocrural muscles, all muscles of the leg and the foot	
Common fibular nerve L4–S2	Biceps femoris, short head	Capsule of the knee joint
Lateral sural cutaneous nerve		Skin of the calf up to the lateral malleolus
Sural communicating branch		Connecting branch to the sural nerve

40 Branches and supplying areas of the lumbosacral plexus (Fig. 595, 1105–1108)

	Motor function	Sensory function
Superficial fibular nerve L4–S2		
Muscular branches	Fibularis (peroneus) longus and brevis	
Medial dorsal cutaneous nerve		Skin of the leg and the back of the foot up to the 1.–3. toe
Intermediate dorsal cutaneous nerve		Skin of the lateral margin of the foot
Dorsal digital nerves of foot		Skin of the back of the toes except for the 1. interdigital space and the lateral side of the 5. toe
Deep fibular nerve L4–S2		
Muscular branches	Tibialis anterior, extensor digitorum longus, extensor hallucis longus, extensor digitorum brevis and extensor hallucis brevis	Periosteum of the bones of the leg and the capsule of the ankle joint
Dorsal digital nerves of foot		Skin of the 1. interdigital space
Tibial nerve L4–S3		
Muscular branches	Triceps surae, plantaris, popliteus, tibialis posterior, flexor digitorum longus, flexor hallucis longus	Capsule of the knee joint
Interosseous nerve of leg		Periosteum of the bones of the leg and the capsule of the ankle joint
Medial sural cutaneous nerve		Skin of the calf up to the medial malleolus, merges with the lateral sural cutaneous nerve to form the sural nerve
Sural nerve		
Lateral dorsal cutaneous nerve		Skin of the lateral margin of the foot up to the 5. toe
Lateral calcaneal branches		Skin of the lateral heel
Medial calcaneal branches		Skin of the medial heel
Medial plantar nerve	Abductor hallucis and flexor digitorum brevis, flexor hallucis brevis (medial head), lumbricals of foot I (II)	Skin of the medial sole
Common plantar digital nerves		Skin of the sole side of the medial $3^1/_2$ toes and the nail areas
Proper plantar digital nerves		
Lateral plantar nerve	Abductor digiti minimi, quadratus plantae,	
Superficial branch		
Common plantar digital nerves	Flexor digiti minimi brevis,	
Proper plantar digital nerves	opponens digiti minimi, interossei of the 4. intermetatarsal space	Skin of the plantar side of the lateral $1^1/_2$ toes and the nail areas
Deep branch	Lumbricals of foot II–IV, adductor hallucis (transverse head), interossei of the 1.–4. intermetarsal space	
Pudendal nerve (S1) S2–S4		
Inferior rectal (anal) nerves S3, S4		Skin of the anal region and the perineum
Perineal nerves		
Posterior scrotal nerves/ Posterior labial nerves		Urethral sphincter, urethral mucosa, dorsal skin of the scrotum or the labia majora and minora, respectively, vestibule
Muscular branches	Superficial and deep transverse perineal muscle, bulbospongiosus and ischiocavernosus, external anal sphincter, deep transverse perineal muscle, urethral sphincter	
Dorsal nerve of penis/ dorsal nerve of clitoris		Skin of the penis, glans/clitoris, prepuce
Coccygeal nerve S4, S5 (Co1)	Ischiococcygeus (coccygeus), levator ani	Skin of the coccygeal region, as well as the skin between the coccyx and the anus
Coccygeal plexus S4, S5 (Co1)		
Anococcygeal nerve		

41 Segmental innervation of the muscles of the lower limb, muscles of diagnostic importance

(According to MUMENTHALER and SCHLIACK; the indicator muscle of each segment is printed in bold.)

Iliopsoas: L1, L2	T12–L3
Tensor fasciae latae	L4–L5
Gluteus medius	L4–S1
Gluteus minimus	L4–S1
Gluteus maximus	L4–S2
Obturatorius internus	L5–S1
Piriformis	L5–S1
Sartorius	L2–L3
Pectineus	L2–L3
Adductor longus	L2–L3
Quadriceps femoris: L3	L2–L4
Gracilis	L2–L4
Adductor brevis	L2–L4
Obturatorius externus	L3–L4
Adductor magnus	L3–L4
Semitendinosus	L4–S1
Semimembranosus	L4–S1
Biceps fermoris	L4–S2

Tibialis anterior: L4	L4–L5
Extensor hallucis longus	L4–S1
Popliteus	L4–S1
Extensor digitorum longus	L4–S1
Soleus L5	L4–S2
Gastrocnemius L5	
Fibulis longus	L5–S1
Fibularis brevis	L5–S1
Tibialis posterior: S1	L5–S2
Flexor digitorum longus	L5–S3
Flexor hallucis longus	L5–S3
Extensor hallucis brevis	L4–S1
Extensor digitorum brevis	L4–S1
Flexor digitorum brevis	L5–S1
Abductor hallucis	L5–S1
Flexor hallucis brevis	L5–S3
Adductor hallucis	S1–S2

42 Ventral muscles of the hip (Fig. 583, 601, 1053, 1055, 1060–1065)

This group only comprises the iliacus and the psoas major, which together form the iliopsoas. These are the only ventral muscles of the hip joint, as all other ventral muscles in front of the hip joint also overstretch the knee joint and are therefore referred to as ventral muscles of the thigh.

Iliacus
Muscular branches (lumbar plexus)

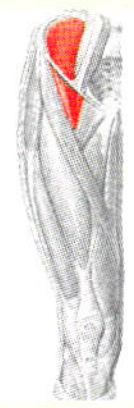

O: Iliac fossa, anterior inferior iliac spine, anterior portion of the capsule of the hip joint

I: Lesser trochanter and adjacent area of the medial lip of the linea aspera

F: Lumbar vertebral column:
lateral flexion,
extension (hyperlordosis)
Hip joint:
flexion,
medial rotation, (lateral rotation only when the glutei are contracted as well)

Psoas major
Muscular branches (lumbar plexus)

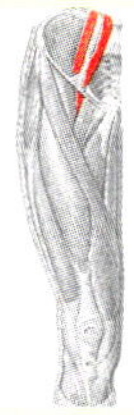

O: Superficial layer: lateral surface of the body of the 12. thoracic – 4. lumbar vertebra, intervetebral discs
Deep layer: Costal process of the 1.–4. lumbar vertebra

I: Lesser trochanter and adjacent area of the medial lip of the linea aspera

F: Lumbar vertebral column:
lateral flexion,
extension (hyperlordosis)
Hip joint:
flexion,
medial rotation, (lateral rotation only when the glutei are contracted as well)

Psoas minor (inconstant muscle; often featuring a long tendinous plate at its insertion
Muscular branches (lumbar plexus)

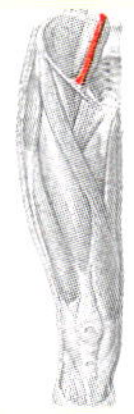

O: Lateral surface of the body of the 12. thoracic and the 1. lumbar vertebra

I: Fascia of the iliopsoas, iliopectineal arch

F: Lumbar vertebral column:
lateral flexion,
extension (hyperlordosis)
Hip joint:
flexion,
medial rotation, (lateral rotation only when the glutei are contracted as well)

43 Dorsal muscles of the hip (Fig. 1054–1056, 1065, 1067–1074)

The gluteus maximus predominantly shapes the surface anatomy of the gluteal region and nearly covers all other muscles of this group. At the ventral and cranial edge, parts of the gluteus medius are visible, which in turn covers the gluteus minimus. Caudally in the deeper layer the following muscles are found: the piriformis, the gemellus superior, the obturatorius internus, the gemellus inferior and the quadratus femoris. The obturatorius internus and the gemelli superior et inferior are also called triceps coxae.

Gluteus maximus (The trochanteric bursa of gluteus maximus is located between the greater trochanter and the iliotibial tract.)
Inferior gluteal nerve (sacral plexus)

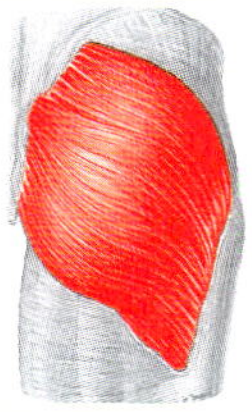

O: Gluteal surface of the ala of ilium dorsal to the posterior gluteal line, posterior surface of the sacrum, thoracolumbar fascia, sacrotuberous ligament

I: Cranial portion via the iliotibial tract tibia just below the lateral condyle,
caudal portion: gluteal tuberosity, lateral femoral intermuscular septum

F: Hip joint:
cranial portion: extension,
lateral rotation,
abduction;
caudal portion: extension,
lateral rotation,
adduction
Knee joint:
cranial portion via iliotibial tract, stabilization when the knee is extended

Gluteus medius
Superior gluteal nerve (sacral plexus)

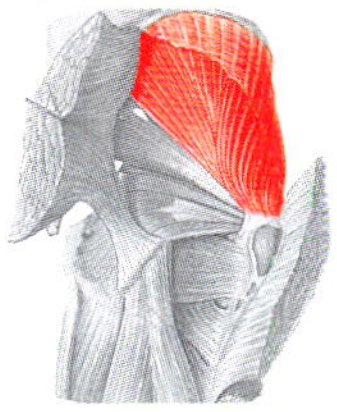

O: Gluteal surface of the ala of ilium beween anterior and posterior gluteal line

I: Tip and lateral margin of the greater trochanter

F: Hip joint:
ventral portion: abduction,
flexion,
medial rotation;
dorsal portion: abduction,
extension,
lateral rotation

Gluteus minimus
Superior gluteal nerve (sacral plexus)

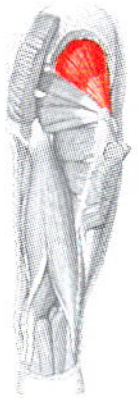

O: Gluteal surface of the ala of ilium beween anterior and inferior gluteal line

I: Tip and lateral margin of the greater trochanter

F: Hip joint:
ventral portion: abduction,
flexion,
medial rotation;
dorsal portion: abduction,
extension,
lateral rotation

Piriformis
Sciatic nerve and/or nerve to piriformis (sacral plexus)

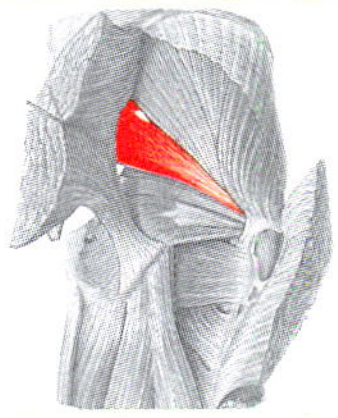

O: Laterally and between the sacral pelvic foramina (3.–5. sacral segment) of the pelvic surface of sacrum, greater sciatic notch close to the sacrum

I: Inner surface of the tip of the greater trochanter

F: Hip joint:
lateral rotation,
extension,
abduction

43 Dorsal muscles of the hip (continuation)

Obturatorius internus
Nerve to obturator internus and muscular branches (sacral plexus)

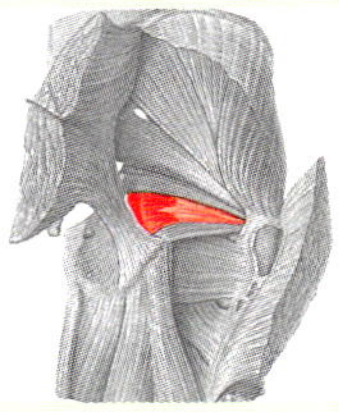

O: Circumference of the obturator foramen, medial surface of the obturator membrane

I: Trochanteric fossa

F: Hip joint:
lateral rotation
extension
adduction

Gemellus superior
Nerve to obturator internus and muscular branches (sacral plexus)

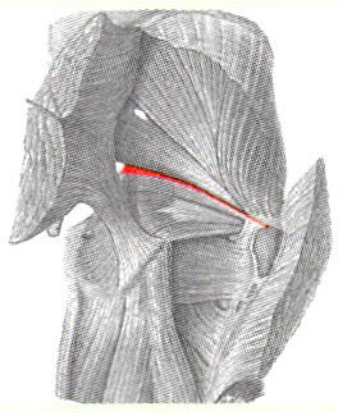

O: Ischial spine

I: Trochanteric fossa

F: Hip joint:
lateral rotation
extension
adduction

Gemellus inferior
Nerve to obturator internus and muscular branches (sacral plexus)

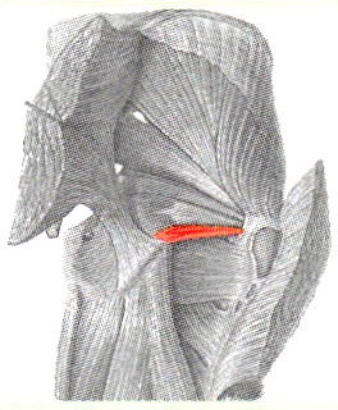

O: Ischial tuberosity

I: Trochanteric fossa

F: Hip joint:
lateral rotation
extension
adduction

Quadratus femons
Nerve to quadratus femoris (sacral plexus)

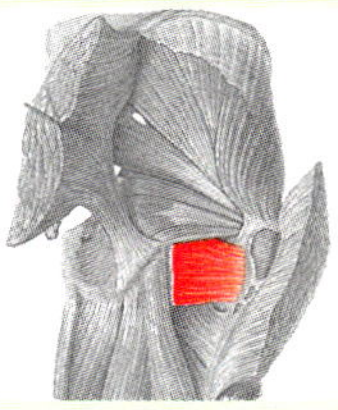

O: Lateral margin of the ischial tuberosity

I: Intertrochanteric crest

F: Hip joint:
lateral rotation
adduction

44 Ventral muscles of the thigh (Fig. 1053, 1055–1058, 1061–1065, 1075–1077)

The sartorius stretches in a spiral-like fashion along the thigh from lateroproximal to mediodistal. With its short muscle belly, the tensor fasciae latae is located most laterally and passes into the iliotibial tract. The major part of the ventral muscle mass of the thigh is formed by the quadriceps femoris.

Quadriceps femoris
Femoral nerve (lumbar plexus)

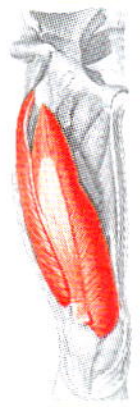

O: Rectus femoris, straight head: Anterior inferior iliac spine
Rectus femoris, reflected head: Cranial margin of the acetabulum
Vastus medialis: Inferior two thirds of the medial lip of the linea aspera
Vastus lateralis: Distal circumference of the greater trochanter, lateral lip of the linea aspera
Vastus intermedius: Upper two thirds of the anterior surface and lateral aspects of the femur
Articularis genus: Distal quarter of the anterior surface of the femur

I: Proximal, lateral and medial margins of the patella, tibial tuberosity via patellar ligament, areas lateral to the tibial tuberosity via the patellar retinacula

F: Hip joint (only rectus femoris): flexion
Knee joint: extension

Sartorius
Femoral nerve (lumbar plexus)

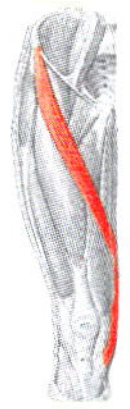

O: Anterior superior iliac spine

I: Medial surface of the tibial tuberosity

F: Hip joint: flexion, lateral rotation, abduction
Knee joint: flexion, medial rotation

Tensor fasciae latae
Superior gluteal nerve (lumbosacral plexus)

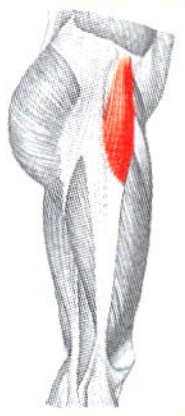

O: Anterior superior iliac spine

I: Tibia below the lateral condyle (via iliotibial tract)

F: Hip joint: flexion, abduction, medial rotation
Knee joint: stabilization when the knee is extended

45 Medial muscles of the thigh (adductors)
(Fig. 1053, 1055, 1056, 1059, 1061–1065, 1071–1077)

Due to their predominant function, the muscles located at the medial side of the thigh are commonly referred to as adductors. In the ventral view, this group appears like a triangular block. The gracilis lies most medially. From proximal to distal follow the pectineus, adductor brevis, adductor longus and the adductor magnus. The obturatorius externus is covered by the pectineus and is juxtaposed to the neck of the femur from inferior.

Pectineus
Femoral nerve and obturator nerve (lumbar plexus)

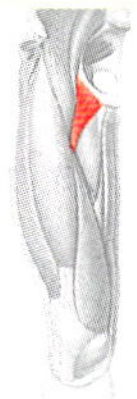

O: Pecten pubis

I: Pectineal line of the femur

F: Hip joint:
adduction,
lateral rotation,
(flexion)

Gracilis
Obturator nerve (lumbar plexus)

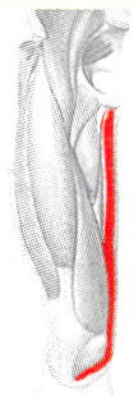

O: Medial edge of the inferior pubic ramus along the symphysis

I: Proximal end of the tibia medial to the tibial tuberosity

F: Hip joint:
adduction,
flexion,
lateral rotation
Knee joint:
flexion,
medial rotation

Adductor brevis
Obturator nerve (lumbar plexus)

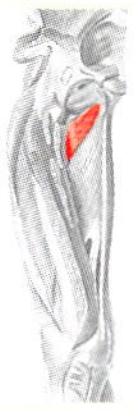

O: Interior pubic ramus closer to the obturator foramen than the adductor longus

I: Proximal third of the medial lip of the linea aspera

F: Hip joint:
adduction,
lateral rotation,
flexion

Adductor longus
Obturator nerve (lumbar plexus)

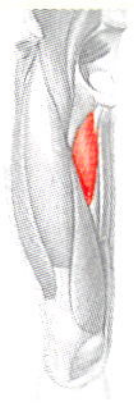

O: Pubis below the pubic crest up to the symphysis

I: Middle third of the medial lip of the linea aspera

F: Hip joint:
adduction,
flexion,
lateral rotation,
(most anterior portion: medial rotation)

Adductor magnus (An incomplete proximal part of the adductor magnus is known as adductor minimus. The opening of the adductor canal is located between the distal insertions of both muscles.)
Obturator nerve (lumbar plexus) and tibial part of the sciatic nerve (sacral plexus)

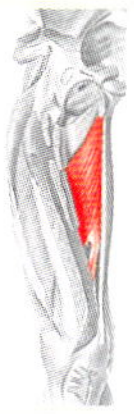

O: Medial margin of the inferior pubic ramus, ramus and tuberosity of ischium

I: Proximal two thirds of the medial lip of the linea aspera, tuberosity, adductor tubercle, adductor minimus: gluteal tuberosity

F: Hip joint:
adduction,
lateral rotation,
(anterior portion: flexion,
posterior portion: extension)

45 Medial muscles of the thigh (adductors) (continuation)

Obturatorius externus
Obturator nerve (lumbar plexus)

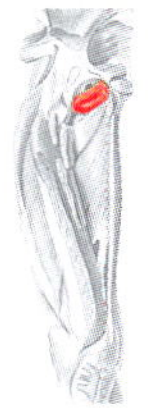

O: Circumference of the obturator foramen,
lateral surface of the obturator membrane

I: Trochanteric fossa

F: Hip joint:
lateral rotation,
adduction

46 Dorsal muscles of the thigh (ischiocrural muscles) (Fig. 1054–1056, 1065, 1066, 1071–1078)

The ischiocrural muscles consist of the biceps femoris, the semitendinosus and the semimembranosus from lateral to medial.

Biceps femoris (The long head stretches over two joints, whereas the short head only spans over one joint.)
Long head: Sciatic nerve, tibial part (sacral plexus)
Short head: Sciatic nerve, fibular part (sacral plexus)

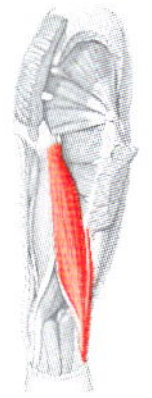

O: Long head: Ischial tuberosity together with the semitendinosus
Short head: Middle third of the lateral lip of the linea aspera

I: Head (ensheaths the fibular collateral ligament), radiates into the deep fascia of leg

F: Hip joint:
extension,
adduction,
(lateral rotation)
Knee joint:
flexion,
lateral rotation

Semitendinosus
Sciatic nerve, tibial part (sacral plexus)

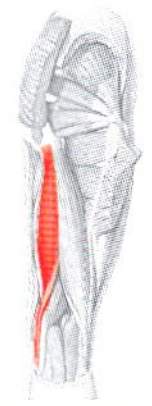

O: Ischial tuberosity together with the long head of the biceps femoris

I: Medial surface of the tibial tuberosity

F: Hip joint:
extension,
adduction,
(medial rotation)
Knee joint:
flexion,
lateral rotation

Semimembranosus (The insertion of the semimembranosus is also referred to as pes anserinus profundus)
Sciatic nerve, tibial part (sacral plexus)

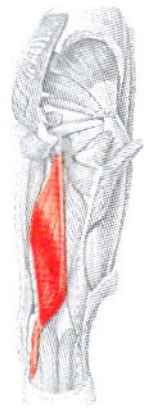

O: Ischial tuberosity

I: Proximal end of the tibia below the medial condyle, posterior capsule of the knee joint, oblique popliteal ligament, fascia of the popliteus

F: Hip joint:
extension,
(adduction),
(medial rotation)
Knee joint:
flexion,
medial rotation

47 Ventral muscles of the leg (Fig. 1053, 1077, 1079, 1083, 1088)

The ventral superficial and medial muscle is the tibialis anterior. It is followd by the extensor digitorum longus, from whose lateral margin the fibularis tertius often originates. The extensor hallucis longus is located most deeply.

Tibialis anterior
Deep fibular nerve (sciatic nerve)

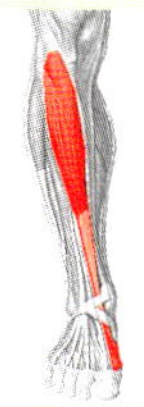

O: Proximal end of the tibia just below the lateral condyle, upper two thirds of the lateral surface of the tibia, deep fascia of leg, (interosseous membrane)

I: Medial margin of the base of metatarsal I, plantar surface of the medial cuneiform

F: Ankle joint: dorsal flexion
Talotarsal joint: supination

Extensor hallucis longus
Deep fibular nerve (sciatic nerve)

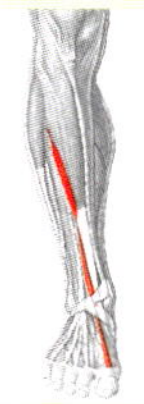

O: Distal two thirds of the medial surface of the fibula, interosseous membrane, deep fascia of leg

I: Base of the distal phalanx and the proximal phalanx of the hallux

F: Ankle joint: dorsal flexion
Talotarsal joint: (supination)
Joints of the great toe: extension

Extensor digitorum longus
Deep fibular nerve (sciatic nerve)

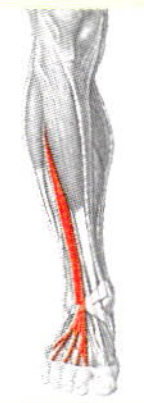

O: Proximal end of the tibia just below the lateral condyle, anterior border of the fibula, interosseous membrane of leg, anterior intermuscular septum of leg, deep fascia of leg

I: Dorsal aponeuroses of the 2.–5. toe

F: Ankle joint: dorsal flexion
Talotarsal joint: (pronation)
Joints of the toes: extension

Fibularis [peroneus] tertius (inconstant muscle)
Deep fibular nerve (sciatic nerve)

See Fig. 1083

O: Distal part of the extensor digitorum longus

I: Base of metatarsal V

F: Ankle joint: dorsal flexion
Talotarsal joint: (pronation)

48 Lateral (fibular) muscles of the leg (Fig. 1053, 1078, 1080, 1083, 1088)

The lateral superficial muscle is the fibularis longus, with the fibularis brevis following in the next deeper layer.

Fibularis [peroneus] longus
Superficial fibular nerve (sciatic nerve)

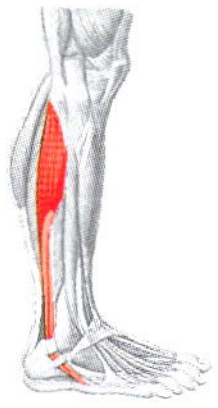

O: Head, proximal two thirds of the lateral surface and the posterior border of the fibula, anterior and posterior intermuscular septum of leg, deep fascia of leg

I: Tuberosity of metatarsal bone (II), plantar surface of the intermediate cune form

F: Ankle joint: plantar flexion
Talotarsal joint: pronation

Fibularis [peroneus] brevis
Superficial fibular nerve (sciatic nerve)

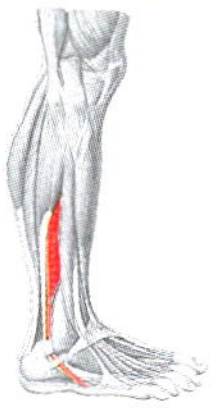

O: Distal half of the lateral surface of the anterior border of the fibula, anterior and posterior intermuscular septum of leg

I: Tuberosity of metatarsal bone V, tendon strips to the little toe

F: Ankle joint: plantar flexion
Talotarsal joint: pronation

49 Superficial dorsal muscles of the leg (Fig. 1054, 1078, 1081, 1084, 1085)

The heads of the gastrocnemius determine the shape of the calf. It is located above the soleus and together these muscles form the triceps surae. The very small plantaris can be considered as a fourth head of this muscle.

Triceps surae (Its broad tendon is also known as Achilles tendon.)
Tibial nerve (sciatic nerve)

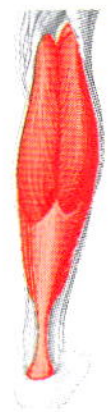

O: Gastrocnemius, medial head: Popliteal surface of the femur proximal to the medial condyle
Gastrocnemius, lateral head: Popliteal surface of the femur proximal to the lateral condyle
Soleus: Head, proximal third of the posterior surface and the posterior border of the fibula, posterior surface of the tibia at and just below the soleal line, tendinous arch of soleus
Plantaris: Popliteal surface of the femur proximal to the lateral condyle

I: Calcaneal tuberosity (via calcaneal tendon)

F: Knee joint: (only gastrocnemius and plantaris): flexion
Ankle joint: plantar flexion
Talotarsal joint: supination

50 Deep dorsal muscles of the leg (Fig. 1078, 1082, 1086, 1087)

The popliteus traverses obliquely in a lateral direction towards the knee joint. Of the muscles running towards the foot the tibialis posterior is located most superficially. The muscle is followed medially by the flexor digitorum longus and laterally by the flexor hallucis longus.

Popliteus
Tibial nerve (sciatic nerve)

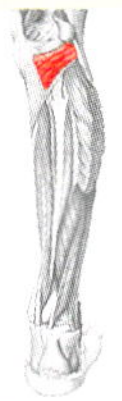

O: Lateral epicondyle of the femur	**I:** Posterior surface of the tibia just above the soleal line	**F:** Knee joint: medial rotation, flexion

Tibialis posterior
Tibial nerve (sciatic nerve)

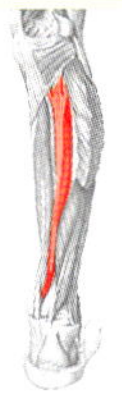

O: Upper three quarters of the interosseus membrane, adjacent areas of the tibia and the fibula	**I:** Tuberosity, plantar surface of cuneiform I–III, base of metatarsals II–IV	**F:** Ankle joint: plantar flexion Talotarsal joint: supination

Flexor digitorum longus
Tibial nerve (sciatic nerve)

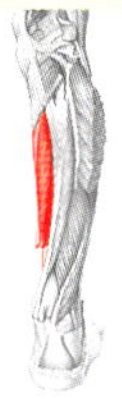

O: Posterior surface of the tibia distal to the soleal line, tendon arcade between the tibia and the fibula proximal to the chiasma crurale	**I:** Distal phalanx of the 2.–5. toe	**F:** Ankle joint: plantar flexion Talotarsal joint: supination Joints of the toes: flexion

Flexor hallucis longus
Tibial nerve (sciatic nerve)

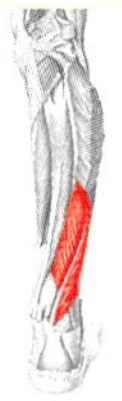

O: Distal two thirds of the posterior surface of the fibula, interosseous membrane, posterior intermuscular septum of leg	**I:** Distal phalanx of the great toe	**F:** Ankle joint: plantar flexion Talotarsal joint: supination Joints of the great toe: flexion

51 Muscles of the back of the foot (Fig. 1088, 1089, 1093, 1094)

Both muscles of the back of the foot only contribute insignificantly to the surface anatomy. The extensor hallucis brevis traverses towards the great toe, whereas the extensor digitorum brevis inserts at the remaining toes.

Extensor digitorum brevis
Deep fibular nerve (common fibular nerve)

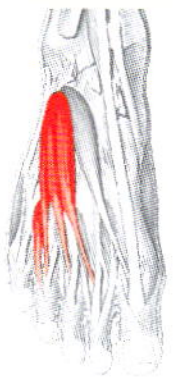

O: Dorsal and lateral surface of the calcaneus

I: Dorsal aponeurosis of the 2.–4. toe

F: Joints of the toes: extension

Extensor hallucis brevis
Deep fibular nerve (common fibular nerve)

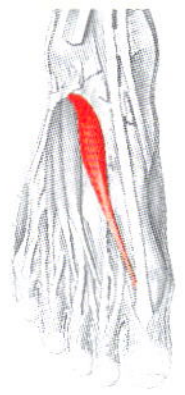

O: Dorsal surface of the calcaneus, tarsal sinus

I: Proximal phalanx of the great toe

F: Metatarsophalangeal joint of the great toe: extension

52 Medial muscles of the sole (Fig. 1096–1099)

The shape of the medial margin of the foot is predominantly formed by the abductor hallucis. The flexor hallucis brevis is juxtaposed just lateral to the former muscle, and is followed laterally by the adductor hallucis.

Abductor hallucis
Medial plantar nerve (tibial nerve

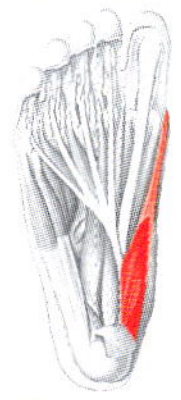

O: Medial process of the calcaneal tuberosity,
plantar aponeurosis, flexor retinaculum

I: Medial sesamoid bone of the capsule of the metatarsophlangeal joint of the great toe,
medial side of the base of the proximal phalanx of the great toe

F: Metatarsophalangeal joint of the great toe:
abduction,
flexion,
opposition

Flexor hallucis brevis
Medial part (medial head): *medial plantar nerve (tibial nerve)*
Lateral part (lateral head): *lateral plantar nerve (tibial nerve)*

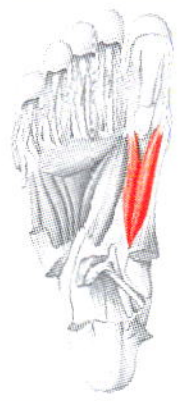

O: Plantar surface of the cuneiforms,
plantar calcaneocuboid ligament,
long plantar ligament,
tendon of the tibialis posterior

I: Medial portion: medial sesamoid bone of the metatarso-phalangeal joint of the great toe,
base of the proximal phalanx I
Lateral portion: lateral sesamoid bone of the metatarsophalangeal joint of the great toe,
base of the proximal phalanx I

F: Metatarsophalangeal joint of the great toe:
flexion

52 Medial muscles of the sole (continuation)

Adductor hallucis
Lateral plantar nerve (tibial nerve)

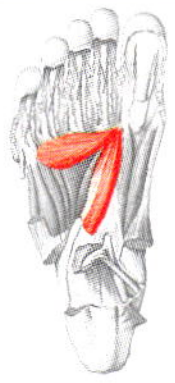

O: Oblique head: Cuboid, lateral cuneiform, long plantar ligament, plantar calcaneocuboid ligament
Transverse head: Capsules of the metatarsophalangeal joints of the toes III–V, deep transverse metatarsal ligament

I: Lateral sesamoid bone of the capsule of the metatarsophalangeal joint of the great toe, base of the proximal phalanx of the great toe

F: Metatarsophalangeal joint of the great toe:
adduction towards the 2. toe, flexion

53 Muscles of the middle of the sole (Fig. 1089, 1093, 1094, 1096–1101)

Several small muscles are located deep within the plantar arch. The flexor digitorum brevis proximally adheres to the plantar aponeurosis. Below this muscle the quadratus plantae is connected to the main tendon of the flexor digitorum longus, of whose four branching tendons the lumbricals I–IV originate. The interossei plantares I–III and the interossei dorsales pedis I–IV fill the spaces between the metatarsals.

Flexor digitorum brevis (Just before the insertion, its tendons are perforated by the tendons of the flexor digitorum longus.)
Medial plantar nerve (tibial nerve)

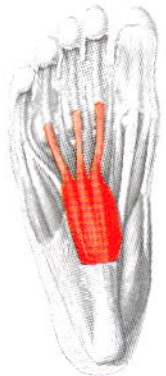

O: Plantar surface of the calcaneal tuberosity, plantar aponeurosis

I: Middle phalanx of the 2.–5. toe

F: Metatarsophalangeal joints:
flexion
Joints of the toes:
flexion

Quadratus plantae (This muscle is also referred to as flexor accessorius.)
Lateral plantar nerve (tibial nerve)

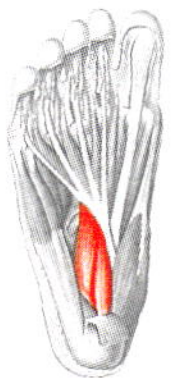

O: Plantar surface of the calcaneus, long plantar ligament

I: Lateral margin of the tendon of the flexor digitorum longus just before its division

F: Shifts the direction of force generated by the flexor digitorum longus towards the longitudinal axis of the foot

Lumbricals I–IV
Medial (I) and lateral (II–IV) plantar nerve (tibial nerve)

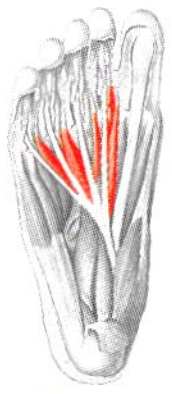

O: Lumbrical I: medial side of the tendon of the flexor digitorum longus to the 2. toe
Lumbrical II–IV: facing sides of the tendons of the flexor digitorum longus to the 3.–5. toe

I: Medial side of the proximal phalanx of the 2.–5. toe, sometimes it radiates into the dorsal aponeurosis

F: Metatarsophalangeal joints:
flexion

Interossei plantares pedis I–III
Lateral plantar nerve (tibial nerve)

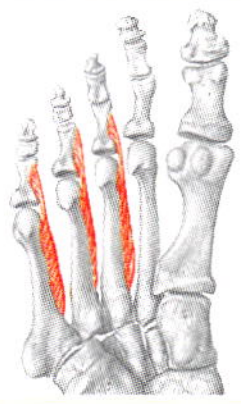

O: Plantar surface of metatarsals III–V, long plantar ligament

I: Medial side of the base of the proximal phalanx of the 3.–5. toe

F: Metatarsophalangeal joints:
flexion,
adduction towards the 2. toe

53 Muscles of the middle of the sole (continuation)

Interossei dorsales pedis I–IV (double headed muscles)
Lateral plantar nerve (tibial nerve)

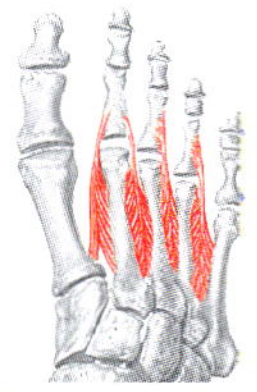

O: Facing sides of metatarsals I–V, long plantar ligament

I: Interosseus dorsalis I: medial side of the base of the proximal phalanx of the 2. toe
Interossei dorsales II–IV: lateral side of the base of the proximal phalanx of the 2.–4. toe, insert into extensor aponeuroses

F: Metatarsophalangeal joints: flexion, medial abduction of the 2. toe, as well as lateral abduction of the 3. and 4. toe
Joints of the toes: (extension)

54 Lateral muscles of the sole (Fig. 1089, 1096–1099)

The abductor digiti minimi is located along the lateral margin of the foot. The flexor digiti minimi brevis and the opponens digiti minimi are situated below its plantar aspect.

Abductor digiti minimi
Lateral plantar nerve (tibial nerve)

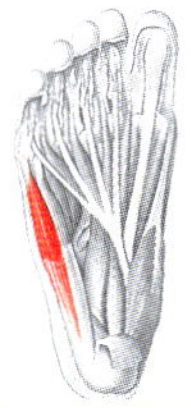

O: Lateral process of the calcaneal tuberosity, plantar aponeurosis, tuberosity of metatarsal bone V

I: Base of the proximal phalanx of the 5. toe

F: Metatarsophalangeal joint of the 5. toe: abduction, flexion, opposition

Flexor digiti minimi brevis
Lateral plantar nerve (tibial nerve)

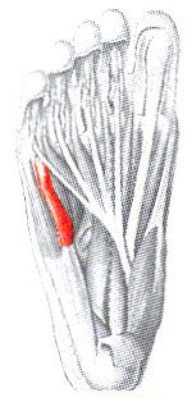

O: Base of metatarsal V, long plantar ligament, tendon sheath of the fibularis longus

I: Proximal phalanx of the 5. toe

F: Metatarsophalangeal joint of the 5. toe: abduction, flexion, (opposition)

Opponens digiti minimi (inconstant muscle)
Lateral plantar nerve (tibial nerve)

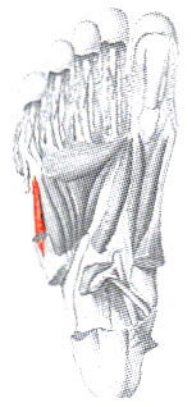

O: Long plantar ligament, tendon sheath of the fibularis longus

I: Lateral margin of metatarsal V

F: Metatarsophalangeal joint of the 5. toe: abduction, flexion, (opposition)

55 Cranial nerves, overview (Fig. 1174)

a	Olfactory nerve [I]
b	Optic nerve [II]
c	Oculomotor nerve [III]
d	Trochlear nerve [IV]
e	Trigeminal nerve [V] – ophthalmic nerve [V/1] – maxillary nerve [V/2] – mandibular nerve [V/3]
f	Abducent nerve [VI]
g	Facial nerve [VII]
h	Vestibulocochlear nerve [VIII]
i	Glossopharyngeal nerve [IX]
j	Vagus nerve [X]
k	Accessory nerve [XI]
l	Hypoglossal nerve [XII]

56 Cranial nerves, functions (different fibre qualities) (Fig. 1188–1191, 1236, 1238)

GSE	General somatic efference: innervation of the skeletal muscles **[III, IV, VI, XII]**
GVE	General visceral efference: innervation of the muscles of the viscera and vessels, and of the glands **[III, VII, IX, X]**
SVE	Specific visceral efference: innervation of the facial muscles, the masticatory muscles, the larynx, the pharynx, the oesophagus, as well as the sternocleidomastoideus and trapezius **[V, VII, IX, X, XI]**
GVA	General visceral afference: information from the internal organs and the blood vessels **[IX, X]**
SVA	Specific visceral afference: sense of taste **[VII, IX, X]**
GSA	General somatic afference: pain, temperature, info. from proprioceptive receptors in the skin and the locomotor systems **[V, VII, IX, X]**
SSA	Specific somatic afference: sense of smell, vision, hearing, sense of balance **[I, II, VIII]**

57 Cranial nerves (Fig. 1174–1194, 1236, 1238)

a Olfactory nerve [I] (Fig. 144, 1174)

All olfactory nerves together are referred to as olfactory nerve, representing the peripheral neuron of the olfactory pathway.

Outset	Olfactory cells in the olfactory region
Passage through the base of skull	Cribriform plate
Passage through the dura mater	Cribriform plate
Entry into the brain	Olfactory bulb
Supplying area	Mucosa (=olfactory mucosa) at the uppermost parts of the nasal cavity, the upper nasal concha and the most cranial parts of the nasal septum

b Optic nerve [II] (Fig. 1174, 1368, 1369)

The optic nerve belongs to the diencephalon and is therefore not really a peripheral nerve

Outset	Optic ganglion of the retina
Course within the dura mater	Sheath of optic nerve
Passage through the base of skull	Optic canal
Further visible course	Optic chiasm with the continuation of its fibres via the optic tract to the lateral geniculate body
Supplying area	Retina

c Oculomotor nerve [III] (Fig. 1175, 1176, 1236, 1238)

Nuclei (fibre quality)	• Nucleus of oculomotor nerve (double main ans single accessory nucleus) (GSE) • Accessory nucleus of oculomotor nerve (GVE) → ciliary ganglion
Exit from the brain	Inner surface of the cerebral peduncle (oculomotor sulcus)
Location in the subarachnoid space	Basal cistern, interpeduncular cistern
Entry into the dura mater	Roof of the cavernous sinus
Exit from the dura mater	Superior orbital fissure
Passage through the base of skull	Superior orbital fissure (medial portion, within the tendinous ring)
Supplying areas	**motor:** levator palpebrae superioris, recti superior, medialis and inferior, obliquus inferior **parasympathetic:** ciliaris, sphincter pupillae (via ciliary ganglion)
Attachment of other nerves	**Sensible** fibres from the nasociliary nerve [V/1] **Sympathetic** fibres from the ophthalmic plexus

d Trochlear nerve [IV] (Fig. 1175, 1176, 1236, 1238)

Nuclei (fibre quality)	• Nucleus of trochlear nerve (GSE)
Exit from the brain	Dorsal/caudal of the inferior colliculus (tectum of midbrain)
Location in the subarachnoid space	Cisterna ambiens, basal cistern
Entry into the dura mater	Between the plica petroclinoidea anterior and posterior
Course within the dura mater	Lateral wall of the cavernous sinus
Exit from the dura mater	Superior orbital fissure
Passage through the base of skull	Superior orbital fissure
Supplying area	**motor:** obliquus superior

e Trigeminal nerve [V] (Fig. 1177–1180, 1236, 1238)	
Nuclei (fibre quality)	• Mesencephalic nucleus of trigeminal nerve (GSA and GVA) • Spinal nucleus of trigeminal nerve (GSA and GVA) • Motor nucleus of trigeminal nerve (SVE)
Exit from the brain	Lateral margin of the pons
Location in the subarachnoid space	Basal cistern, trigeminal cave
Entry into the dura mater	Lateral wall of the cavernous sinus as trigeminal ganglion
Division into three branches	– ophthalmic nerve [V/1] – maxillary nerve [V/2] – mandibular nerve [V/3]
– Ophthalmic nerve [V/1]	
Course within the dura mater	Lateral wall of the cavernous sinus
Exit from the dura mater	Superior orbital fissure
Exit from the base of skull	Superior orbital fissure – nasociliary nerve: medial portion – frontal nerve: lateral portion – lacrimal nerve: lateral portion
Supplying areas	**Sensible:** Dura mater of the anterior cranial fossa, falx cerebri, tentorium cerebelli, forehead, upper eyelid, back of the nose, sclera, cornea, anterior ethmoidal cells, sphenoidal sinus, nasal cavity (anterior part)
Attachment of other nerves	**Parasympathic (secretory) fibres** to the lacrimal nerve for the lacrimal gland (from the superior salivatory nucleus via the facial nerve, greater petrosal nerve to the pterygopalatine ganglion and further on to the zygomatic nerve and communicating branch with zygomatic nerve)
– Maxillary nerve [V/2]	
Course within the dura mater	Lateral wall of the cavernous sinus
Exit from the dura mater	Foramen rotundum
Exit from the base of skull	Foramen rotundum
Supplying areas	**Sensible:** Dura mater of the middle cranial fossa, cheek, lower eyelid, lateral parts of the nose, upper lip, teeth and gingiva of the maxilla, posterior ethmoidal cells, sphenoidal sinus, maxillary sinus, superior and middle nasal concha, palate, palatine tonsil, pharynx (roof)
Attachment of other nerves	**Parasympathetic (secretory) fibres** to the diverse nasal branches to the nasal glands, to the palatine nerves for the palatine glands as well as to the zygomatic nerve for the lacrimal gland (from the superior salivatory nucleus via the facial nerve, greater petrosal nerve and the ganglionic branches to pterygopalatine ganglion)
– Mandibular nerve [V/3]	
Course within the dura mater	Lateral wall of the cavernous sinus
Exit from dura mater	Foramen ovale
Exit from base of skull	Foramen ovale
Supplying areas	**Motor:** masticatory muscles, tensor veli palatini, mylohyoid, digastric (anterior belly), tensor tympani **Sensible:** Dura mater of the middle cranial fossa, mastoid cells, skin of the mandible, temple, cheek, auricle (upper parts), external acoustic meatus, tympanic membrane (externally), teeth and gingiva of the mandible, anterior 2/3 of the tongue, isthmus of fauces, temporomandibular joint
Attachment of other nerves	**Sensory:** anterior 2/3 of the tongue (facial nerve [VII] via chorda tympani to the lingual nerve) **Parasympathetic (secretory) fibres** a) to the lingual nerve for the submandibular and sublingual glands (superior salivatory nucleus via the facial nerve and the chorda tympani to the submandibular ganglion) b) to the auriculotemporal nerve for the parotid gland (inferior salivatory nucleus via the glossopharyngeal nerve, tympanic nerve and the lesser petrosal nerve to the otic ganglion)

f Abducent nerve [VI] (Fig. 1175, 1176, 1236, 1238)

Nuclei (fibre quality)	• Nucleus of abducent nerve (GSE)
Exit from the brain	Between pons and pyramis
Location in the subarachnoid space	Basal cistern
Entry into the dura mater	Upper third of the clivus
Course within the dura mater	Via apex of petrous part, freely through the cavernous sinus, lateral to the internal carotid artery
Exit from the dura mater	Superior orbital fissure
Passage through the base of skull	Superior orbital fissure, medial portion (within the tendinous ring)
Supplying area	**Motor:** rectus lateralis

g Facial nerve [VII] (Fig. 1181, 1182, 1236, 1238)

Nuclei (fibre quality)	• Motor nucleus of facial nerve (GVE) • Superior salivatory nucleus (GVE) → pterygopalatine ganglion → submandibular ganglion • Solitary nucleus (SVA)
Exit from the brain	Cerebellopontine angle
Location in the subarachnoid space	Basal cistern, pontocerebellar cistern
Entry into the base of skull	Porus → internal acoustic meatus
Passage through the dura mater	Fundus of internal acoustic meatus
Course within the base of skull	Facial canal
Exit from the base of skull	Stylomastoid foramen
Supplying areas	**Motor:** facial muscles, auricular muscles, digastric (posterior belly), stylohyoid, stapedius **Sensory:** anterior 2/3 of the tongue (via chorda tympani to the lingual nerve) **Parasympathetic:** lacrimal gland, nasal glands, palatine glands (via pterygopalatine ganglion), submandibular gland, sublingual gland (via submandibular ganglion)
Attachment of other nerves	**Sensible fibres** from the trigeminal nerve to the facial branches of the facial nerve

h Vestibulochochlear nerve [VIII] (Fig. 1183, 1236, 1238)

Nuclei (fibre quality)	• Anterior and posterior chochlear nuclei (SSA) • Medial, lateral, superior and inferior vestibular nuclei (SSA)
Exit from the brain	Cerebellopontine angle
Location in the subarachnoid space	Basal cistern, pontocerebellar cistern
Entry into the base of skull	Porus → internal acoustic meatus
Exit from the dura mater	Fundus of internal acoustic meatus
Course within the base of skull	Directly to the labyrinth of the petrous part of the temporal bone
Supplying areas	**Sensory:** chochlear nerve: organ of hearing (= organ of CORTI) **Sensory:** vestibular nerve: organ of balance

i Glossopharyngeal nerve [IX] (Fig. 1184, 1236, 1238)	
Nuclei (fibre quality)	• nucleus ambiguus (SVE) • spinal nucleus of trigeminal nerve (GVA) • nucleus solitary (SVA) • inferior salivatory nucleus (GVE) → otic ganglion
Exit from the brain	Medulla oblongata, posterolateral sulcus (between the olive and the cuneate tubercle)
Location in the subarachnoid space	Basal cistern
Passage through the dura mater	Jugular foramen
Passage through the base of skull	Jugular foramen
Supplying area	**Motor:** pharyngeal muscles (cranial parts), levator veli palatini, palatoglossus, palatopharyngeus, stylopharyngeus **Sensible:** pharyngeal mucosa (cranial parts), palatine tonsil, posterior third of the tongue, tympanic plexus, tympanic membrane (internally), carotid sinus **Sensory:** tongue (posterior third) **Parasympathetic:** parotid gland (via otic ganglion) lingual glands (posterior)

j Vagus nerve [X] (Fig. 1185, 1236, 1238)	
Nuclei (fibre quality)	• nucleus ambiguus (SVE) • spinal nucleus of vagus nerve (GVA) • solitary nucleus (SVA) • inferior dorsal nucleus of vagus nerve (GVE)
Exit from the brain	Medulla oblongata, posterolateral sulcus (dorsal to the olive)
Location in the subarachnoid space	Basal cistern
Passage through the dura mater	Jugular foramen
Passage through the base of skull	Jugular foramen
Supplying areas	**Motor:** pharyngeal muscles (caudal parts), levator veli palatini, musculus uvulae, laryngeal muscles **Sensible:** dura mater of the posterior cranial fossa, deep parts of the external acoustic meatus, tympanic membrane (externally) **Sensory:** root of the tongue **Parasympathetic:** organs of the neck, thorax and abdomen up to the point of CANNON-BÖHM

k Accessory nerve [XI] (Fig. 1186, 1236, 1238)	
Nuclei (fibre quality)	• nucleus ambiguus (SVE) • nucleus of accessory nerve (SVE)
Exit from the brain	Cranial roots: medulla oblongata, posterolateral sulcus (retro-olivary) Spinal roots: cervical medulla (lateral)
Location in the subarachnoid space	Basal cistern
Entry into the base of skull	Foramen magnum (spinal roots)
Passage through the dura mater	Jugular foramen
Passage through the base of skull	Jugular foramen
Supplying area	**Motor:** sternocleidomastoid, trapezius (together with the cervical plexus)

l Hypoglossal nerve [XII] (Fig. 1187, 1236, 1238)	
Nuclei (fibre quality)	• Nucleus of hypoglossal nerve (GSE)
Exit from brain	Medulla oblongata, anterolateral sulcus
Location in the subarachnoid space	Basal cistern
Passage through the dura mater	Hypoglossal canal
Passage through the base of skull	Hypoglossal canal
Supplying area	**Motor:** inner muscles of the tongue, styloglossus, hyoglossus, genioglossus

Index

The numbers refer to the numbers of the tables.

N

O

P